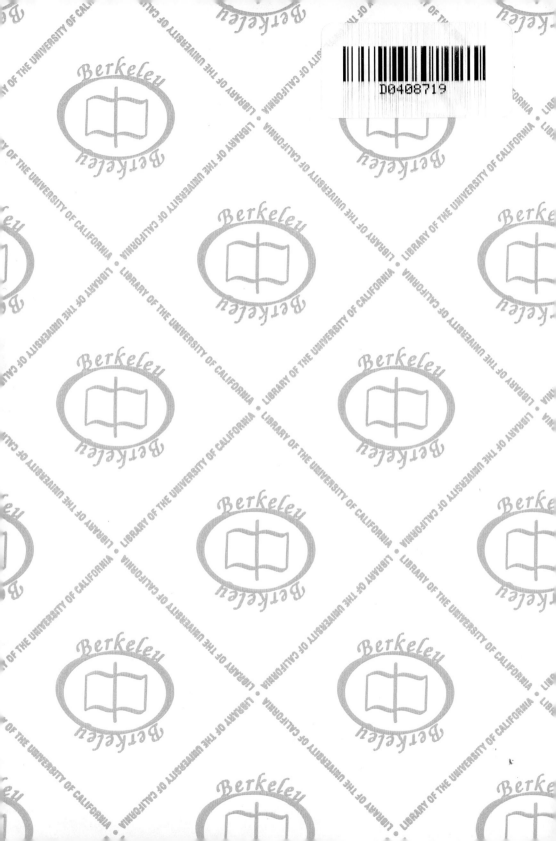

Spanish-English
English-Spanish
Medical Dictionary

Diccionario Médico
Español-Inglés
Inglés-Español

Spanish-English
English-Spanish
Medical Dictionary

Diccionario Médico
Español-Inglés
Inglés-Español

Third Edition

Onyria Herrera McElroy, Ph.D.
Lola L. Grabb, M.A.

Foreword by Vincent A. Fulginiti, M.D.
Emeritus Professor
University of Arizona

Introducción por la Dra. Beatriz Varela
Emeritus Professor of Spanish
University of New Orleans, New Orleans

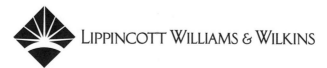

LIPPINCOTT WILLIAMS & WILKINS

A Wolters Kluwer Company
Philadelphia • Baltimore • New York • London
Buenos Aires • Hong Kong • Sydney • Tokyo

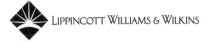

Publisher: Julie K. Stegman
Senior Product Manager: Eric Branger
Associate Managing Editor: Tiffany Piper
Graphic Artist: Susan Caldwell
Production Coordinator: Jason Delaney
Typesetter: Publication Services
Printer: RR Donnelley

LIPPINCOTT WILLIAMS & WILKINS

Copyright 2005
Lippincott Williams & Wilkins
A Wolters Kluwer Health Company
351 West Camden Street
Baltimore, MD 21201-2346
www.stedmans.com
stedmans@lww.com

The authors and publisher have taken care to ensure that the information in this book is true and accurate at the date of going to press. Neither the authors nor the publisher can accept any legal responsibility or liability for any errors or omissions that may be found in this book. However, it is still possible that mistakes have been made. The reader is strongly urged to consult drug companies' printed instructions before administering any of the drugs mentioned in this book, and to consult their physicians to ensure that diagnosis and treatment of any diseases mentioned in this book comply with the latest standards of practice.

Third Edition, 2005

Printed in the United States of America

Library of Congress Cataloging-in-Publication Data

McElroy, Onyria Herrera.
Spanish-English, English-Spanish medical dictionary = Diccionario médico, español-inglés, inglés-español / Onyria Herrera McElroy, Lola L. Grabb; foreword by Vincent A. Fulginiti; introducción por Beatriz Varela.–3rd ed.
      p.; cm.
      ISBN 0-7817-5011-3
      1. Medicine-Dictionaries. 2. English language-Dictionaries-Spanish. 3. Medicine-Dictionaries-Spanish.
      4. Spanish language-Dictionaries-English. I. Grabb, Lola L. II. Title.
      [DNLM: 1. Medicine-Dictionary-English.]
R121.M488 2005
610'.3–dc22
DNLM/DLC
for Library of Congress   2005000455

Contents / Contenido

FOREWORD

Non-Spanish-speaking physicians are frustrated when attempting to communicate with their Spanish-speaking patients. Not only is there an obvious language barrier, but also the precise definitions of some words that the physician may acquire from dictionaries may not be correct in the medical context. Additionally, patients are uncomfortable with those who do not share their language, and facility with the language may be an incentive to full disclosure. Most of us who are not multilingual pick up phrases and terms that we use loosely in attempting to explore history or reactions to our physical examinations. Now McElroy and Grabb have provided us with a handy reference that will facilitate our ability both to understand our patients and to communicate with them with greater precision and ease.

They have assisted us by providing a well-written, well-structured volume that will provide ready reference to the words, phrases, and constructions that we need. Their use of side by side English-Spanish throughout facilitates ready reference in both directions and can help persons other than the health-care worker and the primarily Spanish speaker to move between the two languages. A unique feature is the inclusion of accepted abbreviations, which I have seen in no other text of this type. The abbreviations are placed in context, which makes learning and transition quick and easy. The conversion tables explain the roots of words, meanings of prefixes and suffixes, and orthographic changes in the two languages.

Finally, the appendixes include a matrix for the physician-patient encounter, with very useful phrases that are commonly employed in gathering historical information and in informing patients of the physician's recommendations and interpretations.

A health-care worker armed with this text will find that he or she is more capable of communication than with most other aids to Spanish-English equivalents. I find this a most useful treatment of this important area in medicine for those whose daily professional and personal lives are dependent on accuracy in communication.

Vincent A. Fulginiti, M.D

INTRODUCCIÓN

La importancia del español y del inglés en el mundo de hoy es obvia, no sólo por el número tan considerable de hablantes que posee cada lengua sino también por las contribuciones culturales llevadas a cabo por ambas civilizaciones y con las cuales se ha venido enriqueciendo y beneficiando la humanidad desde hace muchos siglos. La medicina, por ejemplo, se halla entre los campos que cuentan con más adelantos: técnicas nuevas, innovaciones en la cirugía y los tratamientos, conceptos desconocidos que hay que expresar con neologismos y muchas novedades en el diagnóstico y la prevención de enfermedades. Las autoras McElroy y Grabb acertaron, pues, en publicar este diccionario médico-bilingüe en estos momentos tan propicios. Desde luego que la habilidad de escoger el tiempo oportuno no es el único acierto de estas escritoras. Nos encontramos ante un diccionario de calidad, que usa definiciones breves, claras y precisas—en inglés y en español—y que además, en secciones que no he visto en otros diccionarios, estudia las abreviaturas médicas más conocidas, las tablas de conversión con los cambios ortográficos propios de cada lengua y la formación de términos médicos por medio de raíces, prefijos y sufijos. También ofrece orientaciones sencillas para la pronunciación de los sonidos que causan más dificultades al anglo y al hispano respectivamente y una gramática simplificada con las estructuras que contrastan en las dos lenguas. Hay asimismo, cinco apéndices en los cuales se traducen pesos y medidas, la temperatura, los números, las tablas de conversión, las frases más comunes que se emplean en el ejercicio de la medicina y los signos y síntomas del paciente. En todas estas divisiones del contenido, las traducciones de cada voz o frase se encuentran una al lado de la otra, de manera que no hay necesidad de acudir a ninguna otra referencia. Cuando se busca una voz en el diccionario, bien sea en español, bien en inglés, aparece en primer lugar el cognado (cuando lo hay) y después la connotación del mismo, expuesta en forma sencilla para que la entienda tanto el científico como el vulgo que nada sabe de estas voces médicas. Se incluye, además, si existe, el vocablo popular de la enfermedad o el tratamiento.

Lo expuesto comprueba que este diccionario médico-bilingüe ha de ser una fuente indispensable no sólo para médicos, trabajadores sociales y enfermeros dedicados a problemas de la salud, sino también para los pacientes y las personas que deseen documentarse sobre distintos aspectos de la medicina contemporánea. Por último, conviene subrayar que la obra ha de beneficiar lo mismo al ciudadano de una nación anglohablante que al de todo país de habla española.

Dra. Beatriz Varela

PREFACE

The rapid pace of scientific and technological advancements in recent years has greatly benefited many areas of human life, medicine and health care certainly being among them. We therefore have welcomed this opportunity to expand and update our dictionary in a third edition.

Surgical and diagnostic procedures have recently been enhanced by the use of new techniques such as lasers, MRI, and molecular imaging by positron emission tomography. We have thus added terms regarding these procedures; and, in the appendices, as visual aids to our readers, you will find new charts on diagnostic and clinical tests and CT scanning. There are also in the appendices new notes on Alzheimer disease, the warning signs of heart attack and stroke, and expanded vocabularies regarding the newborn and nutrition. New dialogues have been added, along with a list of cognates that are particularly helpful to the reader's formation of an expanded medical vocabulary in the language that is foreign.

Another new feature, in the deluxe version of this edition, is a CD-ROM in which native speakers of each language (English and Spanish) provide the dictionary's users with the actual sounds of English and Spanish words so that they can improve their pronunciation of the other language.

Because more complex rules and regulations have emerged in response to the emphasis now being given the rights of patients and health-care providers, we have added sample forms that will be helpful to diagnostic procedures, surgery, and understanding the responsibilities of both health-care personnel and patients.

The insecurities and fears occasioned by 9/11 has prompted us to add a section that succinctly covers two agents that could be used in a massive terrorist attack. This section gives information on the symptoms that these agents produce, their possible antidotes, and state and federal officials to contact in case of an emergency of this sort.

Another feature in this third edition of our bilingual medical dictionary that should be of particular practical use in acquiring vocabulary and communicating with patients is a colored Anatomy Atlas with bilingual labels, as well as the insertion of many small illustrations throughout the dictionary's two lexicons.

We hope that you will continue to find our efforts to help communication between patients and health-care personnel worthy of your attention and that you will, as in the past, send to our publisher any comments on this edition or suggestions you might wish to make for further improvements.

O.H.M.
L.L.G.

Tucson
November, 2004

PRÓLOGO

La rapidez con que se han desarrollado los avances científicos y tecnológicos en los recientes años ha traído grandes beneficios a muchas esferas de la vida, destacándose entre éstas los campos de la medicina y la atención a la salud. Por lo tanto hemos acogido con entusiasmo la oportunidad de expandir y poner al día nuestro diccionario en una tercera edición.

Procedimientos quirúrugicos y de diagnóstico han sido realzados recientemente mediante el uso de nuevas técnicas tales como los láseres, IRM, e imágenes moleculares de la tomografía de emisión por positron y otras. Por lo tanto hemos añadido términos referentes a estos procedimientos; en los apéndices, como ayuda visual a nuestros lectores, hemos incluído cuadros de pruebas clínicas y de diagnóstico, y de escán de tomografía computerizada. También en los apéndices incluímos nuevas observaciones sobre la enfermedad de Alzheimer, signos que advierten un posible ataque cardíaco o embolia cerebral, y vocabularios más completos sobre nutrición, así como sobre el recién nacido. Se han añadido diálogos y hemos incluído una lista de vocablos cognados que esperamos sea particularmente beneficiosa para el lector que persigue ampliar su vocabulario médico en el otro idioma.

Otra adición en la version "deluxe" de esta edición es un CD-ROM en el cual hablantes nativos de cada idioma (inglés y español) ofrecen a los usuarios del diccionario los sonidos de palabras en inglés y español, para que de esa manera ellos puedan mejorar su pronunciación en el otro idioma.

Debido a las reglas y regulaciones más complejas que han surgido a consecuencia del énfasis que se le da actualmente a los derechos del paciente y los proveedores de salud, hemos añadido muestras de formularios y planillas que servirán de ayuda para procedimientos diagnósticos, cirugía, y comprensión de las responsabilidades tanto del proveedor de salud como del paciente.

La inseguridad y el temor ocasionados por los eventos del 9/11 nos han llevado a añadir una sección que en forma sucinta cubre dos de los agentes que pudieran ser usados en un ataque masivo de terrorismo biológico. Esta sección da información sobre los síntomas que estos agentes pueden causar, posible antídotos y oficinas estatales y federales a las que se puede referir en caso de una emergencia de ese tipo.

También se ha incorporado a esta tercera edición de nuestro diccionario médico bilingüe un Atlas de Anatomía en color con rótulos en ambos idiomas lo cual debe resultar muy práctico para la adquisición de vocabulario y para la comunicación con los pacientes. También se han incluído ilustraciones más pequeñas a través de ambos léxicos.

Esperamos que nuestros esfuerzos para lograr una mejor comunicación entre paciente y personal de salud médica merezca su atención y consideración, y, como lo han hecho anteriormente, le envién a los editores del dicionario comentarios sobre esta edición o sugerencias que puedan servir de ayuda en el futuro.

O.H.M.
L.L.G.

Tucson
Noviembre 2004

ACKNOWLEDGMENTS

The third edition of the dictionary has been a major undertaking which, like the previous two editions, was inspired by the helpful observations of readers and supported by many other persons.

First, we wish to thank Albert G. Grabb, M.D., for his useful feedback to our many inquiries, and Julius Pietrzak, M.D., for the important assistance he has given us. John Harmon McElroy gave us copyediting advice and constant encouragement. To Anita Stone and Lauren McElroy, who assisted us in reviewing the lexicon and the proofreading, and to Beatriz Varela, who contributed Spanish words that have recently been approved by the Real Academia Española, we also extend our gratitude. Acknowledgment is likewise due Julie Stegman, Eric Branger, and Tiffany Piper at Lippincott Williams & Wilkins who have contributed so much to the production of the third edition. And we want to renew our previous expressions of gratitude to Roseann D. González, Leila Catán, and Matilde Sandefur who have always been strongly supportive of the dictionary. Finally, a special thanks is owed Susan Caldwell for her meticulous and beautiful work on the artistic part of the illustrations.

HOW TO USE THE DICTIONARY

MAIN ENTRIES

The main entries are printed in **boldface**, in slightly larger type than the rest of the text set flush to the left hand margin. The main entry may consist of:

1. one word: **abdomen**
2. words joined by a hyphen: **cross-eyed**
3. descriptive phrases: **sympathetic nervous system**

The main entries are listed in alphabetical order according to the initial letter of the entry. Two kinds of entries appear: a) strictly medical words and b) common words related to general communication with patients.

When the main entry is a medical term, a simple definition is given with the most important facts pertaining to it. When the main entry has different meanings which are identified as the same part of speech, they are itemized numerically and labeled with an abbreviation if it is needed for clarification (1). When the main entry is a non-medical word or a common term, synonyms are used to define it. If a main entry has more than one meaning, a word or phrase between brackets is given, in italics, in the same language as the entry to clarify its meaning, or in some cases the entry is used in a phrase to clarify its use (2). We have listed new technical words designating programs, products, instruments, or treatments and defined them by following the general rules of language usage.

> (1) **absorption** *n*. absorción. 1. la acción de un organismo de absorber o pasar líquidos u otras sustancias; 2. ensimismación.

> (2) **fit** *n*. ataque, convulsión; *a*. [*suitable*] adecuado-a; *v*. [*to adjust to shape*] ajustar, encajar.

In some cases, when there is a slight difference in the spelling of words with the same meaning, both spellings are entered together, and the most common one of the two is entered first (3).

> (3) **exophthalmia, exophthalmus** *n*. exoftalmia, exoftalmus, protrusión anormal del globo del ojo.

Only words that would pertain to communication in a medical situation and to needs related to patients or medical personnel are included in the glossary.

SUBENTRIES

Subentries under main entries of medical words in the same language as the entry are printed in **boldface type** (4); subentries under main entries of common words and phrases and idiomatic expressions are printed in **boldface type** (5). A slash (/) separates the translation of the subentries from English to Spanish or Spanish to English, while a double space (__) stands for the main entry. Subentries generally are not defined. Their plural forms are indicated by adding **-s** or **-es** after the double space.

> (4) **dislocation** *n*. luxación, desplazamiento de una articulación; **closed** __ / __ cerrada; **complicated** __ / __ complicada; **congenital** __ / __ congénita.

> (5) **around** *prep*. cerca de; en; *adv*. alrededor de, cerca; a la vuelta; más o menos; __ **here** / __ aquí; *v*. **to look** __ / buscar; **to turn** __ / dar la vuelta; voltear; voltearse.

SYNONYMS

When an entry refers to a sickness which is known by more than one name, only one definition is given. The abbreviation *V.* (See) will guide the reader to the term defined (6).

---

(6) **chickenpox** *n.* varicela. *V.* **varicella**.

PARTS OF SPEECH

All main entries, simple or combined, are identified as to part of speech. When the main entry has more than one word, the combined phrase is also identified (7).

---

(7) **robust** *a.*
  role model *n.*
  radioactive iodine excretion test *n.*

The meanings of a word used as more than one part of speech are indicated in the following order of forms: **noun** *n.*; **adjective** *a.*; **verb** *v.*; **irregular verb** *vi.*; **reflexive verb** *vr.*; **adverb** *adv.* (2).

In the English section of the dictionary, the glossary includes nouns, adjectives, infinitives of verbs, the past participle (classified as an adjective), comparatives and superlatives, prepositions and adverbs. Idiomatic expressions involving the main entry are included following the definitions. Other parts of speech such as pronouns and verb forms can be found in the grammar section of the dictionary.

In the Spanish section nouns and adjectives are identified by their gender (*m.*, *f.*). In the English section, the translations into Spanish of nouns and adjectives indicate their gender (masculine or feminine) by adding the feminine ending **-a**, accordingly, to nouns and adjectives ending in **-o** that are inflected. In example (8) **rápido-a** means that the masculine is **rápido**, and the feminine is **rápida**. When the adverb is indicated by the ending **-mente**, it means that this ending has to be added to the feminine ending of the adjective, or just added to it if the adjective ends in a consonant.

---

(8) **fast** *n. ayuno*; *a.* (*speedy*) rápido-a; ligero-a; **color** __ / resistente a un colorante; *v.* (*not to eat anything*) ayunar; **to break one's** __ / dejar de ayunar; *adv.* aprisa; rápidamente; **to walk** __ / andar __; __ **asleep** / profundamente dormido-a.

HOMOGRAPHS AND EPONYMS

When entries are spelled alike but have a different classification (homographs), the part of speech is indicated by its corresponding abbreviation, definitions follow separated by semicolons without using numerals, as is the case when the entry has the same classification regarding part of speech (1).

---

(9) **mucoid** *n.* mucoide, glucoproteína similar a la mucina; *a.* de consistencia mucosa.

Eponyms are entered alphabetically according to last names (10).

---

(10) **Babinski's reflex** *n.* reflejo de Babinski, dorsiflexión del dedo gordo al estimularse la planta del pie.

PLURALS

Irregular plurals in English, and the plurals of Latin and Greek nouns used in medical terminology are indicated in parentheses after the entry.

---

(11) **woman** *n.* (*pl.* **women**) mujer.

---

(12) **septum** *L.* (*pl.* **septa**) septum, tabique o membrana que divide dos cavidades o espacios.

Consult the grammar section of the dictionary to find the rules that apply to the formation of plurals in each language.

CAPITALIZATION

Most entries in English begin with a lowercase. Capitalization is used in eponyms and trade names of medications; names of plants and animals are capitalized, printed in italics, and given in the singular if referring to the genus, and in the plural if referring to the class, order, family, or phylum (13).

(13) *Salmonella n.* Salmonela, género de bacterias de la familia *Enterobacteriaceae* que causan fiebres entéricas, otras infecciones gastrointestinales y septicemia.

MEDICAL ABBREVIATIONS AND CONVERSION TABLES

To save space and facilitate their use, medical abbreviations and prefixes, suffixes, and roots have been listed in separate sections entitled **Most Common Medical Abbreviations** and **Conversion Tables**.

COMMUNICATING WITH PATIENTS

This section is intended to satisfy the simplest daily communications that a health professional who speaks either Spanish or English may need to have with a patient who speaks the other language. It is also intended that this section will have the effect of increasing the reader's ability to use the other language in non-clinical context.

APPENDIXES

Numerals, measures, words related to time, words related to signs and symptoms, as well as practical charts on contagious diseases, emergency care, medical tests, nutrition, physical fitness, idioms and vocabulary for conducting interviews with patients and giving them instructions are found in separate appendices.

ILLUSTRATIONS

In the third edition, the reader will find a section with an Anatomy Atlas in color and several illustrations throughout the vocabulary pages. The deluxe edition also has a CD-ROM for audiovisual use.

WORD TO THE READER

In the third edition, new additions have been made, some of them following the suggestion of our readers. We hope that our new readers will do the same, forwarding via Lippincott Williams & Wilkins recommendations for improving this dictionary in future editions.

USO DEL DICCIONARIO

ENTRADAS PRINCIPALES

Las entradas principales aparecen impresas en letra **negrita** formando el margen izquierdo. La entrada principal puede consistir en:

1. una sola palabra: **abdomen**
2. una palabra compuesta: **intra-abdominal**
3. una frase descriptiva: **cuello uterino**

Las entradas principales siguen un orden alfabético de acuerdo con la primera letra de la palabra. Hay dos tipos de entradas: (a) palabras estrictamente médicas, (b) palabras del lenguaje común necesarias para la comunicación con los pacientes.

Cuando la entrada principal es un vocablo médico, a éste le sigue una definición simple que señala los aspectos más importantes del mismo. Si el vocablo tiene más de una acepción para una misma parte de la oración (sustantivo, adjetivo, etc.), a cada acepción se le atribuye un número y una abreviatura adicional para mayor claridad (1). Cuando la entrada principal es un vocablo común, no médico, se hace uso de sinónimos para traducirla. Si tiene más de un significado, se hace uso de alguna palabra o frase entre corchetes ([]), en bastardilla y en el mismo idioma de la entrada, para aclarar su significado, o se emplea la misma entrada en una frase para aclarar su uso. (2). En algunos casos incluimos nuevas palabras técnicas que designan programas, productos, instrumentos y tratamientos; estas palabras están definidas de acuerdo con las reglas generales del uso del idioma.

> (1) **absorción** *f.* absorption, uptake. 1. taking up of fluids and other substances by an organism; 2. self-centeredness.

> (2) **apagar** *v.* [*luces*] to turn off; [*fuego*] to put out.

En algunos casos, cuando hay una pequeña diferencia en la forma escrita de dos palabras con el mismo significado, ambas palabras se presentan en la misma entrada, y se registra primero la palabra de uso más común (3).

> (3) **fibrocístico-a, fibroquístico-a** *a.* fibrocystic, cystic and fibrous in nature; **enfermedad __ de la mama /** __ disease of the breast.

En el glosario de este diccionario se han incluido solamente términos relacionados con una situación médica, ya sea para la comunicación con los pacientes o para la atención a sus necesidades.

ENTRADAS SUBALTERNAS

Las entradas subalternas que aparecen bajo la entrada principal están impresas en letra **negrita** si están en el mismo idioma que ésta; asimismo, ya refiriéndose a la terminología no médica o a expresiones idiomáticas en el mismo. Una línea inclinada (/) separa la traducción del español al inglés y del inglés al español en las entradas subalternas, y un doble guión (__) sustituye la entrada principal; el plural se indica con una **-s** o con **-es** después del doble guión. Las entradas subalternas generalmente no se definen (4).

> (4) **cuidado** *m.* care, attention; __ **intensivo** /intensive __; __ **postnatal** /postnatal __; **estar al __de /** to be under the __ of; **tratar con,** __ /to handle with __.
> **febril** *a.* febrile, having a body temperature above normal, **convulsiones __ -es /** __ convulsions.

SINÓNIMOS

Cuando un término médico tiene más de un nombre, solamente se define uno de los términos; la abreviatura *V.* (Véase) en la entrada del otro término, guía al lector a la entrada que aparece definida (5).

> (5) **glucopenia** *f.* *V.* **hipoglicemia.**

PARTES DE LA ORACIÓN

Después de cada entrada, consistente ésta de una o de más palabras, se indica la parte correspondiente de la oración (6).

> (6) **emulsión** *f.*
> **enajenamiento mental** *m.*
> **brazalete de identificación** *m.*

Cuando una misma entrada tiene más de una clasificación como parte de la oración, se sigue el siguiente orden: **nombre** *m., f.*; **adjetivo** *a.*; **verbo** *v.*; **verbo irregular** *vi.*; **verbo reflexivo** *vr.*; **adverbio** *adv.* Las terminaciones **-a** y **-mente** indican la terminación que se añade a la entrada para formar el adjetivo y el adverbio respectivamente (7).

> (7) **elástico** *m.* elastic; **-a** *a.* elastic, that can be returned to its original shape after being extended or distorted.
> **natural** *a.* natural; **-mente** *adv.* naturally.

En la sección del diccionario en español, el glosario incluye sustantivos, adjetivos, infinitivos de verbos, el participio pasado (clasificado como adjetivo), preposiciones y adverbios. Las expressiones idiomáticas aparecen como entradas subalternas a continuación de las definiciones. Otras partes de la oración, pronombres y distintas formas de los verbos aparecen en la sección de gramática del diccionario.

En la sección del diccionario en español, los sustantivos y adjetivos se identifican por su género (*m., f.*). En la sección en inglés, la traducción de sustantivos y adjetivos al español indica el género de los mismos (masculino o femenino) mediante el uso de la terminación **-a** añadida a los sustantivos y adjetivos terminados en **o** (8).

> (8) **métrico-a** *a.* metric, rel. to meter or the metric system.

HOMÓGRAFOS Y EPÓNIMOS

Cuando a una misma entrada se le atribuye más de una clasificación (términos homógrafos) cada parte de la oración se indica con su correspondiente abreviatura, y las definiciones siguen a cada clasificación, separadas por un punto y coma pero sin asignarles números como se hace en los casos en que un mismo término tiene más de una acepción pero mantiene la misma clasificación (véanse ejemplos 1 y 7). Los epónimos están registrados alfabéticamente por apellido (9).

> (9) **Babinski, reflejo de** *m.* Babinski's reflex, dorsiflexion of the big toe on stimulation of the sole of the foot.

PLURALES

Los plurales de vocablos incorporados del latín y del griego, así como los plurales irregulares, se indican entre paréntesis a continuación de la entrada (10).

> (10) **septum** *L.* (pl. **septa**) septum, partition between two cavities.

En la sección de gramática del diccionario se encuentran las reglas que gobiernan la formación de los plurales en cada idioma.

LETRAS MAYÚSCULAS

La mayoría de las entradas en inglés y en español aparecen en letra minúscula. Las letras mayúsculas se usan en los epónimos y en nombres comerciales de medicinas. Los nombres de plantas y animales se presentan con letra mayúscula, en bastardilla, en singular si se refieren al género y en plural si se refieren a la clase, orden, familia o filo (11).

> (11) **Salmonela** *f. Salmonella*, a gram-negative bacteria of the *Enterobacteriaceae* that causes enteric fever, gastrointestinal infection and septicemia.

ABREVIATURAS MÉDICAS Y TABLAS DE CONVERSIÓN

Para abreviar y facilitar su uso, las abreviaturas médicas y los prefijos, sufijos y raíces aparecen en secciones aparte tituladas **Abreviaturas médicas más usuales** y **Tablas de conversión**.

COMUNICACIÓN CON LOS PACIENTES

Esta sección tiene como propósito facilitar la comunicación entre el profesional médico y el o la paciente cuando el inglés o el español no es el idioma común.

APÉNDICES

Los apéndices que se encuentran al final del diccionario comprenden: números, pesos y medidas, palabras relacionadas con el tiempo, síntomas y signos, enfermedades contagiosas, cuidado de emergencia, pruebas médicas, nutrición, acondicionamiento físico, y una sección de vocabulario y frases, **Comunicación con los pacientes**.

ILLUSTRACIONES

En la tercera edición el lector encontrará un Atlas de Anatomia en color y pequeñas ilustraciones que aparecen en el vocabulario. La edición "deluxe" tiene, además un CD-ROM para uso audiovisual.

PALABRAS A LOS LECTORES

En esta tercera edición hemos hecho varias adiciones, algunas de ellas siguiendo la sugerencia de nuestros lectores. Esperamos que los nuevos lectores del diccionario hagan lo mismo, enviándonos sus recomendaciones por vía Lippincott Williams & Wilkins, para seguir mejorando ediciones futuras.

Abbreviations / Abreviaturas

ENGLISH		SPANISH	
a.	adjective	*a.*	adjetivo
abbr.	abbreviation	*abr.*	abreviatura
adv.	adverb	*adv.*	adverbio
approx.	approximate	*aprox.*	aproximadamente
art.	article	*art.*	artículo
aux	auxiliary	*aux.*	auxiliar
Cast.	Castilian	*Cast.*	castellano
comp.	comparative	*comp.*	comparativo
cond.	conditional	*cond.*	condicional
conj.	conjunction	*conj.*	conjunción
cu.	cubic	*cu.*	cúbico
dem.	demonstrative	*dem.*	demostrativo
esp.	especially	*esp.*	especialmente
f.	feminine	*f.*	femenino
		fam.	familiar
Fr.	French	*Fr.*	francés
form.	formal pronoun		
gen.	generally	*gen.*	generalmente
Gr.	Greek	*Gr.*	griego
gr.	grammar	*gr.*	gramática
H.A.	Hispanic America	*H.A.*	Hispanoamérica
imp.	imperative	*imp.*	imperativo
impf.	imperfect	*impf.*	imperfecto
ind.	indicative	*ind.*	indicativo
indef.	indefinite	*indef.*	indefinido
inf.	infinitive	*inf.*	infinitivo
infl.	inflammation	*infl.*	inflamación
int.	interjection	*int.*	interjección
interr.	interrogative	*interr.*	interrogativo
L.	Latin	*L.*	latín
m.	masculine	*m.*	masculino
Mex.	Mexico	*Mex.*	México
Mex.A.	Mexican-American	*Mex.A.*	Mexicano-americano

n.	noun	*n.*	nombre
neut.	neuter	*neut.*	neutro
obj.	object	*obj.*	objeto
pop.	popular	*pop.*	popular
pp.	past participle	*pp.*	participio de pasado
p.p.	present participle	*p.p.*	participio de presente
pref.	prefix	*pref.*	prefijo
prep.	preposition	*prep.*	preposición
pres.	present	*pres.*	presente
pret.	preterite	*pret.*	pretérito
pron.	pronoun	*pron.*	pronombre
psych.	psychology	*psic.*	psicología
ref.	reflexive	*ref.*	reflexivo
rel.	relative	*rel.*	relativo
subj.	subjunctive	*subj.*	subjuntivo
sup.	superlative	*sup.*	superlativo
surg.	surgery	*cirg.*	cirugía
U.S.A.	United States of America	*E.U.A.*	Estados Unidos de América
usu.	usually	*usu.*	usualmente
V.	see	*V.*	véase
v.	verb	*v.*	verbo
vi.	irregular verb	*vi.*	verbo irregular
vr.	reflexive verb	*vr.*	verbo reflexivo

Most Common Medical Abbreviations / Abreviaturas médicas más usuales

In English, abbreviations are commonly used in oral communication as well as in written medical reports. In Spanish, however, they are generally only used in written reports.

Las abreviaturas en inglés se usan comúnmente como medio de expresión oral y escrita. En español, las siglas indicadas sólo se usan general-mente en la forma escrita.

Latin expressions (*in italics*), and abbreviations that are the same in both languages appear only on the left (English column).

Las expresiones en latín (*en letra bastardilla*), y las abreviaturas comunes a ambos idiomas aparecen a la izquierda solamente (columna en inglés).

ABBR.	ENGLISH / INGLÉS	ABREV.	SPANISH / ESPAÑOL
A	accomodation	—	acomodación
A_2	aortic second sound	—	segundo ruido aórtico
AA	Alcoholics Anonymous	—	Alcohólicos Anónimos (asociación de)
AA	auto accident	—	accidente de automóvil
A&B	apnea and bradycardia	—	apnea y bradicardia
A&P	auscultation and percussion	—	auscultación y percusión
AASH	adrenal androgen-stimulating hormone	HASE	hormona andrógena suprarrenal estimulante
Ab	abortion; antibody	aba	aborto; anticuerpo
AB	apical beat	LA	latido apical
ABC	artificial beta cells	CBA	células beta artificiales
abd	abdomen	—	abdomen
ABE	acute bacterial endocarditis	EIA	endocarditis infecciosa aguda
ABG	arterial blood gases	GSA	gases de sangre arterial / gasometria arterial
ABMT	autologous bone marrow transplant	TAMO	trasplante autólogo de médula ósea
abn	abnormal	an	anormal
ABP	androgen-binding protein	PAT	proteína andrógena transportadora
ac (*ante cibum*)	before meals	—	antes de las comidas
ACBP	aortocoronary bypass	DAC	derivación aorto-coronaria
ACE	angiotension-converting enzyme	EAC	enzima de angiotensión y conversión avanzada
ACG	angiocardiography	—	angiocardiografía
ACLS	advanced cardiovascular life support	PCVA	progreso cardiovascular de vida avanzada

ABBR.	ENGLISH / INGLÉS	ABREV.	SPANISH / ESPAÑOL
ACT	activated clotting time	TAC	tiempo activado de coagulación
ACTH	adrenocorticotropic hormone	HACT	hormona adrenocorticotrópina
ad (*ad*)	until	—	hasta
AD	right ear	OD	oído derecho
ADD	attention deficit disorder	DDA	desorden de falta de atención
ad effect (*ad effectum*)	until it is effective	—	hasta que produzca efecto
ADH	antidiuretic hormone	HAD	hormona antidiurética o vasopresina
ADHD	attention deficit hyperactivity disorder	DAHD	desorden de falta de atención por hiperactividad
ADL	activities of daily living	AVD	actividades de la vida cotidiana
AE	above elbow	EC	por encima del codo
AF	auricular fibrillation	FA	fibrilación auricular
AFB	aorto-femoral bypass	DAF	derivación aorto-femoral
Afeb.	afebrile	afeb	afebril
AFP	alphafetoprotein	—	alfafetoproteína
AG	albumin-globulin ratio	IAG	índice de albúmina y globulina
agit (*agitatum*)	shake	—	agítese
AHF	antihemophilic factor VIII	FAH	Factor VIII antihemofílico
AI	aortic insufficiency	IA	insuficiencia aórtica
AICD	automatic implantable cardioverter defibrillator	DCA	autoimplantable defribilador cardiovertedor
A.I.D.	artificial insemination by donor	I.A.D.	inseminación artificial por donante
AIDS	acquired immunodeficiency syndrome	SIDA	síndrome de inmunodeficiencia aquirida
A.I.H.	artificial insemination by husband	I.A.E.	inseminación artificial por esposo
AK	above knee	ER	por encima de la rodilla

ABBR.	ENGLISH / INGLÉS	ABREV.	SPANISH / ESPAÑOL
AL	left ear	AU	oído izquierdo
ALB	albumin	—	albúmina
ALL	acute lymphocytic leukemia	LLA	leucemia linfocítica aguda
ALS	amyotrophic lateral sclerosis	ELA	esclerosis lateral amiotrófica
ALT	serum alanine aminotransferase	ALAT	alanina aminotransferasa sérica
a.m.	routine care in the morning	a.m.	cuidado matutino rutinario del paciente
AMA	against medical advice	CRM	contra recomendación médica
A.M.A.	American Medical Association	A.M.A.	Asociación Médica Americana
AMI	acute myocardial infarction	IGM	infarto grave del miocardio
AML	acute myelogenous leukemia	LAM	leucemia mielógena aguda
amnio	amniocentesis	—	amniocentesis
ANA	antinuclear antibody	—	anticuerpo antinuclear
Anes.	anesthesia	—	anestesia
AO	aorta	—	aorta
AOP	aortic pressure	PAO	presión aórtica
AP	anteroposterior	—	anteroposterior
APTT	activated partial thromboplastin time	APTP	tiempo de tromboplastina activado parcialmente
AR	aortic regurgitation	RA	regurgitación aórtica
ARC	AIDS-related complex	CS	complejo del SIDA
ARDS	acute respiratory distress syndrome	SDE	syndrome disneico extremo
arf	acute rheumatic fever	fra	fiebre reumática aguda
ARF	acute renal failure	IRA	insuficiencia renal aguda
ARM	artificial rupture of membranes	RAM	ruptura artificial de membranas
ART	assessment, review, and treatment	ERT	evaluación, repaso y tratamiento

ABBR.	ENGLISH / INGLÉS	ABREV.	SPANISH / ESPAÑOL
AS	aortic stenosis	EA	estenosis aórtica
AS	left ear	OI	oído izquierdo
ASAP	as soon as possible	LAP	lo antes posible
ASC	ambulatory surgery center	CCA	centro de cirugía ambulatoria
ASCVD, ASVD	arteriosclerotic vascular disease	ASV	arteriosclerosis vascular
ASD	atrial septal defect	DTA	defecto del tabique auricular
ASHD	arteriolsclerotic heart disease	CI	cardiopatía isquémica
AST	aspartate aminotransferase	—	aspartato aminotransferasa
ATB	antibiotic	ATB	antibiótico
ATC	around the clock	—	durante las 24 horas
ATN	acute tubular necrosis	NTA	necrosis tubular aguda
ATP	adenosine triphosphate	TFA	trifosfato de adenosina
ATR	Achilles tendon reflex	RTA	reflejo del tendón de Aquiles
AV	arteriovenous	—	arteriovenoso
AV	atrioventricular	—	auriculoventricular
AVM	arteriovenous malformation	MAV	malformación arteriovenosa
AVR	aortic valve replacement	RVA	reemplazo de la válvula aórtica
AVS	arteriovenous shunt	DAV	derivación arteriovenosa
AZT	Azidothymidine	—	cidovudina
ba	barium	ba	bario
BAO	basic acid output	GAB	gasto de ácido básico
BB	blood bank	BS	banco de sangre
BBB	bundle branch block	BR	bloqueo de rama
BC	blood culture	CH	cultivo hemático
BCG	bacillus Calmette-Guérin	BCG	bacilo de Calmette Guerin
BE	bacterial endocarditis	EB	endocarditis bacteriana
BE	barium enema	EB	enema de bario
BEE	basal energy expenditure	GED	gasto de energía basal

ABBR.	ENGLISH / INGLÉS	ABREV.	SPANISH / ESPAÑOL
BF	breast feeding	LM	lactancia materna
BI	bacterial infection	IB	infección bacteriana
bid (*bis in die*)	twice a day	—	dos veces al día
BIL	bilateral	—	bilateral
BKA	below knee amputation	ADR	amputación debajo de la rodilla
BLT	bleeding time	DS	duración de sangramiento
BM	bowel movement	EF	evacuación, defecación, eliminación fecal
BMR	basal metabolic rate	IMB	índice metabólico basal
BP	blood pressure	PA	presión arterial
BPD	bronchopulmonary dysplasia	DBP	displasia broncopulmonar
BPH	benign prostatic hyperplasia	HBP	hiperplasia benigna de la próstata
BSO	bilateral salpingo-oophorectomy	SOB	salpingo-ooforectomía bilateral
BUN	blood urea nitrogen	US	urea sanguínea
Bx	biopsy	—	biopsia
c.	with	—	con
CA, Ca	cancer, carcinoma	CA	cáncer, carcinoma / marcador tumoral
CAB	coronary artery bypass	DC	derivación coronaria
CABG	coronary artery bypass graft	IDAC	injerto-derivación coronaria
CAD	coronary artery disease	—	enfermedad de la arteria coronaria
CAH	congenital adrenal hyperplasia	HCS	hiperplasia suprarrenal congénita
C&A	carotid arteriectomy	A&C	arterectomía de la carótida
CAPD	continuous ambulatory peritoneal dialysis	DPAC	diálisis peritoneal ambulatoria continua
cap(s)	capsule(s)	cap(s)	cápsula(s)
CAT	computerized axial tomography	TAC	tomografía axial computerizada
CATH	catheterize	CAT	cateterizar

ABBR.	ENGLISH / INGLÉS	ABREV.	SPANISH / ESPAÑOL
CBC	complete blood count	CSC	conteo sanguíneo completo
CBD	common bile duct	CBC	conducto biliar común
CC	chief complaint	QP	queja principal
cc	cubic centimeter	—	centímetro cúbico
CCU	coronary care unit	SCC	sala de cuidado coronario
CDC	Centers for Disease Control	CCE	Centros de Control de Enfermedades
CD4	helper-induced T-cells	CD4	células T cooperadoras-inductoras
CDH	congenital dislocation of the hip	DCC	dislocación congénita de la cadera
CEA	carcinoembryonic antigen	ACE	antígeno carcino-embriónico
CF	cystic fibrosis	FC	fibrosis cística
CFS	chronic fatigue syndrome	SFC	síndrome de fatiga crónica
CHD	coronary heart disease	CP	coronariopatía
CHD	congenital heart disease	CC	cardiopatía congénita
CHF	congestive heart failure	ICC	insuficiencia cardíaca congestiva
CHOL	cholesterol	COL	colesterol
CIN	cervical intraepithelial neoplasia	NIC	neoplasia intraepitelial cervical
cl	clear	—	claro
CM	continuous murmur	—	soplo continuo
CMV	cytomegalovirus	—	citomegalovirus
CNS	central nervous system	SNC	sistema nervioso central
c/o	complains of	q/d	quejas
CO	cardiac output	GC	gasto cardíaco
CO_2	carbon dioxide	CDC	contenido de dióxido de carbono
COPD	chronic obstructive pulmonary disease	NCO	neumopatía crónica obstructiva
C.P.	chest pain	D.P.	dolor de pecho

ABBR.	ENGLISH / INGLÉS	ABREV.	SPANISH / ESPAÑOL
CPR	cardiopulmonary resuscitation	RCP	reanimación cardiopulmonar
CR	cardiorespiratory	CR	cardiorespiratorio
CRF	chronic renal failure	IRC	insuficiencia renal crónica
CRH	corticotropin-releasing hormone	HCTL	hormona corticotrópica liberina
C&S	culture and sensitivity	—	cultivo y sensibilidad
CS	cesarean section	OC	operación cesárea
CSD	cat-scratch disease	ERG	enfermedad de rasguño de gato
CSF	cerebrospinal fluid	LCR	líquido cefalorraquídeo
CSP	carotid sinus pressure	PSC	presión del seno carotenoide
CT	computerized tomography	TC	tomografía computada
CV	cardiovascular	—	cardiovascular
CVA	cerebrovascular accident	AP	apoplejía
CVD	cardiovascular disease	ECV	enfermedad cardiovascular
CVI	cerebrovascular insufficiency	ICV	insuficiencia cerebrovascular
CVP	central venous pressure	PVC	presión venosa central
CVS	chorionic villus sampling	MC	muestra coriónica
CVS	cardiovascular system		aparato circulatorio
CXR	chest X-ray	TXR	radiografía del tórax
cysto	cystoscopic examination	cisto	cistoscopía
d.	dose	—	dosis
D	delivery	P	parto
D&C	dilation and curettage	—	dilatación y curetaje
D&S	dilation and suction	—	dilatación y succión
DAT	diet as tolerated	—	dieta tolerada
DC	discontinue	SP	suspéndase
DD	differential diagnosis	—	diagnóstico diferencial

ABBR.	ENGLISH / INGLÉS	ABREV.	SPANISH / ESPAÑOL
ddC 2', 3	dideoxycytidine	ddc	dideoxitidina
dd in d	from day to day	—	de un día a otro día
dE 2'3	dideoxyinosine	DGI	dideoxiinosina
DFA	direct flourescent antibody	AFD	anticuerpo fluorescente directo
DGI	disseminated gonoccochal infection	IGD	infección gonocócica diseminada
DI	diabetes insipidus	—	diabetes insípida
DIC	disseminated intravascular coagulopathy	CID	coagulopatía intravascular diseminada
DIFF	differential blood count	CSD	conteo sanguíneo diferenciado
dil	dilute	—	diluir
DJC	degenerative joint disease	EDA	emfermedad degenerativa de las articulaciones
DKA	diabetic ketoacidosis	CE	cetoacidosis diabética
DM	diabetes mellitus	—	diabetes mellitus
DM	diastolic murmurs	SD	soplos diastólicos
DNA	deoxyribonucleic acid	ADN	ácido desoxirribonucleico
DNR	do not resuscitate	NR	no reanimar
DOB	date of birth	FDN	fecha de nacimiento
DOE	dyspnea on exertion	DDE	disnea de esfuerzo
DPT	diphtheria-pertussis-tetanus	DPT	difteria, pertusis, tétano
DR	delivery room	SP	sala de partos
DRG	drainage	DRJ	drenaje
DSA	digital subtraction angiography	ADS	angiografía digital de sustracción
DTP	diphtheria, tetanus, and pertussis vaccine	DTP	vacuna contra difteria, tétano y pertusis
DTR	deep tendon reflexes	RTP	reflejos tendinosos profundos
DUB	dysfunctional uterine bleeding	TSU	trastorno de sangrado del útero
DVT	deep vein thrombosis	TVP	trombosis de vena profunda
Dx	diagnosis	—	diagnóstico

Most Common Medical Abbreviations / Abreviaturas médicas más usuales

ABBR.	ENGLISH / INGLÉS	ABREV.	SPANISH / ESPAÑOL
EBL	estimated blood loss	PES	pérdida estimada de sangre
ECF	extended care facility	IAE	instalación para atención extendida
ECG, EKG	electrocardiogram	ECG	electrocardiograma
ECM	erythema chronicum migrans	ECM	eritema crónico migratorio
ECT	electroconvulsive therapy	TEC	terapia electroconvulsiva
EEG	electroencephalogram	EEG	electroencefalograma
EFW	estimated fetal weight	PEF	peso estimado del feto
EIA	enzyme immunoassay	IEE	immunoanálisis de enzimas
ELISA	enzyme-linked immunosorbent assay	ELISA	prueba inmunosorbente enzimática
EM	ejection murmur	SE	ruido de eyección
EMG	electromyogram	EMG	electromiograma
EMS	emergency medical services	SME	servicios médicos de emergencia
ENT	ear, nose, and throat	NGO	nariz, garganta, y oídos
EPA	Environmental Protection Agency	AM	Agencia del Medioambiente
ER	emergency room	SE	sala de emergencia
ES	expulsion sound or click	SE	ruido de expulsión, chasquido o clic
ESR	erythrocyte sedimentation rate	IES	índice de eritrosedi-mentación
ESRD	end-stage renal disease	ERTF	etapa final de enfermedad renal
EST	electric shock therapy	ECH	electrochoque
ESWL	extracorporeal shock wave lithotripsy	LEOCH	litotripsia extracorpórea con ondas de choque
EUA	examination under anesthesia	EBA	exploración bajo anesthesia
EUG	excretory urography	UE	urografía intravenosa
EXT	extremity	EXT	extremidad
f	female	F	sexo femenino
FBS	fasting blood sugar or glucose	GA	glicemia en ayunas

ABBR.	ENGLISH / INGLÉS	ABREV.	SPANISH / ESPAÑOL
FCF	fetal cardiac frequency	—	frecuencia cardíaca del feto
FEV	forced expiratory volume	VEM	volumen expiratorio máximo
FFP	fresh fetal plasma	PFC	plasma fetal recién congelado
FHM	fetal heart monitoring	MCF	monitoreo cardiofetal
FHR	fetal heart rate	FCF	frecuencia cardíaca fetal
fl	fluid	—	fluido liquido
FMH	family medical history	HMF	historia médica de la familia
FSH	follicle-stimulating hormone	HFE	hormona folículo-estimulante
FTND	full term normal delivery	PAT	parto a término (normal)
FTT	failure to thrive	DC	déficit en el crecimiento
FUO	fever of unknown origin	FOD	fiebre de origen desconocido
F/U	follow-up	S/C	seguimiento del caso
Fx	fracture	—	fractura
G	gonorrhea	—	gonorrea
GA	gastric analysis	AG	análisis gástrico
GAD	generalized anxiety disorder	TAG	trastorno generalizado de ansiedad
GB	gallbladder	VB	vesícula biliar
GC	gonococcus	—	gonococo
gen	general	—	general
GEN	genetics	—	genética
GGT	gamma-glutamyl transferase	—	gamma glutamil transferasa
GH	growth hormone	HC	hormona del crecimiento
GI	gastrointestinal	—	gastrointestinal
GIT	gastrointestinal tract	TGI	tracto gastrointestinal
GLUC	glucose	—	glucosa
GnRH	gonadotropin-releasing hormone	HLH	hormona liberadora de gonadotropina
Grx	gravida	Gra	grávida
GSW	gunshot wound	HB	herida de bala

Most Common Medical Abbreviations / Abreviaturas médicas más usuales

ABBR.	ENGLISH / INGLÉS	ABREV.	SPANISH / ESPAÑOL
GTT	glucose tolerance test	PTG	prueba de tolerancia a la glucosa
Gtt., gtt (*guttatim*)	drops	—	gotas
GU	genitourinary	—	genitourinario
GYN	gynecology	GIN	ginecología
h	hour	—	hora
HAV	hepatitis A virus	VHA	virus de hepatitis A
HB	hepatitis B vaccine	VHB	vacuna de hepatitis B
HBV	hepatitis B virus	VHB	virus de hepatitis B
HCG	human chorionic gonadotropin	GCH	gonadotropina coriónica humana
HCT	hematocrit	—	hematócrito
HCVD	hypertensive cardiovascular disease	ECVH	enfermedad cardiovascular hipertensiva
HD	hemodialysis	—	hemodiálisis
HD	hip disarticulation	DC	desarticulación de la cadera
HD	hospital discharge	DDA	dado de alta
HDL	high density lipoprotein	LAD	lipoproteína de alta densidad
HGT	height	—	altura
H/H	hemoglobin/hematocrit	—	hemoglobina/hematocrito
HIB	haemophilus b conjugate vaccine	HBI	vacuna conjugada de hemófilo b
HIV	human immunodeficiency virus	VIH	virus inmunodeficiente humano
HLA	human-leukocyte antigen	ALH	antígeno leucocitado humano
HM	health maintenance	MS	mantenimiento de la salud
H_2O	water	—	agua
HNP	herniated nucleus pulposus	—	hernia del núcleo pulposo
HR	heart rate	IC	índice cardíaco
HRT	hormone replacement therapy	HTR	hormonoterapia restitutiva

ABBR.	ENGLISH / INGLÉS	ABREV.	SPANISH / ESPAÑOL
hs (*hora somni*)	at bedtime	—	a la hora de acostarse
hypo	hypodermically		inyectado
Hyst	hysterectomy	Hist	histerectomía
ICF	intracellular fluid	LIC	líquido intracelular
ICH	intracerebral hematoma	HIC	hematoma intracerebral
ICH	intracraneal hemorrhage	HIC	hemorragia intracraneana
ICSH	interstitial cell-stimulating hormone	HECI	hormona de estimulación de célula intersticial
ICU	intensive care unit	SCI	sala de cuidado intensivo
I&D	incision and drainage	—	incisión y drenaje
ID	identification	—	identificación
ID	intradermal	—	intradérmica
id	infectious disease		enfermedad contagiosa
IDDM	insulin-dependent diabetes mellitus	DMID	diabetes mellitus (sacarina) insulinodependiente
IE	infective endocarditis	EI	endocarditis infecciosa
IFA	immunofluorescent assay	AFI	análisis fluorescente immunológico
IgG	immunoglobulin G	—	inmunoglobulina G
IgM	immunoglobulin M	—	inmunoglobulina M
II	icteric index	—	índice ictérico
IIM	idiopathic inflammatory myopathy	MII	miopatía idiopática inflamatoria
ILD	instersititial lung disease	EPI	enfermedad pulmonar intersticial
im	intramuscular	in	intramuscular
Imp	impression	—	impresión
INFO	information	—	información
I&O	intake and output	AG	absorción y gasto
IOL	intraocular lens	LIO	lente intraocular
IPD	intermittent peritoneal dialysis	DPI	diálisis peritoneal intermitente
IPPB	intermittent positive pressure breathing	RIPP	respiración intermitente con presión positiva

Most Common Medical Abbreviations / Abreviaturas médicas más usuales

ABBR.	ENGLISH / INGLÉS	ABREV.	SPANISH / ESPAÑOL
IPV	polio vaccine shots	VPI	vacunas de polio inyectadas
IQ	intelligence quotient	CI	cociente de inteligencia
ISE	ion-selective electrodes	EIS	electrodos de iones seleccionados
ISG	immune serum globulin	GSI	globulina sérica inmunológica
ITA	ischemic transient attack	AIP	ataque isquémico pasajero
ITP	idiopathic thrombocytopenic purpura	PTI	púrpura trombocitopénica idiopática
IU	international unit	UI	unidad internacional
IUD	intrauterine device	DIU	dispositivo intrauterino
IUM	intrauterine monitoring	—	monitoreo intrauterino
IUP	intrauterine pregnancy	EIU	embarazo intrauterino
IUT	intrauterine transfusion	TIU	transfusión intrauterina
IV	intravenous	VIV	vía intravenosa
IVC	intravenous cholangiogram	CIV	colangiograma intravenoso
IVP	intravenous pyelogram	PIV	pielograma intravenoso
JRA	juvenile rheumatoid arthritis	ARJ	artritis reumatoidea juvenil
JVP	jugular vein pulse	PVY	pulso de la vena yugular
K	potassium	—	potasio
KCL	potassium chloride	CLP	cloruro de potasio
KD	knee disarticulation	DR	desarticulación de la rodilla
KUB	kidney, ureter, bladder	RUV	riñón, uréter, vejiga (placa simple de abdomen)
KVO	keep vein open	MVA	mantener la vena abierta
L	left	Iz.	izquierdo-a
L	leukoplakia	—	leucoplaquia
LA	left atrium	AI	aurícula izquierda
LAB	laboratory	—	laboratorio
LAP	laparotomy	—	laparotomía

ABBR.	ENGLISH / INGLÉS	ABREV.	SPANISH / ESPAÑOL
LBBB	left bundle branch block	BRI	bloqueo de rama izquierda
LBP	low blood pressure	HA	hipotensión arterial
LBW	low birth weight	PBN	peso bajo al nacer
LDH	lactate dehydrogenase	DHL	deshidrogenasa láctica
LDL	low density lipoprotein	LBD	lipoproteína de baja densidad
LE	lupus erythematosus	—	lupus eritematoso
LE	left eye	OI	ojo izquierdo
LES	lower esophageal sphincter	SEI	esfínter esofágico inferior
LFT	liver function test	PFH	prueba de función hepática
LH	luteinizing hormone	HL	hormona luteinizante
LLE	left lower extremity	EIIz	extremidad inferior izquierda
LLL	left lower lobe	LII	lóbulo inferior izquierdo
LLQ	left lower quadrant	CIIz	cuadrante inferior izquierdo
LMP	last menstrual period	UPM	último periodo menstrual
LP	lumbar puncture	PL	punción lumbar
LHRF	luteinizing hormone-releasing factor	FLE	factor luteinizante de descargo
LS	liver scan	EH	escán o barrido del hígado
LS	lumbar spine	EL	espina lumbar
LSD	low salt diet	DH	dieta hiposódica
LUE	left upper extremity	ESIz	extremidad superior izquierda
LUQ	left upper quadrant	CSIz	cuadrante superior izquierdo
LVH	left ventricular hypertrophy	HVI	hipertrofia ventricular izquierda
L&W	living and well	V y S	vivo y saludable
m	murmur	s	soplo
MAE	moves all extremities	MTE	mueve todas las extremidades

ABBR.	ENGLISH / INGLÉS	ABREV.	SPANISH / ESPAÑOL
MAT	multifocal atrial tachycardia	TAM	taquicardia auricular multifocal
max	maximum	max	maximum
mc	millicurie	—	milicurie
MCA	middle cerebral artery	ACM	arteria cerebral media
MCB	medium corpuscular volume	VCM	volumen corpuscular medio
MCH	mean corpuscular hemoglobin	ICH	índice corpuscular de hemoglobina
MCNS	minimal change nephrotic syndrome	SN	síndrome nefrótico de cambio mínimo
MCV	mean corpuscular index	IVC	índice de volumen corpuscular
MD	medical doctor	DM	doctor en medicina
ME	middle ear	OM	oído medio
MED	medicine	—	medicina
MHCM	medium hemoglobin corpuscular concentration	CCHM	media de concentración corpuscular de hemoglobina
MI	myocardial infarction	IC	infarto cardíaco
mi	mitral insufficiency	IM	insuficiencia mitral
min	minute, minimum	—	minuto; mínimo
MM	mucous membrane	—	membrana mucosa
MMR	measles, mumps, and rubella vaccine	VSPR	vacuna triple de sarampión, paperas y rubéola
MR	mitral regurgitation	RM	regurgitación mitral
MRA	magnetic resonance angiography	ARM	angiografía de resonancia magnética
MRI	magnetic resonance imaging	IRM	imagen de resonancia magnética
MS	multiple sclerosis	EM	esclerosis múltiple
MS	mitral stenosis	EM	estenosis mitral
MT	medical technologist	TM	técnico médico
MVI	multivitamins	—	multivitaminas
MVP	mitral valve prolapse	PVM	prolapso de la válvula mitral
mx	mixture	mc	mezcla

ABBR.	ENGLISH / INGLÉS	ABREV.	SPANISH / ESPAÑOL
NA	nursing assistant	AE	asistente de enfermería
N / A	not applicable	—	no aplicable
Na	sodium	—	sodio
NAS	no added sodium	—	no añadir sodio
NEC	necrotizing enterocolitis	EC	enterocolitis necrosante
NCV	nerve conduction velocity	VCN	velocidad de la conducción neural
neurol	neurology	—	neurología
NG	nasogastric	—	nasogástrico
NH	neonatal hyperthyroidism	HN	hipertiroidismo neonatal
NIH	National Institutes of Health	INS	Instituto Nacional de Salud
NKA	no known allergies	SAC	sin alergia conocida
NPO	nothing by mouth	NPB	nada por la boca
NR	neonatal resuscitation	RN	reanimación neonatal
NREM	nonrapid eye movement	MOL	movimiento ocular lento
NS	nephrotic syndrome	SN	síndrome nefrótico
NST	nonstress test	PSE	prueba sin esfuerzo
NSR	normal sinus rhythm	RSN	ritmo sinusal normal
NTG	nitroglycerin	—	nitroglicerina
N&V	nausea and vomiting	—	náusea y vómitos
NVD	neck, vein distention	DVY	distensión de las venas yugulares
OA	osteoarthritis	—	osteoartritis
OB, Obs	obstetrics	Obs	obstetricia
OC	oral contraceptive	AO	anticonceptivos orales
OCD	obsessive-compulsive disorder	TOC	trastorno obsesivo-convulsivo
od	once a day	—	una vez al día
OD	(occulus dexter) right eye		ojo derecho
OD	overdose	SD	sobredosis
omn hor (*omni hora*)	every hour	—	cada hora
on (*omni nocte*)	every night	—	todas las noches
O&P	ova and parasites	P	parásitos y
op	operation	—	operación

Most Common Medical Abbreviations / Abreviaturas médicas más usuales

ABBR.	ENGLISH / INGLÉS	ABREV.	SPANISH / ESPAÑOL
OPV	oral poliovaccine	VPO	vacuna oral de poliomielitis
OR	operating room	Q	quirófano, sala de operaciones
ORTHO	orthopedic	ORTO	ortopédico
OS,RE	right eye	OD	ojo derecho
OS,LE	left eye	OI	ojo izquierdo
OT	occupational therapy	TO	terapia ocupacional
OTC	over-the-counter	SRx	medicinas sin necesidad de receta médica
O2	both eyes	—	ambos ojos
P	prognosis	—	prognosis
P	pulse	—	pulso
p (*post*)	after	—	pasado (el tiempo de), después de
p	plan	p	plan
PA	pernicious anemia	AP	anemia perniciosa
PA	pulmonary artery	AP	arteria pulmonar
PAC	premature atrial contraction	CAP	contracción auricular prematura
PAD	peripheral artery disease	AP	arteriopatía periférica
Pap	Papanicolaou	UN	Papanicolaou
PAR	plasma renin activity	APR	actividad del plasma y la renina
PAT	paroxysmal atrial tachycardia	TAP	taquicardia auricular paroxística
PATH	pathology	PAT	patología
PA view	posteroanterior view (radiology)	VPA	vista postero-anterior (radiología)
PBC	primary biliary cirrhosis	CBP	cirrosis biliar primaria
pc (*post cibus*)	after meals	—	después de las comidas
PCA	passive cutaneous anaphylaxis	ACP	anafilaxis cutánea pasiva
PCA	patient-controlled anesthesia	ARP	anestesia regulada al paciente
PCH	past clinical history	HCP	historia clínica previa
PCO2	carbon dioxide content of blood	—	contenido de dióxido de carbono en la sangre

ABBR.	ENGLISH / INGLÉS	ABREV.	SPANISH / ESPAÑOL
PCP	Pneumocystis Carinii pneumonia	—	neumonía neumocística carinii
PD	pulse deficit	DP	déficit de pulso
PE	physical examination	EF	examen físico
pe	pulmonary embolism	ep	embolia pulmonar
PEG	percutaneous endoscopic gastrectomy	GEP	gastroctomía endoscópica percutánea
PEL	permissible exposure limit	LEP	límite de exposición permitida
PERRLA	pupils equal, round, and equally reactive to light and accommodation	PIRRLA	pupilas iguales y redondas de igual reacción a la luz y acomodación
PET	positron emission tomography		tomografía de emisión por positrón
PFC	persistent fetal circulation	CFP	circulación fetal persistente
PGH	pituitary growth hormone	HPC	hormona pituitaria del crecimiento
pH	hydrogen ion concentration (acidity)	—	concentración de iones de hidrógeno (acidez)
PH	pulmonary hypertension	HP	hipertensión pulmonar
PI	present illness	EF	enfermedad actual
PI	principal investigator	IP	investigador principal
PICU	pediatric intensive care unit	SPCI	sala pediátrica de cuidado intensivo
PID	pelvic inflammatory disease	EIP	enfermedad inflamatoria de la pelvis
PLTS	platelets	—	plaquetas
pm (*post meridiem*)	afternoon	—	pasado meridiano
PMH	past medical history	HM	historia médica previa
PMI	point of maximum impulse	PIM	punto de impulso máximo
PMN	polymorphonuclear	—	polimorfonuclear
PMR	proportional mortality rate	IMP	índice de mortalidad proporcional
PMS	premenstrual syndrome	SPM	síndrome premenstrual

ABBR.	ENGLISH / INGLÉS	ABREV.	SPANISH / ESPAÑOL
PND	paroxysmal nocturnal dyspnea	DPN	disnea paroxística nocturna
PNH	paroxysmal nocturnal hemoglobinuria	HPN	hemoglobinuria paroxística nocturna
PNS	peripheral nervous system	SNP	sistema nervioso periférico
PO (per os)	by mouth	—	por vía oral
PO$_2$	oxygen content of blood	—	contenido de oxígeno en la sangre
POS	positive	—	positivo
Post-OP	after operation	—	post operatorio
p.p.m.	pulses per minute	—	pulsaciones por minuto
PR	per rectum	PVR	por vía rectal
PR	pulse ratio	FP	frecuencia del pulso
PSA	prostatic specific antigen	AEP	antígeno prostático específico
psych	psychiatry	psiq	psiquiatría
PT	physical therapy	TF	terapia física
PT	prothrombin time	TP	tiempo de protrombina
PTA	prior to admission	AI	anterior al ingreso
PTCA	percutaneous transluminal coronary angioplasty	ACPT	angioplastia coronaria percutánea transluminal
PTH	parathyroid hormone	HP	hormona paratiroidea
PTT	partial thromboplastin time	TPT	tiempo parcial de tromboplastina
PUD	peptic ulcer disease	UP	úlcera péptica
PV	peripheral vision	VP	visión periférica
PVC	premature ventricular contraction	CVP	contracción ventricular prematura
q (quaque)	every	—	cada
QA	quality assurance	SC	seguridad de calidad
QC	quality control	CC	control de calidad
q.d. (quaque die)	every day	—	diariamente
q.h. (quaque hora)	every hour	—	cada hora
qhs	at hour of sleep	—	a la hora de dormir

ABBR.	ENGLISH / INGLÉS	ABREV.	SPANISH / ESPAÑOL
qid (*quater in die*)	four times a day	—	cuatro veces al día
qod	every other day	—	días alternos
qns (*quantum non sufficit*)	quantity not sufficient	—	cantidad insuficiente
q.q.h. (*quaque quarta*)	every quarter of an hour	—	cada cuarto de hora
QS (*quantum sufficit*)	a sufficient amount	—	en suficiente cantidad
q 2h	every two hours	—	cada dos horas
R	respiration; radiotherapy	—	respiración; radioterapia
RA	right atrium	AD	aurícula derecha
RACAB	robot-assisted coronary artery bypass	DCAR	derivación coronaria asistida por robot
rad	radiation absorbed dose	dra	dosis de radiación absorbida
RAI	radioactive iodine	YR	yodo radioactivo
RAM	rapid alternating movements	MAR	movimientos alternos rápidos
RAP	recurrent abdominal pain	DAR	dolor abdominal recurrente
RBC	red blood cells	GR	glóbulos rojos (hematíes)
RDS	respiratory distress syndrome	SDR	síndrome de dificultad respiratoria
RDSN	respiratory distress syndrome of newborn	SDN	síndrome disneico neonatal
RE	right eye	OD	ojo derecho
REM	rapid eye movement	MRO	movimientos rápidos oculares
REM$_2$	reticular erythematous mucinosis	MER	mucinosis eritematosa reticular
RF	renal failure	IR	insuficiencia renal
RF	rheumatoid factor	AR	anticuerpos reumatoideos
Rh	blood factor	—	factor sanguíneo
RHD	rheumatic heart disease	CR	cardiopatía reumática
RI	respiratory insufficiency	IR	insuficiencia respiratoria

Most Common Medical Abbreviations / Abreviaturas médicas más usuales

ABBR.	ENGLISH / INGLÉS	ABREV.	SPANISH / ESPAÑOL
RIA	radioimmunoassay	ERI	estudio radioinmunológico
RKS	radial keratotomy surgery	CQR	cirugía de queratotomía radial
RLE	right lower extremity	EID	extremidad inferior derecha
RLL	right lower lobe	LID	lóbulo inferior derecho
RLQ	right lower quadrant	CID	cuadrante inferior derecho
RM	regurgitation murmur	SR	soplo de regurgitación
RM	rigor mortis		rigor mortis
RNA	ribonucleic acid	ARN	ácido ribonucleico
RO	rule out	—	elimínese
ROM	range of motion	AM	alcance movimiento
ROS	review of systems	IS	interrogatorio por sistemas
RPR	rapid plasma reagin test	PRP	prueba plasmática de reagina
RR	respiratory rate	IR	índice respiratorio
RT	radiation therapy	TR	terapia de radiación
RTA	renal tubular acidosis	ATR	acidosis tubular renal
RU	routine urinalysis	AO	análisis de orina
RUL	right upper lobe	LSD	lóbulo superior derecho
RUP	right upper extremity	ESD	extremidad superior derecha
RV	right ventricle	VD	ventrículo derecho
RVH	renovascular hypertension	HRV	hipertensión renovascular
Rx	prescription	—	receta, prescripción
s (*sine*)	without	—	sin
s. (*signetur*)	label	—	desígnese
S&A	sugar and acetone	A&A	azúcar y acetona
SA	spontaneous abortion	AE	aborto espontáneo
SARS	super acute respiratory syndrome	SRSA	síndrome disneico fulminante
SBE	subacute bacterial endocarditis	EBS	endocarditis bacteriana subaguda

ABBR.	ENGLISH / INGLÉS	ABREV.	SPANISH / ESPAÑOL
SBO	spina bifida occulta	EBO	espina bífida oculta
SCD	sequential compression devices	DCS	dispositivos de compresión en secuencia
SE	Status Epilepticus	—	estado o condición epiléptica
SEM	systolic ejection murmur	SSE	soplo sistólico de eyección
S.G.O.	Surgeon General's Office	OCG	Oficina del Cirujano General
SGOT	serum glutamic-oxaloacetic transaminase	TGOS	transaminasa glutámico-oxaloacética sérica
SGPT	serum glutamic-pyruvic transaminase	TGPS	transaminasa glutámico-pirúvica sérica
SH	serum hepatitis	HS	hepatitis sérica
SI	international system of units	—	sistema internacional de unidades
SIADH	syndrome of inappropriate antidiuretic hormone secretion	SSHAI	síndrome de secreción hormonal antidiurética insuficiente
SIDS	sudden infant death syndrome	SMIS	síndrome de muerte infantil súbita
SLUD	salivation, lacrimation, urination, and diarrhea	SLOD	salivación, lagrimeo, orina y diarrea
SM	systolic murmurs	SS	soplos sistólicos
SOB	shortness of breath	FDR	falta de respiración
sol (*solutio*)	solution	—	solución
sp.gr.	specific gravity	gr.esp.	gravedad específica
SRM	systolic regurgitant murmurs	SSR	soplo sistólico regurgitante
ss	half	—	medio-a
staph	staphylococcus	—	estafilococo
stat (*statim*)	immediately	—	inmediatamente
STD	sexually transmitted disease	EV	enfermedad venérea
strep	streptococcus	estrep	estreptococo
s SC	subcutaneously	—	subcutáneo-a

Most Common Medical Abbreviations / Abreviaturas médicas más usuales

ABBR.	ENGLISH / INGLÉS	ABREV.	SPANISH / ESPAÑOL
surg.	surgery, surgical	cirg.	cirugía
SVR	systemic vascular resistance	RVS	resistencia vascular sistémica
SVT	supraventricular tachycardia	TSV	taquicardia supraventricular
Sx	symptoms	—	síntomas
T	temperature	—	temperatura
T&A	tonsillectomy and adenoidectomy	—	tonsilectomía y adenoidectomía
TAB	tablet	tb	tableta
TAH	total abdominal hysterectomy	HAC	histerectomía abdominal completa
TB	tuberculosis	—	tuberculosis
TBG	thyroxine-binding globuline	FGT	fijación de globulina-tiroxina
TFT	thyroid function tests	PFT	pruebas funcionales de la tiroides
THR	total hip replacement	RTC	reemplazo total de la cadera
TI	tricuspid insufficiency	IT	insuficiencia tricuspídea
TIA	transient ischemic attack	AIP	ataque isquémico pasajero
tid (*ter in die*)	three times a day	—	tres veces al día
TORCHES syndrome	toxoplasmosis, rubella, cytomegalovirus, herpes simplex, syphilis	—	síndrome de toxoplasmosis, rubeola, citomegalovirus, herpes simple, sífilis
TPR	temperature, pulse, and respiration	—	temperatura, pulso y respiración
TR	transrectal ultrasonography	UT	ultrasonografía transrectal
TR	tricuspid regurgitation	RT	regurgitación tricuspídea
TRU	transrectal ultrasonography	UTR	ultrasonografía transrectal
TRH	thyrotropin-releasing hormone	HLT	hormona liberadora de tirotropina
TSH	thyroid-stimulating hormone	HTE	hormona tiroestimulante

ABBR.	ENGLISH / INGLÉS	ABREV.	SPANISH / ESPAÑOL
TSS	toxic shock syndrome	SCHT	síndrome de choque tóxico
TURBT	transurethral resection of bladder tumor	RTUTV	resección transuretral de tumor vesical
TURP	transurethral resection of prostate	RTUP	resección transuretral de la próstata
TV	tricuspid valve	VT	válvula tricúspide
TWE	tap water enema	E	enema de agua de pila
TX	transplant	—	trasplante
Tx	treatment	—	tratamiento
U	units	—	unidades
UA	urinalysis	AO	análisis de orina
UC	uterine contractions	CU	contracciones uterinas
UC	ulcerative colitis	—	colitis ulcerativa
UCD	usual childhood diseases	ECI	enfermedades comunes de la infancia
UGI	upper gastrointestinal tract	TGA	tracto gastrointestinal alto
ung	ointment	—	ungüento
ur	urine		orina
URI	upper respiratory infection	ITRS	infección del tracto respiratorio superior
US	ultrasound imaging	IUS	imagen de ultrasonido
UTI	urinary tract infection	IVU	infección de las vías urinarias
Vag	vaginal	—	vaginal
VAIN	vaginal intraepithelial neoplasia	NVI	neoplasia vaginal intraepitelial
VAT	ventricular activation time	TAV	tiempo de activación ventricular
VC	vital capacity	CV	capacidad vital
VD	veneral disease	EV	enfermedad venérea
VHD	ventricular heart disease	EVC	enfermedad ventricular cardíaca
VLDL	very low density lipids	LBD	lípidos de baja densidad

ABBR.	ENGLISH / INGLÉS	ABREV.	SPANISH / ESPAÑOL
VLDL	very low density lipoprotein	LDBD	lipoproteína de muy baja densidad
VLS	ventilation lung scanning	EVP	escán de ventilación pulmonar
VR	ventricular hypertrophy	HV	hipertrofía ventricular
vs	vital signs	sv	signos vitales
VSD	ventricular septal defect	DVS	defecto ventricular septal
WBC	white blood cells	GB	glóbulos blancos
WC	wheel chair	—	silla de ruedas
WNV	West Nile virus	VNO	virus del Nilo occidental
WR	Wassermann reaction	RW	reacción de Wassermann
Wt	weight	P	peso
y / o	years old	Ed	edad
Z	zone	—	zona

CONVERSION TABLES

The **Conversion Tables** facilitate vocabulary building in both languages. They also instruct the reader in the recognition of the fundamental orthographic differences between Spanish and English and in the etymological analysis of words.

Consult the **Conversion Tables** when building a vocabulary of medical words or interpreting medical words either in Spanish or in English.

Table 1: Rules for orthographic changes and differences in spelling between English and Spanish words.
Table 2: Most commonly used roots.
Table 3: Most frequently used prefixes.
Table 4: Most frequently used suffixes in surgical procedures, diagnoses, and symptoms.

The three components listed in Tables 2, 3, and 4 may or may not be together at the same time in a medical term.

Start in Table 1 by learning the orthographic changes and differences in spelling between English and Spanish words. This practice will help you to independently increase your vocabulary in Spanish and English.

When forming or interpreting a medical term it is advisable to find the meaning of the **suffix** first. For example, given the medical term **gastropathy / gastropatía**, the meaning of the suffix (in Table 4) **-pathy / -patía** is **disease / enfermedad**; the root of the term (in Table 2) is **gastr-, stomach / estómago**. The vowel o is added to the root to join another term which begins in a consonant. The interpretation of the medical word results in: **disease of the stomach / enfermedad del estómago.** When interpreting or building a medical term keep in mind that a word root is the main element of the term, often indicating a body part. A medical term may contain more than one root element.

A **prefix** used at the beginning of a medical term either changes its meaning or makes it more specific. In the term **hypodermic**, for example, the three components or elements are present:

prefix	word root	suffix
hypo	derm	-ic (adjective ending)
(under)	(skin)	(pertaining to)

The meaning of the word root becomes more specific after the **prefix**, while the **suffix** indicates, in this case, how the term relates to the root's meaning.

TABLAS DE CONVERSIÓN

Las **Tablas de conversión** facilitan el aprendizaje continuado del vocabulario en ambos idiomas. Al mismo tiempo, enseñan al lector a reconocer las diferencias ortográficas fundamentales entre el español y el inglés, así como a analizar los vocablos etimológicamente.

Consulte las **Tablas** cuando trate de crear nuevos términos médicos o de interpretar el significado de un término no conocido, ya sea en español o en inglés.

Tabla 1: cambios ortográficos y diferencia en la escritura de palabras entre el inglés y el español.
Tabla 2: raíces más comunes.
Tabla 3: prefijos usados con más frecuencia.
Tabla 4: sufijos usados con más frecuencia en cirugía, síntomas y diagnósticos.

Estos tres últimos elementos (raíces, prefijos y sufijos) pueden o no estar presentes al mismo tiempo en un término médico.

Comience en la Tabla 1 para ver los cambios ortográficos que ocurren entre las palabras inglesas y las españolas. Al componer o interpretar un término médico, es aconsejable encontrar primero el significado del sufijo si se está haciendo su composición o interpretación en inglés. Por ejemplo, dado el término médico **gastro-patía / gastropathy**, el significado del sufijo **-patía / -pathy** (V. la Tabla 4) es **enfermedad / disease**, la raíz o radical (V. la Tabla 2) es **gastr-, estómago / stomach**. En este caso, la vocal o se ha añadido a la raíz para unirla a otro vocablo que empieza con una consonante. El significado del término médico es: **enfermedad del estómago / disease of the stomach**. Cuando se crea o interpreta un término médico, se debe tener en cuenta que la raíz es el elemento principal del vocablo y que se refiere generalmente a una parte del cuerpo humano. Un mismo término médico puede tener más de una raíz.

El **prefijo** es un elemento que va delante de la raíz y cuya presencia modifica el significado de la misma o lo hace más específico. Tomemos, por ejemplo, la palabra **hypodermic / hipodérmico**. Si separamos los tres elementos o componentes tendremos:

prefijo	raíz	sufijo
hipo-	derm-	-ico (terminación adjectiva)
(bajo)	(piel)	(referente a)

El **prefijo** hace más específico el significado de la raíz, mientras que el **sufijo** indica a que se refiere el término o simplemente califica la parte definida por la raíz.

Conversion Table 1 / Tabla de conversión 1

ORTHOGRAPHIC CHANGES / CAMBIOS ORTOGRÁFICOS

English / Inglés	Spanish / Español	English / Inglés	Spanish / Español
cc	c	accommodate	acomodar
cc[1]	cc before e and i	accessory	accesorio
		accident	accidente
ch	c	character	carácter
ch before e and i	qui	chemistry	química
		chiropractor	quiropráctico
comm-	com-	commissure	comisura
im-	in-	immersion	inmersión
qu	cu	quart	cuarto
r[2]	l	paper	papel
es[3]	special	especial	
		gastrospasm	gastroespasmo
ph	f	phlebitis	flebitis
pn[4]	pn or n	pneumonia	pneumonía, neumonía
ps	ps or s	psychology	psicología, sicología
rh	r	rheumatic	reumático
th	t	therapy	terapia
y[5]	i	typhoid	tifoidea

[1] In Spanish words only two double consonants are used: **cc** and **nn**. The **ll** and **rr** are considered to be single characters in the Spanish alphabet.
En español sólo hay dos consonantes dobles: **cc** y **nn**. La **ll** y la **rr** se consideran letras en el alfabeto español.

[2] May change to **l** at the end of a word.
Puede combiar a **l** al final de palabra.

[3] Only before consonants **p** and **t**, including compound words.
Sólo delante de las consonantes **p** y **t** incluso en palabras compuestas.

[4] **pn** and **ps** may drop the initial **p** in Spanish.
En español se puede omitir la **p** inicial en las palabras que comienzan en **pn** o **ps**.

[5] When **y** is not at the end of the word.
Cuando la **y** es final.

Conversion Table 1 / Tabla de conversión 1

Orthographic Changes and Cognates / Cambios ortográficos y cognadas

	EXAMPLES	EJEMPLOS
1. There are only two double consonants in Spanish words: **cc** and **nn**		acción
		accidente
		innovación
2. Change **mm** to **m** except when preceded by **i**	com**m**unicate	co**m**unicar
	com**m**unication	co**m**unicación
3. **ch** changes to **c**, except when it is before **e** or **i**, then it changes to **qu**	**m**echanic	**m**ecánico
	choleric	**c**olérico
	chimera	**qui**mera
	chemotherapy	**qui**mioterapia
4. Drop the **h-** inside words except in **alcohol**[a]	t**h**erapy	terapia
	aut**h**orization	autorización
	hemor**rh**age	hemo**rr**agia
5. **ph** becomes **f** The **ph** at the beginning or in the middle of a word corresponds to **f** in Spanish.	**ph**armacy	**f**armacia
	phase	**f**ase
	dip**h**theria	dif**t**eria
6. Drop one **-s**. There are no words with double **ss** in Spanish.	nece**ss**ity	nece**s**idad
	di**ss**ect	di**s**ecar
	fi**ss**ura	fi**s**ura
7. English words that begin in **s + consonant** have corresponding Spanish words beginning in **es-**.	**sp**ecial	**esp**ecial
	scene	**esc**ena
	scan	**esc**án
8. The **y** in the middle of a word may change to **-i**.	cr**y**stal	cr**i**stal
	s**y**philis	s**í**filis
	tr**y**psin	tr**i**psina
9. **Add -a** to words ending in **-gram**: gram + **-a** = **grama**.	diagram	diagram**a**
10. The suffix **-um** drops and is substituted by **-o** in Spanish.	stadi**um**	estadi**o**
	pendul**um**	péndul**o**
	rostr**um**	rostr**o**

[a]and other words of Arabic origin.

11. The suffix **-osis** referring[b] to condition or disease, remains the same in Spanish.	dermat**osis**	dermat**osis**
	lymphocyt**osis**	linfocit**osis**
	anisocyt**osis**	anisocit**osis**
12. **-ty** becomes **-dad**	fideli**ty**	fideli**dad**
Many words in English ending in **-ty** have a corresponding Spanish word ending in **-dad**.	communi**ty**	comuni**dad**
	reali**ty**	reali**dad**
13. **-ous** becomes **-oso** or **-osa**	vigor**ous**	vigor**oso**
For many words ending in **-ous** in English, the corresponding word in Spanish ends in **-oso** or **osa**	numer**ous**	numer**oso**
	por**ous**	por**oso**
14. **-tion** becomes **-ción** in Spanish	educa**tion**	educa**ción**
	communica**tion**	comunica**ción**
	administra**tion**	administra**ción**

15. **Exact cognates.**
Words in Spanish and English that are spelled exactly the same way, have the same root, and mean the same are called exact cognates: **control, factor, local.**
However, there are other cognates that have similar or the same spelling and are misleading, because the meaning could be different: **real** can be translated **real** or **royal**; **actual** can mean **current**; **asistir** can be translated as **to attend** or **to help**; while **atender** in Spanish means to **pay attention** or **to take care of**.

---

[b]See conversion tables 2–4 for other word changes in prefixes and suffixes in English and Spanish.

Conversion Table 2 / Tabla de conversión 2

A root is the main part or element of a term. In medicine, it generally refers to a body part. Compound words (words with more than one root) are common in medical terminology.

La raíz o radical es el elemento principal de la palabra. En medicina la raíz se refiere generalmente a órganos o partes del cuerpo. En la terminología médica abundan palabras compuestas (palabras formadas por más de un elemento o raíz).

Most Commonly Used Roots / Raíces más frecuentes

ENGLISH / INGLÉS	SPANISH / ESPAÑOL	MEANING / SIGNIFICADO	EXAMPLE / EJEMPLO[a]
acou-	acu-	hearing / sonido	acoustics / acústica
aden-	aden-	gland / glándula	adenoids / adenoides
aer-	aer-	air / aire	aerogenic / aerogénico
angi-	angi-	vessel / vaso	angiotitis
ankyl-, anchyl-	anquil-	immobility, stiffness / inmovilidad, rigidez	anchylosis / anquilosis
arth-	art-	joint / articulación	arthritic / artrítico
brachi-	braqui-	arm / brazo	brachialgia / braquialgia
bronchi-	bronqui-	bronchi / bronquios	bronchopathy / broncopatía
bucca-	buca-	mouth / boca	buccal / bucal
cardi-	cardi-	heart / corazón	cardiodynia / cardiodinia
carpo-	carpo-	wrist / carpo	carpal
cephal-	cefal-	head / cabeza	cephalitis / cefalitis
cerebr-	cerebr-	brain / cerebro	cerebral
cerv-	cerv-	neck / cerviz, cuello	cervical
cheil-	queil-	lip / labio	cheilectomy / queilectomía
cost-	cost-	rib / costilla	costal
crani-	crane-	skull / cráneo	cranial / craneal
cysto-	cisto-	bladder / vejiga	cystocele / cistocele
dactyl-	dactil-	finger, toe / dedo	dactylitis / dactilitis
derm-	derm-	dermis / piel	dermatitis
duoden-	duoden-	duodenum / duodeno	duodenohepatic / duodeno-hepático
encephal-	encefal-	brain / cerebro	encephaloma / encefaloma

[a]When the words have an identical spelling and meaning in both languages, the Spanish translation is not given.
Cuando las palabras tienen igual significado y se escriben igual en ambos idiomas, la traducción al español se omite.

enter-	enter-	intestine / intestino	enteritis
fibro-	fibro-	fiber / fibra	fibroma
gastr-	gastr-	stomach / estómago	gastritis
genu-	genu-	knee / rodilla	genuflexion / genuflexión
gloss-	glosa-	tongue / lengua	glossalgia / glosalgia
glyco-	glico-	sugar / glucosa, azúcar	glycogen / glicógeno
hem-, hemo-	hem-, hemo	blood / sangre	hemotoxic / hematóxico
hepat-	hepat-	liver / hígado	hepatitis
histo-	histo-	tissue / tejido	histoma
homo-	homo-	same, equal / igual	homologous / homólogo
hydr-	hidro-	water, liquid / agua, líquido	hydrocele / hidrocele
hypn-	hipno-	sleep / sueño	hypnosis / hipnosis
hyster-	hister-	uterus / útero	hysterectomy / histerectomía
ili-	ili-	flank / ilíaco	iliocostal
leuk-	leuc-	white corpuscle / leucocito	leukemia / leucemia
lingu-	lingu-	tongue / lengua	lingual
lip-	lip-	fat / grasa	lipoid / lipoide
lith-	lit-	stone / cálculo	lithotriptor / litotriturador
mening-	mening-	membrane / membrana	meningitis
metr-	metr-	uterus / útero	metrorrhagia / metrorragia
my-	mi-	muscle / músculo	myocardium / miocardio
myel-	miel-	marrow / médula	myelitis / mielitis
narc-	narc-	sleep / sueño	narcotism / narcotismo
naso-	naso-	nose / nariz	nasopharynx / nasofaringe
ne-, neo-	neo-	new, recent / nuevo, reciente	neonatal
nephr-	nefr-	kidney / riñón	nephritis / nefritis
neur-	neur-	nerve / nervio	neurotripsy / neurotripsia
noct-	noct-	night / noche	nocturia

nucle-	nucle-, nucleo-	nucleus / núcleo	nucleic / nucleico
oculo-	oculo-	eye / ojo	ocular
oo-, ovi-	oo-, ovo-	ovum, egg / óvulo, huevo	ooplasm / ooplasma
oste-	oste-	bone / hueso	osteosis
oto-	oto-	ear / oído	otodynia / otodinia
ovari-	ovari-	ovary / ovario	ovariectomy / ovariectomía
ox-	ox-	oxygen / oxígeno	oxygenation / oxigenación
path(o)-	pato-	disease / enfermedad	pathology / patología
ped-	ped-	child / infante	pediatrics / pediatría
phleb-	fleb-	vein / vena	phlebitis / flebitis
pleur-	pleur-	pleura / pleura	pleuritis
pneum-	pneum-, neum-	air, lung / aire, pulmón	pneumothorax / neumotórax
prostat-	prostat-	prostate / próstata	prostatic / prostático
psych-	psic-, sic-	mind, spirit / mente	psychology / psicología
pupill-	pupil-	pupil / pupila	pupillometer / pupilómetro
pyel-	piel-	renal pelvis / pelvis renal	pyelitis / pielitis
ren-	ren-	kidney / riñon	renal
retin-	retin-	retina / retina	retinitis
rhin-	rin-	nose / nariz	rhinoclesis / rinoclesis
sarco-	sarco-	flesh / carne	sarcoma
semi-	semi-	half, partial / parcial, medio	semiflexion / semiflexión
sinus-	sinus-	cavity / cavidad	sinusitis
spermat-	espermat-	sperm, semen / esperma, semen	spermatoid / espermatoide
spondylo-	espondilo-	vertebra / vértebra	spondylous / espondiloso
strepto-	estrepto-	twisted / torcido	streptococcal / estreptocócico
techno-	tecno-	skill / técnica	technology / tecnología
ten-	ten-	tendon / tendón	tendonitis

thoraco-	torac-	chest, thorax / pecho, tórax	thoracic / torácico
thrombo-	trombo-	clot / coágulo	thrombosis / trombosis
toxic-	toxic-	toxic / tóxico	toxicity / toxicidad
ur-, uro-	ur-, uro-	urine / orina	urinary / urinario
vas-	vas-	vessel, duct / vaso	vascular
ventro-	ventro-	abdomen, anterior part / abdomen, porción anterior	ventroscopy / ventroscopía
xeno-	xeno-	foreign, strange / extranjero, extraño	xenophthalmia / xenoftalmia

Conversion Table 3 / Tabla de conversión 3

Prefixes are placed at the beginning of words; in medical terms the prefix is the element which changes the meaning of the term or makes it more specific. Prefixes are generally formed by one or two syllables. Most medical prefixes, roots, and suffixes are derived from Latin and Greek.

Los prefijos se colocan al principio de la palabra; en términos médicos el prefijo es el elemento que cambia el significado del término y lo hace más específico. Los prefijos tienen generalmente una o dos sílabas. La mayor parte de los prefijos, raíces y sufijos se derivan del latín y del griego.

Most Commonly Used Prefixes / Prefijos de uso más frecuente

ENGLISH / INGLÉS	SPANISH / ESPAÑOL	MEANING / SIGNIFICADO	EXAMPLE / EJEMPLO[a]
a-, an-	a-	lack of, without / falta de, sin	apathy / apatía
ab-	a-	away from / lejos de, sin	abnormal / anormal
ad-	ad-	toward, near to / hacia, con respecto a	adduction / aducción
ambi-	ambi-	both / ambos	ambidextrous / ambidextro
amphi-	anfi-	on both sides, double / en los dos lados, doble	amphibious / anfibio
ana-	ana-	up, back, again / sobre, otra vez, excesivo	anadipsia
ante-	ante-	before / antes de	antenatal
anti-	anti-	against, reversed / contra, reversión	antibiotic / antibiótico
bi-	bi-	twice, double / dos, doble	bifocal
brady-	bradi-	slow / despacio	bradycardia / bradicardia
circum-	circun-	about, around / alrededor de	circumcision / circuncisión
com-	co-	together, with / junto a, con	commisure / comisura
con-	con-	with, together / junto a, con	congenital / congénito
contra-	contra-	against, opposite / opuesto a,en contra de	contraceptive / contraceptivo
de-	de-, des-	away from, to suppress / separación, suprimir	dehydrated / deshidratado-a
dia-	dia-	through, across / por medio, a través	diaphragm / diafragma
diplo-	diplo-	double / doble	diplocardia

dis-	dis-	away, apart / separado	distention / distensión
dys-	dis-	bad, improper / malo, impropio	dysentery / disentería
e-, ex-	ex-	out, away from / fuera, lejos de	excrete / excretar
ecto-	ecto-	external, outside / afuera, sin	ectoderm / ectodermia
em-	em-	in / adentro de	embolic / embólico
endo-	endo-	inside, within / dentro, entre	endometrium / endometrio
epi-	epi-	upon, on / sobre, encima	epidermis
extra-	extra-	outside / fuera de	extracardial / extra-cardíaco
hemi-	hemi-	half / medio	hemisphere / hemisferio
hyper-	hiper-	excessive / excesivo	hypertensive / hipertensivo
hypo-	hipo-	under, deficient / falta de, deficiente	hypoglycemia / hipoglicemia
im-, in-	in-	in, into / dentro, junto	infiltration / infiltración
infra-	infra-	below / debajo	infraorbital
intra-	intra-	between / entre	intraglobular
intro-	intro-	into, within / dentro de	introversion / introversión
lingu-	lingu-	tongue / lengua	lingual
mal-	mal-	bad, abnormal / malo, anormal	malocclusion / maloclusión
meso-	meso-	in the middle / en el medio	mesocardia
meta-	meta-	beyond / más allá	metastasis / metástasis
micro-	micro-	small, minute / pequeño, diminuto	micrococcus / micrococo
neur-	neur-	nerve / nervio	neurosis
para-	para-	beside, near / al lado, cerca	paracardiac / paracardíaco
per-	per-	through, excessive / a través, excesivo	perforation / perforación
peri-	peri-	around / alrededor de	perithelial / peritelial
poly-	poli-	many, several / varios	polyacid / poliácido

post-	post-	after, behind / después, detrás	postfebrile / postfebril
pneum-	neum-	lung / pulmón	pneumonia / neumonía
pre-	pre-	before, in front / antes, en frente	prediastole / prediástole
psych-	psico-	soul, mind / alma, mente	psychotherapy / psicoterapia
pyro-	piro-	heat, fire / calor, fuego	pyrogen / pirógeno
re-	re-	back again / de regreso otra vez	revive / revivir
retro-	retro-	backward, behind / en retroceso, detrás	retrolingual
schizo-	esquizo-	division / división	schizophrenia / esquizofrenia
semi-	semi-	partly, half / medio, parcial	semiflexion / semiflexión
sub-	sub-	under / debajo	subneural
super-	super-	above, upper / encima de, superior	supercentral
supra-	supra-	above / encima de	supranasal
sym-, syn-	sin-	together, with / junto, con	synovia / sinovia
tachy-	taqui-	accelerated, fast / rápido, acelerado	tachycardia / taquicardia
tetra-	tetra-	four / cuatro	tetralogy / tetralogía
therap-	terap-	treatment / tratamiento	therapeutic / terapéutico
thromb-	tromb-	clot / coágulo	thrombosis / trombosis
trans-	trans-, tras-	across, through / transversal, a través	transurethral / transuretral
trauma-	trauma-	wound, trauma / herida, trauma	traumatism / traumatismo
tri-	tri-	three / tres	tridimensional
un-	in-, no	against, reversal / contrario, opuesto	unconscious / inconsciente
ultra-	ultra-	beyond, excess / más allá, excesivo	ultrasonic / ultrasónico

[a]When the words have an identical spelling and meaning in both languages, the Spanish translation is not given. Cuando las palabras tienen igual significado y se escriben igual en ambos idiomas, la traducción al español se omite.

Conversion Table 4 / Tabla de conversión 4

Suffixes are endings attached to the root or stem of a word to modify its meaning. In medical terminology suffixes are added to the root to define terms according to operative, diagnostic, and symptomatic meanings.

Los sufijos son terminaciones que al añadirse a la raíz de una palabra modifican el significado de la misma. En la terminología médica los sufijos se añaden a la raíz para definir términos usados en cirugía, diagnosis y síntomas.

Surgical Procedure Suffixes / Sufijos referentes a procedimientos quirúrgicos

ENGLISH / INGLÉS	SPANISH / ESPAÑOL	MEANING / SIGNIFICADO	EXAMPLE / EJEMPLO
-centesis	-centesis	aspiration, puncture / aspiración, punción	thoracentesis / toracentesis
-cision	-cisión	cut / corte	incision / incisión
-ectomy	-ectomía	excision, removal / excisión, extirpación	tonsillectomy / tonsilectomía
-desis	-desis	binding, fixation / ligar, fijar	arthrodesis / artrodesis
-oclasis	-oclasis	to break down / romper, quebrar	osteoclasis
-olysis	-olisis	separate, destroy / separar, destruir	enterolysis / enterolisis
-ostomy	-ostomía	forming an opening / crear un boquete o abertura	colostomy / colostomía
-otomy	-otomía	incision, cut into / incisión, piquete	lithotomy / litotomía
-pexy	-pexia	suspension, fixation / suspensión, fijación	hysteropexy / histeropexia
-plasty	-plastia	rebuilding, molding / reformando, moldeando	osteoplasty / osteoplastia
-rrhaphy	-rrafia	suture, closure / sutura, cierre	perineorrhaphy / perineorrafia
-tomy	-tomía	incision, section / incisión, sección	laparectomy / laparectomía
-tripsy	-tripsia	to crush / triturar	lithotripsy / litotripsia

Suffixes Relating to Diagnoses and Symptoms / Sufijos referentes a diagnósticos y síntomas

ENGLISH / INGLÉS	SPANISH / ESPAÑOL	MEANING / SIGNIFICADO	EXAMPLE / EJEMPLO
-algia	-algia	pain / dolor	cephalalgia / cefalalgia
-capnia	-capnia	carbon monoxide / monóxido de carbono	hypercapnia / hipercapnia
-cele	-cele	hernia, swelling / hernia, inflamación	metrocele
-chalasis	-calasia	relaxation / relajación	achalasia / acalasia
-dynia	-dinia	pain / dolor	metrodynia / metrodinia
-ectasis	-ectasia	dilation, expansion / dilatación, expansión	bronchiectasis / bronquiectasia
-emesis	-emesis	vomit / vómito	hematemesis / hematemesis
-emia	-emia	blood / sangre	hyperglycemia / hiperglicemia
-iasis	-iasis	condition, presence / condición, presencia	lithiasis / litiasis
-itis	-itis	inflammation / inflamación	dermatitis
-logy	-logía	study of / estudio de	dermatology / dermatología
-malacia	-malacia	softening / reblandecimiento	osteomalacia
-mania	-manía	obsession / obsesión	kleptomania / cleptomanía
-megaly	-megalia	enlargement / engrosamiento	hepatomegaly / hepatomegalia
-oid	-oide	resembling / de tipo similar	lipoid / lipoide
-oma	-oma	tumorous / tumoroso	nephroma / nefroma
-osis	-osis	abnormal condition / condición anormal	dermatosis
-pathy	-patía	disease / enfermedad	gastropathy / gastropatía
-penia	-penia	decrease, deficiency / disminución, deficiencia	leukopenia / leucopenia
-phagia	-fagia	to eat / comer	dysphagia / disfagia

Suffixes Relating to Diagnoses and Symptoms / Sufijos referentes a diagnósticos y síntomas

ENGLISH / INGLÉS	SPANISH / ESPAÑOL	MEANING / SIGNIFICADO	EXAMPLE / EJEMPLO
-phasia	-fasia	speech / habla	aphasia / afasia
-phobia	-fobia	fear / miedo, temor	acrophobia / acrofobia
-plegia	-plejía	paralysis, stroke / parálisis, ataque	hemiplegia / hemiplejía
-poiesis	-poyesis	formation / formación	hematopoiesis / hematopoyesis
-praxia	-praxia	activity, action / actividad, acción	apraxia
-rrhage	-rragia	bursting forth, flooding / derramamiento	hemorrhage / hemorragia
-rrhea	-rrea	discharge / flujo, descarga	diarrhea / diarrea
-sclerosis	-esclerosis	hardening / endurecimiento	arteriosclerosis / arterioesclerosis
-spasm	-espasmo	contraction / contracción	gastrospasm / gastroespasmo
-sthenia	-estenia	strength / fuerza	myasthenia / miastenia
-thymia	-timia	mind / mente	cyclothymia / ciclotimia
-uria	-uria	urine / orina	hematuria / hematuria

Notes:

1. When the suffix begins with a vowel, the word root is directly added to the suffix: **cephalalgia / cefalalgia**.
2. When the suffix begins with a consonant, a connecting vowel is placed between the word root and the suffix (**-o** in the majority of cases): **cardiogram / cardiograma.**

Notas:
1. Cuando el sufijo comienza con una vocal, la raíz se añade directamente al sufijo: **cefalalgia / cephalalgia**.
2. Cuando el sufijo comienza en consonante se coloca una vocal, gen. una **-o-**, entre la raíz y el sufijo: **cardiograma / cardiogram**.

Suffixes that Form a Noun / Sufijos que forman un nombre

ENGLISH / INGLÉS	SPANISH / ESPAÑOL	MEANING / SIGNIFICADO	EXAMPLE / EJEMPLO
-cide	-cidio	destruction, killing / destrucción, muerte	suicide / suicidio
-clysis	-clisis	irrigation / irrigación	venoclysis / venoclisis
-coccus	-coco	berry-shaped / en forma de baya	streptococcus / estreptococo
-cyte	-cito	cell / célula	oocyte / oocito
-gram	-grama	record made by an instrument / trazo de un instrumento	cardiogram / cardiograma
-graph	grafo-a	device for recording / dispositivo para grabar	polygraph / polígrafo
-graphy	-grafía	description made by an instrument / descripción hecha por un instrumento	radiography / radiografía
-ia	-a, -ia, -ía	condition or disease / condición o enfermedad	pneumonia / neumonía
-ician	-ico, -ica	person associated with a given speciality / persona asociada a una especialidad	technician / técnico
-ics	-ia	an art or science / un arte o ciencia	orthopedics / ortopedia
-ine	-ina	substance / sustancia	quinine / quinina
-is, -ism	-is, -ismo	abnormal condition / condición anormal	alcoholism / alcoholismo
-ist	-ista	specialist / especialista	dentist / dentista
-lysis	-lisis	setting free / liberar	dialysis / diálisis
-ologist[a]	-ólogo-a	specialist / especialista	cardiologist / cardiólogo
-ology	-ología	study, knowledge / estudio, conocimiento	pathology / patología
-oma	-oma	tumor	adenoma
-osis	-osis	condition, formation / condición, formación	tuberculosis
-osmia	-osmia	smell / olor	anosmia / anosmia

Suffixes that Form a Noun / Sufijos que forman un nombre

ENGLISH / INGLÉS	SPANISH / ESPAÑOL	MEANING / SIGNIFICADO	EXAMPLE / EJEMPLO
-pathy	-patía	disorder, disease / enfermedad, anomalía	myelopathy / mielopatía
-penia	-penia	deficiency / deficiencia	osteopenia
-phagic	-fágico	rel. to eating / rel. a comer	esophagic / esofágico-a
-philia	-filia	tendency, abnormal liking / tendencia, atracción mórbida	hemophilia / hemofilia
-phylaxis	-filaxis	protection / protección	prophylaxis / profilaxis
-ty	-dad	condition / condición	senility / senilidad
-y	-ia, -ía	condition or process / condición o proceso	myopathy / miopatía

[a]If **-log** precedes **-ist** in English, **-ist** is omitted in Spanish, and the ending **-o** (*m.*) or **-a** (*f.*) is added: **psychologist / psicólogo-a**. **Si en** una palabra inglesa **-log** precede a **-ist**, esta terminación se omite en español y se añade **-o** (*m.*) o **-a** (*f.*) a **log: psicólogo-a / psychologist**.

Suffixes that Form an Adjective / Sufijos que forman un adjetivo

ENGLISH / INGLÉS	SPANISH / ESPAÑOL	MEANING / SIGNIFICADO	EXAMPLE / EJEMPLO
-iac	-iaco, iaca	pertaining to, one affected by / en relación a, afectado por	cardiac / cardíaco[a]
-al	-al	related to / que trata de	visual / visual
-ant	-ante	pertaining to, with characteristics / en relación a, con características	abundant / abundante
-ate	-ado, -ada	condition / condición	delicate / delicado
-cidal	-cida	destructive, that kills / destructivo, que mata	bactericidal / bactericida
-ic	-ico, -ica	affected by / afectado por	asthmatic / asmático
-ile	-il	state of being / estado	senile / senil
-prandial	-prandial	meal / comida	postprandial

[a]Adjectives ending in **-o** change the **-o** to **-a** to form the feminine.
Los adjectiveos que terminan en **-o** cambian la terminación a **-a** para formar el femenino.

Suffixes that Form a Verb / Sufijos que forman un verbo

English / Inglés	Spanish / Español	Example / Ejemplo
-ate	-ar	accommodate / acomodar
-e	-ar	cure / curar
-fy	-ficar	verify / verificar
-ize	-izar	revitalize / revitalizar

SPANISH SOUNDS / SONIDOS DEL ESPAÑOL

The Spanish alphabet has four more characters than the English alphabet: **ch, ll, ñ, rr**. When alphabetizing Spanish words those words beginning with **ch, ll, and ñ**, follow words that begin in **c, l,** and **ñ**. The letter **rr** never begins a word.

Learning to Pronounce Spanish
English equivalents given for Spanish sounds are only approximate.

1. Spanish Vowel Sounds / Sonidos vocálicos en español
a, e, i, o, u and sometimes **y** are single sounds pronounced always clearly whether they are a stressed vowel or not. A tendency by English speakers to slur over the unstressed vowels is a habit that should not be done when Spanish vowels are pronounced. Spanish vowel sounds are short. There are only five vowel sounds in Spanish.

VOWEL /VOCAL	SOUND /SONIDO	EXAMPLE /EJEMPLO	MEANING /SIGNIFICADO
a	ah as in *father*	*a*m**e**ba* (ah-meh-bah)	ameba
e	eh as in *let*	ac**né** (ahk-neh)	acne
i	ee as in *see*	an**e**m*i*a (ah-neh-mee-ah)	anemia
o	oh as in *spoke*	c**a**ll*o* (kah-yoh)	callus
u	oo as in *cool*	ac**ú**stica (ah-coos-tee-kah)	acoustics

The stressed syllable is indicated in bold. Example of vowels are indicated in italics.
*Although these two words are written alike, in the English word the **e** is pronounced like the Spanish **i**.

Note / Nota: The **y** is pronounced like the vowel **i** when it is by itself or at the end of a word: **y** / and; I am / Yo so**y**.

Mute Vowel u and Consonant h / La vocal muda u y la consonante h.
   The **u** is only mute when placed after **g** or **q** preceding **e** or **i** in the syllables **gue, gui**. If **u** has a dieresis (two dots over the **ü**) it is sounded. Examples: silent **u: gu**itarra (ghee-tah-rrah); sounded **u: ungüento (oon-goo-ehn-toh).**
   The consonant **h** is never pronounced in Spanish. The vowel **u** sounds when indicated by a diéresis.

Diphthongs / Diptongos
A diphthong is a combination of two vowels in a syllable. A dipthong is made by two vowels, one of the vowels can be a strong vowel (**a, e, o**) and the other a weak vowel (**i, [y]**, or **u**), or two weak vowels. Two strong vowels together do not form a diphthong. When the combination is that of a strong vowel and a weak vowel, the strong vowel is stressed; if the diphthong is formed by two weak vowels, the second vowel is stressed.

STRONG AND WEAK VOWELS FORMING A DIPHTHONG:

ai	au	ia	ua
ai-re air	**au**-sente absent	v**ia**-ble viable	**cua**-dro picture
ei	eu	ie	ue
rei-no kingdom	**eu**-fórico euphoric	**rie**sgo risk	b**ue**-no good
oi	oy	ey	uo
oi-go I hear	voy	**rey**	c**uo**-ta

Note: The **y** is pronounced like the vowel **i** when it is by itself or at the end of a word: **y** / and; I am / so**y** .

2. Consonant Sounds that Differ Most from English.

Sonidos de las consonantes que más difieren de los sonidos en inglés.

The example consonant is given in bold. / La consonante usada como ejemplo aparece en letra negrita.

LETTER / LETRA	APPROX. ENGLISH SOUND / SONIDO APROX. EN INGLÉS	WORD, PRONUNCIATION AND MEANING / PALABRA, PRONUNCIACIÓN Y SIGNIFICADO
c before e, i (Cast.)	th as in *think* (Castillian Spanish)	círculo (theer-koo-loh) / circle
c before e, i (H.A.)	s as in *sick*	centro (sehn-troh) / center
c before a, o, u	k as in *cancer*	cáncer (kahn-sehr) / cancer
ch	ch as in *check*	leche (leh-cheh) / milk
d between vowels	like th in *weather*	medio (meh-dee-oh) / half
d after n or l	like d in *dart*	donde (dohn-deh) / where
g before e, i	harsher than h in *hemoglobin*	germen (her-men) / germ
gue, gui	hard g as in *guest*	guisado[a] (ghee-sah-doh) / stew
güe, güi	gwe as in *Gwen*	ungüento[b] (oon-goo-en-toh) / ointment
h[c]	always silent as in *hour*	hora (oh-rah) / hour
j	more forcefully than in *ham*	jamón (hah-mohn) / ham
ll (Cast.)	lli as in *million*	millón (mee-llohn) / million
ll (H.A.)	same as y in *yes*	millón (mee-yohn)
ñ	ny as in *canyon*	muñeca (moo-nyeh-kah) / wrist
p	not aspirated, less explosive than in *patient*	paciente (pah-see-enh-teh) / patient
q	always pronounced as k	queso[d] (keh-soh) / cheese
r	1. initial: multiple thrill, roll r more than in *diarrhea*	reuma (reh-oo-mah) / rheum
r	2. not initial, sound produced by tip of the tongue against the alveolar ridge	cirugía / surgery
rr	same as initial r	diarrea (deeah-reh-ah) / diarrhea
v as in b labial	as in *bowl*	vacuna (bah-kooh-nah) (bacuna) / vaccine
x	ks, gs as in *oxygen*	oxígeno / oxygen; excelente (egseh-lehn-teh) / excellent
y	same as y in *yes*; like j in *injection*	yeso (yeh-soh) / plaster; inyección (een-yek-seeohn) / injection
y	by itself or at the end of a word, like e in *me*	soy (soh-eeh) / I am
z (Cast.)	like th in *thumb*	zumo (thoo-moh) / juice
z (H.A.)	as s in *soft*	zumbido (soom-bee-doh) / buzz

[a]Silent u. la u muda
[b]sounded u. la u pronunciada.
[c]the letter h is never pronounced in Spanish. La letra h no se pronuncia nunca en el español.
[d]Silent u.

Note/Nota: The pronunciation of the words in parentheses is the pronunciation of the word in Latin America. The descriptions of sounds in this chart are approximations and do not indicate exact equivalence between English and Spanish sounds. The Royal Academy of the Spanish Language has ruled since 1994, that while **ch** and **ll** are considered letters of the alphabet, for alphabetization purposes only they should not be treated that way. The Spanish alphabet has four more characters than the English alphabet: **ch, ll, ñ, rr.** (In Spanish **rr** never begins a word.) In alphabetizing Spanish words, those beginning with **ch, ll,** and **ñ** follow words that begin in **c, l, n.**

Letter B: b and **v** have the same sound in Spanish. Try to pronounce the **b** in *bacteria.* Imitate this same sound of the **b** or **v** in other Spanish words. After **m** or **n** the sound of the **b** is more like the English **b** as in *imbecil,* or in *invasive,* words that are very similar in Spanish: *imbécil* (eem-**beh**-seehl) stressed in the syllable **be,** and *invasivo* (een-bah-**seeh**-boh) stressed in the syllable **si.**

Letter C: c sounds like **k** or "hard" **c,** as in *cat,* when preceding **a, o, u,** as in *cancer.* This "hard" sound of **c** is not aspirated. Pronounce *cavidad* (kah-bee-**dahd**) as in *cavity;* *costo* (**kohs**-toh) cost; *cuatro* (**kooah**-troh) four. **c** has a different pronunciation when placed before **e** or **i** as in *centro* (**sehn**-troh) center, as pronounced in Latin America; *círculo,* with a **th** sound as in *think* (**theer**-coo-loh) as pronounced in Castillian.

Letter CH: Pronounce **ch** as in *child, leche* (**leh**-sheh).

Note. The Royal Academy of the Spanish Language has ruled since 1994 that **ch** and **ll** are considered combinations of letters of the alphabet (called *dígrafas*); for alphabetization purposes only.

Letter G: g placed before **a, o, u** has a gutural sound as in *gasp, gota* (**goh**-tah) drop. **g** has a different pronunciation when placed before **e** or **i,** in that case it sounds like a harsher **h,** as in *hemoglobin, género* (**heh**-neh-roh) gender.

Letter J: j is pronounced more forcefully than in *ham* as in *jarabe* (jah-**rah**-beh) syrup.

Letter Q: q is always pronounced as **k,** or **c** as in *cut,* *queso* (**keh**-soh) cheese; or *quiste* (**kees**-teh) cyst. **q** is always followed by a silent **u.**

Letter R: r inicial and **rr** in the middle of a word has a multiple thrill as in *hemorrhage / hemorragia* (eh-moh-**rrah**-heeah). Remember that the **h** is always silent. **r** in the middle, or at the end of a word is pronounced as in *heart, mirar* (meeh-**rahr**) to look.

Letter Ñ: ñ (n with a tilde), pronounce this letter as ny in *canyon, niño* (neeh-nyoh) child.

Letter LL: ll is pronounced approximately like in *million,* as in *millón* (meeh-**llóhn**) in Castillian, and like *yes* in Latin America (meeh-**yóhn**).

Letter X: x its approximate sounds are **ks, gs,** as in *oxygen, oxígeno* (ohg-**see**-heh-noh) placed between vowels. It is pronounced like **s** before consonants, as in *see, extraño,* (ehs-**trah**-gnoh) strange.

Letter Y: y with the same sound as **y** in *yes, yeso* (**yeh**-soh) chalk, and like the vowel **i** by itself as the conjunction **y** (meaning and).

Letter Z: z same sound as **th** in *thumb* in Castillian, *zumo* (**thooh**-moh) juice, or like *see* in Latin America, (**sooh**-moh).

3. Rules of Syllabication in Spanish / División de palabras en sílabas.

A Spanish word has as many syllables as it has vowels or diphthongs.

1. The consonants **b, c, f, g, p, t,** combine with **l** or **r** to form a syllable with the following vowel. The letter **d** also combines with **r** but it does not with the letter **l.**

b	c	f
blan-co (**blahn**-coh) white	**cla**-se (**clah**-seh) class	**fla**-co (**flah**-coh) thin, lanky
g	p	
glu-**co**-sa (glooh-**coh**-sah) glucose	**pla**-ca (**plah**-cah), plate, plaque	
c	b	d
cre-ma (**creh**-mah) cream	**bra**-vo (**brah**-voh) brave	**dra**-ma (**drah**-mah) drama
f	g	p
frá-gil (**frah**-geel) fragile	**gran**-de (**grahn**-deh) big	**pre**-cio (**preh**-seeoh) price
t		
trau-ma (**trahooh**-mah) trauma		

2. Any consonant following another (except the combinations described above) mark a division between syllables.
parte: pa**r-t**e (**pahr**-teh), part
bronquitis: bron-**qui**-tis (brohn-**keeh**-teehs), bronchitis
pulso: **pul**-so (**pool**-soh), pulse

3. The vowels that make up a dipthong are never seperated:
malaria: ma-**la**-ria (mah-**lah**-reeah), malaria
tifoidea: ti-**foi**-dea (tee-pho-heeh-deh-hah) typhoid
serie: **se**-rie (**seh**-reeeh) series

4. An accent over a weak vowel (**i** or **u**) dissolves the dipthong and forms a separated syllable:
anatomía: a-na-to-**mí**-a (ah-nah-toh-**mee**-ah) anatomy
oído: o-**í**-do (oh-**eeh**-doh) ear

5. Consecutive strong vowels are separated, forming different syllables:
monitoreo: mo-ni-to-**re**-o (moh-nee-toh-**reh**-oh), monitoring

6. A vowel followed by a consonant at the beginning of a word can make a syllable by itself if the consonant forms a syllable with a following vowel, or if it is part of a combination described in (1).
inexperiencia: **i**-nex-pe-rien-cia (e-negs-peh-**reehn**-see-ah) inexperience
aplicaión: **a**-pli-ca-ción (ah-pleeh-cah-**seeohn**) application

Rules of Accentuation / Reglas de acentuación
STRESS / ACENTO TÓNICO O FUERZA DE VOZ.
Stress is the emphasis given to a certain syllable in a word. The stress establishes a change between different words. (The stress is on the syllable in bold.)

IN-GRE-**SAR**
This word has three syllables. in-gre-**sar** is a verb infinitive. All infinitives in Spanish have the stress on the second to last (penultimate) syllable.
ingre**sa**do in-gre-**sa**-do The stress falls on the syllable **-sa**.
The patient is ad**mit**ted. / El paciente es in-gre-**sa**-do.
ingre**sar** and *ingresado* follow the rules of accentuation:

ENDING / TERMINACIÓN	STRESS / ACENTO	EXAMPLE / EJEMPLO
vowel: **a e i o u**	next-to-the-last syllable	ingre**sa**do (in-gre-**sa**-do)
consonant: **n** or **s**	next-to-the-last syllable	ingre**san** (in-**gre**-san)
consonant other than **n** or **s**	on the last syllable	ingre**sar** (in-gre-**sar**)

Where should a written accent mark be placed?
Any words that do not comply wth the above rules require a written **accent mark / acento escrito** over the vowel as in: caf**é**, atenci**ón**, **rí**gido.

A written accent mark is also used to distinguish two words of different meaning that are written alike, such as demonstrative adjectives, demonstrative pronouns, interrogatives, and relative pronouns.

adjective   **pronoun**
this patient / **este** paciente   this one / **éste**

Adjective: **This** patient is admitted today / **este** paciente es ingre**sa**do hoy
Pronoun: **This one** will be admitted tomorrow / **éste** (this one) será admitido mañana

interrogative what / **¿qué**   **relative pronoun** that / **que**
What patient? / **¿que paciente?**   The patient that will be admitted
                                         El paciente **que** (that) será admitido

Other words that require an accent to differentiate them are:

yes / **sí** to make a difference from if / **si**;

dé / to give a command, and the preposition **de** / of;

he / **él** and the / **el** the definitive article;

the subject pronoun you (familiar) **tú** /, and your / **tu** possessive adjective.

Punctuation / Punctuación

(.) puntos	(ü) diérisis
(;) punto y coma	(*) asterisco
(:) dos puntos	(-) guión
(¿) interrogación abierta	(_) raya
(?) interrogación cerrada	() paréntesis
(¡) admiración abierta	(" ") comillas
(!) admiración cerrada	(. . .) puntos suspensivos

ENGLISH SOUNDS / SONIDOS DEL INGLÉS

A difercia del español, en el que cada letra tiene un sonido más o menos definido, en inglés una misma letra puede tener más de una pronunciación y es esa la mayor dificultad que la persona hispanoparlante confronta al tratar de aprender la pronunciación de la lengua inglesa. La mayoría de los textos lingüísticos recurren al uso de algún alfabeto fonético que sirve de clave para la pronunciación. Para los efectos de este diccionario nos hemos limitado a dar una sencilla orientación que ayude al lector a pronunciar aquellas letras y sonidos que más difieren de la correspondiente pronunciación en español y que, por lo tanto, presentan mayor dificultad al hispanoparlante. Debemos señalar que esta presentatión simplificada de las letras en inglés no abarca todas las posibilidades; las excepciones a las reglas generales son muy numerosas.

El alfabeto inglés tiene veintiséis letras: cinco vocales y veintiuna consonantes. La letra **y**, como en español, puede ser vocal (se pronuncia como la **i** en español) **remedy** / remedio, o puede ser una consonante (se pronuncia como la **y** en *ya*) **yes** / sí.

Vocales / vowels

Las vocales en inglés tienen generalmente dos sonidos, uno breve o corto y otro largo. La **e** puede además ser muda al final de la palabra.

[*Sonido breve o corto*: Ocurre generalmente cuando la vocal es seguida por una consonante en la misma sílaba.]

LETRA	PALABRA EN INGLÉS	*SONIDO APROXIMADO EN ESPAÑOL*
a	**nap** / siesta	sonido intermedio entre la **a** de mano y la **e** de pesa.
	call / llamada	b**o**ca (gen. en palabras que terminan en **ll**).
e	**bed** / cama	fr**e**nte.
	late / tarde	muda (gen. ocurre al final de la palabra).
i	**chill** / enfriamiento	sonido intermedio entre la **i** y la **e** en español.
o	**compare** / comparar	c**o**mparar
	hot / caliente	sonido intermedio entre la **a** y la **o** en español.
	move / mover	c**u**ra
u	**drug** / droga	sonido intermedio entre la **o** y la **u** en español.
	full / lleno	**tú**

[*Sonido largo*: Ocurre generalmente cuando la vocal es la vocal final de una sílaba o cuando va seguida de una **e** muda o de una **e** muda y una consonante. Es un sonido vocálico demorado en el cual algunas veces una vocal sencilla tiene un sonido diptongado.]

a	**basic** / básico	l**ey**
e	**he** / él	s**í**
i	**bite** / picadura	h**ay**
o	**dose** / dosis	sonido equivalente al sonido del diptongo **ou** en español.
oo	**blood** / sangre	p**o**ro
	book / libro	c**u**ra
u	**putrid** / pútrido	c**iu**dad, combinación equivalente al sonido de **iu** en español

DIPTONGOS / DIPHTHONGS

ew: Sonido en inglés corresponde al sonido **iu:**

few / varios.	ciudad

ou: Sonido semejante al diptongo **au** en español o sonido breve semejante a la **o** en español:

mouth / boca	causa
bought / compró	dosis

Consonantes / Consonants

El alfabeto en inglés tiene dos consonantes que casi no se usan en español, la **k** y la **w**; la **ñ,** en cambio, no existe en el alfabeto inglés y las letras **ch, ll,** y **rr** no se consideran caracteres propios, sino combinación de dos letras (letra dígrafa). En general, la pronunciación de la mayoría de las consonantes es semejante en ambos idiomas, aunque en inglés la pronunciación de las mismas es más explosiva.

Consonantes y letras dígrafas que más difieren de la pronunciación española

CONSONANTES	PALABRA EN INGLÉS	SONIDO APROXIMADO EN ESPAÑOL
b	Sonido semejante a la **b** inicial en español; es muda en algunas palabras cuando precede a la letra **t.**	
	Sonido aproximado en español	
	bacillus / bacilo	**b**acilo
	doubt / duda	(muda)
ch	Presenta varios sonidos según su posición en la palabra.	
	child / niño	**ch**ico
	cholera / cólera	cólera
	machine / máquina	**sh**shsh! (*semejante al sonido que se emplea para indicar silencio*)
g	Cuando le sigue una **e** o una **i** tiene un sonido semejante a la **y** en español (*sonido suave*). Esta regla tiene por excepción las palabras monosílabas.	
	general / general	**y**eso (*sonido africado*)
	giant / gigante	**y**eso (*sonido africado*)
	girl / muchacha	**g**ota
	En casi todas las otras situaciones, tiene el mismo sonido que la **g** fuerte en español.	
	gastric / gástrico	**g**ástrico
	gram / gramo	**g**ramo
	guide / guía	**g**uía
gh	En medio de la palabra, esta combinación de letras es generalmente muda.	
	daughter / hija	
h	Sonido aproximado al de la **j** en español, pero algo más suave.	
	hemorrhage / hemorragia	**j**arabe
j	Sonido semejante a la **y** en español.	
	jejunum / yeyuno	**yey**uno (*con africación*)
ll	Sonido igual al de la **l** sencilla.	
	generally / generalmente	genera**l**mente
kn	La **k** es muda.	
	knee / rodilla	**n**uez

mm	Sonido igual a la **m** simple.
	immunology / inmunología a**mm**eba
ph	Sonido de **f.**
	pharmacy / farmacia **f**armacia
r	Sonido articulado en inglés sin trino y con la lengua situada más hacia atrás de la boca y la parte anterior curvada hacia el paladar sin tocarlo.
	surgery / cirugía ci**r**ugía
rr	Sonido igual al del la r sencilla.
	hemorrhage / hemorragia ci**r**ugía
s	Sonido semejante a la **s** sorda en español en la mayoría de los vocablos.
	consult / consultar con**s**ulta
	sperm / esperma e**s**perma

Sonido semejante a la **s** sonora de mi**s**mo o de**s**de cuando está entre vocales o antes de la consonante **m.**

disease / enfermedad mi**s**mo
metabolism / metabolismo de**s**de

Al final de la palabra, puede tener sonido de **s** o de **z** en inglés.
yes / sí sí
is / es (*sonido de z en inglés*)

Cuando está seguida del diptongo **io,** tiene sonido semejante al de la **y** (*sonido de consonante*), muy exagerado, o al de la **j** en francés como en **J**ean.
lesion / lesión le**y**ó

Cuando está seguida de la vocal **u,** tiene un sonido semejante a la **sh** en inglés.
sure / seguro **sh**shsh (*como cuando se está silenciando a alguien*)

ss	Sonido igual al de la **s** en español.
	class / clase cla**s**e
th	Tiene dos sonidos: (1) parecido a la **d;** (2) parecido a la **z** castellana.
	this / este de**d**o
	therapy / terapia **z**apato (*con ceceo castellano*)
w	Sonido semejante al de la **u** en español como en la palabra h**u**eso.
	weight / peso h**u**eso
z	Sonido semejante al que se hace para imitar el zumbido de una abeja.
	zero / cero **z**zzz...

Acentuación de las palabras en inglés

El acento gráfico no existe en inglés. Las reglas a seguir son pocas, pero tienen muchas excepciones.

1. Las palabras de dos sílabas se acentúan generalmente en la penúltima sílaba:
   swollen / hinchado
   abscess / abceso
2. Palabras a las que se le hayan añadido sufijos o prefijos retienen el acento en la misma sílaba acentuada de la raíz o palabra básica:
   normal: abnormal / anormal
   coloration: discoloration / descoloración

3. Palabras de tres o más sílabas generalmente tienen una sílaba que se acentúa más enfáticamente y otra sílaba que lleva un acento menos pronunciado:

rapidly / **rá**pida**men**te

Punctuation / Puntuación

(.) period	(-) the dash
(,) comma	( ) parentheses
(;) semicolon	(" ") quotation marks
(:) colon	([ ]) brackets
(?) the question mark*	(') apostrophe
(!) the exclamation point*	(*) asterisk

*En inglés los signos de interrogación y admiración se usan solamente al final de la oración.

COGNATES / COGNADOS

Cognates are words related in origin, that is, words that have the same origin as other words in another language. The spelling of a word (noun, adjective, or verb) may be identical or almost the same as the other language's word. Cognates follow spelling rules, and may have equivalent endings in both languages. The terminology made up of the "new" terms found, are words made by combining prefixes, roots (stems) and suffixes of Greek and Latin origin. Spelling changes took place in the stem of the word, new word endings were added to the Latin or Greek words, which were substituted by derivatives proper to the many languages of the users.

You will find in the following list some of the variations that have occurred to scientific terms and in common English and Spanish words. These two languages, English and Spanish, have as many as seventy-five percent of scientific words that are common to each other, called **cognates/cognados**. By using the examples of cognates given in the following list and the rules employed in the English words for transformation into Spanish, you will learn to build your own additional vocabulary.

List of Cognates / Lista de cognados[1]
Division into Syllables or Syllabification / División de palabras en sílabas

EW[2]	SB	SW
abdominal	ab-do-mi-**nal**	abdominal
accept	a-cep-**tar**	aceptar
accumulate	a-cu-mu-**lar**	acumular
acidosis	a-ci-**do**-sis	acidosis
Words ending in -**osis**, a suffix referring to condition or disease, do not change in either language.		
action	ac-**ción**	acción
acupuncture	a-cu-pun-**tu**-ra	acupuntura
addict	a-**dic**-to	adicto[3] (f.) adicta
Drop one -**d**; there are no words with double **dd** in Spanish: **addicted** > adicto.		
addiction	a-dic-**ción**	adicción
adhesive	ad-he-**si**-vo	adhesivo
adipose	a-di-**po**-so	adiposo
adjust	a-jus-**tar**	ajustar
adjusted	a-jus-**ta**-do	ajustado
administer	ad-mi-nis-**trar**	administrar
admission	ad-mi-**sión**	admisión
admit	ad-mi-**tir**	admitir
admitted	ad-mi-**ti**-do	admitido
affirm	a-fir-**mar**	afirmar
air	**ai**-re	aire
alienated	a-lie-**na**-do	alienado
alienation	a-lie-na-**ción**	alienación

[1]Cognates divided into syllables.
[2]**EW** English word, **SW** Spanish word, **SB** Syllabification of Spanish words.
[3]The ending of the feminine adjectives (-a) is indicated following the masculine form. To form the feminine, drop the ending **-o**, and add **-a** instead; **hombre adicto** (m.), **una mujer adicta** (f.)

allergic	a-**lér**-gi-co	alérgico (*m.*), alérgica (*f.*)
alter	al-te-**rar**	alterar
altered	al-te-**ra**-do	alterado
amputate	am-pu-**tar**	amputar

> Verbs ending in -**ate** in English have the infinitive ending -**ar** in Spanish, such as **terminate** > terminar.

amputation	am-pu-ta-**ción**	amputación
analyze	a-na-li-**zar**	analizar
analyzed	a-na-li-**za**-do	analizado
anemia	a-**ne**-mia	anemia
angina	an-**gi**-na	angina
annual	a-**nual**	anual
anorexia	a-no-**re**-xia	anorexia
antibiotic	an-ti-**bió**-ti-co	antibiótico
antigen	an-**tí**-ge-no	antígeno
appendicitis	a-pen-di-**ci**-tis	apendicitis

> Words ending in the suffix -**itis** have the same ending in Spanish: **myelitis** > mielitis.

appetite	a-pe-**ti**-to	apetito
application	a-pli-ca-**ción**	aplicación
appreciate	a-pre-**ciar**	apreciar
appreciated	a-pre-**cia**-do	apreciado

> For regular Spanish verbs ending in -**ar**, add the ending -**ado** to the root to make the past participle (p.p.). An English p.p. ending in -**ed** such as **appreciated** changes to **apreciado** in Spanish. (There are no words with double **p** in Spanish.)

arsenic	ar-**sé**-ni-co	arsénico
articulation	ar-ti-cu-la-**ción**	articulación
associate	a-so-**ciar**	asociar
associated	a-so-**cia**-do	asociado
association	a-so-cia-**ción**	asociación
astigmatism	as-tig-ma-**tis**-mo	astigmatismo
attention	a-ten-**ción**	atención
autonomy	au-to-no-**mí**-a	autonomía
autophobia	au-to-**fo**-bia	autofobia
autopsy	au-**top**-sia	autopsia
authorization	au-to-ri-za-**ción**	autorización

> Convert English nouns ending in -**tion** into Spanish by changing -**tion** to -**ción**: reaction > reacción.

authorized	au-to-ri-**za**-do	autorizado
autotoxin	au-to-to-**xi**-na	autotoxina
bacillus	ba-**ci**-lo	bacilo
basic	**bá**-si-co	básico
bilateral	bi-la-te-**ral**	bilateral
billion	bi-**llón**	billón

biology	bio-lo-**gí**-a	biología

English nouns ending in **-y** may change to **-ia** or **-ía** in Spanish: **biopsy** > biopsia; **anatomy** > anatomía.

biomedical	bio-**mé**-di-co	biomédico
biopsy	**biop**-sia	biopsia
biosphere	bios-**fe**-ra	biosfera
bronchitis	bron-**qui**-tis	bronquitis
bronchium	**bron**-quio	bronquio
bulimia	bu-**li**-mia[4]	bulimia
bursitis	bur-**si**-tis	bursitis
calcium	**cal**-cio	calcio

The Latin suffix **-um** drops, and is substitued by **-o** in Spanish: **museum** > museo.

calm	**cal**-ma	calma
cancer	**cán**-cer	cáncer
cancerous	can-ce-**ro**-so	canceroso
capacity	ca-pa-ci-**dad**	capacidad
cape	**ca**-pa	capa
capsule	**cáp**-su-la	cápsula
cardiac	car-**dí**-a-co	cardíaco
cartilage	car-**tí**-la-go	cartílago
catheter	ca-**té**-ter	catéter
cauterize	cau-te-ri-**zar**	cauterizar
center	**cen**-tro	centro

Nouns ending in **-ter** in English change the ending to **-tro** in Spanish: **meter** > metro.

circulation	cir-cu-la-**ción**	circulación
cirrhosis	ci-**rro**-sis	cirrosis
clinic	**clí**-ni-ca	clínica
coagulation	co-a-gu-la-**ción**	coagulación
cocaine	co-ca-**í**-na	cocaína

Nouns ending in **-in** or **-ine** in English change into **-ina** in Spanish: **cocaine** > cocaína.

codeine	co-de-**í**-na	codeína
colitis	co-**li**-tis	colitis
coma	**co**-ma	coma
condition	con-di-**ción**	condición
consult	con-sul-**tar**	consultar
contagious	con-ta-**gio**-so	contagioso
contaminate	con-ta-mi-**nar**	contaminar
contraceptive	con-tra-cep-**ti**-vo	contraceptivo
control	con-**trol**	control
convert	con-ver-**tir**	convertir

[4]A written accent mark on the í (ía) dissolves the diphthong. There is no accent mark on the i in bulimia.

English	Pronunciation	Spanish
converted	con-ver-**ti**-do	convertido
conversion	con-ver-**sión**	conversión
convulsion	con-vul-**sión**	convulsión
cosmetics	cos-**mé**-ti-cos	cosméticos
cost	**cos**-to	costo
cranium	**cra**-nio	cranio
crystal	cris-**tal**	crystal

> The **-y-** in the middle of an English word may change to **-í-** in Spanish: **symptom** > síntoma.

debilitate	de-bi-li-**tar**	debilitar
debilitated	de-bi-li-**ta**-do	debilitado
decide	de-ci-**dir**	decidir
deficiency	de-fi-**cien**-cia	deficiencia
defibrillation	de-fi-bri-la-**ción**	defibrilación
dental	den-**tal**	dental
dentist	den-**tis**-ta	dentista

> The equivalent Spanish ending to the English ending **-ist** is **-ista**, used for both masculine and feminine genders: **pianist** > pianista; **dentist** > dentista.

depression	de-pre-**sión**	depresión
depressor	de-pre-**sor**	depresor
description	des-crip-**ción**	descripción
destroy	des-**truir**	destruir
diarrhea	dia-**rre**-a	diarrea
dictionary	dic-cio-**na**-rio	diccionario

> English nouns ending in **-ary** have the ending **-ario** in Spanish: **vocabulary** > vocabulario.

diet	**die**-ta	dieta
difficulty	di-fi-cul-**tad**	dificultad
dilate	di-la-**tar**	dilatar
direction	di-rec-**ción**	dirección
disc	**dis**-co	disco
disinfect	de-sin-fec-**tar**	desinfectar
diuretic	diu-**ré**-ti-co	diurético
ecology	e-co-lo-**gí**-a	ecología
education	e-du-ca-**ción**	educación
effective	e-fec-**ti**-vo	efectivo
electrocardiogram	e-lec-tro-car-dio-**gra**-ma	electrocardiograma

> Add an **-a** to words ending in **-gram** to form the ending **-grama** in Spanish: **diagram** > diagrama.

elevator	e-le-va-**dor**	elevador
eliminate	e-li-mi-**nar**	eliminar
emergency	e-mer-**gen**-cia	emergencia
emphysema	en-fi-**se**-ma	enfisema

endometrium	en-do-**me**-trio	endometrio
epilepsy	e-pi-**lep**-sia	epilepsia
estrogen	es-**tró**-ge-no	estrógeno
evaluate	e-va-**luar**	evaluar
examine	e-xa-mi-**nar**	examinar
examined	e-xa-mi-**na**-do	examinado
expectorate	ex-pec-to-**rar**	expectorar
expulsive	ex-pul-**si**-vo	expulsivo
extrovert	ex-tro-ver-**ti**-do	extrovertido
facilitate	fa-ci-li-**tar**	facilitado
factor	fac-**tor**	factor
family	fa-**mi**-lia	familia
fantastic	fan-**tás**-ti-co	fantástico
fibroma	fi-**bro**-ma	fibroma
form	**for**-ma	forma
formation	for-ma-**ción**	formación
fracture	frac-**tu**-ra	fractura
generous	ge-ne-**ro**-so	generoso
germ	**ger**-men	germen
gestation	ges-ta-**ción**	gestación
glucose	glu-**co**-sa	glucosa
gonorrhea	go-no-**rre**-a	gonorrea
halitosis	ha-li-**to**-sis	halitosis
hemorrhage	he-mo-**rra**-gia	hemorragia

> In converting to Spanish, the **-h-** in the middle of an English word is usually dropped (except for the **-h-** in **alcohol** and other words of Arabic origin): **hemorrhage** > hemorragia.

hepatitis	he-pa-**ti**-tis	hepatitis
hereditary	he-re-di-**ta**-rio	hereditario
hermetic	her-**mé**-ti-co	hermético (*m.*), hermética (*f.*)
hernia	**her**-nia	hernia
heroine	he-**roí**-na	heroína
herpes	**her**-pes	herpes
homosexual	ho-mo-sex-**ual**	homosexual
hormone	hor-**mo**-na	hormona
humor	hu-**mor**	humor
hydrogen	hi-**dró**-ge-no	hidrógeno
hypothermia	hi-po-**ter**-mia	hipotermia
hysterectomy	his-te-rec-to-**mí**-a	histerectomía
hysteria	his-**te**-ria	histeria
imagine	i-ma-gi-**nar**	imaginar

inflammation	in-fla-ma-**ción**	inflamación

Drop one **m** in **inflammation** to convert: **inflammation** > inflamación.

immunization	in-mu-ni-za-**ción**	inmunización
immune	in-**mu**-ne	inmuno (*m.*), immuna (*f.*)
inclusion	in-clu-**sión**	inclusión
incompetent	in-com-pe-**ten**-te	incompetente
incubation	in-cu-ba-**ción**	incubación
indicate	in-di-**car**	indicar
infancy	in-**fan**-cia	infancia
infect	in-fec-**tar**	infectar
infection	in-fec-**ción**	infección
inflammation	in-fla-ma-**ción**	inflamación
inform	in-for-**mar**	informar
infusion	in-fu-**sión**	infusión
inoculate	i-no-cu-**lar**	inocular
insect	in-**sec**-to	insecto
insecticide	in-sec-ti-**ci**-da	insecticida
inspection	ins-pec-**ción**	inspección
instinct	ins-**tin**-to	instinto
intensity	in-ten-si-**dad**	intensidad

Many nouns in English ending in **-ty** have a corresponding Spanish word ending in **-dad**: **intensity** > intensidad.

intensive	in-ten-**si**-vo	intensivo
intestinal	in-tes-ti-**nal**	intestinal
intestine	in-tes-**ti**-no	intestino
intolerance	in-to-le-**ran**-cia	intolerancia
investigate	in-ves-ti-**gar**	investigar
irrigation	i-rri-ga-**ción**	irrigación
irritable	i-rri-**ta**-ble	irritable
labor	la-**bor**	labor
laboratory	la-bo-ra-**to**-rio	laboratorio
lactose	lac-**to**-sa	lactosa
laparoscopy	la-pa-ros-co-**pí**-a	laparoscopía
laryngitis	la-rin-**gi**-tis	laringitis
lesion	le-**sión**	lesión
local	lo-**cal**	local
lotion	lo-**ción**	loción
lymphatic	lin-**fá**-ti-co	linfático
magic	**má**-gico	mágico
margin	**mar**-gen	margen
mechanical	me-**cá**-ni-co	mecánico

medicine	me-di-**ci**-na	medicina
memory	me-**mo**-ria	memoria
menstruation	mens-trua-**ción**	menstruación
microscope	mi-cros-**co**-pio	microscopio

> The suffix **-scope** is equivalent to the ending **-scopio** in Spanish: **endoscope** > endoscopio.

morphine	mor-**fi**-na	morfina
nasal	na-**sal**	nasal
nausea	**náu**-se-a	náusea
necessity	ne-ce-si-**dad**	necesidad
negative	ne-ga-**ti**-vo	negativo
nervous	ner-**vio**-so	nervioso

> Many adjectives ending in **-ous** in English have a corresponding ending in Spanish: **-oso** (*m.*), or **-osa** (*f.*), as in **nervous** > nervioso.

neurotic	neu-**ró**-ti-co	neurótico
notification	no-ti-fi-ca-**ción**	notificación
notify	no-ti-fi-**car**	notificar
nuclear	nu-**clear**	nuclear
nutrition	nu-tri-**ción**	nutrición
obesity	o-be-si-**dad**	obesidad
observe	ob-ser-**var**	observar
obstruct	obs-**truir**	obstruir

> Verbs ending in **-struct** have the equivalent ending **-struir** in Spanish: **construct** > construir.

omit	o-mi-**tir**	omitir
operate	o-pe-**rar**	operar
operation	o-pe-ra-**ción**	operación
oral	o-**ral**	oral
ovary	o-**va**-rio	ovario
paranoia	pa-ra-**noia**	paranoia
parasite	pa-**rá**-si-to	parásito
passive	pa-**si**-vo	pasivo
paste	**pas**-ta	pasta
paternity	pa-ter-ni-**dad**	paternidad
patient	pa-**cien**-te	paciente
penetrate	pe-ne-**trar**	penetrar
permit	per-mi-**tir**	permitir
person	per-**so**-na	persona
perspire	pers-pi-**rar**	perspirar
pharmacy	far-**ma**-cia	farmacia

> For many English words with **ph** in the beginning or in the middle, one may change the **ph** to **f** in deriving the Spanish equivalent: **pharmacy** > farmacia.

| plasma | **plas**-ma | plasma |
| plastic | **plás**-ti-co | plástico |

pneumonia[6]	pneu-mo-**ní**-a, neu-mo-**ní**-a	pneumonía, neumonía
portion	por-**ción**	porción
positive	po-si-**ti**-vo	positivo
practice	prac-ti-**car**	practicar
prepare	pre-pa-**rar**	preparar
prevent	pre-ve-**nir**	prevenir
problem	pro-**ble**-ma	problema
professor	pro-fe-**sor**	profesor
prohibit	pro-hi-**bir**	prohibir

> In converting the verbs **prohibit** and **exhibit** to their Spanish equivalents, retain the **h** in the middle of the word and change the ending to **-ibir**: **prohibir, exhibir**.

psychology	psi-co-lo-**gí**-a	psicología[7]
pulse	**pul**-so	pulso
pupil	pu-**pi**-la	pupila
pyorrhea	pio-**rre**-a	piorrea
reaction	reac-**ción**	reacción
relation	re-la-**ción**	relación
religion	re-li-**gión**	religión
refrigerate	re-fri-ge-**rar**	refrigerar
respiration	res-pi-ra-**ción**	respiración
saliva	sa-**li**-va	saliva
secretion	se-cre-**ción**	secreción
section	sec-**ción**	sección
sensitive	sen-si-**ti**-vo	sensitivo
separate	se-pa-**rar**	separar
septic	**sép**-ti-co	séptico (*m.*), séptica (*f.*)
serious	**se**-rio	serio
sterilizer	es-te-ri-li-za-**dor**	esterilizador

> For English words beginning in **s + a consonant**, in many cases add an **e** before the initial **s** to form the Spanish equivalent: **special** > especial.

spasm	es-**pas**-mo	espasmo
specialist	es-pe-cia-**lis**-ta	especialista
stimulant	es-ti-mu-**lan**-te	estimulante
stomach	es-**tó**-ma-go	estómago
strict	es-**tric**-to	estricto
stupor	es-tu-**por**	estupor
suppurate	su-pu-**rar**	supurar
syndrome	**sín**-dro-me	síndrome
tachycardia	ta-qui-**car**-dia	taquicardia

---

[6]Pneumonía, neumonía or pulmonía
[7]Another noun that may drop the **-p** in Spanish: sicología

talcum	**tal**-co	talco
temperature	tem-pe-ra-**tu**-ra	temperatura
tendon	ten-**dón**	tendón
tension	ten-**sión**	tensión
therapeutic	te-ra-**péu**-ti-co	terapéutico
therapy	te-**ra**-pia	terapia
thermal	ter-**mal**	termal
thermometer	ter-**mó**-me-tro	termómetro
thorax	**tó**-rax	tórax
thyroid	ti-**roi**-de	tiroide

English nouns ending in **-oid**, add **-e** to this ending in Spanish: In **thyroid** the **h** drops and the **y** changes to **i**: **thyroid** > tiroide.

total	to-**tal**	total
toxic	**tó**-xi-co	tóxico
trachea	**trá**-que-a	tráquea
transfusion	trans-fu-**sión**	transfusión
transmissible	trans-mi-**si**-ble	transmisible
transmission	trans-mi-**sión**	transmisión
transplant	tras-**plan**-te	trasplante
tube	**tu**-bo	tubo
tuberculosis	tu-ber-cu-**lo**-sis	tuberculosis
turn	**tur**-no	turno
ulcer	**úl**-ce-ra	úlcera
ultrasonic	ul-tra-**só**-ni-co	ultrasónico
urethra	u-**re**-tra	uretra
urethritis	u-re-**tri**-tis	uretritis
uterine	u-te-**ri**-no	uterino
vaporizer	va-po-ri-za-**dor**	vaporizador
venereal	ve-**né**-re-o	venéreo
victim	**víc**-ti-ma	víctima
vomit	**vó**-mi-to	vómito
yard	**yar**-da	yarda
zone	**zo**-na	zona

Equivalences in Endings, English / Spanish

ENGLISH	SPANISH	ENGLISH	SPANISH
-ent	-ente	accident	accidente
-ine	-ina	morphine	morfina
-ment	-mento	instrument	instrumento
-ide	-uro	chloride	cloruro

Adjective Endings

ENGLISH	SPANISH	ENGLISH	SPANISH
-ive	-ivo, -iva	active	activo (*m.*), activa (*f.*)
-nal	-no, -na	internal	interno (*m.*), interna (*f.*)
-id	-do	liquid	líquido (*m.*), líquida (*f.*)
-ct	-cto, -cta	perfect	perfecto (*m.*), perfecta (*f.*)

Verb Endings

ENGLISH	SPANISH	ENGLISH	SPANISH
-ce	-zar	commence	comenzar
-iate	-iar	affiliate	afiliar
-ish	-ecer	establish	establecer
-ize	-izar	cauterize	cauterizar

COGNATES AND THEIR PRONUNCIATIONS IN SPANISH
WORDS THAT HAVE THE SAME OR SIMILAR SPELLING[a]

COGNATES	SPANISH PRONUNCIATION
anasarca *f.* anasarca	ah-nah-**sahr'**-kah
abdominal *a.* abdominal	ahb-doh-mee-**náhl'**
abulia *n.* abulia	ah-**boo'**-leeah
acarina *f.* acarina	ah-kah-**ree'**-nah
accidente *m.* accident	ahk-see-**dehn'**-te
acidosis *f.* acidosis	ah-see-**doh'**-sees
bismuto *m.* bismuth	bees-**moo**-toh
benzocaína *f.* benzocaine	behn-zoh-kah-**ee'**-nah
bradicardia *f.* bradycardia	brah-dee-**cahr'**-deeah
cervix[b] *m.* cervix	**sehr'**-beeks
cisterna *f.* cistern	sees-**tehr'**-nah
clavícula *f.* clavicle	klah-**beeh'**-cooh-lah
colon *m.* colon	**koh'**-lohn
color *m.* color	koh-**lohr'**
coma *m.* coma	**koh'**-mah
comensal *m.* commensal	koh-mehn-**sahl**
compacta *a.* compact	kohm-**pahk**-tah
control *m.* control	kohn-**trohl**
gama *f.* gamma	**gah**-mah
gástrico *a.* gastric	**gáhs**-tree-coh
glándula *f.* gland	**gláhn**-doo-lah

[a]The stressed syllable in the Spanish words is indicated by **bold** and the symbol (´).
[b]**Cervix**, a Latin word used in anatomy in both English and Spanish, is pronounced very similarly in both languages. Do not confuse this word, translated as **cuello uterino** (part of the uterus), with the term **cerviz**, nape of the neck.

COGNATES	SPANISH PRONUNCIATION
glaucoma *m.* glaucoma	glahoo-**koh**-mah
gluten *m.* gluten	**gloo**-tehn
hepatitis *f.* hepatitis	eh-pah-**tee**-tees
hospital *m.* hospital	ohs-pee-**tahl'**
hematoma *m.* hematoma	eh-mah-**toh'**-mah
infantil *a.* infantile	eehn-fahn-**teel'**
infección *f.* infection	een-fehk-**seeohn'**
influenza *f.* influenza	een-flooh**ehn'**-zah
lámina *f.* lamina	**lah'**-mee-nah
lanugo *a.* lanugo	lah-**noo'**-goh
medicamento *m.* medicament	meh-dee-kah-**mehn'**-toh
nasal *a.* nasal	nah-**sah'l**
neonatal *a.* neonatal	neh-oh-**nah'**-tahl
neoplasia *f.* neoplasia	neh-oh-**plah'**-seeah
normal *a.* normal	nor-**mahl'**
nuclear *a.* nuclear	noo-kleh-**ahr'**
osmosis *f.* osmosis	ohs-**moh'**-sees
orolingual *a.*orolingual	oh-roh-leen-**gooahl'**
pectoral *a.* pectoral	pehk-toh-**rahl'**
persona *f.* persona	pehr-**soh'**-nah
placenta *f.* placenta	plah-**sehn'**-tah
pneumonía[c]*f.* pneumonia	nehoo-moh-**nee**ah'
podagra *f.* podagra	poh-**dah'**-grah
región *f.* region	reh-hee-**ohn'**
renal *a.* renal	reh-**nahl'**
repulsión *f.* repulsion	reh-pool-**seeohn'**
saliva *f.* saliva	sah-**lee'**-bah
semicircular *a.* semicircular	seh-mee-seer-coo-**lahr'**
senil *a.* senile	seh-**neel'**
sensorial *a.* sensoreal	sehn-soh-**reeahl'**
serositis *f.* serositis	she-roh-**see'**-tees
sexual *a.*sexual	sehg-**sooahl'**
simple *a.* simple	**seem'**-pleh
soda *a.* soda	**soh'**-dah
superior *a.* superior	soo-peh-ree**ohr'**
temporal *a.* temporal	tehm-poh-**rahl'**
tenia *f.* tenia	**teh'**-neeah
tensión *f.* tension	tehn-see**ohn'**
trauma *m.* trauma	**trahw'**-mah

[c]Words beginning in pn- and ps- gen. drop the letter p in Spanish.

Simplified Spanish Grammar

Gramática española simplificada

THE ARTICLE / EL ARTÍCULO

The article (definite or indefinite) precedes the noun. Spanish articles agree with the noun in gender and number.

THE DEFINITE ARTICLE *(THE)*

	FEMININE (1)	MASCULINE (2)
SINGULAR	la	el
PLURAL	las	los

THE ARTICLE

1. the chronic infection / **la infección crónica**
   the chronic infections / **las infecciones crónicas**
2. the extreme case / **el caso extremo**
   the extreme cases / **los casos extremos**

Note: Singular feminine nouns that begin with stressed **a** or **ha** require the masculine form **el.**
   the water / **el agua**
   the speech / **el habla**

When **de** / of precedes **el,** they contract to **del;** and when **a** / to precedes **el,** they contract to **al.**

THE INDEFINITE ARTICLE (A, AN, SOME)

	FEMININE (1)	MASCULINE (2)
SINGULAR	una	un
PLURAL	unas	unos

1. a complicated situation / **una situación complicada**
   some complicated situations / **unas situaciones complicadas**
2. an asthmatic boy / **un niño asmático**
   some asthmatic boys / **unos niños asmáticos**

   In the first two examples of the definite article, the nouns **infección,** which is feminine, and **caso,** which is masculine, determine the gender and number of the article that precedes them. The descriptive adjectives that follow the nouns have the same gender and number as the noun they modify. The same rules of agreement apply in the examples for the indefinite article.

USES OF THE DEFINITE ARTICLE / USOS DEL ARTÍCULO DEFINIDO

1. To refer to parts of the body and articles of clothing.
   Antonia raises her arm. / **Antonia levanta el brazo.**
   The patient puts on her robe. / **La paciente se pone la bata.**
2. To refer to days of the week, dates, and seasons.
   Check into the hospital on Thursday. / **Ingrese en el hospital el jueves.**
3. With nouns of rate, weight, and measure.
   Take half of the pill. / **Tome la mitad de la pastilla.**
4. With titles when speaking about a person or persons.

Dr. Ruiz is famous. / **El doctor Ruiz es famoso.**
5. With cardinal numbers to tell time (feminine forms **la** and **las** only).
I'll see you at one. / **Te veo a la una.**
Come back tomorrow at eleven. / **Vuelva mañana a las once.**

USES OF THE INDEFINITE ARTICLE / USOS DEL ARTÍCULO INDEFINIDO

1. To indicate some, any, a few, about (meaning approximately).
The patient is about twenty years old. / **El paciente tiene unos veinte años.**
2. To stress a person's identity.
Who is he? He is a famous doctor. / **¿Quién es él? Es un médico famoso.**
3. To identify objects or persons after **hay** (there is, there are).
There are a book, a glass, and some medicines on the table. /
Hay un libro, un vaso y unas medicinas en la mesa.

Note: The indefinite article is generally omitted after the verb **ser** with an unmodified noun referring to profession, religion or nationality:
He is a doctor. / **Él es médico.**

NOUNS / NOMBRES
GENDER / GÉNERO

In Spanish, nouns are either masculine or feminine. There are no neuter nouns.
Nouns referring to female beings and certain things are classified as feminine; they have the following endings.

ENDINGS OF FEMININE NOUNS / TERMINACIONES DE NOMBRES FEMENINOS

MOST COMMON	EXAMPLE	EXCEPTION
-a	**hora** / hour	**el día** / day
OTHERS		
-ad	**enfermedad** / sickness	
-ión	**atención** / attention	**el avión** / airplane
-is	**flebitis** / phlebitis	—
-ud	**salud** / health	—
-umbre	**costumbre** / custom	—

Nouns referring to masculine beings, days of the week, and names of languages are usually classified as masculine, as are the names of things having the following endings.

ENDINGS OF MASCULINE NOUNS / TERMINACIONES DE NOMBRES MASCULINOS

MOST COMMON	EXAMPLE	EXCEPTION
-o	**brazo** / arm	**la mano** / hand
OTHERS		
-or	**doctor**	
-ma	**sistema** / system	**la flema** / phlegm
-pa	**mapa** / map	

Only nouns of Greek origin ending in **-ma, -pa** are masculine. This rule applies to most scientific names having these endings.

ADJECTIVES / ADJETIVOS
GENDER / GÉNERO

Adjectives are used in both the masculine and feminine genders. Change the ending **-o** of a masculine adjective to **-a** to form the feminine.

> the anemic boy / **el niño anémico**
> the anemic girl / **la niña anémica**

Add -a to an adjective of nationality ending in a consonant to form the feminine. The written accent on the last syllable drops when the feminine ending is added. However, the stress remains on the vowel **e.**

> **el estudiante francés** / the French student
> **la estudiante francesa** / the French student

Adjectives ending in **-e** or the consonant **l** remain unchanged for both the masculine and feminine forms:

> **la niña inteligente** / the intelligent girl
> **el niño inteligente** / the intelligent boy
> **la pregunta fácil** / the easy question
> **el examen fácil** / the easy examination

Adjectives ending in **-án, -ón,** and **-or** (except comparatives), add **-a** to form the feminine. The written accent is omitted when the feminine ending is added.

> reductor / **reductor, reductora**   lazy / **haragán, haragana**

Note: The adjective may follow or precede the noun; however, nouns and adjectives that have the same endings are inflected alike.

NUMBER / NÚMERO
NOUNS AND ADJECTIVES / NOMBRES Y ADJETIVOS

Plural Endings

add -s	if the noun or adjective ends in an unaccented vowel or diphthong, or stressed **é:**	
	microbio / microbe	**microbios**
	café / coffee	**cafés**
	amargo / bitter	**amargos**
add -es	if the noun or adjective ends in a consonant:	
	pulmón / lung	**pulmones**
	especial / special	**especiales**
add -es	**if the noun or adjective ends in z,** change **z** to **c** before adding **-es.**	
	luz / light	**luces**
	feliz / happy	**felices**

Note: Nouns ending in unstressed **-is** or **-es** remain unchanged in the plural. Their number is indicated by the preceding article.

la crisis	las crisis
el jueves	los jueves
el análisis	los análisis

ADJECTIVES THAT PRECEDE THE NOUN / ADJETIVOS QUE PRECEDEN AL NOMBRE
DEMONSTRATIVES / DEMOSTRATIVOS

Demonstratives indicate location. A demonstrative adjective indicates persons, animals, or objects in relation to the speaker.

NEAR THE SPEAKER

	SINGULAR *this*	PLURAL *these*
MASCULINE	este	estos
FEMININE	esta	estas

this medicine / **esta medicina**   these medicines / **estas medicinas**
this doctor / **este médico**   these doctors / **estos médicos**

NOT FAR FROM THE PERSON ADDRESSED OR THE SPEAKER (IN TIME OR SPACE)

	SINGULAR *that*	PLURAL *those*
MASCULINE	ese	esos

NOT FAR FROM THE PERSON ADDRESSED OR THE SPEAKER (IN TIME OR SPACE)

	SINGULAR *that*	PLURAL *those*
FEMININE	esa	esas

that white robe / **esa bata blanca**   those white robes / **esas batas blancas**
that week / **esa semana**   those weeks / **esas semanas**

DISTANT FROM THE SPEAKER AND PERSON ADDRESSED

	SINGULAR *that*	PLURAL *those*
MASCULINE	aquel	aquellos
FEMININE	aquella	aquellas

that lady (over there) / **aquella señora**   those ladies (over there) / **aquellas señoras**
that case (that was treated) / **aquel caso**   those cases (that were treated) / **aquellos casos**

DEMONSTRATIVE PRONOUNS / PRONOMBRES DEMOSTRATIVOS

Demonstrative adjectives and pronouns have the same form except that the pronouns always carry an accent mark that distinguishes them from the adjectives: **éste, ése, aquél, ésta, ésa, aquélla; éstos, ésos, aquéllos, éstas, éstas, ésas, aquéllas.**

Adjective: This patient has a fever. / **Este paciente tiene fiebre.**
Pronoun: That one is anemic. / **Aquél es anémico.**

When referring to a concept, situation, or object of unknown gender, the forms **esto, eso,** and **aquello** are used:

Why do you say that? / **¿Por qué dice eso?**
What is this? / **¿Qué es esto?**
That was awful! / **¡Aquello fue terrible!**

POSSESSIVE ADJECTIVES / ADJETIVOS POSESIVOS

Possessive adjectives agree in gender and number with the thing possessed (the noun they modify). The following forms precede the noun.

SINGULAR	PLURAL	ENGLISH
mi	mis	my
tu	tus	your (*fam.*)
su	sus	his her its, your (*form.*)
nuestro -a	nuestros -as	our
vuestro -a	vuestros -as	your (*fam. Cast.*)
su	sus	their, your

my patient / **mi paciente**   my patients / **mis pacientes**
our evaluation / **nuestra evaluación**   our patients / **nuestros pacientes**

7

Note: To clarify **su** (which can refer to more than one possessor), substitute the preposition **de** and the subject pronoun for **su:**

> article + noun + **de** + pronoun

> His temperature is normal. /   **Su temperatura es normal.**
>   **La temperatura de él es normal.** [*m. sing.*]
> Their temperature is normal. /   **Su temperatura es normal.**
>   **La temperatura de ellas es normal.** [*f. pl.*]

OTHER POSSESSIVE FORMS

Other possessive forms that are stressed and placed after the noun are inflected in their endings like adjectives.

SINGULAR	PLURAL	ENGLISH
mío -a	míos –as	my, of mine
tuyo -a	tuyos –as	your (*fam.*), of yours
suyo -a	suyos –as	his, her, your, its, of his, of hers, of yours
nuestro -a	nuestros –as	our, of ours
vuestro -a	vuestros –as	your (*fam.*), of yours
suyo -a	suyos –as	their, your, of theirs, of yours

> this patient of mine / **este paciente mío**
> that patient of ours / **ese paciente nuestro**

Note: To clarify the meaning of **suyo, suya** (*sing.* or *pl.*) replace it with the preposition **de** and the corresponding personal pronoun, as explained in the case of **su.**

> her temperature / **la temperatura suya / la temperatura de ella**

The stressed forms of the possessive adjectives can be used as possessive pronouns.

> Adjective: Your medicine is here / **La medicina suya está aquí.**
> Pronoun: Yours is here / **La suya está aquí.**
> Adjective: Our treatment finishes today / **El tratamiento nuestro termina hoy.**
> Pronoun: Ours finishes today / **El nuestro termina hoy.**

LIMITING ADJECTIVES / ADJETIVOS QUE LIMITAN AL NOMBRE

Numbers and indefinite adjectives that indicate quantities usually precede the noun.

SINGULAR	PLURAL	ENGLISH
mucho-a	muchos-as	many, a lot, much
otro-a	otros-as	another
todo-a	todos-as	all, ever
algún, alguna	algunos-as	some, any

SINGULAR	PLURAL	ENGLISH
ningún, ninguno-a	ningunos-as	not any, none
primer, primero-a	primeros-as	first
tercer, tercero-a	terceros-as	third

Note: **Ninguno** changes to **ningún, primero** to **primer,** and **tercero** to **tercer** when placed in front of a masculine singular noun; **ningunos** and **ningunas** are rarely used.

> Go down to the first floor. / **Baje al primer piso.**

DESCRIPTIVE ADJECTIVES / ADJETIVOS DESCRIPTIVOS

In Spanish, descriptive adjectives are most frequently placed after the noun, except adjectives denoting quantity, size, or order, which are generally placed before the noun.

> You have high blood pressure. / **Tiene la presión alta.**
> That sickness has many complications. / **Esa enfermedad tiene muchas complicaciones.**
> It is the third time. / **Es la tercera vez.**

Some descriptive adjectives change in meaning depending on whether they precede or follow the noun:

bueno –a	**un médico bueno** / a good doctor (compared to others)
	un buen médico (he is excellent, worth recommending)
grande	**un hombre grande** / a big man (in a physical sense)
	un gran hombre / a big man (in a moral, spiritual, or intellectual sense)
malo –a	**una dieta mala** / a bad diet (of bad quality)
	una mala dieta / a bad diet (as compared to a good one)

Note: The adjectives **bueno** and **malo** drop the ending **-o** before a masculine singular noun; **grande** drops the ending **-de** before a singular noun, masculine or feminine.

Comparisons of Inequality
más / more + the adjective + **que** / than

> John is taller than Joe. / **Juan es más alto que Pepe.**

menos / less + the adjective + **que** / than

> Joe is shorter than John. / **Pepe es menos alto que Juan.**

Comparisons of Equality
tan / as + an adjective or adverb + **como** / as

> This pill is as effective as that one. / **Esta pastilla es tan eficaz como ésa.**

tanto -a, -os, -as / as much, as many + noun + **como**

> He has as much fever as yesterday. / **Tiene tanta calentura como ayer.**

Irregular Comparatives

ADJECTIVES	COMPARATIVE	SUPERLATIVE
bad / **malo**	worse / **peor**	worst / **el, la peor**
big / **gran, grande**	bigger / **más grande**	the greatest / **el, la mayor**
good / **bueno**	better / **mejor**	the best / **el, la mejor**
young / **joven**	younger / **más joven**	youngest / **el, la menor**
low / **bajo**	lower / **inferior**	the lowest / **ínfimo**
much / **mucho**	more / **más**	the most / **el, la más**
old / **viejo**	older / **más viejo**	oldest / **el, la mayor**

Note: The forms oldest / **mayor** and youngest / **menor** usually refer to persons.
Translate **la mayor parte de** as *most* (*of*).

> **La mayor parte de los pacientes son adultos.** / Most of the patients are adults.

Article and adjective agree with the noun in gender and number.

> This is the best treatment. / **Este es el mejor tratamiento.**
> These are the best pills. / **Estas son las mejores pastillas.**

Note: In Spanish the preposition de is generally used after the superlative; before numerals, de is the translation of the English *than*.

> The sickest of all. / **El más enfermo de todos.**
> There are more than ten cases. / **Hay más de diez casos.**

The absolute superlative refers only to a quality possessed by a person or object to a high degree, without comparison to others. To form the absolute superlative, the ending **-ísimo** or **-ísima** is added to the radical of the adjective:

> mucho → muchísimo   rápido → rapidísimo
> excelente → excelentísimo   inteligente → inteligentísimo

Note: Adjectives ending in **-co** and **-go** change the **c** to **qu** and the **g** to **gu** before adding **-ísimo**:

> poco → po**quí**simo   largo → lar**guí**simo

ADVERBS	SUPERLATIVES
well / **bien**	better, best / **mejor**
bad, badly / **mal**	worse, worst / **peor**
much / **mucho**	more, most / **más**
little / **poco**	less, least / **menos**

> Do you feel well today? / **¿Se siente bien hoy?**
> I feel better. / **Me siento mejor.**
> I feel worse today. / **Me siento peor hoy.**

PRONOUNS / PRONOMBRES

A pronoun is a word that takes the place of a noun. Different types of pronouns may replace the same noun according to how the noun is used.

SUBJECT PRONOUNS / PRONOMBRES PERSONALES

Subject pronouns tell who is performing the action of the verb. They are often omitted in Spanish since the form of the verb indicates person and number. Subject pronouns are used in Spanish for clarification and emphasis. The familiar **tú** is used when speaking to a friend, a relative, or a child. **Vosotros -as** is rarely used in Hispanic America, where **ustedes** is used for the plural of **tú**. There is no translation in Spanish for the English subject pronoun *it*.

> It is a complicated case. / **Es un caso complicado.**
> It is I. / **Soy yo.**

DIRECT OBJECT PRONOUNS / PRONOMBRES DE OBJETO DIRECTO

A direct object pronoun replaces a noun object of the verb:

> Did you bring the sample? / **¿Trajo la muestra?**
> Yes, I brought it. / **Sí, la traje.**

INDIRECT OBJECT PRONOUNS / PRONOMBRES DE OBJETO INDIRECTO

An indirect object pronoun replaces a noun indirect object of the verb.

> Did you give María (to her) the prescription? / **¿Le dio la receta a María?**
> Yes, I gave it to her. / **Sí, se la di.**

Note: When two object pronouns are used together, the indirect object pronoun generally precedes the direct. **Se** replaces **le, les** when preceding **lo, la, los, las.**

FIRST AND SECOND PERSON (FAMILIAR)

SUBJECT PRONOUNS	DIRECT OBJECT PRONOUNS	INDIRECT OBJECT PRONOUNS
I / **yo**	me / **me**	to me, for me / **me**
you / **tú**	you / **te**	to you, for you / **te**
we / **nosotros-as**	us / **nos**	to us, for us / **nos**
you / **vosotros-as**	you / **os**	to you, for you / **os**

Note: Me, te, nos and os may be used as direct and indirect object pronouns, or as reflexive pronouns.

THIRD AND SECOND PERSON (FORMAL)

SUBJECT PRONOUNS	DIRECT OBJECT PRONOUNS	INDIRECT OBJECT PRONOUNS
you / **usted**	you / **lo, la**	to you, for you / **le**
he / **él**	him / **lo**	to him, for him / **le**

SUBJECT PRONOUNS	DIRECT OBJECT PRONOUNS	INDIRECT OBJECT PRONOUNS
she / **ella**	her / **la**	to her, for her / **le**
	it / **lo, la**	to it, for it / **le**
you / **ustedes**	them / **los, las**	to you, for you / **les**
they / **ellos**	them / **los**	to them, for them / **les**
they / **ellas**	them / **las**	to them, for them / **les**

Note: The subject pronoun is sometimes used with the preposition **a** either for emphasis or clarification in addition to the indirect object pronoun.

> **El doctor le recetó esta pastilla a ella.** / The doctor prescribed this pill for her.

Note: **Le** and **les** are also used in Spain as direct object pronouns for the second person: **usted, ustedes,** and for the third person masculine. In Hispanic America this usage is less frequent.

REFLEXIVE PRONOUNS / PRONOMBRES REFLEXIVOS

A reflexive pronoun is used when the subject acts upon itself. The forms **me, te, nos,** and **os,** are also used in the reflexive, meaning myself, yourself, ourselves, and yourselves. For the other persons **se** is used, meaning yourself (for **usted**), herself, and himself for the singular forms; yourselves (for **ustedes**), and themselves for the plural forms.

SUBJECT PRONOUNS	REFLEXIVE PRONOUNS
I / **yo**	myself / **me**
you / **tú**	yourself / **te**
you / **usted**	yourself / **se**
he / **él**	himself / **se**
she / **ella**	herself / **se**
we / **nosotros-as**	ourselves / **nos**
you / **vosotros-as**	yourselves / **os**
you / **ustedes**	yourselves / **se**
they / **ellos-as**	themselves / **se**

> She washed her hands. / **Ella se lavó las manos.**
> They get up early. / **Ellos se levantan temprano.**

RELATIVE PRONOUNS / PRONOMBRES RELATIVOS

A relative pronoun (**que; el (la) cual; quien** / that, who; that, which; who) introduces an adjective clause that refers back to an antecedent noun; it can be the subject or direct object of the clause's verb, or the object of a preposition.

> I know a nurse who can assist you. / **Conozco a una enfermera que puede asistirlo.**
> The medicine (that) you took. / **La medicina que usted tomó.**
> The case which we are talking about... / **El caso del cual estamos hablando...**
> The patient, to whom you gave the pill... / **El paciente, a quien le diste la pastilla...**

Possessive pronouns and demonstrative pronouns were explained under Adjectives.

VERBS / VERBOS

In Spanish as in English, the mood of a verb states
1. a fact.

Indicative

> The doctor is in his office. / **El doctor está en su consulta.**

2. a condition expressed by the speaker involving some doubt, wish, hope, or possibility.

Subjunctive

> I hope you feel better tomorrow. / **Espero que se sienta mejor mañana.**

Expressions of willing that are generally followed by the infinitive in English are followed by the subjunctive in the dependent clause in Spanish:

> I want you to come next week. / **Quiero que venga la semana próxima.**

The subjunctive is generally used when the subject of the dependent clause is not the subject of the main clause. The subjunctive is more frequently used in Spanish than it is in English. It appears in the main clause to express a formal command, after certain adverbs implying uncertainty (**tal vez, quizás**), or after interjections that introduce nonfactual statements.

> Perhaps he can leave tomorrow. / **Quizás él pueda salir mañana.**

3. what might happen, without establishing when it would or could happen:

Conditional

> I would call the doctor. / **Yo llamaría al médico.**

4. a command or a request:

Imperative

> Take the medication now. / **Tome la medicina ahora.**

VERB TENSES / TIEMPOS DEL VERBO

Tense means the time when the action takes place: present, past, or future. See how the verb changes in the following examples using a regular verb in the indicative.

Present	The doctor is speaking to the patient now. / **La doctora habla con el paciente ahora.**
Past	The doctor spoke to the patient. / **La doctora habló con el paciente.**
Future	The doctor will speak to the patient. / **La doctora hablará con el paciente.**

To indicate the tense of the verb in Spanish, add to the stem of the verb—or to its infinitive in the case of the future tense and the conditional mood—the ending that belongs to the appropriate tense, person, and number:

Present	**habl** + **-a** (third person singular) → **habla**
Past	**habl** + **ó** (third person singular) → **habló**
Future	**hablar** (infinitive) + **-á** (third person singular) → **hablará**
Conditional	**hablar** (infinitive) + **-ía** (third person singular) → **hablaría**

The Spanish tenses are divided into simple and compound. The compound tenses of the indicative and subjunctive are formed with a simple tense form of the auxiliary verb **haber** and the past participle of the conjugated verb. In the indicative and the conditional, the compound tenses are generally translated as follows:

Simple Tenses

To examine / **examinar** has the following forms in the third person singular:

Present	**examina**	he, she examines; he, she is examining; he, she does examine
Imperfect	**examinaba**	he, she examined; he, she was examining; he, she did examine
Preterit	**examinó**	he, she examined; he, she did examine
Future	**examinará**	he, she will examine
Conditional	**examinaría**	he, she would (could) examine

Compound Tenses

Perfect	**ha examinado**	he, she has examined
Pluperfect	**había examinado**	he, she had examined
Future perfect	**habrá examinado**	he, she will have examined
Conditional perfect	**habría examinado**	he, she would (could) have examined

Note: See the Verb Tables in Appendix C for complete conjugation of compound tenses of the indicative, subjunctive, and conditional.

CONJUGATION OF VERBS / CONJUGACIÓN DEL VERBO

The infinitive of verbs in Spanish end in: **-ar** (**tomar** / to take, to drink), **-er** (**comer** / to eat), and **-ir** (**admitir** / to admit). The letters preceding the infinitive ending are the root or stem of a Spanish verb. The tenses of regular verbs are formed by adding endings to the root, except for the future and the conditional tenses, which use the whole infinitive as a root. Only the most common verbs and irregularities are shown here.

MOODS / MODOS DEL VERBO
INDICATIVE / INDICATIVO:
PRESENT / PRESENTE

To form the present tense, drop the infinitive ending and add to the root of the verb the following endings:

Verbs Ending in **-ar**

SINGULAR		PLURAL	
I / **yo**	**-o**	we / **nosotros -as**	**-amos**
you / **tú** (*fam.*)	**-as**	you / **vosotros -as**	**-áis**
you / **usted**	**-a**	you / **ustedes**	**-an**
he / **él**	**-a**	they / **ellos**	**-an**
she / **ella**	**-a**	they / **ellas**	**-an**

Example: (tomar)

> **Yo tomo la medicina.** / I take the medication.
> **Tú tomas la medicina.** / You take the medication.

Verbs Ending in **–er**

Using the same procedure, change the vowel **-a** to -e:

Singular: o, es, e; **Plural:** emos, éis, **en.**

Example: (comer)

> **Usted come muy bien.** / You eat very well.
> **Ellos comen muy bien.** / They eat very well.

Verbs Ending in **–ir**

The singular endings are the same as for verbs ending in -er. The plural endings are also the same, except for the first person (nosotros -as) -imos, and the second person (**vosotros -as**) **-ís.**

Example: (vivir)

> **Vivimos en California.** / We live in California.
> **Ella vive en California.** / She lives in California.

IMPERFECT AND PRETERIT / IMPERFECTO Y PRETÉRITO

There are two tenses of the indicative that refer to the past. The imperfect is one of them, frequently called the past descriptive because it describes actions and conditions which took place in a continuous or customary way.

> I used to work from 8 A.M. until 3 P.M. /
> Yo **trabajaba** desde las ocho de la mañana hasta las tres de la tarde.

The preterit refers in a narrative way to an action in the past which ended at a definite time. Historical facts are generally narrated in the preterit.

> Yesterday I worked from 2 P.M. until 10 P.M. /
> Ayer **trabajé** desde las dos de la tarde hasta las diez de la noche.

IMPERFECT / IMPERFECTO

Verbs Ending in **–ar**

SINGULAR		PLURAL	
I / **yo**	-aba	we / **nosotros -as**	-ábamos
you / **tú** (*fam.*)	-abas	you / **vosotros -as**	-abais
you / **usted**	-aba	you / **ustedes**	-aban
SINGULAR		PLURAL	
he / **él**	-aba	they / **ellos**	-aban
she / **ella**	-aba	they / **ellas**	-aban

Example: (tomar)

> **Yo tomaba la medicina.** / I was taking the medication.
> **Tú tomabas la medicina.** / You were taking the medication.

Verbs Ending in **–er**

Using the same procedure, add the following endings.

Singular: ía, ías, ía; **Plural:** íamos, íais, ían.

Example: (comer)

> **Usted comía muy bien.** / You were eating very well.
> **Ellos comían muy bien.** / They were eating very well.

Verbs Ending in **–ir**

The singular and plural endings are the same as for verbs ending in **-er.**

Example: (vivir)

> **Vivíamos en California.** / We were living in California.
> **Ella vivía en California.** / She was living in California.

Note: The only irregular verbs in the imperfect indicative are: ser, ver, and ir: yo era, yo veía, yo iba. See the verb tables in Appendix C for complete conjugation.

PRETERIT / PRETÉRITO

Verbs Ending in **–ar**

SINGULAR		PLURAL	
I / **yo**	-é	we / **nosotros -as**	-amos
you / **tú** (*fam.*)	-aste	you / **vosotros -as**	-asteis
you / **usted**	-ó	you / **ustedes**	-aron

SINGULAR		PLURAL	
he / **él**	**-ó**	they / **ellos**	**-aron**
she / **ella**	**-ó**	they / **ellas**	**-aron**

Example: (tomar)

> **Yo tomé la medicina.** / I took the medication.
> **Tú tomaste la medicina.** / You took the medication.

Verbs Ending in **–er**

Using the same procedure, add the following endings.

Singular: **í, iste,**   **ió;**   **Plural:**   **imos,**   **isteis,**   **ieron.**

Example: (comer)

> **Usted comió muy bien.** / You ate very well.
> **Ellos comieron muy bien.** / They were eating very well.

Verbs Ending in **–ir**

The singular and plural endings are the same as verbs ending in **-er.**

Example: (vivir)

> **Vivimos en California.** / We lived in California.
> **Ella vivió en California.** / She lived in California.

Note: The first person plural of the present and the preterit have the same verb form.

FUTURE / FUTURO

The Spanish future expresses not only actions that will take place in the future, but often probability or speculation.

> She will be here at 9 A.M. / **Estará aquí a las nueve de la mañana.**
> I wonder what time it is? / **¿Qué hora será?**
> It is probably one o'clock. / **Será la una.**
> I wonder if the surgery will take a long time. / **¿Durará mucho la operación?**

The present tense is also used to express the immediate future.

> He will arrive at 10 A.M. / **Llega** a las diez de la mañana.

Note: When translating English expressions in which *will* refers to willingness of someone to do something, use the verb **querer** and not the future tense: Will you please bring me some water? / **¿Quieres traerme agua, por favor?**

All verbs use the same endings to form the future tense. Comer and vivir take the same endings as **tomar,** shown here.

INFINITIVE + ENDINGS	SINGULAR	ENDINGS	
tomar +	I / **yo**	-é	tomaré
comer +	you / **tú** (*fam.*)	-ás	tomarás
admitir +	you / **usted**	-á	tomará
	he, she / **él, ella**	-á	tomará
	PLURAL	ENDINGS	
	we / **nosotros-as**	-emos	tomaremos
	you / **vosotros-as**	-éis	tomaréis
	you / **ustedes**	-án	tomarán
	they / **ellos-as**	-án	tomarán

Conditional

All verbs use the same endings to form the conditional. The conditional is formed by adding to the infinitive the same endings used to form the imperfect indicative of **-er** and **-ir** verbs.

The conditional often refers to probability in the past:

> Joey felt bad last night. Could it be something he ate? /
> Pepito se sintió mal anoche. ¿**Sería** algo que comió?

INFINITIVE + ENDINGS	SINGULAR	ENDINGS	
tomar +	**yo**	-ía	tomaría
comer +	**tú** (*fam.*)	-ías	tomarías
admitir +	**usted**	-ía	tomaría
	él, ella	-ía	tomaría
	PLURAL	ENDINGS	
	nosotros-as	-íamos	tomaríamos
	vosotros-as	-íais	tomaríais
	ustedes	-ían	tomarían
	ellos-as	-ían	tomarían

Note: Use the infinitive to form the future and the conditional. Only twelve verbs have irregularities in their radical in the future and the conditional: **caber / cabr-; haber / habr-; saber / sabr-; poder / podr-; poner / pondr-; salir / saldr-; tener / tendr-; valer / valdr-; venir / vendr-; hacer / har-; decir / dir- querer / querr-.** See the verb tables in Appendix D for complete conjugation.

Present Subjunctive

All persons of the present subjunctive have the same root as the first person singular of the present indicative except for the verbs: **dar, ser, estar, haber, ir, saber.** To form the present subjunctive, drop the -o of the first person singular of the present indicative before adding the endings of the subjunctive.

For verbs ending in **-ar,** start with the first person of the present indicative: **tomo.** Drop the **-o** and add the endings of the present subjunctive.

TOMAR	SINGULAR	ENDINGS	
tom-+	I / **yo**	-e	tome
	you / **tú** (*fam.*)	-es	tomes
	you / **usted**	-e	tome
	he, she / **él, ella**	-e	tome
	PLURAL	ENDINGS	
	we / **nosotros-as**	-emos	tomemos
	you / **vosotros-as**	-éis	toméis
	you / **ustedes**	-en	tomen
	they / **ellos, ellas**	-en	tomen

Verbs ending in **-er** and **-ir** have the same endings in the present subjunctive.

com- + Endings

COMER	SINGULAR ENDINGS	PLURAL ENDINGS	
I / **yo**	coma	we / **nosotros**	com**amos**
you / **tú**	comas	you / **vosotros**	com**áis**
you / **usted**	coma	you / **ustedes**	com**an**
he, she / **él, ella**	coma	they / **ellos, ellas**	com**an**

viv- + Endings

VIVIR	SINGULAR ENDINGS	PLURAL ENDINGS	
I / **yo**	viv**a**	we / **nosotros-as**	viv**amos**
you / **tú** (*fam.*)	viv**as**	you / **vosotros-as**	viv**áis**
you / **usted**	viv**a**	you / **ustedes**	viv**an**
he, she / **él, ella**	viv**a**	they / **ellos, ellas**	viv**an**

Note: Observe that the subjunctive endings are the reverse of the indicative endings, except for the first person singular.

Imperfect Subjunctive / Imperfecto de subjuntivo

The subjunctive has only one simple past tense, **el imperfecto de subjuntivo.** The endings are identical for all the verbs with infinitives ending in **-ar, -er,** or -ir. However, the endings are not added to the root of the verb, but to the third person plural of the preterit indicative, after dropping the ending **-on.**

SINGULAR	ENDINGS	PLURAL	ENDINGS
I / **yo**	**-a**	we / **nosotros-as**	**-amos**
you / **tú** (*fam.*)	**-as**	you / **vosotros-as**	**-ais**
you / **usted**	**-a**	you / **ustedes**	**-an**
he / **él**	**-a**	they / **ellos**	**-an**
she / **ella**	**-a**	they / **ellas**	**-an**

I was hoping that he would eat more. / **Esperaba que él comiera más.**

GIVING AN ORDER OR MAKING A REQUEST

Imperative / El imperative

A command is given generally to a second person, the person spoken to. There are two forms of addressing a second person in Spanish: a familiar way, **tú,** and a formal way, **usted.** A physician or health care professional addresses his or her patients in a formal way unless the patient is a child or a friend. A command is often followed by the polite phrase **por favor** (please).

Command Forms for **usted** and **ustedes** with Regular Verbs

Infinitives ending in **-ar** add **-e** to form the command with **usted** and **-en** to form the command with ustedes. Infinitives ending in **-er** or **-ir** add **-a** to form the command with **usted** and **-an** to form the command with **ustedes.**

INFINITIVE	DROP ENDING	ADD	USTED	USTEDES (+N)
tomar / to take, to drink	-ar	-e	tom**e**	tom**en**
comer / to eat	-er	-a	com**a**	com**an**
vivir / to live	-ir	-a	viv**a**	viv**an**

COMMAND FORMS OF IRREGULAR VERBS

To form the **usted** command of irregular verbs, use the first person singular of the present indicative and drop the **-o** ending. Add **-e** to **-ar** verbs and **-a** to **-er** and **-ir** verbs. To form the ustedes command, add **-n** to the command form of usted.

	COMMAND FORMS		
INFINITIVE	1ST P. SING.	USTED	USTEDES (+n)
to say, tell / **decir**	digo	dig**a**	dig**an**
to do, make / **hacer**	hago	hag**a**	hag**an**
to put / **poner**	pongo	pong**a**	pong**an**
to leave / **salir**	salgo	salg**a**	salg**an**
to have / **tener**	tengo	teng**a**	teng**an**
to bring / **traer**	traigo	traig**a**	traig**an**
to come / **venir**	vengo	veng**a**	veng**an**

COMMAND FORMS

INFINITIVE	1ST P. SING.	USTED	USTEDES (+n)
to think / **pensar**	pienso	piens**e**	piens**en**
to move / **mover**	muevo	muev**a**	muev**an**
to sleep / **dormir**	duermo	duerm**a**	duerm**an**

EXCEPTIONS: SPECIAL FORMS OF COMMANDS

INFINITIVE	USTED	USTEDES
to give / **dar**	dé	den
to be / **estar**	esté	estén
to have / **haber**	haya	hayan
to go / **ir**	vaya	vayan
to know / **saber**	sepa	sepan
to be / **ser**	sea	sean
to see / ver	vea	vean

Formal commands of root-vowel changing verbs (**e-ie, o-ue, e-i**) have the same root form as the first person singular of the present indicative.

> to sleep / **dormir** duerma Ud.   to think / **pensar** piense Ud.

Verbs ending in **-car, -gar,** and **-zar** require spelling changes to keep the same sounds of the **c, g,** and **z** in the infinitive.

c → qu

> to look for / **buscar**   Look for the prescription. / **Busque la receta.**

g → gu

> to pay / **pagar**   Pay the bill / **Pague la cuenta.**

z → c

> to begin / **empezar**   Begin now. / **Empiece ahora.**

Negative Formal Commands

Negative formal commands are formed by placing no before the command.

> Take the medicine. / **Tome la medicina.**   Don't take the medicine. / **No tome la medicina.**

Negative **tú** Commands

> **No + command of usted + s**
> **No + tome + s No tomes** (tú).

Affirmative **tú** Commands

Use an informal command with persons whom you address by their first name, using the same form as the third person singular of the present indicative.

Tomar	Take the medicine. / **Toma (tú) la medicina.**
Comer	Eat less. / **Come (tú) menos.**
Dormer	Sleep more. / **Duerme (tú) más.**

Special Forms of Commands of **tú** in the Affirmative

to say / **decir**	Tell me. / **Dime.**
to do, to make / **hacer**	Do it. / **Hazlo.**
to go / **ir**	Go home. / **Ve a la casa.**
to put / **poner**	Put your hand here. / **Pon la mano aquí.**
to leave / **salir**	Leave now. / **Sal ahora.**
to be / **ser**	Be attentive. / **Sé atento.**

Plural of **tú** Commands

Affirmative commands with **vosotros** are formed by substituting **-d** for the final **-r** of the infinitive. In Hispanic America, the plural form of the formal command is used for the plural of **tú** commands.

Nosotros Commands

Translate let us in either of two ways:
1. **Vamos a** + infinitivo: Let's examine her. / **Vamos a examinarla.**
2. Using the present subjunctive of the first personal plural: Let's study the case. / **Estudiemos el caso.**

ROOT-VOWEL CHANGING VERBS AND SPELLING CHANGE VERBS / VERBOS DE CAMBIO VOCÁLICO Y ORTOGRÁFICO

1. **Root-vowel changing verbs** are classified according to the pattern of changes in the root vowel.
   a. **First class:** Verbs with infinitive ending in **-ar** and **-er.** When the root is stressed, root vowel **e** changes to **ie,** and **o** changes to **ue,** in all the forms of the present indicative and present subjunctive except the first and second person plural. **Apretar, entender, mostrar, volver,** and others belong to this class. See chart for conjugation of these verbs after spelling change verbs.
   b. **Second class:** Verbs with the infinitive ending **-ir.** When the root is stressed the changes occur in the same tenses as verbs in the first class: **e** changes to **ie,** and **o** changes to **ue,** in the singular and the third person plural of the present indicative and the present subjunctive. They also occur in the first and second person plural of the present subjunctive but not the indicative. The **e** changes to **i,** and the **o** to **u,** in the third person singular and plural of the preterit and in the present participle (gerund). Examples of the second class are **sentir (ie)** and **dormir (ue).**
   c. **Third class:** Verbs ending in **-er** and **-ir.** When the root is stressed, the change is **e** to **i,** in the same forms in which changes take place in the second class. See the conjugation of **repetir** as a model verb for this class.

2. **Spelling changing verbs:** Changes in spelling occur in Spanish in certain verbs to keep the sound of the final consonant of the root.

Note: When followed by **e** in the tenses indicated, these verb endings change as shown.

Verbs with Infinitive Ending in **–ar**

ENDING	CHANGE	TENSES
car	c-qu	1st. person pret., and
gar	g-gu	all persons pres. subj.
guar	gu-gü	for all these endings
zar	z-c	

EXAMPLES

VERB	PRETERIT	PRES. SUBJ.
buscar / to look for	bus**qué**	bus**que**
		bus**ques**
		bus**que**
pagar / to pay	pa**gué**	pa**gue**
		pa**gues**
		pa**gue**
averiguar / to find out	averi**güé**	averi**güe**
		averi**gües**
		averi**güe**
abrazar / to embrace, to hug	abra**cé**	abra**ce**
		abra**ces**
		abra**ce**

Note: The following changes occur when the consonant in the ending precedes **a** or **o** or when **i** falls between two vowels in a conjugated form.

Verbs with Infinitive Ending in **-er** and **–ir**

ENDING	CHANGE	TENSES
cer	c-z	1st. person sing. pres. indic.,
cir	c-z	
ger	g-j	all persons pres. subj.,
gir	g-j	
guir	gu-g	3rd person sing. and plural preterit,
eer	i-y	all persons imperf. subj.,

ENDING	CHANGE	TENSES
ocer	+z	before **c** all persons pres. subj.
ucir		

TENSES	CONOCER / TO KNOW	REDUCIR / TO REDUCE	PROTEGER / TO PROTECT	CREER (CREYENDO) / TO BELIEVE
PRESENT INDICATIVE	conozco	reduzco	protejo	
PRETERIT INDICATIVE	—	—	—	creyó
				creyeron
PRESENT SUBJUNCTIVE	conozca	reduzca	proteja	
	conozcas	reduzcas	protejas	
	conozca	reduzca	proteja	
IMPERFECT SUBJUNCTIVE	—	—	—	creyera
				creyeras
				creyera

Note: Tenses not listed are regular. Only the singular forms are given.

Perfect Forms

haber / to have

INDICATIVE TENSES				SUBJUNCTIVE TENSES		
PRESENT	IMPERFECT	PRETERIT	FUTURE	PRESENT	IMPERFECT	CONDITIONAL
he	había	hube	habré	haya	hubiera	habría
has	habías	hubiste	habrás	hayas	hubieras	habrías
ha	había	hubo	habrá	haya	hubiera	habría
hemos	habíamos	hubimos	habremos	hayamos	hubiéramos	habríamos
habéis	habíais	hubisteis	habréis	hayáis	hubiérais	habríais
han	habían	hubieron	habrán	hayan	hubieran	habrían

Combine **haber** with the past participle to form the **perfect tenses.**

Indicative

Present perfect: present of **haber** + past participle of the conjugated verb.	**He tomado**
Past perfect: imperfect of **haber** + past participle of the conjugated verb.	**Había comido**
Preterit perfect: preterit of **haber** + past participle of the conjugated verb.	**Hube venido**
Future perfect: haber in the future + past participle of the conjugated verb.	**Habré dormido**

Note: In spoken Spanish the simple preterit replaces the preterit perfect.

Subjunctive

Present perfect: present of **haber** + past participle of the conjugated verb.	**Yo haya tomado**
Past perfect: imperfect of **haber** + past participle of the conjugated verb.	**Yo hubiera comido**

Conditional

Conditional perfect: conditional form of **haber** + past participle of the conjugated verb.	**Yo habría dormido**

LIST OF USEFUL VERBS / LISTA DE VERBOS ÚTILES

ENGLISH	SPANISH
to abort	abortar, acortar, impedir
to abstain, to refrain	abstenerse de
to accelerate, to speed up	acelerar
to accept	aceptar
to accompany, to go with	acompañar
to accumulate, to gather	acumular
to ache, to hurt	doler (ue)
to acquire	adquirir (ie)[a]
to add	añadir, agregar
to admit	admitir
to advise	aconsejar
to age	envejecer
to affect	afectar
to aggravate	empeorar, agravar
to aid	ayudar
to alleviate	aliviar
to amputate	amputar

ENGLISH	SPANISH
to anesthetize	anestesiar
to announce (*to warn*)[b]	anunciar; informar; avisar
to annoy	molestar
to appear	aparecer
to apply for	solicitar
to approach, to draw near	acercarse
to approve	aprobar (ue)
to arouse	excitar
to arrange	arreglar
to arrest	arrestar; (*to stop*) parar
to arrive	llegar; [*on time*] llegar a tiempo
to ask for (*to request*)	pedir (i)
to ask (*to question*)	preguntar
to aspirate	aspirar
to aspire to	aspirar a
to assimilate	asimilar
to associate	asociar
to assume	asumir
to assure	asegurar
to astonish	asombrar
to attack	atacar
to attend	asistir
to attract	atraer
to bathe	bañarse
to be	estar; ser
to be able, can	poder (ue)
to be absent	estar ausente
to be afraid	tener miedo
to be at fault	tener la culpa
to be born	nacer
to be [*hot, cold*] [*weather*]	tener calor, tener frío hacer (calor, frío)
to be hungry	tener hambre
to be in a hurry	tener prisa

ENGLISH	SPANISH
to be long [*time*]	tardar
to be lucky	tener suerte
to be quiet	callarse; (*to calm down*) calmarse
to be silent	callarse
to be right	tener razón
to be sick	estar enfermo -a
to be sleepy	tener sueño
to be ... years old	tener... años
to become (*adj.*)	hacerse; ponerse (+ *adj.*)
to begin	empezar (ie), comenzar (ie)
to behave	portarse
to belch	eructar
to believe	creer
to bend, to flex	doblar; doblarse
to bite	morder (ue)
to blame	culpar
to bleed	sangrar
to blink	parpadear
to bother, to annoy	molestar
to break	romper; quebrar
to breast-feed	amamantar, dar el pecho
to breathe	respirar
to bring	traer
to buy	comprar
to bruise	magullarse; amoratarse
to brush	cepillar
to burn	quemar; quemarse
to burp	eructar; repetir (i)
to call	llamar
to carry, to wear	llevar
to cause	causar
to change [*one's clothes*]	cambiarse (de ropa)
to chat	charlar
to check [*to examine*]	examinar, revisar
to choke	atragantarse; ahogar; sofocar

List of Useful Verbs / Lista de verbos útiles

ENGLISH	SPANISH
to choose	escoger, elegir (i)
to clean	limpiar
to climb up	subirse
to close	cerrar (ie)
to come	venir
to complain [of, about]	quejarse (de)
to complete	completar
to conceive	concebir (i)
to consider	considerar
to contact	contactar
to contain	contener
to continue	continuar, seguir (i)
to convalesce	convalecer; recuperarse
to cost	costar (ue)
to count	contar (ue)
to cough	toser
to create	crear
to cry	llorar
to cut	cortar
to deliver [to give birth]	dar a luz; estar de parto; pop. aliviarse
to deny	negar (ie)
to depend on	depender de
to develop	desarrollar; [a photo] revelar
to die	morir (ue, u)
to diet	estar a dieta; hacer una dieta
to discharge [secretion]	tener secreciones
to discharge [a patient]	dar te alta
to disinfect	desinfectar
to do, to make	hacer
to doubt	dudar
to dream	soñar (ue)
to dress [with clothes]	vestir; vestirse (i)
to dress [a wound]	vendar
to drink	beber; tomar
to earn	ganar

ENGLISH	SPANISH
to eat	comer
to eat breakfast	desayunar
to eat dinner	cenar
to eat lunch	almorzar (ue)
to ejaculate	eyacular
to enter	entrar
to examine	examinar
to exercise	hacer ejercicio
to exist	existir
to expect	esperar
to explain	explicar
to fail	dejar de, fallar
to fall asleep	dormirse (ue, u)
to fall down	caerse
to fear	temer; tener miedo
to feel	sentir (ie, i)
to follow	seguir (i)
to forget	olvidar
to form	formar
to fracture	fracturar; quebrar; romper
to function	funcionar
to gargle	hacer gárgaras
to get	obtener, conseguir (i)
to get angry	enfadarse, enojarse
to get better	mejorarse
to get up	levantarse
to get well	curarse, sanarse, ponerse bien
to give	dar
to go	ir; salir
to go away	irse
to go to bed	acostarse (ue)
to grow	crecer
to happen, to turn out	suceder
to hand over	entregar
to have	tener; [*aux.*] haber

ENGLISH	SPANISH
to hear	oír
to heat	calentar
to help	ayudar
to hide	esconder; esconderse
to hope	esperar
to hurry	apurarse, darse prisa
to hurt	doler (ue); lastimar
to immobilize	inmovilizar
to improve	mejorar
to incline	inclinar, inclinarse
to increase	aumentar
to inform	informar
to inject	inyectar
to insert	insertar, introducir, meter
to itch	picar
to kill	matar
to know	saber; [to be acquainted with] conocer
to lack	faltar
to leak	gotear
to lean on	apoyarse en
to learn	aprender
to leave	salir
to let	dejar, permitir
to lie	mentir (ie, i)
to lie down	acostarse (ue)
to lift	levantar, alzar
to like	gustar
to listen	escuchar, atender (ie)
to live	vivir
to look at	mirar
to look for	buscar
to lose	perder (ie)
to love	amar; querer (ie)
to lower [arm, leg]	bajar
to marry	casarse

ENGLISH	SPANISH
to masturbate	masturbarse
to menstruate	menstruar
to miscarry	abortar
to move	mover (ue)
to need	necesitar
to nurse [*a baby*]	amamantar
to nurse [*the sick*]	cuidar
to nurture	nutrir
to obtain	conseguir (i), obtener
to obstruct	obstruir
to open	abrir
to oppose	oponerse
to order	ordenar, mandar
to owe	deber
to palpate	palpar
to pant	jadear
to paralyze	paralizar
to participate	participar
to pay	pagar
to penetrate	penetrar
to permit	permitir, dejar
to plan	planear
to practice	practicar
to prefer	preferir (ie)
to prescribe	recetar, prescribir
to promise	prometer
to push [*downward*]	pujar
to put	poner
to put in	poner; meter
to put on [*clothing*]	ponerse
to put to bed	acostar (ue)
to qualify	capacitar
to question	preguntar
to raise	levantar
to react	reaccionar

ENGLISH	SPANISH
to read	leer
to receive	recibir
to recover	recobrar
to recuperate	recuperar, recobrar
to rejuvenate	rejuvenecer
to relax	relajar, aflojar
to release	soltar (ue), librar, desprender
to relieve	aliviar, mejorar
to remain	quedar
to remember	recordar (ue)
to remove, take off	quitar; quitarse
to repeat	repetir (i)
to reply	contestar, responder
to resolve	resolver (ue), solucionar
to respond	responder
to rest	descansar
to restore	restaurar, reparar
to restrict	restringir, confinar
to return	volver (ue)
to run	correr
to say	decir
to scratch	arañar
to seat	sentar
to see	ver
to seem	parecer
to send	mandar
to serve	servir (i)
to shake	agitar
to shout	gritar
to show	mostrar (ue), señalar, enseñar
to shower	ducharse
to sit down	sentarse (ie)
to smoke	fumar
to sneeze	estornudar
to solve	resolver (ue)

ENGLISH	SPANISH
to speak	hablar
to spend	gastar; [time] pasar
to spit	escupir
to sprain	torcer (ue)
to spray	rociar
to stand up	levantarse
to stimulate	estimular
to study	estudiar
to suck	chupar, absorber
to suffer	sufrir
to suppose	suponer
to surprise	sorprender
to swallow	tragar
to sweat	sudar
to sweeten	endulzar
to swell	hinchar
to take	tomar
to take off	quitar, quitarse
to talk	hablar
to teach	enseñar
to tell	decir
to think	pensar (ie)
to throw [into]	echar
to tighten	apretar, ajustar
to try	tratar de; probar (ue)
to turn	virar; virarse
to turn around	dar vuelta; voltearse
to turn down	rechazar
to urinate	orinar
to use	usar, emplear
to visit	visitar
to visualize	visualizar
to vomit	vomitar
to wait	esperar
to wake up	despertarse (ie)

ENGLISH	SPANISH
to want	querer (ie), desear
to wear	llevar
to wheeze	respirar con ruido sibilante
to wish	querer (ie), desear
to work	trabajar
to write	escribir

[a]Vowels between parentheses indicate root-changing verbs.
[b]Brackets clarify the meaning of the verb. Parentheses indicate a synonym.

SPANISH VERBS WITH IRREGULAR PAST PARTICIPLES[1]

Infinitive	Past Participle
SPANISH / ENGLISH	SPANISH / ENGLISH
abrir / to open	**abierto** / opened
absolver / to absolve	**absuelto** / absolved
abstraer / abstract	**abstracto*** / abstracted
atender / to attend	**atento*** / attended
bendecir / to bless	**bendito*** / blessed
comprimir / to compress	**compreso*** / compressed
concluir / to conclude	**concluso*** / concluded
confundir / to confuse	**confuso*** / confused
contradecir / to contradict	**contradicho** / contradicted
corregir / to correct	**correcto*** / corrected
cubrir / to cover	**cubierto** / covered
decir / to say, to tell	**dicho** / said
decomponer / to decompose	**descompuesto** / decomposed
describir / to describe	**descrito** / described
descubrir / to discover	**descubierto** / discovered
deshacer / to undo	**deshecho** / undone
despertar / to awake	**despierto*** / awaken
devolver / to return	**devuelto** / returned
disolver / to dissolve	**disuelto** / dissolved
entreabrir / to half-open	**entreabierto** / half-opened
escribir / to write	**escrito** / written
exponer / to expose	**expuesto** / exposed
freír / to fry	**frito** / fried
hacer / to do, to make	**hecho** / done, made
imponer / to impose	**impuesto** /imposed
imprimir / to print	**impreso** / printed
inscribir / to inscribe	**inscrito** / inscribed
juntar / to join	**junto** / joined
maldecir / to curse	**maldito*** / cursed
oprimir / to oppress	**opreso*** / oppressed
poner / to put	**puesto**[2] / put
predecir / to predict	**predicho** / predicted

Infinitive	Past Participle
SPANISH / ENGLISH	**SPANISH / ENGLISH**
prender / to apprehend, arrest	**preso*** / arrested
proveer / to provide	**provisto** / provided
pudrir / to rot	**podrido**[3] / rotten
revolver / to turn over	**revuelto** / turned over
romper / to break	**roto** / broken
satisfacer / to satisfy	**satisfecho** / satisfied
soltar / to release, free	**suelto*** / released
sujetar / to hold	**sujeto*** / holded
tumefacer[4] / to swell	**tumefacto*** / swollen
ver / to see	**visto** / seen
volver / to return, turn around	**vuelto** /returned
yuxtaponer / to juxtapose	**yuxtapuesto** / juxtaposed

Note: Verbs in **boldface** serve as models for the derivate compound forms that do not appear in this list. / Los verbos en **negrita** sirven de modelo para los derivados que no aparecen en esta lista.

[1]The list includes some past participles that have regular forms as well, and are used in compound tenses with the forms of the verb *haber* as well as with *ser* and *estar*. / La lista incluye varios participios de pasado que tienen también un participio regular usado con los tiempos compuestos del verbo *haber*.

[2]Other verbs that form the past participle with the same ending as poner **–puesto** are: componer, compuesto; disponer, dispuesto; imponer, impuesto; oponer, opuesto; reponer, repuesto; suponer, supuesto.

[3]El verbo podrir o pudrir, se conjuga gen. con el radical del gerundio en las formas del presente y del pretérito, excepto en la primera persona, y en el futuro, las otras formas adoptan la *o* en el radical / *Podrir* or pudrir, is gen. conjugated with the radical *u* in the gerund, present forms and the preterit, except in the first person, the future, other forms adopt the *o* in the radical.

*Past Participles used as adjectives and not with the form *haber* in compound tenses.

*Participios de pasado most commonly used as adjectives.

Spanish-English Glossary

Glosario español-inglés

a

a *abr.* **absoluto** / absolute; **acidez** / acidity; **acomodación** / accommodation; **alergia** / allergy; **anterior** / anterior; **aqua** / aqua; **arteria** / artery.

a *prep.* **[hacia] to, voy ___ la farmacia** / I am going to the drugstore; **[direción] to, ___ la derecha** / to the right; **___ la izquierda** / to the left; **[hora] at, voy___ las tres** / I'm going at three o'clock; **[frecuencia] a, per, tres veces al dia** / three times a day.

abajo *adv.* below, down.

abandonar *v.* to abandon, to neglect.

abarcar *vi.* to contain, to include; **___ mucho** / to cover a lot of ground.

abasia *f.* abasia, uncertainty of movement.

abastecer *v.* to supply.

abastecimiento *m.* supply; **artículos para ___** / supplies.

abatido-a *a.* depressed, dejected.

abdomen *m.* abdomen; *pop.* belly; **___ de péndulo** / pendulous ___; **___ escafoideo** / scaphoid ___ . *V.* ilustración esta página.

abdominal *a.* abdominal, rel. to the abdomen; **cirugía ___ / ___ surgery; cavidad ___ / ___** cavity; **disnea ___ / ___** dysnea; **distensión ___ / ___** distention; **fístula ___ / ___** fistula; **punción ___ / ___** puncture; **respiración ___ / ___** breathing; **retortijón, torsón ___ / ___** cramp; **rigidez ___ / ___** rigidity; **traumatismos ___ - es / ___** injuries; **vendaje ___ / ___** bandage.

abdominocentesis *f.* abdominocentesis, abdominal puncture.

abdominoplastia *f.* abdominoplasty, plastic surgical repair of the abdominal wall.

abdominovaginal *a.* abdominovaginal, rel. to the abdomen and the vagina.

abducción *f.* abduction; separation.

abeja *f.* bee.

aberración *f.* aberration. 1. deviation from the norm; **___ cromática** / chromatic ___; 2. mental disorder; **___ mental** / mental ___ .

aberrante *a.* aberrant, departing from the usual course; wandering.

abertura *f.* opening.

abierto-a *a. pp.* of **abrir,** open.

abiotrofia *f.* abiotrophy, premature loss of vitality.

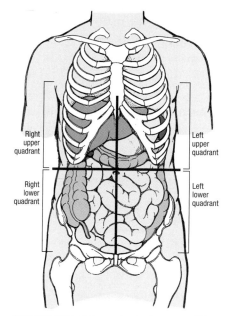

Quadrants of the abdomen: showing the organs within each quadrant

ablación *f.* ablatio, ablation, detachment, removal; **___ de la placenta / ___** placentae; **___ de la retina / ___** retinae.

ablandar *v.* to soften.

abofetear *v.* to slap.

abogado *m.* lawyer, attorney.

aborrecer *vi.* to abhor, to hate.

abortar *v.* to abort, to interrupt the course of a pregnancy or to stop an illness.

abortista *m., f.* abortionist, an individual who interrupts a pregnancy.

abortivo *m.* abortifacient, stimulant to induce abortion.

aborto *m.* abortion; miscarriage; **___ criminal / criminal ___; ___ electivo / elective ___; ___ espontáneo / spontaneous ___; ___ incompleto / incomplete ___; ___ inducido / induced ___; ___ inevitable / imminent ___; ___ por succión / suction ___; ___ provocado / induced ___; ___ terapéutico / therapeutic ___ . *V.* cuadro en la página 298.

abotonar *v.* to button up.

abrasión *f.* abrasion, damage to or wearing away of a surface by injury or friction; **círculo**

de ___ / ___ collar, circular trace left on the skin by gunpowder.

abrasivo-a *a.* abrasive, rel. to or that causes abrasion.

abrazadera *f.* brace.

abrazar *vi.* to embrace.

abrazo *m.* hug, embrace.

abrebocas *m.* gag, jaw-lever, device used to keep the patient's mouth open.

abreviar *v.* to reduce, to shorten; **para** ___ / in short.

abreviatura *f.* abbreviation.

abrigarse *vr., vi.* to put on warm clothing; to keep warm.

abrigo *m.* overcoat; cover; **buscar** ___ / to look for shelter.

abrir *v.* to open; ___ **de nuevo** / to reopen.

abrochar *v.* to fasten.

abrumar *v.* to overwhelm; to tax.

abrupción de la placenta *f.* abruptio placentae, premature detachment of the placenta.

abrupto-a *a.* abrupt, brusque.

absceso *m.* abscess, accumulation of pus gen. due to a breakdown of tissue. *V.* cuadro en la página XX.

absoluto-a *a.* absolute, unconditional.

absorbente *a.* absorbent.

absorber *v.* to absorb, to take in.

absorción *f.* absorption, uptake. 1. taking up of fluids and other substances by an organism;___ **bucal** / mouth ___; ___ **cutánea** / cutaneous ___; ___ **entérica** / intestinal ___; ___ **estomacal** / stomach ___; ___ **externa** / external ___; ___ **parenteral** / parenteral ___; ___ **percutánea** / percutaneous ___; 2. self-centeredness.

abstemio-a *m., f.* abstemious.

abstenerse *vr., vi.* to abstain, to refrain; ___ **de relaciones sexuales** / ___ from sexual intercourse.

abstinencia *f.* abstinence, voluntary restraint.

absurdo-a *a.* absurd.

abuelo-a *m., f.* grandfather; grandmother.

abulia *f.* abulia, loss of will power; ___ **cíclica** / cyclic ___ .

abultado-a *a.* bulky, massive; swollen.

abundancia *f.* abundance.

abundante *a.* abundant, plentiful.

aburrido-a *a.* bored.

aburrirse *vr.* to become bored.

abusado-a *a.* abused; beyond the limits.

abusar *v.* to abuse, to mistreat.

abuso *m.* abuse, overuse; ___ **de medicamento** / overuse of medication; ___ **emocional** /

Absceso	Abscess
agudo	acute
alveolar	alveolar
crónico	chronic
cutáneo	cutaneous
de drenaje	drainage
de la raíz	radicular
de la uña	paronychial
de las amígdalas	peritonsilar
de las encías	gingival
de sutura	suture
dental	dental
enquistado	encysted
facial	facial
fecal	fecal
folicular	follicular
hepático	hepatic
mamario	mammary
mastoideo	mastoid
óseo	osseous
pancreático	pancreatic
pélvico	pelvic
pulmonar	pulmonary
tubárico	tubo-ovarian

emotional ___; ___ **físico** / physical ___; ___ **verbal** / verbal ___ .

acabar *v.* to finish, to complete; ___ **de llegar** / to have just arrived; ___ **con eso** / to put an end to that; **acabarse** / *vr.* to be finished; [*una sustancia*] to run out.

acalasia *f.* achalasia, inability to relax, esp. in reference to the sphincter muscles.

acantoide *a.* acanthoid, thornlike shape.

acantosis *f.* acanthosis, skin condition manifested by thick and warty growth.

acapnia *f.* acapnia, state produced by a decrease of carbon dioxide in the blood.

acariasis *f.* acariasis, skin disease caused by acarids.

ácaro *m.* acarid, parasite, mite.

acatarrarse *vr.* to catch a cold.

acceso *m.* 1. access, attack, seizure; ___ **de asma** / an asthma attack; 2. entrance.

accesorio *m.* accessory.

accidentado-a *m., f.* an injured person.
accidental *a.* accidental, unexpected.
accidente *m.* accident; ___ **automovilístico /** car ___; ___ **de trabajo** / work-related ___; ___ **de tráfico** / traffic ___; **víctima de un** ___ / casualty.
acción *f.* action.
aceite *m.* oil; ___ **de hígado de bacalao** / cod liver ___; ___ **de jojoba** / jojoba ___; ___ **de oliva** / olive ___; ___ **de palmito /** palm ___; ___ **de ricino** / castor ___; ___ **de soya** / soy ___; ___ **graso** / fatty ___ .
aceituna *f.* olive.
aceleración, aceleramiento *f., m.* acceleration.
acelerador *m.* accelerator, substance or agent acting as an accelerant; **-a** / *a.* having the property of accelerating a process.
acelerar *v.* to accelerate, to quicken, to speed up; ___ **la cura** / to speed the healing process.
acelular *a.* acellular, without cells.
acento *m.* accent.
acentuado-a *a.* accented, accentuated.
acentuar *v.* to accentuate, to emphasize.
aceptable *a.* acceptable.
aceptación *f.* acceptance.
aceptar *v.* to accept.
acera *f.* sidewalk.
acerca (de) *adv.* about, concerning; ___ **de eso** / about that.
acercar *vi.* to bring closer; **acercarse /** *vr.* to approach, to get close.
acertado-a *a.* right; **un diagnóstico** ___ / a correct diagnosis.
acertar *vi.* to be right; to guess.
acetábulo *m.* acetabulum, hip socket.
acetato *m.* acetate, salt or ester of acetic acid.
acético-a *a.* acetic, sour, rel. to vinegar or its acid.
acetona *f.* acetone, fragrant substance used as a solvent and found in excessive amount in diabetic urine.
acetonemia *f.* acetonemia, excess acetone in the blood.
acetonuria *f.* acetonuria, excess acetone in the urine.
achacoso-a *a.* sickly, ailing.
achaque *m.* ailment, infirmity.
achicar *vi.* to reduce.
acidemia *f.* acidemia, excess acid in the blood.
acidez *f.* acidity, sourness.
ácido *m.* acid; ___ **acético** / acetic ___; ___ **ascórbico** / ascorbic ___; ___ **bórico /**

boric ___; ___ **butírico** / butyric ___; ___ **clorogénico** / chlorogenic ___; ___ **cólico /** cholic ___; ___ **desoxirribonucleico /** deoxyribonucleic ___; ___ **fólico** / folic ___; ___ **gástrico** / gastric ___; ___ **láctico /** lactic ___; ___ **nicotínico** / nicotinic ___; ___ **nucleico** / nucleic ___; ___ **para-amino benzoico** / para-amino benzoic ___; ___ **resistente /** ___ fast; ___ **ribonucleico /** ribonucleic ___; ___ **salicílico /** salicylic ___; ___**-s grasos** / fatty ___ -s; ___ **sulfónico** / sulfonic ___; ___ **sulfúrico /** sulfuric ___; **a prueba de** ___ / ___ proof; **-a** *a.* bitter.
ácido clorhídrico, hidroclórico *m.* hydrochloric acid, a constituent of gastric juice.
ácido glicocólico *m.* glycocholic acid, a compound of glycine and cholic acid.
ácido glucurónico *m.* glucuronic, glycuronic acid, acid that acts as a disinfectant in human metabolism.
ácido hialurónico *m.* hyaluronic acid, acid present in the substance of the connective tissue that acts as a lubricant and connecting agent.
acidosis *f.* acidosis, excessive acidity in the blood and tissues of the body; ___ **diabética /** diabetic ___; ___ **metabólica** / metabolic ___ .
ácido úrico *m.* uric acid, a product of protein breakdown present in the blood and excreted in the urine.
acinesia *f.* akinesia, acinesia, partial or total loss of movement.
aclaramiento *m.* clearance, elimination of a given substance from the blood plasma of the kidneys.
aclarar *v.* to clarify, to explain.
aclimatación *f.* acclimatization.
aclimatarse *vr.* to acclimate; to get used to a condition or custom; to adjust.
acloropsia *f.* achloropsia, inability to distinguish the color green.
acné *f.* acne, inflammatory skin condition;___ **rosácea /** ___ rosacea; ___ **vulgar o común /** ___ vulgaris, common acne.
acolia *f.* acholia, absence of bile.
acomodación *f.* accomodation, adaptation; the state of adapting to something; ___ **de un nervio** / nerve ___; ___ **histológica /** histologic ___; ___ **negativa** / negative ___; ___ **positiva** / positive ___; **amplitud de** ___ / amplitude of ___; **jerarquía de** ___ / range of ___ .
acomodación del ojo *f.* eye accommodation, coordination process of the eye muscles and the lens to enable the eye to focus in near objects.

acomodar *v.* to accommodate, to adjust.
acompañante *m., f.* companion.
acompañar *v.* to accompany.
acondicionamiento *m.* conditioning; ___ físico / physical fitness.
acondroplasia *f.* achondroplasia, dwarfism, congenital osseous deformity.
aconsejar *v.* to advise, to recommend; ___ mal / to misguide.
acontecer *v.* to transpire, to occur.
acordar *vi.* to agree; **acordarse** / *vr.* to remember, to recall.
acortar *v.* to shorten.
acosamiento *m.* harassment.
acosar *v.* to harass.
acostado-a *a.* reclining; lying down.
acostar *vi.* to lay down, to put to bed; **acostarse** / *vr.* to go to bed, to lie down; **hora de** ___ / bedtime.
acostumbrado-a *a.* accustomed, used to; **no** ___ / unaccustomed.
acostumbrarse *vr.* to get used to.
acre *a.* acrid, sour.
acreción *f.* accretion, growth; accumulation.
acreditado-a *a.* accredited, certified.
acreditar *v.* to credit, to accredit, to certify.
acrilamida *f.* acrylamide, a potencial cancer causing agent.
acrocianosis *f.* acrocyanosis, Raynaud's disease, bluish discoloration and coldness of the extremities due to a circulatory disorder gen. brought about by exposure to cold or by emotional stress.
acrodermatitis *f.* acrodermatitis, infl. of the skin of hands and feet; ___ **crónica atrófica** / ___ chronica atrophicans.
acrofobia *f.* acrophobia, excessive fear of heights.
acromasia *f.* achromasia, lack or loss of pigmentation in the skin, characteristic of albinos.
acromático-a *a.* achromatic, lacking in color.
acromatopsia *f.* achromatopsia, color blindness.
acromegalia *f.* acromegaly, chronic disease common in middle age, manifested by progressive enlargement of the bones of the extremities and of certain head bones, gen. caused by a malfunction of the pituitary gland.
acromion *m.* acromion, part of the scapular bone of the shoulder.
acropustulosis *f.* acropustulosis, pustular eruptions of the hands and feet, often a form of psoriasis.

acrotismo *m.* acrotism, absence or imperceptibility of the pulse.
actina *f.* actin, protein in muscle tissue that together with myosin makes possible muscle contraction.
actitud *f.* attitude, disposition.
activar *v.* to activate.
actividad *f.* activity.
actividades de resistencia *f.* endurance activities.
actividades de la vida diaria *f.* activities of daily living.
activo-a *a.* active.
acto *m.* act; deed; **en el** ___ / right away.
actual *a.* actual, present, true, real; **-mente** *adv.* actually, presently.
actuar *v.* to act.
acuclillarse *vr.* to squat.
acuerdo *m.* agreement; **estar de** ___ / to be in agreement, to agree.
acumulación *f.* accumulation; pile, heap.
acumular *v.* to accumulate, to pile up, to amass.
acuoso-a *a.* aqueous; **humor** ___ / ___ humor; **intoxicación** ___ / water intoxication, condition caused by excessive retention of water in the body.
acupuntura *f.* acupuncture, method of inserting needles into specific points of the body as a means of relieving pain.
acústico-a *a.* acoustic, rel. to sound or hearing.
Adán, nuez de *f.* Adam's apple.
adaptabilidad *f.* adaptability; compliance. 1. the ease with which a substance or structure can change its shape, such as the ability of an organ to distend; 2. the degree to which a patient follows a prescribed regimen.
adaptación *f.* adaptation, adjustment.
adaptar *v.* to adapt, to fit, to accommodate; **adaptarse** *vr.* to adapt oneself.
adaptómetro *m.* adaptometer, instrument that determines the required time of adaptation of the retina.
Addison, enfermedad de *f.* Addison's disease, insufficiency or nonfunction of the adrenal glands.
adecuado-a *a.* adequate, suitable.
adelantado-a *a.* advanced, ahead; **por** ___ / in advance.
adelantar *v.* to advance, to move ahead; ___ **la fecha** / to move up the date.
adelante *adv.* forward, ahead; **más** ___ / later on; **de hoy en** ___ / from now on.
adelanto *m.* improvement, progress.

adelgazar *vi.* to lose weight, to get thin.
además *adv.* besides, in addition.
adenectomía *f.* adenectomy, removal of a gland.
adenitis *f.* adenitis, infl. of a gland.
adenoacanthoma *m.* adenoacanthoma, slow-growing cancer of the uterus.
adenocarcinoma *m.* adenocarcinoma, malignant tumor arising from a gland or organ.
adenocistoma *m.* adenocystoma, benign gland tumor formed by cysts.
adenofibroma *m.* adenofibroma, benign fibrous glandular tumor seen in the breast and uterus.
adenoide *m.* adenoid, gland-like; accumulation of lymphatic tissue located in the throat behind the nose.
adenoidectomía *f.* adenoidectomy, excision of the adenoid.
adenoiditis *f.* adenoiditis, infl. of the adenoid.
adenoma *m.* adenoma, glandular-like tumor; ___ acidófilo / acidophil ___; ___ adrenocortical / adrenocortical ___; ___ basófilo / basophil ___; ___ bronquial / bronchial ___; ___ de la mama / ___ of nipple; ___ embrional / embryonal ___; ___ folicular / follicular ___; ___ hepático / hepatic ___; ___ renal cortical / renal cortical ___; ___ sebáceo / sebaceous ___; ___ tóxico / toxic ___ .
adenomioma *m.* adenomyoma, benign tumor usu. seen in the uterus.
adenopatía *f.* adenopathy, a lymph gland disease.
adenosarcoma *m.* adenosarcoma, malignant tumor.
adenosis *f.* adenosis, enlargement of a gland.
adentro (de) *adv.* inside; inside of.
adherencia *f.* adhesion, attachment.
adherir *vi.* to adhere, to attach.
adhesivo-a *a.* adhesive.
adicción *f.* addiction, dependency, propensity; **dejar la** ___ / *pop.* [*droga*] to kick the habit.
adictivo *m.* addictive, rel. to or causing addiction.
adicto-a *a.* addicted, physically or psychologically dependent on a substance such as alcohol or a narcotic.
adiós *int.* goodbye.
adiposito *m.* adipocyte, adipose cell.
adiposo-a *a.* adipose, fatty; **cirrosis** ___ / ___ cirrhosis; **corazón** ___ / ___ heart; **hernia** ___ / ___ hernia; **riñón** ___ / ___ kidney; **tejido** ___ / ___ tissue.

adjetivo *m.* adjective.
adjuntar *v.* to enclose; to include.
adjutor *m.* adjuvant, helper; substance added to a medication to heighten its action.
administración *f.* administration, management.
administrador-a *m., f.* administrator, manager.
admisión *f.* admission.
admitir *v.* to admit.
ADN recombinante *n.* recombinant DNA, alteration of the DNA in the laboratory by which the genes from one species of an organism are transplanted or spliced to another organism.
adolescencia *f.* adolescence, puberty.
adolescente *m., f.* adolescent.
adolorido-a *a.* sore.
adopción *f.* adoption.
adoptar *v.* to adopt.
adoptivo-a *a.* adoptive.
adormecer *vi.* to put to sleep, [*un nervio*] to deaden; **adormecerse** *vr.* to drowse.
adquirir *vi.* to acquire.
adquisición *f.* acquisition.
adrede *adv.* on purpose.
adrenal *a.* adrenal. suprarenal.
adrenalectomía *f.* adrenalectomy, removal of the adrenal gland.
adrenalina *f.* adrenaline, epinephrin, hormone secreted by the adrenal medulla, commonly used as a cardiac stimulant.
adrenalismo *m.* adrenalism, inadequate function of the adrenal glands.
adrenérgicos *m., pl.* adregenic, blocking agents, rel. to drugs that mimic the actions of the sympathetic nervous system.
adrenocorticotropina *f.* adrenocorticotropin, hormone secreted by the pituitary gland that has a stimulating effect on the adrenal cortex.
adrenogénico-a *a.* adrenogenous, originating in the adrenal glands.
aducción *f.* adduction, 1. movement toward the midline of the body or toward a limb or part; 2. movement toward a common center.
aductor-a *a.* adductor, a muscle that draws a part towards the median line.
adueñarse *vr.* to take possession.
adulterado-a *a.* adulterated, changed from the original; **no** ___ / unadulterated.
adulterar *v.* to adulterate, to change the original.
adulterio *m.* adultery.
adulto-a *a.* adult.
adverbio *m. gr.* adverb.

adverso-a *a.* adverse, unfavorable.
advertencia *f.* warning, forewarning; advice.
advertir *vi.* to warn; to advise.
adyacente *a.* adjacent, next to.
aeróbic *f.* aerobics, a system of physical fitness combining calisthenics and a dance routine intended to promote cardiovascular endurance.
aeróbico-a *a.* aerobic, 1. rel. to an aerobe; 2. rel. to an exercise coordinated as a physical activity; **baile** ___ / ___ dance; **ejercicio** ___ / ___ exercise; 3. that lives or occurs in the presence of oxygen.
aerobio *m.* aerobe, organism that requires oxygen to live.
aeroembolismo *m.* aeroembolism, condition caused by a release of bubbles of nitrogen into the blood gen. due to a sudden change in atmospheric pressure; *pop.* the bends.
aeroenfisema *m.* aeroemphysema, condition caused by a sudden ascent in space without adequate decompression; *pop.* the chokes.
aerofagia *f.* aerophagia, excessive swallowing of air.
aerogénico-a *a.* aerogenic, gas-producing.
afán *m.* eagerness, desire.
afasia *f.* aphasia, inability to coordinate word and thought in speaking. ___ **atáxica** / ataxic ___; ___ **amnésica** / amnesic ___ .
afebril *a.* afebrile, without fever.
afección *f.* affection, fondness; condition, sickness.
afectado-a *a.* affected.
afectar *v.* to affect; to cause change.
afectivo-a *a.* affective; **síntoma** ___ / ___ symptom; **trastornos** ___-s / ___ disorders.
afeitar *v.* to shave; **afeitarse** *vr.* to shave oneself.
afemia *f.* aphemia, loss of speech gen. due to a cerebral hemorrhage, a blood clot or a tumor.
afeminado *a.* effeminate.
aferente *a.* afferent, that moves in a direction toward a center, as in certain arteries, veins, vessels, and nerves.
afibrinogenemia *f.* afibrinogenemia, deficiency of fibrinogen in the blood.
afinidad *f.* affinity; similarity.
afirmación *f.* affirmation.
afirmar *v.* to affirm, to make certain.
aflicción *f.* affliction, sorrow, grief, distress; **reación de** ___ / grief reaction.
afligido-a *a.* afflicted, distressed, sorrowful, grief-stricken, troubled.
afligir *vi.* to afflict, to cause pain; **afligirse** *vr.* to lament, to be grieved.

aflojar *v.* to loosen, to slacken; **aflojarse** *vr.* to become weak; to lose courage.
afonía *f.* aphonia, loss of voice due to an affliction of the larynx.
afónico-a *a.* aphonic, without voice or sound.
afortunado-a *a.* fortunate, lucky.
afrodisíaco *m.* aphrodisiac, any agent that arouses sexual desire.
afrontar *v.* to confront.
afta *f.* aphtha, a small ulcer, sign of fungal infection of the oral mucosa.
afuera *adv.* outside.
agacharse *vr.* to bend; to stoop, to squat.
agallas *f. pl.* tonsils; *pop.* **tener** ___ / to have guts, to be bold.
agalorrea *f.* agalorrhea, cessation or lack of milk in the breasts.
agammaglobulinemia *f.* agammaglobulinemia, deficiency of gamma globulin in the blood.
agarrar *v.* to grab, to grip.
agenesia, agenesis *f.* agenesia, agenesis. 1. congenital failure of an organ to grow or develop; 2. sterility or impotence.
agente *m.* agent, factor.
agentes citotóxicos *m., pl.* cytotoxic agents, chemical compounds used in chemotherapy to destroy cancerous cells.
ágil *a.* agile, nimble; mentally sharp.
agilidad *f.* agility; ___ **mental** / mental ___ .
agitación *f.* excitement, agitation.
agitar *v.* to stir up, to shake; ___ **la botella** / to shake the bottle; **agitarse** *vr.* to become agitated or excited.
aglomeración *f.* agglomeration.
aglutinación *f.* agglutination, the act of binding together.
aglutinante *m.* agglutinant, agent or factor that holds parts together during the healing process.
agnosia *f.* agnosia, disorder or incapacity due to a cerebral lesion by which the person suffers a total or partial loss of the senses and does not recognize familiar persons or objects; ___ **visual** / visual ___ .
agobiar *v.* to weigh down; to burden.
agonía *f.* agony, anguish. 1. extreme suffering; 2. state preceding death.
agonizar *vi.* to agonize.
agorafobia *f.* agoraphobia, fear of being alone in a wide open space.
agotado-a *a.* exhausted, tired.
agotador-a *a.* exhausting, tiring.
agotamiento *m.* exhaustion, extreme fatigue; wasting.

agotar *v.* to exhaust; ___ **todos los recursos** / to ___ all means.

agradable *a.* pleasant.

agradecer *vi.* to be grateful, to be thankful.

agradecido-a *a.* grateful, thankful.

agrafia *f.* agraphia, loss of ability to write due to a brain disorder.

agrandamiento *m.* enlargement.

agrandar *v.* to enlarge.

agranulocitosis *f.* agranulocytosis, acute condition caused by the absence of leukocytes in the blood.

agregar *v.* to add.

agresivo-a *a.* aggressive, hostile.

agriarse *vr.* to turn sour.

agrietado-a *a.* chapped; **labios** ___-s / ___ lips; **manos** ___-as / ___ hands.

agrio-a *a.* sour.

agua *f.* water; **abastecimiento de** ___ / ___ supply; ___ **alcanforizada** / camphor julep; ___ **corriente o de pila** / tap ___; ___ **de rosa** / rose ___; ___ **helada** / ice ___; ___ **oxigenada** / hydrogen peroxide; **bolsa de** ___ **caliente** / hot ___ bottle; **cama de, colchón de** ___ / ___ bed; **contaminación del** ___ / ___ pollution; **ingestión o toma de** ___ / ___ intake; **purificación del** ___ / ___ purification; **soluble en** ___ / ___ soluble.

aguado-a *a.* watered down.

aguantar *v.* to hold; to endure.

agudo-a *a.* acute, piercing, sharp.

agero *m.* omen.

aguja *f.* needle; ___ **hipodérmica** / hypodermic ___ .

agujero *m.* hole.

ahí *adv.* there.

ahijado-a *m., f.* godchild.

ahogamiento *m.* drowning.

ahogar *vi.* to drown; to smother, to extinguish; **ahogarse** *vr.* to drown oneself; to choke.

ahora *adv.* now, presently.

ahorcarse *vr. vi.* to hang oneself.

ahorita *adv.* right away.

ahorrar *v.* to save; to spare; ___ **tiempo** / ___ time.

aire *m.* air, wind; breath; ___ **acondicionado** / ___ conditioned; ___ **contaminado, viciado** / contaminated ___ , pollution; ___ **de ventilación** / ventilated ___; ___ **respiratorio** / tidal ___; ___ **viciado** / viciated ___; **bolsa de** ___ / ___ pocket; **burbujas de** ___ / ___ bubbles; **cámara de** ___ / ___ chamber; **conducto de** ___ /

airway, air passage; **enfriado por** ___ / ___ - cooled; **falta de** ___ / ___ hunger; **falto de** ___ / shortness of breath.

airear *v.* to aerate, to ventilate. 1. to saturate a liquid with air; 2. to change the venous blood into arterial blood in the lungs; 3. to circulate fresh air.

aislado-a *a.* isolated.

aislamiento *m.* isolation, separation of a patient or patients to avoid contagion for his or her own protection. ___ **conductual** / behavioral ___; ___ **infeccioso** / infectious ___; ___ **por exclusión** / exclusion ___; ___ **protector** / protective ___; **sala de** ___ / ___ ward.

aislar *v.* to isolate.

ajo *m.* garlic.

ajustado-a *a.* tight-fitting; adjusted.

ajustar *v.* to tighten; to adjust.

ajuste *m.* adjustment, fit; ___ **oclusivo** / oclussive ___ .

ala *m.* wing.

alambre *m.* wire.

alar *a.* rel. or similar to a wing.

alargado-a *a.* elongated, as the digestive tract.

alargar *vi.* to lengthen; to prolong.

alarma *f.* alarm; danger signal; ___ **de fuego** / fire ___ .

alarmante *a.* alarming.

alarmar *v.* to alarm; **alarmarse** *vr.* to become alarmed.

albahaca *f.* sweet basil.

alberca *f.* swimming pool; pond; tank.

albinismo *m.* albinism, lack of pigment in the skin and hair.

albino-a *m., f.* albino, person afflicted with albinism.

albúmina *f.* albumin, protein component.

albuminuria *f.* albuminuria, presence of albumin or globulin in the urine.

alcaloide *m.* alkaloid, one of a group of organic, basic substances found in plants.

alcalosis *f.* alkalosis, physiological disorder in the normal acid-base balance of the body.

alcance *m.* reach; span; **al** ___ **de** / within ___; ___ **de movimiento** / range of motion.

alcanfor *m.* camphor, camphor julep.

alcanzar *vi.* to reach; to catch up.

alcohol *m.* alcohol; ___ **etílico** / ethyl ___ .

alcohólico-a *m., f.* an alcoholic; **abstinencia** ___ / ___ withdrawal; **detoxificación** ___ / ___ detoxification; **privación** ___ / ___ withdrawal;

alcoholismo *m.* alcoholism, excess intake of alcohol.

aldosterona *f.* aldosterone, hormone produced by the adrenal gland.

aldosteronismo *m.* aldosteronism, anomaly caused by excessive secretion of aldosterone.

alegre *a.* cheerful, joyful, merry.

alelo, alelomorfo *m.* allele, any one of a series of two or more genes situated at the same place in homologous chromosomes that determined alternative characteristics in inheritance.

alentar *vi.* to encourage, to reassure.

alérgenos *m., pl.* allergens, term for any antigen that induces an allergic or hypersensitive response. V. cuadro en la página 305.

alergia *f.* allergy.

alérgico-a *a.* allergic; **reacción** ___ / ___ reaction; **rinitis** ___ / ___ rhinitis.

alergista *m., f.* allergist.

alerta *a.* alert, vigilant, being alert.

aleteo *m.* flutter, cardiac arrhythmia characterized by fast auricular contractions that simulate the flutter of the wings of birds; ___ **auricular** / ___ atrial, auricular; ___ **ventricular** / ___ ventricular; ___ **y fibrilación** / ___ and fibrillation.

aleucemia *f.* aleukemia, absence or deficiency of leukocytes in the blood.

alexia *f.* alexia, inability to understand the written word.

alfiler *m.* pin.

alfombra *f.* rug.

álgido-a *a.* algid, cold.

algodón *m.* cotton.

algor *m.* algor, chill.

algoritmo *m.* algorithm, arithmetical and algebraic method used in the diagnosis and treatment of a disease.

aliento *m.* 1. breath; **mal** ___ / bad ___ ; **sin** ___ / breathless; 2. encouragement.

aligeramiento *m.* lightening, descent of the uterus into the pelvic cavity in the final stage of pregnancy.

aligerar *v.* to lighten, to ease.

alimentación *f.* feeding, alimentation, nourishment; ___ **enteral** / enteral ___ ; ___ **forzada** / forced ___ ; ___ **intravenosa** / intravenous ___ ; ___ **por sonda** / tube ___ ; ___ **rectal** / rectal ___ ; **horario de** ___ / feeding schedule; **requisitos de la** ___ / food requirements.

alimentar *v.* to nourish, to feed.

alimenticio-a *a.* alimentary, nourishing; **aditivos** ___ -s / food additives;

intoxicación ___ / food poisoning; **tracto** ___ / ___ tract.

alimento *m.* food, nourishment, nutrient; ___ **dietético** / dietetic ___ ; ___ **orgánico** / organic ___ ; ___ **sano** / health ___ ; ___ -s **enriquecidos** / ___ supplements; **manipulación de** ___ -s / ___ handling.

alinfocitosis *f.* alymphocytosis, abnormal decrease of lymphocytes.

aliviado-a *a.* relieved, alleviated.

aliviar *v.* to relieve, to alleviate; [*un dolor*] to lessen.

alivio *m.* relief; **,qué** ___ ! / what a relief!

allí *adv.* there.

almacenamiento *m.* storage; [toma] captura y ___ / uptake and ___ .

almanaque *m.* calendar, almanac.

almeja *f.* clam.

almendra *f.* almond.

almidón *m.* starch, main form of storage of carbohydrates.

almohada *f.* pillow.

almohadilla *f.* pad.

almorzar *vi.* to have lunch.

almuerzo *m.* lunch.

alógeno-a *a.* allogenic, having a different genetic constitution from others belonging to the same species; **células** ___ -as / ___ cells; **sistema** ___ / ___ system.

aloinjerto *m.* allograft, homoinjection.

alojamiento *m.* lodging.

alojar *v.* to lodge; to accommodate.

alopecia *f.* alopecia, loss of hair.

alquilar *v.* to rent.

alrededor *adv.* around, about.

alteración *f.* alteration. 1. a change; 2. changing; making different; ___ **cualitativa** / qualitative ___ ; ___ **cuantitativa** / quantitative ___ .

alterar *v.* to alter, to change.

alternar *v.* to alternate.

alternativa *f.* alternative, option.

alto-a *a.* tall.

alto riesgo *m.* high risk; ___ **de contaminación** / ___ contamination; ___ **de infección** / ___ infection; ___ **de lesión** / ___ injury; ___ **de violencia** / ___ violence.

altura *f.* height.

alucinación, alucinamiento *f., m.* hallucination, subjective feeling not related to a real stimulus; ___ **auditiva** / auditory ___ , imaginary perception of sound; ___ **gustativa** / gustatory ___ , imaginary perception of taste; ___ **motora** / motor ___ , imaginary perception of body movements; ___ **olfativa** / olfactory ___ , imaginary perception of odors; ___ **táctil** / haptic ___ , imaginary perception of pain, temperature or other skin sensation.

alucinar *v.* to hallucinate.

alucinógeno *m.* hallucinogen, drug that produces hallucinations, such as LSD, peyote, or mescaline.

alucinosis *f.* hallucinosis, state of persistent hallucinations; ___ **alcohólica** / alcoholic ___ , extreme fear accompanied by auditory hallucinations.

alumbramiento *m.* parturition, the act of giving birth.

alveoalgia *f.* alveoalgia, post-operative complication of tooth extraction.

alveolar *a.* alveolar, rel. to an alveolus.

alveolitis *f.* alveolitis. 1. infl. of lung's alveoli; 2. infl. of a tooth socket.___ **alérgica extrínseca** / extrinsic allergic ___; ___ **fibrosa crónica** / chronic fibrosing ___; ___ **fibrosa criptogénica** / cryptogenic fibrosing ___; ___ **pulmonar aguda** / acute pulmonary ___ .

alvéolo *m.* alveolus, cavity; ___ **pulmonar** / air sac.

alzar *vi.* to raise, to lift; **alzarse** / *vr.* to raise oneself, to get up.

Alzheimer, enfermedad de *f.* Alzheimer's disease, presenile dementia.

amable *a.* kind, nice.

amalgamar *v.* to amalgamate, to mix.

amamantar *v.* to nurse, to suckle, to breast-feed.

amar *v.* to love.

amargado-a *m., f.* a bitter person; *a.* [*persona*] bitter.

amargar *vi.* to make bitter; **amargarse** *vr., vi.* to become bitter.

amargo-a *a.* bitter.

amargura *f.* bitterness.

amarillento-a *a.* yellowish.

amarillo-a *a.* yellow. **atrofia** ___ **del hígado** / ___ atrophy of the liver; **fibras** ___ / ___ fibers; **fiebre** ___ / ___ fever.

amarrar *v.* to tie, to fasten, to bind.

amarre *m.* fastening, binding; ___ **de las trompas** / tubal ligation.

amasadura, amasamiento *f. m.* kneading, methodical rubbing and pressing of muscles.

amastia *f.* amastia, absence of breasts.

amaurosis *f.* amaurosis, blindness without apparent change in the eye, attributed to an injury in the brain.

amaurótico-a *a.* amaurotic, rel. to amaurosis.

ambarino-a *a.* amber-colored.

ambición *f.* ambition.

ambicionar *v.* to aspire.

ambidextro *a.* ambidextrous.

ambiente *m.* environment, ambiance, setting.

ambivalencia *f.* ambivalence.

ambliopía *f.* amblyopia, diminished vision.

ambos-as *a.* both.

ambulancia *f.* ambulance.

ambulante, ambulatorio-a *a.* ambulant, ambulatory.

ameba *m.* amoeba, ameba, one-celled organism.

amebiano-a *a.* amebid, rel. to amebae.

amebiasis *f.* amebiasis, infection by amebae.

amenaza *f.* threat; menace.

amenazar *vi.* to threaten.

ameno-a *a.* pleasant, affable.

amenorrea *f.* amenorrhoea, absence of menstrual period.

americano-a *a.* American.

ametropía *f.* ametropia, poor vision due to an anomaly or disturbance in the refractive powers of the eye.

amígdalas *f. pl.* amygdalae, tonsils.

amigdalitis *f.* tonsillitis, infl. of the tonsils.

amigdalotomía *f.* tonsillectomy, removal of the tonsils.

amigo-a *m., f.* friend.

amiloide *a.* amyloid, starch-like protein. **degeneración** ___ / ___ degeneration; **enfermedad** ___ / ___ sickness; **nefrosis** ___ / ___ nephrosis; **riñón** ___ / ___ kidney.

amiloidosis *m.* amyloidosis, accumulation of amyloid in different tissues of the body.

amina *f.* amine, one of the basic compounds derived from ammonia.

aminoácido *m.* amino acid, an organic metabolic compound that is the end product of protein and necessary for the growth and development of the human body.

amistad *f.* friendship.

amitosis *f.* amitosis, direct division of the nucleus and cell, without the changes in the nucleus that occur in the ordinary process of cell reproduction.

amnesia *f.* amnesia, loss of memory.

amniocentesis *m.* amniocentesis, puncture of the uterus to obtain amniotic fluid.

amnios *m.* amnion, membranous sac surrounding the embryo in the womb.

amnioscopía *f.* amnioscopy, use of the amnioscope to visualize the fetus through the amniotic fluid.

amnioscopio *m.* amnioscope, endoscope used in the study of the amniotic fluid.

amniótico-a *a.* amniotic, rel. to the amnion; **fluido** ___ / ___ fluid; **saco** ___ / ___ sac.

amoldamiento *m.* molding, adjustment of the head of the fetus to the shape and size of the birth canal.

amoníaco *m.* ammonia.

amoniuría *f.* ammoniuria, excretion of urine containing ammonia.

amor *m.* love.

amor propio *m.* self-esteem.

amoratado-a *a.* black and blue, bruised.

amorfo-a *a.* amorphous, without shape.

amparar *v.* to protect; to shelter.

ampicilina *f.* ampicillin, semisynthetic penicillin.

ampliación *f.* amplification.

ampliar *v.* to amplify, to magnify, to enlarge.

amplio-a *a.* wide, large, ample.

ampolla *f.* blister, bulla.

ámpula *f.* ampule, vial, small glass container.

amputación *f.* amputation.

amputar *v.* to amputate.

Amsler, gráfico de *m.* Amsler graphic, useful chart in revealing signs of macular degeneration.

anabólico-a *a.* anabolic, rel. to anabolism; **esteroides** ___-s / ___ steroids.

anabolismo *m.* anabolism, cellular process by which simple substances are converted into complex compounds; constructive metabolism.

anacidez *f.* anacidity, state of being without acid.

anacusia *f.* anacusia, total loss of hearing.

anaeróbico-a *a.* anaerobic, rel. to anaerobes.

anaerobio *m.* anaerobe, germ that multiplies in the absence of air or oxygen.

anafase *f.* anaphase, a stage in cell division.

anafiláctico-a *a.* anaphylactic, rel. to anaphylaxis.

anafilaxis *f.* anaphylaxis, extreme allergic reaction; hypersensitivity.

anal *a.* anal; **fístula** ___ / ___ fistula;

analfabeto-a *a.* illiterate.

analgésico *m.* analgesic, pain reliever.

análisis *m.* analysis, test, assay. *V.* cuadro.

análisis endostático *m.* endostatic assay, a method to determine the diagnosis of anthrax by using a precipitin reaction, which indicates the presence of heat-stable *Bacillus anthracis* antigen in the extracted tissue.

analizar *vi.* to analyze, to examine.

Análisis	Analysis
de acumulacíon	accumulation
de aminoácido	amino acid
de la mordida	bite
del aliento	breath
cefalométrico	cephalometric
del carácter	character
cualitativo	qualitative
cuantitativo	quantitative
de costes	cost
de datos	data
de orina	urinalysis
del pelo	hair
gástrico	gastric
de los sueños	dream

analogía *f.* analogy, similarity.

anaplasia *f.* anaplasia, lack or loss of differentiation of cells.

anaplástico-a *a.* anaplastic, rel. to anaplasia.

anaquel *m.* shelf; shelf-like structure.

anaranjado-a *a.* orange.

anasarca *f.* anasarca, generalized infiltration of edema fluid in subcutaneous connective tissue.

anastomosis *f.* anastomosis, creation of a passage or communication between two or more organs; inosculating.

anastomosis ileoanal *f.* ileoanal anastomosis, removal of the colon and the inner lining of the rectum.

anatomía *f.* anatomy, science that studies the structure of the human body and its organs; ___ **macroscópica** / gross ___ , rel. to structures that can be seen with the naked eye; ___ **topográfica** / topographic ___ , rel. to a specific area of the body.

anatómico-a *a.* anatomic, anatomical, rel. to anatomy.

ancianidad *f.* old age.

anciano-a *m., f.* old man, old woman.

andador *m.* walker, device used to help a person walk.

andar *vi.* to walk; to go; ___ **con cuidado** / to be careful;

andrógeno *m.* androgen, masculine hormone; *a.* androgenic, rel. to the male sexual characteristics.

androginoide *a.* androgynous, having both male and female characteristics.

androtomía *f.* androtomy, dissection of a cadaver.

anejos, anexos *m. pl.* adnexa, appendages such as found in the uterine tubes.

anemia *f.* anemia, insufficiency of blood cells either in quality, quantity or in hemoglobin content; ___ **aplástica** / aplastic ___ , highly deficient production of blood cells; ___ **de glóbulos falciformes** / sickle cell ___ ; ___ **hemorrágica o hemolítica** / hemorrhagic, hemolytic ___ , progressive destruction of red blood cells; ___ **hipercrómica** / hyperchromic ___ , abnormal increase in the hemoglobin content; ___ **hipocrómica y microcítica** / hypochromic and microcytic ___ , small-sized blood cells and insufficient amount of hemoglobin; ___ **macrocítica** / macrocytic ___ , large-sized blood cells, pernicious anemia; ___ **por deficiencia de hierro** / iron deficiency ___ .

anergia *f.* anergy, 1. asthenia, lack of energy; 2. reduction or lack of response to a specific antigen.

anestesia *f.* anesthesia. *V.* cuadro.

anestesiar *v.* to anesthetize.

anestésico *m.* anesthetic.

anestesiólogo-a *m., f.* anesthesiologist.

aneurisma *m.* aneurysm, dilation of a portion of the wall of the artery; ___ **aórtico** / aortic ___ ; ___ **cerebral** / cerebral ___ ; ___ **desecante** / dissecting ___ ; ___ **falso** /

Anestesia	Anesthesia
con hipotensión controlada	hypotensive
en silla de montar	saddle block
endotraqueal	endotracheal
epidural	epidural
general intravenosa	general intravenous
general por inhalación	general by inhalation
general por intubación	general by intubation
intercostal	intercostal
local	local
por hipnosis	hypnosis
tópica	topical
térmica	thermic
raquídea	spinal
regional	regional

false ___ ; ___ **fusiforme** / fusiform ___ ; ___ **saculado** / berry ___ ; ___ **verdadero** / true ___ .

aneurisma de la arteria coronaria *m.* coronary artery aneurysm, gen. caused by atherosclerosis, inflammatory processes, or a coronary fistula.

aneurismal *a.* aneurysmal, rel. to an aneurysm.

aneurismectomía *f.* aneurysmectomy, excision of an aneurysm.

anexo-a *a.* contiguous, annexive.

anfetamina *f.* amphetamine, type of drug used as a stimulant of the nervous system.

angiítis *f.* angiitis, infl. of blood or lymph vessel.

angina *f.* angina, painful constrictive sensation; ___ **inestable** / unstable ___ ; ___ **intestinal** / intestinal ___ , acute abdominal pain caused by insufficient blood supply to the intestines; ___ **laríngea** / laryngeal ___ , infl. of the throat; ___ **pectoris** / ___ pectoris, chest pain caused by insufficient blood supply to the heart muscle.

angiocardiografía *f.* angiocardiography, x-ray of the heart chambers.

angiodisplasia *f.* angiodysplasia, abnormal structural vasculature caused by a degenerative or congenital factor.

angioedema *f.* angioedema, angioneurotic edema, allergic infl., gen. of the face.

angioespasmo *m.* angiospasm, prolonged contraction of a blood vessel.

angioestenosis *f.* angiostenosis, stenosis of a vessel, esp. a blood vessel.

angiogénesis *f.* angiogenesis, the development of the vascular system.

angiografía *f.* angiography, x-ray of the blood vessels after injection of a substance to show their outline.

angiografía coronaria *f.* coronary angiography, images of the circulation of the myocardium taken with a contrast medium, and gen. done through catheterization of each of the coronary arteries.

angiograma *m.* angiogram; visualization of a blood vessel obtained after injecting a radiopaque substance.

angioma *m.* angioma, benign vascular tumor.

angioneurótico *m.* angioneurotic, rel. to angioneurosis.

angioplastia *f.* angioplasty, plastic surgery of the blood vessels; ___ **coronaria percutánea** / percutaneous coronary ___ ; ___ **periférica percutánea** / percutaneous peripheral ___ .

angioplastia transluminal percutánea *f.* percutaneous transluminal angioplasty, process of dilating an artery or vessel by using a balloon that is inflated by pressure.

angiosarcoma *m.* angiosarcoma, a rare malignant neoplasm most often found in soft tissues.

angiotensina *f.* angiotensin, a family of peptides of known and similar sequence, produced by enzymatic action of renin.

angiotensinógeno *m.* angiotensinogen, a protein that when activated by the enzyme renin causes the blood vessels to constrict and raises the blood pressure.

angloparlante *m., f.* English speaker.

angosto-a *a.* narrow; tapered.

ángulo *m.* angle.

angustia *f.* anguish, distress.

angustiado-a *a.* distraught, distressed.

angustiarse *vr.* to be distressed, to feel anguish.

anhidrasa *f.* anhydrase, enzyme that catalyzes the removal of water from a compound; **inhibidores de** ___ **carbónica** / carbonic ___ inhibitors.

anhidrosis *f.* anhidrosis, diminished secretion of sweat.

anillo *m.* ring, margin, verge; ___ **anal** / anal verge.

animal *m.* animal.

animar *v.* to animate, to cheer up; **animarse** *vr.* to become more lively.

ánimo *m.* spirit; **estado de** ___ / mood; **no tener** ___ / to be without spirit.

animosidad *f.* animosity, rancor.

aniquilación *f.* annihilation, total destruction.

anisocitosis *f.* anisocytosis, unequal size of red blood cells.

anisocoria *f.* anisocoria, a condition in which the two pupils are not of equal size. ___ **central-simple** / simple-central ___; ___ **esencial** / essential ___; ___ **fisiológica** / physiologic ___; ___ **simple** / simple ___;

ano *m.* anus.

anoche *adv.* last night.

anodino *m.* anodyne, pain reliever; *-a* / *a.* insipid.

anomalía, anormalidad *f.* anomaly, abnormality, irregularity.

anorexia *f.* anorexia, disorder characterized by total lack of appetite.

anoréxico-a *a.* 1. lacking appetite.*n.* 2. person affected with anorexia nervosa.

anormal *a.* abnormal, irregular.

anosmia *f.* anosmia, lack of the sense of smell.

anotar *v.* to make or take note.

anovulación *f.* anovulation, cessation of ovulation.

anoxemia *f.* anoxemia, insufficient oxygen in the blood.

anoxia *f.* anoxia, lack of oxygen in body tissues. ___ **anémica** / anemic ___; ___ **de altitud** / altitude ___; ___ **de estancamiento** / stagnant ___; ___ **del neonato** / neonatorum ___ .

anóxico *a.* anoxic, rel. to anoxia.

anquilosado-a *a.* ankylosed, immobilized.

anquilosis *f.* ankylosis, immobility of an articulation.

ansiedad *f.* anxiety, anguish, state of apprehension or excessive worry; **estados de** ___ / ___ disorders; **neurosis de** ___ / ___ neurosis.

ansioso-a *a.* anxious, apprehensive.

anteayer *adv.* the day before yesterday.

antebrazo *f.* forearm.

antecubital *a.* antecubital, preceding the elbow.

anteflexión *f.* anteflexion, bending forward.

antemano *adv.* beforehand.

antenatal *a.* antenatal, that occurs or is formed before birth.

anteojos *m. pl.* eyeglasses; binoculars, espejuelos.

antepasados *m. pl.* ancestors.

antepié *m.* ball of the foot.

anterior *a.* preceding, previous; [*tiempo*] before, pre-existing; [*posición*]___ **ventral** / ventral ___ .

anteroposterior *a.* anteroposterior, from front to back.

antes *adv.* before, sooner; ___ **de** / before, prior to; ___ **de las comidas** / ___ meals; **lo** ___ **posible** / as soon as possible.

anteversión *f.* anteversion, turn toward the front.

antiácido *m.* antacid, acidity neutralizer.

antiadrenérgico *m.* antiadrenergic, adrenergic blocking agents, antagonistic to the action of sympathetic or other adrenergic nerve fibers.

antialérgico *m.* antiallergic, drug used to treat allergies.

antiarrítmico-a *a.* antiarrhythmic, that can prevent or be effective in the treatment of arrhythmia; **agentes** ___*-s* / cardiac depressants.

antiartrítico-a *a.* antiarthritic, rel. to medication used in the treatment of arthritis.

antibiótico *m.* antibiotic, antibacterial drug. ___
antineoplásico / antineoplastic ___; ___
bactericida / bactericidal ___; ___ **de amplio**
espectro / broad spectrum ___ .
anticarcinógeno *m.* anticarcinogen, drug used
in the treatment of cancer.
anticipar *v.* to anticipate.
anticoagulante *m.* anticoagulant, substance
used in the prevention of blood clotting.
anticolinérgico-a *a.* anticholinergic, that rel.
to the blockage of the impulses of the
parasympathetic nerves.
anticonceptivo *m.* contraceptive; **-a** / *a.* that
acts as a contraceptive; ___ **oral** / oral ___;
drogas ___-**s** / anovulatory drugs;
injerto ___ / ___ implant.
anticonvulsante, anticonvulsivo *m.*
anticonvulsant, medication used to prevent fits or
convulsions.
anticuerpo *m.* antibody, protein substance
produced by lymph tissue in response to the
presence of an antigen; ___ **monoclónico** /
monoclonal ___ , derived from hybridoma
cells; ___-**s de reacción cruzada** / cross
reacting ___ -s.
antidepresivo *m.* antidepressant, medication or
process used in the treatment of depression.
antidiarreico *m.* antidiarrheal.
antidiurético *m.* antidiuretic, drug that
decreases urine secretion.
antídoto *m.* antidote, substance used to
neutralize a poison; ___ **universal** /
universal ___ .
antiemético *m.* antiemetic, medication used to
treat nausea.
antiespasmódico *m.* antispasmodic, drug used
in the treatment of spasms.
antígeno *m.* antigen, toxic substance which
stimulates formation of antibodies; ___
carcinoembriogénico / carcinoembriogenic ___ .
antígeno B *m.* B antigen, protein present in the
erythrocytes' membranes that could cause a
serious reaction in a transfusion.
antihipertensivo *m.* antihypertensive,
medication to lower elevated blood pressure.
antihistamínico *m.* antihistamine, medication
used in the treatment of some allergies.
antiinflamatorio *m.* anti-inflammatory, agent
used to treat inflammations.
antineoplástico *m.* antineoplastic, drug that
controls or destroys cancer cells.
antipatía *f.* antipathy, aversion.
antipirético *m.* antipyretic, agent that reduces
fever.

antiprurítico *m.* antipruritic, medication used to
reduce itching.
antiséptico *m.* antiseptic, agent that destroys
bacteria.
antisuero anafiláctico *m.* anaphylactic
antiserum.
antitóxico *m.* antitoxin, neutralizer of the effects
of toxins.
antitoxina *f.* antitoxin, antibody that has a
neutralizing effect on a given poison introduced
in the body by a microorganism. ___ **diftérica** /
diphtheria ___; ___ **tetánica** / tetanus ___ .
antivirósico *m.* antiviral, agent that stops the
action of a virus.
antracosis *f.* anthracosis, lung condition due to
prolonged inhalation of coal dust.
ántrax *m.* anthrax, virus caused by the agent
cutaneous anthrax. The *Bacillus anthracis*
develops in infected animals through the skin.
Humans suffering from anthrax experience
symptoms of hemorrhage and serous effusions in
several organ cavities and lethargy; it is not
transmissible by contact, but if transmitted by air
can cause fatal pneumonia. *V.* Apéndice C. ___
cerebral / cerebral ___; ___ **cutáneo** /
cutaneous ___ .
antrectomía *f.* antrectomy, removal of the wall
or walls of an antrum.
antro *m.* antrum, any cavity semi-closed,
particulary one with bony walls; ___ **auris** / ___
auris; ___ **cardíaco** / ___ cardiacum; ___
folicular / follicular ___; ___ **mastoideo** / ___
mastoideum; ___ **maxilar** / maxillary ___; ___
pilórico / ___ pyloricum; ___ **timpánico** /
tympanic ___ .
antropoide *a.* anthropoid, of human
resemblance.
anular *a.* annular, circular, ring-shaped;
erupción ___ / ___ rash; *v.* to cancel, to make
void, to annul.
anuria *f.* anuria, lack of urine production due to
kidney malfunction.
año *m.* year.
aorta *f.* aorta, major artery originating from the
left ventricle; ___ **ascendente** / ascending ___;
cayado de la ___ / aortic arch; **coartación o**
compresión de la ___ / coarctation of the ___;
descendente / descending ___ .
aórtico-a *a.* aortic, rel. to the aorta; **válvula**
semilunar ___ / ___ semilunar valve.
aortocoronaria *a.* aortocoronary, rel. to the
aorta and coronary arteries.
aortografía *f.* aortography, outline of the aorta
on an x-ray.

aortoilíaca *a.* aortoiliac, rel. to the aorta and the illiac arteries.

aortoplastia *f.* aortoplasty, procedure for the repair of the aorta.

apagado-a *a.* turned off; dim, unlit.

apagar *vi.* [*luces*] to turn off; [*fuego*] to put out.

aparato digestivo *m.* digestive system.

aparato eléctrico *m.* electrical appliance.

aparente *a.* apparent, manifest, patent, visible.

apariencia *f.* appearance.

apasionado-a *a.* passionate.

apatía *f.* apathy, lack of interest.

apático-a *a.* apathetic, listless, languid.

apelar *v.* to appeal.

apellido *m.* surname, family name.

apenado-a *a.* grieved.

apenas *adv.* barely; no sooner than; as soon as.

apendectomía *f.* appendectomy, removal of the appendix.

apéndice *m.* appendix.

apendicitis *f.* appendicitis, infl. of the appendix.

apendicular *a.* appendicular, rel. to the appendix.

apepsia *f.* apepsia, poor digestion.

aperitivo *m.* aperitive, aperient. 1. mild laxative, physic; 2. aperitif, agent that stimulates the appetite.

apesadumbrado-a *a.* mournful, grieved.

apetito *m.* appetite.

ápice *m.* apex, the upper or base point of an organ.

apicectomía *f.* apicectomy, surgical removal of a tooth root apex.

apio *m.* celery.

aplanar *v.* to flatten.

aplasia *f.* aplasia, failure of organ development.

aplastamiento *m.* squashing, crushing.

aplastar *v.* to crush, to squash.

aplazar *vi.* to postpone, to put off.

aplicación *f.* application; ___ **de hielo** / ice treatment, icing.

aplicador *m.* applicator; ___ **de algodón /** cotton ___ .

aplicar *vi.* to apply.

apnea *f.* apnea, shortness of breath; ___ **del sueño** / sleep ___ , intermittent apnea that occurs during sleep.

apófisis *f.* apophysis, bony outgrowth.

aponeurosis *f.* aponeurosis, connective tissue that attaches the muscles to the bones and to other tissue.

apoplejía *f.* apoplexy, stroke, cerebrovascular accident.

apósito *m.* dressing. 1. clean or sterile application of material, to a wound for protection, absorbency, drainage, etc. 2. adhesive absorbent dressing.___ **amarrado /** tie-over ___; ___ **antiséptico /** antiseptic ___; ___ **apretado /** pressure ___; ___ **cambiado /** removable ___; ___ **desechable /** removable ___; ___ **fijo /** fixed ___; ___ **humedecido /** wet ___; ___ **oclusivo /** occlusive ___; ___ **seco /** dry ___ .

apoyar *v.* to back, to support; **apoyarse** *vr.* to lean on.

apoyo *m.* backing, support.

apraxia *f.* apraxia, lack of muscular coordination and movement.

apreciar *v.* to appreciate, to value; to be grateful.

aprender *v.* to learn.

aprendizaje *m.* learning. 1. generic term for the relatively permanent change in behavior that occurs as a result of practice or experience; 2. act of acquisition of knowledge; ___ **cognitivo /** cognitive ___; ___ **dependiente de estado /** state-dependent ___; ___ **incidental___ /** incidental ___; ___ **latente /** latent ___; ___ **pasivo /** passive ___ .

apretado-a *a.* tight.

apretar *vi.* to tighten, to squeeze, to press down.

aprisa *adv.* fast.

aprobación *f.* approval, consent, acceptance.

aprobar *v.* to approve; to accept.

apropiado-a *a.* appropriate, adequate.

aprovechar *v.* to make use of; to take advantage of.

aproximado-a *a.* approximate; **-mente** *adv.* approximately.

aptitud *f.* aptitude, capacity, ability; **prueba de** ___ / ___ **test.**

apto-a *a.* competent, apt.

apurado-a *a.* in a hurry; in difficulty.

apurarse *vr.* to hurry.

apuro *m.* need; hurry; **estar en un** ___ / to be in trouble.

aquí *adv.* here; **por** ___ / this way.

aquietar *v.* to calm down.

Aquiles, tendón de *m.* Achilles tendon, the tendon that originates in the muscles of the calf and attaches to the heel.

aracnoide *m.* arachnoid, weblike membrane that covers the brain and spinal cord.

araña *f.* spider; ___ **viuda negra /** black widow ___ .

arañar *v.* to scratch.

arañazo *m.* scratch.

árbol *m.* 1. anatomical structure resembling a tree; 2. tree;___ **bronquial** / bronchial ___; ___ **genealógico** / genealogical ___ .

arcadas *f., pl.* retching, spasmodic abdominal contractions that precede vomiting.

arco *m.* arch. ___ **carotideo** / carotid a; ___ **del paladar** / palate ___; ___ **plantar** / plantar ___ .

arder *v.* to have a burning feeling.

ardor *m.* ardor, burning feeling; ___ **en el estómago** / heartburn.

arena *f.* sand.

arenilla *f.* minute, sandlike particles.

arenoso-a *a.* sandy.

aréola *f.* areola, circular area of a different color around a central point.

Argyll Robertson, pupila de *f.* Argyll Robertson's pupil, a pupil of the eye that accommodates to distance but does not react to the refraction of light.

arma de fuego *m.* firearm.

arma química *f.* chemical weapon, chemical substances that can be delivered by warfare to cause death or severe harm to humans, animals, and plants.

armazón *f.* frame, supportive structure. ___ **de tracción en garra** / claw type traction ___ .

aroma *m.* aroma, pleasant smell.

aromático-a *a.* aromatic, rel. to an aroma.

arqueado-a *a.* arch-like

arquetipo *m.* archetype, original type from which modified versions evolve.

arquiblastoma *m.* archiblastoma, cerebral tumor; a neoplasm composed chiefly or entirely of immature undifferentiated cells.

arraigado-a *a.* deep-rooted.

arrancar *vi.* to tear off; to pull out.

arrebato *m.* fit; temporary insanity.

arreflexia *f.* areflexia, absence of reflexes.

arreglado-a *a.* in order; neat; fixed.

arreglar *v.* to fix, to arrange.

arreglo *m.* settlement, agreement.

arrenoblastoma *m.* arrhenoblastoma.

arrepentido-a *a.* repentant, regretful.

arrepentirse *vr.* *vi.* to regret; to repent.

arriba *adv.* above, upstairs; **de ___ a abajo** / from top to bottom.

arriesgado-a *a.* risky.

arriesgar *vi.* to risk, to imperil; **arriesgarse** *vr.* to take a risk.

arritmia *f.* arrhythmia, irregular heartbeats.

arrodillarse *vr.* to kneel.

arrojar *v.* to throw up, to vomit.

arroz *m.* rice.

arruga *f.* wrinkle.

arrugado-a *a.* wrinkled.

arrugar *vi.* to wrinkle; *arrugarse vr.* to become wrinkled.

arsénico *m.* arsenic; **envenenamiento por ___** / ___ poisoning.

arteria *f.* artery; vessel carrying blood from the heart to tissues throughout the body; ___ **innominada** / innominate ___ .

arterial *a.* arterial, rel. to the arteries; **enfermedades ___ -es oclusivas** / ___ occlusive diseases; **sistema ___** / ___ system.

arterioesclerosis *f.* arteriosclerosis, hardening of the walls of the arteries.

arteriografía *f.* arteriography, x-ray of the arteries.

arteriograma *m.* arteriogram, angiogram of the arteries; ___ **cerebral o carótico** / cerebral or carotid ___; ___ **mesentérico** / mesenteric ___; ___ **periférico** / peripheral ___; ___ **renal** / renal ___ .

arteriola *f.* arteriole, minute artery ending in a capillary.

arteriotomía *f.* arteriotomy, opening of an artery.

arteriovenoso-a *a.* arteriovenous; rel. to an artery and a vein; **anastomosis ___ quirúrgica** / ___ shunt, surgical; **fístula ___** / ___ fistula; **malformaciones ___ -as** / ___ malformations.

arteritis *f.* arteritis, infl. of an artery.

articulación *f.* joint, articulation. 1. joint between two or more bones; ___ **cartilaginosa** / cartilagenous ___; ___ **chasqueante** / snapping ___; ___ **condiloidea** / condyloid ___; ___ **de la cabeza de la cadera** / ___ of head of hip; ___ **de la cadera** / hip ___; ___ **de la falange** / phalangeal ___; ___ **de la mandíbula** / jaw ___; ___ **de la mano** / ___ of hand; ___ **de la pelvis** / pelvic ___; ___ **de la rodilla** / knee ___; ___ **del carpo** / carpal ___; ___ **del codo** / elbow ___; ___ **del hombro** / shoulder ___; ___ **del oído** / ___ of ear bones; ___ **del pie** / foot ___; ___ **del tobillo** / ankle ___; ___ **femuropatelar** / ___ femuropatellar; ___ **fibrosa** / fibrous ___; ___ **inestable** / flail ___; ___ **inmóvil** / immovable ___; ___ **interarticular** / interarticular ___; ___ **intercarpales** / intercarpal ___; ___ **interfalange** / interphalangeal ___; ___ **neurocentral** /

neurocentral ___; ___ **petrooccipital** / petrooccipital ; ___ **radioulnar** / radioulnar ___; ___ **rotatoria** / pivot ___; ___ **seudoartrosis** / false ___; ___ **sinovial** / synovial ___; ___ **tibiofibular** / tibiofibular ___; 2. articulation, distinctive and clear pronunciation of words in speech.

articular *a.* articular, rel. to the articulations; *v.* to articulate, to pronounce words clearly.

artículo *m.* article.

artificial *a.* artificial, substituting that which is natural; **fecundación** ___ / ___ impregnation, fecundation; **respiración** ___ / ___ respiration.

artrítico-a *a.* arthritic, rel. to or suffering from arthritis.

artritis *f.* arthritis, infl. of an articulation or joint; ___ **aguda** / acute ___; ___ **coronaria reumatoide** / rheumatoid coronary ___; ___ **crónica** / chronic ___; ___ **degenerativa** / degenerative ___; ___ **hemofílica** / hemophilic ___; ___ **reumatoidea** / rheumatoid ___; ___ **traumática** / traumatic ___ .

artrodesis *f.* arthrodesis. 1. fusion of the bones of a joint; 2. artificial ankylosis.

artrograma *m.* arthrogram, x-ray of a joint.

artropatía *f.* arthropathy, any disease of the joints.

artroplastia *f.* arthroplasty, reparation of a joint or building of an artificial one.

artroscopía *f.* arthroscopy, examination of the inside of a joint with an arthroscope.

artroscopio *m.* arthroscope, device used to examine the inside of a joint.

artrotomía *f.* arthrotomy, incision of a joint for therapeutic purposes.

asa *f.* loop.

asado-a *a.* roasted.

asbesto *m.* asbestos.

asbestosis *f.* asbestosis, chronic infection of the lungs caused by asbestos.

ascariasis *f.* ascariasis, intestinal infection caused by a worm of the genus *Ascaris*.

ascárido *m.* ascaris, type of worm commonly found in the intestinal tract.

ascendencia *f.* ancestry, genealogy.

ascendiente *m.* ascendent, ancestor.

ascitis *f.* ascites, accumulation of fluid in the peritoneal cavity.

asco *m.* nausea; disgust, loathing; **dar** ___ / to produce nausea.

aseado-a *a.* clean, tidy.

asear *v.* to clean; **asearse** *vr.* to clean oneself.

asegurar *v.* to assure; **asegurarse** *vr.* to make sure.

asentaderas *f. pl.* buttocks.

asepsia *f.* asepsia, total absence of germs.

aséptico-a *a.* aseptic, sterile.

asexual *a.* asexual, having no gender; **reproducción** ___ / ___ reproduction.

asfixia *f.* asphyxia, suffocation; ___ **fetal** / ___ fetalis.

asfixiarse *vr.* to asphyxiate, to suffocate.

así *adv.* like this; ___ **que** / therefore.

asiento *m.* seat, space upon which a structure rests.

asignación *f.* assignment, task, mission.

asignar *v.* to assign.

asilo *m.* nursing home, shelter; ___ **para ancianos** / ___ for the aged.

asimilación *f.* assimilation. 1. integration of digested materials from food into the tissues; 2. restructuring and modification of received information and experiences into a cognitive structure.

asimilar *v.* to assimilate.

asinergia *f.* asynergia, lack of coordination among normally harmonious organs.

asintomático-a *a.* asymptomatic, without symptoms.

asistencia *f.* 1. assistance, care, help; ___ **medico-sanitaria** / health and medical ___; ___ **social** / welfare; ___ **social a la infancia** / child welfare; **recibir** ___ / to be on relief; 2. attendance.

asistente *m., f.* attendant, assistant.

asistir *v.* to attend; to help.

asistolia *f.* asystole, asystolia, absence of heart contractions.

asma *m.* asthma, allergic condition that causes bouts of short breath, wheezing, and edema of the mucosa. ___ **cardíaca** / cardiac ___ .

asmático-a *a.* asthmatic, rel. to or suffering from asthma.

asociación *f.* association.

asociado-a *m., f.* associate.

asombrar *v.* to amaze; **asombrarse** *vr.* to be amazed.

aspartamo *m.* aspartame, low calorie sweetener.

aspartato *m.* aspartate, a salt or ester of aspartic acid.

aspartato amino transferasa *m.* aspartate amino transferase, diagnostic aid in viral hepatitis and in myocardial infarction.

aspecto *m.* appearance, aspect.

aspereza *f.* roughness, harshness.

Asperger, syndrome de *m.* Asperger's disorder, characterized by impairment in social skills, pedantic speech, superficial interests, however having a normal IQ.

aspergiloma *m.* aspergilloma, a mass of *Aspergillus hyphae* colonizing an invaded cavity of the lung.

aspergilosis *f.* aspergillosis, infection caused by the fungi *Aspergillus hyphae* that gen. affects the sense of hearing.

aspermia *f.* aspermia, failure to form or emit semen.

áspero-a *a.* rough, harsh; **piel** ___ / ___ skin.

aspersión nasal *f.* the act of using nasal spray.

aspiración *f.* aspiration, inhalation.

aspirar *v.* to breathe in, to inhale; ___ **por la mucosa nasal** / to snort.

aspirina *f.* aspirin, a derivative of salicylic acid.

astigmatismo *m.* astigmatism, defective curvature of the refractive surfaces of the eye.

astilla *f.* splinter.

astrágalo *m.* astragalus, ankle bone.

astringente *m.* astringent, agent that has the power to constrict tissues and mucous membranes.

astrocitoma *f.* astrocytoma, brain tumor.

asunto *m.* subject, matter; business.

asustado-a *a.* frightened, startled.

asustar *v.* to frighten, to scare; **asustarse** *vr.* to become frightened.

ataque *m.* attack, fit, stroke, bout, seizure; ___ **cardíaco** / heart ___ .

ataraxia *f.* ataraxia, impassiveness.

atareado-a *a.* busy.

ataúd *m.* coffin, casket.

atavismo *m.* atavism, inherited trait from remote ancestors.

ataxia *f.* ataxia, deficiency in muscular coordination; ___ **sifilítica** / tabes dorsal.

atelectasia *f.* atelectasis, partial or total collapse of a lung.

atención *f.* attention; care; courtesy;___ **a largo plazo** / long term ___; ___ **de especialidad** / specialty ___; ___ **del neonato** / newborn ___; ___ **dirigida** / managed ___; ___ **domiciliaria** / home ___; **falta de** ___ / lack of ___; ___ **holística** / holistic ___; ___ **intraparto** / labor ___; ___ **médica** / medical care; ___ **médica laboral** / occupational ___; **prestar** ___ / to pay ___; ___ **temporal** / respite ___; ___ **sanitaria preventiva** / preventive health ___ .

atender *v.* to attend, to look after; to pay attention.

atento-a *a.* attentive; polite; **estar** ___ / to be ___ .

atenuación *f.* attenuation, rendering less virulent.

ateo-a *m., f.* atheist.

aterectomía coronaria *f.* coronary atherectomy, removal of obstructions from the coronary artery by use of a cardiac catheter.

atérmico-a *a.* athermic, without fever.

ateroma *f.* atheroma, fatty deposits in the intima of an artery.

atetosis *f.* athetosis, infantile spasmodic paraplegia.

atleta *m.* athlete.

atlético-a *a.* athletic.

atmósfera *f.* atmosphere.

atmósferico-a *a.* atmospheric.

atolondrado-a *a.* confused, bewildered.

atolondramiento *m.* confusion, bewilderment.

atomizador *m.* atomizer.

átomo *m.* atom.

atonía *f.* atony, lack of normal tone, esp. in the muscles.

atontado-a *a.* stunned, stupefied.

atopía *f.* atopy, type of allergy considered as having a hereditary tendency.

atópico-a *a.* rel. to atopy.

atorarse *vr.* to gag, to choke.

atormentar *v.* to torment.

atrás *adv.* behind; **ir hacia** ___ / to go backwards.

atrasado-a *a.* backward, late, behind; ___ **mental** / mentally retarded.

atravesar *v.* to cross; to go through; ___ **la calle** / ___ the street.

atresia *f.* atresia, congenital absence or closure of a body passage.

atreverse *vr.* to dare, to take a chance.

atrevido-a *a.* daring; insolent.

atrial *a.* atrial, rel. to an atrium; **defecto septal** ___ / ___ septal defect.

atribuir *vi.* to attribute; to confer.

atrio *m.* atrium. 1. cavity that is connected to another structure; 2. upper chamber of the heart that receives the blood from the veins.

atrioventricular, auriculoventricular *a.* atrioventricular, auriculoventricular, rel. to an atrium and a ventricle of the heart, **nudo** ___ / ___ node; **orificio** ___ / ___ orifice.

atrofia *f.* atrophy, deterioration of cells, tissue, and organs of the body. ___ **artrítica** /

arthritic ___; ___ **alveolar** / alveolar ___; ___
amarilla aguda hepática / acute yellow ___ of
the liver; ___ **cerebelosa** / cerebellar ___; ___
cerebelar de tipo nutricional / nutritional type
cerebellar ___; ___ **cerebral progresiva** /
progressive cerebral ___; ___ **de sistema**
múltiple / multiple system ___; ___ **epiléptica** /
epileptic ___; ___ **infantil músculo-espinal**
progresiva / infantile progressive spinal-
muscular ___; ___ **macular primaria de la**
piel / primary macular ___ of skin; ___
muscular espinal juvenil / juvenile spinal
muscular ___; ___ **muscular isquémica** /
ischemic muscular ___; ___ **macular** /
macular ___; ___ **neurogénica** /
neurogenic ___; ___ **periodontal** /
periodontal ___; ___ **postmenopáusica** /
postmenopausal ___; ___ **senil** / senil ___ .
atropellar *v.* to run over, to trample.
atropina *f.* atropine sulphate, agent used as a
muscle relaxer, esp. applied to the eyes to dilate
the pupil and paralyze the ciliary muscle during
eye examination.
atún *m.* tuna fish.
aturdido-a *a.* confused, stunned.
aturdimiento *m.* confusion, bewilderment.
aturdir *v.* to stun; to confuse.
audición *f.* audition, sense of hearing; **pérdida**
de la ___ / hearing loss.
audífono *m.* hearing aid.
audiograma *m.* audiogram, instrument that
records the degree of hearing.
audiovisual *a.* audiovisual, rel. to hearing and
vision.
auditivo-a, auditorio-a *a.* auditory, rel. to
hearing; **conducto** ___ / ___ canal ;
nervio ___ / ___ nerve; **tapón** ___ / ear plug.
aumentar *v.* to increase, to augment, to
magnify; ___ **de peso** / to gain weight.
aumento *m.* increase.
aún *adv.* still, yet; ___ **cuando** / even though.
aunque *conj.* although.
aura *f.* aura, sensation preceding an epileptic
attack.
aurícula *f.* auricle. 1. the outer visible part of the
ear; 2. either of the two upper chambers of the
heart.
auricular *m.* earphone; *a.* 1. rel. to the sense of
hearing; 2. rel. to an auricle of the heart.
auscultación *f.* auscultation, the act of listening
to sounds arising from organs such as the lungs
and the heart for diagnostic purposes.
auscultar *v.* to auscultate, to examine by
auscultation.

ausencia *f.* absence.
ausente *a.* absent; missing.
autismo *m.* autism, behavioral disorder
manifested by extreme self-centeredness; ___
infantil / infantile ___ .
autístico-a *a.* autistic, suffering from or rel. to
autism.
autoclave *f.* autoclave, an instrument for
sterilizing by steam pressure.
autóctono-a *a.* native, autochthonous,
indigenous.
autodigestión *f.* autodigestion, digestion of
tissues by their own enzymes and juices.
autógeno-a *a.* autogenous, produced within the
individual.
autohipnosis *f.* autohypnosis, self-hypnosis.
autoinfección *f.* autoinfection, infection by an
agent from the same body.
autoinjerto *m.* autograft, autogenous implant
taken from another part of the patient's body.
autoinmunización *f.* autoimmunization,
immunity resulting from a substance developed
within the affected person's own body.
autoinoculable *a.* autoinoculable, susceptible
to a germ from within.
autólogo-a *a.* autologous, derived from the same
individual.
automatismo *m.* automatism, behavior not
under voluntary control.
automedicación *f.* self-medication.
automóvil *m.* automobile.
autonomía *f.* autonomy.
autónomo-a *a.* autonomic, autonomous, that
functions independently; **sistema**
nervioso ___ / ___ nervous system.
autoplastia *f.* autoplasty, implantation of an
autograft.
autoplástico-a *a.* autoplastic, rel. to
autoplasty.
autopsia *f.* autopsy, postmortem examination of
the body.
autorización *f.* authorization.
autorizar *vi.* to authorize.
autosugestión *f.* autosuggestion, self-suggested
thought.
autotrasplante *m.* autotransplant, autologous
graft.
auxilio *m.* aid, help; **primeros** ___-s / first ___ .
avanzar *vi.* to advance.
avena *f.* oats; **harina de** ___ / oatmeal.
aventado-a *a.* bloated.
aventarse *vr.* to become bloated.

aversión *f.* aversion, dislike.
aviso *m.* notice; **dar** ___ / to notify.
avispa *f.* wasp; **picadura de** ___ / ___ sting.
avispón *m.* hornet.
avitaminosis *f.* avitaminosis, disorder caused by a lack of vitamins.
avivar *v.* to liven up; to strengthen.
avulsión *f.* avulsion, removal or extraction of part of a structure.
axénico-a *a.* axenic, germ-free.
axial *a.* axial, rel. to the axis.
axila *f.* axilla, armpit.
axilar *a.* axillary, rel. to the axilla.
axis *m.* axis, imaginary central line passing through the body or through an organ.
ayer *adv.* yesterday.

Ayerza, síndrome de *m.* Ayerza's syndrome, syndrome manifested by multiple symptoms, esp. dyspnea and cyanosis, gen. as a result of pulmonary deficiency.
ayuda *f.* help; **sin** ___ / unassisted.
ayudante *m., f.* helper.
ayudar *v.* to help, to assist.
ayunar *v.* to fast.
ayuno *m.* fast.
azoospermia *f.* azoospermia, lack of spermatozoa in the semen.
azotemia *f.* azotemia, excess urea in the blood.
azúcar *m.* sugar, carbohydrate consisting essentially of sucrose; ___ **de la uva** / grape ___ , dextrose.
azufre *m.* sulfur.
azul *a.* blue; **mal** ___ / ___ baby.

b

b *abr.* **bacilo** / bacillus; **bucal** / buccal.
baba *f.* spittle.
babear *v.* to slobber.
babero *m.* bib.
Babinski reflejo de *m.* Babinski's reflex, dorsiflexion of the big toe when the sole of the foot is stimulated.
bacalao *m.* codfish.
bacilar *a.* bacillary, rel. to bacillus.
bacilemia *f.* bacillemia, presence of bacilli in the blood.
bacilo *m. bacilli* bacillus rod-shaped bacteria; ____ **de Calmette-Guérin** / Calmette-Guérin bacillus, bacile bilié; ____ **de Koch** / Koch's ____ , *Mycobacterium tuberculosis*; ____ **de la fiebre tifoidea** / typhoid ____ , Salmonella typhi; **portador de** ____ **-s** / bacilli carrier.
bacilosis *f.* bacillosis, infection caused by bacilli.
baciluria *f.* bacilluria, presence of bacilli in the urine.
bacín *m.* basin, large bowl; bedpan.
bacitracina *f.* bacitracin, antibiotic effective against some staphylococci.
bacteremia *f.* bacteremia, presence of bacteria in the blood.
bacteria *f.* bacterium; germ.
bacteriano-a *a.* bacterial; **infecciones** ____ **-s** / ____ infections; **endocarditis** ____ / ____ endocarditis; **pruebas de sensibilidad** ____ / ____ sensitivity tests.
bactericida *m.* bactericide, agent that kills bacteria.
bacteriógeno *a.* bacteriogenic. 1. of bacterial origin; 2. that produces bacteria.
bacteriolisina *f.* bacteriolysin, antibody that destroys bacterial cells.
bacteriólisis *f.* bacteriolysis, the destruction of bacteria.
bacteriología *f.* bacteriology, the study of bacteria.
bacteriológico-a *a.* bacteriologic, bacteriological, rel. to bacteria.
bacteriólogo-a *m., f.* bacteriologist, specialist in bacteriology.
bacteriosis *f.* bacteriosis, an infection caused by bacteria.

bacteriostático-a *a.* bacteriostatic, that inhibits the growth or multiplication of bacteria.
bacteriuria *f.* bacteriuria, presence of bacteria in the urine.
Bacteroides *m. pl. Bacteroides*, a type of anaerobic bacteria, having gram-negative rods that constitute part of the normal flora of the intestinal tract and is present in less degree in the respiratory and urogenital cavities. Some species are pathogenic.
baipás *m.* bypass; surgically created alternate channel or route; derivación. ____ **aortoilíaco** / aortoiliac ____ ; ____ **aortorrenal** / aortorenal ____ ; ____ **cardiopulmonar** / cardiopulmonary ____ ; ____ **coronario** / coronary ____ ; ____ **extracraneal-intracraneal** / extracranial-intracranial ____ ; ____ **o derivación aortocoronaria** / aortocoronary ____ ; *v.* to move new flow of fluids from one body part to another through a diversionary channel.
bajar *v.* [*escaleras*] to go down; [*movimiento*] to lower; ____ **de peso** / to lose weight; ____ **el brazo** / to lower the arm.
bajo-a *a.* low, short; **presión** ____ / ____ blood pressure; **bajo** *prep.* under; ____ **observación** / ____ observation; ____ **tratamiento** / ____ treatment.
bala *f.* bullet; **herida de** ____ / ____ wound.
balance *m.* balance, equilibrium, quantities and concentrations of parts and fluids that in a normal form constitute the human body; ____ **acidobásico** / acid-base ____ ; ____ **hídrico** / fluid ____ .
balanceado-a *a.* balanced; in a state of equilibrium.
balanitis *f.* balanitis, an infl. of the glans penis, gen. accompanied by infl. of the prepuce.
balanopostitis *f.* balanoposthitis, infl. of the glans penis and prepuce.
balanza *f.* balance, scale, device to measure weights.
balbucear *v.* to babble.
baldado-a *a.* maimed, crippled.
balón *m.* balloon; ____ **insuflable** / ____ tamponade.
balsámico-a *a.* balmy.
bálsamo *m.* balsam, soothing agent.
banana *f.* banana.
banco *m.* bank; bench.
bandeja *f.* tray.
bañar *v.* to bathe. **bañarse** *vr.* to take a bath.
bañadera, bañera *f.* bathtub.
baño *m.* bath, bathroom; ____ **aceitado** / oil ____ ; ____ **antipirético** / antipyretic ____ , to

reduce fever; ___ **aromático** / aromatic ___; ___ **cinetoterapéutico** / kinetotherapeutic ___; ___ **completo** / full ___; ___ **con esponja** / sponge ___; ___ **con inmersión** / immersion ___; ___ **de agua caliente** / hot ___; ___ **de agua fría** / cold ___; ___ **de agua tibia** / warm ___; ___ **de asiento caliente** / Sitz ___ , from the waist down; ___ **de remolino** / whirlpool ___; **cuarto de** ___ / bathroom; **papel de** ___ / toilet tissue.

baragnosis *f.* baragnosis, inability to recognize weight and pressure.

barato-a *a.* inexpensive.

barba *f.* beard.

barbilla *f.* chin, the tip of the chin.

barbituratos *m.* barbiturates, derivatives of barbituric acid.

barbitúrico *m.* barbiturate, hypnotic and sedative agent.

barestesia *f.* baresthesia, the sensation of pressure or weight.

barifonia *f.* baryphonia, thick, heavy voice.

bario *m.* barium, ingested suspension of barium sulfate to be used as a contrast media in a radiography of the hypopharynx and the esophagus.

barorreceptor *m.* baroreceptor, a sensory nerve ending that reacts to changes in pressure.

barotrauma *m.* barotrauma, physical lesion due to a lack of balance between an affected cavity and environmental pressure, as seen in scuba divers affected by decompression sickness (the bends).

barrer *v.* to sweep.

barrera *f.* barrier, obstacle.

barrera hematoencefálica *f.* brain barrier.

barriga *f.* belly; **dolor de** ___ / ___ ache.

barrigón-a *a. pop.* pot-bellied.

barrio *m.* neighborhood.

barro *m.* blackhead, pimple; mud.

bartolinitis *f.* bartholinitis, infl. of Bartholin's vulvovaginal gland.

Bartolino, glándula de *f.* Bartholin's vulvovaginal gland.

basal *a.* basal, pertaining or close to a base; **enfermedad de los ganglios** ___ **-es** / ___ ganglia disease; **metabolismo** ___ / ___ metabolic rate.

basca *f.* náusea.

base *f.* base, foundation.

basial, basilar *a.* basal, basilar, rel. to a base.

básico-a *a.* basic.

basiloma *f.* basiloma, carcinoma composed by basal cells.

basofobia *f.* basophobia, fear of walking.

bastante *a.* sufficient, enough.

bastar *v.* to be enough; **bastarse** *vr.* to be self-sufficient.

bastardo-a *m., f.* bastard; *a.* bastard, illegitimate.

bastón *m.* cane.

bastoncillo *m.* rod; ___ **-s y conos** / ___ -s and cones, sensitive receptors of the retina.

basura *f.* garbage, trash, refuse; **cesto de** ___ / wastebasket.

bata *f.* gown, housecoat.

batalla *f.* battle, struggle.

batallar *v.* to struggle.

batir *v.* to whip; beat; pound.

bazo *m.* spleen, vascular lymphatic organ situated in the abdominal cavity; ___ **accesorio** / accessory ___ .

bebé *m.* baby, infant.

bebedero *m.* drinking fountain.

beber *v.* to drink.

bebida *f.* beverage; **dado a la** ___ / heavy drinker.

beca *a.* scholarship, grant.

bel *m.* bel, a unit of sound intensity.

beligerante *a.* belligerent.

Bell, parálisis de *f.* Bell's palsy, paralysis of one side of the face caused by an affliction of the facial nerve.

belladona *f.* belladona, medicinal herb whose leaves and roots contain atropine and related alkaloids.

bello-a *a.* beautiful.

Bencedrina *f.* Benzedrine, trade name for amphetamine sulfate.

Benedict, prueba de *f.* Benedict's test, chemical analysis to determine the presence of sugar in the urine.

benefactor-a *m., f.* benefactor.

beneficiado-a *a.* beneficiary.

beneficiar *v.* to do good; **beneficiarse** *vr.* to benefit, to profit.

beneficio *m.* benefit; **asignación de** ___ / allocation of ___; ___ **-s de asistencia social** / welfare ___ -s.

benigno-a *a.* benign.

benjuí *m.* benzoin, resin used as an expectorant.

béquico *m.* cough medicine.

beriberi *m.* beriberi, endemic neuritis caused by a deficiency of thiamine in the diet.

berrinche *m.* tantrum, fit of anger.

berro *m.* watercress.

besar *v.* to kiss.

beso *m.* kiss.

bestialidad *f.* bestiality, sexual relations with an animal.

bezoar *m.* bezoar, concretion found in the stomach or the intestines constituted by elements such as hair or vegetable fibers.

biaxial *a.* biaxial, having two axes.

biberón *m.* baby bottle; **suplemento con ___ /** bottle propping.

bibliografía *f.* bibliography.

biblioteca *f.* library.

bicarbonato *m.* bicarbonate, a salt of carbonic acid.

bicarbonato de sodio *m.* baking soda.

bíceps *m.* biceps muscle.

bicicleta *f.* bicycle; **___ estacionaria /** stationary ___ .

bicipital *a.* bicipital. 1. rel. to the biceps muscle; 2. having two heads.

bicóncavo-a *a.* biconcave, having two concave surfaces as in a lens.

biconvexo-a *a.* biconvex, with two convex surfaces as in a lens.

bicúspide *a.* bicuspid, having two points.

bicho *m.* bug, insect.

bien *adv.* well; **todo va o está ___ /** all is well.

bienestar *m.* well-being, welfare, solace.

bienvenida *f.* welcome.

bienvenido-a *a.* welcome, pleasant; well received.

bífido-a *a.* bifid, split in two.

bifocal *a.* bifocal, having two foci.

bifurcación *f.* bifurcation, division into two branches or parts.

bigeminia *f.* bigeminy, two pulse beats occurring in rapid succession.

bigote *m.* moustache.

bilabial *a.* bilabial, having two lips.

bilateral *a.* bilateral, having or rel. to two sides.

bilharziasis *f.* bilharziasis. esquistosomiasis.

biliar *a.* biliary, rel. to the bile, to the bile ducts, or to the gallbladder; **ácidos y sales ___ -es /** acids and salts; **conductos ___ -es /** bile ducts; **cálculo ___ /** gallstone; **enfermedades de los conductos ___ -es /** tract diseases; **obstrucción del conducto ___ /** ___ duct obstruction; **pigmentos ___ -es /** ___ pigments;

bilinge *a.* bilingual.

biliosidad *f.* biliousness, disorder manifested by constipation, headache, and indigestion due to excess secretion of bile.

bilioso-a *a.* bilious, excess bile.

bilirrubina *f.* bilirubin, a red pigment of the bile.

bilirrubinemia *f.* bilirubinemia, presence of bilirubin in the blood.

bilirrubinuria *f.* bilirubinuria, presence of bilirubin in the urine.

bilis *f.* bile, gall, bitter secretion stored in the gallbladder.

bimanual *a.* bimanual, performed with both hands.

binario-a *a.* binary, consisting of two of the same.

biociencia *f.* bioscience, any of the natural sciences that is concerned with the study of behavior and structure of living organisms.

bioensayo *m.* bioassay, sampling the effect of a drug on an animal to determine its potency.

biofísico-a *m., f.* health specialist.

biología *f.* biology, the study of live organisms; **___ celular /** cellular ___ ; **___ molecular /** molecular ___ .

biológico-a *a.* biologic, biological, rel. to biology; **análisis ___ /** ___ assay; **control ___ /** ___ control; **evolución ___ /** ___ evolution; **guerra ___ /** ___ warfare; **indicador ___ /** ___ indicator; **inmunoterapia ___ /** ___ immunotherapy; **semivida ___ /** ___ half-life; **siquiatría ___ /** ___ psychiatry.

biólogo-a *m., f.* biologist.

biomedicina *f.* biomedicine, a branch of medicine that applies biological and physiological norms to clinical practice.

biomédico-a *a.* biomedical, rel. to fields of the natural sciences, esp. the biologic and physiologic sciences that interrelate with medicine.

biométrica *f.* biometrics, a branch of biology concerned with the study of biological phenomena and its observations by using statistical analysis.

biopsia *f.* biopsy, procedure to remove sample tissue for diagnostic examination; **___ abierta por excisión /** open ___ by excision; **___ con cepillo /** brush ___ ; **___ de aguja fina /** fine needle ___ ; **___ de espécimen cuneiforme /** specimen wedge ___ ; **___ de la arteria temporal /** temporal artery ___ ; **___ de la mama /** ___ of the breast; **___ de la médula ósea /** bone marrow ___ ; **___ del cuello uterino /** ___ of the cervix; **___ del ganglio vigilante /** sentinel node ___ ; **___ del nódulo linfático /** ___ of lymph nodes; ___

endoscópica / endoscopic ___; ___ **muscular** / muscle ___; ___ **por ablación** / ___ by ablation; ___ **por aspiración** / aspiration ___ ; needle ___; ___ **por excisión** / excision ___; ___ **por incisión** / incision ___ .

bioquímica *f.* biochemistry, the chemistry of living organisms.

biosíntesis *f.* biosynthesis, formation of chemical substances in the physiological processes of living organisms.

biotipo *m.* biotype, group of individuals with the same genotype.

bípedo *m.* biped, two-legged animal.

birrefringente *a.* birefringent, refracting twice.

bisabuelo-a *m., f.* great-grandfather; great-grandmother.

bisagra *f.* hinge; **movimiento de** ___ / ___ movement.

bisexual *a.* bisexual. 1. having gonads of both sexes, hermaphrodite; 2. having sexual relations with both sexes.

bisinosis *f.* bissinosis, obstructive airway disease suffered by workers of unprocessed cotton, flax, or hemp, caused by reaction to the dust that may include endotoxin from bacterial contamination. Known as "Monday morning asthma" or "cotton-dust asthma."

bisturí *m.* scalpel, surgical knife.

Bitot, manchas de *f., pl.* Bitot spots, small triangular gray spots that appear in the conjunctiva and are associated with a deficiency of vitamin B.

bizco-a *a.* cross-eyed.

biznieto-a *m., f.* great-grandson; great-grand-daughter.

bizquera *f.* squint, the condition of being cross-eyed. estrabismo.

Blalock-Tausig, operación de *f.* Blalock-Tausig operation, surgery to repair a congenital malformation of the heart.

blanco *m.* target. 1. an object or area at which something is directed; 2. a cell or organ that is affected by a particular agent such as a drug or a hormone; 3. the color white. *-a / a.* white.

blancura *f.* whiteness.

blancuzco-a *a.* whitish.

blando-a *a.* soft, bland.

blanquear *v.* to bleach.

blastema *f.* blastema, primitive mass substance from which cells are formed.

blastomicosis *f.* blastomycosis, infectious fungus disease.

blástula *f.* blastula, an early stage of the embryo.

blefarectomía *f.* blepharectomy, excision of a lesion of the eyelid.

blefaritis *f.* blepharitis, infl. of the eyelid.

blefarocalasis *f.* blepharochalasis, relaxation of the skin of the upper eyelid due to loss of interstitial elasticity.

blefaroplastia *f.* blepharoplasty, plastic surgery of the eyelids.

blefaroplejía *f.* blepharoplegia, paralysis of the eyelid.

blenorragia *f.* blennorrhagia. 1. discharge of mucus; 2. gonorrhea.

bloqueado-a *a.* blocked, obstructed.

bloqueador *m.* blocker, ___ **de canal cálcico, antagonista cálcico** / calcium channel ___ .

bloqueo *m.* block, stoppage, obstruction; ___ **atrioventricular** / heart ___ , atrioventricular, interruption in the A-V node; ___ **de rama** / heart ___ , bundle-branch; ___ **interventricular** / heart, ___ interventricular; ___ **senoatrial** / heart ___ , sinoatrial.

blusa *f.* blouse.

bobería *f.* foolishness.

bobo-a *m., f.* fool, simpleton; *a.* silly, foolish.

boca *f.* mouth; ___ **abajo** / face-down; ___ **arriba** / face-up; **por la** ___ / by mouth, orally.

boca de trinchera *f.* trench mouth, infection with ulceration of the mucous membranes of the mouth and the pharynx.

bocado *m.* mouthful, bite.

bochorno *m.* embarrassment.

bocio *m.* goiter, enlargement of the thyroid gland; ___ **coloide endémico** / endemic, colloid ___; ___ **congénito** / congenital ___; ___ **exoftálmico** / exophthalmic ___; ___ **móvil** / wandering ___; ___ **tóxico** / toxic ___ .

bofetada *f.* slap.

bofetón *m.* hard blow, forceful slap.

bola *f.* ball; ___ **adiposa** / fat pad; ___ **de pelo** / hair ___ , a type of bezoar.

bolo *m.* bolus, 1. a specific amount of a given substance administered intravenously; 2. dose in a rounded mass given to obtain an immediate response; 3. mass of soft consistency ready to be ingested; ___ **alimenticio** / alimentary ___; **infusión en** ___ / bolus ___ .

bolsa *f.* sac; bag; handbag, pouch, pocket; ___ **amniótica** (*de agua*) / amniotic ___ (water bag); ___ **de agua caliente** / hot water bottle; ___ **de hielo** / icepack; ___ **de papel** / paper bag; ___ **eléctrica** / heating pad.

bolsillo *m.* pocket.

bomba *f.* pump; ___ **de angioplastia /** angioplasty ___; ___ **desmontable /** detachable ___; ___ **gástrica /** stomach ___; ___ **intravenosa /** intravenous ___; ___ **oxigenadora /** oxygenator ___ .

bomba-balón *f.* belloon-pump.1. an expandable device used to support several body structures; 2. an inflatable device used to widening or stretching a blood vessel.

bombear *v.* to pump; ___ **hacia afuera /** to ___ out.

bombeo *m.* pumping; ___ **del corazón /** heart ___; ___ **estomacal /** stomach ___ .

bombero-a *m., f.* firefighter.

bombilla *f.* light bulb.

bondadoso-a *a.* kind.

boniato *m.* sweet potato.

bonito-a *a.* pretty.

bonito *m.* tuna fish.

boquiabierto-a *a.* open-mouthed.

borato de sodio *m.* borax.

borde *m.* border, rim, edge; ___ **bermellón /** vermillion ___, the exposed pink margin of a lip.

bordeando *a.* bordering.

borrachera *f.* drunken spree.

borracho-a *a.* drunk.

borradura, borramiento *f. m.* effacement, obliteration of an organ, such as the cervix during labor.

borrar *v.* to erase, scrape; wipe out.

bosquejo *m.* profile.

bostezar *vi.* to yawn.

bostezo *m.* yawn; yawning.

bota *f.* boot; ___ **enyesada /** short-leg cast.

botar *v.* to throw away; to hurl.

botella *f.* bottle.

botica *f.* drugstore, pharmacy.

boticario-a *m., f.* druggist, pharmacist.

botiquín *m.* medicine cabinet; ___ **de primeros auxilios /** first aid kit.

botón *m.* button; ___ **para llamar /** push ___ .

botulismo *m.* botulism, food poisoning caused by a toxin that grows in improperly canned or preserved foods.

bóveda *f.* vault, dome-shaped anatomical structure.

bovino *a.* bovine, rel. to cattle.

BRCA 1 cáncer del seno *m.* BRCA 1 acronym for breast cancer, belongs to the gene of the breast cancer found in a low percentage of women descending from relatives who suffered from that type of cancer.

BRCA 2 cáncer uterino *m.* BRCA 2 uterine cancer, acronym of the cancer gene that is found in a low percentage of women descending from relatives who suffered that type of cancer.

bracero *m.* farmhand; laborer.

bradicardia *f.* bradycardia, abnormally slow heart beat.

bradipnea *f.* bradypnea, abnormally slow respiration.

braditaquicardia *f.* bradytachycardia, cardiac frequency alternating from very high to very low cardiac rates.

braguero *m.* truss, binding device used to keep a reduced hernia in place; brace; ___ **de cuello /** neck ___ .

Braille, sistema de lectura *m.* Braille reading system, a method of writing and printing of raised dots that distinguishes letters, numbers, and punctuation and enables the blind to read by touching.

braquial *a.* brachial, rel. to the arm; **músculo** ___ / ___ muscle.

braquidactilia *f.* brachydactyly, abnormally short fingers and toes.

braquiocefálico-a *a.* brachiocephalic, rel. to the arm and the head.

bravo-a *a.* angry; brave.

brazalete de identificación *m.* identification bracelet.

brazo *m.* arm.

brea *f.* tar.

bregma *m.* bregma, the point in the skull at the junction of the sagittal and coronal sutures.

breve *a.* brief; short; **en** ___ / in short, briefly.

Bright, enfermedad de *f.* Bright's disease. glomerulonephritis. V. glomerulonefritis.

brillante *a.* bright.

brincar *vi.* to hop, to skip.

brindar *v.* to offer.

brisa *f.* breeze.

broma *f.* joke; **en** ___ / jokingly, kidding.

bromidrosis *f.* bromhidrosis, fetid perspiration.

bromo, bromuro *m.* bromide, nonmetallic element, member of the halogen group, very irritating to mucous membranes. It is used as oxidant and antiseptic.

bronceado-a *a.* bronzed.

broncoalveolar *a.* bronchoalveolar, *Syn.* **bronchovesicular.**

broncoconstricción *f.* bronchoconstriction, diminution in the caliber of a bronchus.

broncodilatación *f.* bronchodilation, dilation of a bronchus.

broncodilatador *m.* bronchodilator, agent that dilates the caliber of a bronchus; *-a; a.* **agentes** ___ **-es /** ___ agents.

broncoesofagoscopía *f.* bronchoesophagoscopy, examination of the bronchi and esophagus with an instrument.

broncoespasmo *m.* bronchospasm, spasmodic contraction of the bronchi and bronchioles.

broncoespirometría *f.* bronchospirometry, process of measuring the ventilatory function of each lung by using a bronchospirometer.

broncofibroscopía *f.* bronchofibroscopy, test done with a flexible fiberoptic bronchoscope for diagnostic purposes, or to remove foreign bodies from the bronchi.

broncógeno-a *a.* bronchogenic, rel. to or originating in the bronchus. **carcinoma** ___ / ___ carcinoma; **quiste** ___ / ___ cyst.

broncografía *f.* bronchography, x-ray of the tracheobronchial tree using an opaque medium in the bronchi.

broncolito *m.* broncholith, a bronchial calculus.

bronconeumonía *f.* bronchopneumonia, acute infl. of the bronchi and the alveoli of the lungs.

broncopulmonar *a.* bronchopulmonary, rel. to the bronchi and the lungs. **ganglios linfáticos** ___ **-es /** ___ lymph nodes; **lavado** ___ / ___ lavage.

broncoscopía *f.* bronchoscopy, inspection of the bronchi with a bronchoscope.

broncoscopío *m.* bronchoscope, instrument to examine the interior of the bronchi. ___ **de fibra óptica /** fiberoptic ___; ___ **con láser /** laser ___ .

broncostomía *f.* bronchostomy, surgical formation of a new opening into a bronchus.

broncotomograma *m.* bronchotomogram, image taken using computerized tomography of the upper respiratory track from the trachea to the lower inferior bronchi.

broncovesicular *a.* bronchovesicular, rel. to the bronchi and alveoli, esp. in regard to the sounds heard in auscultation. *Syn:* **broncoalveolar.**

bronquial *a.* bronchial, rel. to the bronchi; **adenoma** ___ / ___ adenoma; **árbol** ___ / ___ tree; **arco** ___ / ___ arch; **asma** ___ / ___ asthma ; **bloqueo** ___ / ___ blockade; **espasmo** ___ / ___ spasm; **estenosis** ___ / ___ stenosis; **fisura** ___ / ___ cleft; **glándulas bronquiales /** ___ glands; **lavado** ___ / ___ washing; **lesion del plexo** ___ / ___ plexus injury; **venas bronquiales /** ___ veins.

bronquiectasia *f.* bronchiectasis, chronic dilation of the bronchi due to an inflammatory disease or obstruction.

bronquio *m. bronquios* bronchi, part of the trachea, passageways of the respiratory tract. Both of the bronchi (right and left) resemble the branches of a tree as they subdivide in smaller passways and are called bronchioli or conducting tubes. ___ **intermedio /** intermediate ___; ___ **lobar /** lobar ___; ___ **lobar izquierdo /** left lobar ___; ___ **principal /** main ___; ___ **principal derecho /** right main ___; ___ **principal izquierdo /** left main ___; ___ **superior a una arteria /** eparterial ___; **impacto mucoso del** ___ / mucoid impaction of ___ .

bronquiocele *m.* bronchiocele, a localized dilation of a bronchus.

bronquiolitis *f.* bronchiolitis, infl. of the bronchioles.

bronquiolo *m.* bronchiole, one of the small branches of the bronquial tree.

bronquitis *f.* bronchitis, infl. of the bronchial tubes.

brotar *v.* to flare up.

brote *m.* flare-up, outburst, outbreak, reddening of the skin due to a lesion, infection, or allergic reaction.

brucelosis *f.* brucellosis, Mediterranean fever, undulant fever, disease caused by bacteria obtained through contact with infected animals or their by-products.

Bruck, enfermedad de *f.* Bruck disease, sickness manifested in imperfect osteogenesis, joint ankylosis, and muscular atrophy.

brusco-a *a.* abrupt, rude.

brutal *a.* brutal.

bruto-a *a.* stupid; rough.

bubón *m.* bubo, swelling of one or more lymph nodes, esp. in the axilla or groin.

bucal *a.* buccal, rel. to the mouth; **antiséptico** ___ / mouthwash; **higiene** ___ / oral hygiene; **por vía** ___ / by mouth.

buche *m.* mouthful; **un** ___ **de agua /** a ___ of water.

bucogingival *a.* buccogingival, rel. to the mouth and the gums.

bucolabial *a.* buccolabial, rel. to the lips and the cheeks.

bueno-a *a.* good, kind; **buenas noches /** [*saludo*] good evening, [*despedida*] good night; **buenas tardes /** good afternoon; **buenos días /** good morning ; **de buena fé /** in good faith.

bulbo *m.* bulb, circular or oval expansion of a tube or cylinder; ___ **piloso** / hair ___ .

bulbo cavernoso *m.* bulbocavernosus, located following the spinal cord.

bulbo raquídeo *m.* medulla oblongata, the most vital part of the brain, it lodges the cardiac center, respiratory center, and the vasomotor center. Connected to the medulla oblongata are the twelve pairs of the cranial nerves.

bulbouretral *a.* bulbourethral, rel. to the bulb of the urethra and the penis.

bulimia *f.* bulimia, hiperorexia, exaggerated appetite.

bulto *m.* lump; swelling; bundle, package.

bunio *m.* bunion, swelling of the bursa on the first joint of the big toe.

bunionectomía *f.* bunionectomy, excision of a bunion.

burbuja *f.* bubble.

burdo-a *a.* coarse; rough.

buril *m.* burr, type of drill used to make openings in bones or teeth.

bursa *f. L.* bursa, saclike cavity containing synovial fluid, situated in tissue areas where friction would otherwise occur; ___ **del tendón calcáneo** / Achille's ___; ___ **popliteal** / popliteal ___ .

bursitis *f.* bursitis, infl. of a bursa.

buscar *vi.* to look for, to search.

búsqueda *f.* search; pursuit.

búster *m.* booster shot, reactivation of an original immunizing agent.

busto *m.* bust.

buzo *m.* diver.

buzón *m.* mailbox.

C

C *abr.* **caloría** / calorie; **centígrado** / centigrade; **carbono** / carbon; **Celsius** / Celsius.

c *abr.* **caloría** / calorie; **cobalt** / cobalto; **cocaína** / cocaine; **contracción** / contraction.

cabalgamiento *m.* [*fracturas*] overriding, the slipping of one part of the bone over the other.

caballero *m.* gentleman.

caballo *m.* horse.

caballo de fuerza *m.* horsepower, a unit of power.

cabecear *v.* to nod; to drop one's head as when snoozing; *pop.* to nod off.

cabecera *f.* head of a bed or table.

cabellera *f.* head of hair.

cabello *m.* hair.

caber *vi.* to fit into something; to have enough room.

cabestrillo *m.* sling, bandage-like support. ___ **de restricción** / restraining ___; ___ **de rodilla** / knee ___; ___ **de suspensión** / suspension ___ .

cabeza *f.* head; **caída de la** ___ / ___ drop; **traumatismo del cráneo, golpe en la** ___ / ___ injury; **apoyo de** ___ / ___ rest; **asentir con la** ___ / to nod one's head.

cabezón-a *a.* big-headed; stubborn.

cabizbajo-a *a.* crestfallen, downcast.

cabra *f.* goat; **leche de** ___ / ___ milk.

caca *f.* excrement, stool of a child.

cacao *m.* cacao. 1. plant from which chocolate is derived; 2. diuretic alkaloid.

cacosmia *f.* cacosmia, perception of imaginary disagreeable odors.

cachetada *f.* slap in the face.

cachete *m.* cheek.

cada *a.* each; ___ **día** / every day; ___ **dos, tres horas** / every two, three hours; ___ **uno-a** / ___ one; ___ **vez** / ___ time.

cadáver *m.* cadaver, corpse.

cadavérico-a *a.* cadaverous, rel. to or having the appearance of a cadaver.

cadena *f.* chain; **reacción en** ___ / ___ reaction; **sutura en** ___ / ___ suture.

cadera *f.* hip; **articulación de la** ___ / ___ joint; ___ **de resorte** / ___ snapping; **dislocación congénita de la** ___ / congenital ___ dislocation; **restitución total de la** ___ / total ___ replacement.

cadmio *m.* cadmium, a bivalent metal similar to tin.

caducidad *f.* 1. expiration date; 2. old age.

caer *vi.* to fall; **caerse** *vr.* to fall down; ___ **muerto** / to drop dead.

café *m.* coffee.

cafeína *f.* caffeine, alkaloid present chiefly in coffee and tea used as a stimulant and diuretic.

cafetería *f.* cafeteria.

caída *f.* fall.

caído-a *a., pp.* of **caer,** fallen.

caja torácica *f.* thoracic cage.

cajero-a *m., f.* cashier.

calabaza *f.* pumpkin, squash.

calambre *m.* cramp, painful contraction of a muscle; ___ **muscular localizado** / Charley horse.

calamina *f.* calamine, astringent and antiseptic used for skin disorders.

calavera *f.* skull.

calcáneo *m.* calcaneus, heel bone.

calcáreo-a *a.* calcareous, rel. to lime or calcium.

calcemia *f.* calcemia, presence of calcium in the blood.

calcetines *m.* socks.

cálcico *a.* calcic, rel. to lime.

calciferol *m.* calciferol, derivative of ergosterol, vitamin D_2.

calcificación *f.* calcification, hardening of organic tissue by deposits of calcium salts.

calcificado-a *a.* calcified.

calcinosis *f.* calcinosis, presence of calcium salts in the skin, subcutaneous tissues, or other organs.

calcio *m.* calcium; **antagonista del** ___ / ___ antagonist.

calcitonina *f.* calcitonin, a hormone secreted by the thyroid gland.

calciuria *f.* calciuria, presence of calcium in the urine.

cálculo *m. caluli* calculus, stone; ___ **biliar** / biliary ___ , gallstone; ___ **de cistina** / cystine ___; ___ **de fibrina** / fibrin ___; ___ **de oxalato de calcio** / calcium oxalate ___; ___ **urinario** / urinary ___ .

caldo *m.* broth, stock; ___ **de pollo** / chicken ___ .

calefacción *f.* heating system; heat.

calendario *m.* calendar.

calentador *m.* heater.

calentamiento *m.* [*acondicionamiento físico*] warm-up.

calentar *vi.* to heat; **calentarse** / *vr.* to warm oneself up.

calentura *f.* fever, temperature.

calenturiento-a *a.* feverish.

calibrador *m.* calibrator, gauge, measuring device.

calibrar *v.* to calibrate; to gauge, to measure the diameter of a canal or tube.

calibre *m.* caliber, the diameter of a tube or canal.

caliceal *a.* caliceal, rel. to the calix.

calicreína *f.* kallicrein, an inactive enzyme present in blood, plasma, and urine, that when activated acts as a powerful vasodilator.

calidad *f.* quality, property.

caliente *a.* hot, warm.

calificar *vi.* to qualify; to correct.

caliuresis *f.* kaliuresis, kaluresis, increased urinary excretion of potassium.

cáliz *m.* calyx, a cup-shaped organ, such as the renal calyx.

calma *f.* calm; calmness; **tener** ___ / to be calm;

calmado-a *a.* calm, serene.

calmante *m.* sedative, tranquilizer; *a.* soothing, mitigating.

calmar *v.* to calm down, to soothe; *calmarse vr.* to become calm.

calomel *m.* calomel, mercurous chloride used primarily as a local antibacterial element.

calor *m.* heat; warmth; ___ **de conducción** / ___ conductive; ___ **de convección** / ___ convective; ___ **seco** / dry ___; **hace** ___ / it is hot; **pérdida de** ___ / ___ loss; **tener** ___ / to be hot;

caloría *f.* calorie, a heat unit, commonly referred to as the energy value of a particular food; **gran** ___ / large ___; ___ **pequeña** / small ___;

calórico-a *a.* caloric, rel. to the energy value of food; **ingestión** ___ / ___ intake;

calostro *m.* colostrum, fluid secreted by the mammary glands before the secretion of milk.

calva *f.* bald crown of the head.

calvaria *f.* calvaria, superior portion of the cranium.

calvicie *f.* calvities, baldness.

calvo-a *a.* bald, without hair.

callado-a *a.* quiet, low-key.

callar *v.* to hush, to silence; *callarse vr.* to become quiet.

calle *f.* street.

callo, callosidad *m., f.* callus, corn.

calloso-a *a.* callous, rel. to a callus.

calzoncillos *m., pl.* men's underpants; shorts.

cama *f.* bed; **al lado de la** ___ / at bedside; **estar en** ___ / to be bedridden; **guardar** ___ / to stay in bed, bedrest; **ocupación de** ___ **-s** / ___ occupancy; **orinarse en la** ___ / bedwetting;

recluido en ___ / bed-confined; **ropa de** ___ / bedclothes;

cámara *f.* 1. chamber, cavity; ___ **acuosa** / aqueous ___; ___ **anterior** / anterior ___; ___ **hiperbárica** / hyperbaric ___; ___ **-s oculares** / ___-s of the eye; 2. photographic camera.

camarón *m.* shrimp.

cambiar *v.* to change; **cambiarse** *vr.* to change clothes.

cambio *m.* change; [*posición*] shift.

camilla *f.* stretcher.

caminar *v.* to walk; to hike.

caminata *f.* a walk; a hike.

camino *m.* road; course, way.

camión *m.* truck; *Mex.* bus.

camisa *f.* shirt; ___ **de fuerza** / straightjacket.

camiseta *f.* men's undershirt; T-shirt.

camisón *m.* nightgown.

campanilla *f.* uvula, epiglottis.

campo *m.* field. 1. area or open space; 2. specialization; ___ **de bajo aumento** / low-power ___; ___ **marginal** / fringe ___; ___ **neuromagnético** / neuromagnetic ___; ___ **visual** / visual ___ .

cana *f.* gray hair.

canal *m.* canal, channel, trough, groove, tubular structure; ___ **del parto** / birth ___; ___ **femoral** / femoral ___; ___ **inguinal** / inguinal ___; ___ **radicular** / root ___ .

canalículo *m.* canaliculus, small channel; ___ **biliar** / biliary ___, between liver cells; ___ **lacrimal, lagrimal** / lacrimal ___ .

canasta *f.* basket.

cancelación *f.* cancellation.

cancelar *v.* to cancel, to annul.

canceloso-a *a.* cancellous, spongy, resembling a lattice.

cáncer *m.* cancer, tumor; ___ **colorectal** / colorectal ___; ___ **incipiente** / early ___; **fases o etapes en relación a la extensión del** ___ / ___ staging; **grado de malignidad del** ___ / ___ grading; **supervivientes de** ___ / ___ survivors.

cancerofobia *f.* cancerophobia, morbid fear of cancer.

canceroso-a *a.* cancerous, rel. to or afflicted by cancer.

candela *f.* fire; flame.

candente *a.* red-hot, burning.

candidiasis *f.* candidiasis, skin infection caused by a yeastlike fungus.

canela *f.* cinnamon.

cangrejo *m.* crab.

canilla *f.* shinbone; tibia.

canino *m.* cuspid tooth; *a.* l. to dogs.

cannabis *L.* cannabis, marijuana, plant whose leaves have a narcotic or hallucinatory effect when smoked.

canoso-a *a.* gray-haired.

cansado-a *a.* tired, weary.

cansancio *m.* tiredness, fatigue.

cansar *v.* to tire; **cansarse** *vr.* to get tired.

cantidad *f.* quantity.

canto *m.* canthus. 1. angles at the corner of the eyes formed by the joining of the external and internal eyelids on both sides of the eye; 2. edge, rim.

cánula *f.* cannula, tube through which fluid and gas are put into the body.

canulación *f.* cannulation, the act of introducing a cannula through a vessel or duct; ___ **aórtica** / aortic ___ .

caolín *m.* kaolin, natural hydrated aluminum silicate having absorbing qualities.

caos *m.* chaos.

capa *f.* layer; ___ **del cuello uterino** / cervical layer.

capacidad *f.* capacity. 1. ability to contain; ___ **de difusión de los pulmones** / diffusion ___ of the lungs; ___ **de memoria** / memory storage ___; ___ **de reserva** / reserve ___; ___ **de sustención** / carrying ___; ___ **inspiratoria** / inspiratory ___; ___ **oxigenadora de la sangre** / oxygen ___ of blood; ___ **vital** / vital ___; 2. qualification, competence.

capaz *a.* able, capable.

capilar *m.* capillary, small blood vessel; ___ **arterial** / arterial ___ , tiny channels carrying arterial blood; ___ **linfático** / lymph ___ , minute vessels of the lymphatic system; ___ **venoso** / venous ___ , small channels carrying venous blood; *a.* resembling hair.

capitelum *L.* capitellum. 1. bulb of a hair; 2. part of the humerus.

capítulo *m.* chapter.

caprichoso-a *a.* capricious; stubborn.

cápsula *f.* capsule, membranous enclosure.

cápsula articular *n.* capsular ligament, fibrous structure lined with synovial membrane surrounding the articulations.

capsulación *f.* capsulation, enclosure in a capsule or sheath.

caquéctico-a *a.* cachectic, rel. to cachexia.

caquexia *f.* cachexia, a grave condition marked by great loss of weight and general weakness.

cara *f.* face; ___ **de luna** / moon ___ , round, puffy face usu. characteristic of someone who

has been under steroid treatment for a long period of time; **peladura de** ___ / ___ peeling; *coloq.* **estiramiento de** ___ / facelift.

caracol *m.* snail.

carácter *m.* 1. character; 2. quality, nature; [actuando en el teatro o cine] actor, actress. **tener buen** ___ / to be good-natured; **tener mal** ___ / to be ill-tempered.

característico-a *a.* characteristic.

caramba *int.* good gracious!

caramelo *m.* hard candy.

carbohidrato *m.* carbohydrate, organic substance composed of carbon, hydrogen, and oxygen such as starch, sugar, and cellulose.

carbólico *a.* carbolic, rel. to phenylic acid.

carbón *m.* coal.

carbonatado-a *a.* carbonated.

carbonización *f.* carbonization

carbonizado-a *a.* charred.

carbono *m.* carbon; **dióxido de** ___ / ___ dioxide; **monóxido de** ___ / ___ monoxide;

carboxihemoglobina *f.* carboxyhemoglobin, a combination of carbon monoxide and hemoglobin that impairs the transportation of oxygen in the blood.

carbunco *m.* carbuncle, large boil of the skin that discharges pus.

cárcel *f.* jail.

carcinogénesis *f.* carcinogenesis, production of cancer.

carcinógeno *m.* carcinogen, cancer producing substance; **-a** *a.* carcinogenic.

carcinoma *m.* carcinoma, cancer derived from living cells of organs. *V.* cuadro en la página 329.

carcinoma in situ *m.* carcinoma in situ, localized tumor cells that have not invaded adjacent structures.

carcinomatosis *f.* carcinomatosis, cancer that has spread throughout the body.

carcinosarcoma *m.* carcinosarcoma, malignant neoplasm with mixed characteristics of carcinoma and sarcoma.

cardíaco-a *a.* cardiac, rel. to the heart; **ápex** ___ / ___ apex; **arritmia** ___ / ___ arrythmia; **asma** ___ / ___ asthma; **ataque** ___ / heart attack; **aurícula** ___ / heart atrium; **auscultación** ___ / ___ examination; **cateterización** ___ / ___ catheterization; **edema** ___ / ___ edema; **esfínter** ___ / ___ sphincter; **estimulación** ___ **artificial** / ___ pacing, artificial; **frecuencia** ___ / heart rate; **gasto o rendimiento** ___ / heart output;

generador del impulso ___ / ___ impulse generator; **insuficiencia** ___ , **ventricular derecha** / heart failure, right-sided; **insuficiencia** ___ , **ventricular izquierda** / heart failure, left-sided; **insuficiencia o fallo** ___ **congestivo** / heart failure, congestive; **masaje** ___ / ___ massage; **paro** ___ / heart arrest, standstill; **reanimación** ___ / ___ resuscitation; **reflejo** ___ / heart reflex; **ruptura** ___ / ___ rupture; **taponamiento** ___ / ___ tamponade; **tonos o ruidos** ___ / ___ sounds. *V.* cuadro en la página 329.

cardias *m.* cardia, esophageal orifice of the stomach.

cardioangiograma *m.* cardioangiogram, image by x-rays of the blood vessels and the chambers of the heart taken after injecting a dye.

cardiocentesis, cardiopuntura *f.* cardiocentesis, puncture or incision of a heart chamber.

cardiodinámica *f.* cardiodynamics, the mechanics of the heart action.

cardioespasmo *m.* cardiospasm, contraction or spasm of the cardia.

cardiogénico *a.* cardiogenic, of cardiac origin; **choque** ___ / ___ shock.

cardiografía *f.* cardiography, recording of the movements of the heart by a cardiograph.

cardiógrafo *m.* cardiograph, instrument that traces the movements of the heart.

cardiograma *m.* cardiogram, electrical tracing of the impulses of the heart.

cardiología *f.* cardiology, the study of the heart.

cardiólogo-a *m., f.* cardiologist, specialist in cardiology.

cardiomegalia *f.* cardiomegaly, enlarged heart.

cardiomiopatía *f.* cardiomyopathy, a disorder of the heart muscle; ___ **alcohólica** / alcoholic ___; ___ **congestiva** / congestive ___; ___ **dilatada** / dilated ___; ___ **hipertrófica** / hypertrophic ___; ___ **hipertrófica familiar** / familial hypertrophic ___; ___ **idiopática** / idiopathic ___; ___ **postpartum** / postpartum ___; ___ **primaria** / primary ___; ___ **restrictiva** / restrictive ___; ___ **secundaria** / secondary ___ .

cardiomioplastia dinámica *f.* dynamic cardiomyoplastia, procedure that is done on patients classified as cardiopathy class III that have suffered cardiac failure or that suffered from cardiac ischemia.

cardiopatía *f.* heart disease; ___ **por hipertensión** / hypertensive ___ .

cardioplegia *f.* cardioplegia, heart paralysis.

cardiopulmonar *a.* cardiopulmonary, rel. to the heart and the lungs; **máquina** ___ / heart-lung machine; **puente** ___ / ___ bypass; **resucitación, reanimación** ___ / ___ resuscitation.

cardiotomía *f.* cardiotomy; 1. incision in the cardiac end of the stomach; 2. incision of the heart.

cardiotónico-a *a.* cardiotonic, having a tonic or favorable effect on the heart; **agente** ___ / cardiac stimulant.

cardiovascular *a.* cardiovascular, rel. to the heart and blood vessels.

cardioversión *f.* cardioversion, the act of restoring the heart to a normal sinus rhythm by electrical countershock.

carditis *f.* carditis, infl. of the heart.

carecer *vi.* to lack.

carga *f.* load, burden.

cargar *vi.* to load; to carry.

caridad *f.* charity.

caries *f.* caries, dental cavity. ___ **dental** / dental ___; ___ **distal** / distal ___; ___ **de fisura** / fissure ___ .

cariñoso-a *a.* affectionate.

cariólisis *f.* karyolysis, breakdown of the nucleus of a cell.

cariolítico-a *a.* karyolytic, rel. to or that produces karyolysis.

carión *m.* karyon, cellular nucleus.

cariotipo *m.* karyotype, chromosome characteristics of an individual species.

caritativo-a *a.* charitable.

carmesí, carmín *m.* carmine.

carne *f.* 1. meat; ___ **asada** / roast beef; ___ **de carnero** / lamb; ___ **de puerco** / pork; ___ **de ternera** / veal; 2. flesh, muscular tissue of the body.

carnívoro-a *a.* carnivorous, that eats meat.

carnosidad *f.* carnosity, fleshy excrescence.

caro-a *a.* expensive, costly.

carótida *f.* carotid, main artery of the neck; **arterias** ___ -s / ___ arteries; **seno de la** ___ / ___ sinus; **síncope del seno de la** ___ / ___ sinus syncope.

carotina *f.* carotene, yellow-red pigment found in some vegetables that converts into vitamin A in the body.

carotodinia *f.* carotodynia, pain caused by pressure of the carotid artery.

carpo *m.* carpus, portion of the upper extremity between the hand and the forearm.

carraspera *f.* hoarseness; sore, itchy throat.

carretera *f.* highway.

carro *m.* automobile, car; cart.

carta *f.* letter.

cartera *f.* lady's handbag; wallet.

cartílago *m.* cartilage, elastic, semihard tissue that covers the bones.

carúncula *f.* caruncle, small, irritated piece of flesh; ___ **uretral** / urethral ___ .

casa *f.* house, home; ___ **de socorro** / first aid station.

casado-a *a.* married.

casarse *vr.* to get married.

cáscara *f.* peel, shell.

cáscara sagrada *f.* cascara sagrada, the bark of Rhamus purshiana shrub, commonly used to treat chronic constipation.

caseína *f.* casein, the main protein found in milk.

caseoso-a *a.* caseous, resembling curd or cheese.

casi *adv.* almost.

caso *m.* case, a specific instant of disease; ___ **ambulatorio** / ambulatory ___; **presentación de un** ___ / ___ reporting; **en** ___ **de** / in ___ of; **hacer** ___ / to pay attention; **no viene al** ___ / it is irrelevant.

caspa *f.* dandruff; dander.

castaño-a *a.* brown, chestnut colored.

castigar *vi.* to punish.

castigo *m.* punishment.

castrar *v.* to castrate, to remove the gonads; [*animales hembras*] to spay.

casual *a.* casual, accidental.

casualidad *f.* chance; **de** ___ / by ___; **por** ___ / by ___ .

catabolismo *m.* catabolism, cellular process by which complex substances are converted into simpler compounds; destructive metabolism.

catalepsia *f.* catalepsy, a condition characterized by loss of voluntary muscular movement and irresponsiveness to any outside stimuli, gen. associated with psychological disorders.

catálisis *f.* catalysis, alteration of the velocity of a chemical reaction by the presence of a catalyst.

catalítico-a *a.* catalytic.

catalizador *m.* catalyst, an agent that stimulates a chemical reaction.

cataplasma *f.* poultice.

cataplexia *f.* cataplexy, sudden loss of muscular tone caused by an exaggerated emotional state.

catarata *f.* cataract, opacity of the lens of the eye; ___ **anular** / anular ___; ___ **blanda** / soft ___; ___ **cerúlea** / blue ___; ___ **completa** / complete ___; ___ **congénita** /

congenital ___; ___ **congénita diabética** / congenital diabetic ___; ___ **eléctrica** / electric ___ , caused by high power electric current; ___ **madura** / mature ___; ___ **negra** / black ___; ___ **senil** / senile ___; ___ **verde** / green ___ .

cataratogénico-a *a.* cataractogenic, rel. to a cataract.

catarral *a.* rel. to catarrh.

catarro *m.* catarrh, cold, sniffle; ___ **de pecho, bronquial** / chest cold.

catarsis *f.* catharsis, purification. 1. purging the body of chemical or other material; 2. therapeutic liberation of anxiety and tension.

catártico *m.* cathartic, laxative; **-a** / *a.* cathartic, rel. to catharsis.

catatonía *f.* catatony, a phase of extreme negativism in schizophrenia in which the patient does not speak, remains in a fixed position, and resists any attempts to activate his or her movement or speech. The same symptoms are present in other mental conditions.

catatónico-a *a.* catatonic, rel. to or affected by catatony.

catecolaminas *f., pl.* catecholamines, amines such as norepinephrine, epinephrine, and dopamine that are produced in the adrenal glands and have a sympathomimetic action.

categoría *f.* category; quality.

catéter *m.* catheter, a rubber or plastic tube used to drain fluid from a body cavity such as urine from the bladder, or to inject fluid, as in cardiac catheterization.

catéter permanente *m.* in-dwelling catheter.

cateterización *f.* catheterization, insertion of a catheter.

cateterizar *vi.* to catheterize, to insert a catheter.

catgut *f.* catgut, type of surgical suture made from the gut of some animals.

cauda *f.* cauda, taillike structure.

caudal *a.* caudal, rel. to the tail.

causa *f.* cause, reason; ___ **actual** / existing ___; ___ **constitucional** / constitutional ___; ___ **de factor predisponente** / predisposing ___; ___ **específica** / specific ___; ___ **inmediata** / proximate ___; ___ **necesaria** / necessary ___; **sin** ___ / unreasonable.

causal *a.* causative, ethiologic.

causalgia *f.* causalgia, burning pain in the skin.

causar *v.* to cause.

cáustico *m.* caustic, substance used to destroy tissue.

cautela *f.* caution.

cauterización *f.* cauterization, burning by application of a caustic, heat, or electric current.

cauterizar *vi.* to cauterize, to burn by application of heat or electric current.

cava *f.* cava, hollow organ, cavity. vena cava.

caverna *f.* cavern, cave, pathological cavity or depression.

cavernoso-a *a.* cavernous, having hollow spaces.

cavidad *f.* cavity, hole; ___ **abdominal** / abdominal ___; ___ **-es cardíacas: auricular y ventricular** / heart chambers; ___ **-es craneales** / cranial cavities; ___ **pelviana** / pelvic ___; ___ **torácica** / thoracic ___ .

cebada *f.* barley.

cebolla *f.* onion.

cecostomía *f.* cecostomy, surgical opening into the cecum.

cefalea, cefalalgia *f.* cephalea, cephalalgia, headache.

cefálico-a *a.* cephalic, rel. to the head.

cefalorraquídeo-a *a.* cerebroespinal.

cefalosporina *f.* cephalosporin, wide spectrum antibiotic.

ceguera, ceguedad *f.* blindness; ___ **al color** / color ___; ___ **nocturna** / night ___; ___ **verde** / green ___; ___ **roja** / red ___ .

ceja *f.* eyebrow.

celíaco-a *a.* celiac, rel. to the abdomen.

celiotomía *f.* celiotomy. laparotomía.

célula *f.* cell, structural unit of all living organisms. *V.* ilustración en la página 332.

célula de microglia *f.* microglia cell, small intestinal migrating cell of the nervous system.

célula T4 cooperadora *f.* T cell also called CD4.

célula T8 citotóxica *f.* cell cytotoxica, also called CD8, carries out functions by destroying antigens, and attacks and eliminates cells infected by virus, parasites and fungi.

célula T reguladora *f.* Cell T regulator directing other cells of the immune system to do special functions having as their main target HIV.

célula T8 supresora *n.* T8 Cell suppressor, a group of cells with a function to inhibit the immune response.

celular *a.* cellular, rel. to the cell; **agua** ___ / ___ water; **compartimentos** ___ **-es** / ___ compartments; **crecimiento** ___ / ___ growth; **tejido** ___ / ___ tissue.

celularidad *f.* cellularity, the condition of cells present in a tissue or mass.

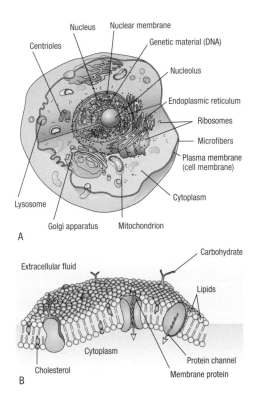

The cell: (A) cell and organelles; (B) typical animal cell and plasma membrane

celulitis *f.* cellulitis, infl. of connective tissue.

celulosa *a.* cellulose.

cementerio *m.* cemetery.

cemento *m.* cement.

cena *f.* evening meal, supper.

cenar *v.* to have dinner or supper.

cenizas *f., pl.* ashes; ___ **radioactivas** / fallout.

censo *m.* census.

centeno *m.* rye.

centígrado *a.* centigrade.

central, céntrico-a *a.* central; **sistema nervioso** ___ / ___ nervous system.

centrífugo-a *a.* centrifugal, going from the center outward.

centrípeto-a *a.* centripetal, going from the outside towards the center.

centro *m.* 1. center; 2. middle, core. ___ **cerebral** / brain ___; ___ **de información** / information ___; ___ **de la micción** / micturation ___; ___ **de la respiración** / respiratory ___; ___ **de la sed** / thirst ___; ___ **del lenguaje** / speech ___; ___ **de percepción**

táctil / perception ___; ___ **de servicio de la salud** / community health ___; ___ **nervioso** / nerve ___ .

ceño *m.* brow; **fruncir el** ___ / to frown.

cepa *f.* strain, group of microorganisms within a species or variety characterized by some particular quality.

cepillo *m.* brush; ___ **de dientes** / toothbrush;

cera *f.* wax. 1. beeswax; 2. waxy secretion of the body; ___ **depilatoria** / depilatory ___ .

cerca *f., adv.* near; **de aquí** / close by.

cercanía *f.* vicinity.

cercano-a *a.* close; neighboring, proximate.

cerclaje *m.* cerclage, procedure that consists of encircling a part with a wire loop or catgut, such as in binding together parts of a fractured bone.

cereal *m.* cereal.

cerebelo *m.* cerebellum, posterior brain mass; **enfermedades del** ___ / cerebellar diseases.

cerebeloso-a *a.* cerebellous, rel. to the cerebrum.

cerebral *a.* cerebral, rel. to the brain; **apoplejía** ___ / cerebrovascular accident; **concusión o conmoción** ___ / ___ concussion; **edema** ___ / ___ edema; **embolismo y trombosis** ___ / ___ embolism and thrombosis; **hemorragia o infarto** ___ / ___ hemorrhage or infarct; **muerte** ___ / brain death; **trauma** ___ / brain injury; **tronco** ___ / brain stem; **tumor** ___ / brain tumor.

cerebro *m.* brain, cerebrum, portion of the central nervous system contained within the cranium that is the chief regulator of body functions; ___ **medio** / midbrain; **escán del** ___ **(gammagrama)** / ___ scan. *V.* ilustración en la página XX.

cerebroespinal, cefalorraquídeo-a *a.* cerebrospinal, rel. to the brain and the spinal cord.

cerebrovascular *a.* cerebrovascular, rel. to the blood vessels of the brain.

cereza *f.* cherry.

cero *m.* zero.

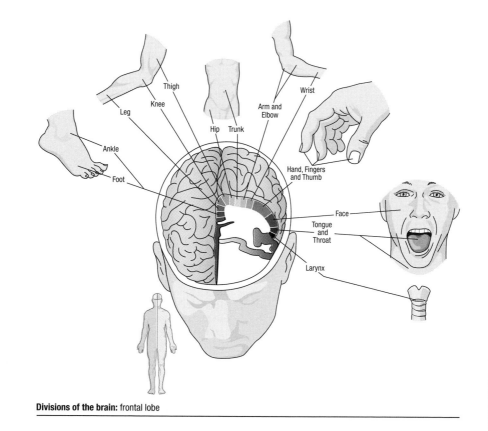

Divisions of the brain: frontal lobe

ceroso-a *a.* waxy.

cerrado-a *a.* closed.

cerradura *f.* lock.

cerrar *vi.* to close; ___ **con llave** / to lock.

certero-a *a.* accurate.

certeza *f.* certainty; accuracy.

certificado *m.* certificate; ___ **de defunción** / death ___ .

cerumen *m.* cerumen, wax that builds up in the ear. ___ **impactado** / impacted ___ .

cerveza *f.* beer.

cervical *a.* cervical. 1. rel. to the cervix; **dilatador** ___ / ___ dilator; 2. rel. to the area of the neck; **displasia** ___ / ___ dysplasia; **erosión** ___ / ___ erosion; **pólipo** ___ / ___ polyp.

cerviz *f.* nape of the neck.

cesar *v.* to cease, to stop.

cesárea *f.* cesarean section.

cese *m.* stoppage.

cesio *m.* cesium, metalic element belonging to the group of alkaline metals.

cetoacidosis *f.* ketoacidosis, acidosis caused by the increase of ketone bodies in the blood.

cetoaciduria *f.* ketoaciduria, acidosis caused by the raise of ketone bodies in the blood.

cetogénesis *f.* ketogenesis, production of acetone.

cetonemia *f.* ketonemia, concentration of ketone bodies in the plasma.

cetosa *f.* ketose.

cetosis *f.* ketosis, excessive production of acetone as a result of incomplete metabolism of fatty acids; acidosis.

ch *f.* fourth letter of the Spanish alphabet.

chalación *f.* chalazion, meibomian cyst, a cyst of the eyelid.

chancro *m.* chancre, the primary lesion of syphilis.

chancroide *m.* chancroid, a nonsyphilitic venereal ulcer.

chaparro-a *a. Mex.* short person.

chaqueta *f.* jacket.

charlatán-a *m., f.* charlatan, a quack, someone claiming knowledge and skills he or she does not have.

chasquido *m.* snap, sharp brief sound related to the abrupt opening of the cardiac valve, gen. the mitral valve; ___ **de apertura** / opening ___ .

chata *f.* bedpan.

cheque *m.* check.

chequear *v.* to check, to verify.

chequeo *m.* checkup, complete medical examination.

Cheyne-Stokes, respiración de *f.* Cheyne-Stokes respiration, respiration manifested by alternating periods of apnea of increased rapidity and depth, gen. associated with disorders of the neurologic respiration center.

chicano-a *a. pop.* (U.S.) Mexican-American.

chícharo *m.* green pea.

chichón *m.* bump in the head.

chico-a *m., f.* young boy; young girl; *a.* small.

chiflado-a *a. pop.* crazy, nuts.

chile *m.* hot pepper.

chillar *v.* to screech, to scream.

chinche *f.* bedbug.

chiquito-a *a.* small.

chochera *f.* senility.

chocho-a *a.* senile.

chocolate *m.* chocolate.

choque *m.* 1. shock; an abnormal state, gen. following trauma, in which insufficient flow of blood through the body can cause reduced cardiac output, subnormal temperature, descending blood pressure and rapid pulse; ___ **alérgico** / allergic ___; ___ **anafiláctico** / anaphylactic ___; ___ **eléctrico** / electric ___; ___ **séptico** / septic ___; 2. collision.

chorizo *m.* sausage.

chorrear *v.* to drip; to spout.

chorro *n.* jet, spurt; stream.

chueco-a *a.* crooked, bent.

chupar *v.* to suck; to absorb; **chuparse el dedo** / thumb sucking.

chupete *n.* pacifier.

churre *m.* dirt, grime.

cianocobalamina *f.* cyanocobalamin, vitamin B_{12}, complex of cyanide and cobalamin used in the treatment of pernicious anemia.

cianosis *f.* cyanosis, purplish blue discoloration of the skin, often as a result of cardiac, anatomic or functional abnormalities.

cianótico-a *a.* cyanotic, rel. to or afflicted by cyanosis.

cianuro *m.* cyanide.

ciática *f.* sciatica, neuralgia along the course of the sciatic nerve.

cibernética *f.* cybernetics, the study of biological systems such as the brain and the nervous system by electronic means.

cicatriz *f.* scar.

cicatrización *f.* cicatrization, scarring.

cicatrizante *m.* cicatrizant, agent that aids the healing process of a wound.

cicatrizar *v.* to scar, the healing process of a wound.

ciclamato *m.* cyclamate, artificial sweetening agent.

ciclectomía *f.* cyclectomy, excision of a portion of the ciliary muscle.

ciclitis *f.* cyclitis, infl. of the ciliary body.

ciclo *m.* cycle, recurring period of time; ___ **gravídico** / pregnancy ___ .

cicloforia *f.* cyclophoria, rotation of the eye due to muscle weakness.

ciclofosfamida *f.* cyclophosphamide, antineoplastic drug also used as an immunosuppressive in organ transplants.

ciclofotocoagulación *f.* cyclophotocoagulation, photocoagulation through the pupil with a laser, gen. used in glaucoma.

cicloplejía *f.* cycloplegia, paralysis of the ciliary muscle.

ciclosporina *f.* cyclosporine, immunosuppressive agent used in organ transplant.

ciclotimía *f.* cyclothymia, disorder manifested by alternate states of agitation and depression.

ciclotímico-a *m., f.* cyclothymic, person afflicted with extreme changes of mood.

ciclotomía *f.* cyclotomy, incision through the ciliary body of the eye.

ciclotropía *f.* cyclotropia, deviation of the eye around the anteroposterior axis.

ciego-a *m., f.* blind person; *a.* blind.

ciego *m.* cecum. 1. cul-de-sac lying below the terminal ileum forming the first part of the large intestine; 2. any cul-de-sac structure.

cielo *m.* sky.

cien, ciento *a., m.* a hundred.

ciencia *f.* science; ___ **médica** / medical ___; **a** ___ **cierta** / for sure.

científico-a *m., f.* scientist; *a.* scientific.

cierto-a *a.* certain, true; **por** ___ / as a matter of fact.

cifosis *f.* kyphosis, exaggerated posterior curvature of the thoracic spine.

cifótico-a *a.* kyphotic, suffering from or rel. to kyphosis.

cigarrillo, cigarro *m.* cigarette.

cigoma, zigoma *m.* zygoma, osseous prominence at the point where the temporal and malar bones join.

cigomático-a *a.* zygomatic, rel. to the zygote; **arco** ___ / ___ arch; **hueso** ___ / ___ bone; **óvulo** ___ / ___ egg.

cigoto *m.* zygote, the fertilized ovum, cell resulting from the union of two gametes.

ciliar *a.* ciliary, rel. to or resembling the eyelash or eyelid.

cilíndrico-a *a.* cylindrical.

cilindro *m.* cylinder. 1. geometrical form resembling a column; 2. cylindrical lens; 3. cylindrical renal cast; ___ **hemático** / blood cast ___;

cilindro granuloso *m.* [*renal*] granular cast, [*ortopedia*] urinary cylinder seen in degenerative or inflammatory nephropathies.

cilindroma *m.* cylindroma, frequently malignant tumor, usu. found in the face or in the orbit of the eye.

cilindruria *f.* cylindruria, presence of cylinders in the urine.

cilio *m.* cilium, eyelid.

cima *f.* summit, top.

cimetidina *f.* cimetidine, antacid used in the treatment of gastric and duodenal ulcers.

cimiento *m.* foundation, base.

cinc *m.* zinc.

cinconismo *m.* cinchonism. quininism.

cinéreo *m.* cinerea, the gray substance of the nervous system.

cinerradiografía *f.* cineradiography, x-ray of an organ in motion.

cinesioterapia *f.* kinesiotherapy, treatment involving physical exercises or specific movements.

cinesis *f.* kinesis, term used to designate physical movements in general, including those that result as a response to a stimulus such as light.

cinestesia *f.* kinesthesia, sensorial experience, sense and perception of a movement.

cinética *f.* kinesics, the study of the body and its static and dynamic positions as a means of communication.

cinético-a *a.* kinetic, rel. to movement or what causes it.

cínico-a *m., f.* cynic; *a.* cynical.

cinta magnética *f.* audiotape.

cinto *m.* belt; waistband.

cintura *f.* waist; waistline.

cinturón *m.* girdle; wide belt; ___ **escapular o torácico** / thoracic ___ .

circinado-a *a.* circinate, ring-shaped.

circuito *m.* circuit.

circulación *f.* circulation; **mala** ___ / poor ___; ___ **periférica** / peripheral ___ .

círculo *m.* circle, a round figure or structure.

circuncidar *v.* to circumcise.

circuncisión *f.* circumcision, removing part or all of the prepuce.

circundar *v.* to encircle, to surround.

circunducción *f.* circumduction, circular movement of the distal end of a limb or part such as the eye, while keeping the proximal end fixed.

circunferencia *f.* circumference.

circunstancia *f.* circumstance; ___ **-s atenuantes** / mitigating ___ -s.

circunvolución *f.* gyrus, elevated portion of the cerebral cortex; ___ **-es de Broca** / ___ , Broca's, third, frontal or inferior; ___ **frontal, superior** / ___ , frontal, superior; ___ **-es occipitales** / ___ , occipital first, superior.

cirrosis *f.* cirrhosis, progressive disease of the liver characterized by interstitial infl. and associated with failure in the function of hepatocytes and resistance to the flow of blood through the liver; ___ **alcohólica** / alcoholic ___; ___ **biliar** / biliary ___ .

ciruela *f.* plum; ___ **pasa** / prune.

cirugía *f.* surgery; the branch of medicine that treats diseases, malformations, and injuries and restores or reconstructs body structures through operative procedures; ___ **ambulatoria** / ambulatory ___; ___ **artroscópica** / arthroscopic ___; ___ **cardiotorácica** / cardiothracic___; ___ **citoreductiva** / cytoreductive ___; ___ **conservadora** / conservative ___; ___ **correctiva** / corrective ___; ___ **cosmética** / cosmetic ___; ___ **endoscópica** / endoscopic ___; ___ **escisión** / excisional ___; ___ **exploretoria** / exploratory ___; ___ **mayor** / major ___; ___ **menor** / minor ___; ___ **oral** / oral ___; ___ **ortopédica** / orthopedic ___; ___ **plástica** / plastic ___; ___ **radical** / radical ___; ___ **reconstructiva** / reconstructive ___; ___ **de sustenso** / sustenance ___; ___ **torácica** / chest or thoracic ___ . *V.* cuadro en la página 529.

cirugía torácica asistida por video *f.* video-assisted thoracic surgery, thoracic surgery performed using endoscopic cameras, optical systems, and display screens; developed new technique making small incisions without spreading of the ribs.

cirujano-a *m., f.* surgeon, specialist in surgery.

cistadenocarcinoma *m.* cystadenocarcinoma, carcinoma and cystadenoma.

cistadenoma *m.* cystadenoma, adenoma that has one or more cysts.

cistectomía *f.* cystectomy, total or partial resection of the urinary bladder.

cisteína *f.* cysteine, amino acid derived from cystine and found in most proteins.

cisterna *f.* cistern, a closed space that serves as a reservoir or receptacle.

cístico-a *a.* cystic, rel. to the gallbladder or the bladder.

cistina *f.* cystine, amino acid that is produced by the digestion of proteins, at times found in the urine.

cistinuria *f.* cystinuria, excessive cystine in the urine.

cistitis *f.* cystitis, infl. of the urinary bladder characterized by frequent urination accompanied by pain and burning.

cistocele *m.* cystocele, hernia of the bladder.

cistofibroma *f.* cystofibroma, fibroma in which cysts or cyst like formations have developed.

cistofibroscopio *m.* cystofibroscope.

cistografía *f.* cystography, x-ray of the bladder using a radiopaque substance.

cistograma *m.* cystogram, x-ray of the bladder using air or a contrasting medium.

cistolitotomía *f.* cystolithotomy, removal of a stone by cutting into the bladder.

cistometría *f.* cystometry, cystometrography, study of the bladder functions through the use of a cystometer.

cistómetro *m.* cystometer, device used to study the pathophysiological functions of the urinary bladder by measuring its capacity and pressure reactions.

cistopexia *f.* cystopexy, fixation of the urinary bladder to the abdominal wall.

cistoscopía *f.* cystoscopy, inspection of the bladder through a cystoscope.

cistoscopio *m.* cystoscope, tube-shaped instrument used to examine the bladder and the urethra.

cistostomía *f.* cystostomy, creation of an opening into the bladder for drainage.

cistotomía *f.* cystotomy, incision in the bladder.

cistouretrografía *f.* cystourethrography, x-ray of the urinary bladder and the urethra.

cistouretroscopio *m.* cystourethroscope, instrument for endoscopic visualization of the bladder and urethra.

cisura *f.* cleft, elongated opening; fissure.

cita *f.* appointment; **hacer una** ___ / to make an ___; **tener una** ___ / to have an ___ .

citocromo *m.* cytochrome, hemochromogen that plays an important part in the oxidation processes.

citolítico-a *a.* cytolytic, having the power to dissolve or destroy a cell.

citología *f.* cytology, the science that deals with the nature of cells.

citomegálico-a *a.* cytomegalic, characterized by abnormally enlarged cells.

citomegalovirus *m.* cytomegalovirus, any of a group of herpes viruses that causes cellular enlargement and is the causative agent of cytomegalic inclusion disease.

citómetro *m.* cytometer, a device used for counting and measuring blood cells.

citopenia *f.* cytopenia, deficiency of cellular elements in the blood.

citoplasma *m.* cytoplasm, protoplasm of a cell with exception of the nucleus.

citotoxicidad *f.* cytotoxicity, the capacity of an agent to destroy certain cells.

citotoxina *f.* cytotoxin, toxic agent that damages or destroys cells of certain organs.

citrato *m.* citrate, salt of citric acid.

cítrico-a *a.* citric, citrous.

cítula *f.* cytula, term used to define the ovum or small impregnated cell.

ciudad *f.* city.

ciudadanía *f.* citizenship.

ciudadano-a *m., f.* citizen.

clara *f.* the white of the egg.

claridad *f.* clarity, brightness.

clarificación *f.* clarification.

clarificar *vi.* to clarify.

claro-a *a.* clear.

clase *f.* class, sort, kind.

clasificación *f.* classification.

clasificar *vi.* to classify, to sort out.

claudicación *f.* claudication, limping; ___ intermitente / intermittent ___ .

clavícula *f.* clavicle, collarbone.

clavo *m.* nail, slender rod of metal or bone used to fasten together parts of a broken bone; ___ ortopédico / orthopedic pin.

cleidocostal *a.* cleidocostal, rel. to the ribs and the clavicle.

cleptomanía *f.* kleptomania, morbid compulsion to steal.

cleptómano-a *m., f.* kleptomaniac, person afflicted with kleptomania.

clérigo *m.* clergyman.

clima *m.* climate.

climaterio *m.* climacteric, termination of the reproductive period in women.

clímax *m.* climax. 1. crisis in an illness; 2. sexual orgasm.

clínica *f.* clinic, a health-care facility; ___ de consulta externa / outpatient ___ .

clínico-a *a.* clinical. 1. rel. to a clinic; 2. rel. to direct observation of patients; **cuadro** ___ / ___ picture; **curso** ___ / ___ progress; **ensayos** ___ -s / ___ trials; **historia** ___ , **expediente médico** / ___ history; **procedimiento** ___ / ___ procedure.

clisis *f.* clisis, the act of supplying fluid to the body by other means than orally.

clitoridectomía *f.* clitoridectomy, excision of the clitoris.

clítoris *m.* clitoris, small protruding body situated in the most anterior part of the vulva.

cloaca *f.* cloaca. 1. common opening for the intestinal and urinary tracts in the early development of the embryo; 2. sewer.

cloasma *f.* chloasma, skin discoloration seen during pregnancy.

clónico-a *a.* clonic, rel. to clonus.

clono *m.* 1. clonus, a series of rapid and rhythmic contractions of a muscle; 2. clone, an individual derived from a single organism through asexual reproduction.

clonorquiasis *f.* chlonorchiasis, parasitic infection that affects the distal bile ducts.

clorambucil *m.* chlorambucil, a form of nitrogen mustard used to combat some forms of cancer.

cloranfenicol *m.* chloramphenicol, chloromycetin, antibiotic esp. effective in the treatment of typhoid fever.

clorhidria *f.* chlorhydria, excess acidity in the stomach.

cloro *m.* chlorine, gaseous element used as a disinfectant and bleaching agent.

clorofila *f.* chlorophyll, green pigment in plants by which photosynthesis takes place.

cloroformo *m.* chloroform, anesthetic.

cloroma *m.* chloroma, green-colored tumor that can occur in different parts of the body.

cloroquina *f.* chloroquine, a compound used in the treatment of malaria.

clorosis *f.* chlorosis, type of anemia usu. seen in women and gen. associated with iron deficiency.

clorotetraciclina *f.* chlortetracycline, antibiotic agent.

clorpromacina *f.* chlorpromazine, tranquilizing and antiemetic agent.

cloruro *m.* chloride, a compound of chlorine.

coaglutinación *f.* coagglutination, group agglutination.

coaglutinina *f.* coagglutinin, agglutinate that affects two or more organisms.

coagulación *f.* coagulation, clot; ___ diseminada intravascular / disseminated intravascular ___; **propiedad de** ___ / blood clotting ability; **tiempo de** ___ / blood ___ time.

coagulante *m.* coagulant, that which causes or precipitates coagulation.

coagular *v.* to coagulate, to clot.

coágulo *m.* coagulation, clot.

coagulopatía *f.* coagulopathy, a disease or condition that affects the coagulation mechanism of the blood.

coalescencia *f.* coalescence, the fusion of parts or elements.

coartación *f.* coarctation, stricture; compression.

cobalto *m.* cobalt.

cobarde *a.* coward.

cobija *f.* cover, blanket.

cobrar *v.* to charge; to collect.

cobre *m.* copper.

coca *f.* coca, plant from which leaves cocaine is extracted.

cocaína *f.* cocaine, addictive narcotic alkaloid derived from coca leaves.

coccidioidina *f.* coccidioidin, a sterile solution used intracutaneously as a test for coccidioidomycosis.

coccidioidomicosis *f.* coccidioidomycosis, valley fever, endemic respiratory infection in the Southwestern United States, Mexico, and parts of South America.

coccigodinia *f.* coccygodynia, pain in the region of the coccyx.

cóccix *m.* coccyx, last bone at the bottom of the vertebral column.

cocer *vi.* to cook; to stew; ___ **a fuego lento** / to simmer.

cociente *m.* quotient; ___ **de inteligencia** / intelligence ___ .

cocimiento *m.* concoction made of medicinal herbs.

cocina *f.* kitchen, stove.

cocinado-a *a.* cooked; **bien** ___ / well-done.

cocinar *v.* to cook.

cóclea *f.* cochlea, spiral tube that forms part of the inner ear.

coco *m.* 1. coccus, bacteria; 2. coconut; **agua de** ___ / ___ milk.

cocoa *f.* cocoa.

coche *m.* automobile.

cochinada *f.* filthy act; dirty trick; filth.

cochino-a *m., f.* pig; *a.* filthy.

codeína *f.* codeine, narcotic analgesic.

codo *m.* elbow; ___ **de tenista** / tennis ___ ; **coyuntura del** ___ / ___ joint.

coenzima *f.* coenzyme, a substance that enhances the action of an enzyme.

coerción *f.* duress, coercion; **bajo** ___ / under ___ .

coger *vi.* to take, to grasp; to get; ___ **un resfriado** / to catch a cold.

cognado *m.* cognate. 1. that which is of the same nature; 2. word that derives from the same root.

cognición *f.* knowledge, the act of knowing.

cognitivo-a *a.* cognitive, rel. to knowledge.

cogote *m.* nape, back of neck.

cohabitar *v.* to live together.

coherencia *n.* coherence, any group designed to be followed or copied for a length of time, such as women with breast cancer in a chosen community.

coherente *a.* coherent.

cohesión *f.* cohesion, the force that holds molecules together.

cohibido *a.* inhibited; uneasy.

coincidencia *f.* coincidence.

coincidir *v.* to coincide.

coito *m.* coitus, sexual intercourse.

cojear *v.* to limp.

cojera *f.* lameness.

cojinete *m.* cushion.

cojo-a *a.* lame, crippled.

col *f.* cabbage.

cola *f.* 1. glue; **inhalar** ___ / ___ sniffing; 2. tail.

colaborar *v.* to collaborate.

colador *m.* sieve, strainer.

colágeno *m.* collagen, the main supportive protein of skin, bone, tendon, and cartilage.

colangiectasia *f.* cholangiectasis, dilation of the biliary ducts.

colangiografía *f.* cholangiography, x-ray of the biliary ducts.

colangiograma *m.* cholangiogram, x-ray of the biliary ducts using a contrast medium.

colangitis *f.* cholangitis, infl. of the biliary ducts.

colapso *m.* collapse, failure; ___ **cardiovascular** / cardiovascular failure ; ___ **circulatorio** / circulatory failure; ___ **nervioso** / nervous breakdown; ___ **parcial del pulmón** / partial lung ___ .

colar *vi.* to strain; to sift.

colateral *a.* collateral. 1. indirect, subsidiary, or accessory to the principal; 2. rel. to a side branch of a nerve axon or blood vessel.

colaterización coronaria *f.* coronary collaterization, expontaneous growth of new blood vessels around the cardiac regions under a restricted blood flow.

colcha *f.* cover, coverlet.

colchón *m.* mattress.

colecistectomía *f.* cholecystectomy, removal of the gallbladder.

colecistitis *f.* cholecystitis, infl. of the gallbladder.

colecistoduodenostomía *f.* cholecystoduodenostomy, anastomosis of the gallbladder and the duodenum.

colecistogastrostomía *f.*
cholecystogastrostomy, anastomosis of the
gallbladder and the stomach.

colecistografía *f.* cholecystography, x-ray of
the gallbladder by administration of a dye, orally
or by injection.

colectar, coleccionar *v.* to collect.

colectomía *f.* colectomy, excision of part or all
of the colon.

colédoco *m.* choledochus, common bile duct,
formed by the union of the hepatic and cystic
ducts.

coledocoduodenostomía *f.*
choledochoduodenostomy, anastomosis of the
choledochus and the duodenum.

coledocolitiasis *f.* choledocholithiasis,
presence of calculi in the common bile duct.

coledocoyeyunostomía *f.*
choledochojejunostomy, anastomosis of the
common bile duct and the jejunum.

colega *m., f.* colleague.

colegio *m.* school.

colelitiasis *f.* cholelithiasis, presence of stones
in the gallbladder or in the common bile duct.

colemia *f.* cholemia, presence of bile in the
blood.

cólera *f.* cholera. 1. acute infectious disease
characterized by severe diarrhea and vomiting; 2.
anger, rage.

colestasis *f.* cholestasis, biliary stasis.

colesteatoma *m.* cholesteatoma, a tumor
containing cholesterol, found most commonly in
the middle ear.

colesteremia, colesterolemia *f.*
cholesteremia, cholesterolemia, excessive
cholesterol in the blood.

colesterol *m.* cholesterol, component of animal
oils, fats, and nerve tissue, a precursor of sex
hormones and adrenal corticoids; **___ alto /**
high ___; **reductor de ___ / ___** reducer.

colesteroluria *f.* cholesteroluria, presence of
cholesterol in the urine.

colgajo *m.* flap, detached tissue.

colgar *vi.* to hang.

cólico *m.* colic, acute spasmodic abdominal pain.

coliflor *f.* cauliflower.

colinesterasa *f.* cholinesterase, a family of
enzymes.

colirio *m.* colyrium, liquid medicinal preparation
for the eye.

colitis *f.* colitis, infl. of the colon; **___ crónica /**
chronic ___; **espasmódica /**
spasmodic ___; **mucomembranosa /**

pseudomembranous ___; **___ mucosa /**
mucous ___; **ulcerativa /** ulcerative ___ .

colmena *f.* beehive.

colmillo *m.* canine tooth; tusk, fang.

colocar *vi.* to place, to set; **colocarse** *vr.* to
position oneself.

colodión *m.* collodion, liquid substance used to
cover or protect skin cuts.

coloide *m.* colloid, gelatin-like substance
produced by some forms of tissue decay.

colon *m.* colon, the portion of the intestine
extending from the cecum to the rectum; **___**
ascendente / ascending ___; **___ descendente /**
descending ___; **neoplasma del ___ /** colonic
neoplasm.

colonia *f.* colony, a group of bacteria in a
culture, all derived from the same organism.

colónico-a *a.* colonic, rel. to the colon.

colonoscopía *f.* colonoscopy, examination of
the inner surface of the colon through a
colonoscope.

colonoscopio *m.* colonoscope, instrument used
to examine the colon.

color *m.* color.___ **-es complementarios /**
complementary ___ s; **___ estructural /**
structural ___; **___ -es extrínsecos /**
extrinsic ___; **___ -es intrínsecos /**
intrinsic ___; **___ primario /** primary ___; **___**
puro / pure ___; **___ reflejado /**

Colores	Colors
amarillo	yellow
ámbar	amber
anaranjado	orange
azul	blue
blanco	white
carmelita	brown
cenizo	ashen
cetrino	greenish yellow
gris	gray
morado	purple, black and blue
pardo	brown
negro	black
rojizo	reddish
rojo	red
rosáceo	pinkish
verde	green

reflected ___; ___ **saturado** / saturated ___; ___ **simple** / simple ___; **confusión de** ___ / ___ confusion; **percepción del** ___ / ___ perception; **tono de** ___ / tone ___ . *V.* ilustración en la página 77.

coloración *f.* coloration, staining.

colorado-a *a.* red; **ponerse** ___ / to blush.

colorante *m.* dye, stain.

colorimétrico-a *a.* rel. to color; **guía** ___ / color index.

colorrectal *a.* colorectal, rel. to the colon and rectum, or to the entire large bowel.

colostomía *f.* colostomy, creation of an artificial anus; **bolsa de** ___ / ___ bag.

colpitis *f.* colpitis, infl. of the vaginal membrane.

colpocele *m.* colpocele, a hernia into the vagina.

colporrafía *f.* colporrhaphy, suture of the vagina.

colporragia *f.* colporrhagia, vaginal hemorrhage.

colposcopía *f.* colposcopy, examination of the vagina and the cervix through a colposcope.

colposcopio *m.* colposcope, endoscopic instrument that allows direct observation of the vagina and the cervix.

colpotomía *f.* colpotomy, incision in the vagina.

columna *f.* column, pillar-like structure.

columna, espina vertebral *f.* spinal column, osseous structure formed by thirty-three vertebrae that surround and contain the spinal cord.

coluria *f.* choluria, presence of bile in the urine.

colutorio *m.* mouthwash, antiseptic solution for rinsing the mouth.

coma *m.* coma, state of unconsciousness.

comadre *f.* godmother; woman friend.

comadrona *f.* woman who specializes in the health of women during pregnancy, delivery, and postpartum, midwife.

comatoso-a *a.* comatose, rel. to or in a state of coma; **estado** ___ / ___ state.

combatir *v.* to combat, to fight.

combinación *f.* combination.

combinar *v.* to combine.

comedón *m.* blackhead, comedo.

comedor *m.* dining room.

comensal *m.* commensal, host, organism that benefits from living within or on another living organism without either benefiting or harming it.

comentar *v.* to comment.

comentario *m.* commentary, remark.

comenzar *vi.* to commence, to begin.

comer *v.* to eat; **dar de** ___ / to feed.

comestible *m.* food; *a.* edible.

cometer *v.* to commit.

comezón *f.* itch.

comida *f.* food; meal; **hora de** ___ / meal time.

comienzo *m.* beginning; start.

comilón-a *a.* big eater.

comisión *f.* commission, assignment.

comisura *f.* commissure, coming together of two parts, such as the labial angles.

comisurotomía *f.* commissurotomy, incision of the fibrous bands of a commissure, such as the labial angles or the commissure of a cardiac valve.

como *adv.* how, as; ___ **quiera** / as you wish; *conj.* like, as; ___ **no** / of course; *prep.* about; **está** ___ **a (una milla)** / it is about (a mile) away; ___ **a (las ocho)** / about (eight o'clock).

cómodo-a *a.* comfortable.

compacto-a *a.* compact.

compadecer *vi.* to pity; **compadecerse** *vr.* to feel sorry for; ___ **a sí mismo** / self-pity.

compadre *m.* godfather; close friend.

compañero *m.* companion, mate.

compañía *f.* company; ___ **de seguros** / insurance ___ .

comparación *f.* comparison.

comparar *v.* to compare.

compartir *v.* to share.

compasión *f.* compassion.

compatible *a.* compatible.

compensación *f.* compensation. 1. that which makes up for a defect or counterbalances some deficiency; 2. defense mechanism; 3. remuneration

compensar *v.* to compensate.

competente *a.* competent, qualified, able to perform well.

complejo *m.* complex, a series of related mental processes that affect behavior and personality; ___ **de castración** / castration ___; ___ **de culpa** / guilt ___; ___ **de Edipo** / Oedipus ___ , morbid love of a son for the mother; ___ **de Electra** / Electra ___ , morbid love of a daughter for the father; ___ **de inferioridad** / inferiority ___; **-a** *a.* complicated; intricate.

complementar *v.* to supplement.

complemento *m.* complement, a serum protein substance that destroys bacteria and other cells that it comes into contact.

completar *v.* to complete.

completo-a *a.* complete.

complexión *f.* complexion, appearance of the facial skin.

complicación *f.* complication.

complicar *vi.* to complicate; **complicarse** *vr.,* to become difficult; to become involved, to get entangled.

componente *m.* component.

componer *vi.* [*una fractura*] to set; to put together; to heal, to restore.

composición *f.* composition.

compostura *f.* composure; serenity.

compota *f.* compote, fruit stew.

comprar *v.* to buy, to purchase.

comprender *v.* to understand.

compresa *f.* compress, pack; ___ **fría** / cold ___ .

compresión *f.* compression, exertion of pressure on a point of the body.

comprimidos *m., pl.* pills.

comprobar *v.* to prove, to verify.

comprometer *v.* to compromise; **comprometerse** *vr.* to commit oneself; to compromise, to become involved.

compromiso *m.* commitment, obligation.

compuesto *m.* compound.

compulsivo-a *a.* compulsive.

computadora *f.* computer.

común *a.* common; **lugar** ___ / ___ place; **nombre** ___ / ___ name; **no** ___ / uncommon; **por lo** ___ / gen; **sentido** ___ / ___ sense.

comunicación *f.* communication.

comunicación privilegiada *f.* privileged communication, such as that between a doctor or psychotherapist and a patient; it is the patient's privilege to keep this information confidential.

comunicar *v.* to communicate, to inform; **comunicarse** *vr.* to communicate with.

comunidad *f.* community.

con *prep.* with, by; ___ **frecuencia** / frequently; ___ **mucho gusto** / gladly; ___ **permiso** / excuse me; ___ **regularidad** / regularly.

cóncavo-a *a.* concave, hollowed.

concebir *vi.* to conceive.

concentración *f.* concentration. 1. increased strength of a fluid by evaporation; 2. the act of concentrating.

concentrado-a *a.* concentrated; ___ **en sí mismo-a** / self-conscious;

concentrar *v.* to concentrate; **concentrarse** *vr.* to concentrate oneself.

concepción *f.* conception.

concepto *m.* concept, idea.

concha *f.* shell; that which resembles a shell.

conciencia *f.* consciousness; conscience, state of awareness.

conciso-a *a.* concise.

concluir *vi.* to conclude; to infer.

conclusión *f.* conclusion.

concreción *f.* concretion, hardening, solidification.

concretio cordis *L.* concretio cordis, partial or complete obliteration of the pericardial cavity due to chronic constrictive pericarditis.

concreto-a *a.* concrete.

concusión *f.* concussion, trauma gen. caused by a head injury and manifested at times by dizziness and nausea; ___ **cerebral** / cerebral ___; ___ **de la médula espinal** / spinal ___ .

condensar *v.* to condense, to make something more dense.

condición *f.* condition, quality; ___ **anterior** / preexisting ___; ___ **sin diagnosticar** / undiagnosed ___ .

condicionar *v.* to condition, to train.

cóndilo *m.* condyle, rounded portion of the bone usu. present at the joint.

condiloma *f.* condyloma, warty growth usu. found around the genitalia and the perineum.

condimentado-a *a.* spicy.

condón *m.* condom, contraceptive device.

condral *a.* chondral, of a cartilaginous nature.

condritis *f.* chondritis, infl. of a cartilage.

condrocalcinosis *f.* chondrocalcinosis, condition that resembles gout, characterized by calcification and degenerative alterations in cartilage.

condrocostal *a.* chondrocostal, rel. to the ribs and the costal cartilages.

condromalacia *f.* chondromalacia, abnormal softening of cartilage.

condrosarcoma *m.* chondrosarcoma, malignant tumor of a cartilage.

conducir *vi.* to conduct; to drive.

conducta *f.* conduct, behavior.

conducto *m.* duct, conduit. *V.* cuadro en la página 80.

conectar *v.* to connect; to switch on.

conejillo de Indias *m.* guinea pig.

conejo *m.* rabbit; **fiebre de** ___ / ___ fever, tularemia; **la prueba del** ___ / ___ test, pregnancy test.

conexión *f.* connection.

conexión con el expediente médico *f.* medical record linkage. 1. any information that connects the patient with his or her medical history; 2. collection of data of the medical history of a patient provided by different

Conducto	Duct
biliar	biliary
cístico	cystic
colédoco	common bile
de Müeller	mullerian
de Wolff	wolffian
deferente	deferent
excretorio	excretory
eyaculatorio	ejaculatory
hepático	hepatic
lacrimal, lagrimal	lacrimal
linfático	lymphatic
nasolagrimal	nasolacrimal
seminal	seminal
seminífero	seminiferous tubule

sources; 3. any data of a participating patient in a clinical study that can reveal his or her identity as a participating subject.

confabulación *f.* confabulation, condition by which the individual fabricates imaginary situations soon to be forgotten.

conferencia *f.* conference, lecture, meeting.

confianza *f.* confidence, trust; ___ **en uno, en sí mismo-a** / self- ___; **falta de** ___ **en sí mismo-a** / lack of self-esteem.

confiar *v.* to entrust, to trust.

confidencial *a.* confidential; **comunicación o información** ___ / privileged communication or information.

confidencialidad *f.* confidentiality.

confinación, confinamiento *f., m.* confinement, restraint.

confinado-a, *a.* confined.

confirmación *f.* confirmation.

confirmar *v.* to confirm.

conflicto *m.* conflict.

confluencia *f.* confluence, meeting point of several channels.

conformar *v.* to conform, to adapt; **conformarse** *vr.* to resign oneself.

confortar *v.* to comfort.

confrontar *v.* to confront.

confundido-a, confuso-a *a.* confused, at a loss; **estar** ___ / to be at a loss.

confundir *v.* to confuse, to mix up; **confundirse** *vr.* to be or to become confused.

confusión *f.* confusion.

congelación *m.* freezing; **corte por** ___ / frozen cut; **punto de** ___ / ___ point; **secar por** ___ / freeze-dry; **sección por** ___ / frozen section, thin specimen of tissue that is frozen quickly and aids in diagnosing malignancies.

congelado-a *a.* frozen; ___ **al instante** / quick-frozen.

congelar *v.* to freeze; **congelarse** *vr.* to become frozen.

congénito-a *a.* congenital, existing since birth; ingrown.

congestión *f.* congestion, excessive accumulation of blood in a given body part or organ. ___ **activa** / active ___; ___ **funcional** / functional ___; ___ **pasiva** / passive ___; ___ **venosa** / venous ___ .

congestionado-a *a.* congested.

conización *f.* conization, removal of a cone shaped tissue such as the mucosa of the cervix.

conjugar *vi.* to conjugate.

conjuntiva *f.* conjunctiva, delicate mucous membrane covering the eyelids and the anterior surface of the eyeball; ___ **bulbar** / bulbar ___; ___ **palpebral** / palpebral ___ .

conjuntivitis *f.* conjunctivitis, infl. of the conjunctiva; ___ **aguda contagiosa** / acute contagious ___; ___ **alérgica** / allergic ___; ___ **catarral** / catarrhal ___; ___ **crónica** / chronic ___; ___ **epidémica** / epidemic ___; ___ **folicular** / follicular ___; ___ **hemorrágica** / hemorrhagic ___; ___ **infantil purulenta** / infantile purulent ___; ___ **vernal** / vernal ___; ___ **viral** / viral ___ .

conjuntivitis vernal o primaveral *f.* vernal or primaveral conjunctivitis, bilateral conjunctivitis accompanied by itching, most likely caused by allergy.

conjunto *m.* whole, sum of parts; a set; **en** ___ / as a whole.

conminuto-a *a.* comminuted, broken in many small fragments as in a fracture.

conmoción *f.* commotion.

cono *m.* cone, sensory organ that together with the rods of the retina receives color stimuli.

conocer *vi.* to know; to know about; **conocerse** *vr.* to know each other; to know oneself.

conocimiento *m.* 1. consciousness; **perder el** ___ / to lose ___; 2. knowledge; **no tener** ___ **de** / to be unaware of.

conque *conj.* so, so then.

consanguíneos *m.* blood relatives.

consciencia, conciencia *f.* conscience.

consciente *a.* conscious, aware.

consecuencia *f.* consequence; aftermath; **a ___ de** / as a result of.

conseguir *vi.* to obtain, to get.

consejero-a *m., f.* counselor.

consejo *m.* counsel, advice.

consenso *m.* consensus.

consentimiento *m.* consent, permission; **___ informado** / informed consent, voluntary permission given by the patient or guardian to perform a medical procedure or study after understanding all the different aspects involved in the procedure.

consentir *vi.* to consent, to permit; to pamper.

conservación *f.* conservation, preservation.

conservar *v.* to keep, to preserve.

consideración *f.* consideration; regard.

considerado-a *a.* considerate.

considerar *v.* to consider.

consistencia *f.* consistency.

consistente *a.* consistent, stable.

consistir *v.* to consist of, to be comprised of.

consolar *v.* to console, to comfort.

consomé *m.* consommé, broth.

constante *a.* constant, invariable.

constitución *f.* constitution, physical makeup.

constituir *vi.* to constitute.

constituyente *a.* constituent.

constricción *f.* constriction, narrowing, contraction.

consulta *f.* consultation; consulting room; **___ particular** / private practice; **horas de ___** / office hours.

consultar *v.* to consult, to confer.

consultor-a *m., f.* consultant, person who acts in an advisory capacity.

consultorio *m.* doctor's office; consulting room.

consumación *f.* consummation, completion.

consumir *v.* to consume; **consumirse** *vr.* to waste away.

consunción *f.* consumption, wasting, general emaciation of the body, as seen in patients with tuberculosis.

contacto *m.* contact; **___ inicial** / initial ___; **lentes de ___** / ___ lenses.

contado-a *a.* numbered; scarce; **al ___** / cash.

contagiar *v.* to transmit, to pass on, to infect.

contagio *m.* contagion, communication of disease.

contagioso-a *a.* contagious, communicable.

contaminación *f.* contamination.

contaminar *v.* to contaminate.

contar *vi.* to count; to tell; **___ con** / to rely on.

contener *vi.* to contain; **contenerse** *vr.* to restrain oneself, to hold back.

contenido *m.* content.

contento-a *a.* happy, content, pleased.

conteo *m.* count; **___ globular o de células sanguíneas** / blood cell ___ .

contestación *f.* answer.

contestar *v.* to answer.

contiguo-a *a.* contiguous, adjacent, next to.

continencia *f.* continence, abstinence, or moderation.

continuación *f.* continuation.

continuar *v.* to continue.

continuidad *f.* continuity.

contorno *m.* contour, outline.

contra *prep.* against.

contracción *f.* contraction, temporary shortening, as of a muscle fiber; **___ de fondo** / deep ___; **___ de hambre** / hunger ___; **___ espasmódica** / twitching; **___ ulterior** / after- ___ .

contracepción *f.* contraception, birth control.

contraceptivo *m.* contraceptive; **métodos ___-s** / methods of contraception.

contráctil *a.* contractile, having the capacity to contract.

contractilidad *f.* contractility, capacity to contract.

contractura *f.* contracture, prolonged or permanent involuntary contraction.

contradecir *vi.* to contradict, to negate.

contradicción *f.* contradiction.

contraer *vi.* to contract, [*una enfermedad*] to catch a sickness; **contraerse** *vr.* to be reduced in size, to shrink up, to crumple up.

contragolpe *m.* countercoup, lesion that occurs as a result of a blow to the opposite point.

contraindicación *f.* contraindication.

contraindicado-a *a.* contraindicated.

contralateral *a.* contralateral, rel. to the opposite side.

contrariado-a *a.* upset.

contrariar *v.* to disappoint, to upset.

contrario-a *a.* contrary; **al ___** / on the ___; **de lo ___** / otherwise.

contrarrestar *v.* to counter, to oppose.

contrastar *v.* to contrast.

contraste *m.* contrast; **medio de ___** / ___ medium.

contraveneno *m.* counterpoison, antidote.

contribución *f.* contribution.

contribuir *vi.* to contribute.

control *m.* control.

controlar *v.* to control, to regulate; **controlarse** *vr.* to control oneself.

contusión *f.* contusion, bruise.

convalecencia *f.* convalescence, period of time between an illness and the return to health.

convaleciente *a.* convalescent.

convencer *vi.* to convince.

conveniente *a.* convenient, handy.

convergencia *f.* convergence, inclination of two elements toward a common point.

conversación *f.* conversation.

conversión *f.* conversion, 1. change, transformation; 2. transformation of an emotion into a physical manifestation.

convertir *vi.* to convert; **convertirse** *vr.* to become.

convexo-a *a.* convex.

convulsión *f.* convulsion, violent involuntary muscular contraction of the muscles; ___ **febril** / febrile ___; ___ **jacksoniana** / Jacksonian ___; ___ **tónico-clónica** / tonic-clonic ___ .

convulsivo-a *a.* convulsive, rel. to convulsions; **actividad** ___ / seizure activity.

cooperación *f.* cooperation.

cooperar *v.* to cooperate.

cooperativo-a *a.* cooperative.

coordinación *f.* coordination; **falta de** ___ / lack of ___ .

coordinar *v.* to coordinate.

copa *f.* cup.

copia *f.* copy, imitation.

copiar *v.* to copy; to imitate.

coproemoliente *m.* stool softener.

coprofagia *f.* coprophagy, disorder that drives a person to eat feces.

coprolito *m.* coprolith, small mass of fecal concretion.

cópula *f.* copulation, sexual intercourse.

coqueluche *m.* whooping cough.

cor *L.* cor, heart; ___ **errante** / ___ mobile; ___ **juvenil** / ___ juvenum; ___ **pulmonar** / ___ pulmonale.

coracoclavicular *a.* coracoclavicular, rel. to the scapula and the clavicle.

coraje *m.* courage; anger.

corazón *m.* heart; hollow, muscular organ situated in the thorax that maintains the circulation of blood; **anormalidades congénitas del** ___ / congenital ___ diseases; **bloqueo del** ___ / ___ block; **bulbo del** ___ / bulbus cordis; **hipertrofia del** ___ / ___ hypertrophy; **latido del** ___ / heartbeat; **operación a** ___ **abierto** / open ___ surgery; **ruido del** ___ / ___ sound; **trasplante del** ___ / ___ transplant; **válvula del** ___ / ___ valve.

corazón artificial *m.* artificial heart, instrument or device that pumps blood with the same capacity as a normal heart.

cordal *a.* **muela** ___ / wisdom tooth.

cordectomía *f.* cordectomy, excision of a vocal cord.

cordel *m.* string, cord.

cordero *m.* lamb; **chuleta de** ___ / ___ chop; **lana de** ___ / ___ 's wool.

cordón *m.* any elongated, rounded structure; cord.

cordón umbilical *m.* umbilical cord, structure that connects the fetus with the placenta during the gestation period.

cordotomía *f.* cordotomy, an operation to cut certain sensory fibers in the spinal cord.

cordura *f.* sanity.

corea *f.* chorea, Huntington's disease, St. Vitus' dance, nervous disorder manifested by involuntary, rapid, and jerky, but well-coordinated movements of the limbs or facial muscles.

coriocarcinoma *m.* choriocarcinoma, malignant tumor found primarily in the testicle and the uterus.

corion *m.* 1. chorion, one of the two membranes that surround the fetus; 2. corium, dermis or true skin.

coriza *f.* coryza, acute or chronic rhinitis; runny nose.

córnea *f.* cornea, transparent membrane on the anterior surface of the eyeball. **injerto de la** ___ / corneal grafting.

córneo-a *a.* corneous, callous.

cornete nasal *m.* nasal concha.

cornezuelo de centeno *m.* ergot, fungus used in dry form or as an extract to induce uterine contractions or stop hemorrhaging after delivery.

coroides *f.* choroid membrane, membrane that supplies blood to the eye.

coroiditis *f.* choroiditis, infl. of the choroid.

corona *f.* corona, circular structure; crown; ___ **artificial** / artificial ___; ___ **en campana** / bell shaped ___; ___ **clínica** / clinical ___ .

coronamiento *m.* crowning.1. the stage of childbirth when the head of the fetus has entered completely the vulvar ring; 2. recovering of the prepared natural tooth with a chosen dental material as a veneer.

coronario-a *a.* coronary, encircling in the manner of a crown; **arteria** ___ / ___ artery; **desviación** ___ / ___ bypass; **trombosis** ___ / ___ thrombosis; **vasoespasmo** ___ / ___ vasospasm.

corporal *a.* corporeal, rel. to the body;
líquido ___ / body fluid; **peso** ___ / body
weight; **temperatura** ___ / body temperature.
corpulento-a *a.* corpulent, stout, robust.
corpus *m.* corpus, the human body.
corpus callosum *L.* corpus callosum, the great
commissure of the brain.
corpúsculo *m.* corpuscle, bud, small mass.
corpus luteum *L.* corpus luteum, yellow body,
yellow glandular mass in the ovary that is
formed by a ruptured follicle and produces
progesterone.
correa *f.* strap, belt.
correctivo-a *m., f.* corrective; antidote.
correcto-a *a.* correct; accurate.
corregir *vi.* to correct, to rectify.
correo *m.* mail.
correr *v.* to run, to jog.
correspondencia *f.* correspondence;
reciprocity.
corriente *f.* current, stream, flow of fluid, air, or
electricity along a conductor; **al** ___ / current,
up-to-date; *a.* current.
corroído-a *a.* corroded.
corromperse *vr.* to be affected with
putrefaction, to be tainted.
corrosión *f.* corrosion, deterioration by chemical
reaction.
corsé *m.* corset, jacket.
cortado-a *a.* cut, incised.
cortadura *f.* cut, slit.
cortar *v.* to cut, to incise; **cortarse** *vr.* to cut oneself.
corte *m.* cut, slit; ___ **transversal** / transection.
corteza *f.* cortex, the outer layer of an
organ; ___ **suprarrenal** / adrenal ___; ___
cerebral / cerebral ___ .
Corti, órgano de *m.* Corti's organ, the organ of
hearing by which sound is perceived.
cortical *a.* cortical, rel. to the cortex.
corticoide, corticosteroide *m.* corticoid,
corticosteroid, a steroid produced by the adrenal
cortex.
corticotropina *f.* corticotropin, hormonal
substance of adrenocorticotropic activity.
cortina *f.* curtain; blinds.
cortisol *m.* cortisol, hormone secreted by the
adrenal cortex.
cortisona *f.* cortisone, glycogenic steroid derived
from cortisol or produced synthetically.
corto-a *a.* short; ___ **de vista** / nearsighted.
cosa *f.* thing.
coser *v.* to sew.

cosmético *m.* cosmetic.
cosquillas *f., pl.* tickle, tickling; **hacer** ___ / to
tickle; **tener** ___ / to be ticklish.
cosquilleo *m.* tingling or prickling sensation.
costado *m.* side, flank; **al** ___ / to the ___ .
costal *a.* costal, rel. to the ribs.
costalgia *f.* costalgia, neuralgia, pain in the ribs.
costar *vi.* to cost; ___ **trabajo** / to be difficult.
costilla *f.* rib. 1. one of the bones of twelve pairs
that form the thoracic cage; 2. chop, a cut of
meat.
costo *m.* cost; ___ **de vida** / ___ of living.
costoclavicular *a.* costoclavicular, rel. to the
ribs and the clavicle.
costocondritis *f.* costochondritis, infl. of one
or more costal cartilages.
costoso-a *a.* costly, expensive.
costovertebral *a.* costovertebral, rel. to the
angle of the ribs and the thoracic vertebrae.
costra *f.* crust, scab; ___ **láctea** / cradle cap.
costumbre *f.* custom, habit; **tener la** ___ / to be
in the habit of.
costura *f.* seam.
cotidiano-a *a.* quotidian, that occurs every day;
malaria ___ / ___ malaria.
cowperitis *f.* cowperitis, infl. of Cowper's
gland.
coxa *f.* coxa, hip.
coxa magna *f.* coxa magna, abnormal widening
of the head of the femur.
coxa valga *f.* coxa valga, hip deformity
resulting in abnormal angulation of the femoral
shaft away from the midline of the body.
coxa vara *f.* coxa vara, hip deformity resulting
in abnormal angulation of the femoral shaft
toward the midline of the body.
coxalgia *f.* coxalgia, pain in the hip.
coxitis *f.* coxitis, infl. of the hip joint.
coyuntura *f.* joint; articulation.
craneal *a.* cranial, rel. to the cranium;
fractura ___ / skull fracture.
craneales, nervios *m., pl.* cranial nerves, each
of the twelve pairs of nerves connected to the
brain; **I. olfatorio** / olfactory; **II. óptico** / optic;
III. motor ocular común / oculomotor; **IV.
troclear** / trochlear; **V. trigémino** / trigeminal;
VI. motor ocular externo, abducente /
abducent; **VII. facial** / facial; **VIII. auditivo** /
auditory; **IX. glosofaríngeo** / glossopharyngeal;
X. neumogástrico, vago / vagus; **XI. espinal** /
accessory; **XII. hipogloso** / hypoglossal.
cráneo *m.* cranium, skull, braincase, the bony
structure of the head that covers the brain; **base
del** ___ / base of the ___ .

craneofaringioma *m.* craniopharyngioma, malignant brain tumor seen esp. in children.

craneoplastia *f.* surgical procedure to repair a defect in the cranium, such as a bone graft.

craneotomía *f.* craniotomy, trepanation of the cranium.

cráter *m.* crater, cavity.

creación *f.* creation.

crear *v.* to create.

creatina *f.* creatine, component of muscular tissue important in the anaerobic phase of muscular contraction.

creatinina *f.* creatinine, end product of the metabolism of creatine present in urine; **depuración de la ___ / ___** clearance, volume of plasma that is clear of creatinine.

crecer *vi.* to grow; **___ hacia adentro /** to grow inward.

crecido-a *a.* grown; large.

crecimiento *m.* growth.

crecimiento cero de población *m.* zero population growth, a demographic condition during a certain period of time, in which a population is stable, neither increasing nor diminishing.

crédito *m.* credit.

creer *vi.* to believe; to think.

crema *f.* cream, ointment.

cremastérico *a.* cremasteric, rel. to the cremaster muscle of the scrotal wall.

creosota *f.* creosote, antiseptic, oily liquid used as an expectorant.

crepitación *f.* crepitation, crackling; **___ pleural / pleural ___ .**

cresta *f.* crest. 1. a bony ridge; 2. the peak of a graph.

cretinismo *m.* cretinism, congenital hypothyroidism due to severe deficiency of the thyroid hormone.

cretino-a *m., f.* cretin, person afflicted with cretinism.

cretinoide *a.* cretinoid, having characteristics similar to cretinism.

crianestesia *f.* cryanesthesia. 1. anesthesia applied by means of localized refrigeration; 2. loss of ability to perceive cold.

cribiforme *a.* cribiform, perforated.

cricoides *a.* cricoid, shaped like a ring.

crimen *m.* crime.

criminal *m.* criminal; felon.

criocirugía *f.* cryosurgery, destruction of tissue through the application of intense cold.

criógeno *a.* cryogenic, that which produces low temperatures.

crioglobulina *f.* cryoglobulin, a serum globulin that crystallizes spontaneously at low temperatures.

crioscopía *f.* cryoscopy, testing and determining the freezing point of a fluid, gen. blood or urine as a sample, and comparing it with that of distilled water.

crioterapia *f.* cryotherapy, therapeutic treatment using a cold medium.

cripta *f.* crypt, small tubular recess.

críptico *m.* cryptic, hidden.

criptococosis *f.* cryptococcosis, a systemic fungus that may affect different organs of the body, esp. the brain.

criptogénico-a *a.* cryptogenic, of an unknown cause.

criptorquidia, criptorquismo*f., m.* cryptorchism, failure of a testis to descend into the scrotum.

crisis *f.* crisis, turning point in a disease; **___ de identidad /** identity **___ ; ___ nerviosa /** nervous breakdown.

crisoterapia *f.* chrysotherapy, treatment with gold salts.

crista *f.* crista, a projecting structure or ridge gen. surmounting a bone.

cristal *m.* crystal.

cristalino *m.* crystalline lens, lens of the eye behind the pupil; **-a** *a.* crystalline, transparent.

cristaloideo-a *a.* crystalloid, resembling crystal.

cromático-a *a.* chromatic, rel. to colors.

cromatina *f.* chromatin, portion of the cell nucleus that stains more readily.

cromocito *m.* chromocyte, a colored or pigmented cell.

cromófobo *m.* chromophobe, a cell or tissue that resists stain.

cromógeno *m.* chromogen, a substance that produces color.

cromosoma *m.* chromosome, part of the nucleus of the cell that contains the genes.

cromosoma x *m.* X-chromosome, differential chromosome that determines the female sex characteristics.

cromosoma y *m.* Y-chromosome, differential chromosome that determines the male sex characteristics.

cromosómico-a *a.* chromosomic, rel. to the chromosome; **aberraciones ___ -s /** chromosome aberrations.

crónico-a *a.* chronic, of long duration, prolonged effect.

cronológico-a *a.* chronological, rel. to the sequence of time.

cronotropismo *m.* chronotropism, modification of the rate of a regular pace or beat such as the heartbeat.

crudo-a *a.* raw; crude; uncooked; **carne ___** / **___** meat.

cruel *a.* cruel.

cruento-a *a.* bloody.

crup *m.* croup, infl. of the larynx in children, usu. accompanied by hoarse coughing, fever, and difficulty in breathing; **___ espasmódico** / spasmodic **___** .

crus *L.* crus, leg or a structure resembling one; **___ del cerebro** / cerebral **___** .

Cruz Roja Internacional *f.* International Red Cross, international organization for medical assistance.

cruzar *vi.* to cross.

cuadra *f.* city block.

cuadrado-a *a.* square, quadrate, that has four equal sides; **lóbulo ___** / **___** lobe.

cuadrángulo *m.* quadrangle.

cuadrante *m.* quadrant, 90°, one-fourth of a circle.

cuadrar *v.* to square; to fit.

cuadriceps *m.* quadriceps, four-headed muscle, extensor of the leg.

cuadriplegia *f.* quadriplegia, paralysis of the four extremities.

cuadriplégico-a *a.* quadriplegic, that is paralyzed in the four extremities.

cuajado-a *a.* curdled; **leche ___** / **___** milk.

cuajar *v.* to curdle; **cuajarse** *vr.* to congeal, to thicken.

cuajo *m.* curd.

cualidad *f.* quality.

cualitativo-a *a.* qualitative, rel. to quality; **prueba ___** / **___** test.

cualquier-a *a.* any.

cuando, cuándo *adv.* when, whenever; **de ___ en ___** / from time to time; **___ usted quiera** / whenever you want; **¿ ___ empezó?** / **___** did it start?

cuantitativo-a *a.* quantitative, rel. to amount.

cuanto, cúanto-a *a., adv.* how much, how many; **¿ ___ tiempo?** / how long?; **___ antes** / as soon as possible; **en ___** / as soon as; **en ___ a** / in regard to; **unos ___ -s** / a few.

cuarentena *f.* quarantine, period of forty days during which a restraint is put on the movement of persons or animals to prevent the spread of a disease.

cuarto *m.* 1. room; **___ de baño** / bathroom; **___ de dormir** / bedroom; **___ de niños** / nursery

room; 2. quart, one-fourth of a whole; **-a** *a.* fourth.

cubeta *f.* basin.

cubierta *f.* covering, sheath, shield.

cubierto-a *a., pp.* of **cubrir,** covered.

cubital *a.* cubital, rel. to the cubital bone or elbow.

cúbito *m.* cubitus, ulna, the inner, long bone of the forearm.

cubreboca *m.* surgical mask.

cubrir *v.* to cover, to drape as with a sterilized cloth.

cucaracha *f.* cockroach.

cuclillas (en) *adv.* in a squatting position.

cuchara *f.* spoon; tablespoon.

cucharada *f.* spoonful; scoop; **___ de postre** / of dessert; **___ de sopa** / **___** of soup.

cucharita *f.* teaspoon; **___ de cafe** / cochleare parvum.

cuchichear *v.* to whisper.

cuchillita *f.* small knife; razor blade.

cuchillo *m.* knife.

cuello *m.* neck; collar. 1. part that joins the head and the trunk of the body; 2. area between the crown and the root of a tooth.

cuello uterino *m.* uterine neck; cervix uteri; **dilatación del ___** / dilation of the cervix; **incompetencia del ___** / cervical incompetence.

cuenta *f.* account, bill; **arreglar la ___** / to settle the **___**; **___ bancaria** / bank **___**; **darse ___** / to realize; **pagar la ___** / to pay the **___**; **tener en ___** / to take into **___** .

cuentacélulas *m.* cell counting device.

cuerda *f.* cord, cordon.

cuerdas vocales *f., pl.* vocal chords, main organ of the voice; **___ superiores o falsas** / false **___**; **___ inferiores o verdaderas** / true **___** .

cuerdo-a *a.* sane; wise.

cuerno *m.* horn.

cuero *m.* skin, hide; **___ cabelludo** / scalp; **en ___ -s** / naked.

cuerpo *m.* body; **___ -s extraños** / foreign bodies. *V.* ilustración en la página 86.

cuerpo amarillo *m.* yellow body; corpus luteum.

cuerpos cetónicos, acetónicos *m., pl.* ketone bodies, known as acetones.

cuestión *f.* question; issue, matter.

cuestionario *m.* questionnaire.

cuidado *m.* care, attention; **___ bajo custodia** / custodial care; **___ intensivo** / intensive **___**; **___ postnatal** /

C

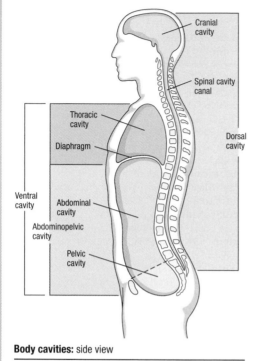

Body cavities: side view

Labels on figure:
- Cranial cavity
- Spinal cavity canal
- Thoracic cavity
- Diaphragm
- Dorsal cavity
- Ventral cavity
- Abdominal cavity
- Abdominopelvic cavity
- Pelvic cavity

postnatal ___; ___ **prenatal** / prenatal ___; ___ **primario** / primary ___; **estar al ___ de** / to be under the ___ of; **negación de ___** / refusal of ___; **nivel de ___ satisfactorio** / reasonable ___; **tratar con ___** / to handle with care.

cuidadoso-a *a.* careful, mindful.

cuidar *v.* to take care, to look after.

cul-de-sac *Fr.* cul-de-sac. 1. blind pouch, cavity closed on one end; 2. rectouterine pouch.

culdoscopía *f.* culdoscopy, viewing of the pelvic and abdominal cavity with a culdoscope.

culdoscopio *m.* culdoscope, an endoscopic instrument inserted through the vagina to do a visual examination of the pelvis and the abdominal cavity.

culebra *f.* snake.

culebrilla *f.* the shingles, herpes zoster, herpes-like cutaneous disease.

culero *m.* diaper.

culpa *f.* guilt; fault, blame; **tener la ___** / to be at fault.

culpar *v.* to blame.

cultivar *v.* to cultivate.

cultivo *m.* culture, artificial growth of microorganisms or living tissue cells in the laboratory; ___ **de orina** / urine ___; ___ **de sangre** / blood ___; ___ **de tejido** / tissue ___; **medio de ___** / ___ medium.

cuna *f.* crib, cradle, bassinet.

cunilinguo-a *a.* cunnilingus, rel. to the practice of oral stimulation or manipulation of the penis or clitoris.

cuña *f.* wedge; bedpan.

cuñado-a *m., f.* brother-in-law; sister-in-law.

cúpula *f.* dome.

cura *f.* 1. cure; *m.* 2. priest.

curable *a.* curable, healable.

curacion *f.* cure; healing process.

curanderismo *m.* faith healing.

curandero *m.* faith healer, medicine man, shaman.

curar *v.* to cure, to heal.

curare *m.* curare, venom extracted from various plants used to provide muscle relaxation during anesthesia.

curativo-a *a.* curative, having healing properties.

cureta *f.* curette, scoop-like instrument with sharp edges used for curettage.

curetaje *m.* curettage, scraping of a surface or cavity with a sharp-edged instrument; ___ **uterino** / D&C, dilation and curettage of the uterine cavity.

curioso-a *a.* curious.

curita *f.* bandaid.

curso *m.* course; direction.

curva *f.* curve, bend.

curvatura *f.* curvature, deviation from a straight line.

Cushing, síndrome de *m.* Cushing's syndrome, adrenogenital syndrome manifested by obesity and muscular weakness gen. associated with an excessive production of cortisol.

cuspideo-a *a.* cuspidal, pointed.

cuspide *f.* cuspid, point.

custodia *f.* custody; **bajo ___ del estado** / ward of the state.

cutáneo-a *a.* cutaneous, rel. to the skin; **absorción ___** / ___ absorption; **glándulas ___-s o sebáceas** / ___ glands; **manifestaciones ___-s** / skin manifestations; **pruebas ___-s** / skin tests; **úlcera ___** / skin ulcer.

cutícula *f.* cuticle, outer layer of the skin.

cutis *m.* cutis, complexion, skin.

cutis colgante *m.* sagging facial skin.

d

d *abr.* **densidad** / density; **difunto** / deceased; **dosis** / dose.

dacriadenitis *f.* dacryadenitis, infl. of the lacrimal gland.

dacriagogo *m.* dacryagogue, an agent that stimulates tear formation.

dacricistalgia *f.* dacrycystalgia, pain in the lacrimal sac.

dacrioadenectomía *f.* dacryoadenectomy, removal of a lacrimal gland.

dacriocistectomía *f.* dacryocystectomy, surgical removal of the lacrimal sac.

dacriocistitis *f.* dacryocystitis, infl. of the lacrimal sac.

dacriocisto *m.* dacryocyst, internal lacrimal sac.

dacriocistotomía *f.* dacryocystotomy, incision of the lacrimal sac.

dacrioestenosis *f.* dacriostenosis, stricture of the lacrimal sac.

dacriolitiasis *f.* dacryolithiasis, stones in the lacrimal apparatus.

dacriopiorrea *f.* dacryopyorrhea, tear excretion containing leukocytes.

dactilitis *f.* dactylitis, infl. of a finger or toe.

dáctilo *m.* dactyl, finger or toe.

dactilocopista *m., f.* fingerprint expert.

dactilología *f.* dactylology, sign language.

dactilografía *f.* dactylography, study of fingerprints.

dactilograma *f.* dactylogram, fingerprint.

dactilomegalia *f.* dactylomegaly, excessive growth of fingers and toes.

dactiloscopia *f.* dactyloscopy, study of fingerprints for the purpose of identification.

dado-a *a. pp.* de **dar,** given; ___ **a** / ___ to; ___ **que** / ___ that.

Dakin, solución de *f.* Dakin's solution, solution used for cleansing wounds.

daltonismo *m.* daltonism, defective perception of the colors red and green.

damiana *f.* damiana, native plant from Mexico the leaves of which are used as a diuretic.

danazol *m.* danazol, Deprancol, Danocrine, synthetic hormone that suppresses the action of the anterior pituitary.

dañado-a *a.* hurt; [*comida*] spoiled; tainted.

dañar *v.* to harm; to hurt; to injure.

dañino-a *a.* harmful; noxious.

daño *m.* harm, [*to an object*] damage, hurt; *v.* **hacer** ___ / to harm, to hurt; **no hace** ___ / it doesn't hurt.

daños y perjuicios *m., pl.* damages.

dapsona *f.* dapsone, sulfone drug used in the treatment of leprosy.

dar *vi.* to give; to minister; ___ **a luz** / to give birth; ___ **de alta** / discharge from the hospital; ___ **de comer** / to feed; ___ **el pecho** / to breast-feed; ___ **lugar a** / to cause; *darse* / *vr.* to give oneself; ___ **por vencido** / to give up; ___ **prisa** / to hurry.

dartos *m.* dartos, a layer of smooth muscle fibers found beneath the skin of the scrotum.

Darvon *m.* Darvon, trade name for dextro propoxyphene hydrochloride, an oral analgesic.

Darwin, reflejo de *m.* Darwinian reflex, tendency of small children to raise themselves holding onto a bar.

dátil *m.* date.

dato *m.* fact, piece of information.

Daviel, operación de *f.* Daviel's operation, extracapsular extraction of a cataract.

de *prep.* of, from; [posesión], **los rayos-x** ___ **la paciente** / the patient's x-rays; [contenido] **bicarbonato** ___ **sodio** / sodium bicarbonate; [procedencia] **vengo** ___ **la consulta** / I am coming from the doctor's office.

debajo *adv.* underneath; ___ **de** / under; **por** ___ / beneath.

deber *v.* to be obligated; to owe.

débil *a.* debilitated, weak, feeble.

debilidad *f.* debility, weakness. ___ **senil** / senility ; ___ **mental** / mental deficiency.

debilitante *a.* debilitating, rel. to a sickness that causes weakness.

debilitar *v.* to weaken; **debilitar(se)** *vr.* to feel weaker.

decaer *vi.* to weaken; [en *ánimo*] to decline.

decaído-a *a.* dispirited, dejected.

decaimiento *m.* dejection.

decalcificación *f.* decalcification, loss or reduction of lime salts from bones or teeth.

decapacitación *f.* decapacitation, process.

decapsulación *f.* decapsulation, incision and extirpation of a capsule.

deceleración *f.* deceleration; diminished velocity, such as of heart frequency.

decepción *f.* deceit; layer of uterine endometrium that is shed during menstruation.

decidido-a *a.* decided; determined.

decidir *v.* to decide; **decidirse** *vr.* to make up one's mind.

decidua *f.* decidua, mucous membrane of the uterus that develops during pregnancy and is discharged after delivery.

deciduo-a *a.* deciduous, of a temporal nature.

decir *vi.* to say; to tell; **querer __ / ** to mean.

decisión *f.* decision, resolution.

declinación *f.* declination, rotation of the eye.

decolesterolización *f.* decholesterolization, therapeutic reduction of cholesterol concentration in the blood.

decorticación *f.* decortication, removal of part of the cortical surface of an organ such as the brain.

decrépito-a *a.* decrepit, worn with age.

decúbito *m.* decubitus, lying down position; **__ dorsal** / dorsal __, on the back; **__ lateral** / lateral __, on the side ; **__ prono** / ventral __; **__ supino** / dorsal __; **__ ventral** / ventral __, on the stomach; **radiografía en __ lateral** / lateral x-ray film.

decusación *f.* decussation, crossing of structures in the form of an x; **__ de las pirámides** / **__** of pyramids, crossing of nervous fibers from one pyramid to the other in the medulla oblongata; **__ óptica** / optic **__**, crossing of the fibers of the optic nerves.

dedalera *f.* foxglove, common name for Digitalis purpurea.

dedo *m.* finger; toe; **caída de los __ -s del pie** / toe drop; **__ del pie** / toe; **__ en garra, en martillo** / hammer, mallet finger or toe; **__ en palillo de tambor** / clubbing; **__ gordo** / hallux; **__ índice** / index **__**, forefinger; **__ meñique** / little **__**; **__ pulgar** / thumb; **desviación de un __** / valgus; **separación de un __** / varus.

deducción *f.* deduction, to reason from the general to the particular.

deducible *a.* deductible.

deducir *vi.* to deduce, to infer.

defecación *f.* defecation, bowel movement.

defecar *vi.* to defecate.

defectivo-a *a.* defective.

defecto *m.* defect; blemish; **__ congénito** / congenital **__** .

defectuoso-a *a.* defective, faulty.

defender *vi.* to defend.

defensa *f.* defense, resistance to a disease; **__ propia** / self-**__**; **mecanismo de __ / __** mechanism.

defensa por demencia *f.* the concept that a defendant who is declared insane cannot be found guilty of the crime committed.

deferente *a.* deferent, conveying away from.

defibrilación *f.* defibrillation, the act of changing an irregular heart beat to a normal rhythm.

deficiencia *f.* deficiency; **__ de lactasa** / lactase **__**; **__ de galactocinasa** / galactokinasa **__**; **enfermedad por __ / __** disease; **__ mental** / mental **__**; **__ mineral** / mineral **__** .

deficiente *a.* deficient, wanting.

déficit *m.* deficit, deficiency.

definición *f.* definition.

definitivo-a *a.* definitive, final; **diagnosis __ / __** diagnosis ; **-mente** *adv.* definitely.

deflexión *f.* deflection, diversion; unconscious diversion of ideas.

deformación *f.* deformation, distortion.

deforme *a.* deformed.

deformidad *f.* deformity, irregularity, a congenital or acquired malformation.

defunción *f.* demise, death.

defurfuración *f.* defurfuration, shedding fine, branlike scales from the skin.

degeneración *f.* degeneration, deterioration.

degenerado-a *a.* degenerate.

degenerar *v.* to degenerate.

deglución *f.* deglutition, the act of swallowing.

deglutir *v.* to swallow.

degradación *f.* degradation, reducing a chemical compound to a simpler one.

dehidroandrosterona *f.* dehydroandrosterone, previously known as dehydroepiandrosterone, androgenic steroid found in the urine.

dehidrocolesterol *m.* dehydrocholesterol, skin substance that becomes vitamin B complex by the action of the sun's rays.

dehidrocorticosterona *f.* dehydrocorticosterone, steroid found in the adrenal cortex.

dehiscencia *f.* dehiscence, splitting open of a wound.

déjá vu *Fr.* déjá vu, an illusory impression of having seen or experienced a new situation before.

dejadez *f.* lassitude, neglect, carelessness.

dejar *v.* to leave; to let, to allow; **__ dicho / __** word; **__ órdenes / __** orders; **__ de / ** to stop from, to quit.

del contraction of the *prep.* **de** and the *art.* **el.**

delante *adv.* in front; before.

deletéreo-a *a.* deleterious, harmful, noxious.

delgado-a *a.* thin, slender, slim.

delgaducho-a *a.* thin; delicate.
delicado-a *a.* delicate, tender.
delicioso-a *a.* delicious.
delicuescencia *f.* deliquescence, condition of a substance when it becomes liquified by absorption of water from the air.
deligación *f.* deligation, art of applying ligatures or binders.
delimitación *f.* delimitation, process of marking the limits or circumscribing.
delincuencia *f.* delinquency; __ **juvenil** / juvenile __ .
delincuente *a.* delinquent.
delirante *a.* delirious, raving.
delirar *v.* to be delirious, to rave.
delirio *m.* delirium, temporary mental disturbance marked by hallucinations and distorted perceptions; __ **agudo** / acute __ ; __ **crónico** / chronic __ ; __ **de control** / __ of control; __ **de grandeza** / __ of grandeur; __ **de negación** / __ of negation; __ **de persecución** / persecution complex; __ **tremens** / __ tremens, a form of alcoholic psychosis.
deltoideo-a *a.* deltoid. 1. rel. to the deltoid muscle that covers the shoulder; 2. shaped like a triangle.
delusión *f.* delusion, false beliefs.
demacrado-a *a.* gaunt, wasted.
demanda *f.* demand; **alimentación por** __ / __ feeding.
demandar *v.* to demand; to sue.
demás *adv.* besides; that which is beyond a certain measure; **lo** __ / the rest.
demasiado-a *a.* excessive; *adv.* too much.
demencia *f.* dementia, dementia praecox, insanity; esquizofrenia; __ **alcohólica** / alcoholic __ ; __ **orgánica** / organic __ ; __ **senil** / senile __ .
demente *a.* demented, one suffering from dementia.
Demerol *m.* Demerol, meperidine hydrochloride, trade name for an analgesic drug with properties similar to morphine.
demora *f.* delay.
demorar *v.* to delay; **demorarse** *vr.* to be delayed, to take too long.
demostración *f.* demonstration.
demostrar *vi.* to demonstrate; to prove.
demulcente *m.* demulcent, agent that soothes and softens the skin or mucosa.
dendrita *f.* dendrite, protoplasmic prolongation of the nerve cell that receives the nervous impulses.

dengue *m.* dengue fever, acute febrile and infectious disease caused by a virus and transmitted by the *Aedes* mosquito.
denominación *f.* denomination, name.
densidad *f.* density; __ **del vapor** / vapor __ ; __ **óptica** / optic __ ; __ **ósea** / bone __ ; __ **urinaria** / urinary __ .
denso-a *a.* dense; thick.
dentado-a *a.* dentiform, toothed. 1. having projections like teeth on the edge; 2. shaped like a tooth.
dentadura *f.* teeth; __ **postiza** / denture.
dental, dentario-a *a.* dental, rel. to the teeth; **absceso** __ / __ abscess; **anquilosis** __ / __ ankylosis; **arco** __ / __ arch; **bulbo** __ / __ bulb; **cavidad** __ / __ cavity; **cirujano** __ / __ surgeon; **cuidado** __ / __ care; **esmalte** __ / __ enamel; **folículo** __ / __ follicle; **hilo** __ / __ floss; **implante** __ / __ implant; **inclusión** __ / __ inclusion; **impacción** __ / __ impaction; **impresión** __ / __ impression; **placa dentaria** / __ plaque; **salud pública** __ / __ public health; **sarro** __ / __ tartar; **servicios de salud** __ / __ health services; **técnico** __ / __ technician; **técnico en profiláctica** __ / __ hygienist; **uso de hilo** __ / flossing.
dentición *f.* dentition, time when children's teeth are cut; __ **primaria** / primary __ , first teeth; __ **secundaria o dientes permanentes** / secondary __ , permanent teeth.
dentilabial *a.* dentilabial, rel. to the teeth and the lips.
dentina *f.* dentin, calcified tissue that constitutes the larger portion of the tooth.
dentinogénesis *f.* dentinogenesis, formation of dentin.
dentinoma *m.* dentinoma, tumor consisting mainly of dentin.
dentista *m., f.* dentist; __ **de niños** / pedodontist.
dentoide *a.* dentoid, tooth-shaped.
dentro *adv.* within; **por** __ / inside.
denudación *f.* denudation, deprival of a protecting surface by surgery, trauma, or pathologic change.
deoxihemoglobina *f.* deoxyhemoglobin, reduced form of hemoglobin that occurs when the oxihemoglobin looses oxygen.
dependencia *f.* dependence, subordination.
depender *v.* to depend; to rely.
dependiente *m., f.* dependent; **drenaje** __ / __ drainage; **edema** __ / __ edema; **personalidad** __ / __ personality.

d

depersonalización *f.* depersonalization, a state of mind in which the subject loses the feeling of his/her own identity in relation to members of groups that he/she is associated with.

depigmentación *f.* depigmentation, partial or complete loss of pigment.

depilación *f.* depilation, removal of hair by the roots.

depilar *v.* to depilate, to remove hair.

depilatorio *m.* depilatory, hair remover.

depleción *f.* depletion; 1. the act of draining; 2. the removal of accumulated liquids or solids to an excess; __ **de fluido** / fluid __; __ **de líquidos del cuerpo, deshidratación** / __ of body liquids, dehydration; __ **de potasio, hipopotasemia** / potassium __, hypopotassemia ; __ **salina** / saline __;

deporte *m.* sports; athletics.

deposición *f.* bowel movement; __ **-es blandas o acuosas** / loose bowels;

depositar *v.* to deposit.

depósito *m.* deposit; precipitate.

depravación *f.* depravation, perversion.

depravado-a *a.* depraved, corrupt; perverted.

depresión *f.* depression. 1. state of sadness and melancholia accompanied by apathy; 2. cavity.

depresor *m.* depressor. 1. agent used to lower an established level of function or activity of the organism; __ **de lengua** / tongue __; 2. tranquilizer; **-a** *a.* producing or rel. to depression.

deprimente *n.* depressing.

deprimido-a *a.* depressed, downcast.

deprimir *v.* to depress; *deprimirse vr.* to become depressed.

depuración *f.* depuration, purification.

depurar *v.* to depurate, to purify.

derecha *f.* right hand side; **a la __** / to the right;

derecho-a *a.* straight, erect; *adv.* straight, straight ahead.

derecho *m.* right; the study of law; **los __-s del paciente** / the patient's __-s; **tener __** / to have the __;

derecho a rehusar tratamiento *m.* the patient's right to refuse treatment.

derecho a tratamiento *m.* right to treatment, the patient's right to receive adequate treatment by a medical facility that has assumed responsibility for the patient's care.

derivación *f.* derivation, bypass. 1. shunt, alternate or lateral course that occurs through anastomosis or through a natural anatomical characteristic; __ **aortocoronaria** / aortocoronary bypass; __ **aortoilíaca** / aortoiliac bypass; __ **portacava** / portacaval shunt; 2. origin or source of a substance.

derivación de flujo lento *f.* low-flow shunt.

derivar *v.* to derive; to infer, to deduce.

dermabrasión *f.* dermabrasion, procedure to remove acne scars, nevi or fine wrinkles of the skin.

dermalgia, dermatalgia *f.* dermalgia, dermatalgia, pain in the skin.

dermático-a *a.* dermal, dermatic, rel. to the skin.

dermatitis *f.* dermatitis, infl. of the skin; __ **actínica** / actinic __, produced by sunlight or ultraviolet light; __ **alérgica** / allergic __; __ **atópica** / atopic __; __ **eritematosa** / erythematous __; __ **gangrenosa** / gangrenous __; __ **medicamentosa** / medicinal __; __ **ocupacional, industrial** / __ occupational; __ **papillaris capilliti** / papillaris capilliti __; __ **por contacto** / contact __; __ **seborréica** / seborrheic __ .

dermatofito *m.* dermatophyte, fungus that attacks the skin.

dermatofitosis *f.* dermatophytosis, athlete's foot, fungal infection of the skin caused by a dermatophyte.

dermatolisis *f.* dermatolysis, loss or atrophy of skin due to sickness.

dermatología *f.* dermatology, the study of skin diseases.

dermatológico-a *a.* dermatological, rel. to the skin.

dermatólogo *m.* dermatologist, specialist in dermatology.

dermatomicosis *f.* dermatomycosis, infl. of the skin by fungi.

dermatomiositis *f.* dermatomyositis, disease of the connective tissue manifested by edema, dermatitis, and infl. of the muscles.

dermátomo, dermatótomo *m.* dermatome, dermatotome, instrument used for cutting skin in thin slices.

dermatoneurosis *f.* dermatoneurosis, any cutaneous eruption or rash due to emotional stimuli.

dermatoplastia *f.* dermatoplasty, surgery of the skin.

dermatosífilis *f.* dermatosyphilis, skin manifestation of syphilis.

dermatosis, dermatopatía *f.* dermatosis, dermatopathy, general term used for skin disease; ___ **eritematosa de los pañales** / diaper rash.

dérmico-a *a.* dermic, rel. to the skin.

dermis *f.* dermis, skin.

dermitis *f.* dermitis, infl. of the skin.

dermoflebitis *f.* dermophlebitis, infl. of superficial veins.

dermoideo-a *a.* dermoid, resembling skin; **quiste** ___ / ___ cyst, congenital, usu. benign.

derramar *v.* to spill.

derrame *m.* spill, overflow, outflow.

derretir *vi.* to melt; **derretirse** *vr.* to become liquified by heat.

desabrido-a *a.* tasteless; insipid.

desabrigado-a *a.* underclothed; too exposed to the elements.

desacostumbrado-a *a.* unaccustomed.

desacuerdo *m.* disagreement.

desadvertidamente *adv.* inadvertently; unintentionally.

desafortunado-a *a.* unfortunate, unlucky.

desagradable *a.* disagreeable, unpleasant.

desagradecido-a *a.* ungrateful.

desahogarse *vr., vi.* to release one's grief; *pop.* to let out steam.

desalentar *v., vi.* to discourage; **desalentarse** *vr.* to become discouraged.

desangramiento *m.* excessive bleeding.

desangrarse *vr.* to bleed excessively.

desanimado-a *a.* downhearted, discouraged.

desaparecer *vi.* to disappear.

desaprobar *vi.* to disapprove; to refute.

desarrollado-a *a.* developed.

desarrollar *v.* [*síntomas*] to develop; to grow.

desarrollo *m.* development; growth; ___ **infantil** / child ___; ___ **físico** / physical ___; ___ **psicomotor y físico** / psychomotor and physical ___ .

desarrollo motor *n.* motor development.

desarticulación *f.* disarticulation, separation or amputation of two or more bones from one joint.

desarticulado-a *a.* disarticulated, rel. to a bone that has been separated from its joint.

desaseo *m.* uncleanliness.

desasosiego *m.* uneasiness, unrest.

desastre *m.* disaster.

desatendido-a *a.* unattended.

desatinado-a *a.* lacking good judgment, wild.

desayunar *v.* to have breakfast.

desayuno *m.* breakfast.

desbridamiento *m.* debridement, removal of foreign bodies or dead or damaged tissue, esp. from a wound.

descafeinado-a *a.* decaffeinated.

descalcificación *f.* decalcification. 1. loss of calcium salts from a bone; 2. removal of calcareous matter.

descalzo-a *a.* barefooted.

descamación *f.* desquamation, the act of shedding scales from the epidermis.

descansado-a *a.* rested, refreshed.

descanso *m.* rest, tranquility.

descarado-a *a.* impudent, shameless.

descarga *f.* discharge, excretion.

descarnado-a *a.* without skin, fleshless; very thin person.

descartar *v.* to reject, to dismiss.

descendente *a.* descending.

descendiente *m.* descendant, offspring.

descentrado-a *a.* decentered, not centered.

descoloramiento *m.* discoloration.

descolorido-a *a.* discolored, washed out.

descompensación *f.* decompensation, inability of the heart to maintain adequate circulation.

descomponerse *vr. vi.* to decompose.

descomposición *f.* decomposition, dissolution of a substance in chemical elements; **índice de** ___ / ___ rate.

descompresión *f.* decompression, lack of air or gas pressure as in deep-sea diving; **cámara de** ___ / ___ chamber; ___ **quirúrgica** / surgical ___; **enfermedad por** ___ / ___ sickness; *pop.* the bends.

desconcierto *m.* uncertainty, confusion.

desconectar *v.* to disconnect; to switch off.

desconfiar *v.* to distrust; to lack confidence.

descongelación *f.* thawing.

descongelar *v.* to defrost; to thaw.

descongestionante *m.* decongestant.

descongestionar *v.* to decongest.

descontaminación *f.* decontamination, the process of freeing the environment, objects, or persons from contaminated or harmful agents such as radioactive substances.

descontaminar *v.* to decontaminate, to free from contamination.

descontento-a *a.* unhappy.

descontinuado-a *a.* discontinued, suspended.

descontinuar *v.* to discontinue.

descoyuntamiento *m.* luxation, dislocation.

descremar *v.* [*leche*] to skim.

describir *v.* to describe.

descripción *f.* description.

descrito-a *a. pp.* de **describir,** described.

descubierto-a *a. pp.* de **descubrir,** uncovered.

d

descubrimiento *m.* discovery.

descubrir *vi.* to discover; to uncover.

descuento *m.* discount.

descuidado-a *a.* careless, negligent.

descuido *m.* carelessness.

desde *prep.* since, from; ___ **ahora en adelante** / from now on; ___ **hace (una semana, un mes)** / it has been (a week, a month) since; ___ **luego** / of course.

desdentado-a *a.* edentulous, toothless.

desdoblamiento *m.* splitting; ___ **de tonos cardíacos** / reduplication of heart sounds.

desear *v.* to wish, to desire.

desecación *f.* desiccation, drying, draining.

desecado-a *a.* desiccated, dried up.

desecante *m.* desiccant, substance that causes dryness.

desecar *vi.* to desiccate, to dry up.

desechable *a.* disposable.

desechar *v.* to discard, to cast aside.

desecho *m.* waste;___ **de efectos medicos** / medical ___ .

desempeñar *v.* to perform a given task or role.

desencadenamiento *m.* trigger, impulse that initiates other events; **puntos de** ___ / ___ points.

desencadenar *v.* to trigger, to initiate a succession of events.

desencajado-a *a.* disengaged; disjointed; gaunt.

desencajar *v.* to disengage.

desenlace *m.* outcome, conclusion.

desensibilizar *v.* to desensitize, to diminish or annul sensibility.

deseo *m.* wish, desire.

deseoso-a *a.* desirous, eager.

desequilibrado-a *a.* imbalanced; ___ **mental** / mentally ___ .

desequilibrio *m.* imbalance;___ **degenerativo** / degenerative ___; ___ **hidroelectrolítico** / hydroelectrolytic ___; ___ **hormonal** / hormonal ___ .

desesperación *f.* desperation, despair, despondency; hopelessness.

desesperado-a *a.* desperate, despairing, despondent.

desesperarse *vr.* to despair, to despond.

desfallecer *vi.* to faint; to become weak.

desfervescencia *f.* defervescence, period of fever decline.

desfibrilación *f.* defibrillation, action of returning an irregular heartbeat to its normal rhythm.

desfibrilador *m.* defibrillator, electrical device used to restore the heart to a normal rhythm.

desfiguración, desfiguramiento *m., f.* defacement; disfigurement.

desfigurar *v.* to disfigure, to distort.

desganarse *vr.* to lose appetite.

desgarradura, desgarro *m. f.* tear, laceration.

desgarrar *v.* to tear, to pull apart; to rip.

desgastado-a *a.* worn; eroded; [*persona*] wasted.

desgastar *v.* to erode; **desgastarse** *vr.* to wear down or away.

desgaste *m.* wearing down.

desgracia *f.* adversity, mishap.

desgraciadamente *adv.* unfortunately.

desgrasar *v.* to degrease, to remove the fat.

deshacer *vi.* to undo.

deshidratado-a *a.* dehydrated, free of water.

deshidratar *v.* to dehydrate, eliminate water from a substance.

deshidratarse *vr.* to dehydrate, to lose liquid from the body or tissues.

deshumanización *f.* dehumanization, loss of human qualities.

deshumectante *m.* dehumidifier, device to diminish humidity.

desierto *m.* desert.

desigual *a.* uneven; unlike, unequal.

desilusión *f.* disillusion, disenchantment.

desilusionar *v.* to disillusion; **desilusionarse** *vr.* to become disenchanted.

desinfección *f.* disinfection; 1. process of extensive cleansing and elimination of pathogens; 2. cleaning for the purpose of daily control of disposal of contaminated organisms, and elimination of microorganisms as done in hospitals.

desinfestación *f.* desinfestation, thorough cleaning and elimination of parasites, rodents, and pests that could bring infestation.

desinfectante *m.* disinfectant, agent that kills bacteria.

desinfectar *v.* to disinfect.

desinflamar *v.* to reduce or remove an inflammation.

desintegración *f.* disintegration; decomposition.

desintoxicar *v.* to detoxicate, to eliminate toxic matter.

deslizamiento *m.* slipping; sliding.

deslizarse *vr. vi.* to glide; **se desliza la mesa dentro del aparato** / the table is slipped into the machine.

deslumbramiento *m.* glare. 1. blurring of the vision with possible permanent damage to the retina; 2. intense light.

desmayarse *vr.* to faint, to pass out; to swoon.

desmayo *m.* fainting.

desmembración, desmembradura *f.* dismemberment.

desmembrar *v.* to dismember, to amputate.

desmielinación, desmielinización *f.* demyelination, demyelinization, loss or destruction of the myelin layer of the nerve.

desmineralización *f.* demineralization, loss of minerals from the body, esp. the bones.

desmoma *f.* desmoma, tumor of the connective tissue.

desmoplásico-a *a.* desmoplastic, that causes adhesions.

desmosis *f.* desmosis, disease of the connective tissue.

desnaturalización *f.* denaturation, change of the usual nature of a substance as by adding methanol or acetone to alcohol.

desnervado-a *a.* denervated, deprived of nerve supply.

desnivel *m.* unevenness.

desnudarse *vr.* to undress.

desnudo-a *a.* naked, bare.

desnutrición *f.* malnutrition, undernutrition; ___ **proteinocalórica** / protein caloric ___ .

desnutrido-a *a.* undernourished, malnourished, underfed.

desobedecer *vi.* to disobey.

desobediencia *f.* disobedience.

desobediente *a.* disobedient.

desodorante *m.* deodorant.

desodorizar *vi.* to deodorize, to remove fetid or unpleasant odors.

desorden *m.* disorder, abnormal condition of the body or mind.

desordenado-a *a.* disorderly, unorganized.

desorganización *f.* disorganization.

desorganizado-a *a.* disorganized, unstructured.

desorientado-a *a.* disoriented, confused.

desosificación *f.* deossification, loss or removal of minerals from the bones.

desoxicorticosterona *f.* deoxycorticosterone, steroid hormone produced in the cortex of the adrenal glands that has a marked effect on the metabolism of water and electrolytes.

desoxigenación *f.* deoxygenation, process of removing oxygen.

desoxigenado-a *a.* deoxygenated, lacking oxygen.

despacio *adv.* slow, slowly.

despejado-a *a.* clear, cloudless; [*persona*] smart, vivacious.

despellejarse *vr.* to peel; to shed skin.

desperdiciar *v.* to waste, to squander.

desperdicio *m.* waste.

despersonalización *f.* depersonalization, loss of identity.

despertarse *vr., vi.* to wake up.

despierto-a *a. pp.* de **despertar,** awake; diligent.

despigmentación *f.* depigmentation, abnormal change in the color of skin and hair.

despiojamiento *m.* delousing, freeing the body from lice.

desplazamiento *m.* 1. displacement; ___ **del cristalino** / dislocation of the lens; 2. transfer of emotion from the original idea or situation to a different one.

desplazar *vi.* to displace.

despliegue *m.* display, exhibition.

desprender *v.* to loosen, to unfasten; **desprenderse** / *vr.* to become loose.

desprendimiento *m.* detachment, separation.

despreocupado-a *a.* unconcerned, carefree.

despreocuparse *vr.* to be unconcerned.

desproporción *f.* disproportion.

desproporcionado-a *a.* disproportionate.

después *adv.* after, afterward.

despuntado-a *a.* [*instrumento*] blunt.

destapar *v.* to uncover.

destemplanza *f.* distemper, indisposition, any disorder with a general feeling of discomfort.

desteñir *vi.* to fade; **desteñirse** *vr.* to become faded.

destetado-a *f.* weanling.

destetar *v.* to wean, to adjust an infant to a form of nourishment other than breast or bottle feeding.

destete *m.* delactation, discontinued breastfeeding; weaning.

destilado-a *a.* distilled; **agua** ___ / ___ water.

destilar *v.* to distil, to create vapor by heat.

destino *m.* fate.

destorsión *f.* detorsion, detortion. 1. surgical correction of a testicular or intestinal torsion; 2. correction of the curvature or malformation of a structure.

destoxicación, destoxificación *f.* detoxification, reduction of the toxic quality.

destreza *f.* skill.

destruido-a *a.* destroyed; exhausted, physically or emotionally.

93

destruir *vi.* to destroy.

destupir *v.* to unclog.

desunión *f.* disengagement. 1. emergence of the fetal head from the vulva; 2. separation.

desvalido-a *a.* destitute, helpless, handicapped.

desvanecerse *vr. vi.* to black out; to swoon.

desvelado-a *a.* unable to sleep, wakeful.

desvelarse *vr.* to stay awake at night.

desvelo *m.* insomnia.

desventaja *f.* disadvantage; diminished capacity.

desvestir *vi.* to strip **desvestirse** *vr.* to undress.

desviación, desvío *f., m.* deviation, shunt. 1. departure from the established path; 2. mental aberration.

desviar *v.* to shunt, to change course; **desviarse** *vr.* to deviate.

detalle *m.* detail.

detectado-a *a.* detected; **no** ___ / undetected.

detectar *v.* to detect.

detector *m.* detector.

detener *vi.* to detain, to stop.

detergente *m.* detergent, cleaning agent.

deterioración, deterioro *f., m.* deterioration, wear, decay.

deteriorarse *vr.* to deteriorate.

determinación *f.* determination; decision; resolution; ___ **propia** / self- ___ .

determinado-a *a.* determined, strong-minded; [*una prueba*] proven.

determinante *m.* determinant, prevailing element; *a.* rel. to a prevailing element or cause.

determinar *v.* to determine.

determinismo *m.* determinism, theory by which all physical or psychic phenomena are predetermined and therefore uninfluenced by the will of the individual.

detestar *v.* to hate, to abhor.

detrás (de) *adv.* behind, in back of.

detrito *m.* debris, detritus, residue of disintegrating matter.

detrusor *m.* detrusor, muscle that expels or projects outward.

deuteranopía *f.* deuteranopia, blindness to the color green.

devitalizar *v.* to devitalize, to debilitate; to deprive from vital force.

devolución *f.* devolution. catabolismo.

devolver *vi.* to return, to give back.

Dexedrina *f.* Dexedrine, amphetamine type drug that stimulates the nervous system.

dextrismo *m.* dextrality, preferred use of the right hand.

dextrocardia *f.* dextrocardia, dislocation of the heart to the right.

dextrómano-a *m.* dextromanual, person who gives preference to the use of the right hand.

dextroposición *f.* dextroposition, displacement to the right.

dextrosa *f.* dextrose, form of glucose in the blood popularly called grape sugar.

dextroversión *f.* dextroversion, turn to the right.

deyección *f.* 1. dejection, state of depression; 2. the act of defecating.

día *m.* day; **de** ___ / daytime, daylight; **(dos, tres) veces al** ___ / (two, three) times a ___ ; **todo el** ___ / all ___ .

diabetes *f.* diabetes, a disease manifested by excessive urination. This term is often used in reference to diabetes mellitus.

diabetes insípida *f.* diabetes insipidus, type of diabetes caused by a deficiency in antidiuretic hormone.

diabetes mellitus *f.* diabetes mellitus, diabetes caused by insufficient production or use of insulin and resulting in hyperglycemia and glycosuria; ___ **con dependencia de insulina** / insulin-dependent ___ ; ___ **sin dependencia de insulina** / noninsulin-dependent ___ .

diabético-a *a.* diabetic, rel. to or suffering from diabetes; **angiopatías** ___ **-s** / ___ angiopathies; **coma** ___ / ___ coma; ___ **inestable** / brittle ___ ; **dieta** ___ / ___ diet; **neuropatía** ___ / ___ neuropathy; **retinopatía** ___ / ___ retinopathy.

diabetogénico-a *a.* diabetogenic, that produces diabetes.

diabetógrafo *m.* diabetograph, instrument used to determine the proportion of glucose in the urine.

diacetemia *f.* diacetemia, presence of diacetic acid in the blood.

diacetilmorfina *f.* diacetylmorphine, heroin.

diadococinesis *f.* diadochokinesis, ability to make opposing movements in rapid succession.

diáfisis *f.* diaphysis, shaft or middle part of a long, cylindrical bone such as the humerus.

diaforesis *f.* diaphoresis, profuse perspiration.

diaforético *m.* diaphoretic, agent that stimulates perspiration; **-a** *a.* sweating profusely.

diafragma *m.* diaphragm. 1. muscle that separates the thorax and the abdomen; 2. contraceptive device.

diagnosticar *vi.* to diagnose.

diagnóstico, diagnosis *m. f.* diagnosis, determination of the patient's ailment; ___

computado / computer ___; ___ **de imágenes por medios radioactivos** / ___ imaging; ___ **diferencial** / differential ___; ___ **equivocado o erróneo** / misdiagnosis; ___ **físico** / physical ___; ___ **propio** / autodiagnosis; **errores de** ___ / diagnostic errors.

diagonal *a.* diagonal.

diálisis *f.* dialysis, procedure used to filter and eliminate waste products from the blood of patients with renal insufficiency; **aparato de** ___ [riñón artificial] / ___ machine; ___ peritoneal / peritoneal ___ .

dializado *m.* dialysate, the part of the liquid that goes through the dialyzing membrane in dialysis; **-a** *a.* dialyzed, having been separated by dialysis.

dializador *m.* dialyzer, device used in dialysis.

dializar *vi.* to dialyze.

diámetro *m.* diameter.

Diana, complejo de *m.* Diana's complex, adoption by a woman of masculine characteristics and conduct.

diapasón *m.* diapason, U-shaped metal device used to determine the degree of deafness.

diapédesis *f.* diapedesis, passage of blood cells, esp. leukocytes, through the intact walls of a capillary vessel.

diaplasis *f.* diaplasis, reduction of a dislocation or fracture.

diapositiva *f.* slide.

diario-a *a.* daily; **-mente** *adv.* daily.

diarrea *f.* diarrhea. V. cuadro.

diartrosis *f.* diarthrosis, articulation that allows ample movement, such as the hip articulation.

diastasa *f.* diastase, enzyme that acts in the digestion of starches and sugars.

Diarrea	Diarrhea
del viajero	traveler's
disentérica	dysenteric
emocional	emotional
estival	summer
infantil	infantile
lientírica	lienteric
mucosa	mucous
nerviosa	nervous
pancreática	pancreatic
purulenta	purulent

diastasis *f.* diastasis. 1. separation of normally attached bones; 2. the rest period of the cardiac cycle, just before systole.

diástole *f.* diastole, dilation period of the heart during which the cardiac chambers are filled with blood.

diastólico-a *a.* diastolic, rel. to the diastole; **presión** ___ / ___ pressure, the lowest pressure point in the cardiovascular system.

diatermia *f.* diathermy, application of heat to body tissues through an electric current.

diatesis *f.* diathesis, organic disposition to contract certain diseases; ___ **hemorrágica** / hemorrhagic ___; ___ **reumática** / rheumatic ___ .

diatrizoato de meglumina *m.* diatrizoate meglumine, radiopaque substance used to visualize arteries and veins of the heart and the brain as well as the gallbladder, kidneys, and urinary bladder.

diazepam *m.* diazepam, Valium, drug used as a tranquilizer and muscle relaxer.

diccionario *m.* dictionary.

dicho *a. pp.* de **decir**, said.

dicigótico-a *a.* dizygotic, rel. to twins derived from two separate fertilized ova.

dicloxacilina *f.* dicloxacillim sodium, semi-synthetic penicillin used against gram-positive organisms.

dicoriónico-a *a.* dichorionic, having two chorions.

dicotomía *f.* dichotomy, dichotomization, process of dividing into two parts.

dicroísmo *m.* dichroism, property of some solutions or crystals to present more than one color in reflected or transmitted light.

dicromatismo *m.* dichromatism, the property of presenting two different colors.

dicrómico-a *a.* dichromic, rel. to two colors.

dicromófilo-a *a.* dichromophil, stainable by both acid and basic dyes.

dicroto-a *a.* dicrotic, having two pulse beats for each heartbeat.

dictioma *m.* dictyoma, a benign tumor of the ciliary epithelium with a structure similar to a net.

didáctico-a *a.* didactic, rel. to teaching through textbooks and lectures as opposed to a clinical or physical approach.

didelfo-a *a.* didelphic, rel. to a double uterus.

didimitis *f.* orquiditis, orquitis.

diembrionismo *m.* diembryony, production of two embryos from a single egg.

diencéfalo *m.* diencephalon, part of the brain.

dienestrol *m.* dienestrol, synthetic nonsteroid estrogen.

diente *m.* tooth (*pl.* teeth); ___ **desviado** / wandering ___; ___ **impactado** / impacted ___; ___ **incisivo** / incisor; ___ **molar** / wall ___; ___ **no erupcionado** / unerupted ___; ___ **-s deciduos, de leche** / deciduous teeth, baby teeth; ___ **-s permanentes** / permanent teeth; ___ **-s postizos** / denture; ___ **-s secundarios** / second teeth.

diestro-a *a.* dexter, rel. to the right side; righthanded.

dieta *f.* diet; ___ **alta en fibra** / high fiber ___; ___ **alta en residuos (fibras celulosas)** / high-residue ___; ___ **baja en grasa** / low in fat ___; ___ **balanceada** / balanced ___; ___ **blanda** / bland ___; ___ **diabética** / diabetic ___; ___ **hospitalaria** / ward ___; ___ **libre de gluten** / gluten-free ___; ___ **líquida** / liquid ___; ___ **macrocítica** / macrocytic ___; ___ **para bajar de peso** / weight reduction ___; ___ **rica en calorías** / high-calorie ___; ___ **sin sal** / salt-free ___.

dietética *f.* dietetics, the science of regulating diets to preserve or recuperate health.

dietético-a *a.* dietetic, rel. to diets.

dietilamida de ácido lisérgico *f.* lysergic acid diethylamide, LSD.

dietilestilbestrol *m.* diethylstilbestrol, synthetic estrogen compound.

dietista *m., f.* dietitian, nutrition specialist.

diezma *f.* decimation, high mortality rate.

difalo *a.* diphallus, partial or complete duplication of the penis.

difamación *f.* defamation.

difásico-a *a.* diphasic, that occurs in two different stages.

difenhidramina *f.* diphenhydramine, Benadryl, antihistamine.

diferencia *f.* difference.

diferenciación *f.* differentiation, distinction of one substance, disease, or entity from another.

diferencial *a.* differential, rel. to differentiation.

diferente *a.* different.

diferido-a *a.* deferred, postponed.

diferir *vi.* to disagree.

difícil *a.* difficult.

dificultad *f.* difficulty.

difonía *f.* diphonia, double voice.

difracción *f.* diffraction, the breaking up of a ray of light into its component parts when it passes through a glass or a prism; **patrón de** ___ / ___ pattern.

difteria *f.* diphtheria, acute infectious and contagious disease caused by the bacillus *Corynebacterium diphtheriae* (Klebs-Loffler bacillus) characterized by the formation of false membranes esp. in the throat; **antitoxina contra la** ___ / ___ antitoxin.

difterotoxina *f.* diphtherotoxin, toxin derived from cultures of diphtheria bacillus.

difundir *v.* to diffuse.

difunto-a *a.* deceased.

difusión *f.* diffusion. 1. the process of becoming widely spread; 2. dialysis through a membrane.

difuso-a *a.* difussed; extended; **absceso** ___ / ___ abscess; **lesión extensa** ___ / ___ injury; **mastocitosis cutánea** ___ / ___ cutaneous mastocytosis.

digerible, digestible *a.* digestible.

digerido-a *a.* digested; **no** ___ / undigested.

digerir *vi.* to digest.

digestión *f.* digestion, transformation of liquids and solids into simpler substances that can be absorbed easily by the body; ___ **gástrica** / gastric ___; ___ **intestinal** / intestinal ___; ___ **pancreática** / pancreatic ___.

digestivo *m.* digestant, digestive, an agent that assists in the digestive process.

digitación *f.* digitation, finger-shaped protrusion as in a muscle.

digitalis *f.* digitalis, cardiotonic agent obtained from the dried leaves of Digitalis purpurea; **intoxicación por** ___ / ___ toxicity, poisoning;

digitalización *f.* digitalization, therapeutic use of digitalis.

digitiforme *a.* finger-shaped.

dígito *m.* digit, digitus, finger or toe.

digitoxina *f.* digitoxin, cardiotonic glycoside obtained from *Digitalis purpurea* used in the treatment of congestive heart failure.

digoxina *f.* digoxin, cardiotonic glycoside obtained from *Digitalis purpurea* used in the treatment of cardiac arrhythmia.

dihidroestreptomicina *f.* dihydrostreptomycin, antibiotic derived from and used more commonly than streptomycin as it causes less neurotoxicity.

dilatación *f.* dilation, stretching; normal or abnormal enlargement of an organ or orifice; ___ **de la pupila** / ___ of the pupil.

dilatador *m.* dilator, stretcher. 1. muscle that on contraction dilates an organ; 2. device used to enlarge cavities or an opening; ___ **de Hegar** / Hegar's ___, used to enlarge the cervical canal.

dilatar *v.* to dilate, to expand.

dilaudid *m.* dilaudid, opium-derived drug that can produce dependence.

diluente *m.* diluent, agent that has the property of diluting.

diluir *vi.* to dilute; ___ **con agua** / to water down; **sin** ___ / undiluted.

dimercaprol *m.* dimercaprol, antidote used in cases of poisoning from heavy metals such as gold and mercury.

dimetilsulfóxido *m.* dimethyl sulfoxide, analgesic and anti-inflammatory agent.

dimetría *f.* dimetria, double uterus.

diminuir, disminuir *vi.* to diminish.

diminuto-a *a.* minute, very small.

dimorfismo *m.* dimorphism, occurring in two different forms; ___ **sexual, hermafroditismo** / sexual ___, hermaphrodism.

dina *f.* dyne, unit of force needed to accelerate one gram of mass one centimeter per second.

dinámica *f.* dynamics, the study of organs or parts of the body in movement.

dinámico-a *a.* dynamic.

dinamómetro *m.* dynamometer. 1. instrument used to measure muscular strength; 2. device that determines the magnifying power of a lens.

dinero *m.* money.

dioptómetro *m.* dioptometer, instrument used to measure ocular refraction.

dioptría *f.* diopter, dioptre, unit of the refracting power of a lens.

dióptrica *f.* dioptrics, the science that studies the refraction of light.

dióptrico-a *a.* dioptric, rel. to the refraction of light.

Dios *m.* God.

dióxido de carbono *m.* carbon dioxide.

diplacusia *f.* diplacusis, hearing disorder characterized by the perception of two tones for every sound produced.

diplejía *f.* diplegia, bilateral paralysis; ___ **espástica** / spastic ___; ___ **facial** / facial ___ .

diplocoria *f.* diplocoria, double pupil.

diploe *m.* diploe, spongy layer that lies between the two flat compact plates of the cranial bones.

diploide *a.* diploid, having two sets of chromosomes.

diplópagos *m.* diplopagus, conjoined twins, each with fairly complete bodies but sharing some organs.

diplopía *f.* diplopia, double vision.

dipsógeno *m.* dipsogen, thirst-causing agent.

dipsomanía *f.* dipsomania, recurring, uncontrollable urge to drink alcohol.

dipsosis *f.* dipsosis, abnormal thirst.

dirección *f.* direction; address.

directo-a *a.* direct, in a straight line; uninterrupted; **-mente** *adv.* directly.

directrices *f.* guidelines.

dirigir *vi.* to direct; to guide.

disacusia, disacusis *f.* dysacusia, dysacousis, difficulty in hearing.

disafea *f.* dysaphia, impaired sense of touch.

disartria *f.* dysarthria, unclear speech due to impairment of the tongue or any other muscle related to speech.

disasimilación *f.* disassimilation, destructive metabolism.

disautonomía *f.* dysautonomy, hereditary disorder of the autonomic nervous system.

disbarismo *m.* dysbarism, condition caused by decompression.

disbasia *f.* dysbasia, difficulty in walking gen. caused by nervous lesions.

disbulia *f.* dysbulia, inability to concentrate.

discalculia *f.* dyscalculia, inability to solve mathematical problems due to brain disease or damage.

discefalia *f.* dyscephalia, malformation of the head and the facial bones.

discinesia *f.* dyskinesia, inability to perform voluntary movements.

disciplina *f.* discipline, strict behavior.

disco *m.* disk; ___ **desplazado** / slipped ___; ___ **óptico** / optic ___; **ruptura de** ___ / ___ rupture.

discógeno-a *a.* discogenic, rel. to an intervertebral disk.

discografía *f.* x-ray of a vertebral disk following injection of a radiopaque substance.

discoide *a.* discoid, shaped like a disk.

discordancia *f.* discordance, the absence of a genetic trait in one of a pair of twins.

discoria *f.* dyscoria, abnormal shape of the pupil.

discrasia *f.* dyscrasia, synonym of disease.

discrepancia *f.* discrepancy.

discreto-a *a.* discrete, moderate, subtle; non-continuous.

discriminación *f.* discrimination, differentiation of race or quality.

discriminar *v.* to discriminate.

discrinismo, disendocrinismo *m.* dyscrinism, abnormal function in the production of secretions, esp. the endocrine glands.

discusión *f.* discussion, argument, debate.

discutir *v.* to discuss; to argue.

disdiadocoquinesia *f.* dysdiadochokinesia, inability to reverse immediately a motor impulse.

disecar *vi.* to dissect, to separate and cut parts and tissues of a body.

disección *f.* dissection, the act of dissecting.

diseminación *f.* dissemination, spreading.

diseminado-a *a.* disseminated, spread out over a large area.

disentería *f.* dysentery, painful infl. of the intestines, esp. of the colon, gen. caused by bacteria or parasites and accompanied by diarrhea; ___ **amebiana** / amebic ___; ___ **bacilar** / bacillary ___ .

disentir *vi.* to disagree, to have an opposite view.

diseño *m.* design.

disergia *f.* dysergia, lack of coordination in muscular voluntary movement.

disestesia *f.* dysesthesia, impaired sense of touch.

disfagia *f.* dysphagia, difficulty in swallowing; ___ **esofágica** / esophageal ___; ___ **orofaríngea** / oropharyngeal ___ .

disfasia *f.* dysphasia, speech impairment caused by a brain lesion.

disfonía *f.* dysphonia, hoarseness.

disforia *f.* dysphoria, severe depression.

disfrutar *v.* to enjoy.

disfunción *f.* dysfunction, malfunction, defective function.

disfuncional *a.* dysfunctional.

disgenesia *f.* dysgenesis, malformation.

disgerminoma *m.* dysgerminoma, malignant tumor in the ovary.

disgnosia *f.* dysgnosia, impairment of the intellectual function.

dishidrosis *f.* dyshidrosis, anomaly of the sweating function.

dislalia *f.* dyslalia, speech impairment due to functional anomalies of the speech organ.

dislexia *f.* dyslexia, reading disorder, sometimes hereditary or caused by a brain lesion.

dislocación, dislocadura *f.* dislocation, displacement; ___ **cerrada** / closed ___, simple; ___ **complicada** / complicated ___; ___ **congénita** / congenital ___ .

dislocado-a *a.* dislocated

dismenorrea, dismenia *f.* dysmenorrhea, painful and difficult menstruation.

dismetría *f.* dysmetria, impaired ability to control range of movement in a coordinated fashion.

dismetropsia *f.* dysmetropsia, disorder that impairs the visual appreciation of size and shape of objects.

disminución *f.* diminution, reducing process; ___ **de lágrimas** / ___ of tears; ___ **del rendimiento urinario** / urine output ___; ___ **de saliva** / saliva ___ .

disminuir *vi.* to diminish, to reduce, to lessen. ___ **la dosis** / to reduce the dosage.

dismiotonía *f.* dysmyotonia, abnormal muscular tonicity.

dismnesia *f.* dysmnesia, impaired memory.

dismorfismo *m.* dysmorphism, capacity of a parasite or agent to change its shape.

disnea, dispnea *f.* dispnoea, dyspnea, shortness of breath; ___ **paroxística nocturna** / paroxysmal nocturnal dyspnea; ___ **por esfuerzo** / exertional ___ .

disneico-a *a.* dyspneic, rel. to or suffering from dyspnea.

disociación *f.* dissociation, split. 1. the action and effect of separating; 2. decomposition of a molecular aggregate in a simpler one; 3. unconscious split of personality, a characteristic of schizophrenia; ___ **atrial** / ___ atrial ; ___ **atrioventricular** / ___ atrioventricular; ___ **de la personalidad** / split personality; ___ **del sueño** / sleep ___; ___ **pupilar** / pupillar ___; ___ **visual quinética** / visual-kinetic ___ .

disoluble *a.* dissoluble.

disolución *f.* dissolution, decomposition; death.

disolvente *m.* dissolvent; *a.* capable of being dissolved.

disolver *vi.* to dissolve, to liquify.

disonancia *f.* dissonance, combination of tones that produces an unpleasant sound.

disosmia *f.* dysosmia, impaired smell.

disostosis *f.* dysostosis, abnormal bone growth.

dispareunia *f.* dispareunia, painful coitus.

disparidad *f.* disparity, inequality.

dispensar *v.* to dispense, to distribute.

dispensario *m.* dispensary, a place that provides medical assistance and dispenses medicines and drugs.

dispepsia *f.* dyspepsia, indigestion characterized by irregularities in the digestive process such as eructation, nausea, acidity, flatulence, and loss of appetite.

dispermia *f.* dyspermia, pain on ejaculation.

dispersar *v.* to disperse, to scatter.

dispigmentación *f.* dyspigmentation, abnormal change in the color of the skin and hair.

displasia *f.* dysplasia, abnormal development of the tissues; ___ **cervical** / cervical ___ .

displásico-a *a.* rel. to dysplasia.

disponer *vi.* to arrange, to prepare.

disponibilidad *f.* availability.

disponible *a.* available.

disposición *f.* disposition, tendency to acquire certain disease.

dispositivo *m.* device, mechanism; ___ **intrauterino** / intrauterine ___ .

dispraxia *f.* dyspraxia, pain or difficulty in performing coordinated movements.

disquiria *f.* dyschiria, inability of a person to distinguish if he or she is being touched on the right or the left side of the body.

disrreflexia *f.* dysreflexia, disruption of the autonomic nervous system causing reactions and stimuli to be inappropriate and out of order.

disrritmia *f.* dysrhythmia, any alteration of a rhythm.

distal *a.* distal, farthermost away from the beginning or center of a structure.

distancia *f.* distance.

distasia *f.* dystasia, difficulty in maintaining a standing position.

distensibilidad *f.* distensibility, capacity of a structure to be extended, dilated, or enlarged in size.

distensión *f.* distension, distention, dilation; ___ **gaseosa** / gas ___, resulting from accumulation of gas in the abdominal cavity.

distinguido-a *a.* [*persona o característica*] distinguished.

distinguir *vi.* to distinguish, to differentiate.

distinto-a *a.* different.

distobucal *a.* distobuccal, rel. to the distal and buccal surfaces of a tooth.

distocia *f.* dystocia, difficult labor.

distoclusión *f.* distoclusion, defective closure, irregular bite.

distonía *f.* dystonia, defective tonicity, esp. muscular.

distorsión *f.* distorsion, bending or twisting out of shape.

distracción *f.* distraction. 1. separation of the surfaces of a joint without dislocation; 2. inability to concentrate or fix the mind on a given experience.

distraído-a *a.* absentminded.

distribución *f.* breakdown, distribution; ___ **detallada** / detailed ___ .

distribuir *vi.* to distribute.

distrofia *f.* dystrophy, degenerative disorder caused by defective nutrition or metabolism.

distrofia muscular *f.* muscular dystrophy, slow, progressive muscular degeneration.

disturbio *m.* disturbance, confusion.

disuelto-a *a. pp.* de **disolver,** dissolved.

disulfiram *m.* disulfiram, Antabuse, drug used in the treatment of alcoholism.

disuria *f.* dysuria, difficult urination.

disyunción *f.* disjunction, chromosome separation at the anaphase state of cell division.

diuresis *f.* diuresis, increased excretion of urine.

diurético *m.* diuretic, agent that causes increased urination; *pop.* water pill.

divergencia *f.* divergence, spreading apart, separation from a common center.

divergente *a.* divergent, moving in different directions.

diverticulectomía *f.* diverticulectomy, removal of a diverticulum.

diverticulitis *f.* diverticulitis, infl. of a diverticulum.

divertículo *m. diverticula* diverticulum, pouch or sac that originates from a hollow organ or structure.

diverticulosis *f.* diverticulosis, presence of diverticula in the colon; ___ **vesical** / vesical ___ .

divertirse *vr. vi.* to have fun.

dividido-a *a.* divided.

dividir *v.* to divide, to disunite; to split.

división *f.* division, separation; split.

divorciado-a *a.* divorced.

divulsión *f.* divulsion, separation or detachment.

doblarse *vr.* to bend; ___ **hacia adelante** / ___ forward; ___ **hacia atrás** / ___ backward.

doble *m.* double; *a.* double; ___ **útero** / ___ uterus.

docena *f.* dozen.

doctor-a *m., f.* doctor.

documentación *f.* documentation.

doler *vi.* to be in pain; to ache.

dolicocefálico-a *a.* dolichocephalic, having a narrow, long head.

dolor *m.* pain. *V.* cuadro en la página 100.

doloroso-a *a.* painful.

doméstico-a *a.* domestic.

domiciliario-a *a.* domiciliary, taking place in the home.

dominancia *f.* dominance, predominance; ___ **cerebral** / cerebral ___; ___ **ocular** / ocular ___ .

dominante *a.* dominant, predominant; **características** ___ -s / ___ characteristics.

donación *f.* donation.

donante *m.* donor; **tarjeta de** ___ / ___'s card.

donante universal *m.* universal donor, individual belonging to blood group O or whose

d

Dolor	Pain
cólico	colicky
constante	constant
fuerte	strong
oprimente	pressing
leve	mild
localizado	localized
opresivo	oppressive
penetrante	piercing
profundo	deep
quemante	burning
referido	referred
sordo	dull
subjetivo	subjective

blood can be given to persons belonging to any other of the AB blood groups with minimal risk of complication.

donde *adv.* where.

dondequiera *adv.* anywhere; everywhere.

Donovanía granulomatosis *f.* Donovania granulomatosis, Donovan's body, bacterial infection that affects the skin and the mucous membranes of the genitalia and the anal area.

dopado *pp.* of **dopar**, doping, to estimate the potency of a drug dose.

dopamina *f.* dopamine, substance synthesized by the adrenal glands that increases blood pressure and is gen. used in shock treatment.

Doppler, técnica de *f.* Doppler's technique, based in the fact that the frequency of the ultrasonic waves changes when these are reflected in a moving surface.

dormido-a *a.* asleep; **profundamente __** / sound __ .

dormir *vi.* to sleep; **dormirse** *vr.* to fall asleep.

dorsal *a.* dorsal, rel. to the back; **fisura o corte __** / **__** slit.

dorsalgia *f.* dorsalgia, backache.

dorsiflexión *f.* dorsiflexion, bending backward.

dorso *m.* dorsum, posterior part, such as the back of the hand or the body.

dorsocefálico-a *a.* dorsocephalic, rel. to the back of the head.

dorsodinia *f.* dorsodynia, pain in the muscles of the upper part of the back.

dorsoespinal *a.* dorsospinal, rel. to the back and the spine.

dorsolateral *a.* dorsolateral, rel. to the back and the side.

dorsolumbar *a.* dorsolumbar, rel. to the lower thoracic and upper lumbar vertebrae area of the back.

dosimetría *f.* dosimetry, precise and systematic determination of doses.

dosímetro *m.* dosimeter, instrument used to detect and measure exposure to radiation; **__ de película** / film badge carrying a film sensitive to x-rays and used to measure the cumulative exposure to the rays.

dosis, dosificación *f.* dose. 1. the giving of medication or other therapeutic agents in prescribed amounts; 2. in nuclear medicine, quantity of radiopharmaco given; **__ acumulada** / cumulative **__**; **__ curativa** / curative **__**; **__ de absorción** / absortion **__**; **__ de bolo, intravenosa** / bolus **__**, intravenous; **__ de exposición** / exposure **__**; **__ de la médula ósea** / bone marrow **__**; **__ de reducción** / reduction **__**; **__ de refuerzo** / booster **__**; **__ dermal** / skin **__**; **__ diaria** / daily **__**; **__ dividida** / divided **__**; **__ efectiva** / effective **__**; **__ equivalente** / equivalent **__**; **__ individual** / unit **__**; **__ inicial** / initial **__**; **__ integral** / integral **__**; **__ máxima** / maximal **__**; **__ mínima letal** / minimal lethal **__**; **__ mínima reactiva** / minimal reacting **__**; **__ óptima** / optimum **__**; **__ preventiva** / preventive **__**; **__ subletal** / sublethal **__**, of insufficient amount to cause death; **__ terapéutica** / therapeutic **__**; **__ tolerada** / tolerance **__**; **__ umbral** / threshold **__**, minimal dose needed to produce an effect; **máxima __ permitida** / maximal permissible **__**; **máxima __ tolerable** / maximum tolerated **__** .

Douglas, placa (saco) de *m.* Douglas cul-de-sac, peritoneal pouch between the uterus and the rectum.

Down, síndrome de *m.* Down syndrome, chromosomal abnormality that causes physical deformity and moderate to severe mental retardation.

dramamina *f.* dramamine, antihistamine used in the prevention and treatment of motion sickness.

dramatismo *m.* dramatism, pompous behavior and language, gen. seen in mental disorders.

drapetomanía, dromomanía *f.* drapetomania, dromomania, abnormal impulse to wander.

drástico *m.* drastic, strong cathartic; **-a** *a.* extreme, very strong.

drenaje *m.* drainage, outlet; ___ **abierto /** open ___; ___ **postural /** postural ___, that allows drainage by gravity; **tubo de** ___ / ___ tube.

drenar *v.* to drain, to draw off fluid or pus from a cavity or an infected wound.

drepanocito *m.* drepanocyte, sickle cell.

droga *f.* drug; medication; **abuso de la** ___ / ___ abuse; **anomalías causadas por la** ___ / ___ anomalies; ___ **adictiva /** dependence producing ___; ___ **de acción prolongada /** long-acting ___; ___ **neuroléptica /** neuroleptic ___, causing symptoms similar to those manifested by nervous diseases; **entregarse a la** ___ / to become ___ addicted; **resistencia microbiana a la** ___ / ___ resistance, microbial.

drogadicción *f.* drug addiction.

drogadicto-a *m., f.* drug addict.

dromotrópico-a *a.* dromotropic, that affects the conductibility of muscular and nervous fibers.

dúctulo *m.* ductule, a very small conduit; *a.* ductile, allowing deformation without breaking.

ductus *m.* ductus, duct.

ducha *f.* douche, jet of water applied to the body for medicinal or cleansing effects; shower; *vr.* **darse una** ___, **ducharse /** to shower.

duda *f.* doubt.

dudar *v.* to doubt, to question.

dudoso-a *a.* doubtful.

duela *f.* fluke, parasitic worm of the *Trematoda* family; ___ **hepática /** liver ___; ___ **intestinal /** intestinal ___; ___ **pulmonar /** lung ___; ___ **sanguínea /** blood ___ .

dulce *a.* sweet.

dulces *m. pl.* [*golosinas*] sweets.

dulcificante *m.* sweetener.

duodenal *a.* duodenal, rel. to the duodenum.

duodenectomía *f.* duodenectomy, partial or total excision of the duodenum.

duodenitis *f.* duodenitis, infl. of the duodenum.

duodeno *m.* duodenum, essential part of the alimentary tract situated between the pylorus and the jejunum.

duodenoenterostomía *f.* duodenoenterostomy, anastomosis between the duodenum and the small intestine.

duodenoscopía *f.* duodenoscopy, endoscopic examination of the duodenum.

duodenostomía *f.* duodenostomy, opening into the duodenum through the abdominal wall to alleviate stenosis of the pylorus.

duodenotomía *f.* duodenotomy, incision of the duodenum.

duodenoyeyunostomía *f.* duodenojejunostomy, creation of a communication between the duodenum and the jejunum.

duplicar *vi.* to duplicate; to double.

durabilidad *f.* durability; duration.

durable *a.* durable, lasting.

duración *f.* duration; continuation.

duramadre, duramáter *f.* dura mater, the outer membrane that covers the encephalum and the spinal cord.

durante *prep.* during; lasting; ___ **los días de invierno /** ___ winter days.

durar *v.* to last; to endure.

durazno *m.* peach.

dureza *f.* hardness.

duro-a *a.* hard, firm.

d

e

E *abr.* **emetropía** / emmetropia; **enema** / enema; **enzima** / enzyme.

e *conj.* and.

ebrio-a *a.* drunk.

ebullición *f.* ebullition, boiling; **punto de ___** / boiling point;

echar *v.* to throw; **___ una carta** / to mail a letter; **___ una mirada** / to give a look; **echarse** *vr.* [food] **echarse a perder** / to go bad.

Echinococcus *L. Echinococcus.* **equinococo.**

Echo, virus *m.* echovirus, any of a group of viruses found in the gastrointestinal tract, associated with meningitis and enteritis.

eclampsia *f.* eclampsia, toxic, convulsive disorder that usu. occurs near the end of pregnancy or right after delivery.

eclámptico-a *a.* eclamptic, rel. to eclampsia.

eco *m.* echo, repercussion of sound.

ecocardiografía *f.* echocardiography, diagnostic procedure that uses sound waves (ultrasound) to visualize the internal structures of the heart; **___ transesofágica** / transesophageal ___ .

ecocardiograma *m.* echocardiogram, ultrasonic record obtained by an echocardiography.

ecoencefalografía *f.* echoencephalography, diagnostic procedure that sends sound waves (ultrasound) to the brain structure and records the returning echoes.

ecografía *f.* echography, ultrasonografía.

ecograma *m.* echogram, graphic representation of an echography.

ecolalia *f.* echolalia, disorder manifested by involuntary repetition of words spoken by another person.

ecología *f.* ecology, the study of plants and animals and their relationship to the environment.

ecológico-a *a.* ecological; **sistema ___** / ___ system.

económico-a *a.* economical, economic.

ecosistema *f.* ecosystem, ecologic microcosm.

ectasia *f.* ectasia, ectasis, expansion of a part of an organ.

ectopia *f.* ectopia, ectopy, displacement of an organ, usu. congenital.

ectópico-a *a.* ectopic, rel. to ectopia.

ectoplasma *m.* ectoplasm, external membrane surrounding the cell cytoplasm.

ectropión *m.* ectropion, eversion of the margin of a body part, such as the eyelid.

ecuador *m.* equator, imaginary line that divides a body in two equal parts.

ecuanimidad *f.* equanimity; steadfastness.

eczema, eccema *m.* eczema, inflammatory, noncontagious skin disease.

edad *f.* age; **___ cronológica** / chronological ___; **de ___ avanzada** / elderly; **mayor de ___** / ___ of consent; **menor de ___** / under ___, a minor.

edad gestacional *f.* gestational age, estimated age of a fetus counted by weeks of gestation.

edema *m.* edema, abnormal amount of fluid in the intercellular tissue; **___ angioneurótico** / angioneurotic ___; **___ cardíaco** / cardiac ___; **___ cerebral** / cerebral ___; **___ de fóvea** / pitting ___; **___ dependiente** / dependent ___; **___ pulmonar** / pulmonary ___ .

edematoso-a *a.* edematous, rel. to or affected by edema.

edetato *m.* edetate, calcium disodium, agent used in diagnosing and treating lead poisoning.

edificio *m.* building.

educación *f.* education.

educar *vi.* to educate.

efectividad *f.* effectiveness.

efectivo-a *a.* effective; **en ___** / cash; **-mente** *adv.* in effect, actually.

efecto *m.* effect, impression; result; **___ secundario** / side ___ .

efector *m.* effector, nerve ending that produces an efferent action on muscles and glands.

efedrina *f.* ephedrine, adrenalinelike drug used chiefly as a bronchodilator.

eferente *a.* efferent, centrifugal, that pulls away from the center.

efervescente *a.* effervescent, that produces gas bubbles.

eficaz, eficiente *a.* efficacious, efficient.

eficientemente *adv.* efficiently.

efímero-a *a.* ephemeral, of brief duration.

efluente *a.* effluent, flowing out.

efusión *f.* effusion, escape of fluid into a cavity or tissue; **___ pericardial** / pericardial ___; **pleural** / pleural ___ .

ego *m.* ego, the self, human consciousness.

egocéntrico-a *a.* egocentric, self-centered.

egoísmo *m.* selfishness, self-centeredness.

egoísta *m., f.* selfish person; *a.* selfish.

egomanía *f.* egomania, excessive self-esteem.

egosintónico-a *a.* ego-syntonic, in harmony with the ego.

egreso *m.* output; [*dar de alta*] discharge; **sumario de** ___ / discharge summary.

eje *m.* axis.

ejemplo *m.* example.

ejercer *vi.* [*una profesión*] to practice; [*autoridad*] to exercise.

ejercicio *m.* exercise; ___ **activo** / active ___; ___ **aeróbico** / aerobic ___; ___ **correctivo** / corrective ___; ___ **de respiración profunda** / deep-breathing ___; ___ **físico** / physical ___; ___ **isométrico** / isometric ___; ___ **isotónico** / isotonic ___; ___ **para adelgazar** / reducing ___; ___ **pasivo** / passive ___ .

elaborado-a *a.* elaborated. 1. rel. to something complex; 2. *pp.* of *to elaborate;* **una operación** ___, **compleja** / a complex operation.

elaborar *v.* to elaborate, to develop fully.

elación *f.* elation, state of jubilation and exaltation characterized by mental and physical excitement.

elastasa *f.* elastase, enzyme that catalyzes the digestion of elastic fibers, esp. of the pancreatic juice.

elasticidad *f.* elasticity, ability to expand easily and resume normal shape.

elástico *m.* elastic; **-a** *a.* elastic, that can be returned to its original shape after being extended or distorted; **tejido** ___ / ___ tissue.

elastinasa *f.* elastinase. elastasa.

electivo-a *a.* elective, optional; **terapia** ___ / ___ therapy; **cirugía** ___ / ___ surgery;

electricidad *f.* electricity.

eléctrico-a *a.* electric, electrical; **corriente** ___ / ___ current;

electrocardiógrafo *m.* electrocardiograph, instrument for recording the electrical variations of the heart muscle in action.

electrocardiograma *m.* electrocardiogram, graphic record of the changes in the electric currents produced by the contractions of the heart muscle; ___ **de esfuerzo** / exercise ___ .

electrocauterización *m.* electrocauterization, destruction of tissues by an electric current.

electrocirugía *f.* electrosurgery, use of electric current in surgical procedures.

electrocución *f.* electrocution, termination of life by electric current.

electrochoque *m.* electroshock, electroconvulsive therapy, treatment of some mental disorders by applying an electric current to the brain.

electrodiagnosis *f.* electrodiagnosis, the use of electronic devices to use for diagnostic purposes.

electrodo *m.* electrode, a medium between the electric current and the object to which the current is applied.

electroencefalografía *f.* electroencephalography, registering of the electrical currents produced in the brain.

electroencefalograma *m.* electroencephalogram, graphic record obtained during an electroencephalography.

electrofisiología *f.* electrophysiology, the study of the relationship between physiological processes and electrical phenomena.

electroforesis *f.* electrophoresis, movement of coloidal particles suspended in a medium charged with an electric current that separates them, such as occurs in the separation of proteins in plasma.

electrólisis *f.* electrolysis, destruction or disintegration by means of an electric current.

electrólito *m.* electrolyte, ion that carries an electrical charge.

electromagnético-a *a.* electromagnetic.

electromiografía *f.* electromyography. 1. recording of muscular activity for diagnostic use; 2. any type of study done in a recording studio including studies on neurologic conduction.

electromiograma *m.* electromyogram, graphic report obtained by electromyography.

electrónico-a *a.* electronic.

electroquirúrgico-a *a.* electrosurgical; **destrucción** ___ **de lesiones** / ___ destruction of lesions.

electroversión *f.* cardioversion, termination of a cardiac dysrhythmia by electric means.

elefantiasis *f.* elephantiasis, chronic disease produced by obstruction of the lymphatic vessels and hypertrophy of the skin and subcutaneous cellular tissue, that affects most frequently the legs and scrotum.

elegible *a.* eligible, qualified for selection.

elegir *vi.* to elect, to choose.

elemental *a.* elemental; rudimentary.

elemento *m.* element.

elemento radiactivo *m.* radioactive element.

elevación *f.* elevation.

elevado-a *a.* elevated, raised.

elevador *m.* elevator. 1. surgical device used for lifting a sunken part or for elevating tissues; 2. elevator.

elevar *v.* to raise, to elevate.

eliminación *f.* elemination, exclusion.

eliminar *v.* to eliminate; to discard waste from the body.

eliptocito *m.* elliptocyte, oval red cell.

eliptocitosis *f.* elliptocytosis, condition of increased number of elliptocytes occurring in certain types of anemia.

elixir *m.* elixir, aromatic, sweet liquor containing an active medicinal ingredient.

emaciación *f.* emaciation, an extreme loss of weight.

embalsamamiento *m.* embalming, treatment of a dead body to retard its decay.

embarazada *a.* pregnant.

embarazo *m.* pregnancy; ___ **de probeta** / test-tube ___; ___ **ectópico** / ectopic ___, extrauterine; ___ **falso** / false ___, enlargement of the abdomen simulating pregnancy; ___ **intersticial** / interstitial ___, located in the part of the uterine tube within the wall of the uterus; ___ **múltiple** / multiple ___, more than one fetus in the uterus at the same time; ___ **prolongado** / prolonged ___, beyond full term; ___ **subrogado** / surrogate ___; ___ **tubárico** / tubal ___, when the egg develops in the Fallopian tube; ___ **tuboabdominal** / tuboabdominal ___; **prueba del** ___ / ___ test.

embarazo ampular *m.* ampular pregnancy. *Syn.* **embarazo tubular.**

embarazo tubárico *n.* tubal pregnancy, fallopian pregnancy, situated near the mid portion of the oviduct.

embolia, embolismo *f., m.* embolism, sudden obstruction of a cerebral artery by a loose piece of clot, plaque, fat, or air bubble; ___ **cerebral** / cerebral ___, stroke; ___ **gaseosa** / air ___; **embolismo pulmonar** / pulmonary ___ .

embolia amniótica *f.* amniotic fluid embolism usually occurring during labor, complication of the gestational cycle that can cause death.

émbolo *m.* embolus, clot of blood or other material that when traveling through the bloodstream becomes lodged in a vessel of lesser diameter.

emborrachamiento, embriaguez *m., f.* intoxication, drunkenness.

emborracharse *vr.* to get drunk.

embotamiento *m.* torpor, sluggishness.

embriología *f.* embryology, study of the embryo and its development up to the moment of birth.

embrión *m.* embryo, primitive phase of an organism from the moment of fertilization to about the second month.

embriónico-a *a.* embryonal, embryonic, rel. to the embryo.

embudo *m.* funnel.

emergencia *f.* emergency, urgency *Syn.* urgencia; ___ **de nacimiento repentino** / sudden childbirth ___; ___ **de un caso extremo** / ___ of an urgent case; ___ **de intervención quirúrgica** / surgical ___; ___ **de una traqueotomía** / ___ of a tracheotomy; **línea telefónica de** ___ / hotline; **servicios de** ___ / ___ medicine.

emético *m.* emetic, agent that stimulates vomiting.

emetina *f.* emetine, emetic and antiamebic.

emigración, migración *f.* emigration, escape, such as of leukocytes, through the walls of capillaries and small veins.

eminencia *f.* eminence, prominence or elevation such as on the surface of a bone.

emisión *f.* emission, discharge; ___ **seminal nocturna** / wet dream, involuntary emission of semen during sleep.

emitir *v.* to emit, to expel; to issue.

emoción *f.* emotion, intense feeling.

emocional, emocionante *a.* emotional, rel. to emotion.

emoliente *a.* emollient, soothing to the skin or mucous membrane.

empachado-a *a.* suffering from indigestion.

empacho *m.* indigestion.

empapar *v.* to soak, to drench; **empaparse** *vr.* to get soaked.

emparejamiento *m.* matching.

emparejar *v.* to match, to pair off.

empaste *m.* [*dientes*] filling.

empatía *f.* empathy, understanding and appreciation of the feelings of another person.

empeine *m.* instep, arched medial portion of the foot.

empeorar *v.* to worsen; **empeorarse** *vr.* to get worse.

empezar *vi.* to begin, to start.

empiema *f.* empyema, presence of pus in a cavity, esp. the pleural cavity.

empírico-a *a.* empiric, empirical, based on practical observations.

empleado-a *m., f.* employee.

emplear *v.* to employ, to use.

empleo *m.* employment, job.

emprender *v.* to undertake.

empujar *v.* to push, to press forward.

empuje *m.* impulse; driving force.

empujón *m.* push, shove.

emulsión *f.* emulsion, distribution of a liquid in small globules throughout another liquid.

emulsionar *v.* to emulsify, to convert into an emulsion.

emulsivo-a *n., a.* emulsifier.

en *prep.* in, on, at; ___ **el hospital** / in the hospital; ___ **la mesa** / on the table; ___ **casa** / at home.

enajenación mental *m.* derangement, mental disorder.

enajenamiento *m.* conversion disorder, the process by which repressed emotions are translated into physical manifestations.

enamorarse *vr.* to fall in love; ___ **de** / ___ with.

enanismo *m.* dwarfism, impaired growth of the body caused by hereditary or physical deficiencies.

enano-a *m., f.* dwarf, individual who is undersized in relation to the group to which he or she belongs; ___ **acondroplástico-a** / achondroplastic ___; ___ **asexual** / asexual ___; ___ **infantil** / infantile ___; ___ **micromélico-a** / micromelic ___ .

encadenamiento *m.* linkage.

encadenar *v.* to link; to chain.

encajamiento *m.* engagement.

encajar *v.* to fit one thing into another; to insert in; to engage; **encajarse** *vr.* to fit in; to become inserted.

encajonamiento *m.* encasement, the act of becoming enclosed in another structure.

encaminar *v.* to put someone or something on the right path.

encapricharse *vr.* to become obstinate or stubborn about something.

encapsulado-a *a.* enclosed in a capsule; walled-off.

encarcelado-a *a.* incarcerated; constricted.

encefalalgia *f.* encephalalgia, intense headache.

encefálico-a *a.* encephalic, rel. to the encephalon.

encefalinas *f.* enkephalins, chemical substances produced in the brain.

encefalitis *f.* encephalitis, infl. of the brain; ___ **alérgica experimental** / experimental allergic ___; ___ **bacteriana** / bacterial ___; ___ **del recién nacido** / neonatorum ___; ___ **epidémica** / epidemic___; ___ **equina del este** / eastern equine ___; ___ **equina del oeste** / western equine ___; ___ **herpética** / herpes ___; ___ **infantil** / infantile ___; ___

letárgica / lethargic ___; ___ **piogénica** / ___ pyogenica; ___ **purulenta** / purulent ___; ___ **severa hemorrágica** / acute hemorrhagic ___; ___ **severa, necronizante** / acute necrotizing ___; ___ **supurativa** / suppurative ___ .

encéfalo *m.* encephalon, portion of the nervous system contained in the cranium.

encefalocele *m.* encephalocele, protrusion of brain matter through a congenital or traumatic defect in the skull.

encefalografía *f.* encephalography, x-ray examination of the brain.

encefaloma *m.* encephaloma, brain tumor.

encefalomalacia *f.* encephalomalacia, softening of the brain.

encefalomielitis *f.* encephalomyelitis, infl. of the brain and the spinal cord.

encefalopatía *f.* encephalopathy, any disease or malfunction of the brain.

encender *vi.* [*una bombilla*] to switch on; [*un fuego*] to kindle.

encerar *v.* to wax, to treat or rub the skin with wax.

encerrar *vi.* to enclose; **encerrarse** *vr.* to lock oneself up.

encía *f.* gum.

encigótico-a, enzigótico-a *a.* enzygotic, rel. to twins developed from the same fertilized ovum.

encima *adv.* on, upon, on top of.

encinta *a.* pregnant.

enclenque *a.* emaciated; feeble.

encogerse *vr. vi.* to shrink.

enconarse *vr.* to fester, to become ulcerated.

encondroma *f.* enchondroma, tumor that develops within a bone.

encontrar *vi.* to encounter, to find; **encontrarse** *vr.* to meet with someone; to find.

encopresis *f.* encopresis, incontinence of feces.

encuesta *f.* inquest, official investigation.

endarterectomía *f.* endarterectomy, excision of the thickened inner lining of an artery.

endarteritis *f.* endarteritis, infl. of the lining of an artery.

endémico-a *a.* endemic, endemical, rel. to a disease that remains for an indefinite length of time in a given community or region; **area** ___ / ___ area; **enfermedad** ___ / ___ sickness.

endentado-a *a.* serrated, teethlike projection.

enderezar *vi.* to straighten out.

endocardio *m.* endocardium, the serous inner lining membrane of the heart.

endocarditis *f.* infl. of the endocardium; ___ **bacteriana** / bacterial ___; ___ **constrictiva** / constrictive ___; ___ **infecciosa** / infectious ___; ___ **maligna** / malignant ___; ___ **mucomenbranosa** / mucomembranous ___; ___ **reumática** / rheumatic ___; ___ **tuberculosa** / tuberculous ___ .

endocervix *m.* endocervix, mucous membrane of the cervix.

endocrino-a *a.* endocrine, rel. to internal secretions and the glands that secrete them; **glándulas** ___ **-s** / endocrine glands, glands that secrete hormones directly into the bloodstream.

endocrinología *f.* endocrinology, the study of the endocrine glands and the hormones secreted by them.

endocrinólogo *m.* endocrinologist.

endodermo *m.* endoderm, the innermost of the three layers of the embryo.

endofítico *a.* endophytic, rel. to an invasive tumor growing internally.

endoflebitis *f.* endophlebitis, infl. of the intima of a vein.

endoftalmitis *f.* endophthalmitis, infl. of the interior tissues of the eyeball, which can be caused by an allergic reaction, a reaction to a drug, or a bacteriologic infection; serious redness of the eye, a probable infection, that in some cases has pus. Other symptoms are vomiting, fever and headache;___ **facoanafiláctica** / ___ phacoanaphylactic; ___ **granulomatosa** / granulomatous ___; ___ **nodosa** / ___ nodosa.

endógeno-a *a.* endogenous; **infección** ___ / ___ infection.

endolinfa *f.* endolymph, fluid contained in the membranous labyrinth of the ear.

endometrial *a.* endometrial, rel. to the endometrium; **biopsia** ___ / ___ biopsy.

endometrio *m.* endometrium, inner mucous membrane of the uterus.

endometrioma *f.* endometrioma, mass containing endometrial tissue.

endometriosis *f.* endometriosis, disorder by which endometrial-like tissue is found in areas outside the uterus.

endometritis *f.* endometritis, infl. of the mucous membrane.

endomiocardial *a.* endomyocardial, rel. to the endocardium and the myocardium; **biopsia** ___ / ___ biopsy; **fibrosis** ___ / ___ fibrosis.

endomiocarditis *f.* endomyocarditis, infl. of the internal layers of the heart, the endocardium, and the myocardium.

endomorfo *m.* endomorph, person whose body is more heavily developed in the torso than in the limbs.

endoplásmico-a *a.* endoplasmic, rel. to endoplasma.

endorfinas *f.* endorphins, chemical substances produced in the brain that have the property of easing pain.

endoscopía *f.* endoscopy, examination of a cavity or conduit using an endoscope.

endoscópico-a *a.* endoscopic, rel. to endoscopy.

endoscopio *m.* endoscope, instrument used to examine a hollow organ or cavity.

endosteo *m.* endosteum, cells located in the central medullar cavity of the bones.

endostio *m.* endosteum, tissue that covers the medullar cavity of the bone.

endotelial *a.* endothelial, rel. to the endothelium.

endotelio *m.* endothelium, thin layer of cells that form the inner lining of the blood vessels, the lymph channels, the heart, and other cavities.

endotérmico-a *a.* endothermic, that absorbs heat.

endotoxemia *f.* endotoxemia, presence of endotoxins in the blood.

endotoxina *f.* endotoxin, venous toxin-free after the organism dies; with less potency than the exotoxin; the infected person may have symptoms of fever, chills, and shock.

endotraqueal *a.* endotracheal, within or through the trachea; **tubo** ___ **con manguito** / ___ tube, cuffed.

endulzar *vi.* to sweeten.

endurecer *vi.* to harden; **endurecerse** *vr.* to become hardened.

endurecimiento *m.* hardening.

enema *f.* enema; ___ **de bario** / barium ___; ___ **de contraste doble** / double-contrast ___ .

energía *f.* energy, the capacity to work, to move, and to exercise with vigor; ___ **cinética** / kinetic ___; ___ **de activación** / ___ of activation; ___ **de fusión** / fusion ___; ___ **interna** / internal ___; ___ **latente** / latent ___; ___ **nuclear** / nuclear ___; ___ **nutritiva** / nutritional ___; ___ **potencial** / potential ___; ___ **química** / chemical ___; ___ **síquica** / psychic ___; ___ **solar** / solar ___; ___ **total** / total ___ .

enérgico-a *a.* energetic, vigorous.

enfadar *v.* to make angry, to upset; **enfadarse** *vr.* to become angry.

énfasis *m.* emphasis; **hacer** ___ / to emphasize.

enfermar *v.* to cause disease; **enfermarse** *vr.* to become ill, to get sick.

enfermedad *f.* sickness, illness, disease, infirmity; **control de** ___ **-es contagiosas** / communicable ___ control; ___ **africana aguda del sueño** / acute African sleeping ___; ___ **ambulante** / walking ___; ___ **biliar** / gall ___; ___ **cardíaca** / cardiac disease; ___ **concomitante** / companion ___; ___ **de la altura** / high altitude sickness, caused by diminished oxygen; ___ **de los buzos** / decompression ___; ___ **de los mineros** / coal miner's ___; ___ **de red o cadena** / heavy chain ___; ___ **de viajeros** / motion ___; ___ **funcional** / functional ___, of unknown origin; ___ **ósea** / bone ___; ___ **por radiación** / radiation ___; ___ **pulmonar crónica obstructiva** / chronic obstructive pulmonary disease; ___ **renal** / renal ___; ___ **respiratoria crónica** / chronic respiratory ___; ___ **sanguínea** / blood ___; ___ **venérea** / venereal ___; **licencia por** ___ / sick leave.

enfermería *f.* infirmary, a place used for treatment of the sick.

enfermero-a *m., f.* nurse; **asistente de** ___ / orderly; ___ **anestesista** / ___ anesthetist; ___ **de cirugía** / scrub ___, surgical ___; ___ **de salud pública** / community or public health ___; ___ **graduado-a** / trained ___; ___ **práctico-a** / practical ___; ___ **privado-a** / private duty ___; ___ **registrado-a** / registered ___; **jefe-a de** ___ **-s** / chief or head ___ .

enfermizo-a *a.* sickly; predisposed to become ill.

enfermo-a *m., f.* sick person; **cuidado de** ___ **-s** / nursing.

enfisema *m.* emphysema, chronic lung condition that causes distension of the small air sacs (alveoli) in the lungs and atrophy of the tissue between them, impairing the respiratory process.

enfisematoso-a *a.* emphysematous, affected by emphysema.

enfocar *vi.* to focus.

enfrente *adv.* across from; in front of.

enfriamiento *m.* cold, chill; [*acondicionamiento físico*] cool-down.

enfriar *v.* to cool down.

engañar *v.* to deceive; to fool; **engañarse** *vr.* to deceive oneself.

engordar *v.* to gain weight; to get fat.

engorroso-a *a.* cumbersome, troublesome.

engrama *f.* engram. 1. permanent mark or trace left in the protoplasm by a passing stimulus; 2. a latent permanent picture produced by a sensorial experience.

engrasar *v.* to grease; to oil.

engurgitado-a *a.* engorged, distended by excess of liquid.

enjabonar *v.* to soap; **enjabonarse** *vr.* to soap oneself.

enjambrazón *f.* swarming, the act of multiplying or spreading, such as bacteria over a culture.

enjuagar *v.* to rinse; **enjuagarse** *vr.* to rinse oneself out.

enjuague *m.* rinse, mouthwash.

enoftalmia *f.* enophthalmos, receded eyeball.

enojado-a *a.* angry, fretful.

enojar *v.* to anger; **enojarse** *vr.* to get angry.

enorme *a.* enormous, huge.

enquistado-a *a.* encysted, enclosed in a sac or cyst.

enredadera *f.* vine.

enredado-a *a.* tangled; [*situación médica*] complicated.

enredar *v.* to tangle; to make things more difficult; **enredarse** *vr.* to become tangled up or complicated.

enriquecer *vi.* to enrich; **enriquecerse** *vr.* to be enriched; to become rich.

enriquecido-a *a.* enriched; of increased value.

enriquecimiento *m.* enrichment.

enrojecer *vi.* to redden.

enrojecimiento *m.* redness.

ensalada *f.* salad.

ensanchar *v.* to widen.

ensangrentado-a *a.* bloody, stained with blood.

ensartar *v.* to thread.

ensayo *m.* assay.

enseñado-a *a.* taught.

enseñar *v.* to teach; to show; to instruct.

ensimismado-a *a.* absorbed in thought, pensive.

ensordecedor-a *a.* deafening; **ruido** ___ / ___ noise.

ensuciar *v.* to dirty; to defecate.

entablillar *v.* to splint.

entamebiasis *f.* entamebiasis, infestation by an ameba.

ente *m.* entity, being.

entender *vi.* to understand, to comprehend.

entendido-a *a.* understood; agreed; informed; wise, learned.

enteralgia *f.* enteralgia, neuralgia of the intestine.

entérico-a, enteral *a.* enteral, rel. to the intestine; **cubierta ___ / ___** coated.

enteritis *f.* enteritis, infl. of the intestine, esp. the small intestine.

entero-a *a.* whole; undiminished.

enterocele *n.* enterocele, a hernial protrusion through a defect in the rectovaginal or vesicovaginal pouch.

enteroclisis *f.* enteroclysis, irrigation of the colon.

enterococo *m.* enterococcus, a streptococcus that inhabits the intestinal tract.

enterocolecistostomía *f.* enterocholecystostomy, opening between the gallbladder and the small intestine.

enterocolitis *f.* enterocolitis, infl. of both the large and small intestine.

enterocutáneo-a *a.* enterocutaneous, that communicates between the intestines and the cutaneous surface.

enteropatía *f.* enteropathy, any anomaly or disease of the intestines.

enteropatógeno-a *a.* enteropathogenic, rel. to a microorganism causing an intestinal disease.

enterostomía *f.* enterostomy, opening or communication between the intestine and the abdominal wall skin; **revisión de una ___ / ___** revision.

enterotoxina *f.* enterotoxin, a toxin produced by or originating in the intestines.

enterovirus *m.* enterovirus, a group of viruses that infect the human gastrointestinal tract, and can cause respiratory diseases and neurological anomalies.

enterrar *vi.* to bury.

entibiar *v.* to make lukewarm.

entidad *f.* entity, that which constitutes the essence of something.

entierro *m.* burial.

entonces *adv.* then, at that time.

entorno *m.* environment, setting, ambiance.

entrada *f.* entrance; entry; inlet; access to a cavity.

entrañas *f.* entrails, bowels; insides.

entrar *v.* to go in; to come in.

entre *prep.* between.

entrenamiento *m.* training.

entrenar *v.* to train; **entrenarse** *vr.* to receive training.

entrevista *f.* interview.

entropía *f.* entropy, in thermodynamics, diminished capacity to convert internal energy into work.

entropión *m.* entropion, inversion or turning inward such as that of the eyelid.

entuerto *m.* afterbirth pains.

entumecido-a *a.* numb.

entumecimiento *m.* numbness; torpor.

entusiasmo *m.* enthusiasm.

enucleación *f.* enucleation, removal of a tumor or a structure.

enuclear *v.* to enucleate. 1. to remove a tumor without causing it to rupture; 2. to destroy or take out the nucleus of a cell; 3. to remove the eyeball.

enuresis, enuresia *f.* enuresis, incontinence; bed-wetting; **___ nocturna /** nocturnal **___** .

envejecer *vi.* to grow old.

envejecido-a *a.* grown old, looking old.

envenenado-a *a.* poisoned.

envenenamiento *m.* poisoning.

envenenar *v.* to poison; **envenenarse** *vr.* to poison oneself.

envenomación *m.* envenomation, the act of injecting by stinging, biting, or any other designed apparatus or form, a poisonous material or venom to a victim.

enviar *v.* to send.

envidia *f.* envy.

enviudar *v.* to become a widow or a widower.

envoltura *f.* pack, cold or hot wrapping.

envolver *vi.* to wrap; to wrap around.

enyesar *v.* to make a cast using plaster of Paris; to plaster.

enzima *f.* enzyme, protein that acts as a catalyst in vital chemical reactions; **___ mucomembranosa /** mucomembranous **___**; **___ tuberculosa /** tuberculous; **grupos de ___ -s /** enzyme groups.

enzimología *f.* enzymology, the study of enzymes.

eosina *f.* eosin, insoluble substance used as a red dye for coloring tissue in microscopic studies.

eosinofilia *f.* eosinophilia, presence of a large number of eosinophilic leukocytes in the blood.

eosinófilo-a *a.* eosinophilic, that stains readily with eosin.

eosinopenia *f.* eosinopenia, deficiency of eosinophilic cells in the blood.

eosinopénico-a *a.* eosinopenic, rel. to eosinopenia.

ependimario-a *a.* ependymal, rel. to the ependyma; **membrana ___ / ___** layer, one of the interior membranes of the neural tube of the embryo.

ependimitis *f.* ependymitis, infl. of the ependyma.

epéndimo *m.* ependyma, membrane that lines the ventricles of the brain and the central canal of the spinal cord.

ependimoma *f.* ependymoma, a tumor of the central nervous system that contains fetal ependymal cells.

epicardio *m.* epicardium, visceral surface of the pericardium.

epicondilitis humeral lateral *f.* lateral humeral epycondilitis, *pop.* tennis elbow.

epicóndilo *m.* epicondyle, a projection or eminence above the condyle of a bone.

epidemia *f.* epidemic, disease that affects a large number of people in a region or community at the same time.

epidémico-a *a.* epidemic; **brote** ___ / ___ outbreak.

epidemiología *f.* epidemiology, the study of epidemic diseases.

epidérmico-a *a.* epidermal, epidermic, rel. to the epidermis.

epidermis *f.* epidermis, external epithelial covering of the skin.

epidermoide *m.* epidermoid, tumor that contains epidermal cells; *a.* 1. resembling the dermis; 2. rel. to a tumor that has epidermal cells.

epidermólisis *f.* epidermolysis, loosening of the epidermis.

epididimitis *f.* epididymitis, infection and infl. of the epididymis.

epidídimo *m.* epididymis, a tube along the back side of the testes that collects the sperm from the testicle to be transported by the vas deferens to the seminal vesicle.

epidural *a.* epidural, situated above or outside of the dura mater.

epifisario-a *a.* epiphysial, epiphyseal, rel. to the epiphysis.

epífisis *f.* epiphysis, the end of a long bone, usu. wider than the diaphysis.

epifisitis *f.* epiphysitis, infl. of an epiphysis.

epifora *f.* epiphora, watering of the eye.

epigástrico-a *a.* epigastric, rel. to the epigastrium; **reflejo** ___ / ___ reflex.

epigastrio *m.* epigastrium, upper back portion of the abdomen.

epiglotis *f.* epiglottis, cartilage that covers the entrance to the larynx and prevents food or liquid from entering it during swallowing.

epiglotitis *f.* epiglottitis, infl. of the epiglottis and adjacent tissues.

epilación *f.* epilation, removal of hair by electrolysis.

epilepsia *f.* epilepsy, grand mal, neurological disorder, gen. chronic and in some cases hereditary, manifested by periodic convulsions and sometimes by loss of consciousness.

epilepsia jacksoniana *f.* Jacksonian epilepsy, partial epilepsy without loss of consciousness.

epiléptico-a *m., f.* person affected with epilepsy; *a.* epileptic, rel. to or suffering from epilepsy; **ataque o crisis** ___ / ___ seizure; **ausencia** ___ / ___ absentia epileptica, momentary loss of consciousness during an epileptic seizure; **demencia** ___ / ___ dementia; **espasmo** ___ / ___ spasm.

epileptógeno *m.* epileptogenic, epileptogenous, agent that causes epileptic seizures.

epinefrina *f.* epinephrine. **adrenalina**.

epiploico-a *a.* epiploic, rel. to the epiploon; **foramen** ___ / ___ foramen, opening that connects the greater and the lesser peritoneal cavities.

epiplón *m.* epiploon, pad of fat that covers the intestines.

episiotomía *f.* episiotomy, incision of the perineum to avoid tearing during parturition.

episodio *m.* episode, non-regulated event as part of a physical or mental condition, or both, and that manifests itself in some illnesses such as epilepsy.

epispadias *m.* epispadias, abnormal congenital opening of the male urethra on the upper surface of the penis.

epistaxis *f.* epistaxis, nosebleed.

epitálamo *m.* epithalamus, the uppermost portion of the diencephalon.

epitelial *a.* epithelial, rel. to the epithelium.

epitelio *m.* epithelium, the outer layer of mucous membranes; ___ **ciliado** / ciliated ___; ___ **columnar** / columnar ___; ___ **cuboidal** / cuboidal ___; ___ **de transición** / transitional ___; ___ **escamoso** / squamous ___; ___ **estratificado** / stratified ___ .

epitelioma *f.* epithelioma, carcinoma consisting mainly of epithelial cells.

epitelización *f.* epithelization, growth of epithelium over an exposed surface, such as a wound.

epitímpano *m.* epitympanum, upper back portion of the eardrum.

epónimo *m.* eponym, a noun that names a medical disorder or device after the name of its discoverer or inventor, such as Down syndrome.

epoxia *f.* epoxy, compound characterized by its adhesiveness.

e

Epsom, sales de *f.* Epsom salts, magnesium sulfate, used as laxative.

Epstein-Barr, virus de *m.* Epstein-Barr virus, virus thought to be the causative agent of infectious mononucleosis.

equilibrado-a *a.* balanced.

equilibrar *v.* to equilibrate, to balance.

equilibrio *m.* equilibrium. 1. the condition of being evenly balanced between opposite forces or effects. An object is in state of equilibrium if forces acting upon it are in equilibrium; 2. a state of apparent repose sometimes indicated by two opposing arrows that refer to two balanced chemical reactions in opposite directions at the same speed.

equimosis *f.* ecchymosis, bruise, gradual blue-black discoloration of the skin due to blood filtering into the cellular subcutaneous tissue.

equinococo *m.* echinococcus, a genus of tapeworm.

equinococosis *f.* echinococcosis, infestation by echinococcus; ___ **hepática** / hepatic ___; ___ **pulmonar** / pulmonary ___ .

equinovaro *m.* equinovarus, congenital deformity of the foot.

equitativo-a *a.* equitable.

equivalencia *f.* equivalence.

equivalente *a.* equivalent.

equivocación *f.* mistake, error.

equivocado-a *a.* mistaken, in error.

equivocarse *vr.; vi.* to make a mistake; to be in error; to miscalculate.

erección *f.* erection, state of rigidity or hardening of erectile tissue when it is filled with blood, such as the penis.

eréctil *a.* erectile, capable of erection or dilation.

erector *m.* erector, a structure that erects, such as a muscle.

ergonomía *f.* ergonomics, branch of ecology that studies design and operations of machines and the physical environment as related to humans.

ergotamina *f.* ergotamine, alkaloid used chiefly in the treatment of migraine headaches.

ergotismo *m.* ergotism, chronic poisoning due to excessive intake of ergot.

erina *f.* dissecting hook.

erisipela *f.* erysipelas, cutaneous infection of cellulites by the streptococcus B-hemolytic characterized by a reddish or brown eruption, defined in size; ___ **ambulante** / ambulant ___; ___ **interna** / internum ___; ___ **migrante** / migrant ___; ___ **pustulosa** / pustulosum; ___ **quirúrgica** / surgical ___ .

eritema *f.* erythema, redness of the skin due to congestion of the capillaries; ___ **de los pañales** / diaper rash; ___ **solar** / sunburn.

eritematoso-a *a.* erythematic, erythematous, rel. to erythema.

eritremia *f.* erythremia, increase of red blood cells due to an excessive production of erythroblasts by the bone marrow.

eritroblasto *m.* erythroblast, primitive red blood cell.

eritroblastosis *f.* erythroblastosis, excessive number of erythroblasts in the blood.

eritrocito *m.* erythrocyte, red blood cell made in the bone marrow that serves to transport oxygen to tissues; **índice de sedimentación de** ___ **-s** / ___ sedimentation rate.

eritrocitopenia *f.* erythrocytopenia, deficiency in the number of erythrocytes present in the blood.

eritrocitosis *f.* erythrocytosis, increase in the number of erythrocytes in the blood.

eritroide *a.* erythroid, reddish.

eritroleucemia *f.* erythroleukemia, malignant blood disease caused by abnormal growth of both red and white blood cells.

eritromelia *f.* erythromelia, cutaneous disorder of the lower extremities with erythema of unknown origin and atrophy of the skin.

eritromelalgia *f.* erythromelalgia, disorder involving the extremities, characterized by paroxysmal attacks of severe burning pains, reddening, sweating, most common in middle age.

eritromicina *f.* erythromycin, antibiotic used chiefly in infections caused by gram-positive bacteria.

eritrón *m.* erythron, system formed by erythrocytes circulating in the blood and the organ from which they arise.

eritropoyesis *f.* erythropoiesis, red blood cell production.

eritropoyetina *f.* erythropoietin, a non-dialyzable protein that stimulates red blood cell production.

erógeno-a *a.* erogenous, that which produces erotic sensations; **zona** ___ / ___ zone.

erosión *f.* erosion, the act of wearing out or away.

erosivo-a *a.* erosive, that causes erosion.

erótico-a *a.* erotic, rel. to eroticism or having the power to arouse sexual impulses.

erotismo *m.* eroticism, erotism, lustful sexual impulses.

erradicar *vi.* to eradicate, to remove, to extirpate.

errante, errático-a *a.* wandering, deviating from the normal course; **exantema** ___ / ___ rash; **neumonía** ___ / ___ pneumonia.

error *m.* error, mistake.

eructación *f.* eructation, belching.

eructar, erutar *v.* to eructate, to belch.

eructo, eruto *m.* eructation, belch.

erupción *f.* eruption, rash, skin outbreak; ___ **escamosa** / squamous ___; ___ **maculopapular** / maculopapular ___ .

escafoide *a.* scaphoid, shaped like a boat, esp. in reference to the bone of the carpus or the tarsus.

escala *f.* scale; ___ **de diferenciación** / range.

escaldadura *f.* scald, skin burn caused by boiling liquid or vapor.

escaldar *v.* to scald; to burn.

escalera *f.* staircase; ladder; ___ **de escape** / fire escape.

escalofrío *m.* chill, a cold, shivering sensation.

escalonar *v.* to stagger; to distribute in sequence.

escalpelo, escarpelo *m.* scalpel, surgical blade, dissecting knife.

escama *f.* scale, a thin, small lamina shed from the epidermis.

escamoso-a *a.* squamous, scaly.

escán *m.* scan, the process of producing an image of a specific organ or tissue by means of a radioactive substance that is injected as a contrasting element; ___ **cardíaco** / heart ___; ___ **de la tiroides** / thyroid ___; ___ **de los huesos** / bone ___; ___ **del cerebro** / brain ___; ___ **pulmonar** / lung ___ .

escáner *m.* scanner, exploratory device.

escán radioisótopo*m.* radioisotope scanning, scan that makes use of radioisotopes for theurapeutic of diagnostic purposes.

escápula *f.* scapula, shoulder blade.

escara *f.* eschar, dark-colored scab or crust that forms in the skin after a burn.

escarificación *f.* scarification, the act of producing a number of small superficial scratches or punctures on the skin.

escarlatina *f.* scarlatina, scarlet fever, an acute contagious disease characterized by fever and a bright red rash on the skin and tongue.

escasez *f.* scarcity, shortage, lack.

escaso-a *a.* scarce, scanty, in short supply.

escatología *f.* scatology. 1. the study of feces; 2. a morbid preoccupation with feces and filth.

escenario *m.* scenario; scene.

escindir *v.* to excise, to cut, to divide.

escintigrama *f.* scintigram, radionucleid imaging, procedure that uses radioisotopes to obtain a two-dimensional image of the distribution of bodily radiation, previously administered as a radiopharmaceutical agent.

escintilador *m.* scintillator.

escintiscan *m.* scintiscan.

escirro *m.* scirrhus, hard cancerous tumor.

escirroso-a *a.* scirrhous, hard, rel. to a scirrhus.

escleritis *f.* scleritis, infl. of the sclera.

esclerodermia *m.* scleroderma, a chronic illness that can cause atrophy of the skin, more common in middle aged women than in men.

escleroma *m.* scleroma, a hardened, circumscribed area of granulation tissue in the skin or in the mucous membrane.

esclerosis *f.* sclerosis, progressive hardening of organs or tissues; ___ **arterial** / arterial ___; ___ **de Alzheimer** / Alzheimer's ___; ___ **lateral amiotrófica** / amyotrophic lateral ___ .

esclerosis múltiple *f.* multiple sclerosis, slow, progressive disease of the central nervous system caused by a loss of the protective myelin covering of the nerve fibers of the brain and spinal cord.

esclerosis tuberosa *f.* tuberous sclerosis, familial disease manifested by convulsive seizures, progressive mental deficiency, and multiple tumor formations in the skin and the brain.

escleroterapia *f.* sclerotherapy, the process of injecting chemical solutions to treat varices in order to produce sclerosis.

esclerótica *f.* sclera, sclerotica, the hard, white exterior part of the eye made of fibrous tissue.

esclerótico-a *a.* sclerotic, rel. to or afflicted by sclerosis.

escobillón *m.* swab.

escoger *vi.* to choose, to elect.

escoliosis *f.* scoliosis, pronounced lateral curvature of the spine.

esconder *v.* to hide, to conceal.

escorbuto *m.* scurvy, disease caused by lack of vitamin C and manifested by anemia, bleeding gums, and a general state of inanition.

escorpión *m.* scorpion; **picadura de** ___ / ___ sting.

escotadura *f.* notch; ___ **supraesternal** ___ / suprasternal ___;

escotoma *m.* scotoma, area of lost or diminished vision within the visual field.

escotopía *f.* scotopia, adjustment to nocturnal vision.

escotópico-a *a.* scotopic, rel. to scotopia; **visión** ___ / ___ vision.

escribir *v.* to write.

escrito-a *a. pp.* of **escribir,** written.

escrófula *f.* scrofula, tuberculosis of the lymphatic glands.

escrofuloderma *m.* scrofuloderma, a type of scrofula with skin lesions.

escrotal *a.* scrotal, rel. to the scrotum.

escroto *m.* scrotum, the sac surrounding and enclosing the testes.

escrúpulo *m.* scruple.

escrupuloso-a *a.* scrupulous.

escrutinio *m.* scrutiny; screening.

escudo *m.* shield, a protective covering.

escupir *v.* to spit.

esencial *a.* essential, indispensable.

esfacelo *m.* slough, mass of dead tissue that has been shed or fallen off from live tissue.

esfenoidal *a.* sphenoidal, rel. to the sphenoid bone.

esfenoides *m.* sphenoid bone, large bone at the base of the skull.

esfera *f.* sphere. 1. a structure shaped like a globe or ball; 2. sociological environment.

esférico-a *a.* spherical, rel. to a sphere.

esferocito *m.* spherocyte, sphere-shaped erythrocyte.

esferocitosis *f.* spherocytosis, presence of spherocytes in the blood.

esferoide *a.* spheroid, shaped like a sphere.

esférula *f.* spherule, minute sphere.

esfigmomanómetro *m.* sphygmomanometer, instrument for determining blood pressure.

esfínter *m.* sphincter, circular muscle that opens and closes an orifice.

esfinteroplastia *f.* sphincteroplasty, plastic surgery of a sphincter muscle.

esfinterotomía *f.* sphincterotomy, cutting of a sphincter muscle.

esfuerzo *m.* effort; ___ **coordinado** / teamwork; ___ **excesivo** / overexertion, strain; **prueba de** ___ / stress test; **sin** ___ / effortless.

esguince *m.* sprain. **torcedura.**

eslabón *m.* link.

esmalte *m.* enamel, hard substance that covers and protects the dentin of a tooth.

esmegma *m.* smegma, thick cheesy substance secreted by sebaceous glands, esp. seen in the external genitalia.

esofagectomía *f.* esophagectomy, excision of a portion of the esophagus.

esofágico-a *a.* esophageal, rel. to the esophagus; **cintigrafía** ___ / ___ scintigraphy; **dilatación** ___ / ___ dilatation; **disfagia** ___ / ___ dysphagia; **espasmo** ___ / ___ spasm; **obstrucción** ___ / ___ obstruction.

esofagitis *f.* esophagitis, infl. of the esophagus.

esófago *m.* esophagus, portion of the alimentary tract between the pharynx and the stomach.

esofagodinia *f.* esophagodynia, pain in the esophagus.

esofagogastritis *f.* esophagogastritis, infl. of the stomach and the esophagus.

esofagogastroduodenoscopía *f.* esophagogastroduodenoscopy, examination of the esophagus, the stomach, and the duodenum by means of an endoscope.

esofagogastroscopía *f.* esophagogastroscopy, endoscopic examination of the esophagus and the stomach.

esofagoscopía *f.* esophagoscopy, interior inspection of the esophagus by using an endoscope.

esoforia *f.* esophoria, crossed eyes, inward deviation of the eyes.

esotropía *f.* esotropia.

espacial *a.* spatial, rel. to space.

espacio *m.* space, area.

espalda *f.* back; **dolor de** ___ / backache.

espanto *m.* fright, excessive fear.

español *m.* [*idioma*] Spanish; [*nativo-a*] Spanish; **-a** *a.* Spanish.

esparadrapo *m.* adhesive tape.

esparcido-a *a.* spread out; scattered.

esparcir *vi.* to scatter, to spread.

espárrago *m.* asparagus.

espasmo *m.* spasm, twitch, involuntary muscular contraction.

espasmódico-a *a.* spasmodic, rel. to spasms; **crup** ___ / ___ croup.

espasticidad *f.* spasticity, increase in the normal tension of a muscle resulting in stiffness and difficult movement.

espástico-a *a.* spastic. 1. resembling, or of the nature of spasms; 2. afflicted with spasms.

espátula *f.* spatula, palette-knife.

especia *f.* spice.

especial *a.* special, especial, unique; **-mente** *adv.* specially.

especialidad *f.* specialty. *V.* cuadro en la página 113.

especialista *m., f.* specialist.

especialización *f.* specialization.

Especialidades	Specialties
anestesiología	anesthesiology
cirugía cardiotorácica	cardiothoracic surgery
cirugía general	general surgery
cirugía plástica	plastic surgery
dermatología	dermatology
gastroenterología	gastroenterology
medicina de emergencia o de urgencia	emergency medicine
medicina general	family practice
medicina interna	internal medicine
medicina nuclear	nuclear medicine
nefrología	nephrology
neurología	neurology
neurocirugía	neurosurgery
obstetricia y ginecología	obstetrics and gynecology
oftalmología	ophthalmology
oncología	oncology
ortopedia	orthopedics
otolaringología	otolaryngology
patología	pathology
pediatría	pediatrics
perinatología	perinatology
psiquiatría	psychiatry
radiología	radiology
urología	urology

especializarse *vr. vi.* to specialize.

especie *f.* species, kind, class of organisms belonging to a biological category.

especificar *vi.* to specify.

específico-a *a.* specific; determined; precise; **no** ___ / nonspecific.

espécimen *m.* specimen, sample.

espectro *m.* spectrum. 1. range of activity of an antibiotic against a variety of microorganisms; 2. series of images resulting from the refraction of electromagnetic radiation; 3. series of colors of refracted sunlight that can be seen with the naked eye or with the help of a sensitive instrument.

espectro electromagnético *m.* electromagnetic spectrum.

especular *v.* to speculate.

espéculo *m.* speculum, instrument used for dilating a conduit or cavity; ___ **rectal** / proctoscope.

espejo *m.* mirror.

espejuelos *m. pl.* eyeglasses, spectacles; ___ **bifocales** / bifocal ___; ___ **para leer** / reading ___; ___ **trifocales** / trifocal ___ .

espera *f.* wait; **salón de** ___ / waiting room.

esperanza *f.* hope; **perder la** ___ / to give up ___; **tener** ___ / to have ___ .

esperar *v.* to wait; to hope; to expect.

esperma *f.* sperm, semen; **conteo disminuído de** ___ / reduced ___ count.

esperma de ballena *m.* whale sperm, called in Spanish spermaceti, a lipid substance extracted from the head of a whale.

espermaticida, espermicida *m.* spermatocide, spermicidal, agent that destroys spermatozoa; *a.* spermatocidal, that kills spermatozoa.

espermático-a *a.* spermatic; rel. to sperm or semen.

espermatocele *m.* spermatocele, a cystic tumor of the epididymis containing spermatozoa.

espermatogénesis *f.* spermatogenesis, the process of formation and development of spermatozoa.

espermatoide *a.* spermatoid, resembling spermatozoa.

espermatorrea *f.* spermatorrhea, involuntary loss of semen.

espermatozoide *m.* sperm cell; the male sperm that fertilizes the female egg.

espermiograma *m.* spermiogram, evaluation of spermatozoa as an aid to determine sterility.

espesar *v.* to thicken; to condense; **espesarse** *vr.* to become thicker; to become condensed.

espeso-a *a.* thick, condensed.

espesor *m.* thickness, consistency.

espica *f.* spica, a type of bandage.

espícula *f.* spicule, a body shaped like a small needle.

espicular *a.* spicular, needle-shaped.

espiga *f.* spike, sharp rise in a curve, such as in the tracing of brain waves.

espín *m.* spin, auricular rotation; *v.* to gyrate, to extend, to prolong.

espina *f.* 2. spina; thorn; fishbone.

espina bífida *f.* spina bifida, congenital anomaly of the spine with a gap; ___ **oculta** / ___ occulta, without protrusion, gen. at the lumbar level.

espina dorsal *f.* columna. columna vertebral.

espinaca *f.* spinach.

espinal *a.* spinal, rel. to the spine or the spinal cord; **atrofia muscular** ___ / ___ muscular atrophy; **canal** ___ / ___ canal; **choque** ___ / ___ shock; **fusión** ___ / ___ fusion; **médula** ___ / ___ cord; **nervio accesorio** ___ / ___ accessory nerve; **nervios** ___-es / ___ nerves; **punción** ___ / ___ puncture.

espinazo *m.* spine, *pop.* backbone.

espinilla *f.* 1. blackhead; 2. shinbone, anterior edge of the tibia.

espinoso-a *a.* spinous, acanthoid, spine-shaped.

espiral *f.* spiral. 1. sphere-like arrangement of cardiac muscular fibers; 2. a type of fingerprint; *a.* coiled; winding around a center or axis.

espirar *v.* to exhale.

espíritu *m.* spirit. 1. alcoholic solution of a volatile substance; 2. soul; **tranquilidad de** ___ / peace of mind.

espiritual *a.* spiritual, rel. to the soul; **cura** ___ / ___ healing.

espirometría *f.* spirometry, the act of measuring the breathing capacity through the use of a spirometer.

espirómetro *m.* spirometer, device used to measure the amount of inhaled and exhaled air.

espiroqueta *f.* spirochete, spinal microorganism that belongs to the order *Spirochaetales* that includes the syphilis causing agent.

espiroquetósico-a *a.* spirochetal, rel. to spirochetes.

esplácnico-a *a.* splanchnic, rel. to or that reaches the viscera; **nervios** ___ -s / ___ nerves.

esplenectomía *f.* splenectomy, excision of the spleen.

esplénico-a *a.* splenic, rel. to the spleen.

esplenoportografía *f.* splenoportography, x-ray of the splenic and portal veins following injection of a radiopaque dye into the spleen.

esplenorrenal *a.* splenorenal, rel. to the spleen and the kidneys; **derivación** ___ / ___ shunt, anastomosis of the splenic veins or artery to the renal vein, esp. used in the treatment of portal hypertension.

espolón *m.* spur, pointed projection, as of a bone; ___ **calcáneo** / calcaneal ___ .

espondilitis *f.* spondylitis, infl. of one or more vertebrae.

espondilitis anquilosa *f.* ankylosing spondylitis, arthritis of the spine, resembling rheumatoid arthritis.

espondilólisis *f.* spondylolysis, dissolution or destruction of a vertebra.

espondilolistesis *f.* spondylolisthesis, forward displacement of one vertebra over another, usu.

the fourth lumber over the fifth or the fifth over the sacrum.

espondilopatía *f.* spondylopathy, any disease or disorder of a vertebra.

espondilosis *f.* spondylosis. 1. vertebral ankylosis; 2. any degenerative condition affecting the vertebrae.

esponja *f.* sponge.

esponjar *v.* to sponge, to soak with a sponge.

esponjoso-a *a.* spongy, porous.

espontáneo-a *a.* spontaneous.

espora *f.* spore, unicellular reproductive cell.

esporádico-a *a.* sporadic, occurring irregularly.

esporicida *m.* sporicide, agent that destroys spores.

esposo-a *m., f.* husband; wife.

esprue *m.* sprue, chronic disease that affects the ability to absorb dietary gluten.

espulgar *vi.* to cleanse of lice or fleas.

espuma *f.* froth, foam; scum.

espurio-a *a.* spurious, false.

esputo *m.* sputum, spittle; ___ **sanguinolento** / bloody ___ .

esquelético-a *a.* skeletal, rel. to the skeleton.

esqueleto *m.* skeleton, the bony structure of the body.

esquema *f.* schema; outline, plan.

esquemático-a *a.* schematic, rel. to a schema.

esquina *f.* corner.

esquirla *f.* bone splinter.

esquistosoma *m. Schistosoma,* blood fluke, a trematode larva that enters the blood through the digestive tract or through the skin by contact with contaminated water.

esquistosomiasis *f.* schistosomiasis, infestation with blood flukes.

esquizofrenia *f.* schizophrenia, a breaking down of the mental functions with different psychotic manifestations such as delusion, withdrawal, and distorted perception of reality.

esquizofrénico-a *a.* schizophrenic, rel. to or suffering from schizophrenia.

esquizoide *a.* schizoid, resembling schizophrenia.

estabilidad *f.* stability, permanence.

estabilización *f.* stabilization, the act of making stable.

estabilizar *vi.* to stabilize, to eliminate fluctuations.

estable *a.* stable, nonfluctuating.

establecer *vi.* to establish.

estación *f.* station. 1. status of condition; 2. stopping place such as a nurse's station; 3. season of the year.

estacionario-a *a.* stationary, in a fixed position.

estadificación *f.* staging, classification in the process of the degree of an illness. ___ **clínica** / clinical ___ .

estadío *m.* stage or transition period during the evolution of an illness.

estadística *f.* statistics; statistic, figure.

estado *m.* state, condition; ___ **asmaticus** / status asthmaticus; ___ **crepuscular** / twilight ___ ; ___ **de gestación** / pregnancy; ___ **nutricional** / nutritional ___ .

estado epiléctico *m.* status epilepticus, repeated epileptic episodes without regaining consciousness between attacks.

estafilococemia *f.* staphylococcemia, presence of staphylococci in the blood.

estafilocócico-a *a.* staphylococcal, staphylococcic, rel. to or caused by staphylococci; **infecciones** ___ / ___ infections.

estafilococo *m.* staphylococcus, any pathological micrococci; **intoxicación alimentaria por** ___ **-s** / staphylococcal food poisoning.

estafilotoxina *f.* staphylotoxin, toxin produced by staphylococci.

estancación, estancamiento *m., f.* stagnation, lack of movement or circulation in fluids.

estancia *f.* stay; ___ **breve en el hospital** / short ___ in the hospital.

estándar *a.* standard, normal established way; **atención o cuidado** ___ / ___ of care; **desviación** ___ / ___ deviation; **error** ___ / ___ error; **procedimiento** ___ / ___ procedure.

estandarización *f.* standardization, uniformity; normalcy.

estanolona *f.* stanolone, anabolic steroid drug.

estapedectomía *f.* stapedectomy, excision of the stapes of the ear to improve hearing.

estar *vi.* to be; ___ **de guardia** / to be on call.

estasis *f.* stasis, stagnation of a body fluid such as blood or urine.

estático-a *a.* static, without movement.

estatura *f.* stature, height.

estatutorio *n.* statutory.

este *m.* [*punto cardinal*] east; **al** ___ **de** / to the ___ of; **-a** *a.* this; **estos-as** *pl.* / these; **éste-a** *dem. pron.* / this, this one; **éstos-as** *pl.* / these; **esto** *neut.* / this, this one.

estearina *f.* stearine, white crystalline component of fats.

esteatorrea *f.* steatorrhea, excess fat in the stool.

estenia *f.* sthenia, normal strength and vigor.

estenosado-a *a.* stenosed, rel. to stenosis.

estenósico-a *a.* stenotic, produced or characterized by stenosis.

estenosis *f.* stenosis, constriction or abnormal narrowing of a passageway; ___ **aórtica** / aortic ___ ; ___ **espinal** / spinal ___ ; ___ **pilórica** / pyloric ___ ; ___ **traqueal** / tracheal ___ .

estepaje *m.* steppage, alteration in the gait as a result of the pendular fall of the foot forcing the lifting of the knee and flexing the muscle over the pelvis.

éster *m.* ester, compound formed by the combination of an organic acid and alcohol.

estereorradiografía *a.* stereoradiography, a three-dimensional x-ray.

estereotaxia *f.* stereotaxis, technique used in neurological procedures to locate with precision an area in the brain.

estereotipia *f.* stereotype, a type that represents a whole group.

estereotípico-a *a.* stereotypic, rel. to a stereotype.

esterificación *f.* esterification, transformation of an acid into ester.

estéril *a.* sterile. 1. aseptic, free of germs; 2. incapable of producing offspring.

esterilidad *f.* sterility. 1. the condition of being sterile; 2. inability to reproduce.

esterilización *f.* sterilization. 1. procedure to prevent reproduction; 2. total destruction of microorganisms; ___ **por calor** / thermosterilization; ___ **por gas** / gas ___ ; ___ **por vapor** / steam ___ .

esterilizador *m.* sterilizer.

esterilizar *vi.* to sterilize.

esternal *a.* sternal, rel. to the sternum; **punción** ___ / ___ puncture.

esternocostal *a.* sternocostal, rel. to the sternum and the ribs.

esternón *m.* sternum, breastbone.

esternotomía *f.* sternotomy, cutting through the sternum.

esteroide *a.* steroid, rel. to steroids.

esteroides *m.* steroids, complex organic compounds that resemble cholesterol and of which many hormones such as estrogen, testosterone, and cortisone are made.

estertor *m.* rale, stertor, an abnormal rattle-like sound heard on ausculation; ___ **agónico** / death rattle; ___ **áspero** / coarse; ___ ; ___ **crepitante** / crepitant ___ ; ___ **crujiente** /

crackling ___; ___ **húmedo** / moist ___; ___
roncus / rhonchus ___, rattling in the throat; ___
seco / dry ___ .

estesia *f.* esthesia, perception or sensation, or any anomaly affecting them.

estetoscopio *m.* stethoscope, instrument used for auscultation.

estigma *m.* stigma. 1. a specific sign of a disease; 2. a mark or sign on the body.

estilete *m.* style, stylet, stylus; [*cirugía*] flexible probe.

estiloide *a.* styloid, long and pointed.

estimado *m.* estimate, evaluation.

estimulación *f.* stimulation; motivation.

estimulador cardíaco *m.* pacemaker.

estimulante *m.* stimulant, agent that incites a reaction; *pop.* upper.

estimular *v.* to stimulate; to motivate, to animate to action, to boost, to prompt.

estímulo *m.* stimulus, agent or factor that produces a reaction; ___ **condicionado** / conditioned ___; ___ **subliminal** / subliminal ___ .

estíptico *m.* styptic, agent with astringent power.

estirado-a *a.* extended, elongated.

estirar *v.* to stretch, to extend.

estirón *m.* stretch, forceful pull.

estoma *m.* stoma, artificial permanent opening, esp. in the abdominal wall.

estomacal *a.* stomachic, rel. to the stomach.

estómago *m.* stomach, sac-like organ of the alimentary canal; ___ **en cascada** / cascade ___; ___ **en bota de vino** / leather bottle ___; **lavado de** ___ / ___ pumping.

estomal *a.* stomal, rel. to a stoma.

estomatitis *f.* stomatitis, infl. of the mucosa of the mouth; ___ **aftosa** / aphthous ___ .

estornudar *v.* to sneeze.

estornudo *m.* sneeze.

estrabismo *m.* strabismus, squint, abnormal alignment of the eyes due to muscular deficiency.

estradiol *m.* estradiol, steroid produced by the ovaries.

estrangulación *f.* strangulation. 1. asphyxia or suffocation gen. caused by obstruction of the air passages; 2. constriction of an organ or structure due to compression.

estrangulado-a *a.* strangulated; constricted.

estrangular *v.* to strangle.

estratificación *f.* stratification; arrangement in layers.

estratificado-a *a.* stratified, arranged in layers; **epitelio** ___ / ___ epithelium.

estrato *m.* stratum, layer.

estrechamiento *m.* narrowing; tightness.

estrechar *v.* to make narrower.

estrechez, estrechura *f.* stricture, narrowness, closeness.

estrecho-a *a.* narrow.

estrella *f.* star; star-shaped body.

estrellado-a *a.* stellate, shaped like a star.

estremecerse *vr., vi.* to shudder, to tremble.

estreñido-a *a.* constipated; hard bound.

estreñimiento *m.* constipation; infrequent or incomplete bowel movements.

estreptococcemia *f.* streptococcemia, blood infection caused by the presence of streptococci.

estreptocócico-a *a.* streptococcal, rel. to or caused by streptococci; **infecciones** ___ -s / ___ infections.

estreptococo *m.* streptococcus, organism of the genus *Streptococcus.*

estreptomicina *f.* streptomycin, antibiotic drug used against bacterial infections.

estrés *m.* stress.

estría *f.* stria, streak.

estriado-a *a.* striated, striate, marked by streaks; **músculo** ___ / ___ muscle.

estribo *m.* stapes, the innermost of the auditory ossicles shaped like a stirrup.

estricnina *f.* strychnine, highly poisonous alkaloid.

estricto-a *a.* strict; exact.

estricturotomía *f.* stricturotomy, the cutting of strictures.

estridor *m.* stridor, whoop, harsh sound during respiration such as following an attack of whooping cough.

estrinización *m.* estrinization, epithelial changes of the vagina due to stimulation by estrogen.

estrogénico-a *a.* estrogenic, rel. to estrogen.

estrógeno *m.* estrogen, female sex hormone produced by the ovaries; **receptor de** ___ / ___ receptor.

estroma *m.* stroma, the supporting tissue of an organ.

estrona *f.* estrone, oestrone, estrogenic hormone.

estroncio *m.* strontium, chemical element with properties similar to those of calcium that is used as an antiseptic and as a gastric tonic.

estropear *v.* to spoil; to maim; to cripple.

estructura *f.* structure; order.

estudiante *m., f.* student.

estudiar *v.* to study.

estudio *m.* study.

estudios cruzados *m. pl.* cross studies.

estupefaciente *m.* stupefacient. 1. agent causing stupor; 2. narcotic analgesic that alters the physiological conditions and produces euphoria.

estupidez *f.* stupidity, foolishness.

estúpido-a *a.* stupid, foolish.

estupor *m.* stupor, daze, state of lethargy.

etapa *n.* stage; ___ -s de la enfermedad / ___ of the illness.

etapas del parto *f., pl.* stages of labor. First, stage uterine contractions; second, stage dilation of the cervix; third, stage expulsion of the infant, expulsion of the placenta and membranes.

éter *m.* ether, chemical liquid used as a general anesthetic through inhalation of its vapor.

eternal, eterno-a *a.* eternal.

ética *f.* ethics, norms and principles that rule professional conduct.

etileno *m.* ethylene, anesthetic.

etiología *f.* etiology, branch of medicine that studies the cause of diseases.

etiológico-a *a.* etiologic, rel. to etiology.

etiqueta *f.* label, tag.

etmoidectomía *f.* ethmoidectomy, removal of ethmoid cells or part of the ethmoid bone.

etmoideo-a *a.* ethmoid, sievelike; seno ___ / ___ sinus, air cavity within the ethmoid bone.

etmoides *m.* ethmoid bone, spongy bone located at the base of the cranium.

eubolismo *m.* eubolism, normal metabolism.

eucalipto *m.* eucalyptus tree.

euforia *f.* euphoria, an abnormal or exaggerated state of well-being.

eugenesia *f.* eugenics, the science that deals with improving and controling procreation to achieve more desirable herediatry characteristics.

eunuco *m.* eunuch, castrated male.

euploidia *f.* euploidy, complete set of chromosomes.

Eustaquio, catéter de *m.* Eustaquian catheter, catheter used through the Eustaquian tube to the middle ear.

Eustaquio, trompa de *m.* Eustachian tube, part of the auditory conduit.

eutanasia *f.* euthanasia, mercy killing.

eutiroideo-a *a.* euthyroid, rel. to the normal function of the thyroid gland.

evacuación *f.* evacuation. 1. act of emptying or evacuating esp. the bowels; 2. the act of making a vacuum.

evacuante *m.* evacuant, an agent that stimulates bowel movement.

evacuar *v.* to evacuate, to empty; to void.

evaginación *f.* evagination, protrusion of some part or organ from its normal position.

evaluación *f.* evaluation, assessment, rating, score; weighing the physical and mental state and capabilities of an individual; ___ **clínica** / clinical assessment; ___ **del estado de salud** / health assessment; ___ **del proceso evolutivo** / follow-up assessment.

evaluar *v.* to evaluate.

evanescente *a.* evanescent, of brief duration.

evaporación *f.* evaporation, conversion of a liquid or a solid into vapor.

eversión *f.* eversion, outward turning, esp. of the mucosa surrounding a natural orifice.

evidencia *f.* evidence, manifestation; [*legal*] evidence; testimony.

evisceración *f.* evisceration, removal of the viscera or contents of a cavity; disembowelment.

evitar *v.* to avoid.

evocar *vi.* to evoke.

evolución *f.* evolution, gradual change.

evulsión *f.* evulsion, tearing away, pulling out.

exacerbación *f.* exacerbation, increase in the severity of a symptom or disease.

exacto-a *a.* exact; **-mente** *adv.* exactly.

exageración *f.* exaggeration.

exagerar *v.* to exaggerate.

exaltación *f.* exaltation, state of jubilation.

examen *m.* exam, examination; evaluation; investigation; ___ **físico completo** / complete physical checkup.

examinar *v.* to examine, to view and study the human body to determine a person's state of health; to look into, to investigate.

exantema *f.* exanthema. 1. cutaneous rash, sign of an acute viral or coccal disease as in scarlet fever or measles; 2. cutaneous eruption; ___ **epidémico** / epidemic ___; ___ **keratoideo** / keratoid ___; ___ **súbito** / ___ subitum.

exasperado-a *a.* exasperated.

exasperar *v.* to exasperate, to aggravate.

exceder *v.* to exceed; to outweigh; to surpass; **excederse** *vr.* to go too far, *pop.* to go overboard.

excéntrico-a *a.* eccentric, odd, different from the norm.

excepción *f.* exception, outside of the rule; **a** ___ **de** / with the ___ of.

excesivo-a *a.* excessive, too much.

exceso *m.* excess; **en** ___ / excessively.

excisión *f.* excision, removal, ablation.

excitación *f.* excitation, reaction to a stimulus.

excitado-a *a.* excited, worked up.

excitante *m.* stimulant, *pop.* upper; *a.* stimulating, exciting.

excitar *v.* to stimulate; to provoke.

excluir *vi.* to exclude, to leave out.

excoriación *f.* excoriation, abrasion of the skin.

excrecencia *f.* excrescence, tumor protruding from the surface of a part or organ.

excreción *f.* excretion, elimination of waste matter.

excremento *m.* excrement, feces.

excreta *f.* excreta, all waste matter of the body.

excretar *v.* to excrete, to eliminate waste from the body.

excusa *f.* excuse.

excusado *m.* outside toilet; privy.

excusar *v.* to excuse.

exenteración *f.* exenteration, V. **evisceration**.

exfoliación *f.* exfoliation, shedding or peeling of tissue.

exhalación *f.* exhalation, the act of breathing out.

exhalar *v.* to exhale.

exhausto-a *a.* exhausted, fatigued.

exhibicionismo *m.* exhibitionism, obsessive drive to expose one's body, esp. the genitals.

exhibicionista *m., f.* exhibitionist, one who practices exhibitionism.

exhumación *f.* exhumation, disinterment.

exigir *vi.* to demand; to require.

existente *a.* existent, on hand.

existir *v.* to exist, to be.

éxito *m.* success; good result.

exocrino-a *a.* exocrine, rel. to the external secretion of a gland.

exoftalmia *f.* exophthalmia, exophthalmos, exophthalmus, abnormal protrusion of the eyeball.

exoftálmico-a *a.* exophthalmic, rel. to or suffering from exophthalmia.

exógeno-a *a.* exogenous, originating outside the organism.

exostosis *f.* exostosis, cartilaginous osseus hypertrophy that projects outward from a bone, or the root of a tooth.

exótico-a *a.* exotic.

exotoxina *f.* exotoxin, toxic substance secreted by bacteria.

exotropía *f.* exotropia, a type of strabismus, outward turning of the eyes due to muscular imbalance.

expandir *v.* to expand, to dilate; **expandirse** *vr.* to become expanded.

expansión *f.* expansion, extension.

expansivo-a *a.* expansive; [*persona*] outgoing.

expectoración *f.* expectoration, the expulsion of mucus or phlegm from the lungs, trachea or bronchi.

expectorante *m.* expectorant, an agent that stimulates expectoration.

expediente *m.* medical record; file; **sumario del** ___ / summary of hospital records.

experiencia *f.* experience, knowledge gained by practice.

experimental *a.* experimental, rel. to or known by experiment.

experimentar *v.* to experiment.

experimento *m.* experiment.

experto-a *m., f.* expert.

expiración *f.* expiration, termination; death.

expirar *v.* to expire, to die.

explicación *f.* explanation; interpretation.

explicativo-a *a.* explanatory.

exploración *f.* exploration, search, investigation.

exploratorio-a *a.* exploratory, rel. to exploration.

exponer *vi.* to expose.

exposición *f.* exposition, demonstration, display.

expresión *f.* expression, facial appearance.

expresividad *f.* expressivity, degree of manifestation of a given hereditary trait in the individual that carries the conditioning gene.

exprimir *v.* to squeeze; to extrude.

expuesto-a *a. pp.* of **exponer,** exposed.

expulsar *v.* to expel, to eject forcefully.

expulsión *f.* expulsion; ___ **de la placenta** / ___ of the placenta; ___ **del recién nacido** / ___ of the infant.

exsanguinación *f.* exsanguination, severe blood loss.

exsanguinotransfusión *f.* exsanguino-transfusion, exchange transfusion, gradual and simultaneous withdrawal of a recipient's blood with transfusion of a donor's blood.

éxtasis *m.* ecstasy, trance accompanied by a pleasurable feeling.

extendedor *m.* stretcher.

extender *vi.* to extend, to stretch out; **extenderse** *vr.* to spread out.

extendido-a *a.* extended; widespread.

extensión *f.* extension, prolongation, straightening of a contracted finger or limb or aligning a dislocated or fractured bone.

extensor-a *a.* extensor, having the property of extending.

extenuado-a *a.* extenuated, exhausted.

exterior *a.* exterior.

exteriorizar *v.* to exteriorize, to temporarily expose a part or organ.

externo-a *a.* external, outer.

extinción *f.* extinction, cessation.

extinguir *vi.* to extinguish, to put out.

extirpación *f.* extirpation, removal of a part or organ.

extirpar *v.* to eradicate, to remove.

extracción *f.* extraction, the process of removing, pulling, or drawing out.

extracelular *a.* extracellular, occurring outside a cell.

extracorporal *a.* extracorporeal, occurring outside the body.

extracto *m.* extract, a concentrated product;___ **alcohólico** / alcoholic ___; ___ **alérgico** / allergic ___; ___ **de belladona** / belladonna ___; ___ **equivalente** / equivalent ___; ___ **líquido** / fluid ___; ___ **hidroalcólico** / hydroalcoholic ___ .

extradural *a.* extradural. V. **epidural**.

extraer *vi.* to extract, to remove; to dig out.

extrañarse *vr.* to wonder, to question.

extraño-a *a.* extraneous. 1. unrelated to or outside an organism; 2. strange, rare; 3. foreign.

extraocular *a.* extraocular, outside the eye.

extrapancreático *a.* extrapancreatic, not connected with the pancreas.

extrasístole *f.* extrasystole, arrhythmic beat of the heart; *pop.* skipped beat.

extrauterino *a.* extrauterine, that occurs or is found outside the uterus.

extravasado-a *a.* extravasated, rel. to the escape of fluid from a vessel or organ into the surrounding tissue.

extravascular *a.* extravascular, outside a vessel.

extremidad *f.* extremity. 1. the end portion; 2. a limb of the body; **amputación de una** ___ / limb amputation; **rigidez de una** ___ / limb rigidity.

extremo-a *a.* extreme, excessive.

extrínseco-a *a.* extrinsic, that comes from without.

extrofia *f.* extrophy, **eversion**.

extrovertido-a *a.* extroverted, excessive manifestation and attention outside the self.

extubación *f.* extubation, removal of a tube, as the laryngeal tube.

exuberante *a.* exuberant, excessive proliferation; overabundant.

exudación *f.* exudation. V. **exudado**.

exudado *m.* exudate, inflammatory fluid such as pus or serum.

exudar *v.* to exude, to ooze out gradually through the tissues.

eyaculación *f.* ejaculation, sudden and rapid expulsion, such as the emission of semen.

eyacular *v.* to ejaculate, to expel fluid secretions such as semen.

eyección *f.* ejection, throwing out with force.

e

f

F *abr.* **Fahrenheit** / Fahrenheit.

f *abr.* **fallo** / failure; **femenino** / feminine; **fórmula** / formula; **función** / function.

fabela *f.* fabella, sesamoid fibrocartilage that can develop in the head of the gastrocnemius muscle.

fabricación *f.* fabrication. confabulación.

faceta *f.* facet, facette *Fr.* small, smooth area on the surface of a hard structure such as a bone.

facetectomía *f.* facetectomy, removal of the auricular facet of a vertebra.

facial *a.* facial, rel. to the face; **arteria** ___ / ___ artery; **axis** ___ / ___ axis; **canal** ___ / ___ canal; **espasmo** ___ / ___ spasm; **hemiplejía** ___ / ___ hemiplegia; **huesos** ___ -es / ___ bones; **nervios** ___ -es / ___ nerves; **parálisis** ___ / ___ paralysis; **reflejo** ___ / ___ reflex; **tic** ___ / ___ tic; **vena** ___ / ___ vein.

facies *f. facies* expression or appearance of the face; ___ **inexpresiva** / masklike ___; ___ **leontina** / ___ leontina.

fácil *a.* easy; **-mente** / *adv.* easily.

facilitar *v.* to facilitate, to make easier.

facioplastia *f.* facioplasty, plastic surgery of the face.

facioplejía *f.* facioplegia, facial paralysis.

facticio-a *a.* factitious, not natural, artificial.

factor *m.* factor, element that contributes to produce an action; ___ **angiogenético tumoral** / tumor angiogenetic ___; ___ **antihemofílico** / antihemophilic ___; ___ **de coagulación de la sangre** / clotting ___; ___ **de crecimiento fibroblástico** / fibroblast growth___; ___ **dominante** / dominant ___; ___ **liberador** / releasing ___; ___ **Rh [erre-ache]** / Rh ___; ___ **reumatoideo** / rheumatoid ___ .

facultad *f.* faculty. 1. capability to perform a normal function; 2. professional staff.

facultativo-a *a.* facultative. 1. not obligatory, voluntary; 2. of a professional nature; **asistencia** ___ **médica** / professional medical help; **cuidado** ___ / professional care.

Faget, signo de *m.* Faget, sign of, low point in relation to the present high temperature.

fagocitario-a, fagocítico-a *a.* phagocytic, rel. to phagocytes.

fagocito *m.* phagocyte, cell that ingests and destroys microorganisms or other cells and foreign particles.

fagocitosis *f.* phagocytosis, the process of ingestion and digestion by phagocytes.

Fahrenheit, escala de *f.* Fahrenheit scale, a temperature scale with a freezing point of water at 32 and a normal boiling point at 212.

faja *f.* girdle; band.

fajero *m.* swaddling band, strip of cloth used to restrain an infant's movements.

falange *f.* phalanx, any of the long bones of the fingers or toes.

falciforme *a.* falciform, shaped like a sickle; **ligamento** ___ / ___ ligament; **ligamento** ___ **del hígado** / ___ ligament of the liver; **proceso** ___ / ___ process.

falda *f.* skirt.

fálico-a *a.* phallic, rel. to or resembling the penis.

falla *f.* defect, deficiency.

fallar *v.* to miss, to fail.

fallecer *vi.* to die, to pass away.

fallecimiento *m.* death.

fallo *m.* failure; insufficiency; ___ **cardíaco** / heart ___; ___ **renal** / renal ___; ___ **respiratorio** / respiratory ___ .

Fallot, tetralogía de *f.* tetralogy of Fallot, congenital deformity of the heart involving defects in the great blood vessels and the walls of the heart chambers.

falo *m.* phallus, the penis.

Falopio, trompas de *f.* Fallopian tubes, tubes leading from the uterus to the ovaries.

falsificación *f.* falsification, distortion or alteration of an event or object.

falsificador-a *m., f.* forger.

falsificar *vi.* to forge; to simulate.

falso-a *a.* false, untrue; **anemia** ___ / ___ anemia; **aneurisma** ___ / ___ aneurysm; **anquilosis** ___ / ___ ankylosis; **articulación** ___ / ___ joint; **blefaroptosis** ___ / ___ blepharoptosis; **costillas falsas** ___ / ribs; **cuerdas vocales** ___ / ___ vocal chords; **divertículo** ___ / ___ diverticulum; **embarazo** ___ / ___ pregnancy; ___ **negativo** / ___ negative; ___ **positivo** / ___ positive; **hematuria** ___ / ___ hematuria; **hermafroditismo** ___ / ___ hermaphroditism; **imagen** ___ / ___ image; **lumen** ___ / ___ lumen; **membrana** ___ / ___ membrane; **neuroma** ___ / ___ neuroma; **poliposis adenomatosa** ___ / ___ adenomatous polyposis; **sutura** ___ / ___ suture; **síndrome** ___ **de la memoria** / ___ memory syndrome.

falta *f.* lack, fault, error; ___ **de alimentos** / ___ of food; ___ **de orientación** / ___ of orientation; **sin** ___ / without fail; for sure.

faltar *v.* to be lacking or wanting; to be absent.

famélico-a *a.* famished.

familia *f.* family; **práctica de** ___ / ___ practice; **terapia de** ___ / ___ therapy.

familiar *m.* family member; *a.* familiar, familial; **bocio** ___ / ___ goiter; **degeneración macular pseudoinflamatoria** ___ / ___ pseudoinflammatory macular degeneration; **descendencia** ___ / kinship; **disautonomía** ___ / ___ dysautonomy; **escrutinio** ___ / ___ screening; **hipercolesteremia** ___ / ___ hypercholesteremia; **ictericia** ___ / ___ jaundice; **neuropatía amiloide** ___ / ___ amyloid neuropathy; **parálisis periódica** ___ / ___ periodic paralysis; **poliposis adenomatosa** ___ / ___ adenomatous polyposis.

fanático-a *m., f.* fanatic; *a.* fanatic, fanatical.

Fanconi, síndrome de *m.* Fanconi's syndrome, congenital hypoplastic anemia.

fantasear *v.* to fantasize, to fancy, to imagine.

fantasía *f.* fantasy, the use of the imagination to transform an unpleasant reality into an imaginary, satisfying experience.

fantasma *f.* phantasm, optical illusion, apparition.

fantoma *m.* phantom. 1. mental image; 2. a transparent model of the human body or any of its parts.

farina *f.* farina, corn flour.

faringe *f.* pharynx, part of the alimentary canal extending from the base of the skull to the esophagus.

faríngeo-a *a.* pharyngeal, rel. to the pharynx.

faringitis *f.* pharyngitis, infl. of the pharynx.

farmacéutico-a *m., f.* pharmacist, specialist in pharmacy; *a.* pharmaceutical, rel. to pharmacy.

farmacia *f.* pharmacy. 1. the study of drugs and their preparation and dispensation; 2. drugstore.

farmacocinética *f.* pharmacokinetics, the study *in vivo* of the metabolism and action of drugs.

farmacodependencia *f.* drug dependence.

farmacodinamia *f.* pharmacodynamics, the study of the effects of medication.

farmacogenética *f.* pharmacogenetics, the study of genetic factors as related to drug metabolism.

farmacología *f.* pharmacology, the study of drugs and their effect on living organisms.

farmacólogo-a *m., f.* pharmacologist, pharmacist, specialist in pharmacology.

farmacopea *f.* pharmacopeia, a publication containing a listing of drugs and formulas as well as information providing standards for their preparation and dispensation.

farmacoterapia *f.* pharmacotherapy, treatment of a disease with the use of medications.

fascia *L.* fascia, fibrous connective tissue that envelops the body beneath the skin and encloses muscles, nerves, and blood vessels; ___ **aponeurótica** / aponeurotic ___, provides muscle protection; ___ **de Buck** / Buck's ___, covers the penis; ___ **de Colles** / Colle's ___, inner layer of the perineal fascia; ___ **lata** / lata ___, protects the muscles of the thigh; ___ **transversalis** / transversalis ___, between the transversalis muscle of the abdomen and the peritoneum; **injerto de una** ___ / ___ graft.

fascial *a.* fascial, rel. to a fascia.

fasciculación *f.* fasciculation. 1. formation of fascicles; 2. involuntary contraction of muscle fibers.

fascicular *a.* fascicular, rel. to a fascicle; **degeneración** ___ / ___ degeneration; **injerto** ___ / ___ graft.

fascículo *m.* fascicle, fasciculus, a bundle of muscular and nervous fibers.

fasciectomía *f.* fasciectomy, partial or total removal of a fascia.

fasciodesis *f.* fasciodesis, procedure to adhere a tendon to a fascia.

fasciola *f.* fasciola, small group of fibers.

fascioplastia *f.* fascioplasty, plastic surgery of a fascia.

fasciorrafia *f.* fasciorrhaphy, suture of a fascia.

fasciotomía *f.* fasciotomy, incision or partition of a fascia.

fascitis *f.* fascitis, infl. of a fascia.

fase *f.* phase, stage.

fásico-a *a.* phasic, rel. to a phase.

fastidioso-a *a.* fastidious, in bacteriology, rel. to complex nutritional demands.

fatal *a.* fatal, deadly, mortal.

fatalidad *f.* fatality.

fatiga *f.* fatigue, extreme tiredness.

fatigarse *vr., vi.* to become fatigued, to get tired.

fauces *f. pl.* fauces, the passage from the mouth to the pharynx.

favor *m.* favor, good deed.

favorable *a.* favorable, advantageous.

faz *f.* face.

fe *f.* faith; **de buena** ___ / in good ___ .

fealdad *f.* ugliness.

febril *a.* febrile, having a body temperature above normal; **convulsiones** ___ **-es** / ___ convulsions.

fecal *a.* fecal, containing or rel. to feces; **absceso** ___ / ___ abscess; **examen** ___ / ___ examination; **fístula** ___ / ___ fistula.

fecalito *m.* fecalith, intestinal concretion of fecal material.

fecaloide *a.* fecaloid, resembling fecal material.

fecaloma *m.* fecaloma, tumor-like accumulation of feces in the colon or rectum.

fecaluria *f.* fecaluria, presence of fecal material in the urine.

fecha *f.* [*día, mes o año*] date; ___ **de defunción** / ___ of death; ___ **del espécimen** / specimen ___ or sample ___; ___ **de nacimiento** / birth ___; ___ **de vigencia** / effective ___ .

fécula *f.* starch.

feculento-a *a.* starchy; **alimentos** ___ **-s, almidones** / ___ foods.

fecundación *f.* fecundation, the act of fertilizing.

fecundidad *f.* fecundity, fertility.

fecundo-a *a.* fruitful; fertile; abundant.

felación *f.* fellatio. cunilinguo-a.

felino-a *a.* feline, rel. to or resembling a cat.

feliz *a.* happy; felicitous.

femenino-a *a.* feminine.

feminidad *f.* femininity; **complejo de** / ___ complex.

feminismo *m.* feminism.

feminista *m., f.* feminist, one who fosters feminism.

feminización *f.* feminization, development of feminine characteristics.

femoral *a.* femoral, rel. to the femur; **arco** ___ **profundo** / deep ___ arch; **arteria** ___ / ___ artery; **arteria nutricional** ___ / ___ nutrient artery; **canal** ___ / ___ canal; **capa** ___ / ___ sheath; **hernia** ___ / ___ hernia; **nervio** ___ / ___ nerve; **triángulo** ___ / ___ triangle; **vena** ___ / ___ vein.

femorotibial *a.* femorotibial, rel. to the femur and the tibia; **capilar** ___ / ___ capillary; **membrana** ___ / ___ membrane.

fémur *m.* femur, the thighbone.

fenestración *f.* fenestration. 1. creation of an opening in the inner ear to restore lost hearing; 2. the act of perforating.

fenestrado-a *a.* fenestrated, having openings.

fénico, fenol *a.* phenic, carbolic.

fenobarbital *m.* phenobarbital, barbiturate used as a hypnotic or sedative.

fenómeno *m.* phenomenon. 1. objective symptom of a disease; 2. event or manifestation; 3. *pop.* freak.

fenotipo *m.* phenotype, characteristics of a species produced by the environment and heredity.

feo-a *a.* ugly.

fermentación *f.* fermentation, splitting a complex compound into simpler ones by the action of enzymes or ferments.

fermentar *v.* to ferment, to produce fermentation.

fermentativo-a *a.* fermentative, that has the property of causing fermentation.

fermento *m.* ferment, the product of fermentation.

ferritina *f.* ferritin, an iron complex that provides a way to store iron in the body.

ferroproteína *f.* ferroprotein, protein combined with a radical containing iron.

ferruginoso-a, ferrugíneo-a *a.* ferruginous. 1. that contains iron; 2. that has the color of oxidated iron.

fértil *a.* fertile, fruitful.

fertilidad *f.* fertility, fruitfulness.

fertilización *f.* fertilization.

fertilizante *m.* fertilizer.

férula *f.* splint, device made of any material such as wood, metal, or plaster, used to immobilize or support a fractured bone or a joint.

festinante *a.* festinant, accelerating, hastening.

fetal *a.* fetal, rel. to the fetus; **circulación** ___ / ___ circulation; **desperdicio** / ___ wastage; **distocia** ___ / ___ dystocia; **hidropesía** ___ / ___ hydrops; **latido del corazón** ___ / ___ heart tone; **medicina** ___ / ___ medicine; **membrana** ___ / ___ membrane; **membranas** ___ **-es** ___ / ___ membranes; **muerte** ___ / ___ death; **monitorización** ___ / ___ monitoring; **placenta** ___ / ___ placenta; **retardo del crecimiento** ___ / ___ growth retardation; **síndrome de aspiración** ___ / ___ aspiration syndrome; **viabilidad** ___ / ___ viability.

feticidio *m.* feticide, destruction of the fetus in the uterus.

fetiche *m.* fetish.

fetidez, fetor *f. m.* stench, offensive odor.

fétido-a *a.* fetid, having a very bad odor.

feto *m.* fetus, phase of gestation between three months and the moment of birth; **presentación frontal del** ___ / brow presentation of ___ .

fetometría *f.* fetometry, estimate of the size of the fetus before birth, esp. of the head.

fetoplacental *a.* fetoplacental, rel. to the fetus and the placenta.

fetoproteína *f.* fetoprotein, an antigen present in the human fetus.

fetoscopía *f.* fetoscopy, antenatal inspection of the fetus by introducing a fetoscope transabdominaly in the mother's womb with the purpose of diagnosis.

fetoscopio *m.* fetoscope, instrument used to visualize the fetus *in utero* to facilitate prenatal diagnosis.

fetotóxico-a *a.* fetotoxic, that can toxify the fetus.

fiasco *m.* fiasco; gross failure.

fibra *f.* fiber, filament; _____ -s amarillas / yellow ___ -s; ___ -s ópticas / fiberoptics.

fibrilación *f.* fibrillation. 1. involuntary or abnormal muscular contraction; ___ **auricular** / atrial, auricular ___, irregular movement of the atria; ___ **ventricular** / ___ ventricular; 2. formation of fibrils.

fibrilación-aleteo *f.* flutter-fibrillation, auricular activity that shows signs of flutter and fibrillation.

fibrilar *a.* fibrillar, fibrillary, rel. to a fibril; **astrocito** ___ / ___ astrocyte; **contracciones** ___ **-es** / ___ contractions.

fibrilla *f.* fibril, a very small fiber.

fibrina *f.* fibrin, insoluble protein that is essential to the coagulation of blood.

fibrinogenemia *f.* fibrinogenemia, presence of fibrinogen in the blood.

fibrinogénico-a *a.* fibrinogenic, fibrinogenous, that produces fibrin.

fibrinógeno *m.* fibrinogen, protein present in blood plasma that converts into fibrin during blood clotting.

fibrinogenólisis *f.* fibrinogenolysis, the dissolution of fibrinogen in the circulating blood.

fibrinoide *a.* fibrinoid, that resembles fibrin.

fibrinólisis *f.* fibrinolysis, the dissolution of fibrinogen by the action of enzymes.

fibrinoso-a *a.* fibrous, fibrinous, of the nature of fibers; **bronquitis** ___ / ___ bronchitis; **inflamación** ___ / ___ inflammation; **pericarditis** ___ / ___ pericarditis; **pleuresía** ___ / ___ pleurisy; **pólipo** ___ / ___ polyp.

fibrinuria *f.* fibrinuria, presence of fibrin in the urine.

fibroadenoma *f.* fibroadenoma, a benign tumor composed of fibrous and glandular tissue.

fibroadiposo-a *a.* fibroadipose, that contains fibrous and adipose tissue.

fibroblasto *m.* fibroblast, a cell from which connective tissue develops.

fibrocartílago *m.* fibrocartilage, a type of cartilage in which the matrix contains a large amount of fibrous tissue.

fibrocelular *a.* fibrocellular, that is of fibrous and cellular composition.

fibrocístico-a, fibroquístico-a *a.* fibrocystic, cystic and fibrous in nature; **enfermedad** ___ **de la mama** / ___ disease of the breast.

fibrocondritis *a.* fibrochondritis, infl. of a fibrocartilage.

fibrocondroma *m.* fibrochondroma, benign tumor made of fibrous and cartilaginous connective tissue.

fibroide *a.* fibroid, rel. to or of a fibrinous nature; **adenoma** ___ / ___ adenoma; **catarata** ___ / ___ cataract.

fibroidectomía *f.* fibroidectomy, excision of a fibroid tumor.

fibrolipoma *m.* fibrolipoma, tumor that contains fibrous and adipose tissue.

fibroma *m.* fibroma, a benign tumor composed of fibrous tissue.

fibromatosis *f.* fibromatosis, production of multiple fibromas on the skin or the uterus.

fibromialgia *f.* fibromyalgia, generalized chronic condition which results in pain and rigidity in the muscles and in the soft tissues.

fibromioma *m.* fibromyoma, tumor that contains muscular and fibrous tissue.

fibromuscular *a.* fibromuscular, of a fibrous and muscular nature.

fibroneuroma *m.* fibroneuroma, tumor of the conjunctive tissue of the nerves.

fibroplasia *f.* fibroplasia, formation of fibrous tissue as seen in the healing of a wound; ___ **retrolental** / retrolental ___ .

fibrosarcoma *m.* fibrosarcoma, malignant tumor of fusiform cells, collagen, and reticulin fibers. Syn. **neurofibroma.**

fibrosis *f.* fibrosis, abnormal formation of fibrous tissue; ___ **cística** / cystic ___; ___ **intersticial del pulmón** / diffuse interstitial pulmonary ___; ___ **proliferativa** / proliferative ___; ___ **pulmonar** / pulmonary ___; ___ **retroperitoneal** / retroperitoneal ___ .

fibroso-a, fibrinoso-a *a.* fibrous, fibrinous. 1. rel. to or of the nature of fibrin; **anquilosis** ___ / ___ ankylosis; **articulación** ___ / ___ joint; **bocio** ___ / ___ goiter; **defecto cortical** ___ / ___ cortical defect; **degeneración** ___ / ___ degeneration; **tejido** ___ / ___ tissue; **tubérculo** ___ / ___ tubercule; 2. threadlike.

fibrótico-a *a.* fibrotic, rel. to fibrosis.

fibular *a.* fibular, rel. to the fibula; **arteria** ___ / ___ artery; **vena** ___ / ___ vein.

ficticio *a.* fictitious, false.

fidelidad *f.* fidelity; loyalty.

fideo *m.* noodle.

fiebre *f.* fever; **ampollas de** ___ / ___ blisters; ___ **de conejo** / rabbit ___, tularemia; ___ **de origen desconocido** / ___ of unknown origin; ___ **del heno** / hay ___; ___ **de trinchera** / trench ___; ___ **entérica** / enteric ___, intestinal; ___ **familiar del Mediterráneo** / familiar Mediterranean ___; ___ **intermitente** / intermittent ___; ___ **ondulante** / undulant ___, brucellosis; ___ **recurrente** / relapsing ___; ___ **remitente** / remittent ___; ___ **reumatoidea** / rheumatoid ___; ___ **tifoidea** / typhoid ___; **tener** ___ / to run a temperature.

fiebre aftosa *f.* aphthous fever, foot and mouth disease, illness caused by a virus found in ruminants and pigs that can be transmitted to humans, and is characterized by an eruption of small vesicles in the tongue and fingers.

fiebre amarilla *f.* yellow fever, endemic disease of tropical areas, transmitted by the bite of a female mosquito, *Aedes aegypti*, and manifested by fever, jaundice, and albuminuria.

fiebre del valle *f.* valley fever, coccidiomicosis.

fiebre manchada de las Montañas Rocosas *f.* Rocky Mountain spotted fever, acute febrile disease caused by a germ transmitted by infected ticks.

fiebre reumática *f.* rheumatic fever, a fever that gen. follows a streptococcal infection manifested by acute generalized pain of the joints, often with cardiac arrythmia and renal disorders as residual effects.

figura *f.* form, shape; figure.

fijación *f.* fixation. 1. immobilization; 2. the act of focusing the eyes directly upon an object; 3. the act of being strongly attached to a particular person or object; 4. interruption of the development of the personality before reaching maturity.

fijador *m.* fixative, a substance used to harden and preserve pathological specimens.

fijar *v.* to fix, to affix, [*una fractura*] to set.

filamento *m.* filament, strand, delicate fiber or fine thread.

film *m.* film; thin layer.

filtración *f.* filtration, the act of straining through a filter impeding passage of certain molecules; **operación de** ___ / ___ operation.

filtrar *v.* to strain; **filtrarse** *vr.* to filter through, to filtrate.

filtro *m.* filter, any device used to strain liquids.

fimbria *f.* fimbria. 1. fingerlike structure; 2. appendage of certain bacteria; ___ **ovárica** / ovarian ___; ___ **de la trompa de Falopio** / ___ of the uterine tube; ___ **del hipocampo** / hippocampal ___ .

fimosis *f.* phimosis, narrowness of the orifice of the prepuce that prevents its being drawn back over the glans penis.

fin *m.* end, conclusion; **¿con qué** ___? / for what purpose?; **a** ___ **de** / in order to.

fin de semana *m.* weekend.

final *m.* end; **al** ___ / at the end; *a.* final, conclusive.

financiero-a *a.* financial, monetary; **gastos** ___ **-s** / ___ expenses.

fingir *vi.* to fake, to malinger.

finito-a *a.* finite, having limits.

Finney, operación de *f.* Finney operation, gastroduodenostomy that creates a large opening to ensure that the stomach empties fully.

fino-a *a.* fine, as opposed to thick or coarse.

firma *f.* signature.

firmar *v.* to sign, to subscribe.

firme *a.* firm, secure.

física *f.* physics, the study of matter and its changes.

físicamente *adv.* physically, referring to the body as opposed to the mind.

físico *m.* 1. physique, appearance, figure; **-a** *m.*, 2. physicist, specialist in physics; *a.* physical, rel. to the body and its condition; **examen** ___ / ___ examination; **terapia** ___ / ___ therapy.

fisicoquímico-a *a.* physicochemical, rel. to physics and to chemistry.

fisiología *f.* physiology, the study of the physical and chemical processes affecting organisms.

fisiológico-a *a.* physiologic, physiological, rel. to physiology; **no** ___ / unphysiological.

fisiólogo-a *m., f.* physiologist, a specialist in physiology.

fisión *f.* fission, a breaking up into parts; ___ **nuclear** / nuclear ___ .

fisioterapia *f.* physiotherapy, treatment by means of physical manipulation and agents such as heat, light, and water.

fisonomía *f.* physiognomy, facial features.

fístula *f.* fistula, abnormal passage from a hollow organ to the skin or from one organ to another; ___ **arteriovenosa** / arteriovenous ___; ___ **biliar** / biliary ___; ___ **del ano** / anal ___ .

fistular, fistuloso-a *a.* fistular, fistulous, rel. to or resembling a fistula.

fistulización *f.* fistulization, pathological or surgical formation of a fistula.

fisura *f.* fissure, cleft, a longitudinal opening.

fitobezor *m.* phytobezoar, a concretion of undigested vegetable fiber that forms in the stomach or intestine.

flácido-a *a.* flaccid, limber, lax.

flaco-a *a.* very thin, lanky.

flagelado-a *a.* flagellated, provided with flagella.

flageliforme *a.* flagelliform, shaped like a whip.

flagelo *m.* flagellum, prolongation or tail in the cells of some protozoa or bacteria.

flanco *m.* flank, loin, part of the body situated between the ribs and the upper border of the ilium.

flato *m.* flatus, gas or air in the stomach or intestines.

flatulencia *f.* flatulence, condition marked by distention and abdominal discomfort due to excessive gas in the gastrointestinal tract.

flebitis *f.* phlebitis, infl. of a vein.

flebograma *m.* phlebogram, venogram, a tracing of the venous pulse.

flebolito *m.* phlebolith, phlebolite, a calcareous deposit in a vein.

flebotomía *f.* phlebotomy, venotomy, incision into a vein for the purpose of drawing blood.

flegmasia *f.* phlegmasia, inflammation.

flegmasia cerúlea dolorosa *f.* milk leg, phlegmasia cerulea dolens, thrombosis of one of the veins of the leg, gen. the femoral vein, that is manifested by acute pain, infl., cyanosis and edema, and that can cause a severe circulatory problem.

flema *f.* phlegm. 1. thick mucus; 2. one of the four humors of the body.

flemático-a *a.* phlegmatic. 1. that produces phlegm; 2. apathetic.

flemón *m.* phlegmon, an infl. of the cellular tissue.

flexibilidad *f.* flexibility, pliability, the capability to flex.

flexible *a.* flexible, bendable, able to change.

flexión *f.* flexion, flexure, the act of bending.

flexionar *v.* to flex, to bend.

flexor *m.* flexor, a muscle that can flex a joint.

flexura *f.* flexure, fold, curvature, bend; ___ **esplénica** / splenic ___, left curvature of the colon; ___ **hepática** / hepatic ___, right curvature of the colon; ___ **sigmoidea** / sigmoid ___, curved part of the colon that precedes the rectum.

floculación *f.* flocculation, precipitation and agglomeration of very small invisible particles into large visible flakes.

flogosis *f.* phlogosis.flegmasia.

flojera *f.* weakness.

flojo-a *a.* weak, flaccid; sluggish.

flor *f.* flower.

flora *f.* flora, group of bacteria within a given organ; ___ **intestinal** / intestinal ___ .

florido-a *a.* florid, showing a bright red coloring of the skin.

flotador *m.* floater, macule, specks in the vision.

flotante *a.* floating, free, not adhered.

flotar *v.* to float.

fluctuación *f.* fluctuation, wavering, wavelike movements produced by vibrations of body fluids on palpation.

fluctuar *v.* to fluctuate, to waver, to go back and forth.

fluidez *f.* fluidity, liquidity.

fluído *m.* fluid, liquid; ___ **amniótico** / amniotic ___; ___ **cefalorraquídeo** / cerebrospinal; ___ **extracelular** / extracellular ___; ___ **extravascular** / extravascular ___; ___ **intersticial** / interstitial ___; ___ **intracelular** / intracellular ___; ___ **seminal** / seminal ___; ___ **seroso** / serous ___; ___ **sinovial** / synovial___ . *V.* cuadro en la página 385.

fluir *vi.* to flow.

flujo *m.* afflux, flow, flux. 1. large amount of fluid discharge from a cavity or surface of the body; ___ **laminar** / laminar ___; ___ **turbulento** / turbulent ___; **medidor de** ___ / flowmeter; 2. the rush of blood or liquid; 3. menstruation.

flúor *m.* fluorine, gaseous chemical element.

fluoresceína *f.* fluorescein, red dye.

fluorescencia *f.* fluorescence, the property of a substance to emit light when exposed to certain types of radiation such as x-rays.

fluorescente *a.* fluorescent, rel. to fluorescence; **anticuerpo** ___ / ___ antibody; **técnica del anticuerpo** ___ / ___ treponemal antibody absorption test.

fluoridación *f.* fluoridation, fluoridization, addition of fluorides to water.

fluoroscopía *f.* fluoroscopy, examination of tissues and structures of the body using the fluoroscope.

fluoroscopio *m.* fluoroscope, instrument that makes x-rays visible on a fluorescent screen.

fluorosis *f.* fluorosis, excess fluoride content.

fluoruro *m.* fluoride, combination of fluorine with a metal or a metalloid.

fobia *f.* phobia, abnormal irrational fear.

fóbico-a *a.* phobic, rel. to phobia.

focal *a.* focal, rel. to focus.

foco *m.* focus, the main point or principal spot.

fofo-a *a.* flabby, soft.

fogaje *m.* hot flash.

folicular *a.* follicular, rel. to a follicle; **fase** ___ / ___ phase.

foliculitis *f.* folliculitis, infl. of a follicle, usu. in reference to a hair follicle.

folículo *m.* follicle, sac or pouchlike secretory depression or cavity; ___ **atrésico** / atretic ___; ___ **de Graaf, ovárico** / Graafian, ovaric ___; ___ **gástrico** / gastric ___; ___ **piloso** / hair ___; ___ **tiroideo** / thyroid ___ .

folleto *m.* pamphlet, brochure.

fomento *m.* hot compress.

fomes *L. fomites* fomes, an element that can absorb and transmit infectious agents.

fonación *f.* phonation, emission of the voice.

fondillo *m.* buttocks.

fondo *m.* bottom; ___ **del ojo** / eyeground.

fonética *f.* phonetics, the study of speech and prounciation.

fonético-a *a.* phonetic, rel. to the voice and articulated sounds.

foniatra *m., f.* phoniatrist, specialist in voice treatment.

fonatría *f.* phoniatrics, treatment and study of voice defects.

fonograma *m.* phonogram, a graphic that indicates the intensity of a sound.

fonoscopio *m.* phonoscope, a device that registers heart sounds.

fontanela *f.* fontanel, fontanelle, soft spot in the skull of a newborn that closes as the cranial bones develop; **caída de la** ___ / fallen ___.

foramen *m.* foramen, orifice, passage, opening; ___ **intervertebral** /

intervertebral ___; ___ **óptico** / optic ___; ___ oval / oval ___ ; ___ **sacrociático mayor** / sciatic, greater ___ ; ___ **yugular** / jugular ___ .

fórceps *m.* forceps, a surgical, tonglike instrument used to grasp, pull, or manipulate tissues or body parts.

forense *a.* forensic, rel. to the courts; **laboratorio** ___ / ___ laboratory; **médico** ___ / ___ physician.

forma *f.* form, shape; established manner of doing something; ___ **frustrada** / forme fruste, *Fr.,* an aborted or atypical form of a disease.

formación *f.* formation, the manner in which something is arranged.

formaldehído *m.* formaldehyde, antiseptic.

formalina *f.* formalin, formaldehyde compound.

formar *v.* to form, to shape.

formicación *f.* formication, skin sensation comparable to one produced by crawling insects.

fórmula *f.* formula, a prescribed way or model.

formulario *m.* 1. form, [*planilla*] blank; 2. formulary, prescription tablet, a book of formulas.

fórnix *m.* fornix, vaultlike structure such as the vagina.

fortalecer *vi.* to fortify, to strengthen.

fortificar *vi.* to fortify.

forúnculo *m.* boil.

fosa *f.* fossa, cavity, depression, hole; ___ **etmoidal** / ethmoid ___; ___ **glenoidea** / glenoid ___; ___ **interpenduncular** / interpenduncular ___; ___ **mandibular** / mandibular ___; ___ **nasal** / nasal ___; ___ **navicular** / navicular ___; ___ **supraclavicular** / supraclavicular ___; ___ **yugular** / jugular ___ .

fósforo *m.* phosphorus.

fotocoagulación *f.* photocoagulation, localized tissue coagulation by an intense controlled ray of light or laser beam, esp. used in surgery of the eye.

fotofobia *f.* photophobia, fear of light.

fotólisis *f.* photolysis, disintegration by rays of light.

fototerapia *f.* phototherapy, light therapy, exposure to sun rays or to an artificial light for therapeutic purposes.

fóvea *f.* fovea, small depression, esp. used in reference to the central fossa of the retina.

fracaso *m.* failure; **neurosis del** ___ / ___ neurosis.

fracción *f.* fraction, separable part of a unit.

fractura *f.* fracture, breaking or separation of a bone; ___ **abierta** / open ___; ___ **cerrada** /

closed ___; ___ **conminuta** /
comminuted ___; ___ **completa** /
complete ___; ___ **con luxación** /
dislocation ___; ___ **con hundimiento** /
depressed ___; ___ **de línea fina** /
hairline ___; ___ **en caña o tallo verde** /
greenstick ___; ___ **en cuña** / wedge ___; ___
en mariposa / butterfly ___; ___ **en martillo** /
mallet___; ___ **en T** / T ___; ___ **espiral** /
spiral ___; ___ **impactada** / impacted ___; ___
incompleta / incomplete___; ___ **patológica** /
pathologic ___; ___ **perforante** /
perforating___; ___ **por avulsión** /
avulsion ___; ___ **por compresión** /
compression ___; ___ **por estallamiento** / blow-
out ___; ___ **por herida de bala** /
gunshot ___; ___ **por sobrecarga** / stress ___ .
V. cuadro en la página 388.

fracturar *v.* to fracture, to break a bone.

frágil *a.* fragile, brittle; breakable.

fragilidad *f.* fragility, disposition to tear or break
easily.

fragmentación *f.* fragmentation, splitting.

fragmento *m.* fragment, small piece of a whole.

frambesia *f.* framboesia, yaws, pian, infectious
tropical disease caused by a spirochete of the
genus *Treponema pertenue* and manifested by a
primary cutaneous lesion followed by raspberry-
like ulcers that spread to different areas of the
body.

francés *m.* [*idioma*] French; [*nativo-a*]; *francés,
francesa a.* French.

frasco *m.* flask, bottle.

frase *f.* phrase.

frazada *f.* blanket.

frecuencia *f.* frequency; rate; **con** ___ /
frequently; ___ **cardíaca fetal** / baseline fetal
heart ___; ___ **de filtración** / filtration ___; ___
de goteo / drip ___; ___ **del pulso** /
pulse ___; ___ **glomerular** /
glomerular ___; ___ **intrínseca** /
intrinsic ___; ___ **respiratoria** / breathing ___ .

frecuente *a.* frequent; **-mente** *adv.* frequently.

freír *vi.* to fry.

frémito *m.* fremitus, a vibration that can be
detected during auscultation or on palpation,
such as the chest vibrations during coughing.

frenectomía *f.* frenectomy, removal of the
frenum.

frenesí *m.* frenzy; madness.

frenético-a *a.* phrenetic, frantic, raving,
maniacal.

frenillo *m.* frenum of the tongue; **con** ___ /
tongue-tied.

frente *f.* forehead, brow; *prep.* in front; **en** ___
de / in ___ of; ___ **a** ___ / face to face; ___ **a** /
across from.

frenulum *f.* frenulum, frenum, small membranous
fold that limits the movement of an organ or
part.

fresa *f.* bur, burr. 1. [*dental*] dental drill; ___**de
fisura** / fissure ___; 2. strawberry; **marca
en** ___ / ___ mark.

fresco *m.* refreshing air; **hace** ___ / it is cool.

freudiano-a *a.* Freudian, rel. to the doctrines of
Sigmund Freud, Viennese neurologist, father of
psychoanalysis, (1856-1939).

friable *a.* friable, that pulverizes easily.

fricción *f.* friction, rub; ___**de alcohol** / alcohol
rub; **roce de** ___ / ___ rub.

frigidez *f.* frigidity, coldness, inability to respond
to sexual arousement.

frígido-a *a.* frigid, cold.

frigolábil *a.* frigolabile, that can easily be
destroyed by cold.

frigorífico *m.* cold-storage place; *a.* frigorific,
that generates cold.

frigoterapia *f.* frigotherapy, therapy by using
cold.

frijol *m.* bean.

frío-a *a.* cold; [*persona*] without warmth or
affection; **hace** ___ / it is cold.

friolento-a *a.* chilly; too sensitive to cold.

frito-a *a. pp.* of **freír,** fried.

Frohlich, síndrome de *m.* Frohlich's
syndrome, adiposogenital dystrophy, manifested
by obesity and sexual infantilism.

frontal *a.* frontal, rel. to the forehead;
hueso ___ / ___ bone; **músculo** ___ / ___
muscle; **senos** ___ **-es** / ___ sinuses.

frotar *v.* to rub; ___ **suavemente** / to stroke.

frote *m.* rub. 1. friction; massage; 2. sound heard
on ausculation, produced by two dry surfaces
rubbing against each other.

frotis *m.* smear, sample of blood or a secretion
for the purpose of microscopic study.

fructosa *f.* fructose, sugar of fruits; levulose;
intolerancia a la ___ / ___ intolerance.

fructosuria *f.* fructosuria, presence of fructose
in the urine.

frustración *f.* frustration, disappointment due to
failure to attain complete satisfaction.

frustrado-a *a.* frustrated.

fruta *f.* fruit.

ftiriasis *f.* phthiriasis. V. **pediculosis.**

fuego *m.* fire.

fuente *f.* source, origin; fountain.

fuera *adv.* out, outside; **estar** ___ / to be ___ or away; ___ **de sí** / beside oneself; **hacia** ___ / outward.

fuerte *a.* strong, vigorous; hard.

fuerza *f.* force, strength; power; ___ **catabólica** / catabolic ___; ___ **de gravedad** / ___ of gravity; **no tengo** ___ / I feel weak.

fuga *f.* flight; ___ **de ideas** / ___ of ideas; interrupted line of thought and talk.

fulguración *f.* fulguration, use of electric current to destroy or coagulate tissue.

fulminante *a.* fulminant, appearing suddenly and with great intensity, esp. in reference to a disease or pain.

fumador-a *m., f.* person who smokes heavily.

fumador-a pasivo-a *m., f.* passive smoker, person who does not smoke but is exposed to other people smoking, thus inhaling the emanating smoke.

fumante *a.* fuming, that gives forth a visible vapor.

fumar *v.* to smoke.

fumigación *f.* fumigation, extermination, or disinfection through the use of vapors.

fumigante *m.* fumigant, agent used in fumigation.

función *f.* function.

funcional *a.* functional, having practical use or value.

funcionamiento *m.* performance; functioning, working.

funcionar *v.* to function, to work.

funda *f.* pillowcase; covering.

fundectomía *f.* fundectomy, excision of the base of the uterus or of any other organ.

fundir *v.* to fuse, to liquefy with heat.

funeral *m.* funeral.

funeraria *f.* funeral parlor, mortuary; **empresario de** ___ / mortician;

fungemia *f.* fungemia, presence of fungi in the blood.

fungicida *m.* fungicide, agent that destroys fungi.

fungiforme *a.* fungiform, in the shape of a fungus.

fungistasis *f.* fungistasis, the action of thwarting the growth of fungi.

fungitóxico-a *a.* fungitoxic, that causes a toxicity in fungi.

fungoso-a *a.* fungous, fungal, rel. to fungi.

funicular *a.* funicular, rel. to the umbilical or spermatic chord.

funiculitis *f.* funiculitis, infl. of the spermatic chord.

furfuráceo-a *a.* furfuraceous, that resembles scales.

furioso-a *a.* furious, frantic.

furor *m.* furor, extreme anger.

furosemida *f.* furosemide, diuretic agent.

furunculosis *f.* furunculosis, condition resulting from the presence of boils.

fusiforme *a.* fusiform, spindle shaped.

fusión *f.* fusion, the act of melting; ___ **nuclear** / nuclear ___ .

futuro *m.* future; **-a** *a.* future.

g

g *abr.* **género** / gender; **glucosa** / glucose; **gramo** / gram; **grano** / grain.

gabinete *m.* cabinet.

Gaenslen, examen de *m.* Gaenslen sign, test, procedure used to determine sacroiliac dysfunction.

gafas *f.* spectacles, eyeglasses.

gago-a *m., f.* stutterer.

gaguear *v.* to stutter.

galactagogo, galactógeno *m.* galactagogue, agent that stimulates the flow of milk.

galactasa *f.* galactase, enzyme present in milk.

galactocele *m.* galactocele, breast cyst containing milk.

galactoforitis *f.* galactophoritis, infl. of the lacteal ducts.

galactopoyesis *f.* galactopoyesis, production of milk.

galáctoro-a *a.* galactophorous, that conducts or carries milk.

galactorrea *f.* galactorrhea. 1. milk secretion or discharge resembling milk; 2. continuation of milk secretion at intervals after the period of lactation has ended.

galactosa *f.* galactose, monosaccharide derived from lactose by the action of an enzyme or mineral acid; **catarata** ___ / ___ cataract.

galactosemia *f.* galactosemia, congenital absence of the enzyme necessary to convert galactose to glucose and its derivatives.

galactosuria *f.* galactosuria, milk-like urine due to the presence of galactose.

galactoterapia *f.* galactotherapy. 1. the treatment of breast-fed infants by the administration of medication to the nursing mother; 2. therapeutic use of milk in the diet.

galacturia *f.* galacturia, milk-like urine.

galio *m.* gallium, metallic element.

galope *m.* gallop, cardiac rhythm resembling the gallop of a horse that indicates heart failure; **ritmo de** ___ / ___ rhythm.

galvánico-a *a.* galvanic, rel. to galvanism; **batería** ___ / ___ battery; **célula** ___ / ___ cell; **corriente** ___ / ___ current.

galvanismo *m.* galvanism, therapeutic use of a direct electrical current.

galvanocauterización *f.* galvanocautery.electrocauterización.

galvanómetro *m.* galvanometer, instrument that measures currents by electromagnetic action.

galleta *f.* cracker.

gallina *f.* hen.

gallo *m.* cock, rooster.

gama *f.* range;___ **de colores** / color ___;

gameto *m.* gamete, sexual cell, masculine or feminine.**transferencia de g. a la trompa de falopio** / ___ intrafallopian transfer;

gametocida *m.* gametocide, agent that kills gametes.

gametocito *m.* gametocyte, a cell that divides to produce gametes, such as the malarial parasite when taken into the mosquito host.

gametogénesis *f.* gametogenesis, development of gametes.

gamma globulina *f.* gamma globulin, a class of antibodies produced in the lymph tissue or synthetically.

gammagrama *m.* scintiscan, a two-dimensional image representation of the interior distribution of a radiopharmaceutical in a previously selected area for diagnostic purposes.

gamopatía *f.* gammopathy, disorder manifested by an excessive amount of immunoglobulins due to an abnormal proliferation of lymphoid cells.

gana *f.* desire, inclination; **de buena** ___ / willingly; **de mala** ___ / unwillingly; **tener** ___ **-s de** / to desire, to want to.

ganancia *f.* gain; advantage.

ganar *v.* to win; to earn.

gancho *m.* hook; clasp; **-s** [*dental*] braces.

gangliectomía, ganglionectomía *f.* gangliectomy, ganglionectomy, excision of a ganglion.

ganglio *m.* ganglion, collection of nerve cells resembling a knot; ___ **basal** / basal ___; ___ **carotídeo** / carotid ___; ___ **celíaco** / celiac ___ .

gangliocito *m.* gangliocyte, a ganglion cell.

ganglioctomía *f.* ganglioctomy, excision of a ganglion.

glanglioglioma *m.* ganglioglioma, tumor with a large number of ganglionic cells.

ganglioma *m.* ganglioma, tumor of a ganglion, esp. a lymphatic ganglion.

ganglión *m.* ganglion, a cystic tumor that develops in a tendon or an aponeurosis, often seen in the wrist, the heel or the knee.

ganglionar *a.* ganglionic, rel. to a ganglion; **bloqueo** ___ / ___ blockade.

ganglioneuroma *m.* ganglioneuroma, benign tumor composed by ganglionic neurons.

ganglios basales *m. pl.* basal ganglia, gray matter localized in the low portion of the brain stem that takes part in muscular coordination.

gangrena *f.* gangrene, local death, destruction and putrefaction of body tissue due to interrupted blood supply.

gangrenoso-a *a.* gangrenous, rel. to gangrene.

Gantrisin *f.* Gantrisin, trade name for sulfisoxazole, an antibacterial agent used in the treatment of urinary infections.

garabato *m.* scribble.

garantía *f.* guarantee, warranty.

garantizar *vi.* to guarantee, to warrant.

garbanzo *m.* chickpea.

Gardner, síndrome de *m.* Gardner's syndrome. 1. multiple polyps of the colon associated with risk of colon carcinoma; 2. soft-tissue tumors of the skin.

garganta *f.* throat, the area of the larynx and the pharynx; anterior part of the neck; **dolor de** ___ / sore ___ .

gárgara, gargarismo *f., m.* gargarism, gargle, gargling, rinsing of the throat and the mouth; **hacer** ___ **-s** / to gargle.

gargolismo *m.* gargoylism, hereditary condition characterized by skeletal abnormalities and sometimes mental retardation.

garra *f.* claw; **mano en** ___ / ___ hand; **pie en** ___ / ___ foot.

garrapata *f.* tick, bloodsucking acarid that transmits specific diseases; **picadura de** ___ / ___ bite.

garrotillo *m.* croup.

gas *m.* gas; ___ **-es arteriales** / arterial blood ___ -es; ___ **-es en la sangre** / blood ___-es; ___ **lacrimógeno** / tear ___; ___ **mostaza** / mustard ___; ___ **neurotóxico** / nerve ___ .

gasa *f.* gauze; **compresa de** ___ / ___ compress; ___ **antiséptica** / antiseptic ___ .

gaseoso-a *a.* gaseous, of the nature of gas.

gasolina *f.* gasoline; **envenenamiento por** ___ / ___ poisoning.

gastado-a *a.* worn out.

gastar *v.* [*dinero*] to spend; **gastarse** *vr.* to wear out.

gasto *m.* [*cardíaco*] output; costs, expense(s); expenditure; waste; ___ **cubiertos** / covered ___ .

gastralgia *f.* gastralgia, stomachache.

gastrectomía *f.* gastrectomy, removal of part or all of the stomach.

gástrico-a *a.* gastric, rel. to the stomach; **alimentación** ___ / ___ feeding; **arteria** ___

___ **-s** / ___ arteries; **derivación** ___ / ___ by-pass; **digestión** ___ / ___ digestion; **fístula** ___ / ___ fistula; **glándulas** ___ / ___ glands; **jugo** ___ / ___ juice; **lavado** ___ / ___ lavage; **vaciamiento** ___ / ___ emptying; **vértigo** ___ / ___ vertigo.

gastrina *f.* gastrin, hormone secreted by the stomach.

gastritis *f.* gastritis, infl. of the stomach; ___ **aguda** / acute ___; ___ **crónica** / chronic ___ .

gastroadenitis *f.* gastroadenitis, infl. of the stomach glands.

gastroanálisis *m.* gastric analysis, analysis of the stomach contents.

gastroanastomosis *f.* gastroanastomosis, anastomosis between two parts of a clock-shaped stomach.

gastrocele *m.* gastrocele, stomach hernia.

gastrocnemio *m.* gastrocnemius, large calf muscle.

gastrocolitis *f.* gastrocolitis, infl. of the stomach and the colon.

gastrocolostomía *f.* gastrocolostomy, anastomosis of the stomach and the colon.

gastroduodenal *a.* gastroduodenal, rel. to the stomach and the duodenum.

gastroduodenitis *f.* gastroduodenitis, infl. of the stomach and the duodenum.

gastroduodenoscopía *f.* gastroduodenoscopy, visual examination of the stomach and the duodenum with an endoscope.

gastroectasia *f.* gastroectasis, gastroectasia, dilation of the stomach.

gastroenteritis *f.* gastroenteritis, infl. of the stomach and the intestine.

gastroenteroanastomosis *f.* gastroenteroanastomosis, anastomosis of the stomach and the small intestine.

gastroenterocolitis *f.* gastroenterocolitis, infl. of the stomach and the small intestine.

gastroenterostomía *f.* gastroenterostomy, anastomosis of the stomach and the small bowel.

gastroepiploico-a *a.* gastroepiploic, rel. to the stomach and the epiploon.

gastroesofágico-a *a.* gastroesophageal, rel. to the stomach and the esophagus; **enfermedad de reflujo** ___ / ___ reflux disease; **hernia** ___ / ___ hernia.

gastroesofagitis *f.* gastroesophagitis. esofagogastritis.

gastroespasmo *m.* gastrospasm, spasmodic contractions of the stomach walls.

gastrogavage *m.* gastrogavage, artificial feeding into the stomach through a tube.

gastroileostomía *f.* gastroileostomy, anastomosis of the stomach and the ileum.

gastrointestinal *a.* gastrointestinal, rel. to the stomach and the intestine;
decompresión ___ / ___ decompression;
examen ___ **superior** / upper ___ examination;
sangramiento ___ / ___ bleeding;
tracto ___ / ___ tract.

gastrolitiasis *f.* gastrolithiasis, calculi in the stomach.

gastrolito *m.* gastrolith, stomach concretion.

gastromalacia *f.* gastromalacia, softening of the stomach walls.

gastromegalia *f.* gastromegaly, enlargement of the stomach.

gastroplicación *f.* gastroplication, suture of a stomach wall to reduce its size.

gastrorrafía *f.* gastrorrhaphy, suture or perforation of the stomach.

gastrorragia *f.* gastrorrhagia, hemorrhaging from the stomach.

gastroscopía *f.* gastroscopy, examination of the stomach and the abdominal cavity with a gastroscope.

gastroscopio *m.* gastroscope, endoscope for visualizing the inside of the stomach.

gastrosquisis *f.* gastroschisis, congenital fissure in the abdominal wall due to a rupture of the amniotic membrane.

gastrostaxis *f.* gastrostaxis, bleeding of the mucous membrane of the stomach.

gastrostomía *f.* gastrostomy, creation of a gastric fistula through the abdominal wall.

gastrotópico-a *a.* gastrotopic, afflicting the stomach.

gastroyeyunostomía *f.* gastrojejunostomy, anastomosis of the stomach and the jejunum.

gástrula *f.* gastrula, an early stage in embryonic development.

gatear *v.* to crawl on all fours, such as babies.

gato-a *m., f.* cat.

Gauss, signo de *m.* Gauss sign, marked mobility in the uterus in early pregnancy.

gelatina *f.* gelatin.

gelatinoso-a *a.* gelatinous, having the consistency of or rel. to gelatin.

gemación *f.* gemmation, method of fission by which the parent cell produces a button containing chromatin that loosens from the cell to create a gemmule.

gemelo-a *m., f.* twin, either of two offspring born of the same pregnancy; ___ **dicigótico-a** / dizygotic ___; ___ **encigótico-a** /

enzygotic ___; ___ **fraternal** / fraternal ___; ___ **idéntico-a** / identical ___; ___ **monocigótico-a** / monozygotic ___; ___ **siamés, siamesa** / Siamese ___; ___ **verdadero-a** / true ___ .

gemido *m.* groan, moan.

gemir *vi.* to groan, to moan.

gémula *f.* gemmule, small button, product of the gemmation process.

gen, gene *m.* gene, basic unit of hereditary traits; ___ **dominante** / dominant ___; ___ **letal** / lethal ___; ___ **ligado al sexo** / sex-linked ___; ___ **recesivo** / recessive ___ .

generación *f.* generation, procreation. 1. the act of creating a new organism; 2. the whole body of individuals born within a time span of approximately thirty years.

generador *m.* generator.

general *a.* general; **estado** ___ / ___ condition; **tratamiento** ___ / ___ treatment; *adv.* **-mente** generally.

generalización *f.* generalization.

generalizar *v.* to generalize.

genérico-a *a.* generic, rel. to the gender; **nombre** ___ / ___ name, not protected by a trademark.

género *m.* 1. gender, sex of an individual; **identidad de** ___ / ___ identity; **papel de** ___ / ___ role; 2. genus, a category of biological classification.

generoso-a *a.* generous.

génesis *f.* genesis, origin, beginning; reproduction.

genética *f.* genetics, branch of biology that studies heredity and the laws that govern it; ___ **médica** / medical ___ .

genético-a *a.* genetic, rel. to heredity or genetics; **acondicionamiento** ___ / ___ fitness; **amplificación** ___ / ___ amplification; **asesoramiento** ___ / ___ counseling; **asociación** ___ / ___ association; **carga** ___ / ___ load; **determinante** ___ / ___ determinant; **epidemiología** ___ / ___ epidemiology; **ingeniería o construcción** ___ / ___ engineering; **marcador** ___ / ___ marker; **patrón** ___ / ___ code; **sustrato** ___ / ___ substratum.

geniculado-a *a.* geniculate. 1. bent as the knee; 2. rel. to the ganglion of the facial nerve.

genicular *a.* genicular, rel. to the knee.

genio *m.* genius, extraordinary mental power or faculties.

geniplastia *f.* genyplasty, reconstructive surgery of the jaw.

genital *a.* genital, rel. to the genitals; **ambigüedad** ___ / ___ ambiguity; **cordón** ___ / ___ cord; **corpúsculos** ___ / ___ corpuscles; **fase** ___ / ___ phase; **herpes** ___ / ___ herpes; **surco** ___ / ___ furrow; **tracto** ___ / ___ tract; **verruga** ___ / ___ wart.

genitales *m. pl.* genitals, genitalia, reproductive organs; *pop.* privates; ___ **externos** / ___ externalia.

genitourinario-a *a.* genitourinary, rel. to the reproductive and urinary organs.

genocidio *m.* genocide, systematic extermination of an ethnic or social group of people.

genodermatosis *f.* genodermatosis, genetic condition of the skin.

genoma *m.* genome, the complete basic haploid set of chromosomes of an organism.

genómico-a *a.* genomic, rel. to a genome; **clon** ___ / ___ clone.

genotipo *m.* genotype, the basic genetic constitution of an individual.

genotóxico-a *a.* genotoxic, rel. to a substance toxic to DNA that may affect the cells causing cancer.

gentamicina *f.* gentamicin, antibiotic that acts effectively against many gram-negative bacteria.

gente *f.* people, persons in general.

genuflexión *f.* genuflexion, bending of the knee.

genuino-a *a.* genuine, authentic, real.

genu valgum *L.* genu valgum, abnormal inward curvature of the knees that begins at infancy as a result of osseus deficiency, *pop.* knock-knee.

genu varum *L.* genu varum, abnormal outward curvature of the knees, *pop.* bowleg.

geofagia, geofagismo *f., m.* geophagia, geophagism, geophagy, propensity to eat soil or similar substances.

geográfico-a *a.* geographic; **atrofia retinal** ___ / ___ retinal atrophy; **queratitis** ___ / ___ keratitis.

geriatra *m., f.* geriatrician, specialist in geriatrics.

geriatría *f.* geriatrics, a branch of medicine that deals with the problems of aging and the treatment of diseases and ills of old age.

germen *m.* germ. 1. microorganism or bacteria, esp. one that causes disease; 2. a substance that can develop and form an organism.

germicida *m.* germicide, germicidal, agent that destroys germs.

germinal *a.* germinal, rel. to or of the nature of germs; **célula** ___ / ___ cell; **disco** ___ / ___ disk; **epitelio** ___ / ___ epithelium; **localización** ___ / ___ localization.

germinoma *m.* germinoma, neoplasm of germinal cells in the testis or ovaries.

geromorfismo *m.* geromorphism, premature senility.

gerontología *f.* gerontology.geriatría.

gerundio *m., gr.* gerund, the present participle of the verb.

gestación *f.* gestation, childbearing, pregnancy; ___ **abdominal** / abdominal ___; ___ **abdominal secundaria** / abdominal secondary ___; ___ **ectópica** / ectopic ___; ___ **intersticial** / interstitial ___; ___ **multiple** / multiple ___; ___ **prolongada** / prolonged ___; ___ **secundaria** / secondary ___; ___ **tubárica** / tubal ___; ___ **tubo-ovárica** / tubo-ovarian ___; ___ **uterotubárica** / uterotubaric ___ .

gestacional *a.* rel. to gestation; **edad** ___ / fetal maturity, chronologic.

Gestalt *m.* Gestalt, a school of thought that explains behavior as an integrated response to a situation as a whole.

gesticular *v.* to gesticulate, to communicate or express by means of gestures or signs.

gesto *m.* gesture.

Ghon, foco, lesión, tubérculo de *m.* Ghon's primary lesion, tubercule, first tubercular lesion in children.

giardiasis *f.* giardiasis, common intestinal infection with *Giardia lamblia* that spreads by contaminated food or water or through direct contact.

gibosidad *f.* gibbosity, the condition of having a hump.

giboso-a *a.* gibbous, humpbacked.

Giemsa, coloración de *f.* Giemsa's stain, stain used for blood smears in lab tests.

Gifford, reflejo de *m.* Gifford reflex, pupil contraction caused by trying to close the eyelids that are held open.

gigante *m.* giant; *a.* giant, unnaturally large.

gigantismo *m.* gigantism, excessive development of the body or some of its parts; ___ **acromegálico** / acromegalic ___; ___ **eunocoide** / eunochoid ___; ___ **normal** / normal ___ .

Gilles de la Tourette, síndrome de *m.* Tourette syndrome, a childhood disease affecting boys more frequently than girls, thought to be of a neurological nature and manifested by muscular anomalies; sometimes accompanied at puberty by involuntary uttering of obscenities and swearing.

Gillies, operación de *f.* Gillies operation, surgical technique to reduce the fracture of the zygoma and the zygomatic arch.

Gimbernat, ligamento de *m.* Gimbernat's ligament, membrane attached to the inguinal ligament on one end and the pubis on the other.

gimnasia, gimnástica *f.* gymnastics.

ginandroide *a.* gynandroid, having enough hermaphroditic characteristics to give the appearance of the opposite sex.

ginecología *f.* gynecology, the study of the female reproductive organs.

ginecológico-a *a.* gynecologic, gynecological, rel. to gynecology.

ginecólogo-a *m., f.* gynecologist, specialist in gynecology.

ginecomastia *f.* gynecomastia, excessive development of the mammary glands in the male.

gingiva *L.* gingiva, gum, tissue around the neck of the teeth.

gingival *a.* rel. to the gums.

gingivectomía *f.* gingivectomy, resection of the gingiva.

gingivitis *f.* gingivitis, infl. of the gums.

girar *v.* to rotate, to revolve.

glacial *a.* glacial, resembling or rel. to ice.

glande *m.* glans, gland-like mass located at the distal end of the penis (glans penis), or clitoris (glans clitoridis).

glándula *f.* gland, an organ that secretes or excretes substances that have specific functions or that eliminate products from the organism; ___ **inflamada** / swollen ___ .

glándulas endocrinas *f. pl.* endocrine glands, glands that secrete hormones directly absorbed into the blood or lymph such as the gonads and the pituitary and adrenal glands.

glándulas exocrinas *f. pl.* exocrine glands, glands that discharge their secretion through a duct, such as the mammary and sweat glands.

Glanzmann, trombastenia de *f.* Glanzmann's thrombasthenia, rare congenital disease caused by platelet abnormality.

Glasgow, escala de *f.* Glasgow's scale, instrument used to evaluate the degree of coma.

glaucoma *m.* glaucoma, eye disease caused by intraocular hypertension that results in hardening of the eye, atrophia of the retina, and sometimes blindness; ___ **absoluto** / absolutum ___ , final stage of acute glaucoma; ___ **infantil** / infantile ___ , between birth and three years of age; ___ **juvenil** / juvenile ___ , in older children and young adults without enlargement of the eyeball.

glenohumeral *a.* glenohumeral, rel. to the humerus and the glenoid cavity; **articulación** ___ / ___ joint; **ligamentos** ___ -es / ___ ligaments.

glenoideo-a *a.* glenoid, socket-like cavity; **cavidad** ___ / ___ cavity; **fosa** ___ / ___ fossa.

glía *f.* glia. neuroglia.

gliacito *m.* gliacyte, neuroglia cell.

glicemia, glucemia *f.* glycemia, concentration of glucose in the blood.

glicerina, glicerol *f.* glycerine, glycerol, an alcohol found in fats.

glicina *f.* glycine, a nonessential amino acid.

glicógeno, glucógeno *m.* glycogen, polysaccharide usu. stored in the liver that converts into glucose as needed.

glicogenólisis, glucogenólisis *f.* glycogenolysis, the breakdown of glycogen into glucose.

glicólisis *f.* glycolysis, breakdown of sugar into simpler compounds.

glicosuria *f.* glycosuria.glucosuria.

glioblastoma *f.* glioblastoma, a type of brain tumor.

glioma *m.* glioma, malignant brain tumor composed of neuroglia cells.

glioneuroma *f.* glioneuroma, a glioma combined with a neuroma.

gliosarcoma *m.* gliosarcoma, glioma abundant in fusiform cells of sarcoma.

globina *f.* globin, protein that is a part of hemoglobin.

globo *m.* globe, spherical body.

globular *a.* globular, spherical.

globulina *f.* globulin, one of a class of simple proteins that is insoluble in water but soluble in moderately concentrated salt solutions; **gamma** ___ / gamma ___ , a family of proteins capable of carrying antibodies; ___ **antilinfocítica** / antilymphocyte ___ , immunosuppressant.

globulina de enlace esteroide córtico suprarrenal *f.* corticosteroid-binding globulin.

globulinuria *f.* globulinuria, presence of globulin in the urine.

glóbulo *m.* globule, small spherical mass; ___ **blanco** / white blood cell, leukocyte; ___ **rojo** / red blood cell, erythrocyte.

globus *L.* globus, spheric body; ___ **histérico** / ___ hystericus, sensation of having a lump in the throat.

glomerular *a.* glomerular, rel. or resembling a glomerulus; cluster-like; **índice de**

filtración ___ / ___ filtration rate; **nefritis** ___ / ___ nephritis; **quiste** ___ / ___ cyst.

glomerulitis *f.* glomerulitis, infl. of the glomeruli, esp. the renal glomeruli.

glomérulo *m.* glomerulus, collection of capillaries in the shape of a tiny ball, present in the kidney.

glomeruloesclerosis *f.* glomerulosclerosis, degenerative process within the renal glomeruli that occurs in renal arteriosclerosis and diabetes.

glomerulonefritis *f.* glomerulonephritis, Bright's disease, infl. of the kidney glomeruli.

glomo *m.* glomus, small mass of arterioles rich in nerve supply and connected directly to veins.

glosa *f.* glossa, tongue.

glosalgia *f.* glossalgia, pain in the tongue.

glosectomía *f.* glossectomy, partial or total excision of the tongue.

glositis *f.* glossitis, infl. of the tongue; ___ aguda / acute ___ , associated with stomatitis.

glosodinia *f.* glossodynia. glosalgia.

glosoplastia *f.* glossoplasty, plastic surgery of the tongue.

glosoplejía *f.* glossoplegia, partial or total paralysis of the tongue.

glosorrafía *f.* glossorrhaphy, surgical suture of the tongue.

glosotomía *f.* glossotomy, incision in the tongue.

glotis *f.* glottis, opening in the upper part of the larynx between the vocal cords; vocal apparatus of the larynx.

glotitis *f.* glottitis, infl. of the glottis.

glucagón *m.* glucagon, one of the two hormones produced by the islets of Langerhans that increase the concentration of glucose in the blood and also have an anti-inflammatory effect.

glucagonoma *a.* glucagonoma, malignant glucagon secreting tumor.

glucocorticoide *a.* glucocorticoid, adrenal cortical hormones active in protecting against stress and affecting carbohydrate and protein metabolism.

glucofilia *f.* glycophilia, the propensity to develop hyperglycemia when even a small amount of glucose is ingested.

glucofosfato deshidrogenasa *m.* glucose-6-phosphate dehydrogenase, enzyme found in the liver and kidney, important in the conversion of glyceryl to glucose.

glucogénesis *f.* glucogenesis, formation of glucose from glycogen.

glucogenólisis *f.* glycogenolysis, chemical process that takes place in the liver and the muscles converting glycogen into glucose.

glucolítico-a *a.* glycolytic, that disintegrates or digests sugars.

gluconeogénesis *f.* gluconeogenesis, glyconeogenesis, formation of glycogen in the liver from noncarbohydrate sources.

glucopenia *f.* glycopenia. hipoglicemia.

glucopéxico-a *a.* glycopexic, that stores sugar.

glucoproteína *f.* glycoprotein, a protein belonging to a compound made of linked carbohydrates of which mucins, amyloid and mucoid are the most important.

glucorraquia *f.* glycorrhachia, presence of glucose in the cerebrospinal fluid.

glucosa *f.* glucose, dextrose, the main source of energy for living organisms; **nivel de** ___ **en la sangre** / blood level of ___; **prueba de tolerancia a la** ___ / ___ tolerance test.

glucósido *m.* glucoside, glycoside, natural or synthetic compound that liberates sugar upon hydrolysis.

glucosuria *f.* glucosuria, glycosuria, abnormal amount of sugar in the urine; ___ **diabética** / diabetic ___; ___ **pituitaria** / pituitary ___; ___ **renal** / renal ___ .

glutamato *m.* glutamate, salt of glutamic acid.

gluten *m.* gluten, albuminoid vegetable matter.

glúteo-a *a.* gluteal, rel. to the buttocks; **pliegue** ___ / ___ fold; **reflejo** ___ / ___ reflex.

gnation *m.* gnathion, the lowest point in the middle line of the jaw.

gnatoplastia *f.* gnathoplasty, plastic surgery of the jaw.

gnosia *f.* gnosia, ability to perceive and recognize people and things.

gola *f.* throat; *pop.* gullet.

goloso-a *m., f.* person very fond of sweets and snacks; *a.* fond of snacking; sweet tooth.

golpe *m.* blow; bruise; bang; ___ **en la cabeza** / ___ to the head.

golpear *v.* to beat, to hit.

goma *f.* 1. gumma, syphilitic tumor; 2. gum rubber; [*de borrar*] eraser; glue.

gónada *f.* gonad, a gland that produces sex cells (gametes). In males the gonads are the testes, in females, the ovaries.

gonadal *a.* gonadal, rel. to a gonad gland; **disgenesia** ___ / ___ dysgenesis, malformation.

gonadectomía *f.* gonadectomy, excision of a sexual gland.

gonadopatía *f.* gonadopathy, disease of the gonad glands.

gonadotropina *f.* gonadotropin, gonad stimulating hormone; ___ **coriónica** /

chorionic ____ , present in the blood and the urine of the female during pregnancy and used in the pregnancy test; **hormona que estimula la secreción de** ____ / ____ releasing hormone.

gonalgia *f.* gonalgia, pain in the knee.

gonartritis *f.* gonarthritis, infl. of the knee joint.

gonión *m.* gonion, the most inferior, posterior, and lateral point on the external angle of the mandible.

goniopuntura *f.* goniopuncture, puncture of the anterior chamber of the eye as a means to treat glaucoma.

goniotomía *f.* goniotomy, procedure to relieve congenital glaucoma.

gonocócico-a *a.* gonoccal, rel. to gonococci; **arthritis** ____ / ____ arthritis; **conjuntivitis** ____ / ____ conjunctivitis.

gonococo *m.* gonococcus, microorganism of the species *Neisseria gonorrhoeae* that causes gonorrhea.

gonorrea *f.* gonorrhea, highly contagious catarrhal bacterial infection of the genital mucosa, sexually transmitted.

gonorreico-a *a.* gonorrheal, rel. to gonorrhea; **artritis** ____ / ____ arthritis; **oftalmia** ____ / ____ ophthalmia.

Goodell, signo de *m.* Goodell sign, a softening of the cervix, and possible indication of pregnancy.

gordiflón-a *m., f.* fat, flabby person.

gordo-a *a.* fat, overweight.

gordura *f.* fatness, corpulence.

gorra *f.* cap, head covering.

gota *f.* gout. 1. a hereditary disease caused by a defect in uric acid metabolism; 2. drop, a very small portion of a liquid.

gotear *v.* to drip; to leak.

goteo *m.* drip, dripping; ____ **postnasal** / postnasal ____ .

gotero *m.* dropper; ____ **para los ojos** / eye ____ .

gotica *f.* droplet.

gozar *vi.* to enjoy, to rejoice.

grabadora *f.* tape recorder.

grabar *v.* to record.

gracias *f. pl.* thanks; **muchas** ____ / thank you very much.

gracilis *m.* gracilis, long internal muscle of the thigh.

gradiente *a.* gradient, index or curve representing the increase or decrease of a variable.

grado *m.* [*temperatura*] degree; [*evaluación*] grade. 1. measurement or standard evaluation; 2. in cancer pathology, indication of the stage of the disease.

gradual *a.* gradual; **-mente** / *adv.* gradually.

Graefe, operación de *f.* Graefe operation. 1. cataract operation by incision of the sclera, separation of the capsula and iridectomy; 2. iridectomy for glaucoma.

Graefe, signo de *m.* Graefe sign, failure of the upper eyelid to follow the downward movement of the eyeball.

gráfica, gráfico *f., m.* graph, chart, diagram.

grafología *f.* graphology, the study of handwriting as an indication of an individual's character, also used as an aid in diagnosis.

Gram, método de *m.* Gram's method, a system of coloring bacteria for the purpose of identifying them on analysis.

gramática *f.* grammar.

gramicidina *f.* gramicidin, antibacterial substance produced by *Bacillis brevis*, active locally against gram-positive bacteria.

gramnegativo *m.* gram-negative, bacteria or tissue that loses coloration when subjected to Gram's method.

gramo *m.* gram, unit of weight in the metric system.

grampositivo *m.* gram-positive, bacteria or tissue that retains coloration when subjected to Gram's method.

gran, grande *a.* big, large.

grano *m.* grain, granum, a small spherical mass; bead.

granulación *f.* granulation, round, small, fleshy masses that form in a wound.

granular, granuloso-a *a.* granular, made up or marked by grains; **cilindro** ____ / ____ cast, urinary cast seen in degenerative and inflammatory nephropathy; **conjunctivitis** ____ / ____ conjunctivitis; **córtex** ____ / ____ cortex; **distrofia** ____ **de la córnea** / corneal dystrophy; **leucocito** ____ / ____ leukocyte; **oftalmia** ____ / ____ ophthalmia; **retículo endoplásmico** ____ / ____ endoplasmic reticulum; **tumor celular** ____ / ____ cell tumor.

gránulo *m.* granule, small grain or particle; ____ **acidófilo** / acidophil ____ , a stain with acid dyes; ____ **basófilo** / basophil ____ , a stain with basic dyes.

granulocito *m.* granulocyte, leukocyte containing granules.

granulocitopenia *f.* granulocytopenia, deficiency in the number of granulocytes in the blood.

granulocitosis *f.* granulocytosis, excessive increase of granulocytes in the blood.

granuloma *m.* granuloma, tumor or neoplasm of granular tissue; ___ **de cuerpo extraño** / foreign body ___; ___ **infeccioso** / infectious ___; ___ **inguinal** / inguinal ___; ___ **ulcerativo de los genitales** / venereum ___ .

granulomatosis *f.* granulomatosis, multiple granuloma.

granulomatoso-a *a.* granulomatous, with the characteristics of a granuloma; **colitis** ___ / ___ colitis; **encefalomielitis** ___ / ___ encephalomyelitis; **enteritis** ___ / ___ enteritis; **inflamación** ___ / ___ inflammation.

granulopenia *f.* granulopenia. granulocitopenia.

granulosa *f.* granulosa, ovarian membrane of epithelial cells; **tumor de células de la** ___ / ___ cell tumor; **tumor de la** ___ **teca** / ___ teca cell tumor.

grapar *v.* to staple; surgical procedure.

grasa *f.* fat, adipose tissue.

grasiento-a, grasoso-a *a.* fatty, greasy; **degeneración** ___ / ___ degeneration.

gratificación *f.* gratification, reward.

gratificar *vi.* to gratify, to reward.

gratis *adv.* gratis, free.

grave *a.* critically ill; of a serious nature.

Grave, enfermedad de *f.* Grave's disease, exophthalmic goiter.

gravedad *f.* gravity. 1. seriousness; **estado de** ___ / critical condition; 2. force of gravity.

grávida *f.* gravida, pregnant woman.

grieta *f.* crevice, cleft, fissure; ___ **-s en las manos** / chapped hands.

gripe *f.* grippe, flu; ___ **asiatica** / Asiatic flu;

griposis *f.* gryposis, abnormal curvature, esp. as seen in nails.

gris *a.* gray; **catarata** ___ / ___ cataract; **columnas** ___ **-es** / ___ columns; **degeneración** ___ / ___ degeneration; **fibras** ___ **-es** / ___ fibers; **hepatización** ___ / ___ hepatizatión; **induracion** ___ / ___ induration; **sustancia** ___ / ___ matter.

gris, materia o sustancia *f.* gray matter, highly vascularized gray tissue of the central nervous system made up primarily of nerve cells and unmyelinated nerve fibers.

griseofulvina *f.* griseofulvin, antibiotic used in fungus skin diseases.

gritar *v.* to scream, to cry out.

grito *m.* scream, cry; *pop.* **estar en un** ___ / to be in great pain.

grosero-a *a.* gross, coarse.

grosor *m.* thickness; density.

grueso-a *a.* heavy; thick.

grumoso-a *a.* grumose, grumous, lumpy, clotted.

grupo *m.* group, cluster; team, an associated group; ___ **de soporte, de apoyo** / support ___ .

grupo sanguíneo *m.* blood group, the different types of human erythrocytes, genetically determined and differentiated immunologically; ___ **RH** / Rh ___ .

guanetidina *f.* guanethidine, agent used in the treatment of hypertension.

guante *m.* glove; ___ **-s de goma** / rubber ___ -s.

guardar *v.* to put away; to keep.

guardería infantil *f.* nursery; children's day care center.

guardián *m.* guardian; custodian.

guayaco *m.* guaiac, substance used in tests as a reagent to detect the presence of blood.

guayacol *m.* guaiacol, antiseptic; expectorant.

gubernaculum *L.* gubernaculum, direction, guidance.

guerra *f.* war.

guía *m., f.* guide, director; ___ **de teléfono** / telephone directory.

guiar *v.* to guide, to direct.

Guillain-Barre, síndrome de *m.* Guillain-Barre syndrome, rare neurological disease evidenced by ascending paralysis that starts in the extremities and can rapidly include the respiratory muscles causing respiratory failure.

guillotina *f.* guillotine, surgical instrument.

guiñar *v.* to wink.

guisado *m.* stew.

guisar *v.* to stew.

gusano *m.* earthworm, maggot, caterpillar; ___ **nematodo que infesta los pulmones** / lungworm; ___ **plano** / flatworm, intestinal worm.

gustar *v.* to like, to enjoy.

gustativo-a *a.* gustatory, rel. to taste; **agnosia** ___ / ___ agnosia; **aura** ___ / ___ aura; **hiperhidrosis** ___ / ___ hyperhidrosis; **rinorrea** ___ / ___ rhinorrhoea.

gusto *m.* the sense of taste; taste; **buen** ___ / good taste; **mal** ___ / bad taste.

gutapercha *f.* gutta-percha, dried and purified latex of some trees that is used in medical and dental treatments.

gutta *L. guttae* gutta, drop.

gutural *a.* guttural, pronounced in the throat.

h

H *abr.* **heroína** / heroin; **hidrógeno** / hydrogen; **hipermetropía** / hypermetropia; **hipodérmico-a** / hypodermic.

h *abr.* **hora** / hour; **horizontal** / horizontal.

haba *f.* lima bean.

haber *vi. aux.* to have.

habichuela *f.* string bean.

hábil, habilidoso-a *a.* able, skillful.

habilidad *f.* ability, aptitude.

habilitar *v.* to habilitate; to equip.

habitación *f.* room.

hábito *m.* habit. ___ -s sanitarios / health ___ .

habitual *a.* habitual, customary; **-mente** *adv.* habitually.

habla *m.* [*locución*] speech; **defecto del** ___ / ___ defect; **patología del** ___ / ___ pathology; **trastorno del** ___ / ___ disorder.

hablar *v.* to speak.

hacer *vi.* to do, to make; ___ **caso** / to mind, to pay attention; ___ **daño** / to harm or hurt; ___ **hincapié** / to emphasize; ___ **lo mejor posible** / to do one's best.

hacia *prep.* towards; ___ **acá** / this way; ___ **allá** / that way; ___ **adelante** / forward; ___ **atrás** / backwards.

hachís *m.* hashish, euphoria producing narcotic extracted from marijuana.

halar *v.* to pull.

hálito *m.* halitus, breath.

halitosis *f.* halitosis, bad breath.

hallar *v.* to find; **hallarse** *vr.* [*en un lugar o condición*] to find oneself.

hallazgos *m. pl.* findings, results of an investigation or inquiry.

hallux valgus *L.* hallux valgus, inward turning of the big toe.

hallux varus *L.* hallux varus, separation of the big toe from the others.

haloide *m.* haloid, salt resulting from the combination of a halogen element and a metal.

halótano *m.* halothane, Fluothane, anesthetic administered by inhalation.

hamartoma *m.* hamartoma, nodule simulating a tumor, usu. benign.

hambre *m.* hunger; **tener** ___ / to be hungry.

hambriento-a *a.* hungry, starved, famished.

Hanot, enfermedad de *f.* Hanot's disease, hypertrophic cirrhosis of the liver accompanied by jaundice; biliary cirrhosis.

Hansen, enfermedad de *f.* Hansen's disease. V. **leprosy**.

haploide *a.* haploid, a sex cell that has half the number of chromosomes characteristic of the species.

haptoglobina *f.* haptoglobin, mucoprotein that links itself to the released hemoglobin in the plasma.

haptómetro *m.* haptometer, device used to measure the acuteness of the sense of touch.

haragán-a *m., f.* lazy person; *a.* lazy.

harina *f.* flour, cornmeal.

harmonía, armonía *f.* harmony, congenial communication.

harmonizar, armonizar *v.* to harmonize.

hartarse *vr.* to overeat, to stuff oneself.

hasta *prep.* until; up to; as far as; ___ **ahora** / heretofore, so far; ___ **aquí** / up to this point; ___ **luego** / goodbye, see you later.

haustrum *L.* haustrum, cavity or pouch, esp. in the colon.

Havers, sistema de *m.* Haversian system, concentric formation of small conduits that constitute the base of the compact bone.

hay *v.* there is, there are; ___ **que** / it is necessary; **no** ___ **remedio** / it can't be helped.

haz *m.* bundle; ___ **ascendente** / ascending tract.

heces *f. pl.* feces.

hecho-a *a. pp.* of **hacer**, done, made; **bien** ___ / well ___; **mal** ___ / badly ___; **de** ___ / as a matter of fact.

Heimlich, maniobra de *f.* Heimlich maneuver, technique applied to force the expulsion of a foreign body that is blocking the passage of air from the trachea or pharynx.

helado *m.* ice cream; *a.* **-a** frozen.

helicoideo-a *a.* helical, in the shape of a helix or a spiral.

helicóptero *m.* helicopter.

helio *m.* helium, gaseous inert chemical element mixed with air or oxygen to be used in the treatment of some respiratory disorders.

heliofobia *f.* heliophobia, excessive fear of the sun.

helioterapia *f.* heliotherapy, sunbathing as therapy.

helmintiasis *f.* helminthiasis, intestinal infection with worms.

helminticida *m.* helminthicide, agent that kills parasites; vermicide.

helminto *m.* helminth, worm found in the human intestines.

hemafecia *f.* hemafecia, presence of blood in the feces.

hemaglutinación, hemoaglutinación *f.* hemagglutination, agglutination of red cells.

hemaglutinina, hemoaglutinina *f.* hemaglutinin, antibody that causes agglutination of red cells.

hemangioma *m.* hemangioma, benign tumor formed by clustered blood vessels that produce a reddish birth mark.

hemangiosarcoma *m.* hemangiosarcoma, malignant tumor of the vascular tissue.

hemartrosis *f.* hemarthrosis, extravasation into a joint cavity.

hematemesis *f.* hematemesis, vomiting of blood.

hematerapia, hemoterapia *f.* hematherapy, hemotherapy, therapeutic use of blood.

hemático *m.* drug used in the treatment of anemia; *a.* **-a** rel. to blood; **biometría** ___ / complete blood count (CBC).

hematocolpos *m.* hematocolpos, retention of menstrual blood in the vagina due to an imperforated hymen.

hematócrito *m.* hematocrit. 1. centrifuge that is used for separating cells and particles in the blood from the plasma; 2. the volume percentage of erythrocytes in the blood.

hematogénesis *f.* hematogenesis. hematopoyesis.

hematógeno-a *a.* hematogenous. 1. rel. to the production of blood and to its constituents; 2. originating in the blood.

hematología *f.* hematology, the study of the blood and the organs that intervene in its formation.

hematológico-a *a.* hematologic, hematological, rel. to blood; **estudios** ___ **-s** / ___ studies. *V.* cuadro en la página 405.

hematólogo-a *m., f.* 1. hematologist, specialist in hematology;2. a specialist in diagnostic blood tests and treating blood diseases.

hematoma *m.* hematoma, localized collection of blood that has escaped from a blood vessel into an organ, space, or tissue; ___ **pélvico /** pelvic ___; ___ **subdural** / subdural___, under the dura mater.

hematomielia *f.* hematomyelia, bleeding into the spinal cord.

hematopoyesis, hemopoyesis *f.* hematopoiesis, hemopoiesis, formation of blood.

hematoquezia *f.* hematochezia, presence of blood in the stool.

hembra *f.* the female of a species.

hemianalgesia *f.* hemianalgesia, insensitivity to pain in one side of the body.

hemianopia, hemanopsia *f.* hemianopia, hemanopsia, loss of vision in one half of the visual field of the left or right eye, or of both.

hemiataxia *f.* hemiataxia, lack of muscular coordination in one side of the body.

hemiatrofia *f.* hemiatrophy, atrophy of half of an organ or half of the body.

hemibalismo *m.* hemiballism, hemiballismus, brain lesion that causes involuntary and rapid movements in half of the body.

hemicolectomía *f.* hemicolectomy, removal of one half of the colon.

hemihipertrofia *f.* hemihypertrophy, hypertrophy of one half of the body.

hemilaminectomía *f.* hemilaminectomy, removal of the vertebral lamina on one side.

hemiparálisis *f.* hemiparalysis, paralysis of one side of the body.

hemiparesia, hemiparesis *f.* hemiparesia, hemiparesis, paralysis affecting one side of the body.

hemiparético-a *a.* hemiparetic, rel. to hemiparesia.

hemiplejía *f.* hemiplegia, paralysis of the side of the body opposite to the affected cerebral hemisphere. ___ **alternante /** alternating ___; ___ **cerebral** / cerebral ___; ___ **cruzada** / crossed ___; ___ **doble /** double ___; ___ **espástica** / spastic ___; ___ **facial** / facial ___ .

hemipléjico-a *a.* hemiplegic, affected or rel. to hemiplegia.

hemisferio *m.* hemisphere, half of a spherical structure or organ.

hemitórax *m.* hemithorax, each side of the thorax.

hemobilia *f.* hemobilia, bleeding in the bile ducts.

hemoblastosis *f.* hemoblastosis, proliferative disorders of the blood tissues.

hemocitoblasto *m.* hemocytoblast, primordial blood cell from which all others are derived.

hemocitómetro *m.* hemocytometer, instrument used for the count of red globules in a given blood volume.

hemoclasis, hemoclasia *f.* hemoclasis, hemoclasia, rupture, [*hemolysis*] dissolution or other type of destruction of red blood cells.

hemoconcentración *f.* hemoconcentration, concentration of red blood cells due to a decrease of liquid elements in the blood.

hemoconcentrar *v.* hemoconcentrate, to concentrate red blood cells.

hemocromatosis *f.* hemochromatosis, iron storage disease, bronze diabetes, disorder of iron metabolism due to excess deposition of iron in the tissues accompanied by anomalies such as bronze skin pigmentation, cirrhosis of the liver, diabetes mellitus, and malfunction of the pancreas.

hemocultivo *m.* blood culture.

hemodiálisis *f.* hemodialysis, dialysis process used to eliminate toxic substances from the blood in cases of acute renal disorders.

hemodializador *m.* hemodializer, artificial kidney machine used in the dialysis process.

hemodilución *f.* hemodilution, increase in the proportion of plasma to red cells in the blood.

hemodinamia *f.* hemodynamics, the study of the dynamics of blood circulation.

hemofilia *f.* hemophilia, inherited disease characterized by abnormal clotting of the blood and propensity to bleed.

hemofílico-a *m., f.* hemophiliac, person who suffers from hemophilia; *a.* hemophiliac, rel. to or suffering from hemophilia.

hemófilo *m.* hemophilus, haemophilus, one of a group of gram-negative aerobic bacteria.

hemofobia *f.* hemophobia, pathologic fear of blood.

hemoglobina *f.* hemoglobin, important protein element of the blood that gives it its red color and participates in the transportation of oxygen; **índice corpuscular de** ___ / mean corpuscular ___ .

hemoglobinemia *f.* hemoglobinemia, presence of freed hemoglobin in the plasma.

hemoglobinuria *f.* hemoglobinuria, presence of hemoglobin in the urine. ___ **de la postparturienta** / postparturient ___; ___ **en malaria** / malarial ___; ___ **epidémica** / epidemic ___; ___ **intermitente** / intermittent ___; ___ **paroxística fría** / paroxysmal cold ___; ___ **paroxística nocturna** / paroxysmal nocturnal ___ .

hemograma *m.* hemogram, graphic representation of the differential blood count.

hemólisis *f.* hemolysis, rupture of erythrocytes with release of hemoglobin into the plasma;___ **del recién nacido** / hemolytic disease of the newborn, gen. caused by incompatibility of the Rh factor; ___ **inmune** / immune ___; ___ **venenosa** / venomous ___ .

hemolítico-a *a.* hemolytic, rel. to or that causes hemolysis; **anemia** ___ / ___ anemia, red cells that rupture easily due to a congenital condition

caused by toxic agents; **trastorno** ___ / ___ disorder.

hemolito *m.* hemolith, concretion in a blood vessel.

hemopneumotórax *m.* hemopneumothorax, accumulation of blood and air in the pleural cavity.

hemoptisis *f.* hemoptysis, bloody expectoration.

hemorragia *f.* hemorrhage, profuse bleeding;___ **cerebral** / cerebrovascular accident; ___ **intracraneana** / intracranial ___; ___ **intraventricular** / intraventicular ___; ___ **nasal** / nasal ___; ___ **oculta** / concealed ___; ___ **petequial** / petechial ___; ___ **puerperal** / postpartum ___ .

hemorrágico-a *a.* hemorrhagic, rel. to hemorrhage.

hemorroide(s) *f.* hemorrhoid, pile, a mass of dilated veins in the inferior anal or rectal wall; ___ **de prolapso** / prolapsed ___, that protrudes outside the anus; ___ **externa** / external ___, outside the anal sphincter; ___ **interna** / internal ___, hidden, proximal to the anorectal line.

hemorroidectomía *f.* hemorrhoidectomy, removal of hemorrhoids.

hemosálpinx *m.* hemosalpinx, accumulation of blood in the fallopian tubes.

hemosiderina *f.* hemosiderin, insoluble iron compound stored in the body for use in the formation of hemoglobin as needed.

hemosiderosis *f.* hemosiderosis, hemosiderin deposit in the liver and the spleen.

hemostasia, hemostasis *f.* hemostasis, cessation of bleeding, natural or otherwise.

hemóstato *m.* hemostat, a surgical clamp or a medication used to suppress bleeding.

hendidura *f.* fissure, crack, cleavage.

heparina *f.* heparin, anticoagulant.

heparinización *f.* heparinization, process of administering heparin.

heparinizar *vi.* heparinize, to avoid coagulation by the use of heparin.

hepatectomía *f.* hepatectomy, removal of a part or all of the liver.

hepático-a *a.* hepatic, rel. to the liver; **circulación** ___ / liver circulation; **cirrosis** ___ / liver cirrhosis; **coma** ___ / ___ coma; **conducto** ___ / ___ duct; **fallo** ___ / liver failure; **lesión** ___ / liver damage; **lóbulos o subdivisiones** ___ -s / ___ lobes; **manchas** ___ -s / liver spots; **pruebas funcionales** ___ -s / liver function tests; **venas** ___ -s / ___ veins.

hepatitis *f.* hepatitis, infl. of the liver; ___
amébica / amebic ___; ___ **colestásica** /
cholestatic ___; ___ **crónica activa** / chronic
active ___; ___ **crónica persistente** / chronic
persistent ___; ___ **epidémica** /
epidemic ___; ___ **inducida por droga** / drug-
induced ___; ___ **infecciosa** /
infectious ___; ___ **no A-no B** / non A-non
B ___ , linked to blood transfusion; ___ **sérica** /
serum ___; ___ **tipo A, viral** ___ / type A,
viral ___; ___ **tipo B, viral** / type B , viral ___ .

hepatocito *m.* hepatocyte, liver cell.

hepatoentérico-a *a.* hepatoenteric, rel. to the
liver and the intestines.

hepatoesplenomegalia *f.*
hepatosplenomegaly, enlargement of the liver
and the spleen.

hepatolenticular *a.* hepatolenticular, rel. to the
lenticular nucleus of the eye and the liver;
degeneración ___ / ___ degeneration.

hepatologia *f.* hepatology, the study of the
liver.

hepatólogo-a *m., f.* hepatologist, specialist in
liver diseases.

hepatomegalia *f.* hepatomegaly, enlargement
of the liver.

hepatorrenal *a.* hepatorenal, rel. to the liver
and the kidneys.

hepatotoxicidad *f.* hepatotoxicity, the
propensity of a medication or toxic product to
harm the liver.

hepatotoxina *f.* hepatotoxin, toxin that destroys
liver cells.

heredado-a *a.* inherited.

heredar *v.* to inherit

hereditario-a *a.* hereditary, inherited.

herencia *f.* heredity, inheritance, transmission of
genetic traits from parents to children; ___
familiar / heredofamilial, rel. to a disease or
condition that is inherited.

herida *f.* wound, injury; ___ **contusa** /
contused ___ , subcutaneous lesion; ___ **de**
perforación / puncture ___; ___ **de bala** /
gunshot ___; ___ **penetrante** / penetrating ___ .

herido-a *a.* wounded; hurt.

herir *vi.* to injure, to hurt.

hermafrodita *f.* hermaphrodite, an individual
that has both ovaric and testicular tissue
combined in the same organ or separately.

hermafroditismo *m.* hermaphroditism,
condition of being a hermaphrodite.

hermano-a *m., f.* brother; sister.

hermético-a *a.* hermetic, airtight.

hernia *f.* hernia, abnormal protrusion of an organ
or viscera through the cavity wall that encloses
it; ___ **escrotal** / scrotal ___ , that descends into
the scrotum; ___ **estrangulada** /
strangulated ___ , obstructing the intestines; ___
femoral / femoral ___ , protruding into the
femoral canal; ___ **hiatal** / hiatus ___ ,
protruding through the esophagic hiatus of the
diaphragm; ___ **incarcerada** / incarcerated ___ ,
frequently caused by adherences; ___ **inguinal** /
inguinal ___ , protruding from the viscera into
the inguinal canal; ___ **lumbar** / lumbar ___ , in
the loin; ___ **por deslizamiento** / sliding ___ ,
of the colon; ___ **reducible** / reducible ___ , that
can be treated by manipulation; ___ **umbilical** /
umbilical ___ , occuring at the navel; ___
ventral / ventral ___ , protrusion through the
abdominal wall; **saco de la** ___ / hernial sac,
peritoneal sac into which the hernia descends. *V.*
cuadro.

herniación *f.* herniation, development of a
hernia.

herniado-a *a.* herniated, hernial, rel. to or
having a hernia.

herniografía *f.* herniography, x-ray of a hernia
with the use of a contrasting medium.

herniorrafía *f.* herniorrhaphy, reparation or
reconstruction of a hernia.

heroico-a *a.* heroic, rel. to very strong
medication or extreme medical procedures.

heroína *f.* heroin, diacetylmorphine, addictive
narcotic derived from morphine; **adicto-a a**
la ___ , **heroinómano-a** / ___ addict.

Hernia	Hernia
abdominal	abdominal
cerebral	cerebral
cística	cystic
congénita-diafragmática	congenital-diaphragmatic
escrotal	scrotal
estrangulada	strangulated
hiatus	hiatal
incarcerada	incarcerated
lumbar	lumbar
por deslizamiento	sliding
reducible	reducible
umbilical	umbilical
ventral	ventral

heroinismo, heroinomanía *m.* heroinism, addiction to heroin.

herpangina *f.* herpangina, infectious disease (epidemic in the summer) that affects the mucous membranes of the throat.

herpes *m.* herpes, inflammatory, painful viral disease of the skin manifested by the formation of small, clustered, blisterlike eruptions; ___ **genital** / ___ genitalis; ___ **ocular** / ocular ___; ___ **simple** / ___ simplex, simple vesicles that keep recurring in the same area of the skin; ___ **zóster [culebrilla]** / ___ zoster; *pop.* shingles, painful eruption along the course of a nerve.

herpético-a *a.* herpetic, rel. to herpes or similar in nature.

hervido-a *a.* boiled.

hervir *vi.* to boil.

heterogéneo-a *a.* heterogeneous, dissimilar, not alike.

heteroinjerto *m.* heterograft, graft that comes from a donor of a different species or type than that of the recipient.

heterólogo-a *a.* heterologous. 1. formed by foreign cell tissue; 2. derived or obtained from a different species.

heteroplasia *f.* heteroplasia, presence of tissue in areas foreign to its normal location.

heteroplastia *f.* heteroplasty, transplant of tissue from an individual of a different species.

heteroplástico-a *a.* heteroplastic, rel. to heteroplasia.

heterosexual *a.* heterosexual, attracted to the opposite sex.

heterosexualidad *f.* heterosexuality.

heterotaxia *f.* heterotaxis, abnormal or irregular position of some organs or parts of the body.

heterotopia *f.* heterotopia, displacement or deviation of an organ or part of the body from its normal position.

heterotópico-a *a.* heterotopic, rel. to heterotopia.

hético-a *a.* hectic, febrile.

heurístico-a *a.* heuristic, rel. to empirical discoveries or investigations.

hexacloruro de gamma-benceno *m.* gamma-benzene hexachloride, powerful insecticide used in the treatment of scabies.

hialina *f.* hyalin, protein that results from the degeneration of amyloids, colloids, and hyaloids.

hialinización *f.* hyalinization, degenerative process by which functioning tissue is replaced by a firm, glasslike material.

hialino-a *a.* hyaline, glasslike, or almost transparent; **cilindro** ___ / ___ cast, found in the urine; **enfermedad de la membrana** ___ / ___ membrane disease, respiratory disorder of the newborn.

hialoide, hialoideo-a *a.* hyaloid, resembling glass.

hiatus *m.* hiatus, opening, orifice, fissure.

hibernoma *m.* hibernoma, benign tumor localized in the hip or the back.

híbrido-a *a.* hybrid, resulting from the crossing of different species of animals or plants.

hibridoma *m.* hybridoma, hybrid cell capable of producing a continuous supply of antibodies.

hidátide *m.* hydatid, cyst found in tissues, esp. in the liver.

hidatídico-a *a.* hydatid, rel. to a hydatid; **enfermedad** ___ / ___ disease, echinococcosis; **quiste** ___ / ___ mole, uterine cyst that produces hemorrhaging.

hidradenitis *f.* hidradenitis, infl. of the sweat glands.

hidramnios *m.* hydramnion, excess of amniotic fluid.

hidratado-a *a.* hydrated, that is moist or contains water.

hidratar *v.* to hydrate, to combine a body with water.

hídrico-a *a.* hydric, rel. to water.

hidrocefalia *f.* hydrocephaly, hydrocephalus, abnormal accumulation of cerebrospinal fluid within the ventricles of the brain.

hidrocefálico-a *a.* hydrocephalic, rel. to hydrocephaly.

hidrocele *m.* hydrocele, an accumulation of serous fluid esp. in the vaginal tunic of the testes.

hidrocelectomía *f.* hydrocelectomy, removal of a hydrocele.

hidrocortisona *f.* hydrocortisone, corticosteroid hormone produced by the adrenal cortex.

hidroeléctrico-a *a.* hydroelectric, rel. to water and electricity; **equilibrio** ___ / water-electrolyte balance; **desequilibrio** ___ / water-electrolyte imbalance.

hidrofílico-a *a.* hydrophilic, having a propensity to attract and retain water.

hidrofobia *f.* hydrophobia. 1. fear of water; 2. rabies, nervous disorder transmitted by an infected animal.

hidrógeno *m.* hydrogen; **concentración de** ___ / ___ concentration.

hidrólisis *f.* hydrolysis, dissolution of a compound by the action of water.

h

hidrolizar *vi.* to hydrolyze.

hidromielia *f.* hydromyelia, increase of fluid in the central canal of the spinal cord.

hidronefrosis *f.* hydronephrosis, distension of the renal pelvis and calices due to obstruction.

hidroneumotórax *m.* hydropneumothorax, presence of gas and fluids in the pleural cavity.

hidropesía, hidropsia *f.* hydropsy, dropsy, accumulation of serous fluid in a cavity or cellular tissue.

hidrópico-a *a.* hydropic, rel. to hydropsy.

hidrosálpinx *m.* hydrosalpinx, accumulation of watery fluid in the fallopian tubes.

hidrosis *f.* hidrosis, hydrosis, abnormal sweating.

hidrostático-a *a.* hydrostatic, rel. to the equilibrium of liquids.

hidroterapia *f.* hydrotherapy, therapeutic use of applied external water in the treatment of diseases.

hidrotórax *m.* hydrothorax, collection of fluid in the pleural cavity without inflammation.

hidrouréter *m.* hydroureter, abnormal distension of the ureter due to obstruction.

hidroxiapatita *f.* hydroxyapatite, calcium phosphate, inorganic compound found in teeth and bones.

hiel *f.* bile; gall.

hielo *m.* ice.

hierro *m.* iron.

hifema *f.* hyphema, bleeding in the anterior chamber of the eye.

hígado *m.* liver, largest gland of the body, located in the upper right part of the abdominal cavity. It secretes bile, stabilizes and produces sugar, enzymes, and cholesterol, and eliminates toxins from the body.

higiene *f.* hygiene, the study and practice of health standards; ___ **dental** / dental ___; ___ **mental** / mental ___; ___ **oral** / oral ___; ___ **pública** / public ___ .

higiénico-a *a.* hygienic, sanitary; rel. to hygiene; **absorbente** ___ / sanitary napkin.

higienista *m., f.* hygienist, specialist in hygiene; ___ **dental** / dental ___ , technician in dental profilaxis.

higroma *m.* hygroma, liquid containing sac.

hijastro-a *m., f.* stepson; stepdaughter.

hijo-a *m., f.* son; daughter.

hilio *m.* hilum, hilus, depression or opening in an organ from which blood vessels and nerves enter or leave.

hilo *m.* thread. 1. material used in sutures; 2. filament-like structure.

himen *m.* hymen, membranous fold that covers partially the entrance of the vagina.

himenectomía *f.* hymenectomy, excision of the hymen.

himenotomía *f.* hymenotomy, incision in the hymen.

hinchado-a *a.* swollen, bloated.

hinchar *v.* to swell, to inflate; **hincharse** *vr.* to become swollen or bloated.

hinchazón *f.* swelling.

hioides *m.* hyoid bone, horseshoe-shaped bone situated at the base of the tongue.

hipalgesia, hipalgia *f.* hypalgia, diminished sensitivity to pain.

hiperacidez *f.* hyperacidity, excessive acidity.

hiperactividad *f.* hyperactivity, excessive activity; *psych.,* excessive activity manifested in children and adolescents, usu. accompanied by irritability and inability to concentrate for any length of time.

hiperalbuminosis *f.* hyperalbuminosis, excess albumin in the blood.

hiperalimentación *f.* hyperalimentation, supplemental intravenous feeding; ___ **intravenosa** / parenteral ___ .

hiperbilirrubinemia *f.* hyperbilirubinemia, excessive bilirubin in the blood.

hipercalcemia *f.* hypercalcemia, excessive amount of calcium in the blood.

hipercalemia, hiperpotasemia *f.* hyperkalemia, hyperpotasemia, abnormal elevation of potassium in the blood.

hipercapnia *f.* hypercapnia, excessive amount of carbon dioxide in the blood.

hipercinesia *f.* hyperkinesia, abnormal increase of muscular activity.

hipercloremia *f.* hyperchloremia, excess of chlorides in the blood.

hipercloridia *f.* hyperchlorhydria, excessive secretion of chloric acid in the stomach.

hipercoagulabilidad *f.* hypercoagulability, abnormal increase in the coagulability of the blood.

hipercolesterolemia *f.* hypercholesterolemia, V. **cholesteremia, cholesterolemia**.

hipercromático-a *a.* hyperchromatic, having excessive pigmentation.

hiperemesis *f.* hyperemesis, excessive vomiting.

hiperemia *f.* hyperemia, excessive blood in an organ or part.

hiperesplenismo *m.* hypersplenism, exacerbation of spleen function.

hiperestesia *f.* hyperesthesia, abnormal increased sensitivity to sensorial stimuli.

hiperflexión *f.* hyperflexion, exaggerated flexion of a limb, gen. caused by trauma.

hiperfunción *f.* hyperfunction, excessive function.

hipergammaglobulinemia *f.* hypergamma-globulinemia, excess gamma globulin in the blood.

hiperglucemia *f.* hyperglycemia, excessive amount of sugar in the blood, such as in diabetes.

hiperglucémico-a *a.* hyperglycemic, rel. to or suffering from hyperglycemia.

hiperglucosuria *f.* hyperglycosuria, excessive amount of sugar in the urine.

hiperhidratación *f.* hyperhydration, abnormal increase of water content in the body.

hiperhidrosis *f.* hyperhidrosis, excessive perspiration.

hiperinsulinismo *m.* hyperinsulinism, excessive secretion of insulin in the blood resulting in hypoglycemia.

hiperlipemia *f.* hyperlipemia, excessive amount of fat in the blood.

hiperlipidemia *f.* hyperlipidemia, excess of lipids in the blood.

hipermenorrea *f.* hypermenorrhea, heavy period, excessive and long menstruation.

hipermetropía *f.* hypermetropia, farsightedness, visual defect in which the rays of light come to focus behind the retina making distant objects better seen than closer ones.

hipermovilidad *f.* hypermobility, excessive mobility.

hipernatremia *f.* hypernatremia, excessive amount of sodium in the blood.

hipernefroma *m.* hypernephroma, Grawitz tumor, neoplasm of the renal parenchyma.

hiperopía *f.* hyperopia.hypermetropia.

hiperópico-a *a.* farsighted.

hiperorexia *f.* hyperorexia, excessive appetite.

hiperosmia *f.* hyperosmia, increased sensitivity of smell.

hiperostosis *f.* hyperostosis, excessive growth of a bony tissue.

hiperpirexia *f.* hyperpyrexia, abnormally high body temperature.

hiperpituitarismo *m.* hyperpituitarism, excessive activity of the pituitary gland.

hiperplasia *f.* hyperplasia, excessive proliferation of normal cells of tissues.

hiperpnea *f.* hyperpnea, increase in the depth and rapidity of breathing.

hiperreflexia *f.* hyperreflexia, exaggerated reflexes.

hipersalivación *f.* hypersalivation, excessive secretion of saliva.

hipersecreción *f.* hypersecretion, excessive secretion.

hipersensibilidad *f.* hypersensibility, excessive sensitivity to the effect of a stimulus or antigen.

hipertelorismo *m.* hypertelorism, excessive distance between two parts or organs.

hipertensión *f.* hypertension, high blood pressure; ___ **benigna** / benign ___; ___ **esencial** / essential ___; ___ **maligna** / malignant ___; ___ **portal** / portal ___; ___ **renal** / renal ___ .

hipertenso-a *a.* hypertensive, rel. to or suffering from hypertension.

hipertermia *f.* hyperthermia.hiperpirexia.

hipertermia maligna *f.* malignant hyperthermia, onset of high fever that can reach 106F or 41C. *Sin.* **hiperpirexia fulminante**.

hipertiroidismo *m.* hyperthyroidism, excessive activity of the thyroid gland.

hipertónico-a *a.* hypertonic, rel. to increased tonicity or tension.

hipertrofia *f.* hypertrophy, abnormal growth or development of an organ or structure; ___ **cardíaca** / cardiac ___ , enlarged heart; ___ **compensadora** / compensatory ___ , resulting from a physical defect.

hipertropía *f.* hypertropia, a form of strabismus.

hiperuricemia *f.* hyperuricemia, excessive amount of uric acid in the blood.

hiperventilación *f.* hyperventilation, extremely rapid and deep inspiration and expiration of air.

hiperviscosidad *f.* hyperviscosity, excessive viscosity.

hipnagógico-a *a.* hypnagogic. 1. that induces sleep; **estado** ___ / ___ state, between wakefulness and sleep; 2. rel. to an hallucination or daydream as sleep begins.

hipnosis *f.* hypnosis, an artificially induced passive state during which the subject is responsive to suggestion.

hipnotismo *m.* hypnotism, the practice of hypnosis.

hipnotizar *vi.* to hypnotize, to put a subject under hypnosis.

hipo *m.* hiccups, involuntary contraction of the diaphragm and the glottis.

hipoadrenalismo *m.* hypoadrenalism, condition caused by diminished activity of the adrenal gland.

hipoalbuminemia *f.* hypoalbuminemia, low level of albumin in the blood.

hipocalcemia *f.* hypocalcemia, low amount of calcium in the blood.

hipocalemia, hipopotasemia *f.* hypokalemia, hypopotassemia, deficiency of potassium in the blood.

hipocampo *m.* hippocampus, curved elevation localized in the inferior horn of the lateral ventricle of the brain.

hipocapnia *f.* hypocapnia, deficiency of carbon dioxide in the blood.

hipociclosis *f.* hypocyclosis, deficiency in eye accommodation; ___ **ciliar** / ciliary ___ , weakness of the ciliary muscle; ___ **lenticular** / lenticular ___ , rigidity of the crystalline lens.

hipocinesia *f.* hypokinesia, diminished motor movement.

hipoclorhidria *f.* hypochlorhydria, deficiency of hydrochloric acid in the stomach, which can be a manifestation of cancer or anemia.

hipocolesteremia *f.* hypocholesteremia, diminished presence of cholesterol in the blood.

hipocondria *f.* hypochondria, obsessive concern over one's mental and physical health.

hipocondríaco-a *a.* hypochondriac, rel. to or suffering from hypochondria.

hipocondrio *m.* hypochondrium, upper abdominal region on either side of the thorax.

hipocromatismo *m.* hypochromatism, lack of pigmentation, esp. in the cell nucleus.

hipocromía *f.* hypochromia, abnormally pale erythrocytes.

hipocrómico-a *a.* hypochromic, rel. to hypochromia.

hipodérmico-a *a.* hypodermic, beneath the skin.

hipofaringe *f.* hypopharynx, portion of the pharynx situated under the upper edge of the epiglottis.

hipofibrinogenemia *f.* hypofibrinogenemia, low content of fibrinogen in the blood.

hipofisectomía *f.* hypophysectomy, removal of the pituitary gland.

hipófisis *f.* hypophysis, pituitary gland, epithelial body situated at the base of the sella turcica.

hipofunción *f.* hypofunction, deficiency in the function of an organ.

hipogammaglobulinemia *f.* hypogammaglobulinemia, low level of gamma globulin in the blood; ___ **adquirida** / acquired ___ , manifested after infancy.

hipogastrio *m.* hypogastrium, anterior, middle and inferior portion of the abdomen.

hipoglicemia, hipoglucemia *f.* hypoglycemia, abnormally low level of glucose in the blood.

hipoglicémico-a, hipoglucémico-a *a.* hypoglycemic, rel. to or that produces hypoglycemia.

hipoglosal *a.* hypoglossal, rel. to the hyoid bone and the tongue.

hipogloso *m.* hypoglossus, muscle of the tongue that has retractive and lateral action; hypoglossal nerve; *-a a.* hypoglossal, beneath the tongue.

hipoinsulinismo *m.* hypoinsulinism, deficient insulin secretion in the blood. diabetes mellitus.

hipolipoproteinemia *f.* hypolipoproteinemia, increase in the lipoprotein of the blood.

hipomanía *f.* hypomania, moderate form of manic-depressive illness.

hiponatremia *f.* hyponatremia, sodium deficiency in the blood.

hipopituitarismo *m.* hypopituitarism, pathological condition due to diminished secretion of the pituitary gland.

hipoplasia *f.* hypoplasia, defective, or incomplete development of an organ or tissue.

hipoplástico-a *a.* hypoplastic, rel. to or suffering from hypoplasia.

hiporreflexia *f.* hyporeflexia, weak reflexes.

hipospadias *m., f.* hypospadias, congenital anomaly by which the wall of the urethra remains open in different degrees in the undersurface of the penis. In the female the urethra opens into the vagina.

hipotálamo *m.* hypothalamus, portion of the diencephalon situated beneath the thalamus at the base of the cerebrum.

hipotensión *f.* hypotension, low blood pressure.

hipotenso-a *a.* hypotensive, rel. to or suffering from low blood pressure.

hipotermia *f.* hypothermia, low body temperature.

hipótesis *f.* hypothesis, a proposition to be proven by experimentation; ___ **nula** / null ___ .

hipotiroideo-a *a.* hypothyroid, rel. to or suffering from hypothyroidism.

hipotiroidismo *m.* hypothyroidism, condition due to a deficiency in the production of thyroxin.

hipotónico-a *a.* hypotonic. 1. rel. to a deficiency in muscular tonicity; 2. having a lower osmotic pressure as compared to another element.

hipotrombinemia *f.* hypothrombinemia, deficiency of thrombin in the blood, which can cause a propensity to bleed.

hipoventilación *f.* hypoventilation, reduction of air entering the alveoli.

hipovolemia *f.* hypovolemia, decreased volume of blood in the body.

hipoxemia, hipoxia *f.* hypoxemia, hypoxia, diminished availability of oxygen to the blood.

hirviente *a.* boiling; **agua** ___ / ___ water.

hispano-a *m., f.* Hispanic person; *a.* Hispanic.

hispanoamericano-a *m., f.* Spanish-American person, latinoamerican; *a.* Hispanic.

histamina *f.* histamine, substance that acts as a dilator of blood vessels and stimulates gastric secretion.

histerectomía *f.* hysterectomy, partial or total removal of the uterus; ___ **abdominal** / abdominal ___ , through the abdomen; ___ **total** / total ___ , removal of the uterus and the cervix; ___ **vaginal** / vaginal ___ , through the vagina.

histerectomía abdominal completa *f.* total abdominal hysterectomy.

histeria *f.* hysteria, extreme neurosis.

histérico-a *a.* hysteric, hysterical, rel. to or suffering from hysteria.

histerismo *m.* hysterics, hysteria.

histerosalpingografía *f.* hysterosalpingography, x-ray of the uterus and fallopian tubes after injecting a radiopaque substance.

histerosalpingooforectomía *f.* hysterosalpingoophorectomy, excision of the uterus, ovaries, and oviducts.

histeroscopía *f.* hysteroscopy, endoscopic examination of the uterine cavity.

histeroscopio *m.* hysteroscope, endoscope used in the examination of the uterine cavity.

histerotomía *f.* hysterotomy, incision of the uterus.

histidina *f.* histidine, amino acid essential in the growth and restoration of tissue.

histiocito *m.* histiocyte, large interstitial phagocytic cell of the reticuloendothelial system.

histocompatibilidad *f.* histocompatibility, state in which the tissues of a donor are accepted by the receiver; **complejo de** ___ **mayor** / major ___ complex.

histología *f.* histology, study of organic tissues.

histólogo-a *m., f.* histologist, specialist in histology.

histoplasmina *f.* histoplasmin, substance used in the cutaneous test for histoplasmosis.

histoplasmosis *f.* histoplasmosis, respiratory disease caused by the fungus *Histoplasma capsulatum.*

histriónico-a *a.* histrionic, dramatic.

Hodgkin, enfermedad de *f.* Hodgkin's disease, malignant tumors in the lymph nodes and the spleen.

hogar *m.* home.

hoja *f.* leaf; [*de papel o metal*] sheet; ___ **clínica** / medical chart.

hola *int.* hi, hello.

holgazán-a *m., f.* lazy person, loafer; *a.* lazy.

holístico-a *a.* holistic, rel. to a whole or unit.

holocrino-a *a.* holocrine, rel. to the sweat glands.

holodiastólico-a *a.* holodiastolic, rel. to a complete diastole.

holografía *f.* holography, tridimensional representation of a figure by means of a photographic image.

holograma *m.* hologram, production of a holography.

holosistólico-a *a.* holosystolic, rel. to a complete systole.

hombre *m.* man, male.

hombro *m.* shoulder, the union of the clavicle, the scapula, and the humerus.

homeopatía *f.* homeopathy, cure by means of administering medication diluted in minute doses that are capable of producing symptoms of the disease being treated.

homeopático-a *a.* homeopathic, rel. to homeopathy.

homicidio *m.* homicide; ___ **sin premeditación** / manslaughter.

homocigótico-a *a.* homozygotic, homozygous, rel. to twins that develop from gametes with similar alleles in regard to one or all characters.

homofobia *f.* homophobia, fear of or revulsion regarding homosexuals.

homofóbico-a *a.* fearful of or having an aversion to homosexuals.

homogéneo-a *a.* homogeneous, similar in nature.

homoinjerto *m.* homograft, transplant from a subject of the same species or type.

homólogo-a *a.* homologous, similar in structure and origin but not in function.

homosexual *a.* homosexual, sexually attracted to persons of the same sex.

homotónico-a *a.* homotonic, having the same tension.

homotopico-a *a.* homotopic, rel. to or occurring in the same corresponding parts.

homúnculo-a *m., f.* homunculus, dwarf with no deformities and with proportionate parts of the body.

hondo-a *a.* deep.

honesto-a, honrado-a *a.* honest.

hongo *m.* fungus; mushroom; ___ **venenoso /** toadstool.

honorario *m.* fee, charges; ___ **-s razonables /** reasonable charges.

hora *f.* hour, time; **a cada___ /** hourly; ___ **de acostarse /** bedtime; **¿qué ___ es? /** what time is it?; **a qué ___ /** at what time?

horario *m.* schedule; timetable.

horizontal *a.* horizontal, parallel to the floor.

hormiga *f.* ant.

hormigueo *m.* tingling sensation.

hormona *f.* hormone, natural chemical substance in the body that produces or stimulates the activity of an organ; ___ **del crecimiento /** growth ___; ___ **estimulante /** stimulating ___ .

hormona eritropoyética *f.* erythropoietic hormone, any protein hormone that participates in the formation of erythrocytes.

hormona luteinizante *f.* luteinizing hormone produced by the anterior pituitary gland. It stimulates the secretion of sex hormones by the testis (testosterone) and the ovaries (progesterone) and also acts in the formation of sperm and ova.

hormona paratiroidea *f.* parathormone, parathyroid hormone, a hormone that regulates calcium in the body.

hormonal *a.* hormonal, rel. to or acting like a hormone; **receptor ___ /** hormone ___; **terapia ___ /** hormone therapy.

hornear *v.* to bake.

Horner, síndrome de *m.* Horner's syndrome, sinking of the eyeball with accompanying eye and facial disorders due to paralysis of the cervical sympathetic nerve.

horno *m.* oven.

horquilla *f.* fourchette, posterior junction of the vulva.

horrible *a.* horrible; abominable, hideous.

hospedar *v.* to host; to lodge.

hospicio *m.* hospice, nursing facility.

hospital *m.* hospital.

hospitalizacion *f.* hospitalization.

hospitalizar *vi.* to hospitalize.

hostil *a.* hostile, unfriendly.

hostilidad *f.* hostility, animosity.

hotel *m.* hotel.

hoy *adv.* today; **de ___ en adelante /** from now on; ___ **en dia /** nowadays.

hoyo *m.* pit, hole.

hoyuelo *m.* dimple, dimple sign; small hole.

hueco *m.* depression, socket; hole; **-a /** *a.* hollow.

huella *f.* impression; print; ___ **-s dactilares /** fingerprints; ___ **del pie /** footprint.

huérfano-a *m., f.* orphan.

huesecillo *m.* bonelet.

hueso *m.* bone; ___ **compacto /** hard ___; ___ **esponjoso /** spongy ___; ___ **quebrado /** fractured ___ .

huésped *m.* [*parasito*] host; **defensas del ___ /** defenses; guest.

Huésped definitivo *m.* definitive host.

huesudo-a *a.* bony.

huevo *m.* egg, ovum, female sexual cell; **cáscara de ___ /** eggshell; **clara de ___ /** ___ white; ___ **duro /** hard-boiled ; ___ **frito /** fried ___; ___ **pasado por agua /** soft-boiled ___; **yema de ___ /** ___ yolk.

humanidad *f.* humanity.

humano-a *a.* human; humane; rel. to humanity.

humear *v.* to fume; to emit vapor or gas.

humectante *m.* humidifier, device that controls and maintains humidity in the air within a given area.

humedad *f.* humidity.

humedecer *v.* to moisten, to dampen.

húmedo-a *a.* humid, damp.

húmero *m.* humerus, long bone of the upper arm.

humo *m.* smoke.

humor *m.* humor. 1. any liquid form in the body; ___ **acuoso /** aqueous ___ , clear fluid in the eye chambers; ___ **cristalino /** crystalline ___ , substance that constitutes the lens of the eye; ___ **vítreo /** vitreous ___ , clear, semifluid substance between the lens and the retina; 2. secretion; 3. disposition, mood; **buen ___ /** good ___; **estar de buen ___ /** to be in a good ___; **estar de mal ___ /** to be in a bad mood; **mal ___ /** bad ___ .

humoral *a.* humoral, rel. to the body fluids.

hundido-a *a.* sunken.

Hunt, neuralgia de *f.* Hunt's neuralgia or syndrome. V. **neuralgia.**

Huntington, corea de *f.* Huntington's chorea.corea.

huso *m.* spindle. 1. structure or cell shaped like a round pin with tapered ends; 2. achromatic arrangements of chromosomes in the nuclear cell during mitosis and meiosis.

huy! *int.* ouch!

i

I *abr.* **iodo, yodo** / iodine.

iátrico-a *a.* iatric, rel. to medicine, the medical profession, or physicians.

iatrogénico-a, iatrógeno-a *a.* iatrogenic. yatrogénico, yatrógeno; **pneumotórax** ___ / ___ pneumothorax; **transmisión** ___ / ___ transmission.

ibuprofen *m.* ibuprofen, anti-inflammatory, antipyretic, and analgesic agent used in the treatment of rheumatoid arthritis.

ictericia *f.* jaundice, disorder caused by excessive bilirubin in the blood and manifested by a yellow-orange coloring of the skin and other tissues and fluids of the body; ___ **del neonato** / icterus gravis neonatorum.

ictérico-a *a.* icteric, jaundiced, or rel. to jaundice.

icterogénico-a *a.* icterogenic, agent that causes jaundice.

icterohepatitis *f.* icterohepatitis, hepatitis associated with jaundice.

icterus *L.* icterus. V. **ictericia.**

ictiosis *f.* ichthyosis, dry and scaly skin.

ictus *L.* ictus, sudden attack.

id *m.* id. 1. name given by Freud to the real unconscious where tendencies of autopreservation and instincts reside; 2. in psychiatry, one of the three divisions of the psyche; 3. -id, suffix denoting secondary eruptions of the skin that appear in areas away from the primary infection.

idea *f.* idea, concept, thought; ___ **fija** / fixed ___ , idée fixe.

ideación *f.* ideation, process by which ideas are formed; ___ **paranoide** / paranoid ___ .

ideal *a.* ideal.

idem *L.* idem, the same.

idéntico-a *a.* 1. identical, same; 2. rel. to twins that result from the fertilization of only one ovum.

identidad *f.* identity, self-recognition.

identificación *f.* identification, unconscious process of identifying oneself with another person or group and assuming its characteristics.

identificar *vi.* to identify.

ideocracia *f.* ideocracy, tendency to submit oneself to certain habits and drugs.

ideología *f.* ideology, a set of concepts and ideas.

ideomoción *f.* ideomotion, muscular activity directed by a prevailing idea.

idiograma *f.* idiogram, graphic representation of the chromosomes of a given cell.

idioma *m.* language.

idiopatía *f.* idiopathy, disease or morbid state of unknown origin.

idiopático-a *a.* 1. rel. to idiopathy; 2. of a spontaneous nature. **aldosteronismo** ___ / ___ aldosteronism; **fibrosis pulmonar** ___ / ___ pulmonary fibrosis; **estenosis subglótica** ___ / ___ subglottic stenosis; **hipercalcemia** ___ **de los niños** / ___ hypercalcemia of children; **neuralgia** ___ / ___ neuralgia.

idiosincracia *f.* idiosyncrasy. 1. set of individual characteristics; 2. an individual's own reaction to a given action, idea, medication, treatment or food.

idiota *m., f.* idiot, fool.

idiotez *f.* idiocy, mental deficiency.

idiotrópico-a *a.* idiotropic.egocéntrico.

idioventricular *a.* idioventricular, rel. to that which affects ventricles only.

ido-a *a.* absentminded, distracted.

ignorante *a.* ignorant.

ignorar *v.* to ignore.

igual *a.* equal, even, same; **-mente** *adv.* equally.

igualar *v.* to equate.

ileal *a.* ileal, rel. to the ileum; **arterias** ___ -es / ___ arteries; **orificio** ___ / ___ orifice; **uréter** ___ / ___ ureter; **venas** ___ -es / ___ veins.

ileectomía *f.* ileectomy, total or partial surgical removal of the ileum.

ilegal *a.* illegal, illicit.

ilegítimo-a *a.* illegitimate, bastard.

ileítis *f.* ileitis, infl. of the ileum; ___ **regional** / regional ___ .

ileocecal *a.* ileocecal, rel. to the ileum and the cecum; **válvula** ___ / ___ valve.

ileocecostomía *f.* ileocecostomy, surgical anastomosis of the ileum to the cecum.

ileocistoplastia *f.* ileocystoplasty, anastomosis of a segment of the ileum to the bladder in order to increase the bladder's capacity.

ileocolitis *f.* ileocolitis, infl. of the mucous membrane of the ileum and the colon.

ileocolostomía *f.* ileocolostomy, surgical anastomosis from the ileum to the colon.

íleon *m.* ileum, distal portion of the small intestine extending from the jejunum to the cecum; **desviación quirúrgica del** ___ / ileal bypass.

ileoproctostomía *f.* ileoproctostomy, anastomosis of the ileum and the rectum.

ileosigmoidostomía *f.* ileosigmoidostomy, anastomosis of the ileum and the sigmoid colon.

ileostomía *f.* ileostomy, anastomosis of the ileum and the anterior abdominal wall.

ileotransversostomía *f.* ileotransversostomy, anastomosis of the ileum and the transverse colon.

ilíaco-a *a.* iliac, rel. to the ilium; **colon** ___ / ___ colon; **cresta** ___ / ___ crest; **hueso** ___ / ___ bone; **músculo** ___ / ___ muscle.

ilimitado-a *a.* unlimited, boundless.

iliofemoral *a.* iliofemoral, rel. to the ilium and the femur.

iliohipogástrico-a *a.* iliohypogastric, rel. to the ilium and the hypogastrium.

ilioinguinal *a.* ilioinguinal, rel. to the iliac and inguinal regions.

iliolumbar *a.* iliolumbar, rel. to the iliac and lumbar regions; **arteria** ___ / ___ artery; **vena** ___ / ___ vein.

ilión *m.* ilium, hip bone.

Ilizarov, técnica de *f.* Ilizarov technique, technique for enlarging the bone and correcting the angular and rotating deformities by cutting the exterior layer of the bone without entering the medullary cavity.

iluminación *f.* illumination; ___ **lateral o indirecta del campo oscuro** / lateral or indirect dark field ___ .

ilusión *f.* illusion, false interpretation of sensory impressions.

iluso-a *a.* deluded.

ilusorio-a *a.* illusory, illusional or rel. to an illusion.

ilustración *f.* illustration, graph.

imagen *f.* image; ___ **de espejo** / mirror ___; ___ **del cuerpo** / body ___; ___ **directa** / direct ___; ___ **doble** / double ___; ___ **eléctrica** / electric ___; ___ **invertida** / inverted ___; ___ **latente** / latent ___; ___ **óptica** / optic ___; ___ **radiográfica** / radiographic ___; ___ **real** / real ___ .

imagen virtual *f.* virtual image.

imágenes por resonancia magnética *f. pl.* magnetic resonance imaging, procedure based in the quantitative analysis of the chemical and biological structure of a tissue.

imágenes por ultrasonido *f. pl.* ultrasound imaging, creation of images of organs or tissues through the use of reflex techniques (echogram).

imaginar *v.* to imagine.

imaginario-a *a.* imaginary, illusory; unreal.

imán *m.* magnet, a body that has the property of attracting iron.

imbécil *m., f.* imbecile. *a.* imbecilic, stupid.

imbibición *f.* imbibition, absorption of a liquid.

imbricado-a *a.* imbricate, imbricated, in layers.

imitación *f.* imitation.

imitar *v.* to imitate.

impacción *f.* impaction. 1. the condition of being lodged or wedged within a given space; 2. impediment of an organ or part.

impacientarse *vr.* to become impatient.

impaciente *a.* impatient.

impactado-a *a.* impacted; **diente** ___ / ___ tooth.

impalpable *a.* impalpable, incorporeal, intangible.

impedimento *m.* impediment; handicap; obstacle.

impedir *vi.* to impede, to prevent; to impair.

impenetrable *a.* impenetrable.

imperativo *m.* rupturing *gr.* imperative mood; *a. -a* imperative.

imperdible *m.* safety pin.

imperfección *f.* imperfection; defect.

imperfecto-a *m., gr.* past tense; *a.* imperfect; defective.

imperforado-a *a.* imperforate, abnormally closed; **himen** ___ / ___ hymen.

impermeable *a.* impermeable, not allowing passage, such as fluids; waterproof.

impersonal *a.* impersonal.

impétigo *m.* impetigo, bacterial skin infection marked by vesicles that become pustular and form a yellow crust on rupturing; ___ **contagioso** / ___ contagious; ___ **del nenonato** / ___ neonatorum; ___ **vulgar** / ___ vulgaris.

ímpetu *m.* impetus, impulse.

impetuoso-a *a.* impetuous, violent.

implacable *a.* implacable, not able to be appeased.

implantación *f.* implantation, insertion and fixation of a part or tissue in an area of the body.

implantar *v.* to implant; to insert.

implante *m.* implant, any material inserted or grafted into the body.

implementación *f.* implementation.

implicación *f.* implication.

implicar *vi.* to imply.

implosión *f.* implosion. 1. violent collapse inward as it occurs in the evacuation of a vessel; 2. method to treat a fear caused by a phobia.

imponer *vi.* to impose; to tax; **imponerse** *vr.* to prevail.

importancia *n.* importance, significance; **sin** ___ / of no significance.

importante *a.* important.

importar *v.* to matter.

imposible *a.* impossible.

impotencia *f.* impotence, inability to have or maintain an erection.

impotente *a.* impotent, rel. to or suffering from impotence.

impráctico-a *a.* impractical.

impregnar *v.* to impregnate; to saturate.

imprescindible *a.* indispensable.

impresión *f.* 1. surface track; 2. an effect upon the mind by external stimuli; 3. copy of the configuration of part or the totality of the dental arch, individual teeth or cavity preparation for the purpose of dental restoration.

impresionante *a.* impressive.

imprevisto-a *a.* unexpected, unforeseen.

improbable *a.* improbable, unlikely.

improvisado-a *a.* improvised.

improvisar *v.* to improvise.

impúbero-a *a.* below the age of puberty.

impuesto *m.* tax; **exempto de** ___ / ___ exempt, free of ___ .

impular *v.* to impel; to accelerate.

impulsivo-a *a.* impulsive; driven.

impulso *m.* drive, thrust; sudden pushing force; ___ **cardíaco** / cardiac ___; ___ **excitante** / excitatory ___; ___ **inhibitorio** / inhibitory ___; ___ **nervioso** / nervous ___; ___ **vital** / élan vital.

impuro-a *a.* impure, contaminated, adulterated.

inaccesible *a.* inaccessible.

inacción *f.* inaction, failure to respond to a stimulus.

inaceptable *a.* unacceptable.

inactividad *f.* inactivity; ___ **física** / physical ___ .

inactivo-a *a.* inactive, passive; in a state of rest.

inadaptado-a *a.* maladjusted, unable to adjust to the environment or to endure stress.

inadecuado-a *a.* inadequate.

inanición *f.* inanition, starvation, hunger.

inanimado-a *a.* inanimate, without animation, lacking life.

inarticulado-a *a.* inarticulate. 1. unable to articulate words or syllables; 2. disjointed.

in articulo mortis *L.* in articulo mortis, at the moment of death.

incandescente *a.* incandescent, glowing with light.

incansable *a.* tireless, untiring.

incapacitado-a *a.* disabled; unable.

incapaz *a.* incapable, unable.

incendio *m.* fire.

incentivo *m.* incentive.

incertidumbre *f.* uncertainty.

incesante *a.* incessant; continuous.

incesto *m.* incest.

incestuoso-a *a.* incestuous.

incidencia *f.* incidence.

incidental *a.* incidental.

incinerar *v.* to incinerate; to cremate.

incipiente *a.* incipient, just coming into existence.

incisión *f.* incision; surgical cut.

incisura *f.* slit; notch.

inclinación *f.* slant, slope, tilt; inclination, predisposition.

inclinado-a *a.* inclined.

incluído *a.* included; enclosed.

incluir *vi.* to include; to embed, to surround a tissue specimen in a firm medium to keep intact in preparation for cutting sections for examination.

inclusión *f.* inclusion, the act of enclosing one thing in another; **cuerpos de** ___ / ___ bodies, present in the cytoplasm of some cells in cases of infection;

incoherencia *f.* incoherence, lack of coordination of ideas.

incoherente *a.* incoherent.

incoloro-a *a.* colorless; achromatic.

incomodar *v.* to disturb, to annoy.

incómodo-a *a.* uncomfortable; annoyed.

incompatibilidad *f.* incompatibility.

incompatible *a.* incompatible.

incompetente *a.* incompetent.

incompleto-a *a.* incomplete, unfinished.

inconsciencia *f.* unconsciousness, impaired consciousness or the loss of it; unawareness.

inconsciente *a.* unconscious. 1. that has lost consciousness; 2. that does not respond to sensorial stimuli.

inconsistencia *f.* inconsistency.

inconsistente *a.* inconsistent.

incontinencia *f.* incontinence, inability to control the emission or expulsion of urine or feces; ___ **fecal** / fecal ___; ___ **intestinal** / bowel ___; ___ **por rebozamiento** / ___ overflow; ___ **por reflejo** / reflex ___; ___ **urinaria** / urinary ___; ___ **urinaria de esfuerzo** / ___ urinary stress.

incontinente *a.* incontinent, rel. to incontinence.

inconveniencia *f.* inconvenience, hardship.
inconveniente *m.* difficulty, obstacle; *a.* inconvenient.
incorporar *v.* to incorporate, to include.
incorrecto-a *a.* incorrect, inaccurate; **acción** ___ / improper action.
incredulidad *f.* disbelief, skepticism.
incremento *m.* increment.
incresión *f.* incretion, internal or endocrine secretion.
incrustación *f.* 1. incrustation, formation of a crust or scab; 2. inlay.
incubación *f.* incubation.1. latent period of a disease before its manifestation; **período de** ___ / ___ period; 2. care of a premature infant in an incubator.
incubadora *f.* incubator, device used to keep optimal conditions of temperature and humidity, esp. in the care of premature infants.
incudectomía *f.* incudectomy, excision of the incus.
incurable *a.* incurable, not subject to healing.
incus *L.* incus, small bone of the middle ear.
indeciso-a *a.* undecided, undecisive, hesitant.
indefinido-a *a.* indefinite, undefined.
independiente *a.* independent, self-sufficient.
indeseable *a.* undesirable.
indeterminado-a *a.* undetermined; undefined.
indicación *f.* indication; suggestion; hint.
indicado-a *a.* indicated; appropriate.
indicador *m.* marker, indicator.
indicar *vi.* to indicate; to point out.
índice *m.* rate, index; mean; ___ **de aborto** / abortion ___; ___ **de edad específica** / age specific ___; ___ **de letalidad de casos** / case fatality ___; ___ **de mortalidad, de mortandad** / death ___; ___ **de mortinatalidad** / birth-death rate; ___ **de natalidad** / birth ___; ___ **de natalidad cero** / zero population growth; ___ **de reproducción** / gross reproduction ___; ___ **medio (de)** / average flow ___ .
indiferenciación *f.* undifferentiation.anaphasia.
indiferente *a.* indifferent.
indiferención *f.* undifferentiation.
indígena *m., f.* native, aboriginal; *a.* indigenous.
indigestarse *vr.* to suffer from indigestion.
indigestión *f.* indigestion, maldigestion.
indirecto-a *a.* indirect; **bilirubina reactiva** ___ / ___ reacting bilirubin; **division nuclear** ___ / ___ nuclear division; **fractura** ___ / ___ fracture; **inmunoflorescencia** ___ / ___

immunofluorescence; **laringoscopía** ___ / ___ laryngoscopy; **prueba de hemaglutinación** ___ / ___ hemagglutination test; **transfusión** ___ / ___ transfusion; **visión** ___ / ___ vision.
indispensable *a.* indispensable, necessary.
indisponer *vi.* to indispose; to make ill.
indispuesto-a *a. pp. de* **indisponer,** indisposed, ill; upset.
individual *a.* individual.
individualidad *f.* individuality.
individuo *m.* individual, person; fellow.
inducido-a *a.* induced.
inducir *vi.* to induce; to force; to provoke.
induración *f.* induration, the process of hardening such as it happens to soft tissues as with the mucous membranes.
ineficiente *a.* inefficient, ineffective.
inercia *f.* inertia, stillness; lack of activity.
inerte *a.* inert, rel. to inertia.
inervación *f.* innervation, distribution of nerves or nervous energy in an organ or area.
inervar *v.* to innervate, to stimulate a nerve.
inesperado-a *a.* unexpected, occurring without warning.
inestabilidad *f.* instability.
inestable *a.* unstable, fluctuating; **angina** ___ / ___ angina; **vejiga** ___ / ___ bladder.
inevitable *a.* inevitable, unavoidable.
inexperiencia *f.* inexperience.
infancia *f.* infancy, period of time from birth to one or two years of age; early age.
infantil *a.* 1. rel. to infancy; 2. childish; **acropustulosis** ___ / ___ acropustulosis; **atrofia muscular espinal** ___ / ___ spinal muscular atrophy; **autismo** ___ / ___ autism; **conjuntivitis purulenta** ___ / ___ purulent conjunctivitis; **eczema** ___ / ___ eczema; **escorbuto** ___ / ___ scurvy; **hipotiroidismo** ___ / ___ hypothyroidism; **osteomalacia** ___ / ___ osteomalacia.
infantilismo *m.* infantilism, infantile characteristics carried into adult life.
infarto *m.* infarct, infarction, necrosis of a tissue area due to a lack of blood supply; ___ **blando** / bland ___; ___ **cardíaco** / myocardial ___; ___ **cerebral** / cerebral ___; ___ **hemorrágico** / hemorrhagic ___; ___ **pulmonar** / pulmonary ___ .
infección *f.* infection, invasion of the body by pathogenic microorganisms and the reaction of

Infección	Infection
aerógena	airborne
aguda	acute
contagiosa	contagious
crónica	chronic
de hongos	fungus
hidrica	waterborne
hospitalaria	cross
inicial o primaria	initial or primary
intrahospitalaria	hospital acquired
masiva	massive
piógena	pyogenic
secundaria	secondary
sistémica	systemic
subclínica	subclinical

tissue to their presence and effect; ___ **inicial o primaria** / initial or primary ___; ___ **intrahospitalaria** / hospital acquired ___ .

infección oportunista *f.* opportunistic infection, caused by an organism, gen. harmless, that can become pathogenic when resistance to disease is impaired, such as occurs in AIDS.

infeccioso-a *a.* infectious, rel. to an infection; **agente** ___ / ___ agent; **enfermedad** ___ / ___ disease.

infectado-a *a.* infected.

infectar *v.* to infect; **infectarse** *vr.* to become infected.

infectivo-a *a.* infectious.

infecundarse *vr.* to become sterile.

infecundidad *f.* infecundity, sterility.

infecundo-a *a.* sterile; barren.

infeliz *a.* unhappy.

inferior *a.* inferior, lower; **esfínter esofágico** ___ / lower esophageal sphincter; **extremidad** ___ / lower extremity.

inferir *vi.* to infer, to surmise.

infertilidad *f.* infertility, inability to conceive or procreate.

infestación *f.* infestation, invasion of the body by parasites.

infibulación *f.* infibulation, female circumcision.

infiltración *f.* infiltration, the accumulation of foreign substances in a tissue, organ, or cell.

infiltrar *v.* to infiltrate, to penetrate.

inflación *f.* inflation, distension.

inflamación *f.* inflammation, reaction of a tissue to injury.

inflamarse *vr.* to become inflamed.

inflamatorio-a *a.* inflammatory, rel. to inflammation; **enfermedad** ___ **de los intestinos** / ___ bowel disease.

inflexible *a.* inflexible.

inflexión *f.* inflection, inflexion, the act of bending inward.

influencia *f.* influence.

influenza *f.* influenza, acute contagious viral infection of the respiratory tract.

influjo *m.* influx.

información *f.* information.

informar *v.* to inform; **informarse** *vr.* to become informed.

informe *m.* report; account.

informe de consentimiento *m.* informed consent.

infraclavicular *a.* infraclavicular, under the clavicle.

infradiafragmático-a *a.* infradiaphragmatic, under the diaphragm.

infraescapular *a.* infrascapular, situated below the scapula.

infraorbitario *a.* infraorbital, situated under the floor of the orbit.

infrarrojo-a *a.* infrared; **rayos** ___ **-s** / ___ rays.

infrecuente *a.* infrequent.

infundíbulo *m.* infundibulum, funnel-like structure. 1. structure shaped like a funnel; 2. any one of the divisions of the renal pelvis; 3. short extension of the right ventricle from which the pulmonary artery begins.

infusión *f.* infusion. 1. slow gravitational introduction of fluid into a vein; 2. the steeping of an element in water to obtain its soluble active principles.

ingerir *vi.* to ingest, to take in.

ingesta *f.* ingesta, ingestant; oral feeding.

ingestión *f.* ingestion, the amount of liquids and substances taken into the body by mouth or parenterally; ___ **calórica** / caloric ___ .

ingle *f.* groin.

inglés *m.* [*idioma*] English; inglés *m.*, *f.* inglesa *f.* [*nativo*] English; *a.* English.

ingravidez *f.* weightlessness.

ingrávido-a *a.* weightless.

ingrediente *m.* ingredient, component.

ingresar *v.* [*en un hospital*] to be admitted.

ingreso *m.* income; *v.* **dar** ___ / to admit.

inguinal *a.* inguinal, rel. to the groin; **anillo** ___ / ___ ring; **canal** ___ / ___ canal;

hernia ___ / ___ hernia; **ligamento** ___ / ___ ligament.

ingurgitado-a *a.* engorged, distended by excess fluid.

inhábil *a.* unfit.

inhabilidad *f.* inability, incapacity.

inhabilidad de desarrollo *f.* developmental disability, loss or impairment of an acquired function due to pre- or postnatal events, such as the acquisition of language, a social or motor skill.

inhalación *f.* inhalation, aspiration; the act of drawing air or other vapor into the lungs; ___ **de humo** / smoke ___ .

inhalación pasiva de humo *f.* passive smoking, the act of inhaling smoke that comes from a person smoking nearby.

inhalante *m.* inhalant, medication administered by inhalation.

inhalar *v.* to inhale, to draw in air or vapor.

inherente *a.* inherent, innate, natural to an individual or thing.

inhibición *f.* inhibition, interruption or restriction of a process.

inhibidor *m.* inhibitor, agent that causes inhibition; ___ **de fusión** / fusion ___ .

inhibir *v.* to inhibit; *vr.* **inhibirse** to restrain from.

inicial *a.* initial.

iniciar *v.* to initiate, to start.

inicio *m.* beginning, start.

injertable *a.* graftable.

injertar *v.* to graft, to implant.

injerto *m.* graft, implant, inlay, any tissue or organ used for transplanation or implantation; ___ **alogénico** / allogenic ___ , taken from a genetically nonidentical donor; ___ **autógeno, autoinjerto** / autogenous ___ , taken from the same patient; ___ **cutáneo** / skin ___ , as in burns; ___ **cutáneo de capa gruesa partida** / thick-split ___ , thick layer of skin used to cover a bare area; ___ **de derivación** / bypass ___; ___ **dermoepidérmico** / full thickness ___ , entire layer of the skin without the subcutaneous fat; ___ **óseo** / bone ___; **rechazo de** ___ / ___ rejection. *V.* cuadro en ;a página 398.

inmaduro-a *a.* immature.

inmediato-a *a.* immediate, close; *adv.* **-mente;** immediately.

inmersión *f.* immersion, submersion of a body in a liquid.

inmigrante *m., f.* immigrant.

inminente *a.* imminent, about to happen.

inmoderado-a *a.* immoderate, without moderation.

inmoral *a.* immoral, corrupt.

inmóvil *a.* immobile, motionless.

inmovilización *f.* immobilization.

inmovilizar *vi.* to immobilize.

inmundicia *f.* filth, dirt; garbage.

inmune *a.* immune, resistant to contracting a specific disease; **adherencia** ___ / ___ adherence; **adsorción** ___ / ___ adsorption; **complejo** ___ / ___ complex; **parálisis** ___ / ___ parálisis; **respuesta** ___ / ___ response.

inmunidad *f.* immunity. 1. condition of the organism to resist a particular antigen by activating specific antibodies; 2. resistance to contracting a specific disease; ___ **activa** / active ___; ___ **adoptiva** / adoptive ___; ___ **adquirida** / acquired ___; ___ **antivírica** / antiviral ___; ___ **antiviral** / antiviral ___; ___ **artificial** / artificial ___; ___ **bacteriófaga** / bacteriophage ___; ___ **concomitante** / concomitant ___; ___ **de grupo** / group ___; ___ **general** / general ___; ___ **innata** / innate ___; ___ **maternal** / maternal ___; ___ **nata** / inborn ___; ___ **natural** / natural ___; ___ **pasiva** / passive ___ .

inmunización *f.* immunization, making the organism immune to a given disease. *V.* cuadro en ;a página 417.

inmunizar *vi.* to immunize.

inmunoanálisis *m.* immunoassay, the process of identifying a substance by its capacity to act as an antigen and antibody in a tissue; ___ **enzimático** / enzyme ___ .

inmunocito *m.* immunocyte.linfocito.

inmunocompetencia *f.* immunocompetency, the process of becoming immune following exposure to an antigen.

inmunocomprometido-a *a.* immunocompromised, rel. to a person with a deficient immunologic system.

inmunodeficiencia *f.* immunodeficiency, inadequate cellular immunity reaction that diminishes the ability to respond to antigenic stimuli; **enfermedad grave de** ___ **combinada** / severe combined ___ disease.

inmunoelectroforesis *f.* immunoelectrophoresis, the use of electrophoresis as a technique of finding the amount and type of proteins and antibodies in body fluids.

inmunoestimulante *m.* immunostimulant, agent that can stimulate an immune response.

inmunofluorescencia *f.* immunofluorescence, method that uses antibodies labeled with fluorescein to locate antigen in tissues.

inmunógeno *m.* immunogen, stimulator that produces an antibody; *a.* immunogenic; that produces immunity; ___ **específico** / targeted ___ .

inmunoglobulina *f.* immunoglobulin. 1. one of a group of proteins of animal origin that participates in the immune reaction; 2. one of the five types of gamma globulin capable of acting as an antibody.

inmunología *f.* immunology, the study of the body's response to bacteria, virus, or any other foreign invasion, such as transplanted tissue or organ.

inmunológico-a *a.* immunologic, rel. to immunology; **competencia** ___ / ___ competence; **deficiencia** ___ / ___ deficiency; **mecanismo** ___ / ___ mechanism; **parálisis** ___ / ___ paralysis; **prueba** ___ **del embarazo** / ___ pregnancy test; **realce** ___ / ___ enhancement; **respuesta o reacción** ___ / immune response; **tolerancia** ___ / ___ tolerance.

inmunólogo-a *m., f.* immunologist, specialist in immunology.

inmunoproteína *f.* immunoprotein, protein that acts as an antibody.

inmunoquimioterapia *f.* immunochemotherapy, combined process of immunotherapy and chemotherapy used in the treatment of some malignant tumors.

inmunoreacción *f.* immunoreaction, immune reaction between antigens and antibodies.

inmunosupresivo *m.* immunosuppressant, agent capable of suppressing an immune response.

inmunoterapia *f.* immunotherapy, prevention or treatment of a disease using passive immunization of agents such as serum or gamma globulin.

innato-a *a.* inborn; congenital; ingrown.

innecesario-a *a.* unnecessary.

inocente *a.* innocent.

inoculable *a.* inoculable, that can be transmitted by inoculation.

inoculación *f.* inoculation, immunization, administration of a serum, vaccine, or some other substance to increase immunization to a given disease.

inocular *v.* to inoculate, to administer an inoculation.

inóculo *m.* inoculum, substance that is inoculated.

inocuo-a *a.* innocuous, that does no harm.

inodoro *m.* toilet, commode; **-a** / *a.* odorless.

inofensivo-a *a.* harmless.

inoperable *a.* inoperable, lacking potential for surgical treatment.

inoportuno-a *a.* untimely, inopportune.

inorgánico-a *a.* inorganic, independent of living organisms.

inotrópico-a *a.* inotropic, affecting the intensity or energy of muscular contractions.

inquieto-a *a.* uneasy, restless, jumpy.

inquietud *f.* unrest, restlessness.

insalubre *a.* insalubrious, unsanitary.

inscribirse *v.* to register.

insecticida *m.* insecticide.

insecto *m.* insect.

inseguridad *f.* insecurity.

inseminación *f.* insemination, fertilization of an ovum.

insensible *a.* insensible, without sensibility.

inseparable *a.* inseparable.

inserción *f.* insertion. 1. the act of inserting; 2. the place where a muscle attaches to the bone.

insertar *v.* to insert.

inservible *a.* useless, unserviceable.

insidioso-a *a.* insidious, rel. to a disease that develops gradually and subtly without warning or early symptoms.

insignificante *a.* insignificant.

insípido-a *a.* insipid, tasteless.

insistir *v.* to insist.

in situ *L.* in situ. 1. in its normal place; 2. that does not extend beyond the place of origin.

insolación *f.* insolation, sunstroke, heat exhaustion, disorder caused by the effect of prolonged exposure to the rays of the sun; ___ **con colapso** / heat prostration.

insoluble *a.* insoluble, that does not dissolve.

insomne *a.* insomnia, insomnious, rel. to or suffering from insomnia.

insomnio *m.* insomnia, inability to sleep.

insoportable *a.* unbearable.

inspección *f.* inspection.

inspiración *n.* inspiration; **capacidad de** ___ / inspiratory capacity.

inspiratorio-a *a.* inspiratory, rel. to inspiration; **capacidad** ___ / ___ capacity; **estridor** ___ / ___ stridor; **reserva de volumen** ___ / ___ reserve volume.

instalación *f.* installation; facility.

instalar *v.* to install.

instante *m.* instant; **en este** ___ / right now.

instilación *f.* instillation, dripping of a liquid into a cavity or onto a surface.

instintivo-a *a.* instinctive.

instinto *m.* instinct.

institución *f.* institution, establishment; ___ **benéfical** / charity ___ .

instrumento *m.* instrument.

insuficiencia *f.* insufficiency, lacking; ___ **cardíaca** / heart failure; ___ **coronaria** / coronary ___ ; ___ **hepática** / hepatic ___ ; ___ **mitral** / mitral ___ ; ___ **pulmonar-valvular** /

pulmonary valvular ___; ___ **renal** /
renal ___; ___ **respiratoria** / respiratory ___; ___
suprarrenal / adrenal ___; ___ **valvular** /
valvular ___; ___ **venosa** / venous ___ .

insuficiencia coronaria *f.* coronary
insufficiency, deficiency in coronary circulation
with risk of suffering pain caused by angina,
thrombosis, or atheroma that can result in a
myocardial infarct.

insuficiente *a.* insufficient.

insuflar *v.* to insufflate, to blow into a tube, cavity,
or organ of the body.

insufrible *a.* insufferable, unbearable.

ínsula *f.* insula, central lobe of the cerebral hemisphere.

insulina *f.* insulin, hormone secreted by the pancreas.

insulinemia *f.* insulinemia, excess amount of
insulin in the blood.

insulinochoque *m.* insuline shock, severe
hypoglycemia that is manifested by sweating,
shaking, anxiety, vertigo, diplopia, and can be
followed by delirium, convulsions, and collapse.

insulinodependiente *a.* insulin-dependent.

insulinogénesis *f.* insulinogenesis, production
of insulin.

integración *f.* integration. 1. anabolic activity; 2. the
process of combining into a being or total entity.

integridad *f.* integrity.

inteligente *a.* intelligent; smart.

intención *f.* intention. 1. goal, purpose. **con** ___ /
purposely; 2. natural healing process of a wound.

intensidad *f.* intensity.

intensificar *vi.* to intensify.

intensivo-a *a.* intensive.

intenso-a *a.* intense.

intentar *v.* to attempt, to try.

interacción *f.* interaction; ___ **de**
medicamentos / drug ___ .

intercalado-a *a.* intercalated, situated or placed
between two parts or elements.

intercostal *a.* intercostal, between two ribs;
espacio ___ / ___ space; **membranas** ___
-es / ___ membranes; **nervios** ___ / ___ nerves.

intercurrente *a.* intercurrent, that appears during
the course of another disease modifying it in some
way.

interdigitación *f.* interdigitation, interlocking of
parts like the fingers of folded hands.

interés *m.* interest.

interferencia *f.* interference, mutual annulment
of, or collision between two parts.

interferir *vi.* to interfere.

interferona *f.* interferon, a natural protein
released by cells exposed to viruses that can be
used in the treatment of infections and neoplasms.

interfibrilar *a.* interfibrillar, between fibrils.

ínterin *m.* interim, meantime.

interior *a.* interior.

interlobitis *f.* interlobitis, infl. of the pleura that
separates two pulmonary lobules.

interlobular *a.* interlobular, occurring between
lobules of an organ.

intermediario-a *a.* intermediary, situated
between two bodies.

intermedio-a *a.* intermediate, situated between
two extremes.

interminable *a.* endless.

intermitente *a.* intermittent, not continuous;
pulso ___ / ___ pulse; **ventilación** ___ **bajo presión**
positiva / ___ positive-pressure ventilation.

internacional *a.* international; **unidad** ___ / ___
unit, accepted measured amount of a substance as
defined by the International Conference of
Unification of Formulae.

internado *m.* internship.

internalización *f.* internalization, unconscious
process by which an individual adopts the beliefs,
values, and attitudes of another person or of the
society in which she or he lives.

internista *m., f.* physician specializing in internal
medicine.

interno-a *m., f.* intern; *a.* internal, inside the body;
hemorragia ___ / ___ bleeding.

interóseo-a *a.* interosseous, between bones or
connecting them.

interpretación *f.* interpretation.

interpretar *v.* to interpret.

interrogatorio *m.* questioning.

interrumpir *v.* to interrupt.

intersección *f.* intersection, common point of
two traversing lines.

intersticial *a.* interstitial, rel. to spaces within an
organ, cell, or tissue; **cistitis** ___ / ___ cystitis;
crecimiento ___ / ___ growth;
embarazo ___ / ___ pregnancy;
enfermedad ___ / ___ disease;
enfisema ___ / ___ emphysema; **fluido** ___ / ___
fluid; **gastritis** ___ / ___ gastritis;
hernia ___ / ___ hernia; **nefritis** ___ / ___
nephritis; **hormona** ___ **estimulante de**
células / ___ cell stimulating hormone.

intértrigo *m.* intertrigo, irritating dermatitis that
occurs between or under the folds of the skin.

intervalo *m.* interval, period of time.

intervención *f.* surgical intervention, operation.

intervenir *vi.* to intervene; to assist; to supervise.

interventricular *a.* interventricular, between the
ventricles; **defecto del tabique** ___ / ___ septal
defect; **tabique** ___ **del corazón** / ___ septum.

intervertebral *a.* intervertebral, between the vertebrae; **disco** ___ / ___ disk.

intestinal *a.* intestinal, rel. to the intestines; **desviación quirúrgica** ___ / ___ bypass surgery; **flora** ___ / ___ flora; **jugo** ___ / ___ juice; **obstrucción** ___ / ___ obstruction; **perforación** ___ / ___ perforation.

intestino *m.* intestine, the alimentary canal extending from the pylorus to the anus; ___ **delgado** / small ___; ___ **grueso** / large ___; ___ **medio del embrión** / midgut.

íntima *f.* intima. 1. the innermost of the three layers of a blood vessel; 2. the innermost layer of several organs or parts.

intimal *a.* intimal, rel. to the intima.

intolerancia *f.* intolerance, inability to withstand pain or the effects of drugs.

intorsión *f.* intorsion, rotation of the eye inwards.

intoxicación *f.* intoxication; poisoning, food poisoning, toxic state produced by the intake of a drug or toxic substance; ___ **de pescado** / fish poisoning. *V.* cuadro en; a página 424.

intoxicar *vi.* to intoxicate, to poison; **intoxicarse** *vr.* to become intoxicated; to become poisoned.

intra-abdominal *a.* intra-abdominal, within the abdominal cavity.

intra-aórtico-a *a.* intra-aortic, within the aorta.

intra-arterial *a.* intra-arterial, within an artery.

intra-articular *a.* intra-articular, within an articulation or joint.

intracapsular *a.* intracapsular, within a capsule.

intracelular *a.* intracellular, within a cell.

intracraneal *a.* intracranial, within the cranium.

intracutáneo-a *a.* intracutaneous, within the dermis.

intrahepático-a *a.* intrahepatic, within the liver; **colestasis** ___ **del embarazo** / ___ cholestasis of pregnancy.

intralobular *a.* intralobular, within a lobule.

intraluminal *a.* intraluminal, within the lumen of a tube.

intramuscular *a.* intramuscular, within a muscle.

intranquilidad *f.* restlessness, uneasiness.

intranquilo-a *a.* restless, uneasy.

intraocular *a.* intraocular, within the eye; **presión** ___ / ___ pressure.

intraoperatorio-a *a.* intraoperative, within the time frame of a surgical procedure.

intraóseo-a *a.* intraosseous, within the bone substance.

intrarrenal *a.* intrarenal, within the kidney; **fallo** ___ / ___ failure.

intrauterino-a *a.* intrauterine, within the uterus; **dispositivo** ___ / ___ device, coil.

intravenoso-a *a.* intravenous, within a vein; **infusión** ___ / ___ infusion; **inyección** ___ / ___ injection.

intraventricular *a.* intraventricular, within a ventricle.

intrínseco-a *a.* intrinsic, inherent; **factor** ___ / ___ factor, protein normally present in the gastric juice of humans.

introducir *vi.* to introduce.

introductor, intubador *m.* introducer, intubator, device used to intubate.

introitus *L.* introitus, an entrance or opening to a canal or cavity.

introspección *f.* introspection, self-analysis.

introversión *f.* introversion, the act of turning one's interests inward with diminished interest in the outside world.

introvertido-a *m., f.* introvert; *a.* rel. to introversion.

intubación *f.* intubation, insertion of a tube into a conduit or cavity of the body.

intuición *f.* intuition.

intumescencia *f.* intumescence, thickening.

intumescer *v.* to intumesce, to swell up, to enlarge.

intususcepción *f.* intussusception, invagination of one part of the intestine into the lumen of the adjoining part causing obstruction.

in utero *L.* in utero, within the uterus.

inútil *a.* useless; ineffective.

invadir *v.* to invade, to take over.

invaginación *f.* invagination, process of inclusion of one part into another.

invaginar *v.* invaginate, to introduce one part of a structure into another part of the same structure.

invalido-a *m., f.* invalid; *a.* crippled; void.

invariable *a.* invariable.

invasión *f.* invasion, the act of invading.

invasivo-a, invasor-a *a.* invasive, rel. to a germ or substance that invades adjacent tissues; **procedimiento no** ___ / non ___ procedure.

inversión *f.* inversion, process of turning around; ___ **de cromosomas** / ___ of chromosomes; ___ **del utero** / ___ of the uterus; ___ **paracéntrica** / paracentric ___; ___ **pericéntrica** / pericentric ___; ___ **visceral** / visceral ___ .

inverso-a, invertido-a *a.* inverse, inverted.

investigación *f.* research; ___ **clínica** / clinical ___; ___ **de laboratorio** / laboratory ___ .

investigar *vi.* to investigate, to research.

invisible *a.* invisible, that cannot be seen with the naked eye.

in vitro *L.* in vitro, rel. to laboratory tests or biological experimentation occurring outside the

living body esp. in a test-tube;
fertilización ___ / ___ fertilization.

in vivo *L.* in vivo, within the body of living organisms.

involución *f.* involution, a retrogressive change.

involucrado-a *a.* involved; **estar** ___ / to be ___ ; to become ___ .

involuntario-a *a.* involuntary.

inyección *f.* injection, shot; ___ **de depósito** / deposit ___; ___ **de refuerzo** / booster shot; ___ **de insulina** / insulin ___; ___ **de prueba** / test ___; ___ **de sensibilización** / sensitizing ___; ___ **hipodérmica subcutánea** / hypodermic ___; ___ **intraarticular** / intraarticular ___; ___ **intradérmica** / intradermic ___; ___ **intrafecal** / intrafecal ___; ___ **intravenosa** / intravenous ___; ___ **selectiva** / selective ___ . *V.* cuadro en la página 422.

inyectar *v.* to inject, to introduce fluid in a tissue, cavity, or blood vessel with an injector.

inyector *m.* injector, device used to inject; syringe.

iodo, yodo *m.* iodine, nonmetallic element used as a germicide and as an aid in the development and function of the thyroid gland.

ión *m.* ion, an atom or group of atoms carrying a charge of electricity.

ionización *f.* ionization, dissociation of compounds into their constituent ions; **radiación por** ___ / ionizing radiation.

ipeca, jarabe de, *m.* syrup of ipecac, an emetic and expectorant agent.

ipsolateral *a.* ipsolateral, on the same side.

ir *vi.* to go; **irse** *vr.* to go away, to leave.

irascible *a.* irascible, easily angered.

iridectomía *f.* iridectomy, removal of a part of the iris.

iridología *f.* iridology, study of the changes suffered by the iris during the course of an illness.

iris *m.* iris, contractile membrane situated between the lens and the cornea in the aqueous humour of the eye which regulates the entrance of light.

iritis *f.* iritis, infl. of the iris.

irracional *a.* irrational.

irradiación *f.* irradiation, therapeutic use of radiation.

irradiar *v.* to irradiate, to expose to or treat by radiation; to emit rays.

irreducible *a.* irreducible, that cannot be reduced.

irregular *a.* irregular.

irrigación *f.* irrigation, the act of washing out; flushing.

irrigar *vi.* to irrigate, to wash out.

irritabilidad *f.* irritability, property of an organism or tissue to react to its environment.

irritable *a.* irritable, that reacts to a stimulus.

irritación *f.* irritation, intense reaction to a pain or pathological condition.

iscuria *f.* ischuria, retention or suspension of urine.

isla *f.* island, isolated piece of tissue or group of cells.

islote *m.* islet, group of isolated cells of a different structure from the one of surrounding cells.

isométrico-a *a.* isometric, of equal dimensions.

isometropía *f.* isometropia, same refraction on both eyes.

isoniacida *f.* isoniazid, antibacterial medication used in the treatment of tuberculosis.

isostenuria *f.* isosthenuria, renal insufficiency.

isotónico-a *a.* isotonic, having equal tension.

isótopo *m.* isotope, one of a group of chemical elements that present almost identical qualities but differ in atomic weight.

isquemia *f.* ischemia, lack of blood supply to a given part of the body; ___ **silenciosa** / silent ___;

isquemico-a *a.* ischemic, rel. to or suffering from ischemia; **ataque** ___ **transitorio** / transient ___ attack, temporary stoppage of blood supply to the brain;

isquion *m.* ischium, posterior part of the pelvis.

istmectomia *f.* isthmectomy, excision of the middle part of the thyroid.

istmo *m.* isthmus. 1. narrow conduit that connects two cavities or two larger parts;2. constriction between two parts of an organ or structure.___ **del encéfalo** / ___ of the encephalon; ___ **del tubo auditivo** / ___ of auditory tube; ___ **del útero** / ___ of the uterus; ___ **de la aorta** / aortic ___; ___ **de la faringe** / pharyngeal ___; ___ **de la trompa de Eustaquio** / ___ of the Eustachian tube; ___ **de la trompa de Falopio** / ___ of the Falopian tube; ___ **de las fauces** / ___ of the fauces;

ixodes *L.* genus that includes ticks and other acarids.

ixodiasis *f.* ixodiasis, cutaneous lesions due to the bite of a certain type of tick.

izquierda *f.* left; left hand; **a la** ___ / to the ___;

izquierdo-a *a.* left.

j

jabón *m.* soap.

Jackson, membrana de *f.* Jackson membrane, thin vascular membrane that covers the anterior surface of the ascending colon.

jadear *v.* to pant.

jadeo *m.* panting, gasping, shortness of breath; wheeze.

Jaeger, examen de *m.* Jaeger test, chart of lines with different types and sizes of letters used to determine visual acuity.

jalea *f.* jelly; ___ **anticonceptiva** / contraceptive ___; ___ **vaginal** / vaginal ___ .

jamais vu *Fr.* jamais vu, the perception of familiar surroundings as a new experience.

jamás *adv.* never, ever.

jamón *m.* ham.

jaqueca *f.* severe headache.

jarabe *m.* syrup; ___ **de ipecacuana** / ipecac syrup; ___ **para la tos** / cough.

jarra *f.* jar, pitcher; ___ **de agua** / pitcher of water.

jazmín *m.* jasmine; **té de** ___ / ___ tea.

jején *m.* gnat.

jengibre *m.* ginger.

jeringa, jeringuilla *f.* syringe; ___ **de aguja hueca** / hollow needle ___; ___ **con tubo de cristal** / glass cylinder ___; ___ **desechable** / disposable ___; ___ **hipodérmica** / hypodermic ___ .

jimaguas *m., pl. Cuba* twins.

joroba *f.* hump.

jorobado-a *m., f.* hunchback; crooked. *a.* hunchbacked; crooked.

joven *m., f.* (**el joven, la joven**) young person; *a.* young.

jovencito-a *a.* youngster.

juanete *m.* bunion.hallux valgus.

jubilado-a *m., f.* retiree; *a.* retired.

juez-a *m., f.* judge.

jugar *vi.* to play.

jugo *m.* juice; ___ **gástrico** / gastric ___; ___ **intestinal** / intestinal ___; ___ **pancreático** / pancreatic ___; ___ **de ciruela** / prune ___; ___ **de manzana** / apple ___; ___ **de naranja** / orange ___; ___ **de piña** / pineapple ___; ___ **de tomate** / tomato ___; ___ **de toronja** / grapefruit ___; ___ **de uva** / grape ___; ___ **de zanahoria** / carrot ___ .

jugoso-a *a.* juicy.

juguete *m.* toy.

junta *f.* meeting, gathering, board.

juntar *v.* to join, to gather together.

junto-a *a.* together.

juntura *f.* joint, juncture.

jurado *m.* jury.

juramento *m.* oath; ___ **hipocrático** / Hippocratic ___ , medical oath.

jurisprudencia médica *f.* medical jurisprudence, the law as applied to the practice of medicine.

Jurkat, células de *f. pl.* Jurkat cells, line of T cells that is used in immunology investigations.

justicia *f.* justice.

justificar *vi.* to justify.

justo-a *a.* just, fair; **-mente** *adv.* justly.

juvenil *a.* juvenile; **artritis** ___ / ___ arthritis; **catarata** ___ / ___ cataract; **delincuencia** ___ / ___ delinquency; **dermatitis plantar** ___ / ___ plantar dermatitis; **epilepsia mioclónica** ___ / ___ myoclonic epilepsy; **principio de diabetes** ___ / ___ on-set diabetes; **periodontitis** ___ / ___ periodontitis.

juventud *f.* youth.

juzgar *vi.* to judge; **a** ___ **por** / judging by.

k

K *abr.* **potasio** / kalium, potassium.

k *abr.* **kilogramo** / kilogram.

kala-azar *m.* kala-azar, *Hindi* black fever, visceral infestation by a protozoa.

Kanner, síndrome de *m.* Kanner syndrome, child autism.

Kaposi, enfermedad de *f.* Kaposi's disease, malignant neoplasm found on the skin of the lower extremities of adult males, very prevalent among individuals suffering from AIDS.

Karvonen, método de *m.* Karvonen method, a sequence to calculate the widest spectrum of cardiac rate during physical tolerance tests.

Katz, fórmula de *f.* Katz formula, formula to obtain the medium velocity of the sedimentation of erythrocytes.

Kawasaki, enfermedad de *f.* Kawasaki disease, acute febrile child disease, characterized by symptoms of conjunctivitis, lesions of the mouth, redness, infl. and peeling of the skin in hands and feet. These symptoms distinguish this disease from others such as scarlet fever and toxic shock syndrome.

Kegel, ejercicios de *m. pl.* Kegel exercises, exercises that consist in alternating contractions and relaxation of the perineal muscles for better control of incontinence.

Kelly, operación de *f.* Kelly operation. 1. subtotal abdominal hysterectomy; 2. surgical procedure to correct urinary incontinence placing sutures in the vagina under the bladder neck.

kernicterus *m.* kernicterus, type of jaundice found in the newborn.

kerosen, kerosene *m., f.* kerosene.

kilómetro *m.* kilometer.

Klebsiella *m.* Klebsiella, gram-negative bacilli associated with respiratory and urinary tract infections.

Klebs-Löffler, bacilo de *m.* Klebs-Löffler bacillus, the diphtheria bacillus.

Koch, bacilo de *m.* Koch's bacillus, *Mycobacterium tuberculosis* the cause of tuberculosis in mammals.

Koplic, manchas de *f.* Koplic spots, small whitish spots surrounded by a red ring that appear in the inner cheek during the early stage of the measles.

Krukenberg, tumor de *m.* Krukenberg's tumor, malignant tumor of the ovary, gen. bilateral and frequently secondary to malignancy in the gastrointestinal tract.

Kussmaul, respiracion de *f.* Kussmaul's breathing, deep and gasping respiration seen in cases of diabetic acidosis.

kwashiorkor *m.* kwashiorkor, severe protein deficiency seen in infants after weaning, esp. in tropical and subtropical areas.

l

l *abr.* **letal** / lethal; **ligero** / light.

L *abr.* **litro** / liter.

laberintectomía *f.* labyrinthectomy, excision of a labyrinth.

laberíntico-a *a.* labyrinthine, rel. to a labyrinth; **arteria** ___ / ___ artery; **fístula** ___ / ___ fistula; **nistagmo** ___ / ___ nystagmus; **punto** ___ / ___ punctum; **vena** ___ / ___ vein; **vértigo** ___ / ___ vertigo.

laberintitis *f.* labyrinthitis. 1. acute or chronic infl. of the labyrinth; 2. internal otitis.

laberinto *m.* labyrinth, maze. 1. communicating channels of the internal ear that function in relation to hearing and to body balance; 2. channels and cavities that communicate forming a system.

labial *a.* labial, rel. to the lips; **férula** ___ / ___ splint; **glándulas** ___ **-es** / ___ glands, situated between the labial mucosa and the orbicular muscle of the mouth; **hernia** ___ / ___ hernia; **oclusión** ___ / ___ occlusion; **ramas del nervio mentoniano** ___ / branches of the ___ mental nerve; **venas** ___ / ___ veins.

labihendido-a *a.* harelipped.

lábil *a.* labile, unstable, fragile, changeable or easily altered.

labilidad *f.* lability, instability.

labio *m. labios*lip. 1. fleshy border; 2. liplike structure; ___ **mayores y menores de la vagina** / *sing.* labia majora and labia minora of the vagina.

labiocorea *f.* labichorea, chronic spasm of the lips that cause language disorders.

labio leporino *m.* harelip, cleft lip, congenital anomaly at the level of the upper lip, caused by faulty fusion of the upper jaw and the nasal processes; **cirugía del** ___ / ___ suture.

labioversión *f.* labioversion, incorrect position of a tooth that does not follow the normal line of occlusion towards the lips.

laboratorio *m.* laboratory; ___ **de trabajo** / workshop.

laboratorista *m., f.* medical laboratory technician.

laborioso-a *a.* labored, laborious; difficult.

laceración *f.* laceration; tear.

lacerar *v.* to lacerate.

lacrimal, lagrimal *a.* lacrimal, lachrymal, rel. to tears or to tear ducts; **conducto** ___ / ___ duct; **hueso** ___ / ___ bone; **saco** ___ / ___ sac.

lacrimógeno-a *a.* lachrymogenous, that produces tears.

lacrimotomía *f.* lacrimotomy, incision of the lacrimal duct or sac.

lactacidemia *f.* lactacidemia, excessive lactic acid in the blood.

lactancia, lactación *f.* lactation, secretion of milk; ___ **materna** / breast-feeding;

lactar *v.* to nurse; to suckle.

lactasa *f.* lactase, intestinal enzyme that hydrolizes lactose producing dextrose and galactose.

lácteo-a *a.* lacteal, rel. to milk; **productos** ___ **-s** / dairy products.

lactífero-a *a.* lactiferous, that secretes and conducts milk; **conductos** ___ / ___ ducts; **senos** ___ **-s** / ___ sinus.

lactoalbúmina *f.* milk albumina.

lactocele *m.* lactocele. galactocele.

lactógeno *m.* lactogen, agent that stimulates the production or secretion of milk.

lacto-ovovegetariano-a *m., f.* lacto-ovovegetarian, person whose diet consists of vegetables, eggs, and dairy products.

lacto-vegetariano-a *a.* lacto-vegetarian, that follows a diet of vegetables and dairy products.

lactosa, lactina *f.* lactose, lactin, milk sugar; **intolerancia a la** ___ / ___ intolerance, characterized by gastrointestinal disorders.

lado *m.* side; **al** ___ / alongside; **al** ___ **de** / next to; **de** ___ / sideways.

lagaña, legaña *f.* lema, gummy secretion of the eye.

lágrima *f.* tear.

lagrimal *a.* lacrimal, lachrymal, rel. to tears or to the lacrimal apparatus; **aparato** ___ / ___ apparatus; **arteria** ___ / ___ artery; **canículo** ___ / ___ canaliculus; **fosa** ___ / ___ fosa; **nervio** ___ / ___ nerve; **papila** ___ / ___ papilla; **punto** ___ / ___ punctum; **vena** ___ / ___ vein.

lagrimear *v.* to shed tears.

lagrimeo *m.* lacrimation, tearing.

lagrimoso-a *a.* tearful.

laguna *f.* lacuna, small cavity or depression such as those found in the brain.

lalación, lambdacismo *f., m.* lallation. 1. phonetic disorder by which the letter *r* is pronounced as *l*; 2. infantile babbling.

Lamaze, método de *m.* Lamaze technique or method, method of natural childbirth by which the mother is trained in techniques of breathing and relaxation that facilitate the process of delivery.

lamentable *a.* regrettable.

lamentar *v.* to regret; **lamentarse** *vr.* to lament, to complain.

lamento *m.* lament, complaint.

lámina *f.* lamina, thin sheath or layer; ___ **anterior clásica de la córnea** / ___ limitans anterior cornea; ___ **basal de la coroide** / ___ basalis choroidae; ___ **del arco vertebral** / ___ arcus vertebrae; ___ **elástica posterior de la cornea** / ___ limitans posterior corneae; ___ **multiforme del cortex del cerebro** / ___ cerebral cortex multiformis.

laminado-a *a.* laminated, formed by one or more laminae.

laminar *a.* laminar, rel. to a lamina; *v.* to laminate, to roll.

laminectomía *f.* laminectomy, removal of one or more vertebral laminae.

laminilla *f.* lamella. 1. thin layer; 2. disk that is inserted in the eye to apply a medication.

lámpara *f.* lamp; ___ **de hendidura** / slit ___; ___ **infrarroja** / infrared ___; **luz de una** ___ / lamplight.

lana *f.* wool.

lanceta *f.* lancet, lance, surgical instrument.

lancinante *a.* lancinating, rel. to an acute, piercing pain.

Landry, parálisis de *f.* Landry paralysis. Guillain Bareé, síndrome de.

Landsteiner, clasificación de *f.* Landsteiner's classification, differentiation of blood types: O-A-B-AB.

langosta *f.* lobster.

languidez *f.* languor, languidness, exhaustion, lack of energy.

lánguido-a *a.* languid, weak.

lanolina *f.* lanolin, purified substance obtained from lamb's wool and used in ointments.

lanugo *m.* lanugo, soft fine hair that covers the body of the human fetus.

laparocele *m.* laparocele, abdominal hernia.

laparoendoscopía *f.* laparoendoscopy, introduction of a laparoscopy in the abdomen to conduct different procedures.

laparoscopía *f.* laparoscopy, examination of the peritoneal cavity with a laparoscope.

laparoscopio *m.* laparoscope, instrument used to visualize the peritoneal cavity.

laparotomía *f.* laparotomy, incision and opening of the abdomen.

lápiz *m.* pencil.

lapso *m.* lapse, span, time interval.

largo-a *a.* long.

laringe *f.* larynx. 1. part of the respiratory tract situated in the upper part of the trachea; 2. voice organ.

laringectomía *f.* laryngectomy, removal of the larynx.

laríngeo-a *a.* laryngeal, rel. to the larynx; **estenosis** ___ / ___ stenosis; **papilomatosis** ___ / ___ papillomatosis; **prominencia** ___ / ___ prominence; **red** ___ / ___ web; **reflejo** ___ / ___ reflex, cough produced by irritation of the larynx; **síncope** ___ / ___ syncope; **ventrículo** ___ / ___ ventricle.

laringitis *f.* laryngitis, infl. of the larynx.

laringoespasmo *m.* laryngospasm, spasm of the laryngeal muscles.

laringofaringe *f.* laryngopharynx, inferior portion of the larynx.

laringofaringitis *f.* infl. of the larynx and the pharynx.

laringoplastia *f.* laryngoplasty, plastic reconstruction of the larynx.

laringoscopia *f.* laryngoscopy, examination of the larynx; ___ **directa** / direct ___ , by means of a laryngoscope; ___ **indirecta** / indirect ___ , by means of a mirror.

laringoscopio *m.* laryngoscope, instrument used to examine the larynx.

larva *f.* larva, maggot, early stage of some organisms such as insects.

larvado-a *a.* larvate, masked, rel. to an insidious or atypical symptom.

larval *a.* larval, rel. to larvae.

larvicida *m.* larvicide, agent that exterminates larvae.

lascivo-a *a.* lascivious, salacious, lustful.

láser *m.* laser. 1. acronym for Light Amplification by Stimulated Emission of Radiation; 2. micro-surgical scalpel used in the cauterization of tumors.

laser, rayos de *m., pl.* laser beams, radiation rays applied for the purpose of destroying tissue or separating parts.

LASIK *abbr.* LASIK, laser assisted in-situ keratomileusis.

lasitud *f.* lassitude, languor.

lástima *f.* pity, compassion; *v.* **tener** ___ / to feel sorry, to pity; **¡qué** ___**!** / what a ___ !

lastimado-a *a.* injured, hurt.

lastimadura *f.* injury, hurt.

lastimar *v.* to hurt, to injure; **lastimarse** *vr.* to get hurt.

lata *f.* [*metal*] tin; [*de alimento*] can.

latencia *f.* latency, the condition of being latent; **período de __ / __** period.

latente *a.* latent, present but not active; with no apparent symptoms or manifestations.

lateral *a.* lateral, rel. to a side.

lateroflexión *f.* lateroflexion, lateral flexion.

látex *m.* latex, substance derived from a seed plant that contains an element of natural rubber; in many cases it can be an allergen.

latido *m.* beat; throb; **__ del corazón /** heart **__; __ ectópico /** ectopic **__** .

latir *v.* to beat, to throb.

lavabo *m.* washstand, basin.

lavado *m.* lavage, enema, irrigation of a cavity.

lavado de cerebro *m.* brain washing.

lavadora *f.* washing machine.

lavamanos *m.* washstand, washbowl.

lavaojos *m.* eyecup.

lavar *v.* to wash; **lavarse** *vr.* to wash oneself.

lavativa *f.* enema.

laxante *m.* laxative, mild physic.

laxitud *f.* laxity, relaxation; weakness.

laxo-a *a.* lax, relaxed, loose.

Leber, enfermedad de *f.* Leber disease, hereditary type of atrophy that causes degeneration of the optic nerve and that affects males.

lección *f.* lesson.

leche *f.* milk; **__ condensada /** condensed **__; __ cuajada /** curd milk; **__ de magnesia /** milk of magnesia; **__ descremada /** skim **__; __ en polvo /** dry milk; **__ evaporada /** evaporated **__; __ hervida /** boiled **__; __ materna /** mother's **__; __ pasteurizada /** pasteurized **__** .

lecitina *f.* lecithin, essential substance in the metabolism of fats found in animal tissue, esp. in the nervous tissue.

lectura *f.* reading; **impedimentos de la __ / __** disorders; **__ labial /** lip **__** .

lechoso-a *a.* milky.

lechuga *f.* lettuce.

leer *vi.* to read.

legal *a.* legal, legitimate, according to the law; **ceguera __ / __** blindness; **pleito __ /** lawsuit.

legaña *f.* lema, gummy secretion of the eye.

Legionarios, enfermedad de los *f.* Legionnaires disease, serious infectious disease that could be lethal and is characterized by pneumonia, a dry cough, muscular ache, and sometimes gastrointestinal symptoms.

legislación médica *f.* medical legislation.

legitimidad *f.* legitimacy.

legítimo-a *a.* legitimate, that goes by the law; authentic.

lego-a *a.* lay, secular.

legumbre *f.* legume, vegetable.

leiomiofibroma *m.* leiomyofibroma, benign tumor of essentially connective fibrous and smooth muscular tissue.

leiomioma *m.* leiomyoma, benign tumor of essentially smooth muscular tissue.

leiomiosarcoma *f.* leiomyosarcoma, combined tumor of leiomyoma and sarcoma.

lejía *f.* lye, bleach; **envenenamiento por __ / __** poisoning.

lejos *adv.* far, afar; **de __ / __** away; **desde __ /** from afar.

Lenegre, síndrome de *f.* Lenegre syndrome, fibrosis of the intracardiac conductive system that is gen. characterized as idiopathic fibrosis of the atrioventricular nodule.

lengua *f.* 1. tongue, lingua; **depresor de __ / __** depressor; 2. language; **__ materna /** native **__** .

lengua geográfica *f.* geographic tongue, tongue characterized by bare patches surrounded by thick epithelium, resembling a geographic map.

lenguaje *m.* language; **__ hablado /** spoken **__** .

lente *m.* lens; **__ acromático /** achromatic **__; __ bicóncavo /** biconcave **__; __ cilíndrico /** cylindrical **__; __ de aumento /** magnifying glass; **__ -s bifocales /** bifocal **__; __ -s de contacto /** contact lens; **__ -s intraoculares / __** implantation, intraocular; **__ -s trifocales /** trifocal **__** .

lenteja *f.* lentil.

lentes correctores *m. pl.* corrective lenses.

lenticular *a.* lenticular. 1. rel. to a lens; 2. rel. to the lens of the eye.

lentiforme *a.* lentiform, in the shape of a lens.

lentiginosis *f.* lentiginosis, presence of a large number of lentigos.

léntigo *m.* lentigo, skin macule; **__ maligno /** malignant **__; __ múltiple /** multiple **__; __ senil /** senile **__** .

lento-a *a.* slow; sluggish, inactive; **-mente** *adv.* slowly.

lepra *f.* leprosy, Hansen's disease, infectious disease caused by the *Mycobacterium leprae* and characterized by more or less severe skin lesions.

leprecaunismo *m.* leprechaunism, hereditary condition with characteristics of dwarfism accompanied by mental and physical retardation, endocrine disorders, and susceptibility to infections.

leproso-a *m., f.* leper, person suffering from leprosy.
leptomeninges *f.* leptomeninges, the thinnest of the cerebral membranes: the pia madre and the arachnoid.
lesbiana *f.* lesbian, homosexual female.
lesbianismo *m.* lesbianism, feminine homosexuality.
lesión *f.* injury, lesion, contusion, wound. V. cuadro en esta página.
letal *a.* lethal, mortal, that causes death; **dosis** ___ / ___ dose; **factor** ___ / ___ factor; **gene** ___ / ___ gene; **mutación** ___ / ___ mutation.
letárgico-a *a.* lethargic, lethargical.
letargo *m.* lethargy, torpor.
letra *f.* [*del alfabeto*] letter; [*escritura*] handwriting.
leucaferesis *f.* leukapheresis, separation of leukocytes from a patient's blood and transfusion of the treated blood back into the patient.
leucemia *f.* leukemia, blood cancer; ___ **aleucémica** / aleukemic ___; ___ **crónica** / chronic ___; ___ **eosinofílica** / eosinophilic ___; ___ **granulocítica crónica** / chronic granulocytic ___; ___ **linfocítica** / lymphocytic ___; ___ **mieloide crónica** / chronic myeloid ___; ___ **monocítica** / monocytic ___ .
leucémico-a *a.* leukemic, rel. to or suffering from leukemia.
leucemoide *a.* leukemoid, with leukemia-like signs and symptoms.
leucina *f.* leucine, amino acid that is essential to the growth and metabolism of humans.

Lesión	Lesion
de latigazo	whiplash
degenerativa	degenerative
depresiva	depressive
difusa	diffuse
funcional	functional
grosera	gross
periférica	peripheral
precancerosa	precancerous
sistémica	systemic
tóxica	toxic
traumática	traumatic
vascular	vascular

leucinuria *f.* leucinuria, presence of leucine in the urine.
leucoblasto *m.* leukoblast, immature leukocyte.
leucocis *f.* leucosis, abnormal formation of leukocytes.
leucocito *m.* leukocyte, white blood cell, element of the blood important in the defensive and reparative functions of the body; ___ **acidófilo** / acidophil ___ , that changes color with acid dye; ___ **basófilo** / basophil ___ , that changes color with basic dye; ___ **eosinofílico** / eosinophilic ___ , that stains readily with eosin; ___ **linfoide** / nongranular lymphoid ___; ___ **neutrófilo** / neutrophil ___ , that has an affinity for neutral stains; ___ **polimorfonucleado** / polymorphonuclear ___ , having multilobed nuclei.
leucocitosis *f.* leukocytosis, an abnormally increase of leukocytes in the blood, gen. occurring during severe infections; ___ **absoluta** / absolute ___; ___ **mononuclear** / mononuclear ___; ___ **polinuclear** / polynuclear ___; ___ **relativa** / relative ___ .
leucocoria *f.* leukokoria, leucocoria, white appearance of the pupil due to a cataract.
leucoencefalitis *f.* leucoencephalitis, infl. of the white matter.
leucoencefalopatía *f.* leucoencephalopathy, white matter changes first discovered in children suffering from leukemia, associated with radiation and chemotherapy lesions.
leucopatía *f.* leukopathia, albinism, lack of pigmentation.
leucopenia *f.* leukopenia, below normal number of leukocytes in the blood.
leucoplasia *f.* leukoplakia, opalescent, precancerous patches of the mucous membrane of the mouth or tongue.
leucorrea *f.* leukorrhea, whitish vaginal discharge.
leucotriquia *f.* leukotrichia, white hair.
levadura *f.* yeast, leaven, minute fungi capable of producing fermentation; used in nutrition as a source of protein and vitamin.
levantar *v.* to raise, to lift, to pull up; **levantarse** *vr.* to get up.
leve *a.* light, slight.
levocardia *f.* levocardia, transposition of the abdominal viscera with normal position of the heart on the left side of the thorax.
levodopa *f.* levodopa, *L.* dopa, chemical substance used in the treatment of Parkinson's disease.

levulosa *f.* levulose. fructosa.

léxico-a *a.* lexical, rel. to the vocabulary.

ley *f.* law; ___ **del buen Samaritano** / good Samaritan ___ , legal protection to a professional who gives aid in an emergency.

liberación *f.* liberation.

liberado-a *a.* freed.

liberar, librar *v.* to liberate, to free, to release.

libertad *f.* liberty; *v.* **tener** ___ **para** / to be free to.

líbido *m.* libido. 1. sexual impulse, conscious or unconscious; 2. in pychoanalysis, the force or energy that determines human behavior.

libidinoso-a *a.* libidinous, rel. to the libido.

Libman-Sacks, enfermedad de *f.* Libman-Sacks endocarditis, Libman-Sacks syndrome, non-bacterial verrucose endocarditis that is associated with disseminated erythematous lupus.

libre *a.* free; **asociación** ___ / ___ association.

librería *f.* bookstore.

libreta *f.* notebook.

libro *m.* book.

licencia *f.* license, permit, licensure, authorization; ___ **para ejercer la medicina** / medical ___ .

licenciado-a *m., f.* attorney, licentiate.

licopenemia *f.* lycopenemia, increase of lycopene in the blood that results in a yellow-orange color of the skin.

licopina *f.* lycopene, vegetable pigment abundant in tomatoes and carrots.

licor *m.* liquor; 1. watery solution that contains a medicinal substance; 2. general term used for some body fluids.

licuar *v.* to liquify, to dissolve.

lidocaína *f.* lidocaine, anesthetic.

lien *m.* lien.bazo.

lientería *f.* lientery, diarrhea which shows particles of non-digested food.

Liga de la Leche, La *f.* La Leche League, an organization that promotes breast-feeding.

ligadura *f.* ligature, tie, affixture; linkage.

ligamento *m.* ligament. 1. bands of connective tissue fibers that protect the joints;___ **acromioclavicular** / acromioclavicular ___ , extending from the clavicle to the acromion; ___ **alveolodentario** / alveolo-dental ___ ; ___ **ancho uterino** / broad uterine ___ , peritoneal fold that extends laterally from the uterus to the pelvic wall; ___ **anococcígeo** / anococcygeal ___ ; ___ **braquicubital** / brachiocubital ___ ; ___ **capsular** / capsular ___ ; **desgarre del** ___ / ___ tear; ___ **esternoclavicular** / sternoclavicular ___ ; ___ **gastrocólico** / gastrocholic ___ ; ___ **glosoepiglótico** / glossoepiglotic ___ ; ___ **hepatoduodenal** / hepatoduodenal ___ ; ___ **iliofemoral** / iliofemoral ___ ; ___ **largo del plantar** / long plantar ___ ; ___ **palmar** / palmar ___ ; ___ **radiocubital** / radiocubital ___ ; ___ **trapezoide** / trapezoid ___ ; ___ **Y,** ___ **iliofemoral** / Y ligament, iliofemoral ___ ; 2. protective band of fascia and muscles that connect or support viscerae.

ligar *vi.* to tie, to apply a ligature; to attach; ___ **las trompas** / ___ the tubes.

ligazón *f.* binding, bandage.

ligero-a *a.* light, slight; *adv.* **-mente** lightly, slightly.

lima *f.* [*fruta*] lime; **jugo de** ___ / ___ juice; [*instrumento*] file.

limar *v.* to file; to smooth.

límbico-a *a.* limbic, marginal; **sistema** ___ / ___ system, group of cerebral structures.

limbo *m.* limbus, the edge or border of a part; ___ **de la córnea** / ___ cornea.

liminal *a.* liminal, almost imperceptible.

limitación *f.* limitation; restriction.

limitado-a *a.* limited, restricted; **movimiento** ___ / restricted motion.

limitar *v.* to limit, to restrict.

límite *m.* limit; ___ **de asimilación** / assimilation ___ ; ___ **de percepción** / ___ of perception; ___ **de saturación** / saturation ___ .

limón *m.* lemon.

limonada *f.* lemonade.

limpiar *v.* to clean; to wipe; *vr.* **limpiarse,** to clean oneself

limpieza *f.* cleaning; cleanliness.

limpio-a *a.* clean.

linaje *m.* pedigree, ancestral line of descent.

lindo-a *a.* pretty.

línea *f.* line; wrinkle; guide.

linear *a.* lineal, resembling a line.

linfa *f.* lymph, clear fluid found in lymphatic vessels.

linfadenectomía *f.* lymphadenectomy, removal of lymphatic channels and nodes.

linfadenitis *f.* lymphadenitis, infl. of the lymphatic ganglia.

linfadenopatía *f.* lymphadenopathy, any disease affecting the lymph nodes; ___ **axilar** / axillary ___ ; ___ **biliar** / portal ___ ; ___ **cervical** / cervical ___ ; ___ **generalizada** / generalized ___ ; ___ **mediastínica** / mediastinal ___ ; ___ **supraclavicular** / supraclavicular ___ .

linfangiectasis *f.* lymphangiectasis, dilation of the lymphatic vessels.

linfangiograma *m.* lymphangiogram, x-ray of the lymph nodes and vessels obtained with the use of a contrasting medium.

linfangitis *f.* lymphangitis, infl. of the lymphatic vessels.

linfático-a *a.* lymphatic, rel. to lymph; **ganglios** ___ **-s** / lymph nodes; **sistema** ___ / ___ system.

linfedema *m.* lymphedema, edema caused by blockage of the lymph vessels.

linfemia *f.* lymphemia, high number of lymphocytes or its precursors or both in the circulating blood.

linfoblasto *m.* lymphoblast, early stage of a lymphocyte.

linfoblastoma *m.* lymphoblastoma, malignant lymphoma formed by lymphoblasts.

linfocito *m.* lymphocyte, lymphatic cell; ___ **B** / B cell, important in the production of antibodies;

linfocitopenia, linfopenia *f.* lymphocytopenia, lymphopenia, diminished number of lymphocytes in the blood.

linfocitos T *m. pl.* T cells, lymphocytes differentiated in the thymus that direct the immunological response and alert the B cells to respond to antigens; ___ **inductores, (ayudantes)** / helper ___ , enhance production of antibody forming cells from B cells; ___ **citotóxicos** / cytotoxic ___ , kill foreign cells (as in rejection of transplanted organs); ___ **supresores** / suppressor ___ , suppress production of antibody forming cells from B cells.

linfocitosis *f.* lymphocytosis, excessive number of lymphocytes in the blood.

linfogranuloma venéreo *f.* lymphogranuloma venereum, viral disorder that may lead to elephantiasis of the genitalia and rectal stricture.

linfogranulomatosis *f.* lymphogranulomatosis. V. **Hodgkin, enfermedad de**.

linfohistiocitosis *f.* lymphohistyocitosis, proliferation or infiltration of lymphocytes and histyocytes.

linfoide *a.* lymphoid, that resembles the lymphatic tissue.

linfoma *m.* lymphoma, any neoplasm of the lymphatic tissue.

linfomatoide *a.* lymphomatoid, rel. to or resembling a lymphoma.

linfopenia, linfocitopenia *f.* lymphopenia, lymphocytopenia, diminished number of lymphocytes in the blood.

linforreticular *a.* lymphoreticular, rel. to reticuloendothelial cells of the lymph nodes.

linfosarcoma *m.* lymphosarcoma, malignant neoplasm of the lymphoid tissue.

lingual *a.* lingual, rel. to the tongue.

língula *f.* lingula, tongue-like projection or structure.

linimento *m.* liniment, liquid substance for external use.

linitis *f.* linitis. gastritis.

lino *m.* linen.

linterna *f.* flashlight.

lío *m.* mess, confusion.

liodermia *f.* glossy skin, a sign of atrophy or traumatism of the nerves.

liofilización *f.* freeze-drying.

lipectomía *f.* lipectomy, removal of fat tissue; ___ **submental** / submental ___ , under the chin.

lipedema *m.* lipedema, chronic infl. of the lower extremities in women due to an excess of fat and liquids in the subcutaneous tissues.

lipemia *f.* lipemia, abnormal presence of fat in the blood.

lipidemia *f.* lipidemia, excess lipids in the blood.

lípido *m.* lipid, lipide, organic substance that does not dissolve in water but is soluble in alcohol, ether, or chloroform.

lipoartritis *f.* lipoarthritis, infl. of fatty tissues in the knee.

lipodistrofia *f.* lipodystrophy, metabolic disorder of fats; ___ **cefalotorácica** / cephalothoracic ___; ___ **insulínica** / insulin ___; ___ **intestinal** / intestinal ___ .

lipofuscinosis *f.* lipofuscinosis, abnormal storage of any of a group of adipose pigments.

lipogénesis *f.* lipogenesis, production of fat.

lipoinfiltración *f.* lipoinfiltration, surgical procedure that consists in infiltration of fat in depressed or deficient areas.

lipólisis *f.* lipolysis, decomposition of fat.

lipoma *m.* lipoma, adipose tissue tumor.

lipomatosis *f.* lipomatosis. 1. condition caused by excessive accumulation of fat in a given area; 2. multiple lipomas.

lipopenia *f.* lipopenia, decrease of fat in the blood and in the organism.

lipoproteínas *f., pl.* lipoproteins, proteins combined with lipid compounds that contain a high concentration of cholesterol; ___ **de alta densidad** / high-density___; ___ **de densidad baja** / low-density___ .

liposarcoma *m.* liposarcoma, malignant tumor containing fatty elements.

liposis *f.* liposis, obesity, excessive accumulation of fat in the body.

liposoluble *a.* liposoluble, that dissolves in fatty substances.

liposucción *f.* liposuction, process of extracting fat by high vacuum pressure.

lipotrofia *f.* lipotrophy, increase of fat in the body.

lipuria *f.* lipuria, presence of lipids in the urine.

liquen *m.* lichen, noncontagious papular skin lesion;___ **de urticaria** / ___ urticatus; ___ **escleroso atrófico** / ___ sclerosus and atrophicus; ___ **escrofularia** / ___ scrofulosorum; ___ **plano** / ___ planus; ___ **ulcerativo** / ___ erosive.

líquido *m.* fluid, liquid; ___ **amniótico** ___ / amniotic ___; ___ **articular** / joint ___; ___ **cefalorraquídeo** / cerebrospinal ___; ___ **corporal** / body ___; ___ **espeso** / heavy liquid; ___ **extracelular** / extracellular liquid; ___ **intersticial** / interstitial ___; ___ **intracelular** / intracellular ___; ___ **peritoneal** / peritoneal ___; ___ **seminal** / seminal liquid; ___ **sérico** / serous ___; ___ **sinovial** / synovial ___ .

lisiado-a *a.* crippled.

lisina *f.* lysin, antibody that dissolves or destroys cells or bacteria.

lisinógeno *m.* lysinogen, agent with the property of producing lysine.

lisis *f.* lysis. 1. destruction or dissolution of red cells, bacteria, or any antigen by lysin; 2. gradual cessation of the symptoms of a disease.

lista *f.* list; ___ **de accidentados** / casualty ___ .

listo-a *a.* ready; clever.

litiasis *f.* lithiasis, formation of calculi, esp. in the biliary and urinary tracts.

litio *m.* lithium, metallic element used as a tranquilizer in severe cases of psychosis.

litotomía *f.* lithotomy, incision in an organ or conduit to remove stones.

litotripsia *f.* lithotripsy, crushing of calculi present in the kidney, ureter, bladder, or gallbladder.

litotriturador *m.* lithotriptor, machine or device used to crush calculi; ___ **extracorporal con ondas de choque** / extracorporeal shock wave ___ .

lituresis *f.* lithuresis, sandy urine.

livedo *m.* livedo, a stain in the skin, often blue or purple like in a bruise.

lividez *f.* lividity, discoloration resulting from the gravitation of blood; ___ **cadavérica** / postmortem lividity.

lívido-a *a.* livid, [*una persona*] ash blue.

LL *m.* fourteenth letter of the Spanish alphabet.

llaga *f.* sore, ulcer, blain.

llamada *f.* call; ___ **de teléfono** / telephone ___ .

llave *f.* key.

llegada *f.* arrival; coming.

llegar *vi.* to arrive; to reach; to attain; ___ **a ser** / to become; **llegarse** / *vr.* to approach.

llenar *v.* to fill; to complete.

lleno-a *a.* full, complete.

llenura *f.* fullness, plenty, abundance; **tener** ___ / to be very full.

llevar *v.* to carry; to take; to transport; ___ **puesto** / to be wearing; ___ **a cabo** / to carry out; **llevarse** / *vr.* to take away; ___ **a cabo** / to take place; ___ **bien** / to get along well; ___ **mal** / not to get along.

llorar *v.* to cry.

lloradera *f.* weeping.

llover *vi.* to rain.

lluvia *f.* rain.

lluvioso-a *a.* rainy.

lobar *a.* lobar, rel. to a lobe; **pulmonía** ___ / ___ pneumonia.

lobectomía *f.* lobectomy, excision of a lobe.

lobotomía *f.* lobotomy, incision of a cerebral lobe to correct certain mental disorders; ___ **completa** / complete ___; ___ **izquierda anterior** / left lower ___; ___ **parcial** / partial ___ .

lobular *a.* lobular, rel. to a lobule.

lobulillo *m.* lobule, small lobe.

lóbulo *m.* lobe, rounded, well-defined portion of an organ.

local *a.* local, rel. to an isolated area, such as local anesthesia; **aplicación** ___ / ___ application; **reaparición** ___ / ___ recurrence.

localización *f.* localization, location. 1. reference to the point of origin of a sensation; 2. determination of the origin of an infection or lesion.

localizar *vi.* to localize; to locate.

loción *f.* lotion.

loco-a *m., f.* insane person; *a.* mad, insane.

locomoción *f.* locomotion.

locular *a.* locular, loculated, rel. to loculus.

lóculo *m.* loculus, small cavity.

locura *f.* madness, insanity, lunacy.

locus *L.* locus, localization of a gene in a chromosome.

logafasia *f.* logaphasia, motor aphasia gen. caused by a cerebral lesion.

logagrafia *f.* logographia, inability to express thoughts in writing.

logamnesia *f.* logamnesia, sensorial aphasia, inability to recognize written or spoken words.

lógico-a *a.* logic, logical; reasonable.

logopedia *f.* logopedics, study and treatment of speech defects.

logoplejía *f.* logoplegia, paralysis of the organs of speech.

lograr *v.* to achieve; to reach.

lombriz *f.* earthworm; ___ **intestinal** / pinworm, belly worm; ___ **solitaria** / tapeworm.

lonche *m.* H.A. lunch, midday meal.

longevidad *f.* longevity. 1. long duration of life; 2. life span.

longitudinal *a.* longitudinal, lengthwise.

loquios *m.* lochia, bloody, serosanguineous discharge from the uterus and the vagina during the first few weeks after delivery.

lordosis *f.* lordosis, abnormally increased curvature of the lumbar spine; saddle back.

Lou Gehrig, enfermedad de *f.* Lou Gehrig disease, amyotrophic lateral sclerosis; progressive muscular atrophy.

lubricación *f.* lubrication.

lubricante *m.* lubricant, oily agent that when applied diminishes friction between two surfaces; ___ **oleaginoso** / oil-based ___ .

lubricar *vi.* to lubricate, to apply a lubricant to a surface.

lucha *f.* struggle; fight.

luchar *v.* to struggle; to fight.

lucidez *f.* lucidity.

lúcido-a *a.* lucid, clear of mind.

luego*adv.* in a while; then; **conj.** therefore; **desde** ___ / of course; **hasta** ___ / so long, good-bye.

luético-a *a.* luetic, syphilitic, rel. to or suffering from syphilis.

lugar *m.* place, space; **en** ___ **de** / in ___ of; *v.* **poner en su** ___ / to put in ___; **tener** ___ / to take ___ .

lujuria *f.* lust, lewdness, lasciviousness.

lujurioso-a *a.* lustful, lewd, libidinous.

lumbago *m.* lumbago, pain in the lower portion of the back.

lumbalgia *f.* low backache.

lumbar *a.* lumbar, rel. to the part of the back between the thorax and the pelvis; back; **punción** ___ / ___ puncture, spinal tap; **vértebras** ___ **-es** / ___ vertebrae.

lumbricosis *f.* lumbricosis, infestation by earthworms.

lumen *m.* lumen. 1. space in a cavity, conduit, or organ; 2. unit of light.

Luminal *m.* Luminal, trade name for a compound containing phenobarbital and used as a sedative.

luminal *a.* luminal, rel. to light in a conduit or canal.

luminiscencia, luminosidad *f.* luminescence, luminosity, emission of light without production of heat.

luminoso-a *a.* luminous, rel. to luminosity.

luna *f.* moon.

lunar *m.* mole; blemish; *a.* rel. to the moon.

lunático-a *m., f.* lunatic, crazy person.

lupa *f.* magnifying glass.

lupa binocular *f.* loupe, convex magnifying lens used esp. by surgeons and ophthalmologists.

lupus *L.* lupus, chronic skin disease of unknown origin that causes degenerative local lesions;___ **anticoagulante** / anticoagulant ___; ___ **eritematoso discoide** / ___ erythematous, discoid, disease that causes irritation of the skin and is characterized by squamous plaques with reddish borders; ___ **eritematoso sistémico** / ___ erythematous, systemic, characterized by febrile episodes affecting the viscera and the nervous system; ___ **marginado** / marginal ___; ___ **vulgar** / ___ vulgaris.

luteína *f.* lutein, yellow pigment that derives from the corpus luteum.

luteo-a, luteínico-a *a.* luteal, rel. to the corpus luteum.

luteoma *f.* luteoma, tumor of the corpus luteum.

luto *m.* mourning; **estar de** ___ / to mourn.

luxación *f.* dislocation, luxation;___ **cerrada** / closed ___; ___ **cervical** / cervical ___; ___ **complicada** / complicated ___; ___ **congénita** / congenital ___; ___ **congénita de la cadera** / congenital ___ of hip; ___ **recidivante** / habitual ___ .

luz *f.* light; *v.* **dar a** ___ / to give birth; **adaptación a la** ___ / ___ adaptation; ___ **del día** / daylight; ___ **deslumbrante** / glare.

Lyme, enfermedad de *f.* Lyme disease, multisystem inflammatory disorder caused by a deer tick; gen. occurs in the eastern part of the United States during spring and summer; the immediate recommendation is to remove the ticks from the body to avoid contagion.

m

M *abr.* **maduro** / mature; **maligno-a** / malignant; **minuto** / minute; **morfina** / morphine.

maceración *f.* maceration. 1. decomposition and softening of organs and tissues by soaking in water or other liquids; 2. fragmentation of the skin through exposure to humidity for a long period of time.

macerar *v.* to macerate, to soften by soaking.

macho *m.* male; *a.* male; manly.

macizo-a *a.* compact, solid.

macroblefaria *f.* macroblepharia, abnormally large eyelid.

macrocefalia *f.* macrocephalia, abnormally large head.

macrocefálico-a *a.* macrocephalic, having an abnormally large head.

macrocitemia, macrocitosis *f.* macrocythemia, macrocytosis, larger than normal erythrocytes in the blood.

macrocosmo *m.* macrocosm. 1. the universe considered as a whole; 2. the total or entire structure of something.

Macrodantina *f.* Macrodantin, trade name for furantoin, bactericide used in the treatment of urinary infections.

macrófago *m.* macrophage, mononuclear phagocytic cell; **migración de __ -s / __** migration.

macroglosia *f.* macroglossia, enlargement of the tongue.

macrognatia *f.* macrognathia, enlargement of the jaw.

macromolécula *f.* macromolecule, a large molecule such as a protein.

macroscópico-a *a.* macroscopic, visible to the naked eye.

macrospora *f.* macrospore, large spore.

mácula *f.* macula, macule, speck, small discolored spot on the skin; **__ lútea / __** lutea, small, yellowish area next to the center of the retina.

maculado-a *a.* maculate.

macular *a.* macular, rel. to macules.

maculopapular *a.* maculopapular, rel. to macules and papules.

madera *f.* wood

madrastra *f.* stepmother.

madre *f.* mother; **__ soltera** / unwed **__** .

madrugada *f.* daybreak; **de __** / at dawn.

madrugar *vi.* to rise early.

madurar *v.* to mature; to ripen.

madurez *f.* maturity; ripeness, stage of full development.

maduro-a *a.* mature, ripened.

magistral *a.* magistral, rel. to medication prepared according to the physician's indications.

magma *f.* magma. 1. suspension of particles in a small amount of water; 2. viscous mass composed of organic material.

magnesia *f.* magnesia, magnesium oxide; **leche de __** / milk of **__** .

magnesio *m.* magnesium; **sulfato de __ / __** sulfate.

magnético-a *a.* magnetic, magnetical, rel. to or that has the properties of a magnet; **campo __ / __** field.

magnetismo *m.* magnetism, the property of attracting or repelling.

magnetoelectricidad *f.* magnetoelectricity, electricity induced by a magnet.

magnífico-a *a.* superb, wonderful.

magnitud *f.* magnitude.

magulladura *f.* bruise, contusion.

majadero-a *a.* spoiled, cranky.

mal *m.* malady, illness, disease.

mal, malo-a *a.* bad; evil; **__ genio** / ill temper; *mal adv.* badly; wrongly; **de __ en peor** / from bad to worse; *v.* **hacer __** / to harm, to hurt.

malabsorción *f.* malabsorption, inadequate absorption of nutrients from the intestinal track.

malacia *f.* malacia, softening or loss of consistency of organs or tissues.

malacoplaquia *f.* malacoplakia, formation of soft patches in the mucous membrane of a hollow organ.

malagradecido-a *a.* ungrateful.

malar *a.* malar, rel. to the cheek or the cheekbone.

malaria *f.* malaria. V. **paludismo**.

malcriado-a *a.* ill-mannered, spoiled.

maleable *a.* malleable.

maléolo *m.* malleolus, hammerlike protuberance, such as the ones on either side of the ankle.

malestar *m.* malaise, discomfort, uneasiness.

maleta *f.* valise, suitcase.

malformación *f.* malformation, anomaly, or deformity, esp. congenital.

malfuncionamiento *m.* malfunction, disorder.

malhumor *m.* bad temper.

malhumorado-a *a.* sullen, bad-tempered.

malignidad *f.* malignancy. 1. quality of being malignant; 2. cancerous tumor.

maligno-a *a.* malignant, virulent, pernicious, having a destructive effect.

malnutrición *f.* malnutrition, deficient nutrition.

maloclusión *f.* malocclusion, defective bite.

malpresentación *f.* malpresentation, abnormal presentation of the fetus at the time of delivery.

malrotación *f.* malrotation, abnormal or defective rotation of an organ or part during embryonic development.

malta *f.* malt.

maltosa *f.* maltose, a type of sugar.

maltratar *v.* to abuse, to mistreat, to manhandle; ___ **maltrato de palabra** / verbal abuse.

malunión *f.* malunion, imperfect union of a fracture.

malleus *L. mallei*malleus, one of the three ossicles of the middle ear.

mama *f.* mamma, breast, milk-secreting gland in the female; **enfermedad benigna de la** ___ / benign breast disease.

mamá *f.* mom, term of endearment for mother.

mamalgia *f.* mammalgia, pain in the [*breast*] mamma.

mamaplastia, mamoplastia *f.* mammaplasty, mammoplasty, plastic surgery of the breast; ___ **de aumento** / augmentation ___; ___ **de reconstrucción** / reconstructive ___; ___ **de reducción** / reduction ___ .

mamar *v.* to suckle, to draw milk from the breast; **dar de** ___ / to breastfeed.

mamario-a *a.* mammary, rel. to the mamma; **glándulas** ___ **-s** / ___ glands.

mamectomía *f.* mammectomy, mastectomy.

mamífero *m.* mammal.

mamilado-a *a.* mammillated, presenting small protuberances that resemble nipples.

mamilar *a.* mammillary, resembling a nipple.

mamiliplastia *f.* mammilliaplasty, plastic surgery of the nipple.

mamilitis *f.* mammillitis, infl. of the nipple.

mamitis, mastitis *f.* mammitis, mastitis, infl. of the mammary gland.

mamograma *m.* mammogram, x-ray of the breast.

mancha *f.* spot, blemish, macula, stain.

manchado-a *a.* spotted, soiled.

manchar *v.* to soil, to spot; to stain; **mancharse** *vr.* to become stained or spotted.

manco-a *m., f.* one-handed person.

mandar *v.* to order, to command; to send.

mandato *m.* order, command.

mandíbula *f.* mandible, mandibula, horseshoe-shaped bone that constitutes the lower jaw; ___ **inferior** / lower ___; ___ **superior** / upper ___ .

mandibular *a.* mandibular, rel. to the mandible.

manejable *a.* manageable.

manejar *v.* to conduct, to drive.

manera *f.* manner, method, way.

manerismo *m.* mannerism, a distinctive trait in dress, speech, or action.

manga *f.* sleeve.

mango *m.* mango. 1. tropical fruit; 2. handle.

manguito *m.* cuff, bandlike fibrous tissue surrounding a joint; ___ **rotador** / rotator ___ ; musculotendinous; **ruptura del** ___ **rotador** / rotator tear.

maní *m.* peanut; **mantequilla de** ___ / ___ butter.

manía *f.* mania, emotional disorder characterized by extreme excitement, exalted emotions, rapid succession of ideas, and fluctuating moods.

maníaco-a, maniático-a *a.* maniac, maniacal, afflicted by mania; **maníacodepresivo** / manic-depressive;

manicomio *m.* insane asylum, madhouse.

manifestación *f.* manifestation, revelation.

manifestar *vi.* to manifest, to express; *manifestarse vr.* to appear, [*enfermedad*] to reveal itself.

maniobra *f.* maneuver, skillful manual procedure such as executed by the obstetrician in the delivery of a baby.

manipulación *f.* manipulation, professional treatment involving the use of hands.

manipular *v.* to manipulate, to handle.

maniquí *m.* mannequin, representative figure of the human body.

mano *f.* hand; **apoyo de la** ___ / ___ rest; **deformidades adquiridas de la** ___ / acquired ___ deformities; **hecho a** ___ / handmade.

manómetro *m.* manometer, device used to measure the pressure of liquids or gases.

manteca *f.* lard, animal fat.

mantener *vi.* to sustain, to support; **mantenerse** *vr.* to hold or keep up; to support oneself.

mantenimiento *m.* maintenance, sustenance.

mantequilla *f.* butter.

manto *m.* mantle, covering.

manual *a.* manual.

manubrium *L.* manubrium, handle-shaped structure.

manutención *f.* maintenance, child care support.

manzana *f.* apple.

manzanilla *f.* chamomile, sedative tea used to alleviate gastrointestinal discomfort.

maña *f.* bad habit.

mañana *f.* morning; tomorrow; **muy de** ___ / very early in the morning; **por la** ___ / in the morning.

máquina *f.* machine, apparatus.

mar *m.* sea.

marasmo *m.* marasmus, extreme malnutrition, emaciation, esp. in young children.

maravilloso-a *a.* marvelous, wonderful.

marca *f.* mark, sign, brand; ___ **de la viruela** / pockmark; ___ **de nacimiento** / birthmark; ___ **enfresa** / strawberry ___; ___ **registrada** / trademark.

marcador *m.* marker, indicator.

marcapaso, marcapasos *m.* pacemaker, electronic cardiac pacer; pacer, regulator of cardiac rhythm; ___ **de ritmo fijo** / fixed rate ___; ___ **ectópico** / ectopic ___; ___ **interno** / internal ___; ___ **temporal** / temporary ___ .

marcar *vi.* to mark; to brand; to point out.

marcha *f.* gait, walk; ___ **anserina** / waddling ___, widespread walk; ___ **atáxica** / ataxic ___, staggering; ___ **cerebelosa** / cerebellar ___; ___ **espástica** / spastic ___; ___ **hemipléjica** / hemiplegic ___, circular movement of one of the lower extremities.

mareado-a *a.* dizzy, light-headed.

marearse *vr.* to get motion sickness; to become dizzy.

mareo *m.* dizziness; motion sickness; ___ **de altura** / altitude sickness.

margarina *f.* margarine.

margen *m.* margin, border.

marginación *f.* margination, accumulation and adhesion of leukocytes to the epithelial cells of the blood vessel walls at the beginning of an inflammatory process.

marginal *a.* marginal, rel. to a margin; **caso** ___ / ___ case.

marido *m.* husband.

mariguana, marihuana *f. Cannabis sativa*, marihuana, marijuana.cannabis.

marisco *m.* shellfish.

marital *a.* marital, rel. to marriage.

marsupialización *f.* marsupialization, conversion of a closed cavity into an open pouch.

martillo *m.* hammer. 1. common name for maleus, small bone of the middle ear; 2. instrument used in physical examination.

más *adv.* more, to a greater degree; **a** ___ **tardar** / at the latest; ___ **allá** / beyond; ___ **que** / more than; ___ **vale** / better to; **por** ___ **que** / however much.

masa *f.* mass, body formed by coherent particles.

masaje *m.* massage, process of manipulation of different parts of the body by rubbing or kneading; ___ **cardíaco** / cardiac ___, resuscitation.

masajista *m., f.* masseur, masseuse, person who performs massage.

mascar, masticar *vi.* to chew.

máscara *f.* mask. 1. covering of the face; 2. appearance of the face, esp. as a pathological manifestation.

mascarilla *f.* death mask.

masculinización *f.* masculinization.

masculino-a *a.* masculine, rel. to the male sex.

masetero *m.* masseter, principal muscle in mastication.

masivo-a *a.* massive.

masoquismo *m.* masochism, abnormal condition by which sexual gratification is obtained from self-inflicted pain or pain inflicted by others.

massa *L.* massa, middle commissure of the brain.

mastadenitis *f.* mastadenitis.mastitis.

mastaligia *f.* mastaligia. V. **mamalgia**.

mastectomía *f.* mastectomy, plastic surgery of the breast.

masticación *f.* mastication, the act of chewing.

mastitis *f.* mastitis, mastadenites, fibrocystic disease of the mama; ___ **cística** / cystic ___; ___ **cística crónica** / chronic cystic ___; ___ **del neonato** / neonatorum ___; ___ **glandular** / glandular ___; ___ **granulomatosa** / granulomatous ___; ___ **láctea** / lacteal ___; ___ **por estasis** / caked breast; ___ **puerperal** / puerperal ___; ___ **supurativa** / suppurative ___ .

mastocitoma *f.* mastocytoma, mast cells accumulation resembling a neoplasm.

mastocitosis *f.* mastocytosis, a condition in which neoplastic mast cells appear in several tissues as urticaria pigmentosa.

mastoideo-a *a.* mastoid. 1. rel. to the mastoid process; **antro** ___ / ___ antrum; **células** ___ -s / ___cells, air spaces in the mastoid process; 2. that resembles a breast or nipple.

mastoides *m.* mastoid process, rounded apophysis of the temporal bone.

mastoiditis *f.* mastoiditis, infl. of the air cells of the mastoid process.

mastopatía *f.* mastopathy, any disorder of the mammary glands.

mastopexia *f.* mastopexy, correction of a pendulous breast.

masturbación *f.* masturbation, autostimulation and manipulation of the genitals to achieve sexual pleasure.

matar *v.* to kill.

materia *f.* matter, substance.

material *m.* material; *a.* material.

maternidad *f.* maternity; **hospital de ___ / ___** hospital.

materno-a *a.* maternal, rel. to the mother; **línea ___ /** matrilineal, tracing descendency to the mother;

matidez *f.* dullness, diminished resonance to palpation.

matriz *f.* womb. 1. matrix, basic material; 2. cast.

matutino-a *a.* of the morning, rel. to the early hours of the day; **enfermedad ___ del embarazo /** morning sickness; **rigidez ___ muscular y de las articulaciones /** morning stiffness.

maxilar *a.* maxillary, rel. to the maxilla; **hueso ___ de la mandíbula /** jawbone.

maxilla *L.* maxilla, bone of the upper jaw.

mayonesa *f.* mayonnaise.

mayor *a.* greater, [*edad*] older; **-mente** *adv.* mostly, mainly.

mayoría *f.* majority.

máximo-a *a.* maximum, the most.

meatal *a.* meatal, rel. to a meatus.

meato *m.* meatus, passage or channel in the body.

mecánico-a *m., f.* mechanic; *a.* mechanical

mecanismo *m.* mechanism. 1. involuntary response to a stimulus; **___ de defensa /** defense ___; **___ de ejecución /** implementation ___; **___ del dolor /** pain ___; 2. machine-like structure.

meconio *m.* meconium. 1. first feces of the newborn; greenish in color

media *f.* mean. 1. average; 2. middle coat of a blood vessel or artery.

mediador-a *m., f.* mediator, entity or person that mediates.

medial *a.* medial, rel. to or situated towards the middle.

medianoche *f.* midnight.

mediante *adv.* by means of.

mediar *v.* to mediate.

medias *f. pl.* socks, stockings; **___ elásticas /** elastic stockings.

mediastinitis *f.* mediastinitis, infl. of the tissues of the mediastinum.

mediastino *m.* mediastinum. 1. mass of tissues and organs separating the lungs; 2. cavity between two organs.

mediastinoscopía *f.* mediastinoscopy, endoscopic examination of the mediastinum.

medicación, medicamento *f., m.* medication, medicine; **medicamento de patente /** patent medicine.

Medicaid *m.* Medicaid, U.S. government program to provide health care for the poor.

Medicare *m.* Medicare, U.S. government program that subsidizes health care esp. for the elderly and the disabled.

medicina *f.* 1. medicine, the healing arts; **___ clínica /** clinical ___; **___ comunal, al servicio de la comunidad /** community ___; **___ del espacio /** aerospace ___; **___ deportiva /** sports ___; **___ ecológica /** environmental ___; **___ familiar /** family practice; **___ forense /** forensic ___; **___ industrial /** industrial ___; **___ interna /** internal ___; **___ legal /** legal ___; **___ nuclear /** nuclear ___; **___ ocupacional /** occupational ___; **___ preventiva /** preventive ___; **___ socializada /** socialized ___; **___ tropical /** tropical ___; **___ veterinaria /** veterinary ___; 2. medication, medicine, drug; **estudiante de ___ /** medical student.

medicina holística *f.* holistic medicine, an approach to medicine that considers the human being as an integral functional unit.

medicinal *a.* medicinal, rel. to medicine or having medical properties.

médico-a *m., f.* physician, doctor; **cuerpo ___ /** medical staff; **___ consultante, asesor /** consulting ___; **___ de asistencia primaria /** primary ___; **___ de cabecera o primario /** primary ___; **___ de familia /** family ___; **___ de guardia /** doctor on call; **___ forense /** coroner; **___ interno /** intern; **___ recomendante /** referring ___; **___ residente /** resident, physician serving a residency; *a.* medical, medicinal, rel. to medicine or that cures; **asistencia ___ / ___** assistance; **atención ___ / ___** care.

medicolegal *a.* medicolegal, the practice of medicine as related to law.

medida *f.* measure; measurement; **con ___ /** moderately;

medida de salvación *f.* life-saving measure.

medidor de ritmo de dosis *m.* dose rate meter.

medio *m.* medium. 1. means to attain an effect; 2. substance that transmits impulses; 3. substance used in the culture of bacteria; **en ___ de /** in the middle of; **por ___ de /** by means of; **medio-a** *a.* half; in part; **línea ___ -a /** medial line; **punto ___ /** medium.

medioambiental *a.* environmental, rel. to the environment.

medio ambiente *m.* environment; **peligros del ___ /** environmental hazards;

mediodía *m.* noon.

medir *vi.* to measure; **cinta de ___ /** measuring tape; **taza de ___ /** measuring cup.

médula espinal *f.* spinal cord, a column of nervous tissue that extends from the medulla oblongata to the first or second lumbar vertebrae, and from which arise all the nerves that go to the trunk of the body and to the extremities.

meduloblastoma *m.* medulloblastoma, a malignant neoplasm located in the fourth ventricle and the cerebellum, or the spinal cord that can also invade the meninges. This type of neoplasm is seen most frequently in children.

médula oblongata *f.* medulla oblongata, portion of the medulla located at the base of the brain.

médula ósea *f.* bone marrow, spongelike tissue present in the cavities of bones; **fallo de la ___ / ___ failure; punción y aspiración de la ___ / ___ puncture and aspiration; transplante de la ___ / ___ transplant.

medular *a.* medullary, rel. to the medulla; **celularidad ___ / ___ cellularity; infiltración ___ / ___ infiltration; insuficiencia ___ / ___ failure; lesión ___ / ___ injury;

megacéfalo-a *a.* megalocephalic.macrocefalia.

megacolon *m.* megacolon, abnormally large colon.

megadosis *f.* megadose, a nutrient dose that is much greater than the recommended daily allowance.

megaesófago *m.* megaesophagus, abnormally large dilation of the inferior portion of the esophagus.

megalofobia *f.* megalofobia, a fear of large objects.

megalomanía *f.* megalomania, delusions of grandeur.

megalómano-a *a.* megalomaniac, suffering from megalomania.

megacariocito *m.* megacaryocyte, a large bone marrow cell essential in the production of platelets.

megavitamina *f.* megavitamin, a dose of vitamin that exceeds the daily requirement.

meiosis *f.* meiosis, process of cell division that results in the production of gametes.

mejilla *f.* cheek.

mejor *a.* [*comp. of bueno*] better; best; **la ___ medicina /** the best medication; *sup.* **es el, la ___ /** it is the best; *adv.* better; *v.* **estar ___ /** to be ___; *vr.* **ponerse ___ /** to get ___; **tanto ___ /** so much the ___ .

mejoramiento, mejoría *m., f.* improvement, amelioration.

mejorana *f.* marjoram.

mejorar *v.* to improve; **mejorarse** *vr.* to get better.

mejoría *f.* improvement, amelioration.

melancolía *f.* melancholia, marked depression.

melancólico-a *a.* rel. to or suffering from melancholia.

melanina *f.* melanin, dark pigmentation of the skin, hair, and parts of the eye.

melanocito *m.* melanocyte, melanine-producing cell.

melanoma *m.* melanoma, malignant tumor made of melanocytes that has the capacity to metastasize rapidly to another part of the skin, lymph, lungs, liver and brain.

melanoma maligno *m.* malignant melanoma, pigmented neoplasm.that can originate in any part of the skin, rarely found in the mucose; it has the capacity to metatazise rapidly in other parts of the lympha, lungs, liver and brain.

melanosis *f.* melanosis, condition characterized by an unusual deposit of dark pigmentation in various tissues or organs.

melanuria *f.* melanuria, presence of dark pigmentation in the urine.

melasma gravídico *m.* melasma gravidarum. *pop.* pregnancy mask.

melena *f.* melena, abnormally dark and pasty stool containing digested blood.

melocotón *m.* peach.

mellizos-as *m., f., pl.* twins.gemelo-a.

membrana *f.* membrane, web, thin layer of tissue that covers or protects an organ or structure; **___ de la placenta /** placental ___; **___ mucosa /** mucous ___; **___ nuclear /** nuclear ___; **___ permeable /**

permeable ___; ___ -s arteriopulmonares / pulmonary arterial webs; ___ **semipermeable /** semipermeable ___; ___ **sinovial /** synovial ___; ___ **timpánica /** tympanic ___ .

membranoso-a *a.* membranous, rel. to or of the nature of a membrane.

memorando *m.* memorandum.

memoria *f.* memory, faculty that allows the registration and recall of experiences; ___ **inmediata /** short-term ___ .

memorizar *vi.* to memorize.

menarca *m.* menarche, first onset of menstruation.

mendelismo *m.* Mendelism, set of principles that explains the transmission of certain genetic traits.

menguar *v.* to subside, to diminish.

meníngeo-a *a.* meningeal, rel. to the meninges.

meninges *f.* meninges, three layers of connective tissue that surround the brain and the spinal cord.

meningioma *m.* meningioma, a slow-growing vascular neoplasm arising from the meninges.

meningismo *m.* meningism, meningismus, congestive irritation of the meninges, gen. of a toxic nature, that presents symptoms similar to those of meningitis but without infl., seen esp. in children.

meningitis *f.* meningitis infl. of the meninges; ___ **criptocóccica /** cryptoccocal ___; ___ **viral /** viral ___ .

meningocele *m.* meningocele, protrusion of the meninges through a defect in the skull or the vertebral column.

meningococo *m. meningocci* V. **meningococcus,** microorganism that causes epidemic cerebral meningitis.

meningoencefalitis *f.* meningoencephalitis, cerebromeningitis, infl. of the encephalum and the meninges.

meningoencefalocele *m.* meningoencephalocele, protrusion of the encephalum and the meninges through a defect in the cranium.

meningomielitis *f.* meningomyelitis, infl. of the spinal cord and the membranes that cover it.

meningomielocele *m.* meningomyelocele, protrusion of the spinal cord and meninges through a defect of the vertebral column.

meniscectomía *f.* meniscectomy, excision of a meniscus.

menisco *m.* meniscus, crescent-shaped, cartilaginous, interarticular structure.

menometrorragia *f.* menometrorrhagia, abnormal bleeding during and between menstruation.

menopausia *f.* menopause, cessation of the fertility stage of adult women, accompanied by a decrease in hormone production.

menor *a.* smaller, less, lesser, [*comp. of pequeño*] younger; smallest, [*sup. of pequeño*] youngest; **el hijo** ___ / the youngest son.

menorragia *f.* menorrhagia, excessive bleeding during menstruation.

menorralgia *f.* menorrhalgia, painful menstruation.

menorrea *f.* menorrhea, normal menstrual flow.

menos *adv.* less; **a** ___ **que** / unless; **poco más o** ___ / more or less; **por lo** ___ / at least.

menospreciar *v.* to underestimate; to hold in low esteem.

mensaje *m.* message.

menstruación *f.* menstruation, periodic flow of bloody fluid from the uterus; **trastornos de la** ___ / menstrual disorders.

menstrual *a.* menstrual, rel. to menstruation; **ciclo** ___ / cycle.

menstruar *v.* to menstruate.

menstruo *m.* menses, menstruation, period.

mensual *a.* monthly; **-mente;** *adv.* monthly.

menta *f.* mint.

mental *a.* mental, rel. to the mind; **actividad** ___ / ___ activity, mentation; **deficiencia** ___ / ___ deficiency; **edad** ___ / ___ age; **enfermedad** ___ / ___ illness; **higiene** ___ / ___ hygiene; **retraso** ___ / ___ retardation; **trastorno** ___ / ___ disorder; **-mente** *adv.* mentally.

mentalidad *f.* mentality, mental capacity.

mente *f.* mind, intellectual power.

mentecato-a *m., f.* numbskull.

mentir *vi.* to lie.

mentira *f.* lie, falsehood.

mentol *m.* menthol, an alcohol obtained from peppermint oil and used for its soothing effects.

mentón *m.* mentus, chin.

meñique *m.* fifth finger.

meralgia *f.* pain in the thigh; ___ **parestética /** ___ paresthetica.

merbromina *f.* merbromin, odorless red powder, soluble in water, used to kill germs.

mercurial *a.* mercurial, rel. to mercury.

mercurio *m.* mercury, volatile liquid metal.

merecer *vi.* to deserve.

merergacia *f.* merergacia, type of simple psychic disorder characterized by anxiety and emotional instability.

meridiano *m.* meridian, an imaginary circular line through the poles of a spherical body which connects the opposite ends of its axis.

mermelada *f.* marmalade.

mes *m.* month.

mesa *f.* table; ___ **de operaciones** / operating ___; ___ **de reconocimiento** / examination ___ .

mescalina *f.* mescaline, poisonous alkaloid with hallucinatory properties.

mesectodermo *m.* mesectoderm, mass of cells that combine with others to form the meninges.

mesencéfalo *m.* mesencephalon, the midbrain of the embrionary stage.

mesénquima *m.* mesenchyme, embryonic tissue from which the connective tissue and the lymph and blood vessels arise in the adult.

mesentérico-a *a.* mesenteric, rel. to the mesentery.

mesenterio *m.* mesentery, peritoneal folds that fix parts of the intestine to the posterior abdominal wall.

mesial *a.* mesial. V. **medial**.

mesión *f.* mesion, imaginary midlongitudinal plane that divides the body in two symmetric parts.

mesmerismo *m.* mesmerism, therapy by hypnotism.

mesocardia *f.* mesocardia, displacement of the heart toward the center of the thorax.

mesocolon *m.* mesocolon, mesentery that fixes the colon to the posterior abdominal wall.

mesodermo *m.* mesoderm, middle germ layer of the embryo, between the ectoderm and the endoderm, from which bone, connective tissue, muscle, blood, blood vessels, and lymph tissue, as well as the membranes of the heart and abdomen, arise.

mesotelio *m.* mesothelium, cell layer of the embryonic mesoderm that forms the epithelium covering the serous membrances in the adult.

mestizo-a *m., f. a.* mestizo, half-breed; crossbred, hybrid.

meta *f.* goal, objective.

metabólico-a *a.* metabolic, rel. to metabolism; **índice** ___ / ___ rate;

metabolismo *m.* metabolism, physiochemical changes that take place following the digestive process; ___ **basal** / basal ___, lowest level of energy waste; ___ **de proteína** / metabolic protein, digestion of proteins as amino acids.

metabolito *m.* metabolite, substance produced during metabolism or essential to the metabolic process.

metacarpiano-a *a.* metacarpal, rel. to the metacarpus.

metacarpo *m.* metacarpus, the five small metacarpal bones of the hand.

metadona *f.* methadone, highly potent habit-forming synthetic drug with narcotic action weaker than that of morphine.

metafase *f.* metaphase, one of the phases of cell division.

metáfisis *f.* metaphysis, the growing portion of a bone.

metal *m.* metal.

metálico-a *a.* metallic, rel. to or composed of metal.

metamorfosis *f.* metamorphosis. 1. change of form or structure; 2. degenerative process.

metanefrina *f.* metanephrine, a catabolite of epinephrine found in the urine.

metanol *m.* methanol, methyl alcohol, wood alcohol.

metástasis *f.* metastasis, extension of a pathological process from a primary focus to another part of the body through blood or lymph vessels, as occurs in some types of cancer.

metastatizar *vi.* to metastasize, to spread by metastasis.

metatálamo *m.* metathalamus, part of the diencephalon.

metatarsiano-a *a.* metatarsal, rel. to the metatarsus.

metatarso *m.* metatarsus, the five small metatarsal bones located between the tarsus and the toes.

meteorismo *m.* meteorism, bloated abdomen due to gas in the stomach or the intestines.

meter *v.* to put in; to put one thing into another.

meticuloso-a *a.* meticulous, scrupulous.

método *m.* method, procedure, process, treatment.

metópico-a *a.* metopic, frontal, rel. to the forehead.

metria *f.* metria, puerperal infl. of the uterus.

métrico-a *a.* metric, rel. to meter or the metric system; **sistema** ___ / ___ system.

metritis *f.* metritis, infl. of the walls of the uterus.

metro *m.* meter.

metrorragia *f.* metrorrhagia, uterine bleeding other than menstruation.

mezcla *f.* mixture, compound.

mezclar *v.* to mix, to blend.

mialgia *f.* myalgia, muscle pain.

miastenia *f.* myasthenia, muscle weakness; ___ **grave** / ___ gravis.

miatonía *f.* myatonia, deficiency or loss of muscle tone.

micción *f.* urination.

micetoma *m.* mycetoma, severe infection caused by fungi that affects the skin, the connective tissue, and the bone.

micología *f.* mycology, the study of fungi and the diseases caused by them.

micoplasmas *m. pl.* mycoplasmas, the smallest free-living organisms, some of which produce diseases such as a type of viral pneumonia and pharyngitis.

micosis *f.* mycosis, general term used for any disease caused by fungi.

micótico-a *a.* mycotic, rel. to or affected by mycosis.

micotoxicosis *f.* mycotoxicosis, systemic toxic condition caused by toxins produced by fungi.

micotoxina *f.* mycotoxin, a fungal toxin.

micrencefalia *f.* micrencephaly, abnormal smallness of the brain.

microabsceso *m.* microabscess, very small abscess.

microanatomía *f.* microanatomy, histology.

microbacterium *L.* microbacterium, gram-positive bacteria resistant to high temperatures.

microbiano-a *a.* microbic, microbial, rel. to microbes.

microbicida *m.* microbicide, agent that destroys microbes.

microbio *m.* microbe, minute living organism.

microbiología *f.* microbiology, science that studies microorganisms.

microcefalia *f.* microcephalia, microcephaly, congenital abnormally small head.

microcirugía *f.* microsurgery, surgery performed with the aid of special operating microscopes and very small precision instruments.

micrococo *m.* micrococcus, microorganism.

microcolon *m.* microcolon, abnormally small colon.

microcosmo *m.* microcosm, a world in miniature.

microcurie *m.* microcurie, a measurement of radiation.

micrófago *m.* microphage.fagocito.

microfalo *m.* microphallus, abnormally small penis.

microficha *f.* microfiche, small film capable of storing a large amount of data.

microfilm, microfilme *m.* microfilm, film that contains information reduced to a minimal size.

microgenitalia *m.* microgenitalia, underdevelopment of the external genitalia.

microgiria *f.* microgyria, underdevelopment of the cerebral gyri.

micrognatia *f.* micrognathia, congenital smallness of the lower jaw.

microgotero *m.* microdrip, an instrument used to administer a small, precise amount of a substance intravenously.

micrografía *f.* micrography, microscopic study.

microinvasión *f.* microinvasion, invasion of the cellular tissue adjacent to a localized carcinoma that cannot be seen with the naked eye.

microlitiasis *f.* microlithiasis, minute concretions discharged in certain organs.

micromelia *f.* micromelia, abnormally small limbs.

micromélico-a *a.* micromelic, rel. to micromelia.

micronúcleo *m.* micronucleus, the smallest nucleus in a cell that has more than one.

microonda *f.* microwave, electromagnetic short wave with a very high frequency.

microorganismo *m.* microorganism, an organism that cannot be seen with the naked eye.

microqueiria *f.* microcheiria, disorder in which the hands are abnormally small.

microscopía *f.* microscopy, microscopic examination.

microscópico-a *a.* microscopic, rel. to microscopy.

microscopio *m.* microscope, optical instrument used to amplify objects that cannot be seen with the naked eye; ___ **de luz** / light ___; ___ **electrónico** / electron ___ .

microsoma *m.* microsome, a fine granular element of the protoplasm.

microsomía *f.* microsomia, condition of having an abnormally small body with otherwise normal structure as in dwarfism.

microtomía *f.* microtomy, cutting thin sections of tissue.

micrótomo *m.* microtome, instrument used to prepare thin sections of tissue for microscopic study.

midriasis *f.* mydriasis, dilation of the pupil of the eye.

midriático *m.* mydriatic, agent used to dilate the pupil of the eye; **-a** *a.* causing dilation of the pupil of the eye.

miectomía *f.* myectomy, excision of a portion of a muscle.

miedo *m.* fear, apprehension.

miel *f.* honey.

mielatelia *f.* myelatelia, developmental defect of the spinal cord.

mielauxa *f.* myelauxe, hypertrophy of the spinal cord.

mielina *f.* myelin, the fat-like substance that forms a covering around certain nerve fibers.

mielinación, mielinización *f.* myelination, myelinization, growth of a myelin sheath around a nerve fiber.

mielinolisis *f.* myelinolysis, disease that destroys the myelin cover; ___ **aguda** / acute ___ .

mielitis *f.* myelitis, infl. of the spinal cord.

mieloblastemia *f.* myeloblastemia, the presence of myeloblasts in the blood.

mieloblasto *m.* myeloblast, an immature cell in the granulocyte series, generally present in bone marrow.

mielocele *m.* myelocele, hernia of the spinal cord through a defect in the vertebral column.

mielocítico-a *a.* myelocytic, rel. to myelocytes; **leucemia** ___ / ___ leukemia.

mielocito *m.* myelocyte, a large, granular leukocyte in the bone marrow that is present in the blood in certain diseases.

mielocitoma *m.* myelocytoma, an accumulation of myelocytes in certain tissues, present in certain illnesses.

mieloclasto *m.* myeloclast, a cell that destroys the myelin sheaths of the nerves of the central nervous system.

mielodisplasia *f.* myelodysplasia, abnormal formation of the spinal cord.

mielofibrosis *f.* myelofibrosis, fibrosis of the bone marrow.

mielógeno-a *a.* myelogenic, myelogenous, produced in the bone marrow.

mielografía *f.* myelography, x-ray of the spine after injection of a contrast medium.

mielograma *m.* myelogram, x-ray of the spinal cord with the use of a contrasting medium.

mieloide *a.* myeloid, rel. to or resembling the spinal cord or the bone marrow; **médula** ___ / ___ tissue.

mieloleucemia *f.* myeloleukemia, a form of leukemia in which abnormal cells are derived from myelopoietic tissue.

mieloquiste *m.* myelocyst, a cyst composed of nerve cells that develops in a canal of the central nervous system.

mieloma *m.* myeloma, tumor formed by a type of cells usu. found in the bone marrow; ___ **múltiple** / multiple ___ .

mielomeningocele *m.* myelomeningocele, hernia of the spinal cord and its meninges through a defect in the vertebral canal.

mielopatía *f.* myelopathy, pathological condition of the spinal cord.

mieloproliferativo-a *a.* myeloproliferative, characterized by proliferation of bone marrow inside or outside of the medulla.

mielosquisis *f.* myeloschisis, spina bifida.

mielosupresión *m.* myelosuppression, decreased production of erythrocytes and platelets in the bone marrow.

miembro *m.* member. 1. organ or limb of the body; 2. person affiliated with an organization; *vr.* **hacerse** ___ / to become a ___ .

mientras *adv.* meanwhile; ___ **que** / while.

miestesia *f.* myesthesia, any type of sensation in a muscle.

migración *f.* migration, movement of cells from one place to another.

migraña *f.* migraine, severe headache usu. unilateral, accompanied by disturbed vision and in some cases by nausea and vomiting.

migratorio-a *a.* migratory, rel. to migration.

miiasis *f.* myasis, infection due to the presence of larvae from the diptera family.

milagro *m.* miracle.

milagroso-a *a.* miraculous.

milia neonatorum *n.* *L.* milia neonatorum, small, non-pathogenic cysts sometimes found on newborns.

miliar *a.* miliary, characterized by the presence of small tumors.

miliaria *f.* miliaria, prickly heat, noncontagious cutaneous eruption caused by the obstruction of sweat glands and characterized by small red vesicles and papules accompanied by itching and prickling.

milieu *Fr.* milieu, environment, surroundings.

milla *f.* mile.

mimado-a *a.* pampered.

mimar *v.* to pamper.

mimético-a *a.* mimetic, mimic, that imitates.

minar *v.* to undermine.

mineral *m.* mineral, inorganic element; *a.* rel. to a mineral; **agua** ___ **efervescente** / carbonated ___ water.

mineralización *f.* mineralization, abnormally large deposition of mineral in tissues.

mineralocorticoide *m.* mineralocorticoid, hormone released by the adrenal cortex involved in the regulation of fluids and electrolytes.

m

minero-a *m., f.* miner.

minilaparotomía *f.* minilaparotomy, a type of pelvic surgery performed for the purpose of diagnosis or sterilization by tubal ligation.

mínimo-a *a.* minimal, least, smallest; **dosis** ___ / ___ dose, smallest amount needed to produce an effect; **dosis letal** ___ / ___ lethal dose, smallest amount needed to cause death.

ministro-a *m., f.* minister, pastor.

minoría *f.* minority.

minucioso-a *a.* thorough, detailed; **examen** ___ / ___ exam; **-mente** *adv.* very carefully; thoroughly.

minusvalía mental *f.* mental handicap

minusválido *m.* a handicapped person.

minuto *m.* minute, fraction of time.

miocárdico-a *a.* myocardial, myocardiac, rel. to the myocardium.

miocardio *m.* myocardium, the middle and thickest muscular layer of the heart wall; **contracción del** ___ / myocardial contraction;

miocardiopatías *f. pl.* myocardial diseases.

miocarditis *f.* myocarditis, infl. of the myocardium.

miocito *m.* myocyte, cell of the muscular tissue.

mioclonus *m. L.* myoclonus, a spasm of a muscle or a group of muscles, as seen in epilepsy.

miodistrofia *f.* myodystrophy, muscular dystrophy.

mioespasmo *m.* myospasm, spasmodic contractions of a muscle.

miofibrilla *f.* myofibril, myofibrilla; minute, slender fiber of the muscle tissue.

miofibroma *m.* myofibroma, tumor containing muscle tissue elements.

miofilamento *m.* myofilament, microscopic element that makes up myofibrils in muscles.

miogénico-a *a.* myogenic, originating in or starting from the muscle.

mioglobina *f.* myoglobin, muscle tissue pigment that participates in the transport of oxygen.

miografía *f.* myography, a recording of muscular activity.

miolisis *f.* myolysis, destruction of muscle tissue.

mioma *m.* myoma, benign tumor of muscle tissue; ___ **previo** / previous ___ .

miomectomía *f.* myomectomy. 1. excision of a portion of a muscle or of muscular tissue; 2. excision of a myoma, esp. one localized in the uterus.

miometrio *m.* myometrium, muscle wall of the uterus.

miometritis *f.* myometritis, infl. of the muscular wall of the uterus.

mionecrosis *f.* myonecrosis, necrosis of muscle tissue.

mioneural *a.* myoneural, rel. to muscles and nerves; **unión** ___ / ___ junction, a nerve ending in a muscle.

miopatía *f.* myopathy, muscle disease; ___ **facial** / facial ___ ; ___ **ocular** / ocular ___ ; ___ **tirotóxica** / thyrotoxic ___ .

miope *a.* myopic. 1. nearsighted; 2. rel. to myopia.

miopía *f.* myopia, nearsightedness, a defect in the eyeball that causes parallel rays to be focused in front of the retina.

miorrexia *f.* myorrhexis, rupture of any muscle.

miosina *f.* myosin, the most abundant protein in muscle tissue.

miosinógeno *m.* myosinogen, a protein present in the muscle tissue.

miosis *f.* miosis, excessive contraction of the pupil.

miositis *f.* myositis, infl. of a muscle or group of muscles.

miotomía *f.* myotomy, dissection of muscles.

miotonía *f.* myotonia, increased rigidity of a muscle following muscle contraction, with diminished power of relaxation.

mirar *v.* to look, to view; ___ **fijamente** / to stare; **mirarse** *vr.* to look at oneself.

miringectomía *f.* myringectomy, myringodectomy, excision of part or all of the tympanic membrane.

miringitis *f.* myringitis, infl. of the eardrum.

miringoplastia *f.* myringoplasty, plastic surgery of the tympanic membrane.

miringotomía *f.* myringotomy, incision of the tympanic membrane.

misantropía *f.* misanthropy, abhorrence of mankind.

miscegenación *f.* miscegenation, sexual relations between individuals of different races.

miscible *a.* miscible, capable of mixing or dissolving.

mismo-a *a.* same; **dominio de sí** ___ / self-control; **sí** ___ / oneself.

misogamia *f.* misogamy, aversion to marriage.

misoginia *f.* misogyny, hatred of women.

mitad *f.* half, each of the two equal parts in which a whole is divided; **a la** ___ / in half.

mitigado-a *a.* mitigated, diminished, moderated.

mitigar *vi.* to mitigate, to alleviate.

mitocondrias *f., pl.* mitochondria, microscopic filaments of the cytoplasm that constitute the main source of energy in cells.

mitogenesia, mitogénesis *f.* mitogenesia, mitogenesis, the process of cell mitosis.

mitógeno *m.* mitogen, substance that induces cell mitosis.

mitosis *f.* mitosis, cell division process that results in new cells and replacement of injured tissue.

mitral *a.* mitral, rel. to the mitral valve;
estenosis ___ / ___ stenosis, a narrowing of the left atrioventricular orifice;
incompetencia ___ / ___ insufficiency;
regurgitación ___ / ___ regurgitation, the flow of blood back from the left ventricle into the left atrium due to a lesion of the mitral valve;
soplo ___ / ___ murmur.

mittelschmerz *m.* mittelschmerz, lower abdominal pain related to ovulation and occuring midway in the menstrual cycle.

mixedema *m.* myxedema, condition caused by deficient thyroid gland function.

mixoma *m.* myxoma, a tumor of the connective tissue.

mixto-a *a.* mixed.

mixtura *f.* mixture.

mnemónica *f.* mnemonics, recall of memory through free association of ideas and other techniques.

moción *f.* motion, movement.

moco *m.* mucus, viscid matter secreted by the mucous membranes and glands.

modalidad *f.* modality, any form of therapeutic application.

moderación *f.* moderation.

moderado-a *a.* moderate, temperate; **-mente** *adv.* moderately.

modesto-a *a.* modest.

modificación *f.* modification, change.

modificar *vi.* to modify, to change.

modo *m.* mode. 1. manner, way; 2. in a series, the value that is repeated most frequently; **de cualquier** ___ / in any way; **de ningún** ___ / in no way.

modulación *f.* modulation, the action of adjusting or adapting, such as occurs with the inflection of the voice.

moho *m.* mildew, mold caused by a fungus.

mojado-a *a.* wet.

mojar *v.* to wet, to dampen; **mojarse** *vr.* to get wet.

molar *m.* molar, any of the twelve molar teeth.

molde *m.* 1. cast, hardened bandage made stiff; 2. template, pattern, mold.

moldear *v.* to cast.

molécula *f.* molecule, the smallest unit of a substance above the atomic level.

molécula gramo *m.* gram molecule, weight in grams equal to the molecular weight.

molecular *a.* molecular, rel. to molecules.

moler *vi.* to grind.

molestar *v.* to annoy, to bother.

molestia *f.* discomfort, annoyance.

molesto-a *a.* annoyed.

momentáneo-a *a.* momentary, of short duration.

momento *m.* moment, fraction of time.

momentum *L.* momentum, impetus, a force of motion.

momificación *f.* mummification, conversion into a state that resembles that of a mummy, as occurs in dry gangrene or in a dead fetus that dries up in the uterus.

moniliasis *f.* moniliasis. V. **candidiasis**.

monitor *m.* monitor. 1. electronic device used to monitor a function; 2. person who oversees an activity or function.

monitorear *v.* to monitor, to check systematically with an electronic device an organic function such as the heartbeat.

monitoreo, monitorización *m., f.* monitoring; ___ **cardíaco** / cardiac ___; ___ **de presión arterial** / blood pressure ___; ___ **fetal** / fetal ___ .

monitoreo de Holter *m.* Holter monitoring, ambulatory electrocardiography.

monitorización glucosa *f.* glucose monitorization, close observation by periodic testing of the glucose percentage in the blood.

monja *f.* nun.

monoarticular *a.* monoarticular, rel. to only one joint.

monocigótico-a *a.* monozygotic, rel. to twins that have identical genetic characteristics.

monocito *m.* monocyte, large, granular, mononuclear leukocyte.

monoclonal *a.* monoclonal, rel. to a single group of cells; **anticuerpos** ___ **-es** / ___ antibodies.

monocromático-a *a.* monochromatic, having only one color.

monocular *a.* monocular, rel. to only one eye.

monogamia *f.* monogamy, legal marriage to or sexual relationship with only one person.

mononuclear *a.* mononuclear, having one nucleus; **célula** ___ / ___ cell.

mononucleosis *f.* mononucleosis, presence of an abnormally large number of monocytes in the blood; ___ **infecciosa** / infectious ___, acute febrile infectious disease.

monosacárido *m.* monosaccharide, simple sugar.

monotonía *f.* monotony; monotone.

monótono-a *a.* monotonous.

monstruo *m.* monster.

montar *v.* to ride; ___ **en bicicleta** / ___ a bicycle; to set up; ___ **una consulta** / ___ to assemble, to fit, to adjust a doctor's office.

montón *m.* heap, pile.

morado *m.* bruise, black and blue mark; the color purple; **-a** *a.* purple.

mórbido-a, morboso-a *a.* morbid, rel. to disease.

morbilidad *f.* morbidity. 1. an illness or disorder; 2. the incidence of a disease in a given population or locality.

morbo *m.* illness.

mordedura *f.* 1. bite; 2. a wound caused by a bite.

morder *vi.* to bite.

mordida *f.* 1. bite; 2. the mark left in the skin by the teeth of an animal; 3. forced occlusion of the inferior jaw on the upper teeth; ___ **cruzada** / cross-bite; ___ **de perro** / dog bite.

mordido-a *pp.* de **morder,** bitten; *a.* bitten.

moretón *m.* bruise, black and blue mark.

morfina *f.* morphine, the main alkaloid of opium, used as a narcotic analgesic.

morfinismo *m.* morphinism, condition caused by addiction to morphine.

morgue *Fr.* morgue, place for temporarily holding dead bodies.

moribundo-a *a.* moribund, dying, on the verge of death.

morir *vi.* to die; ___ **con dignidad** / to die with dignity.

morón, morona *m., f.* moron, a mentally retarded person with an IQ of 50 to 70.

mortal *m.* mortal, a human being; *a.* deadly, mortal; **herida** ___ / fatal wound; **veneno** ___ / ___ poison.

mortalidad, mortandad *f.* mortality, death rate; **índice de** ___ / death rate; ___ **fetal** / fetal ___; ___ **infantil** / infant ___; ___ **materna** / maternal ___; ___ **neonatal** / neonatal ___; ___ **perinatal** / perinatal ___ .

mortífero-a *a.* deadly, that can cause death.

mortinatalidad *f.* natimortality, index of still-births.

mortinato-a *m., f.* stillborn.

motor *f.* morula, solid, spheric mass of cells that results from the cell division of a fertilized ovum.

mosaicismo *f.* mosaicism, as in a mosaic, genetically multiple mutated chromosomes determining different characteristics, such as in female physiognomy.

mosaico *m.* 1. mosaic, the presence in one individual of different cell populations derived from just one cell as a result of mutation; 2. mosaic, inlaid artwork combining different small pieces forming a composition.

mosca *f.* fly.

moscardón *m.* gadfly.

mosquito *m.* mosquito.

mostaza *f.* mustard.

mostaza nitrogenada *f.* nitrogen mustard, HG_2, used in the treatment of leukemia and lymphatic neoplasms.

mostrar *vi.* to show, to point out.

moteado-a *a.* mottling, mottled, discolored.

motilidad gástrica *f.* gastric motility, the normal peristaltic movements of the stomach that facilitate the function of digestion.

motivación *f.* motivation, driving force.

motivar *v.* to motivate, to animate.

motivo *m.* motive, cause, driving force.

motocicleta *f.* motorcycle.

motor *m.* motor, agent that causes or induces movement; **-a** *a.* that causes movement.

mover *vi.* to move, to put in motion; **moverse** *vr.* to move oneself.

movible, móvil *a.* mobile, able to move or be moved.

movilidad *f.* mobility, motility.

movilización *f.* mobilization.

movimiento *m.* movement, move, motion; **alcance de** ___ / range of motion; ___ **corporal** / body ___ .

mucina *f.* mucin, glycoprotein that is the chief ingredient of mucus.

mucocele *m.* mucocele, dilation of a cavity due to accumulated mucous secretion.

mucocutáneo-a *a.* mucocutaneous, rel. to the mucous membrane and the skin.

mucoide *m.* mucoid, glycoprotein similar to mucin; *a.* having the consistency of mucus.

mucomembranoso-a *a.* mucomembranous, rel. to the mucous membrane.

mucosa *f.* mucosa, mucous membrane, thin sheets of tissue cells that line openings or canals of the body that communicate to the outside;___ **alveolar** / alveolar ___; ___ **bronquial** / bronchial ___; ___ **de la boca o bucal** / ___ oral; ___ **de la pelvis renal** / ___ of the renal pelvis; ___ **de la vagina** / vaginal ___; ___ **de la vejiga urinaria** / ___ of (*urinary*) bladder; ___ **del colon** / ___ of colon; ___ **del estómago o estomacal** / ___ of stomach; ___ **del intestino delgado** / ___ of small intestine; ___ **esofágica** / esophageal ___; ___ **faringea** / gastric ___; ___ **gástrica** / gastric ___; ___ **laríngea** / laryngeal ___; ___ **lingual** / lingual ___; ___ **nasal** / nasal ___; ___ **olfatoria** / olfactory ___ .

mucoso-a *a.* mucous, mucosal, rel. to or of the nature of the mucosa; **membrana** ___ / ___ membrane, mucosa.

muchacho-a *m., f.* boy; girl.

mudar *v.* to move; ___ **los dientes** / to get one's second teeth; ___ **la piel** / to shed skin.

mudo-a *m., f.* mute.

mueca *f.* grimace.

muela *f.* molar tooth, grinder; **dolor de** ___ **-s** / toothache; ___ **-s del juicio** / wisdom teeth.

muerte *f.* death; ___ **aparente** / apparent ___; ___ **cerebral** / brain ___; ___ **legal** / legal; ___ **por piedad** / mercy killing, euthanasia.

muerte de cuna *f.* crib-death; sudden infant death syndrome.

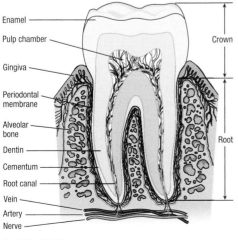

Enamel
Pulp chamber
Gingiva
Periodontal membrane
Alveolar bone
Dentin
Cementum
Root canal
Vein
Artery
Nerve
Crown
Root

A molar tooth

muerte súbita *m.* sudden death, occurring without having a known cause.

muerto-a *m., f.* a dead person; *a.* dead.

muestra *f.* sample; **tomar** ___ **-s** / sampling; **tomar** ___ **-s al azar** / random sampling.

muestreo *m.* sampling; ___ **al azar** / random ___ .

mugre *f.* grime.

muguet *Fr.* thrush, fungus infection of the oral mucosa, manifested by white patches on the lips, tongue, and the interior surface of the cheek.

mujer *f.* woman.

muletas *f. pl.* crutches.

multicelular *a.* multicellular, having many cells.

multifactorial *a.* multifactorial, rel. to many factors.

multifocal *a.* multifocal, rel. to many foci.

multiforme *a.* multiform.

multilocular *a.* multilocular.multicelular.

multípara *f.* multiparous, a woman who has given birth to more than one infant.

multiparidad *f.* multiparity. 1. condition of having borne more than one child; 2. multiple birth.

múltiple *a.* multiple, more than one; **fallo** ___ **de órganos** / ___ organ failure; **personalidad** ___ / ___ personality.

mundo *m.* world.

muñeca *f.* 1. wrist; ___ **caída** / drop ___; carpo. 2. doll.

muñón *m.* stump.

mural *a.* mural, rel. to the walls of an organ or part.

muriático-a *a.* muriatic, derived from common salt; **ácido** ___ / ___ acid.

murino-a *a.* murine, rel. to rodents, esp. mice and rats.

murmullo *m.* murmur, bruit, gen. in reference to an abnormal heart sound.

murmullo vesicular *m.* vesicular breath sound.

muscular, musculoso-a *a.* muscular, rel. to the muscles; **atrofia** ___ / ___ atrophy; **contracción** ___ **brusca** / jerk; **desarrollo** ___ / muscle building; **distensión** ___ / muscle strain; **pérdida de la tonicidad** ___ / loss of muscle tone; **relajador** ___ / muscle relaxant; **rigidez** ___ / ___ rigidity; **tonicidad** ___ / muscle tone.

muscularis *L.* muscularis, muscular layer of an organ or tubule.

musculatura *f.* musculature, the total muscular system.

músculo *m.* muscle, a type of fibrous tissue that has the property to contract allowing movement of the parts and organs of the body; ___ **estriado voluntario** / striated voluntary ___; ___ **flexor** / flexor ___; ___ **visceral involuntario** / visceral involuntary ___ .

musculoesquelético-a *a.* musculoskeletal, rel. to the muscles and the skeleton.

musculotendinoso-a *a.* musculotendinous, having both muscle and tendons.

muslo *m.* thigh, the portion of the lower extremity between the hip and the knee.

musofobia *f.* musophobia, fear of mice.

mutación *f.* mutation, spontaneous or induced change in genetic structure.

mutágeno *m.* mutagen, substance or agent that causes mutation.

mutante *a.* mutant, rel. to an individual or organism with a genetic structure that has undergone mutation.

mutilación *f.* mutilation, castration.

mutilado-a *a.* mutilated.

mutilar *v.* to mutilate, to maim; to cut in pieces.

mutismo *m.* mutism.

mutuo-a *a.* mutual, reciprocal.

muy *adv.* very.

Mycobacterium *L. Mycobacterium,* gram-positive, rod-shaped bacteria, including species that cause leprosy and tuberculosis.

n

N *abr.* **nasal** / nasal; **nervio** / nerve; **nitrógeno** / nitrogen; **normal** / normal; **número** / number.

Naboth, quistes de *m.* nabothian cysts, small, usu. benign cysts that form in one of many small mucus-secreting glands of the neck of the uterus due to obstruction.

nacer *vi.* to be born.

nacido-a *a. pp.* de **nacer,** born; ___ **vivo** / ___ alive; **recién** ___ / newly ___ .

naciente *a.* nascent, incipient. 1. just born; 2. liberated from a chemical compound.

nacimiento *m.* birth; **certificado de** ___ / ___ certificate; ___ **prematuro** / premature ___ ; ___ **tardío** / post-term ___ ; ___ **sin vida** / stillbirth.

nacionalidad *f.* nationality.

nada *f.* nothing, nothingness; *indef. pron.* (after thanks) **de** ___ / Don't mention it!; not at all; by no means.

nadie *pron.* nobody, no one.

nalgas *f. pl.* buttocks.

nanismo *m.* nanism.enanismo.

nanocefalia *f.* nanocephaly, abnormal smallness of the head.

nanocormia *f.* nanocormia. microsomía.

nanomelia *f.* nanomelia. micromelia.

naranja *f.* orange.

narcisismo *m.* narcissism. 1. excessive love of self; 2. sexual pleasure derived from contemplation and admiration of one's own body.

narcoanálisis *m.* narcoanalysis, applied method of narcotherapy; originally used in cases of war psychosis, and later in the treatment of infantile trauma.

narcohipnosis *f.* narcohypnosis, hypnosis induced by the use of narcotics.

narcolepsia *f.* narcolepsy, chronic uncontrollable disposition to sleep.

narcoléptico-a *a.* narcoleptic, rel. to or that suffers from narcolepsia.

narcosis *f.* narcosis, unconsciousness caused by a narcotic. 1. lethargy and alleviation of pain by the effect of narcotics; 2. drug addiction.

narcoterapia *f.* narcotherapy, psychotherapy applied under the effect of a sedative or anarcotic.

narcótico *m.* narcotic, substance with potent analgesic effects that can become addictive;

bloqueo ___ / ___ blockade; **reversión** ___ / ___ reversal.

narcotismo *m.* narcotism, the stuporous state caused by narcotics.

naris *L. nares*naris, nostril.

nariz *f.* nose; **sangramiento por la** ___ / nosebleed; *vr.* **sonarse la** ___ / to blow one's nose.

nasal *a.* nasal, rel. to the nose; **cavidad** ___ / ___ cavity; **congestión** ___ / ___ congestion; **fosa** ___ / nostril; **goteo** ___ / ___ drip; **hemorragia** ___ / ___ hemorrhage; **instilación** ___ / ___ instillation; **meato** ___ / ___ meatus; **pólipo** ___ / ___ polyp; **secreción** ___ / ___ discharge; **tabique** ___ / ___ septum.

nasión *f.* nasion, middle point in the nasofrontal suture.

nasofaringe *f.* nasopharynx, portion of the pharynx that lies above the soft palate. *V.* ilustración en la página 182.

nasogástrico-a *a.* nasogastric, rel. to the nose and the stomach; **tubo** ___ / ___ tube.

nasolabial *a.* nasolabial, rel. to the nose and the lip.

nata *f.* cream.

natal *a.* natal, rel. to birth.

natalidad *f.* natality; **control de la** ___ / birth control; **índice de la** ___ / birth rate.

natilla *f.* custard.

natimortalidad *f.* natimortality, proportion of the death rate of perinatal and natal deaths as to the natality rate. *V.* **natimortality**.

nativo-a *a.* native. 1. in its natural state; 2. indigenous.

natremia *f.* natremia, presence of sodium in the blood.

natriurético *m.* natriuretic. *V.* **diuretic**.

natural *a.* natural; **derechos** ___ -es / birth rights; *v.* **ser** ___ **de** / to be from; **-mente** / *adv.* naturally.

naturaleza *f.* nature.

naturópata *m.* naturopath, practitioner of naturopathy.

naturopatía *f.* naturopathy, therapeutic treatment by natural means.

náusea *f.* nausea, nauseousness; seasickness; *v.* **dar, provocar** ___ / to nauseate; **tener** ___ **-s** / to be nauseated.

nauseabundo-a *a.* nauseous, that causes nausea.

nauseado-a *a.* nauseated.

nauseoso-a *a.* nauseous, that causes nausea.

navicular *a.* navicular. 1. scaphoid bone; 2. boat-shaped; **abdomen** ___ / ___ abdomen;

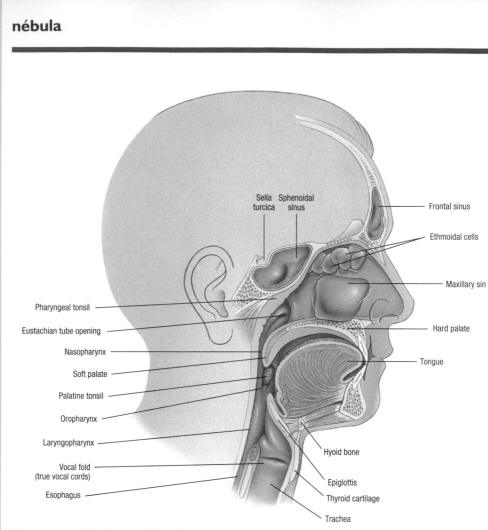

Sella turcica   Sphenoidal sinus   Frontal sinus

Ethmoidal cells

Maxillary sin

Pharyngeal tonsil

Eustachian tube opening   Hard palate

Nasopharynx

Tongue

Soft palate

Palatine tonsil

Oropharynx

Laryngopharynx

Vocal fold
(true vocal cords)   Hyoid bone

Esophagus

Epiglottis

Thyroid cartilage

Trachea

Nasopharyngeal structures: sagittal section

---

fosa ___ **de la uretra** / ___ fossa of the urethra; **hueso** ___ / ___ bone.

nébula *f.* nebula, slight opacity of the eye.

nebulización *f.* nebulization, conversion of liquid into spray or mist.

nebulizador *m.* nebulizer, device used to produce spray or mist from liquid.

nebuloso-a *a.* nebulous.

necesario-a *a.* necessary; **lo** ___ / what is ___; *v.* **ser** ___ / to be ___ .

necesidad *f.* necessity, need; *v.* **tener** ___ / to need.

necesitado-a *a.* needy; **los** ___ **-s** / the needy;

necesitar *v.* to need.

necrobiosis *f.* necrobiosis, gradual degeneration of cells and tissues as a result of changes due to development, aging, and use.

necrocomio *m.* morgue, place to store dead bodies temporarily.

necrofilia *f.* necrophilia. 1. morbid attraction to corpses; 2. sexual intercourse with a corpse.

necrofobia *f.* necrophobia, morbid fear of death and corpses.

necrógeno-a *a.* necrogenic. 1. rel. to death; 2. formed or composed of dead matter.

necrología *f.* necrology, the study of mortality statistics.

necropsia, necroscopia *f.* necropsy. autopsia.

necrosar *v.* to necrose, necrotizing, to cause or undergo necrosis.

necrosis *f.* necrosis, death of some or all of the cells in a tissue such as occurs in gangrene; ___ **aguda de la retina** / acute retinal ___; ___

aséptica / aseptic ___; ___ **caseosa** / caseous ___; ___ **central** / central ___; ___ **cística media** / cystic medial ___; ___ **de coagulación** / coagulation ___; ___ **de tejidos grasos subcutáneos del neonato** / subcutaneous fat ___ of the newborn; ___ **externa progresiva de la retina** / progressive outer retinal ___; ___ **focal** / focal ___; ___ **grasa** / fat ___; ___ **isquémica** / ischemic ___; ___ **laminal cortical** / laminal cortical ___; ___ **progresiva enfisematosa** / progressive emphysematous ___; ___ **renal papilar** / renal papillary ___; ___ **simple** / simple ___; ___ **supurativa** / suppurative ___; ___ **total** / total ___ .

necrótico-a *a.* necrotic, rel. to necrosis.

nefrectomía *f.* nephrectomy, removal of a kidney.

néfrico-a *a.* nephric, renal.

nefrítico-a *a.* nephritic, rel. to or affected by nephritis. **cólico** ___ / ___ colic.

nefritis *f.* nephritis, infl. of a kidney; ___ **aguda** / acute ___; ___ **analgésica** / analgesic ___; ___ **crónica** / chronic ___; ___ **de complejo inmune** / immune complex ___; ___ **focal** / focal ___; ___ **glomerular** / glomerular ___; ___ **hemorrágica** / hemorrhagic ___; ___ **hereditaria** / hereditary ___; ___ **intersticial** / interstitial ___; ___ **lipomatosa** / lupus ___; ___ **sifilítica** / syphilitic ___; ___ **supurativa** / suppurative ___ .

nefrocalcinosis *f.* nephrocalcinosis, renal calcium deposits in the tubules of the kidney that may cause renal insufficiency.

nefrocele *m.* nephrocele, kidney hernia.

nefroesclerosis *f.* nephrosclerosis, hardening of the arterial system and the interstitial tissue of the kidney.

nefrograma *m.* nephrogram, kidney x-ray.

nefrolitiasis *f.* nephrolithiasis, presence of kidney stones.

nefrolitotomía *f.* nephrolithotomy, incision in the kidney to remove kidney stones.

nefrología *f.* nephrology, the study of the kidney and the diseases affecting it.

nefroma *m.* nephroma, kidney tumor.

nefromegalia *f.* nephromegaly, extreme hypertrophy of the kidney.

nefrona *f.* nephron, the functional and anatomical unit of a kidney.

nefropatía *f.* nephropathy, disease of the kidney.

nefropexia *f.* nephropexy, fixation of a floating kidney.

nefrosis *f.* nephrosis, degenerative renal disorder associated with large amounts of protein in the urine, low levels of albumin in the blood, and marked edema.

nefrostomía *f.* nephrostomy, creation of a fistula in the kidney or renal pelvis.

nefrotomía *f.* nephrotomy, surgical incision into the kidney.

nefrotomografía *f.* nephrotomography, tomography of the kidney.

nefrotóxico-a *a.* nephrotoxic, that destroys kidney cells.

nefrotoxina *f.* nephrotoxin, agent that destroys kidney cells.

negación *f.* negation, denial.

negar *vi.* to deny.

negativismo *m.* negativism, behavior characterized by acting in a manner opposite to the one suggested.

negativo-a *a.* negative; **cultivo** ___ / ___ culture; **-mente** *adv.* negatively.

negligencia *f.* negligence; ___ **profesional** / malpractice.

negligente *a.* negligent.

negro-a *m., f.* 1. a black person; 2. the color black; *a.* black.

nematelminto *m.* nemathelminth, roundworm, intestinal worm of the phylum *Nemathelminthes*.

nematocida *m.* nematocide, agent that kills nematodes.

Nematoda *Gr.* Nematoda, class of worms of the phylum *Nemathelminthes*; nematode.

nematodiasis *f.* nematodiasis, infection by nematode parasites.

nemátodo *m.* nematode, worm of the class *Nematoda*.

nematología *f.* nematology, the study of worms of the class *Nematoda*.

nene-a *m., f.* baby.

neoartrosis *f.* nearthrosis, neoarthrosis, false or artificial joint.

neologismo *m.* neologism. 1. word or phrase to which a mentally disturbed individual attributes a meaning unrelated to its real meaning; 2. new word or phrase or an old one to which a new meaning has been attributed.

neomicina *f.* neomycin, broad-spectrum antibiotic.

neonatal *a.* neonatal, rel. to the first four to six weeks after birth.

neonato-a *a.* 1. neonate, newborn; 2. infant born 37 weeks into normal gestation.

neonatología *f.* neonatology, specialty that studies the care and treatment of newborns.

neonatólogo-a *m., f.* neonathologist, specialist in neonatology.

neoplasia *f.* neoplasia, formation of neoplasms.

neoplasma *m.* neoplasm, abnormal growth of new tissue such as a tumor.

neoplástico-a *a.* neoplastic, rel. to a neoplasm.

neovascularización *f.* neovascularization, abnormal proliferation of new blood vessels as a reaction to ischemia.

nervio *m.* nerve, one or more bundles of fibers that connect the brain and spinal cord with other parts and organs of the body; **bloqueo del** ___ / ___ block; **degeneración del** ___ / ___ degeneration; ___ **pellizcado** / pinched ___; **terminación del** ___ / ___ ending.

nervio ciático *m.* sciatic nerve, nerve that extends from the base of the spine down to the thigh with branches throughout the lower leg and the foot.

nerviosismo *m.* nervousness; *pop.* jitters.

nervioso-a *a.* nervous, rel. to the nerves; **crisis** ___ / ___ breakdown, collapse; **fibra** ___ / nerve fiber; **impulso** ___ / nerve impulse; **tejido** ___ / nerve tissue.

nestiatría *f.* nestiatria, fasting therapy.

neumático-a *a.* pneumatic, rel. to air or respiration.

neumatización *f.* pneumatization, formation of air cavities in a bone, esp. the temporal bone.

neumatocele *m.* pneumatocele. 1. hernial protuberance of lung tissue; 2. a tumor or sac containing gas.

neumococal, neumocócico-a *a.* pneumococcal, rel. to or caused by pneumococci.

neumococo *m.* pneumococcus, one of a group of gram-positive bacteria that cause acute pneumonia and other infections of the upper respiratory tract.

neumoencefalografía *f.* pneumoencephalography, x-ray of the brain by previous injection of air or gas allowing visualization of the cerebral cortex and ventricles.

neumonía *f.* pneumonia, infectious disease of the upper respiratory tract caused by bacteria or virus that affect the lungs; ___ **doble** / double ___; ___ **estafilocócica** / staphylococcal ___; ___ **lobar** / lobar ___ .

neumonía migratoria *f.* migratory pneumonia, type of pneumonia that appears in different parts of the lung.

neumonía neumocística carinii *f.* pneumocystis pneumonia carinii, a type of acute pneumonia caused by the bacillus *Pneumocystis carinii* and one of the opportunistic diseases seen in cases of AIDS.

neumónico-a *a.* pneumonic, rel. to the lungs or to pneumonia.

neumonitis *f.* pneumonitis. neumonía.

neumopatía *f.* lung disease.

neumotórax *m.* pneumothorax, accumulation of gas or air in the pleural cavity that results in the collapse of the affected lung; ___ **espontáneo** / spontaneous ___; ___ **por tensión** / tension ___ .

neural *a.* neural, rel. to the nervous system; **arco** ___ / ___ arch; **cresta** ___ / ___ crest; **pliegues neurales** / ___ folds; **placa** ___ / ___ plate; **quiste** ___ / ___ cyst.

neuralgia *f.* neuralgia, pain along a nerve;___ **facial** / facial ___; ___ **facial atípica** / atypical facial ___; ___ **glosofaríngea** / glossopharyngeal ___; ___ **halucinatoria** / hallucinatory ___; ___ **trigeminal atípica** / atypical trigeminal ___ .

neurálgico-a *a.* neuralgic, rel. to neuralgia; **puntos** ___ -s / tender points.

neurapraxia *f.* neurapraxia, temporary paralysis of a nerve without degeneration.

neurastenia *f.* neurasthenia, term usu. associated with increased irritability, tension, and anxiety, accompanied by physical exhaustion; ___ **angiopática** / angiopathic ___; ___ **grave** / ___ gravis; ___ **precoz** / praecox ___; ___ **primaria** / primary ___; ___ **pulsativa** / pulsating ___ .

neurasténico-a *a.* neurasthenic, rel. to or afflicted by neurasthenia.

neurectomía *f.* neurectomy, excisíon or resection of a nerve.

neurilema *f.* neurilemma, thin membranous covering that encloses a nerve fiber.

neurinoma *m.* neurinoma, benign neoplasm of the sheath surrounding a nerve.

neuritis *f.* neuritis, infl. of a nerve.

neuroanatomía *f.* neuroanatomy, the study and practice of the anatomy of the nervous system.

neuroblasto *m.* neuroblast, the immature nerve cell.

neuroblastoma *m.* neuroblastoma, malignant tumor of the nervous system formed mostly of neuroblasts.

neurocirugía *f.* neurosurgery, the study and practice of surgery of the nervous system.

neurocirujano-a *m., f.* neurosurgeon, specialist in neurosurgery.

neurodermatitis *f.* neurodermatitis, chronic skin disease of unknown origin manifested by intense itching in localized areas.

neuroectodermo *m.* neuroectoderm, embryonary tissue from which the nerve tissue derives.

neuroendocrinología *f.* neuroendocrinology, the study of the nervous system as it relates to hormones.

neurofarmacología *f.* neuropharmacology, the study of drugs and medications as they affect the nervous system.

neurofibroma *m.* neurofibroma, tumor of the fibrous tissue of a peripheral nerve.

neurofibromatosis *f.* neurofibromatosis, disease characterized by the presence of multiple neurofibromas along the peripheral nerves.

neurofisiología *f.* neurophysiology, the study of the physiology of the nervous system.

neurogenético-a *a.* neurogenic, neurogenetic. 1. that originates in the nervous tissue; 2. due to nervous impulses; **atrofia** ___ / ___ atrophy.

neuroglia *f.* neuroglia, connective, supportive cells that constitute the interstitial tissue of the nervous system.

neurohipófisis *f.* neurohypophysis, posterior and nervous portion of the pituitary gland.

neurolepsia *f.* neurolepsia, agitated state of consciousness due to drugs; patient shows signs of anxiety and indifference.

neuroléptico *m.* neuroleptic, tranquilizer; it belongs to the psycotropic group of drugs used in the treatment of psychosis, esp. schizophrenia; **-a** *a.* **anestesia** ___ / ___ anesthesia;

neurolisina *f.* neurolysin, injectable antibody that is obtained from a cerebral substance. *Syn.* **neurotoxina**.

neurolisis *f.* neurolysis, process of liberating a nerve from inflammatory adnexa.

neurología *f.* neurology, the study of the nervous system.

neurólogo-a *m., f.* neurologist, specialist in neurology.

neuroma *f.* neuroma, tumor composed mainly of nerve cells and fibers; ___ **acústico** / acoustic ___ .

neuromalacia *f.* neuromalacia, pathologic softening of nervous tissue.

neuromarcapaso *m.* neuropacemaker, instrument used to stimulate the spinal cord electrically.

neuromatosis *f.* neuromatosis, the presence of multiple neuromas.

neuromeníngeo-a *a.* neuromeningeal, rel. to the nervous tissues and the meninges.

neuromuscular *a.* neuromuscular, rel. to the nerves and the muscles; **agentes bloqueadores** ___ -es / ___ blocking agents; **relajador** ___ / ___ relaxant; **sistema** ___ / ___ system.

neurona *f.* neuron, nerve cell, the basic functional and structural unit of the nervous system; ___ **motor** / motor ___ , carries the impulses that initiate muscle contraction.

neuro-oftalmología *f.* neuro-ophthalmology, the study of the relationship between the nervous and visual systems.

neuropatía *f.* neuropathy, a disorder or pathological change in the peripheral nerves.

neurópilo *m.* neuropil, network of nervous fibers (neurites, dendrites, and glia cells) that concentrate in different parts of the nervous system.

neuroporo *m.* neuropore, embryonic aperture to the exterior of the neural canal.

neuroradiología *f.* neuroradiology, x-ray study of the nervous system.

neurorregulador *m.* neurotransmitter, a chemical substance that affects the transmission of impulses across a synapse between nerves or between a nerve and a muscle.

neurosarcoclesis *f.* neurosarcoclesis, surgical intervention to alleviate neuralgia consisting in the resection of a wall of the osseous canal, and transposition of the nerve to soft tissues.

neurosicofarmacología *f.* neuropsychopharmacology, the study of drugs as they affect the treatment of mental disorders.

neurosífilis *f.* neurosyphilis, syphilis that affects the nervous system; ___ **tabética** / tabetic ___ .

neurosis *f.* neurosis, condition manifested primarily by anxiety and the use of defense mechanisms; ___ **accidental** / accident ___; ___ **cardíaca** / cardíac ___; ___ **compulsiva** / compulsive ___; ___ **de ansiedad** / anxiety ___; ___ **de compensación** / compensation ___; ___ **de guerra** / combat ___; ___ **del carácter** / character ___; ___ **depresiva** / depressive ___; ___ **hipocondríaca** / hypochondriacal ___; ___ **histérica** / hysterical ___; ___ **obsesiva** / obsessional ___; ___ **obsesiva-compulsiva** / obsessive-compulsive ___; ___ **ocupacional** / occupational ___; ___ **post-traumática** / post-traumatic ___ . *V.* cuadro en la página 465.

neurótico-a *a.* neurotic, rel. to or suffering from neurosis.

neurotomía *f.* neurotomy, dissection or division of a nerve.

neurotoxicidad *f.* the capacity of a substance or agent to destroy or harm the nervous tissue.

neurotóxico-a *a.* neurotoxic, that has a toxic effect on the nervous system; **agente** ___ / ___ agent;

neurotoxina *f.* neurotoxin, any toxin that sets itself specifically over the nervous tissue.

neurotrasmisor *m.* neurotransmitter, chemical substance that modifies the transmission of impulses through a synapse between nerves or between a nerve and a muscle; ___ **adrenérgico** / adrenergic ___; ___ **colinérgico** / cholinergic ___ .

neurovascular *a.* neurovascular, rel. to the nervous and vascular systems.

neutral, neutro-a *a.* neutral.

neutralización *f.* neutralization, process that annuls or counteracts the action of an agent.

neutralizar *vi.* to neutralize, to counteract.

neutrofilia *f.* neutrophilia, increase in number of neutrophils in the blood.

neutropenia *f.* neutropenia. agranulocitosis.

neutrotaxis *f.* neutrotaxis, stimulation of neutrophils by a substance that either attracts or repels them.

nevar *vi.* to snow.

nevo *m.* nevus, mole, birthmark; ___ **comedónico** / comedonicus ___; ___ **compuesto** / compound ___; ___ **de cola de fauno** / faun tail ___; ___ **de displasia** / dysplastic ___; ___ **de Ota** / Ota's ___; ___ **de unión** / junction, junctional ___; ___ **melanocítico** / melanocytic ___; ___ **sebáceo** / sebaceous ___ .

nexo *m.* nexus, connection.

ni *conj.* neither, nor; ___ **bueno** ___ **malo** / neither good nor bad; ___ **siquiera** / not even.

niacina *f.* niacin, nicotinic acid.

nicotina *f.* nicotine, toxic alkaloid that is the main ingredient of tobacco causing ill effects on smokers.

nictalopía *f.* nyctalopia, night blindness.

nictitación *f.* nictitation, the act of winking.

nicturia, nocturia *f.* nocturia, nycturia, frequent urination during the night.

nicho *m.* niche, small defect or depression esp. in the wall of a hollow organ.

nidación *f.* nidation, implantation of the fertilized ovum into the uterine endometruim.

nido *m.* nest, small cellular mass resembling a bird's nest.

niebla *f.* fog.

nieto-a *m., f.* grandson, granddaughter.

nieve *f.* snow; *Mex.* ice cream.

nigua *f.* chigger, chigoe.

nihilismo *m.* nihilism, in psychiatry an illusory idea that nothing is real or existent.

ninfa *f.* nympha, inner lip of the vulva.

ninfectomía *f.* nymphectomy, partial or total excision of the labium.

ninfomanía *f.* nymphomania, excessive sexual desire in the female.

ninfomaníaca *f.* nymphomaniac, rel. to or suffering from nymphomania.

ningún, ninguno-a *a.* not one, not any; **de** ___ **modo, de ninguna manera** / in no way; *pron.* nobody; none, no one; neither.

niña del ojo *f.* pupil of the eye.

niñez *f.* childhood.

niño-a *m., f.* child; ___ **maltratado-a** / battered ___ .

nistagmo *m.* nystagmus, involuntary spasm of the eyeball; ___ **palatino** / palatal ___ .

nistagmografía *f.* nystagmography, technique to register nystagmus.

nitrato *m.* nitrate, chemical agent.

nitrógeno *m.* nitrogen; ___ **auténtico, legítimo** / authentic, legitimate ___; ___ **ilegítimo** / illegitimate ___; ___ **monóxido** / monoxide ___; ___ **no protéico** / non protein ___; ___ **residual** / residual ___; ___ **uréico** / urea ___ .

nitroglicerina *f.* nitroglycerine, a nitrate of glycerin used in medicine as a vasodilator, esp. in angina pectoris.

nivel *m.* level.

nivelación *f.* levelling.

no *adv.* no, not; ___ **importa** / it doesn't matter; ___ **obstante** / nevertheless.

Nocardia *f.* Nocardia, gram-positive microorganism, cause of nocardiasis.

nocardiasis *f.* nocardiasis, infection caused by the species *Nocardia* that gen. affects the lungs but can also expand to other parts of the body.

noche *f.* night; **de** ___ / at ___; **buenas** ___ **-s** / good evening, good night; **por la** ___ / in the evening.

nocivo-a *a.* noxious, harmful, pernicious.

nocturno-a *a.* nocturnal; **emisión** ___ / ___ emission.

nodal *a.* nodal, rel. to a node.

nodular *a.* nodular, rel. to or resembling a nodule.

nódulo *m.* nodule, small node; ___ **linfático** / lymphatic ___; ___ **solitario** / solitary ___; ___ **subcutáneo** / subcutaneous ___ .

noma *f.* noma, ulcer, gangrenous stomatitis usually beginning in the corner of the mouth or interior cheek, progressing to the lips; gen. following a debilitating sickness.

nómada *a.* nomadic, free, wandering.

nombre *m.* name; ___ **genérico** / generic ___ , common name of a drug or medication that is not registered commercially; ___ **de pila** / given ___ .

nomenclatura *f.* nomenclature, terminology.

nominal *a.* nominal, rel. to the noun; **afasia** ___ / ___ aphasia, inability to name objects.

nonato-a *m., f.* 1. unborn; 2. born by Cesarean section.

non compos mentis *L.* non compos mentis, mentally incompetent.

norepinefrina *f.* norepinephrine, vasoconstrictor agent produced in the adrenal gland.

norma *f.* norm, model, standard.

normal *a.* normal.

normalización *f.* normalization, return to a normal state.

normoblasto *m.* normoblast, red blood cell, a precursor of erythrocytes in humans.

normocalcemia *f.* normocalcemia, normal level of calcium in the blood.

normoglicemia *f.* normoglycemia, normal concentration of glucose in the blood.

normopotasemia *f.* normokalemia, normal level of potassium in the blood.

normotenso-a *a.* normotensive, having a normal blood pressure.

normotermia *f.* normothermia, normal temperature.

normovolemia *f.* normovolemia, normal blood volume.

norte *m.* north; **al** ___ / to the ___ .

nosocomial *a.* nosocomial, rel. to a hospital or infirmary; **infección** ___ / ___ infection, acquired in a hospital.

nostalgia *f.* nostalgia, homesickness.

nota *f.* note; remark.

notable *a.* remarkable.

notalgia *f.* notalgia, back ache.

notar *v.* to note; to become aware of something.

noticias *f. pl.* news.

notificación *f.* notification, notice.

notificar *vi.* to notify, to make known.

notocordio *m.* notochord, the axial fibrocellular cord in the embryo that is replaced by the vertebral column.

novocaína *f.* novocaine, anesthetic.

núbil *a.* nubile, rel. to female sexual maturity.

nublado-a *a.* bleary; cloudy; **vista** ___ / ___ eyed.

nuca *f.* nucha, nape, posterior part of the neck.

nucal *a.* nuchal, rel. to the nape.

nuclear *a.* nuclear. 1. rel. to the nucleus; **envoltura** ___ / ___ envelope, the two parallel membranes surrounding the nucleus, as seen under an electron microscope; 2. rel. to atomic power; **desecho** ___ / ___ waste.

núcleo *m.* nucleus, the essential part of the cell; ___ **pulposo** / ___ pulpous, central gelatinous mass within an intervertebral disk.

nucleolo *m.* nucleolus, small spherical structure found in the nucleus of cells.

nucleópeto-a *a.* nucleopetal, that moves towards the nucleus.

nucleotido *m.* nucleotide, the structural unit of nucleic acid.

nudillo *m.* knuckle.

nudo *m.* node, knotlike mass of tissue; knot; ___ **de los ordeñadores** / milker's ___; ___ **del vermis** / vermis ___; ___ **sifilítico** / syphilitic ___; ___ **vocal o de los cantantes** / vocal or singer's ___ .

nudoso-a *a.* nodose, that has nodules or protuberances.

nuevo-a *a.* new.

nuez *f.* walnut; nut.

nuez de Adan *f.* Adam's apple.

nuligrávida *f.* nulligravida, a woman who has never conceived.

nulípara *f.* nullipara; nullipara, a woman who has never borne a living child; *a.* nulliparous, nonparous.

nulo-a *a.* null, void.

número *m.* number; figure.

numeroso-a *a.* numerous.

nunca *adv.* never; at no time; **casi** ___ / hardly ever.

nutrición *f.* nutrition, nourishment.

nutriente *m.* nutrient, nutritious substance; *a.* nourishing.

nutritivo-a *a.* nutritious, providing nourishment.

Ñ

Ñ *m.* seventeenth letter of the Spanish alphabet.

ñame *m.* yam.

ñoco-a *a. pop.* missing, **la mano-** (*le falta un dedo*), he has lost a finger in his hand.

ñoñería *f.* childishness; simplemindedness.

ñoño-a *a.* childlike; simple-minded.

O

O *abr.* **ojo** / oculus; **oral, oralmente** / oral, orally; **oxígeno** / oxygen.

o *conj.* either, or; ___ **bien** ___ **mal** / one way or another, anyway.

obedecer *vi.* to obey.

obediente *a.* obedient, compliant.

obesidad *f.* obesity, excess fat; ___ **alimentaria** / alimentary ___; ___ **endógena** / endogenous ___; ___ **exógena** / exogenous ___ .

obeso-a *a.* obese, excessively fat.

objetivo *m.* objective, goal; target; **-a** *a.* rel. to the perception of any happening or phenomenon as it is manifested in real life; **-mente** *adv.* objectively.

oblicuidad *f.* obliquity, the state of being slanted.

oblicuo-a *a.* oblique, diagonal; skewed.

obligación *f.* obligation, duty.

obligar *vi.* to obligate, to force, to compel.

obliteración *f.* obliteration, destruction, occlusion by degeneration or by surgery.

obliterar *v.* to obliterate, to annul, to destroy.

obrar *v.* to act, to work; *Mex.* to have a bowel movement.

obscuridad, oscuridad *f.* darkness.

obscuro-a, oscuro-a *a.* dark.

observación *f.* observation; remark.

observar *v.* to observe.

obsesión *f.* obsession, abnormal preoccupation with a single idea or emotion; *pop.* hang-up.

obsesivo-compulsivo-a *a.* obsessive-compulsive, rel. to an individual that is driven to repeat actions excessively as a relief of tension and anxiety.

obseso-a *a.* possessed, dominated by an idea or passion.

obsoleto-a *a.* obsolete, outdated; inactive.

obstáculo *m.* obstacle, hurdle.

obstetra *m., f.* obstetrician.

obstetricia *f.* obstetrics, the study of the care of women during pregnancy and delivery.

obstétrico-a *a.* obstetric, rel. to obstetrics.

obstinado-a *a.* obstinate, headstrong, opinionated, stubborn.

obstipación *f.* obstipation, severe constipation.

obstrucción *f.* obstruction, blockage; ___ **crónica del pulmón** / obstructive lung disease, chronic condition caused by the physical or functional narrowing of the bronchial tree; ___ **en el conducto aéreo superior** / upper airway ___; ___ **intestinal** / ___ intestinal blockage.

obstruído-a *a.* obstructed, blocked; **no** ___ / unobstructed.

obstruir *vi.* to obstruct, to block, to impede.

obtener *vi.* to obtain, to attain, to achieve.

obturación *f.* obturation, occlusion.

obturador-a *a.* obturator, that obstructs an opening.

obtuso-a *a.* obtuse. 1. lacking mental acuity; 2. [*filo*] blunt, dull.

obvio-a *a.* obvious, evident.

ocasión *f.* occasion.

ocasionar *v.* to cause.

occipital *a.* occipital, rel. to the back part of the head; **hueso** ___ / ___ bone; **lóbulo** ___ / ___ lobe.

occipitofrontal *a.* occipitofrontal, rel. to the occiput and the forehead.

occipitoparietal *a.* occipitoparietal, rel. to the occipital and parietal bones and lobes.

occipitotemporal *a.* occipitotemporal, rel. to the occipital and temporal bones.

occipucio *m.* occiput, posteroinferior part of the skull.

oclusión *f.* occlusion, obstruction; ___ **coronaria** / coronary ___; ___ **de la pupila** / pupillar ___ .

octogenario-a *m., f.* octogenarian, individual that is about eighty years old.

ocular *a.* ocular, visual, rel. to the eyes; **cuerpo extraño** ___ / ___ foreign body; **globo** ___ / eyeball; **movimientos** ___ **-es** / ___ movements; **ataxia** ___ / ___ ataxia; **cono** ___ / ___ cone; ___ [de un aparato óptico] / ___ eyepiece; **órbita** ___ / ___ eyesocket; **traumatismo** ___ / ___ eye injury; **vértigo** ___ / ___ vertigo.

oculista *m., f.* oculist. oftalmólogo.

oculógiro-a *a.* oculogyric, rel. to the rotation of the eyeball.

oculografía *f.* oculography, method of registering the position and movement of the eyes.

oculomotor *a.* oculomotor, rel. to the movement of the eyeball.

ocultar *v.* to conceal, to hide.

oculto-a *a.* occult, concealed, not visible.

oculus *L.* oculus, eye.

ocupación *f.* occupation.

ocupacional *a.* occupational, rel. to an occupation; **lesiones ocupacionales** / ___ injuries; **salud** ___ / ___ health; **terapista** ___ / ___ therapist.

ocupado-a *a.* busy; occupied.

Oddi, esfínter de *m.* Oddi's sphincter, circular contractile muscle located at the level of the angular notch of the stomach and the pancreatic ducts.

odiar *v.* to hate.

odinofobia *f.* odynophobia, morbid fear of pain.

odio *m.* hate, hatred.

odontalgia *f.* odontalgia, toothache.

odontectomía *f.* odontectomy, tooth extraction.

odontogénesis *f.* odontogenesis, tooth development.

odontoideo-a *a.* odontoid, dentiform, resembling a tooth.

odontología *f.* odontology, the study of dentistry.

odontólogo-a *m., f.* odontologist, dentist or oral surgeon.

odontoplastia *f.* odontoplasty, surgical procedure used to improve plaque control and gingival care.

oeste *m.* west; **al** ___ / to the ___ .

oficial *a.* official, authorized; **no** ___ / unofficial, rel. to medication not listed in the Pharmacopeia or standard formulary.

oficina *f.* office.

oftalmia *f.* ophthalmia. 1. severe conjunctivitis; 2. internal infl. of the eye.

oftálmico-a *a.* ophthalmic, rel. to the eye; **nervio** ___ / ___ nerve; **solución** ___ / ___ solution.

oftalmitis *f.* ophthalmitis, infl. of the eye.

oftalmología *f.* ophthalmology, the study of the eye and its disorders.

oftalmólogo-a *m., f.* ophthalmologist, oculist, specialist in eye disorders.

oftalmopatía *f.* ophthalmopathy, eye disorder.

oftalmoplastia *f.* ophthalmoplasty, plastic surgery of the eye.

oftalmoplejía *f.* ophthalmoplegia, paralysis of an eye muscle.

oftalmoscopía *f.* ophthalmoscopy, examination of the eye with an ophthalmoscope.

oftalmoscopio *m.* ophthalmoscope, instrument for viewing the interior of the eye.

oído *m.* ear. 1. hearing organ formed by the inner, middle, and external ear; 2. the sense of hearing; **dolor de** ___ / earache; ___ **tapado con cerumen** / ___ covered with earwax; **zumbido en los** ___ -s / ringing ___ -s.

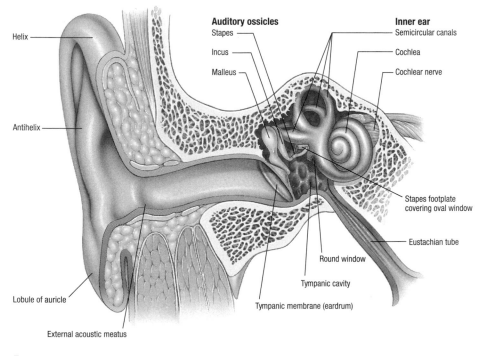

Helix

Antihelix

Lobule of auricle

External acoustic meatus

Auditory ossicles
Stapes
Incus
Malleus

Inner ear
Semicircular canals
Cochlea
Cochlear nerve

Stapes footplate covering oval window

Eustachian tube

Round window

Tympanic cavity

Tympanic membrane (eardrum)

Ear structures

oír *vi.* to hear.

ojeada *f.* glance; **dar una** ___ / to glance.

ojeras *f. pl.* dark circles under the eyes.

ojeroso-a *a.* haggard, referring to someone with dark circles under their eyes.

ojo *m.* eye; **banco de** ___ **-s** / ___ bank; **cuenca del** ___ / ___ socket; **fondo del** ___ / eyeground; **gotas para los** ___ **-s** / ___ drops; ___ **de vidrio** / glass ___; ___ **-s inyectados** / bloodshot ___ **-s**; ___ **-s llorosos** / watery ___ **-s**; ___ **-s saltones** / goggle-eyed. *V.* ilustración en la página 192.

oleada *f.* tide, a space of time; rise and fall.

oleaginoso-a *a.* oleaginous, oily, unctuous.

oleomargarina *f.* oleomargarine.

oler *vi.* to smell, to scent.

olfacción *f.* olfaction. 1. the act of smelling; 2. the sense of smell.

olfatear *v.* to sniff.

olfato *m.* 1. the sense of smell; 2. odor.
  olfatorio-a *a.* olfactory, rel. to smell.

oligodactilia *f.* oligodactyly, less than the normal number of toes or fingers.

oligodendrocito *m.* oligodendrocyte, neuroglia cell that participates in few and delicate processes.

oligodendroglia *f.* oligodendroglia, a neuroglia cell that forms or maintains the tissue of the central nervous system.

oligodoncia *f.* oligodontia, hereditary condition consisting in fewer teeth than normal.

oligohemia *f.* oligemia, hyphemia.hipovolemia.

oligohidramnios *m.* oligohydramnios, low level of amniotic fluid.

oligomenorrea *f.* oligomenorrhea, deficient or infrequent menstruation.

oligospermia *f.* oligospermia, diminished number of spermatozoa in the semen.

oliguria *f.* oliguria, diminished formation of urine.

oliva *f.* olive. 1. gray body behind the medulla oblongata; 2. green olive color; 3. the olive tree.

olor *m.* odor, smell, scent; ___ **penetrante** / penetrating smell.

oloroso-a *a.* odorous.

olvidadizo-a *a.* forgetful.

olvidar *v.* to forget.

omalgia *f.* omalgia, pain in the shoulder.

ombligo *m.* umbilicus, navel, a depression in the center of the abdomen at the point of insertion of the uterine canal at the time of birth; *pop.* belly button.

omental *a.* omental, rel. to or formed from omentum.

omentectomía *f.* omentectomy, partial or total removal of the omentum.

omentitis *f.* omentitis, infl. of the omentum.

omento *m.* omentum, a fold of the peritoneum that connects the stomach with some abdominal viscera.

omisión *f.* omission.

omitir *v.* to omit.

onanismo *m.* onanism, coitus interruptus, interrupted coitus.

oncogénesis *f.* oncogenesis, formation and development of tumors.

oncogénico-a *a.* oncogenic, rel. to oncogenesis.

oncólisis *f.* oncolysis, destruction of tumor cells.

oncología *f.* oncology, the study of tumors.

oncótico-a *a.* oncotic, rel. to or caused by swelling.

onda *f.* wave. 1. ondulant movement or vibration that travels along a fixed direction; 2. ondulant graphic representation of an activity, such as seen in an electroencephalogram; **guía de** ___ **-s** / waveguide; **longitud de** ___ / wavelength; ___ **pulsátil** / pulse ___; ___ **Q** / Q ___; ___ **R** / R ___; ___ **-s cerebrales** / brain ___ **-s**; ___ **-s de excitación** / excitation ___ **-s**; ___ **sonora** / sound ___; ___ **-s ultrasónicas** / ultrasound ___ **-s**.

onda T *f.* T wave, part of the electrocardiogram that represents the repolarization of the ventricles.

onda V *f.* V wave, positive wave that follows the T wave in an electrocardiogram.

ondulado-a *a.* ondulant, having an irregular or wavy border.

onfalectomía *f.* omphalectomy, removal of the umbilicus.

onfálico-a *a.* omphalic, rel. to the umbilicus.

onfalitis *f.* omphalitis, infl. of the umbilicus.

onfalocele *m.* omphalocele, umbilical hernia.

onicopatía *f.* onicopathy, any disease of the nail.

onicosis *f.* onychosis, deformity or sickness of a nail.

oniomanía *f.* oniomania, pathological urge to spend money.

oniquectomía *f.* onychectomy, excision of a nail.

oniquia *f.* onychia, infl. of a nailbed.

onírico-a *a.* oneiric, rel. to dreams.

onirismo *m.* oneirism, dreamlike state while awake.

onomatonamía *f.* onomatonamia, obsessive urge to repeat words.

oocinesis *f.* ookinesis, mitosis of the egg in the embryonic ovary during maturation and fertilization.

oocito, ovocito *m.* oocyte, female ovum before maturation.

ooforectomía *f.* oophorectomy, partial or total excision of an ovary.

ooforitis *f.* oophoritis, infl. of an ovary.

ooforocistosis *f.* oophorocystosis, formation of an ovarian cyst.

ooforopexia *f.* oophoropexy, fixation or suspension of a displaced ovary.

oogénesis, ovogénesis *f.* oogenesis, ovogenesis, formation and development of an ovum.

oospermo *m.* oosperm, a fertilized ovum.

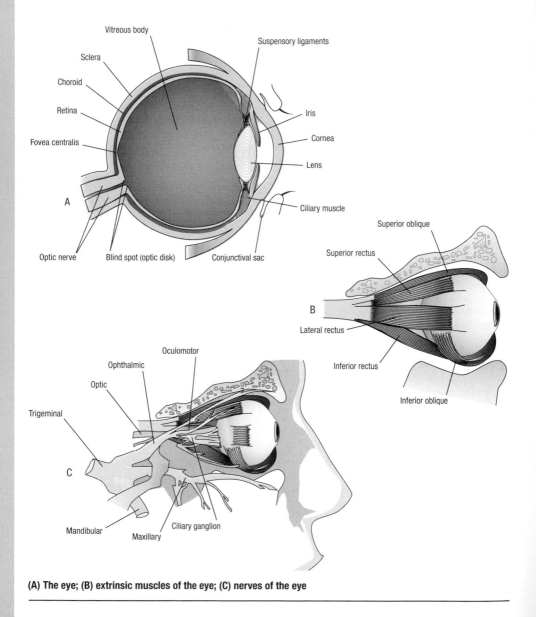

(A) The eye; (B) extrinsic muscles of the eye; (C) nerves of the eye

opacidad *f.* opacity, dimness, lack of transparency.

opacificación *f.* opacification, process of rendering something opaque.

opaco-a *a.* opaque, that does not filter light.

operable *a.* operable, that can be treated by surgery.

operación *f.* operation, surgical procedure.

operar *v.* to operate, to intervene surgically.

opérculo *m.* operculum. 1. covering or lid; 2. any of the several parts of the cerebrum covering the insula.

operón *m.* operon, a system of linked genes in which the operator gene regulates the remaining structural genes.

opiáceo *m.* opiate, opium-derived drug.

opinar *v.* to express an opinion.

opinión *f.* opinion, judgment.

opio *m.* opium, *Papaver somniferum,* narcotic, analgesic, alucinogen, stimulant, addictive

opistótonos *m.* opisthotonos, tetanic spasm of the muscles of the back in which the heels and head bend backward and the trunk projects forward.

oponer *vi.* to oppose; *vr.* **oponerse,** to be against, to oppose.

oportunidad *f.* opportunity, chance.

oportunista *a.* opportunistic; opportune.

oportuno-a *a.* timely, opportune.

oposición *f.* opposition; objection.

opresión *f.* oppression; heaviness; ___ **en el pecho** / an ___ in the chest.

opresivo-a *a.* oppressive; overwhelming.

oprimir *v.* to oppress.

opsoclono *m.* opsoclonus, irregular movement of the eyes, esp. seen in some cases of brain lesion.

opsonina *f.* opsonin, antibody that combines with a specific antigen and makes it more susceptible to phagocytes.

óptica *f.* optics, the study of light and its relation to vision; *a.* **óptico-a,** optic, optical, rel. to vision; **disco** ___ / ___ disk, blind spot of the retina; **ilusión** ___ / ___ illusion; **nervio** ___ / ___ nerve.

óptimo-a *a.* optimum, the best, the ideal.

optómetra, optometrista *m., f.* optometrist, professional who practices optometry.

optometría *f.* optometry, the practice of examining the eyes for visual acuity and prescribing corrective lenses and other optical aids.

optómetro *m.* optometer, instrument used to measure eye refraction.

opuesto-a *a.* opposite; opposed.

oral *a.* oral, delivered or taken by mouth.

orbicular *a.* orbicular, circular; **músculo** ___ / ___ muscle, that surrounds a small opening such as the orbicular muscle of the mouth; ___ **de los labios** / ___ oris; ___ **de los párpados** / ___ ciliaris.

órbita *f.* orbit, bony cavity that contains the eyeball and associated structures.

orbital *a.* orbital, rel. to the orbit.

orden *m.* order, arrangement; regulation.

ordenar *v.* to order; to arrange.

ordeño *m.* milking, maneuver to force material out of a tube.

ordinario-a *a.* ordinary, usual, common.

oreja *f.* external ear; **lóbulo de la** ___ / ear lobe.

orejera *f.* ear protector.

orejuela *f.* auricle, flop of tissue that partially covers the atrium.

orexígeno-a *a.* orexigenic, that stimulates appetite.

organelo, organito *m.* organelle, minute organ of unicellular organisms.

orgánico-a *a.* organic. 1. rel. to an organ; 2. rel. to organisms of vegetable or animal origin; **enfermedad** ___ / ___ disease.

organismo *m.* organism, a living being.

organización *f.* organization, association.

organizar *vi.* to organize, to arrange.

órgano *m.* organ, part of the body with a specific function; **desplazamiento de** ___ / ___ displacement; ___ **terminal** / end ___; **transplante de un** ___ / ___ transplant.

organogénesis *f.* organogenesis, growth and development of an organ.

organomegalia *f.* organomegaly, abnormal enlargement of the visceral organs. *Syn.* visceromegaly.

orgasmo *m.* orgasm, sexual climax.

orgulloso-a *a.* proud.

orientación *f.* orientation, direction.

orientacion a la realidad *f.* reality orientation, the patient remains turned inward and in contact with his or her own environment.

orificio *m.* orifice, aperture, opening.

origen *m.* origin, source, beginning.

original *a.* original.

orín, orina *m., f.* urine, the clear fluid secreted by the kidneys, stored in the urinary bladder, and discharged by the urethra; **cultivo de** ___ / ___ culture; **especimen de** ___ **a mitad de chorro** / midstream ___ specimen; **muestra de** ___ / ___ sample; ___ **claro-a** / clear ___; ___ **lechoso-a** /

milky ___; ___ **turbio-a** / hazy ___; **sedimento de** ___ / ___ sediment. *V.* cuadro en la página 553.

orinal *m.* urinal, chamber pot, container or receptacle for urine.

orinar *v.* to urinate, to micturate; **ardor al** ___ / burning on urination; ___ **a menudo** / frequent urination; ___ **con dificultad** / difficult urination; ___ **con dolor** / painful urination; *vr.* **orinarse,** to wet oneself; ___ **en la cama** / bedwetting.

ornitina *f.* ornithine, an amino acid not present in proteins, but an important element in the urea cycle.

orofacial *a.* orofacial, rel. to the mouth and the face.

orofaringe *m.* oropharynx, central part of the pharynx.

Oroya, fiebre de *f.* Oroya fever, Carrión disease, found in Peru, characterized by very high fever, pernicious anemia and great sensitivity of the hemopoietic tissues.

orquidectomía, orquiectomía *f.* orchidectomy, orchiectomy, removal of a testicle.

orquiditis, orquitis *f.* orchiditis, orchitis, infl. of a testicle.

orquidopexia, orquiopexia *f.* orchidopexy, orchiopexy, procedure by which an undescended testicle is lowered into the scrotum and sutured to it.

orquiotomía *f.* orchiotomy, incision in a testicle.

ortocefálico-a *a.* orthocephalic, having a normal head with a cephalic index between 70 and 75.

ortocromático-a *a.* orthochromatic, of natural color or that accepts coloration.

ortodiágrofo *m.* orthodiagraph, radiographic apparatus that accurately records the form, size, and position of the internal organs and of any foreign objects in the body.

ortodigita *f.* orthodigita, correction of malformations of fingers and toes.

ortodoncia *f.* orthodontics, the study of irregularities and corrective procedures of teeth.

ortodoncista *m., f.* orthodontist, specialist in orthodontics.

ortógrado-a *a.* orthograde, that walks in an erect position.

ortomixovirus *m.* orthomyxoviridae, family of viruses to which belong the three groups of influenza viruses.

ortopedia *f.* orthopedics, the study of bones, joints, muscles, ligaments, and cartilages and the preventive and corrective procedures that deal with their related disorders.

ortopédico-a, ortopedista *m., f.* orthopedist, specialist in orthopedics; *a.* **orthopedic,** rel. to orthopedia; **calzado** ___ / ___ shoes.

ortopnea *f.* orthopnea, difficulty in breathing except when in an upright position.

ortóptica *f.* orthoptics, the study and correction of disorders of binocular vision and of the movements of the eye.

ortosiquiatría *f.* orthopsychiatry, a branch of psychiatry that embraces child psychiatry, pediatrics, developmental psychology and family care and is concerned with the prevention and treatment of psychological disorders in children and adolescents.

ortostático-a *a.* orthostatic, rel. to an erect position.

ortótonos *m.* orthotonos, orthotonus, a tetanic spasm which provokes rigidity in a straight line to the neck, limbs and body.

ortotópico-a *a.* orthotopic, in the normal or correct position.

orzuelo *m.* sty, stye, infl. of the sebaceous glands of the eyelid.

os *L.* os, bone.

oscilación *f.* oscillation, a pendulum-like motion.

oscilatorio *a.* oscillatory, that oscillates.

oscilopsia *f.* oscillopsia, oscilating vision during the advance stage of multiple sclerosis.

óseo-a *a.* osseous, rel. to bone; **desarrollo** ___ / bone development; **lesiones** ___ **-s** / bone lesions; **placa** ___ / bone plate.

Osgood-Schlatter, enfermedad de *f.* Osgood-Schlatter disease, infl. of the tibial apophysis.

osículo *m.* ossicle, small bone.

osificación *f.* ossification. 1. conversion of a substance into bone; 2. bone development.

osificar *vi.* to ossify, to turn into bone.

osífico-a *a.* ossific, rel. to the formation of bone tissue.

osmolar, osmótico-a *a.* osmolar, osmotic, rel. to or of the nature of osmosis.

osmología *f.* osmology, the study of odors.

osmorreceptor *m.* osmoreceptor. 1. a group of cells in the brain that receive olfactory stimuli; 2. a group of cells in the hypothalamus that respond to changes in the osmotic pressure of the blood.

osmosis *f.* osmosis, diffusion of a solvent through a semipermeable membrane separating two solutions of different concentration.

osmótico-a *a.* osmotic, rel. to or of the nature of osmosis.

osteítis, ostitis *f.* osteitis, ostitis, infl. of a bone; ___ **fibrosa quistica** / ___ fibrosa cystica, with cystic and nodular manifestations.

osteoaneurisma *m.* osteoaneurysm, aneurysm that occurs within a bone.

osteoartritis *f.* osteoarthritis, degenerative hypertrophy of the bones and joints.

osteoartropatía *f.* osteoarthropathy, disease of a joint and a bone, gen. accompanied by pain.

osteoblasto *m.* osteoblast, a cell that forms bone tissue.

osteoblastoma *m.* osteoblastoma. osteoma.

osteocarcinoma *m.* osteocarcinoma, bone cancer.

osteocartilaginoso-a *a.* osteocartilaginous, rel. to or formed by bone and cartilage.

osteocito *m.* osteocyte, a mature osteoblast that has become isolated in a lacuna of the bone substance.

osteoclasto *m.* osteoclast, giant multinuclear cell that participates in the formation of bone tissue and replaces cartilage during ossification.

osteocondral *a.* osteochondral, rel. to or made of bone and cartilage.

osteocondritis *f.* osteochondritis, infl. of bone and cartilage.

osteocondroma *f.* osteochondroma, tumor of both of osseous and cartilaginous elements.

osteodistrofia *f.* osteodystrophia, osteodystrophy, defective bone formation.

osteófito *m.* osteophyte, bony outgrowth.

osteogénesis *f.* osteogenesis. osificación.

osteoide *a.* osteoid, rel. to or resembling bone.

osteología *f.* osteology, the study of bones.

osteoma *m.* osteoma, a tumor of bone tissue.

osteomalacia *f.* osteomalacia, softening of the bones due to loss of calcium in the bone matrix.

osteomielitis *f.* osteomyelitis, infection of bone and bone marrow.

osteomielodisplasia *f.* osteomyelodysplasia, disease causing osseous displacement characterized by thinning of the osseous layer, an increase of the marrow cavities of the bones, leukopenia, and fever.

osteonecrosis *f.* osteonecrosis, destruction and death of bone tissue.

osteópata *m., f.* osteopath, specialist in osteopathy.

osteopatía *f.* osteopathy. 1. an approach to medicine that places emphasis on a favorable environment and on normal structural relationships of the musculoskeletal system, using extensive manipulation as a corrective tool; 2. any sickness of the bones.

osteopenia *f.* osteopenia, diminished calcification of the bones.

osteoplástico-a *a.* osteoplastic. 1. rel. to bone formation; 2. plastic surgery of a bone.

osteoporosis *f.* osteoporosis, loss of bone density.

osteosarcoma *m.* osteosarcoma, osseous sarcoma, the most common malignant sarcoma of the long bones.

osteosíntesis *f.* osteosynthesis, surgical fixation of a bone by mechanical means such as a plate or nail.

osteotomía *f.* osteotomy, the cutting or sawing of a bone.

ostial *a.* ostial, rel. to an opening or orifice.

ostium *L.* (*pl. ostia*) ostium, small opening.

ostium primum *n. L.* ostium primum, opening that communicates the two auricles of the fetal heart and that gradually becomes smaller and closes after birth.

ostomía *f.* ostomy, creation of an artificial opening between the bowel or intestine and the skin, as in ileostomy and colostomy.

ostra *f.* oyster.

otalgia, otodinia *f.* otalgia, otodynia, earache.

otectomía *f.* otectomy, excision of the structural contents of the middle ear.

ótico-a *a.* otic, rel. to the ear.

oticodinia *f.* oticodinia, vertigo caused by an ear disorder.

otitis *f.* otitis, infl. of the external, middle, or inner ear; ___ **del nadador** / swimmer's ear.

otolaringología *f.* otolaryngology, the study of the ear, nose and throat.

otolaringólogo-a *m., f.* otolaryngologist, specialist in otolaryngology.

otología *f.* otology, the study of the ear and its disorders.

otoneurología *f.* otoneurology, the study of the inner ear as related to the nervous system.

otoplastia *f.* otoplasty, plastic surgery of the ear.

otorragia *f.* otorrhagia, bleeding from the ear.

otorrea *f.* otorrhea, purulent discharge from the ear.

otosclerosis *f.* otosclerosis, progressive deafness due to formation of spongy tissue in the labyrinth of the ear.

otoscopia *f.* otoscopy, examination of the ear with an otoscope.

otoscopio *m.* otoscope, instrument to examine the ear.

ototóxico-a *a.* ototoxic, having toxic effects on the eighth pair of cranial nerves or on the hearing organs.

otro-a *a.* other; *pron.* another; **el** ___, **la** ___ / the ___ one; **los** ___ **-s, las** ___ **-s** / the others.

oval *a.* oval. 1. rel. to an ovum; 2. in the shape of an egg; **ventana** ___ / ___ window, membrane that separates the middle and the inner ear.

ovárico-a *a.* ovarian, rel. to the ovaries.

ovariectomía *f.* ovariectomy, ooforectomy.

ovario *m.* ovary, female reproductive organ that produces the ova.

oviducto *m.* oviduct, uterine conduit.

ovoide *a.* ovoid, egg-shaped.

ovotestis *f.* ovotestis, hermaphroditic gland that contains both ovarian and testicular tissue.

ovulación *f.* ovulation, periodic release of the ovum from the ovary.

óvulo *m.* ovum, egg cell.

oxidación *f.* oxidation, the chemical change resulting from the combination of oxygen with another substance.

oxidado-a *a.* rusty.

oxidante *m.* oxidant, agent that causes oxidation.

oxigenación *f.* oxygenation, saturation with oxygen.

oxigenado-a *a.* oxygenated.

oxigenador *m.* oxygenator, device that oxygenates blood, gen. used during surgery.

oxígeno *m.* oxygen, free element found in the atmosphere as a colorless, tasteless, and odorless gas; **cámara de** ___ / ___ tent; **distribución de** ___ / ___ distribution; **falta de** ___ / ___ deficiency; **tratamiento de** ___ / ___ treatment.

oxigenoterapia *f.* oxygenotherapy, therapeutic use of oxygen.

oxihemoglobina *f.* oxyhemoglobin, bright red substance that forms when the red cells combine permanently with oxygen.

oxímetro *m.* oximeter, instrument used to measure the amount of oxygen in the blood.

oxitocina *f.* oxytocin, pituitary hormone that stimulates uterine contraction.

p

P *abr.* **plasma** / plasma; **positivo-a** / positive; **posterior** / posterior; **presión** / pressure; **psiquiatría** / psychiatry; **pulso** / pulse.

pábulum *L.* pabulum, nutrient.

paciencia *f.* patience; **con** ___ / patiently.

paciente *m., f.* patient; **alta del** ___ / patient's discharge; **cuidado del** ___ / ___ 's care; ___ **externo, no hospitalizado** / outpatient; ___ **privado** / private ___; ___ **solvente** / self-paying ___; *a.* patient.

padecer *vi.* to be afflicted by a sickness or injury; ___ **de** / to suffer from.

padecimiento *m.* suffering; affliction.

padrastro *m.* stepfather.

padre *m.* father; **-s** / the parents, mother and father.

pagado-a *a.* paid, *pp.* of **pagar.**

pagar *vi.* to pay; ___ **al contado** / ___ in cash.

pago *m.* payment; ___ **compartido** / copayment; ___ **de una vez de la suma total** / lump sum ___ .

palabra *f.* word.

paladar *m.* palate, the roof of the mouth; ___ **blando** / soft ___; ___ **duro** / hard ___; ___ **hendido** / cleft ___, congenital fissure; ___ **óseo** / bony ___ .

palatino-a *a.* palatine, rel. to the palate.

paliativo-a *a.* palliative, that mitigates.

palidecer *vi.* to become pale.

palidez *f.* pallor.

pálido-a *a.* pallid, pale, sallow.

paliza *f.* beating.

palma *f.* 1. palm, palm of the hand; 2. palm tree; **aceite de** ___ / ___ oil.

palmacristi *f.* castor oil.

palmar *a.* palmar, rel. to the palm of the hand.

palpable *a.* palpable, that can be touched.

palpación *f.* palpation, examination with the hands.

palpar *v.* to palpate, to feel, to touch.

palpitación *f.* palpitation, rapid pulsation or throbbing.

palpitante *a.* throbbing.

palpitar *v.* to palpitate; to pant.

palúdico-a *a.* rel. to or afflicted by malaria.

paludismo *m.* malaria, paludism, highly infectious, febrile, and often chronic disease caused by the bite of an infected *Anopheles* mosquito.

pampiniforme *a.* pampiniform, simulating the structure of a vine.

pan *m.* bread; ___ **y mantequilla** / ___ and butter.

panacea *f.* panacea, a remedy to cure all ills.

panadizo *m.* felon, painful abscess of the distal phalanx of a finger.

panarteritis *f.* 1. panarteritis, infl. of the layers of an artery. 2. infl. of the arteries of the body.

panartritis *f.* panarthritis. 1. infl. of some joints of the body; 2. infl. of all the tissues of a joint.

pancitopenia *f.* pancytopenia, abnormal decrease in the number of blood cells.

páncreas *m.* pancreas, gland of the digestive system that externally secretes the pancreatic juice, and internally secretes insulin and glucagon.

pancreatectomía *f.* pancreatectomy, partial or total removal of the pancreas.

pancreático-a *a.* pancreatic, rel. to the pancreas; **conducto** ___ / ___ duct; **jugo** ___ / ___ juice; **quiste** ___ / ___ cyst.

pancreaticoenterostomía *f.* pancreaticoenterostomy, creation of a passage between the pancreatic duct and the intestines.

pancreatina *f.* pancreatin, digestive enzyme obtained from the pancreas.

pancreatitis *f.* pancreatitis, infl. of the pancreas; ___ **aguda** / acute ___; ___ **hemorrágica aguda** / acute hemorrhagic ___ .

pandémico-a *a.* pandemic, that occurs over a wide geographical area.

panendoscopio *m.* panendoscope, optical instrument used to examine the urethra and the bladder.

panfleto *m.* pamphlet.

panglosia *f.* panglossia, excessive talking.

panhidrosis *f.* panhidrosis, generalized sweating.

panhipopituitarismo *m.* panhypopituitarism, deficiency of the anterior pituitary gland.

panhisterectomía *f.* panhysterectomy, total excision of the uterus.

pánico *m.* panic, excessive fear; **ataques de** ___ / ___ attacks; **trastornos de** ___ / ___ disorder; *v.* **tener** ___ / to panic.

paniculitis *f.* paniculitis, infl. of the panniculus adiposus.

paniculo *m.* panniculus, layer of tissue; ___ **adiposo** / ___ adiposus; ___ **carnoso** / ___ carnosus.

pannus *L.* pannus, a membrane of granulation tissue covering a normal surface.

pansinusitis *f.* pansinusitis, infl. of all the paranasal sinuses in one or both sides.

pantalones *m.* pants, slacks.

pantalla *f.* screen.

pantorrilla *f.* calf of the leg.

panza *f.* belly.

panzudo-a *a. pop.* potbellied.

pañal *m.* diaper; ___ -es desechables / disposable ___ -s.

papa, patata *m.* potato.

papá *m.* dad.

papada *f.* double chin.

Papanicolau, prueba de *f.* Papanicolau's test, Pap smear, sample of mucus from the vagina and the cervix for the purpose of early detection of cancer cells.

papaya *f.* papaya.

papel *m.* paper; ___ higiénico / toilet ___; role; *v.* hacer el ___ de / to play the ___ of.

paperas *f.* mumps, acute, febrile, highly contagious disease characterized by swelling of the salivary glands.

papila *f.* papilla, bud, small, nipple-like eminence of the skin, esp. seen in the mouth;___ acústica / acoustic ___; ___ dérmica / dermal ___; ___ duodenal / duodenal ___; ___ filiforme / filiform ___; ___ gustativa / taste bud; ___ lagrimal / lacrimal ___; ___ lingual / lingual ___ .

papilar *m.* papillary, rel. to a papilla.

papiledema *m.* papilledema, edema of the optic disk.

papiliforme *a.* papilliform, resembling a papilla.

papilitis *f.* papillitis, infl. of the optic disk.

papiloma *m.* papilloma, benign epithelial tumor.

papilomatosis *f.* papillomatosis. 1. the development of numerous papillomas; 2. papillary projections.

papovavirus *m.* papovavirus, type of virus used in the study of cancer.

pápula *f.* papule, small, hard eminence of the skin.

papular *a.* papular, rel. to papules.

papuloescamoso-a *a.* papulosquamous, rel. to papules and scales; enfermedades cutáneas ___ / ___ skin diseases.

paquete celular *m.* packed cells, red blood cells that have been separated from the plasma.

paquidermia *f.* pachydermia. V. **elefantiasis**.

paquigiria *f.* pachygyria, thick convolutions of the cerebral cortex.

par *m.* pair, couple.

para *prep.* to, for; for the purpose of; in order to; ___ siempre / forever; ¿ ___ qué / what for?

paracentesis *f.* paracentesis, puncture to obtain or remove fluid from a cavity.

parado-a *a.* in a standing position.

paraesternal *a.* parasternal, adjacent to the sternum.

parafasia *f.* paraphasia, type of aphasia manifested by inability to use words coherently.

parafimosis *f.* paraphimosis. 1. retraction or constriction of the prepuce behind the glans penis; 2. retraction of the eyelid behind the eyeball.

parafina *f.* paraffin.

parainfluenza, virus de *m.* parainfluenza virus, any of several viruses associated with some respiratory infections, esp. in children.

paralaje *m.* parallax, the apparent displacement of an object according to the position of the viewer.

parálisis *f.* palsy, paralysis, partial or total loss of function of a part of the body; ___ alcohólica / alcoholic ___; ___ alterna / alternative ___; ___ amiotrófica / amyotrophic ___; ___ ascendente / ascending ___; ___ central / central ___; ___ cerebral / cerebral ___ , partial paralysis and lack of muscular coordination due to a congenital brain lesion; ___ cerebral atáxica infantil / infantile cerebral ataxic ___; ___ de acomodación / accommodation ___; ___ de los buzos / diver's paralysis, decompression sickness (bends); ___ facial / facial ___; ___ facial periférica / peripheral facial ___; ___ galopante / rapidly progressive gen. ___; ___ histérica / hysterical ___; ___ infantil / infantile paralysis; ___ motora / motor ___; ___ por enfriamiento / cold-induced ___ .

parálisis cerebral *f.* cerebral paralysis, partial paralysis and lack of muscular coordination due to a congenital brain lesion.

paralítico-a *a.* paralytic, invalid, rel. to or suffering from paralysis; íleo ___ / ___ ileus, paralysis of the intestines.

paralizar *vi.* to paralyze.

paramagnético-a *a.* paramagnetic, rel. to substances that are susceptible to magnetism.

paramédico-a *m., f.* paramedic, individual trained and certified to offer emergency medical assistance.

parametrio *m.* parametrium, loose cellular tissue around the uterus.

paramiotonía *f.* paramyotonia, atypical myotonia, characterized by muscle spasms and abnormal muscular tonicity; ___ atáxica /

ataxic ___; ___ **congenital** / congenital ___; ___ **sintomática** / symptomatic ___; **trastornos de** ___ / ___ disorders.

paranasal *a.* paranasal, adjacent to the nasal cavity.

paraneumonía *f.* parapneumonia, illness with clinical characteristics resembling pneumonia.

paranoia *f.* paranoia, mental disorder characterized by delusions of persecution and grandeur.

paranoico-a *a.* paranoid, rel. to or afflicted with paranoia.

parapancreático-a *a.* parapancreatic, adjacent to the pancreas.

paraparesia *f.* paraparesis, partial paralysis esp. of the lower limbs.

paraplejía *f.* paraplegia, paralysis of the legs and the lower half of the body; ___ **cerebral infantil** / cerebral infantile ___; ___ **espasmódica familiar** / familiar, spasmodic ___; ___ **espasmódica, espástica** / spasmodic, spastic ___; ___ **flácida** / flaccid ___ .

parapléjico-a *a.* paraplegic, rel. to or affected with paraplegia.

parapsicología *f.* parapsychology, the study of psychic phenomena such as mental telepathy and extrasensory perception.

parar *v.* to stop, to halt; **pararse** *vr.* to stand up; ___ **de puntillas** / to stand on tiptoe.

pararrectal *a.* pararectal, adjacent to the rectum.

parasimpático-a *a.* parasympathetic, rel. to one of two branches of the autonomic nervous system.

parasístole *f.* parasystole, an irregularity in cardiac rhythm.

parasítico-a *a.* parasitic.

parasitismo *m.* parasitism, infestation with parasites.

parásito *m.* parasite, organism that lives upon another one.

parasitología *f.* parasitology, the study of parasites.

parasomnia *f.* parasomnia, term used to designate any disorder suffered during sleep, enuresis, nightmares, sleepwalking, etc.

paratífica, fiebre *f.* paratyphoid fever, a fever that simulates typhoid fever.

paratiroidectomía *f.* parathyroidectomy, removal of one or more of the parathyroid glands.

paratiroideo-a *a.* parathyroid, located close to the thyroid gland.

paratiroides *f.* parathyroid, group of small endocrine glands situated behind the thyroid gland.

paraumbilical *a.* paraumbilical, close to the navel.

paravertebral *a.* paravertebral, adjacent to the vertebral column.

parcial *a.* partial; **-mente** *adv.* partially.

parco-a *a.* sparing, scanty, moderate.

parche *m.* patch, piece of cloth or adhesive used to protect wounds; **prueba del** ___ / ___ test, for allergies.

parecer *vi.* to seem, to appear; **parecerse** *vr.* to look alike, to resemble.

parecido-a *a.* resembling.

pared *f.* wall; partition.

paregórico *m.* paregoric, sedative derived from opium.

pareja *f.* pair, couple.

parejo-a *a.* even, equal.

parénquima *m.* parenchyma, the functional elements of an organ.

parenteral *a.* parenteral, that is introduced in the body in a way other than the gastrointestinal route.

parentesco *m.* kindred, family relationship.

paresia *f.* paresis, slight or partial paralysis.

parestesia *f.* paresthesia, sensation of pricking, tingling, or tickling, gen. associated with partial damage to a peripheral nerve.

parético-a *a.* paretic, rel. to or afflicted by paresis.

pariente-a *m., f.* family relative; ___ **consanguíneo** / blood relation.

parietal *m.* parietal bone; *a.* parietal. 1. rel. to the parietal bone; 2. rel. to the wall of a cavity.

parir *v.* to give birth.

Parkinson, enfermedad de *f.* Parkinson's disease, degenerative process of the brain nerves characterized by tremor, progressive muscular weakness, blurred speech, and shuffling gait.

paro *m.* standstill, arrest.

parodinia *f.* parodynia, difficult or abnormal delivery.

paroniquia *f.* paronychia, infl. of the area adjacent to a fingernail.

parótida *f.* parotid, gland that secretes saliva, situated near the ear.

parotiditis, parotitis *f.* parotiditis, parotitis. paperas.

paroxismal, paroxístico-a *a.* paroxysmal, rel. to paroxysm.

paroxismo *m.* paroxysm. 1. attack, spasm, or convulsion; 2. recurring intensified symptoms.

parpadear *v.* to blink.
parpadeo *m.* blinking; flicker.
párpado *m.* eyelid; cilium.
parrilla *f.* grill; **a la ___** / grilled.
pars *L.* part, portion.
parte *f.* part, portion; **por todas ___ -s /** everywhere.
partenogénesis *f.* parthenogenesis, unusual reproductive process in which the ovum develops without being fertilized by a spermatozoon; **___ artificial** / artificial ___ .
partición *f.* partition, sectioning, division.
participar *v.* to participate.
partícula *f.* particle, one of the minute parts that form matter.
particular *a.* particular; **-mente** / *adv.* particularly.
particularidad *f.* peculiarity.
partir *v.* to sever, to break; to divide.
parto *m.* labor, delivery, parturition; **antes del, después del ___** / before, after delivery; **canal del ___** / birth canal; **dolor de ___ / ___ pains; estar de ___** / to be close to delivery; **etapas del ___** / stages of ___; **___ activo /** active ___; **___ de un feto sin vida /** stillbirth; **___ falso** / false ___; **___ inducido /** induced ___; **___ laborioso** / hard, difficult ___; **___ natural** / natural childbirth; **___ normal** / normal delivery; **___ prematuro** / premature___; **___ prolongado, tardío** / prolonged ___; **___ seco** / dry ___ .
parturienta *f.* parturient, a woman in the act of delivering or who has just delivered.
parturifaciente *m.* parturifacient, an agent that induces parturition.
párulis *f.* gumboil, an abscess of the gums.
parvovirus *m.* parvovirus, any of a group of viruses that cause diseases in animals but not in humans.
pasa *f.* raisin.
pasado *m.* the past tense; **-a** *a.* past; **___ mañana** / the day after tomorrow; **la semana ___** / last week.
pasaje *m.* passage. 1. conduit or meatus; 2. evacuation of the bowels.
pasajero-a *a.* fleeting, that doesn't last.
pasar *v.* to pass, to pass by; to happen.
pasear *v.* to go for a stroll or outing.
paseo *m.* a stroll; an outing.
pasillo *m.* hall, hallway, corridor; covered way.
pasión *f.* passion, intense emotion.
pasividad *f.* passivity, abnormal dependency on others.

pasivo-a *a.* passive, not spontaneous or active; **ejercicio ___ / ___** exercise.
paso *m.* step, pace.
pasta *f.* pasta; paste; **___ de dientes** / toothpaste.
pasteurización *f.* pasteurization, the process of destroying microorganisms by applying regulated heat.
pasteurizar *vi.* to pasteurize, to perform pasteurization.
pastilla *f.* pill, tablet; lozenge; **___ para dormir** / sleeping ___; **___ para el dolor** / pain ___ .
pastoso-a *a.* clammy; doughy.
patada *f.* hard kick.
patear *v.* to kick.
patelectomía *f.* patellectomy, excision of the patella.
patelofemoral *a.* patellofemoral, rel. to the patella and the femur.
patella *L.* patella, kneecap.
patente *m.* 1. patent, exclusive right or privilege; **medicina de ___ / ___** medicine; *a.* 2. patulous; open, not obstructed; evident.
paternidad *f.* paternity; **prueba de ___ / ___** test.
paterno-a *a.* paternal, rel. to the father.
patético-a *a.* pathetic.
patizambo-a *a.* pigeon-toed, feet turned inward.
patofisiología *f.* pathophysiology, the study of the effects of a disease on the physiological processes.
patogénesis *f.* pathogenesis, origin and development of a sickness.
patógeno *m.* pathogen, agent that causes disease; **-a** *a.* pathogenic, that can cause a disease.
patognomónico-a *a.* pathognomonic, rel. to a sign or symptom characteristic of a given disease.
patología *f.* pathology, the study of the origin and nature of disease.
patológico-a *a.* pathologic, pathological, rel. to disease.
patólogo-a *m., f.* pathologist, specialist in pathology.
patrón *m.* pattern, model, type.
pausa *f.* pause, rest; interruption; **___ compensadora** / compensatory ___ , long interval of time, following a heartbeat.
pausado-a *a.* slow, deliberate.
pavo *m.* turkey.
paz *f.* peace; *v.* **dejar en ___** / to leave alone; **en ___ / at ___** .

peau d'orange *Fr.* peau d'orange, skin condition resembling that of the peel of an orange, an important sign in breast cancer.

peca *f.* freckle, spot, small discoloration of the skin.

pecho *m.* chest; ___ **de paloma** / pigeon breast; *v.* **dar el** ___ / to breast-feed.

pechuga *a.* breast or white meat of a fowl.

pecoso-a *a.* freckled.

pectina *f.* pectin, carbohydrate obtained from the peel of citrus fruits or apples.

pectus *L. (pl. pectora)* pectus, breast, chest.

peculiar *a.* peculiar.

pedal *a.* pedal, rel. to the foot.

pedazo *m.* piece, part of a whole.

pederastia *f.* pederasty, anal intercourse between males, esp. between an adult and a young boy.

pediatra *m., f.* pediatrician, specialist in pediatrics.

pediatría *f.* pediatrics, the study of the care and development of children and the treatment of diseases affecting them.

pediátrico-a *a.* pediatric, rel. to pediatrics.

pedículo *m.* pedicle, narrow, stemlike part of a tumor that connects it with its base.

pediculosis *f.* pediculosis, infestation with lice.

pedir *vi.* to ask for something, to request.

pedofilia *f.* pedophilia, morbid sexual attraction to children.

pedunculado-a *a.* pedunculate, pedunculated, rel. to, or having peduncles.

pedúnculo *m.* peduncle, stemlike connection.

pedunculus *L. (pl. pedunculi)* pedunculus, peduncle.

pegajoso-a *a.* sticky, gummy.

pegar *vi.* to stick together, to glue, to adhere.

peinar *v.* to comb; **peinarse** *vr.* to comb one's hair.

peine *m.* comb.

peladura *f.* peeling, scaling, exfoliation; ___ **química** / chemical ___ .

pelagra *f.* pellagra, illness caused by deficiency of niacin and characterized by dermatitis, gastrointestinal, and mental disorders.

pelar *v.* to peel; to give a haircut; **pelarse** *vr.* to get a haircut.

pelea *f.* fight, quarrel.

pelear *v.* to fight, to quarrel.

película *f.* 1. film, movie; 2. thin layer or membrane.

peligro *m.* danger, risk; hazard; peril; *v.* **estar en** ___ / to be in ___; **poner en** ___ / to endanger, to jeopardize.

peligroso-a *a.* dangerous, risky, hazardous.

pellejo *m.* peel, hide; *pop.* skin.

pellizcar *vi.* to pinch.

pellizco *m.* pinch.

pelo *m.* hair; **raíz del** ___ / ___ root; **bola de** ___ / ___ ball, type of bezoar; **transplante de** ___ / ___ transplant.

pelota *f.* ball.

peloteo *m.* ballottement, maneuver used during examination of the abdomen and pelvis to determine the presence of tumors or enlargement of organs; ___ **renal** / renal ___ .

peluca *f.* wig.

peludo-a *a.* hairy.

pélvico-a, pelviano-a *a.* pelvic, rel. to the pelvis.

pelvis *f.* pelvis. 1. cavity in the lower end of the trunk formed by the hip bone, the sacrum, and the coccyx; **enfermedad inflamatoria de la** ___ / pelvic inflammatory disease; 2. basin-shaped cavity.

pelvis menor, verdadera *f.* true pelvis, the inferior and contractile part of the pelvis.

pena *f.* sorrow, affliction.

penacho *m.* tuft, a small cluster or mass.

pendiente *a.* pending, unfinished.

pendular *a.* pendulous, oscillating or hanging.

pene *m.* penis, the external part of the male reproductive organ that contains the urethral orifice through which urine and semen pass.

peneal, peneano-a *a.* penile, rel. to the penis.

penetración *f.* penetration. 1. the act of penetrating; 2. the capacity of radiation to go through a substance.

penetrante *a.* penetrating; piercing.

penetrar *v.* to penetrate, to go through.

pénfigo *m.* pemphigus, a variety of dermatosis characterized by the presence of blisters that can become infected upon rupturing.

penfigoideo-a *a.* pemphigoid, similar to pemphigus but having clinical differences.

penicilina *f.* penicillin, antibiotic derived directly or indirectly from cultures of the fungus *Penicillium*.

pensar *vi.* to think.

peor *a., comp.* worse; *sup.* worst; *adv.* worse.

pepino *m.* cucumber.

pepsina *f.* pepsin, the main enzyme of the gastric juice.

péptico-a *a.* peptic, rel. to the action or the digestion of gastric juices.

pequeño-a *a.* small in size.

pera *f.* pear; ___ **de goma** / bulb syringe.

p

percepción *f.* perception. 1. the conscious mental recognition of a sensory stimulus; ___ **extrasensorial** / extrasensory ___; 2. understanding or comprehension of an idea.

percibir *v.* to perceive, to realize.

percusión *f.* percussion, procedure that consists in tapping the surface of the body with the fingers or a small tool, in order to produce sounds or vibrations that indicate the condition of a given part of the body; ___ **auscultatoria** / auscultatory ___ .

percutáneo-a *a.* percutaneous, applied through the skin.

percutir *v.* to percuss, to use percussion.

perder *vi.* to lose, to forfeit; ___ **sangre** / to bleed; ___ **la oportunidad** / to miss an opportunity; ___ **tiempo** / to waste time; ___ **un turno** / to miss an appointment.

pérdida *f.* loss; ___ **de sangre** / ___ of blood; ___ **del conocimiento** / ___ of consciousness; ___ **del contacto con la realidad** / ___ of contact with reality; ___ **del equilibrio** / ___ of balance; ___ **del movimiento** / ___ of motion; ___ **de la audición** / ___ of hearing; ___ **de la memoria** / ___ of memory; ___ **de la tonicidad muscular** / ___ of muscle tone; ___ **de la visión** / ___ of vision; ___ **neural de la audición** / neural hearing ___ .

perdido-a *a.* lost.

perfeccionismo *m.* perfectionism, excessive drive to attain perfection, regardless of the importance of the task.

perfeccionista *m., f.* perfectionist.

perfecto-a *a.* perfect; **-mente** *adv.* perfectly.

perfil *m.* profile, side view; outline; ___ **bioquímico** / biochemical ___; ___ **físico** / physical ___ .

perforación *f.* perforation, hole.

perforar *v.* to perforate; to pierce.

perfusión *f.* perfusion, passage of a liquid through a conduit.

periamigdalino-a *a.* peritonsillar, close to the tonsils.

perianal *a.* perianal, located around the anus.

pericardial, pericárdico-a *a.* pericardiac, pericardial, rel. to the pericardium; **derrame** ___ , **efusión** ___ / ___ effusion; **vibración** ___ / ___ fremitus.

pericardiectomía *f.* pericardiectomy, partial or total excision of the pericardium.

pericardio *m.* pericardium, saclike, double-layered membrane that surrounds the heart and the origins of the large blood vessels.

pericarditis *f.* pericarditis, infl. of the pericardium; ___ **constrictiva** / constrictive ___; ___ **localizada** / localized ___; ___ **reumática** / rheumatic ___ .

periferia *f.* periphery, part of a body or organ away from the center.

periférico-a *a.* peripheral, rel. to or occurring in the periphery; **sistema nervioso** ___ / ___ nervous system, the group of nerves situated outside the central nervous system.

perilla *f.* rubber bulb.

perinatal *a.* perinatal, rel. to or occurring before, during, or right after birth.

perinatología *f.* perinatology, study of the fetus and newborn during the perinatal period.

perinatólogo-a *m., f.* perinatologist, specialist in perinatology.

perineal *a.* perineal, rel. to the perineum.

perinéfrico-a *a.* perinephric, close to the kidney.

perineo *m.* perineum, the pelvic outlet bounded anteriorly by the scrotum in the man and the vulva in the woman, and posteriorly by the anus.

perineural *a.* perineural, around the nerve.

periódico *m.* newspaper; **-a** *a.* periodic; **-mente** *adv.* periodically.

período *m.* period. 1. interval of time, epoch; ___ **de tiempo** / time span.

periodo *m.* menstruation.

periodoncia *f.* periodontics, branch of odontology dealing with areas surrounding the teeth.

periodoncio *m.* periodontium, support tissue surrounding a tooth.

periodoncista *m., f.* periodontist, specialist in periodontics.

periodontal *a.* periodontal, surrounding the tooth.

periodontitis *f.* periodontitis, infl. of the periodontium.

periostio *m.* periosteum, thick fibrous membrane that covers the entire surface of the bone except the articular surface.

peristalsis *f.* peristalsis, wavelike contractions that occur in a tubular structure such as the alimentary canal, by which the contents are forced onward.

peristáltico-a *a.* peristaltic, rel. to peristalsis.

peritoneal *a.* peritoneal, rel. to the peritoneum.

peritoneo *m.* peritoneum, serous membrane that lines the abdominopelvic walls and the viscera.

peritoneoscopía *f.* peritoneoscopy, examination of the abdominopelvic cavity with a peritoneoscope or laparoscope passed through the abdominal wall.laparoscopía.

peritoneoscopio *m.* peritoneoscope, an endoscope used to examine the peritoneal cavity. *Sin.* **laparoscopio.**

peritonitis *f.* peritonitis, infl. of the peritoneum.

periungual *a.* periungual, around the nail.

periuretral *a.* periurethral, around the urethra.

perjudicial *a.* detrimental, damaging.

perleche *Fr.* perleche, disorder manifested by fissures at the corner of the mouth, seen esp. in children and gen. as a result of malnutrition.

permanecer *vi.* to remain; to last.

permanente *a.* permanent, lasting; **-mente** *adv.* permanently.

permeabilidad *f.* permeability, the quality of being permeable, not obstructed; ___ **capilar** / capillary ___ .

permeable *a.* permeable, allowing passage through structures such as a membrane.

permiso *m.* permit; consent.

permitido-a *a.* permissible; permitted.

permitir *v.* to allow, to consent, to agree.

pernicioso-a *a.* pernicious, noxious, harmful.

pero *conj.* but.

peroné *m.* perone, fibula, calf bone, the outer and thinner of the two lower leg bones.

perpendicular *a.* perpendicular.

per rectum *L.* per rectum, by the rectum.

perro *m.* dog.

persecución *f.* persecution.

perseveración *f.* perseveration, mental disorder manifested by the abnormal repetition of an idea or action.

persistir *v.* to persist, to persevere.

persona *f.* person. 1. individual; 2. outward personality that conceals the real one.

personal *m.* personnel; ___ **médico** / medical ___ ; *a.* personal, rel. to a person.

personalidad *f.* personality, traits, characteristics, and individual behavior that distinguish one person from another; ___ **anal** / anal ___ ; ___ **antisocial** / antisocial ___ ; ___ **compulsiva** / compulsive ___ ; ___ **esquizoide** / schizoid, split ___ ; ___ **extravertida** / extroverted ___ ; ___ **intravertida** / introverted ___ ; ___ **neurótica** / neurotic ___ ; ___ **paranoica** / paranoid ___ ; ___ **psicopática** / psychopathic ___ .

perspectiva *f.* perspective.

perspiración *f.* perspiration, exudation.

persuadir *v.* to persuade.

persuasión *f.* persuasion, therapeutic treatment that tries to deal with the patient through the use of reason.

pertenecer *vi.* to belong.

perteneciente *a.* pertaining or rel. to.

pertinente *a.* pertinent, relevant.

perturbación *f.* perturbation. 1. feeling of uneasiness; 2. abnormal variation from a regular state.

perturbar *v.* to perturb, to disrupt, to disturb.

pertussis *L.* pertussis, whooping cough.

perversión *f.* perversion, deviation from socially accepted behavior; ___ **sexual** / sexual ___ .

pervertido-a *m., f.* pervert, individual given to sexual perversion.

pervio-a *a.* pervious, permeable.

pes *L.* pes, the foot or a structure resembling it.

pesa *f.* weighing scale.

pesadez *f.* heaviness.

pesadilla *f.* nightmare.

pesado-a *m., f.* a boring person; *a.* heavy; [*conducta*] boring; **sueño** ___ / deep sleep.

pésame *m.* condolences.

pesar *m.* grief, sorrow; *v.* to weigh; **a** ___ **de** / in spite of.

pesario *m.* pessary, a rubber cup-shaped device that is introduced into the vagina to be used as a support to the uterus.

pescado *m.* fish.

pescuezo *m.* neck.

pesimismo *m.* pessimism, an inclination to see and judge situations in their most unfavorable light.

pesimista *m., f.* pessimist; *a.* pessimist, rel. to, or that manifests pessimism.

peso *m.* weight; **aumento de** ___ / ___ gain; **falto de, bajo de** ___ / underweight; **pérdida de** ___ / ___ loss; ___ **al nacer** / birth ___ .

pestañas *f. pl.* eyelashes.

pestañear *v.* to blink, to wink.

pestañeo *m.* blink; blinking.

peste *f.* 1. bubonic plague, an epidemic infectious disease transmitted by the bite of infected rats or fleas; 2. plague, any epidemic contagious disease with a high rate of mortality; 3. foul smell.

peste neumónica *f.* pneumonic plague, pulmonary plague, a form of plague with symptoms of bloody sputum, chills and high fever that can be lethal.

pesticida *m.* pesticide, chemical agent that kills insects and other pests.

petequia *f.* petechiae, minute hemorrhagic spots in the skin and the mucosa that can appear in connection with some severe fevers such as typhoid.

petición *f.* petition, request; claim; **proceso para revisión de ___ -es** / claim review procedure.

petit mal *Fr.* petit mal, benign epileptic attack with loss of consciousness at times, but with no convulsions.

petrificado-a *a.* petrified. 1. made rigid like stone; 2. terrified.

peyote *m.* peyote, plant from which the hallucinatory drug mescaline is obtained.

pezón *m.* nipple; ___ **agrietado** / cracked ___ ; ___ **enlechado** / engorged ___ ; ___ **umbilicado** / retracted ___ .

pH *m.* Potential of Hydrogen. Indicates the degree of acidity or alkalinity of a substance; ___ **cutáneo** / cutaneous ___ ; ___ **sanguíneo** / blood ___ .

piamadre *f.* pia mater, thin vascular membrane, the innermost of the three cerebral meninges.

pica *f.* pica, a craving for inedible substances.

picada, picadura *f.* sting, bite.

picante *a.* piquant, highly seasoned.

picar *vi.* to bite; to pierce, to prick; to itch.

picazón *f.* itching.

pie *m.* foot; ___ **de atleta** / athlete's ___ , dermatofitosis; ___ **en extensión** / footdrop; ___

plano / flatfoot; **planta del ___** / sole; *v.* **estar de ___** / to be standing; **ir a ___** / to go on foot; *vr.* **ponerse de ___** / to stand up.

pie de trinchera *m.* trench foot, infectious condition of the feet resulting from long exposure to cold.

piedra *f.* stone, calculus.

piel *f.* skin; hide, epidermis; **cáncer de la ___ / ___** cancer; **fricción de la ___** / skin chafing; **injerto de ___ / ___** graft. *V.* ilustración en la página 519.

pielografía *f.* pyelography. pielograma.

pielograma *m.* pyelogram, x-ray of the renal pelvis and the ureter using a contrasting medium.

pielolitotomía *f.* pyelolithotomy, incision to remove a calculus from the renal pelvis.

pielonefritis *f.* pyelonephritis, infl. of the kidney and renal pelvis.

pieloplastia *f.* pyeloplasty, plastic surgery of the renal pelvis.

pielostomía *f.* pyelostomy, creation of an opening in the renal pelvis to divert the urine to the exterior.

pielotomía *f.* pyelotomy, incision of the renal pelvis.

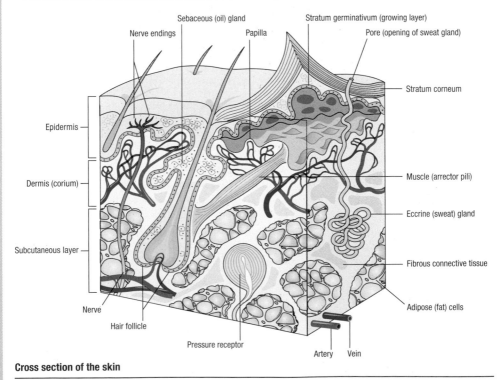

Cross section of the skin

pierna *f.* leg, lower extremity that extends from the knee to the ankle; ___ **arqueada** / bowleg, genu varum; **traumatismo de la** ___ / ___ injury.

pigmentación *f.* pigmentation.

pigmento *m.* pigment, coloring element.

pijama, piyamas *f.* pajamas.

pila *f.* faucet; battery.

píldora *f.* pill; ___ **de control del embarazo** / birth control ___ .

piliación *f.* piliation, formation and development of hair.

pilórico-a *a.* pyloric, rel. to the pylorus.

píloro *m.* pylorus, the lower aperture of the stomach that opens into the duodenum.

piloroplastia *f.* pyloroplasty, plastic surgery to repair the pylorus.

pilus *L.* (*pl. pili*) pilus, hair.

pimienta *f.* pepper.

pincelación *f.* penciling, application of a medical solution to an area of the skin or to a cavity with a medicated pencil, brush, or cotton swab.

pinchar *v.* to prick.

pinchazo *m.* prick, jab; cut.

pinna *L.* pinna, ear lap.

pinocitosis *f.* pinocytosis, absorption of liquids by cells.

pintar *v.* to paint; to apply a medication to the skin.

pinzas *f. pl.* clip, forceps, pincers, tweezers, devices used to assist in the extraction process; ___ **de secuestro** / sequestrum forceps.

piocito *m.* pyocite, a pus corpuscle.

piógeno-a *a.* pyogenic, that produces pus.

piojo *m.* louse, parasite that is the primary transmitter of some diseases such as typhus.

piorrea *f.* pyorrhea. periodontitis.

pipeta *f.* pipette, a narrow glass tube.

pirámide *f.* pyramid, a cone-shaped structure of the body such as the medulla oblongata.

pirético *m.* pyretic, rel. to fever.

pirexia *f.* pyrexia, high temperature; fever.

pirógeno *m.* pyrogen, agent that elevates a fever.

piromanía *f.* pyromania, obsession with fire.

piscina *f.* swimming pool.

piso *m.* floor; ground.

pistola *f.* pistol, handgun.

pituitaria, glándula *f.* pituitary gland.

piuria *f.* pyuria, presence of pyocites in the urine.

pivote *m.* pivot, part used to support the artificial crown of a tooth.

placa *f.* 1. plate, flat structure such as a thin layer of bone; 2. plate, thin layer of metal used to support a structure; 3. plaque, a patch on the skin or mucous membrane; 4. x-ray

placebo *m.* placebo, harmless substance of no medical value, gen. used for experimental purposes.

placenta *f.* placenta, vascular organ that develops in the wall of the uterus, through which the fetus derives its nourishment; ___ **previa** / ___ previa, placenta situated before the fetus in relation to the cervical opening, that may cause severe hemorrhaging.

placentario-a *a.* placental, rel. to the placenta; **insuficiencia** ___ / ___ insufficiency.

plaga *f.* plague, epidemic infectious disease.

plan *m.* plan; design.

planeamiento *m.* planning.

planear *v.* to plan.

planificación familiar *f.* family planning.

planilla *f.* [*formulario*] form.

plano *m.* plane. 1. flat surface; 2. a relatively smooth surface formed by making an imaginary or real cut through a part of the body; ___ **axial** / axial ___ ; ___ **coronal** / coronal ___ ; ___ **frontal** / frontal ___ ; ___ **horizontal** / horizontal ___ ; ___ **medio** / midplane; ___ **sagital** / sagittal ___ .

planta *f.* plant; ___ **del pie** / sole of the foot; ___ **-s medicinales** [*hierbas*] / medicinal ___ -s or herbs.

plantar *a.* plantar, rel. to the sole of the foot; **reflejo** ___ / ___ reflex, Babinski's reflex.

plaqueta *f.* platelet, thrombocyte, an element of the blood in the form of minute disks, essential to coagulation; **conteo de** ___ **-s** / ___ count.

plasma *m.* plasma, liquid component of the blood and lymph, made of 91 percent water and 9 percent of a combination of elements such as proteins, salts, nutrients, and vitamins.

plasticidad *f.* plasticity, the capacity to be molded.

plástico *m.* plastic; **-a** *a.* plastic.

plata *f.* silver; **nitrato de** ___ / ___ nitrate.

plátano *m.* banana.

platicar *vi.* to converse, to talk.

plegado-a *a.* plicate, folded.

pleomorfismo *m.* pleomorphism, the quality of assuming various forms.

pletismografía *f.* plethysmography, the recording of the changes in size of a part of the body as affected by circulation.

plétora *f.* plethora, an excess of any one of the body fluids.

pleura *f.* pleura, doublefold membrane that covers each lung; ___ **parietal** / parietal ___ ; ___ **visceral** / visceral ___ .

pleural *a.* pleural, rel. to the pleura; **cavidad___ / ___** cavity; **derrame ___ / ___** effusion.

pleuresía *f.* pleurisy, infl. of the pleura.

pleurítico-a *a.* pleuritic, rel. to pleurisy.

pleuritis *f.* pleuritis infl. of the pleura.

pleuroscopía *f.* pleuroscopy, inspection of the pleural cavity through an incision into the thorax.

plexiforme *a.* plexiform, in the shape of a plexus or net.

plexo *m.* plexus, an interlacing of nerves, blood, or lymphatic vessels.

plica *f.* plica, fold, crease.

pliegue *m.* fold.

plomo *m.* lead; **delantal de ___ / ___** apron; **envenenamiento por ___ / ___** poisoning; **sonda de ___ / ___** probe.

pluma *f.* pen.

plumbismo *m.* plumbism, chronic lead poisoning.

plural *m.* plural, the presence of more than one.

pluripotencial *a.* pluripotent, pluripotential, able to take more than one course of action.

población *f.* population.

pobre *a.* poor.

pobreza *f.* poverty.

poción *f.* draft, potion, a single dose of liquid medicine.

poco-a *a.* little, in small quantity; *adv.* little, small; **dentro de ___ /** in a short while; **___ a ___ /** little by little; **por ___ /** almost.

poder *m.* power, strength; *vi.* to be able to; to have the power to.

podíatra *m., f.* podiatrist, specialist in podiatry.

podiatría *f.* podiatry, the diagnosis and treatment of conditions affecting the feet.

podrido-a *a.* rotten, decomposed.

polar *a.* polar, rel. to a pole.

polaridad *f.* polarity. 1. the quality of having two poles; 2. the quality of presenting opposite effects.

polen *m.* pollen.

poli *m.* poly, polymorphonuclear leukocyte.

poliarticular *a.* polyarticular, affecting more than one joint.

poliartritis *f.* polyarthritis, infl. of more than one joint.

policístico-a *a.* polycystic, composed of many cysts; **enfermedad ___ del riñón / ___** kidney disease; **síndrome ___ ovárico / ___** ovarian síndrome.

policitemia *f.* polycythemia, excess of red blood cells; **___ primaria /** primary **___ ,** vera; **___**

rubra / ___ rubra, vera; **___ secundaria /** secondary ___ , erythrocythemia; **___ vera /** ___ vera, erythremia.

policlínica *f.* polyclinic, a general hospital.

polidactilia *f.* polydactylia, polydactyly, the presence of more than five fingers or toes.

polidipsia *f.* polydipsia, excessive thirst.

poligamia *f.* polygamy, the practice of having more than one spouse at the same time.

polígrafo *m.* polygraph, device that registers simultaneously the arterial and venous pulsations.

polihidramnios *m.* polyhydramnios, an excess of amniotic fluid.

poli-insaturado-a *a.* polyunsaturated, denoting a fatty acid.

polimialgia *f.* polymyalgia, condition characterized by pain affecting several muscles.

polimiositis *f.* polymyositis, dermatomyositis.

polimorfonucleado-a, polimorfonuclear *a.* polymorphonuclear, having a deeply lobed nucleus; **granulocito ___ / ___** granulocyte, having a nucleus with multiple lobes.

polineuropatía *f.* polyneuropathy, any disease that affects several nerves at one time.

polio, poliomielitis *f.* polio, poliomyelitis, contagious disease that attacks the central nervous system and causes paralysis of the muscles, esp. of the legs.

poliomiopatía *f.* polymyopathy, any disease that affects several muscles at the same time.

poliovirus *m.* poliovirus, causative agent of poliomyelitis.

polipectomía *f.* polypectomy, excision of a polyp.

pólipo *m.* polyp, tag, mass, or growth protruding from a mucous membrane.

poliposis *f.* polyposis, formation of multiple polyps.

poliquístico-a *a.* polycystic, having many cysts.

polisacárido *m.* polysaccharide, a carbohydrate capable of hydrolysis.

polivalente *a.* polyvalent, having an effect against more than one agent.

póliza de seguro *f.* insurance policy.

pollo *m.* chicken.

polo *m.* pole, each of the two opposite extremes of a body, organ, or part.

polución *f.* pollution.

polución de ruido *f.* noise pollution.

polvo *m.* dust; powder; **en ___ /** powdered.

pomada *f.* ointment, pomade, salve, semisolid medicinal substance for external use; **___**

contraceptiva / contraceptive jelly; ___ **facial** / cold cream; ___ **vaginal** / vaginal jelly.

pomo *m.* jar; bottle.

pómulo *m.* molar bone, cheekbone.

poner *vi.* to put, to set, to lay down; **ponerse** *vr.* [*vestido*] to put on; to become; ___ **viejo** / to grow or become old.

pons *L.* pons, tissue formation that connects two separate parts of an organ.

poplíteo-a *a.* popliteal, rel. to the area behind the knee.

por *prep.* for, by, through, from; ___ **ahora** / for the time being; ___ **atrás** / from or through the back; ___ **delante** / from or through the front; ___ **eso** / because of that; ___ **lo tanto** / therefore.

porcentaje *m.* percentage, percent.

porcino-a *a.* porcine, rel. to swine.

porción *f.* portion.

porfiria *f.* porphyria, congenital defect in metabolism manifested by the presence of great amounts of porphyrin in the blood, urine, and stools causing physical and psychiatric disorders.

porfirina *f.* porphyrin, compound occurring in the protoplasm, basis of the respiratory pigments.

poro, porus *m.* pore, porus, minute opening of the skin such as the duct of a sweat gland.

poroso-a *a.* porous, permeable.

porque *conj.* because, for the reason that; *interr.* **¿por qué?** / why?, for what reason?

porta *L.* porta, opening or entry, esp. one through which blood vessels and nerves penetrate into an organ.

porta, vena *f.* portal vein, short, thick trunk formed by branches of many veins leading from abdominal organs.

portacatéter *m.* catheter holder.

portacava *a.* portacaval, rel. to the porta and the inferior vena cava.

portador *m.* carrier, a disease causing agent that can be transmitted to other individuals; ___ **de bacilos** / bacillicarrier.

portal *m.* portal, entryway; *a.* rel. to the portal system.

portal, circulación *f.* portal circulation, flow of blood into the liver via the portal vein and out via the hepatic vein.

portal, hipertensión *f.* portal hypertension, increase in pressure in the portal vein due to an obstruction in blood circulation in the liver.

portaobjeto *m.* slide, specimen holder for microscopic examination.

poseer *vi.* to possess.

poseído-a *a., pp.* de **poseer**, possessed, dominated by an idea or passion.

posesivo *m., gr.* possessive; **-a** *a.* possessive.

posibilidad *f.* possibility.

posible *a.* possible; **-mente** *adv.* possibly.

posición *f.* position; ___ **anatómica** / anatomic ___; ___ **de litotomía** / lithotomy ___; ___ **distal** / distal ___; ___ **dorsal recumbente** / dorsal recumbent ___; ___ **erecta** / upright ___; ___ **genucubital** / genocubital ___ , knee-elbow; ___ **genupectoral** / knee-chest ___; ___ **inadecuada** / malposition; ___ **lateral** / lateral ___; ___ **prona** / prone ___ , face down; ___ **supina, yacente** / supine ___ , face up.

positividad *f.* positivity, manifestation of a positive reaction.

positivo-a *a.* positive; certain, without doubt.

posponer *vi.* to postpone, to delay.

posterior *a.* posterior. 1. rel. to the back or the back part of a structure; 2. following in sequence.

posthipnótico-a *a.* posthypnotic, following the hypnotic state.

postictal *a.* postictal, following a seizure or attack.

postmaduro *a.* postmature, rel. to an infant born after the forty-first week of gestation.

post mortem *L.* postmortem, occurring after death; autopsy.

postnasal *a.* postnasal, behind the nose.

postparto *m.* postpartum, period of time following childbirth; **depresión del** ___ / ___ depression; **insuficiencia pituitaria del** ___ / ___ pituitary insufficiency; **psicosis del** ___ / ___ psychosis.

postoperatorio-a *a.* postoperative, following surgery; **complicación** ___ / ___ complication; **cuidado** ___ / ___ care.

postprandial *a.* postprandial, after a meal.

postración *f.* prostration, exhaustion, extreme fatigue.

postrado-a *a.* prostrate. 1. in prone position; 2. exhausted, debilitated.

postre *m.* dessert.

póstumo-a *a.* posthumous, occurring after death; **examen** ___ / postmortem examination.

postura *f.* posture, position of the body.

postural *a.* postural, rel. to position or posture; **hipotensión** ___ / ___ hypotension, decrease in blood pressure in an erect position.

potable *a.* potable, drinkable, that can be drunk without harm.

p

potasemia *f.* kalemia, presence of potassium in the blood.

potasio *m.* potassium, mineral which, combined with others in the body, is essential in the transmission of nerve impulses and in muscular activity.

potencia *f.* potency, strength.

potencial *m.* potential, electric pressure or tension; *a.* having a ready disposition or capacity.

potente *a.* potent, strong.

práctica *f.* practice.

practicar *vi.* to practice.

práctico-a *a.* practical.

prandial *a.* prandial, rel. to meals.

preagónico-a *a.* preagonal, rel. to a condition preceding death.

preanestésico *m.* preanesthetic, preliminary agent given to ease the administration of general anesthesia.

precanceroso-a *a.* precancerous, tending to become malignant.

precario-a *a.* precarious, uncertain.

precaución *f.* precaution.

precavido-a *a.* cautious, on guard.

preceder *v.* to precede.

precio *m.* price, cost.

precipitado *m.* precipitate, deposit of solid particles that settles out of a solution; **-a** *a.* that occurs suddenly.

precisión *f.* precision, exactness.

precocidad *f.* precocity, early development of physical or mental adult traits.

precoz *a.* precocious.

precursor *m.* precursor, something that precedes, such as a symptom or sign of a disease; **-a** *a.* introductory, preliminary.

predecir *vi.* to predict.

predisposición *f.* predisposition, propensity to develop a condition or illness, caused by environmental, genetic, or psychological factors.

predispuesto-a *a.* predisposed, prone or susceptible to develop a disease or any other condition.

predominante *a.* predominant.

predominio *m.* predominance.

preeclampsia *f.* preeclampsia, a toxic condition of late pregnancy, manifested by hypertension, albuminuria, and edema.

preferencia *f.* preference.

preferible *a.* preferable.

preferir *vi.* to prefer, to favor one thing, person, or condition over another.

prefijo *m., gr.* prefix.

pregunta *f.* question; *v.* **hacer una ___** / to ask a ___ .

preguntar *v.* to ask, to inquire.

prejuicio *m.* prejudice, bias.

preliminar *a.* preliminary.

premadurez *f.* prematurity, the condition of a viable infant born prior to completion of the thirty-seventh week of gestation.

prematuro-a *m., f.* premature baby; *a.* 1. born prior to the thirty-seventh week of gestation; 2. *pop.* preemie.

premedicación *f.* premedication.

premenstrual *a.* premenstrual; **tensión ___** / **___** tension;

premonición *f.* premonition, forewarning.

premonitorio-a *a.* premonitory; **advertencia o señal ___** / **___** signal; **síntoma ___** / **___** symptom.

premunición *f.* premunition, immunity to a given infection established by the previous presence of the causative agent.

prenatal *a.* prenatal, prior to birth; **cuidado ___** / **___** care.

prensil *a.* prehensile, adapted or shaped for grasping or lifting.

preñada *a. pop.* pregnant.

preocupación *f.* preoccupation, concern.

preocupado-a *a.* concerned, worried.

preocuparse *vr.* to worry, to be preoccupied; **no se preocupe, no te preocupes** / don't worry.

preoperativo-a *a.* preoperative; **cuidado ___** / **___** care.

preparación *f.* preparation. 1. the act of making something ready; 2. a medication ready for use.

preparar *v.* to prepare, to make ready.

preposición *f., gr.* preposition.

prepubescente *a.* prepubescent, before puberty.

prepucio *m.* prepuce, foreskin, loose fold of skin that covers the glans penis.

prerrenal *a.* prerenal. 1. in front of the kidney; 2. that occurs in the circulatory system before reaching the kidney.

presacro-a *a.* presacral, in front of the sacrum.

presbiopía *f.* presbyopia, farsightedness that occurs with increasing age due to the loss of elasticity of the lens of the eye.

prescribir *vi.* to prescribe.

prescripción *f.* prescription.

prescrito-a *a., pp.* de **prescribir**, prescribed, ordered.

presencia *f.* presence.

presentación *f.* presentation. 1. position of the fetus in the uterus as detected upon examination; 2. position of the fetus in reference to the birth canal at the time of delivery; ___ **cefálica** / cephalic ___; ___ **de cara** / face ___; ___ **de nalgas** / breech ___; ___ **transversa** / transverse ___; 3. oral report.

presente *a.* present, manifest.

preservación *f.* preservation, conservation.

preservar *v.* to preserve.

preservativo *m.* preservative. 1. agent that is added to food or medication to destroy or impede multiplication of bacteria; 2. condom.

presilla *f.* staple.

presión *f.* pressure, stress, strain, tension; ___ **arterial** / arterial ___, pressure exerted by the blood in the arteries; ___ **atmosférica** / atmospheric ___, pressure exerted by the mass of air surrounding the earth; ___ **central venosa** / central venous ___, blood pressure of the right atrium of the heart; ___ **del pulso** / pulse ___, the difference between sistolic and diastolic pressure; ___ **diastólica** / diastolic ___, lowest arterial blood pressure during diastole of the heart; ___ **intracraneana** / intracranial ___, pressure exerted within the cranium; ___ **osmótica** / osmotic ___; ___ **parcial** / partial___, pressure exerted by a single gas component in a single, mixed composition; ___ **sistólica** / systolic ___, arterial blood pressure during contraction of the ventricles; ___ **venosa** / venous ___, pressure exerted by the blood on the walls of the veins; *v.* **hacer** ___ / to exert pressure.

presión sanguínea *f.* blood pressure, pressure by the blood on the arteries, produced by the action of the left ventricle, the resistance of the arterioles and capillaries, the elasticity of the arterial walls, and the viscosity and volume of the blood expressed in relation to the atmospheric pressure; ___ **alta** / high ___; ___ **baja** / low ___; ___ **normal** / normal ___ .

presionar *v.* to exert pressure.

presor *a.* pressor, that tends to raise the blood pressure.

pretender *v.* to attempt, to try.

pretérito *m., gr.* preterite.

pretérmino *m.* preterm, occurring during the period of time prior to the thirty-seventh week in a pregnancy.

prevaleciente *a.* prevailing.

prevalencia *f.* prevalence, the total number of cases of a specific disease present in a given population at a certain time.

prevención *f.* prevention.

prevenir *vi.* to prevent, to forestall.

preventivo-a *a.* preventive; **servicios de salud** ___ / ___ health services.

prever *vi.* to foresee.

prevertebral *a.* prevertebral, in front of a vertebra.

previo-a *a.* previous, prior.

previsto-a *a., pp.* de **prever,** foreseen.

priapismo *m.* priapism, painful and continued erection of the penis as a result of disease.

primario-a *a.* primary, initial; chief, principal.

primavera *f.* springtime.

primer, primero-a *a.* first, prime.

primeriza *f.* primipara, a woman who has given birth to a child for the first time.

primeros auxilios *m. pl.* first aid.

primitivo-a *a.* primitive; embryonic.

primo-a *m., f.* cousin.

primogénito-a *a.* first-born.

primordial *a.* primordial, essential.

principal *a.* main, principal, foremost; **-mente** *adv.* primarily, mainly.

principiante *m.* beginner, novice.

principio *m.* 1. beginning, start; 2. principle, chief ingredient of a medication or chemical compound; 3. principle, rule.

principio del placer *m.* pleasure principle, behavior directed at obtaining immediate gratification and avoiding pain.

principio de la realidad *m.* reality principle, orientation to reality and self-gratification through awareness of the outside world.

prioridad *f.* priority, precedence.

prisa *f.* haste, rush; **a toda** ___ / right away; *vr.* **darse** ___ / to hurry; *v.* **tener** ___ / to be in a hurry.

privación *f.* privation, hardship; withdrawal.

privado-a *a.* private; **cuarto** ___ / private room; **-mente** *adv.* privately.

privilegio *m.* privilege.

probabilidad *f.* probability.

probable *a.* probable; **-mente** *adv.* probably.

probador *m.* tester.

probar *vi.* [*esfuerzo*] to try; [*gusto*] to taste; [*comprobar*] to prove; to sample.

probeta *f.* pipette, glass tube.

problema *m.* problem; trouble.

problemático-a *a.* problematic, disputable.

procedente *a.* originating.

proceder *v.* to proceed, to continue.

procedimiento *m.* procedure; ___ **clínico** / clinical ___; ___ **quirúrgico** / surgical ___; ___ **terapéutico** / therapeutic ___ .

P

proceso *m.* process, method, system.

procrear *v.* to procreate, to beget.

proctalgia *f.* proctalgia, pain in the rectum and anus.

proctitis *f.* proctitis, infl. of the rectum and the anus.

proctología *f.* proctology, the branch of medicine that studies the colon, rectum, and anus, and the treatment of the diseases affecting them.

proctólogo-a *m., f.* proctologist, specialist in proctology.

proctoscopio *m.* proctoscope, endoscope used to examine the rectum.

procurar *v.* to procure; to try.

prodrómico-a *a.* prodromal, rel. to the initial stages of a disease.

pródromo *m.* prodrome, a premonitory symptom.

producción *f.* production, rendering.

producir *vi.* to produce.

productivo-a *a.* productive.

producto *m.* product; result or effect.

profase *f.* prophase, first stage of cell division.

profesión *f.* profession.

profesional *m., f.* professional; *a.* professional.

profiláctico-a *a.* prophylactic. 1. agent or method used to prevent infection; 2. condom.

profilaxis *f.* prophylaxis, preventive treatment.

profunda *L.* profunda, deep, esp. in reference to the location of some arteries.

profundidad *f.* depth.

profundo-a *a.* deep; **anillo inguinal** ___ / ___ inguinal ring; **arteria** ___ **del brazo** / ___ artery of the arm; **arteria** ___ **del clítoris** / ___ artery of the clitoris; **arteria** ___ **del pene** / ___ artery of the penis; **trombosis venenosa** ___ / ___ venous thrombosis; **venas cerebrales** ___ / ___ cerebral veins; **venas cervicales** ___ / ___ cervical veins; **vena facial** ___ / ___ facial vein.

profuso-a *a.* profuse, plentiful; **-mente** *adv.* profusely.

progesterona *f.* progesterone, steroid hormone secreted by the ovaries.

prognato-a *a.* prognathous, having a pronounced jaw.

programar *v.* to schedule; to program.

progresar *v.* to advance; to improve; to thrive.

progresivo-a *a.* progressive, advancing.

progreso *m.* progress.

prohibir *v.* to forbid, to prohibit, to ban.

prolapso *m.* prolapse, the falling down or slipping of a body part from its usual position.

proliferación *f.* proliferation, multiplication, esp. of similar cells; ___ **excesiva** / overgrowth.

prolífico-a *a.* prolific, that multiplies readily.

prólogo *m.* preface.

prolongación *f.* prolongation, extension.

prolongar *vi.* to prolong, to delay.

promedio *m.* average.

promesa *f.* promise.

prometer *v.* to promise, to give one's word.

prominencia *f.* prominence, elevation of a part; projection.

promontorio *m.* promontory, elevation; projection.

pronar *v.* to pronate, to put the body or a body part in a prone position.

prono-a *a.* prone, lying in a face down position.

pronombre *m., gr.* pronoun.

pronosticar *vi.* to prognosticate, to predict.

pronóstico *m.* prognosis, evaluation of the probable course of an illness.

pronto *adv.* soon, fast, quickly; **por lo** ___ / for the time being.

pronunciar *v.* to pronounce, to articulate sounds.

propagación *f.* propagation, reproduction.

propagar *vi.* to propagate.

propenso-a *a.* predisposed to; ___ **a** / inclined to.

propiedad *f.* property. 1. possessions; 2. quality that distinguishes a person, specie, or object from another. *V.* cuadro en la página 211.

propio-a *a.* proper, naturally suiting, complying with, relevant to.

propioceptivo-a *a.* proprioceptive, capable of receiving stimulations originating within the tissues of the body.

propioceptor *m.* proprioceptor, sensory nerve ending that reacts to stimuli and gives information concerning movements and position of the body.

proporción *f.* proportion.

proporcionado-a *a.* proportionate.

propósito *m.* purpose; **a** ___ / on purpose, by the way.

proptosis *f.* proptosis, forward displacement of a part, such as the eyeball.

prosencéfalo *m.* prosencephalon, anterior portion of the primary cerebral vesicle from which the diencephalon and the telencephalon develop.

próstata *f.* prostate, male gland that surrounds the bladder and the urethra; **hipertrofia de la** ___ / prostatic hypertrophy, benign enlargement of the prostate.

Propiedades	Properties
abundante	abundant
ácido	acid
afilado	[*instrumento*] sharp
agrio	sour
alto	tall
amargo	bitter
bajo	[*estatura*] short
caliente	hot
claro	clear
deficiente	deficient
desabrido	tasteless
dulce	sweet
esbelto	slender, svelte
espeso	thick
fresco	cool
frío	cold
fuerte	strong
grasoso	fatty
grueso, gordo	heavy, fat
húmedo	humid, moist
insípido	tasteless
largo	long
ligero	light
líquido	liquid
mojado	wet
pesado	[*peso*] heavy
pobre	poor
rico	rich
seco	dry
sólido	solid
sucio	dirty
tibio	lukewarm

prostatectomía *f.* prostatectomy, partial or total excision of the prostate.
prostático-a *a.* prostatic, rel. to the prostate.
prostatismo *m.* prostatism, disorder resulting from obstruction of the bladder neck by an enlarged prostate.
prostatitis *f.* prostatitis, infl. of the prostate.
prostitución *f.* prostitution.
protección *f.* protection.

protector-a *a.* protective.
proteger *vi.* to protect.
proteico-a *a.* protean, that has various forms of manifestation.
proteína *f.* protein, nitrogen compound essential in the development and preservation of body tissues.
proteináceo-a *a.* proteinaceous, of the nature of or resembling protein.
proteinemia *f.* proteinemia, concentration of proteins in the blood.
proteínico-a *a.* proteinic, rel. to protein; **balance** ___ / protein balance.
proteinosis *f.* proteinosis, excess protein in the tissues.
proteinuria *f.* proteinuria, the presence of protein in the urine.
prótesis *f.* prosthesis, artificial replacement of a missing part of the body, such as a limb.
protética *f.* prosthetics. 1. the art of manufacturing and adjusting artificial parts for the human body; 2. branch of surgery concerned with the replacement of parts of the body.
protocolo *m.* protocol. 1. a record taken from notes; 2. a written proposal of a procedure to be performed; ___ **toxicológico** / toxicology screen.
protoplasma *m.* protoplasm, essential part of the cell that includes the cytoplasm and the nucleus.
prototipo *m.* prototype, role-model, example.
protozoario-a *a.* protozoan, rel. to protozoa.
protozoo *m.* protozoan, unicellular organism.
protracción *f.* protraction, extension of teeth or other structures of the jaw into a position anterior to their normal position.
protrombina *f.* prothrombin, one of the four major plasma proteins along with albumin, globulin, and fibrinogen.
protuberancia *f.* protuberance, prominence.
provechoso-a *a.* beneficial.
proveer *vi.* to provide, to administer.
provisional *a.* provisional, temporary.
provisiones *f. pl.* provisions, supplies.
proximal *a.* proximal, closest to the point of reference.
próximo-a *a.* next to, close by.
proyección *f.* projection. 1. protuberance; 2. a mechanism by which one's own unacceptable ideas or traits are attributed to others.
prueba *f.* test, proof, trial; indication; **a** ___ **de agua** / waterproof; **a** ___ **de fuego** / fireproof; ___ **antinuclear de anticuerpo** / antinuclear antibody ___; ___ **controlada por**

placebo / placebo-controlled ___; ___ **cutánea** / skin ___; ___ **de aclaramiento de creatinina** / creatinine clearance ___; ___ **de ciego simple** / single-blind trial; ___ **de coagulación sanguínea** / blood coagulation ___; ___ **de control sin método** / random controlled trial; ___ **de doble incógnita** / double-blind trial; ___ **de esfuerzo** / stress ___ , treadmill; ___ **de función hepática** / liver function ___; ___ **de función respiratoria** / respiratory function ___; ___ **de función tiroidea** / thyroid function ___; ___ **de grasa fecal** / stool fat ___; ___ **de rasguño** / scratch ___ ,allergy ___; ___ **de resistencia** / endurance ___; ___ **de tiempo limitado** / timed ___; ___ **de tipo** / type ___; ___ **de tolerancia** / tolerance ___; ___ **de tolerancia a la glucosa** / glucose tolerance ___; ___ **del embarazo** / pregnancy ___; ___ **eliminatoria** / screening ___; **hay** ___ / there is an indication; **resultado de la** ___ / results of the ___; ___ **-s sanguíneas cruzadas** / crossmatching ___ -s; ___ **serológica** / serology ___; ___ **sin pronóstico o tratamiento cierto** / double-blind technique; ___ **subsecuente, de seguimiento** / follow-up ___; ___ **visual de campimetría** / visual field ___; ___ **visual de letras** / visual ___ .

prueba del funcionamiento del páncreas f. pancreatic function test.

pruriginoso-a a. pruriginous, rel. to prurigo.

prurigo m. prurigo, chronic inflammatory condition of the skin characterized by small papules and severe itching.

prurito m. pruritus, severe itching.

pseudoaneurismo m. pseudoaneurysm, an aneurysm-like dilation in a vessel.

pseudociesis f. pseudocyesis, false pregnancy.pseudoembarazo.

pseudoembarazo m. pseudopregnancy, false or imaginary pregnancy.

pseudoquiste m. pseudocyst, cyst-like formation.

psicoactivo-a a. psychoactive, affecting the mind.

psicoanálisis m. psychoanalysis, branch of psychiatry founded by Sigmund Freud that endeavors to make the patient conscious of repressed conflicts through techniques such as interpretation of dreams and free association of ideas.

psicoanalista m., f. psychoanalyst, one who practices psychoanalysis.

psicobiología f. psychobiology, the study of the mind in relation to biological processes.

psicodélico-a a. psychedelic, rel. to a substance that can induce pathological states of altered perception such as hallucinations and delusions.

psicodrama m. psychodrama, the psychiatric method of diagnosis and therapy by which the patient acts out conflicting situations of his or her real life.

psicofarmacología f. psychopharmacology, the study of the effect of drugs on the mind and behavior.

psicofisiológico-a a. psychophysiologic, rel. to the mind's influence on bodily processes, as manifested in some disorders or diseases.

psicofisiológicos, desórdenes m. pl. psycho-physiologic disorders, disorders that result from the relation between psychological and physiological processes.

psicología f. psychology, the study of mental processes, esp. as related to the individual's environment.

psicología del desarrollo mental f. psychology of mental development.

psicológico-a a. psychological, rel. to psychology.

psicólogo-a m., f. psychologist, person who practices psychology.

psicomotor-a a. psychomotor, rel. to motor actions that result from mental activity.

psicópata m., f. psychopath, sociopath, person suffering from an antisocial personality disorder.

psicopatología f. psychopathology, the branch of medicine that deals with the causes and nature of mental illness.

psicosis f. psychosis, severe mental disorder of organic or emotional origin in which the patient loses touch with reality and suffers hallucinations and mental aberrations; ___ **alcohólica** / alcoholic ___; ___ **depresiva** / depressive ___; ___ **maniacodepresiva** / manic-depressive ___; ___ **orgánica** / organic ___; ___ **por droga** / drug-related ___; ___ **senil** / senile ___; ___ **situacional** / situational ___; ___ **tóxica** / toxic ___; ___ **traumática** / traumatic ___ .

psicosocial a. psychosocial, rel. to both psychological and social factors.

psicosomático-a a. psychosomatic, rel. to both mind and body; **síntoma** ___ / ___ symptom.

psicoterapia f. psychotherapy, the treatment of mental or emotional disorders through psychological means, such as psychoanalysis.

psicótico-a *a.* psychotic, rel. to or suffering from psychosis.

psicotrópicas, drogas *f.* psychotropic drugs, drugs capable of affecting mental functions or behavior.

psique *f.* psyche, conscious and unconscious mental life.

psiquiatra *m., f.* psychiatrist, specialist in psychiatry.

psiquiatría *f.* psychiatry, the study of the psyche and its disorders.

psiquiátrico-a *a.* psychiatric, rel. to psychiatry.

psíquico-a *a.* psychic, rel. to the psyche.

psoas *Gr.* psoas, one of the two muscles of the loin.

psoriasis *f.* psoriasis, chronic dermatitis manifested chiefly by red patches covered with white scales.

ptosis *Gr.* ptosis, prolapse of an organ or part, such as the upper eyelid.

púbero-a *a.* pubescent, having reached puberty.

pubertad *f.* puberty, the period of adolescence that marks the development of the secondary sexual characteristics and the beginning of reproductive capacity.

pubescencia *f.* pubescence. 1. beginning of puberty; 2. covering of soft, fine hair, lanugo.

púbico-a *a.* pubic, rel. to the pubis; **pelo** ___ / ___ hair.

público-a *a.* public.

pudendum *L. pudenda*pudendum, external sexual organs, esp. the female.

pudrirse *vr.* to rot; to decay.

puente *m.* bridge; ___**coronario** / coronary ___; ___**dental** / dental ___ .

puerco *m.* pig, pork.

pueril *a.* puerile. 1. rel. to a child; 2. childish.

puerperal *a.* puerperal, rel. to the puerperium.

puerperio *m.* puerperium, the period of approximately six weeks following childbirth during which the organs of the mother return to normalcy.

puerta *f.* door.

pues *conj.* therefore; then; so.

puesto-a *a., pp.* de **poner**, placed, put.

pujar *v.* to bear down.

pulga *f.* flea, blood-sucking insect.

pulgada *f.* inch.

pulgar *m.* the thumb.

pulmón *m.* lung, respiratory organ situated inside the pleural cavity of the thorax, connected to the pharynx through the trachea and the larynx; **cáncer del** ___ / ___ cancer; **colapso del** ___ / collapse of the ___ .

pulmón de granjero *m.* farmer's lung, hypersensitivity of the pulmonary alveoli caused by exposure to fermented hay.

pulmón de hierro *m.* iron lung, machine used to produce artificial respiration.

pulmonar *a.* pulmonary, pulmonic, rel. to the lungs or to the pulmonary artery; **absceso** ___ / lung abscess; **arteria** ___ / ___ artery; **elasticidad** ___ / lung elasticity; **embolismo** ___ / ___ embolism; **enfisema** ___ / ___ emphysema; **estenosis** ___ / ___ stenosis; **hemorragia** ___ / ___ hemorrhage; **insuficiencia** ___ / ___ insufficiency; **presión diferencial de la arteria** ___ / ___ artery wedge pressure; **proteinosis alveolar** ___ / ___ alveolar proteinosis; **válvula** ___ / ___ valve; **vena** ___ / ___ vein; **volumen** ___ / lung capacity.

pulmonía *f.* pneumonia. neumonia.

pulpa *f.* pulp. 1. soft part on an organ; 2. chyme; 3. soft inner part of a tooth.

pulsación *f.* pulsation, throbbing, rhythmic beat such as that of the heart.

pulsátil *a.* pulsatile, having a rhythmic pulsation.

pulsímetro *m.* pulsimeter, instrument for measuring the force of the pulse.

pulso *m.* pulse, rhythmic arterial dilation gen. coinciding with the heartbeat. *V.* cuadro.

pulverizar *vi.* to pulverize, to reduce a substance to powder.

punción *f.* puncture, perforation, the act of perforating a tissue with a sharp instrument.

Pulso	Pulse
alternante	alternating
bigeminado	bigeminal
de la arteria dorsal del pie	dorsalis pedis
en martillo de agua	water hammer
femoral	femoral
filiforme	filiform
irregular	irregular
lleno	full
periférico	peripheral
radial	radial
rápido	rapid
regular	regular
saltón	bounding

pungente *a.* pungent, sharp.

punta *f.* tip, point, sharp end of an instrument.

punteado *m.* stippling, the condition of being spotted such as seen in red corpuscles.

puntiagudo-a *a.* sharp, pointed.

punto *m.* 1. stitch; 2. point, a position in time or space; *v.* **estar a** ___ **de** / to be on the verge of; 3. spot; ___ **ciego** / blind ___; 4. *gr.* period.

puntos de presión *m. pl.* pressure points, points in an artery where the pulse can be felt or where pressure can be exerted to control bleeding.

puntual *a.* punctual, prompt, on time.

punzada *f.* twinge; sharp, sudden pain; jab.

punzante *a.* piercing, sharp.

punzar *vi.* to puncture; to tap, to perforate.

puñal *m.* dagger.

puñalada *f.* stab.

puño *m.* fist; **cerrar el** ___ / to make a fist.

pupila *f.* pupil, contractile opening of the iris of the eye that allows the passage of light; ___ **saltona** / bounding ___; ___ **fija** / fixed ___.

pupilar *a.* pupillary, rel. to the pupil.

puré *m.* puree; ___ **de papas** / mashed potatoes.

purga *f.* cathartic medication.

purgación *f.* purgation, evacuation of the bowels using a medical purgative.

purgante *m.* purgative, laxative, agent used to cause evacuation of the intestines; ___ **de sal** / saline cathartic.

purgar *v.* 1. to purge, to clean; 2. to force intestinal evacuation by means of a purgative.

purificación *f.* purification.

purificar *vi.* to purify.

purificado-a *a.* purified; **agua** ___ / ___ water.

puro-a *a.* pure, uncontaminated.

púrpura *L.* purpura, condition characterized by reddish or purple spots that result from the escape of blood into tissues; ___ **trombocitopénica** / thrombocytopenic ___.

purulencia *f.* purulence, the condition of being purulent.

purulento-a *a.* purulent, containing pus, pus-like.

pus *f.* pus, thick, yellowish fluid that results from inflammation; **supuración de** ___ / pus discharge.

pústula *f.* pustule, sore, small elevation of the skin filled with pus.

putrefacción *f.* putrefaction, the process of decomposing.

putrefacto-a, pútrido-a *a.* putrid, rotten, foul.

q

q *abr. L.* **quaque** / cada; **quaque** / every.

quadratus *L.* quadratus. 1. four-sided muscle; 2. four-sided figure.

Quant, signo de *m.* Quant sign, a T-shaped depression that appears in the occipital bone, mostly seen in cases of rachitism.

quantum *L.* quantum, a unit of energy.

quaque *L.* quaque, each; every.

quebradizo-a *a.* brittle, that breaks easily.

quebradura *f.* split; break.

quebrar *vi.* to break, to crack.

Queckenstedt, signo de *m.* Queckenstedt's sign, little or no increase in the pressure of the cerebrospinal fluid when there is compression of the veins of the neck; in healthy persons the pressure rises rapidly on compression.

quedarse *vr.* to stay, to remain in one place; ___ **atrás** / to lag behind.

queilectomía *f.* cheilectomy, partial excision of the lip.

queilitis *f.* cheilitis, infl. of the lip.

queiloplastia *f.* cheiloplasty, plastic surgery of the lip.

queilosis *f.* cheilosis, disorder caused by a deficiency of vitamin B$_2$ complex (riboflavin) and marked by fissures at the angles of the lips.

queilosquisis *f.* cheiloschisis. labio leporino.

queirología *f.* cheirology. 1. the study of the hand; 2. sign language.

queja *f.* complaint, grievance; ___ **principal** / chief ___ .

quejarse *vr.* to complain; to whine.

quejido *m.* groan, moan, whimper, whine.

quelis *m.* kelis, keloid.

queloide *m.* keloid, thick, reddish scar formation following a wound or surgical incision.

quemadura *f.* burn; ___ **de primer, segundo, tercer grado** / first-, second-, third-degree ___ ; ___ **de sol** / sunburn; ___ **por frío** / frostbite; ___ **por radiación** / radiation ___ ; ___ **por viento** / windburn.

quemar *v.* to burn, to scorch; **quemarse** *vr.* to get burned.

quemazón *m.* burning; [comezón], itching.

queratina *f.* keratin, organic, insoluble protein component of nails, skin, and hair.

queratinización *f.* keratinization, process by which cells become horny due to a deposit of keratin.

queratinoso-a *a.* keratinous, rel. to or of the nature of keratin.

queratitis *f.* keratitis, infl. of the cornea; ___ **intersticial** / interstitial ___ ; ___ **micótica** / mycotic ___ , caused by fungus; ___ **trófica** / trophic ___ , caused by the herpes virus.

queratocele *m.* keratocele, hernia of the innermost layer of the cornea.

queratoconjuntivitis *f.* keratoconjunctivitis, simultaneous infl. of the cornea and the conjunctiva.

queratocono *m.* keratoconus, corneal deformity in the shape of a cone.

queratoderma, queratodermia *f.* keratoderma, hypertrophy of the corneal layer of the skin, esp. in the palms of the hands and the soles of the feet.

queratoideo-a *a.* keratose, resembling the cornea.

queratólisis *f.* keratolysis. 1. exfoliation of the skin; 2. congenital anomaly that causes the skin to shed periodically; ___ **neonatal** / ___ neonatorum.

queratolítico-a *a.* keratolytic, agent that causes exfoliation of the skin.

queratomalacia *f.* keratomalacia, degeneration of the cornea due to a deficiency of vitamin A.

queratoplastia *f.* keratoplasty, plastic surgery of the cornea.

queratorrexis *f.* keratorrhexis, rupture of the cornea caused by a perforating ulcer or trauma.

queratosis *f.* keratosis, horny condition of the skin; ___ **actínica** / actinic ___ , precancerous lesion; ___ **blenorrágica** / ___ , blenorrhagica, manifested by a scaly rash, esp. on the palms or the soles of the feet.

queratotomía *f.* keratotomy, surgical incision of the cornea.

querer *vi.* to want, to desire; to love.

querido-a *a.* dear, beloved.

querubismo *m.* cherubism, fibro-osseous disease in children that causes enlargement of the jaw bones.

queso *m.* cheese.

quetoacidosis *f.* ketoacidosis, acidosis caused by an increase in the ketone bodies.

quiasma *m.* chiasm, chiasma, the crossing of two elements or structures; ___ **óptico** / optic ___ , the point at which the fibers of the optic nerve cross.

quiescente *a.* quiescent, inactive; latent.

quieto-a *a.* quiet, still; *v.* **estar** ___ / to be still.

quijada *f.* jaw, osseous structure of the mouth.

quilemia *f.* chylemia, presence of chyle in the blood.

quilo *m.* chyle, milky fluid that results in the absorption and emulsification of fats in the small intestine.

quilocele *m.* chylocele, presence of chyle within the tunica vaginalis of the testis.

quilomicrón *m.* chylomicron, microscopic particle of fat found in the blood.

quilorrea *f.* chylorrhea, discharge of chyle due to a rupture of the thoracic duct.

quiloso-a *a.* chylous, rel. to or that contains chyle.

quilotórax *m.* chylothorax, accumulation of chyle in the thoracic cavity.

quiluria *f.* chyluria, passage of chyle into the urine.

quimera *f.* chimera, an organism containing cells derived from different zygotes as in the case of twins.

química *f.* chemistry, the science that studies the composition, structure, and properties of matter, and the transformations that they may undergo.

químico-a *m., f.* chemist; *a.* chemical, rel. to chemistry.

quimiocirugía *f.* chemosurgery, removal of diseased tissue through the use of chemicals.

quimiocoagulación *f.* chemocoagulation, coagulation that results from the use of chemicals.

quimionucleolisis *f.* chemonucleolysis, dissolution of the nucleus pulposus of a hernia by injection of a proteolytic enzyme.

quimioprofilaxis *f.* chemoprophylaxis, drug used as a preventive agent.

quimiorreceptor *m.* chemoreceptor, a cell or a receptor that can be excited by chemical change.

quimiotaxis *m.* chemotaxis, movement by a cell or an organism as a reaction to a chemical stimulus.

quimioterapia *f.* chemotherapy, treatment of a disease by chemical agents.

quimo *m.* chyme, semiliquid substance that results from the gastric digestion of food.

quimografía *f.* kymography, technique or method used to register involuntary movement of an organ or structure, esp. the heart and the diaphragm.

quimotripsina *f.* chymotrypsin, pancreatic enzyme.

quimotripsinógeno *m.* chymotrypsinogen, pancreatic enzyme, precursor of chymotrypsin.

Quincke, edema de *m.* Quincke's edema. angioedema.

quinidina *f.* quinidine, alkaloid derived from the bark of the cinchona tree, used in the treatment of cardiac arrhythmia.

quinina *f.* quinine, the most important alkaloid obtained from the cortex of the cinchona, used as an antipyretic in the treatment of malaria and typhoid fever.

quininismo *m.* quininism, cinchonism, quinine poisoning.

quintana *f.* quintan, fever occurring every fifth day.

quíntuple *m., f.* quintuplet, any of a set of five children born at one birth.

quiropráctica *f.* chiropractic, therapeutic treatment that consists of manipulation and adjustment of body structures, esp. of the spinal column in relation to the nervous system.

quirúrgico-a *a.* surgical, rel. to surgery; **colgajo** ___ / ___ flap; **equipo** ___ / ___ equipment; **instrumento** ___ / ___ instrument; **malla** ___ / ___ mesh.

quiste *m.* cyst, sac, or pouch containing a fluid or semifluid substance; ___ **pilonidal** / pilonidal ___ , containing hair and gen. occurring in the dermis of the sacrococcygeal area; ___ **sebáceo** / sebaceous ___ , gen. localized on the scalp.

quitar *v.* to take away, to remove.

quizás *adv.* perhaps.

r

R *abr.* **radioactivo-a** / radioactive; **resistencia** / resistance; **respiración** / respiration; **respuesta, reacción** / response.

rabadilla *f.* coccyx, the extremity of the backbone.

rábano *m.* radish.

rabdomioma *m.* rhabdomyoma, benign tumor composed of striated muscle fiber.

rabdomiosarcoma *m.* rhabdomyosarcoma, malignant tumor of striated muscle fibers affecting primarily the skeletal muscles.

rabdosarcoma *m.* rhabdosarcoma. rabdomiosarcoma.

rabia *f.* rabies. 1. hydrophobia; 2. rage, anger; *v.* **tener ___** / to be enraged.

rabieta *f.* tantrum.

rabino *m.* rabbi.

rabioso-a *a.* rabid. 1. rel. to or afflicted by rabies; 2. enraged.

rabo *m.* tail.

racemoso-a, racimoso-a *a.* racemose, resembling a cluster of grapes.

racial *a.* racial, ethnic, rel. to race; **inmunidad ___** / ___ immunity, natural immunity of the members of a race; **prejuicio ___** / ___ prejudice.

ración *f.* ration, food portion.

racional *a.* rational, reasonable, based on reason.

racionalización *f.* rationalization, defense mechanism by which behavior or actions are justified by explanations that may seem reasonable but are not necessarily based on reality.

racionar *v.* to ration.

rad *L.* rad. 1. unit of absorbed radiation; 2. *abr.* radix, root.

radiación *f.* radiation. 1. emission of particles of radioactive material; 2. propagation of energy; 3. emission of rays from a common center; **enfermedad por ___** / ___ sickness, radiation syndrome, illness caused by overexposure to x-rays or radioactive materials; **___ electromagnética** / electromagnetic ___; **___ ionizante** / ionizing ___; **___ por rayos infrarrojos** / infrared ___; **___ por rayos ultravioletas** / ultraviolet ___ .

radiación oncológica *n.* 1. the use of radiation for the treatment of neoplasms; 2. radiation therapy.

radiactividad, radioactividad *f.* radioactivity, property of some elements to produce radiation.

radiactivo-a *a.* radioactive, rel. to or having radioactivity; **medio de contraste ___** / ___ contrast medium.

radial *a.* radial. 1. rel. to the radius; 2. that radiates from a center in all directions.

radiante *a.* radiant, that emits rays.

radical *a.* radical. 1. aimed at eradicating the root of a disease or all the diseased tissue; 2. rel. to the root; **-mente** *adv.* radically.

radicular *a.* radicular, rel. to the root or source.

radiculectomía *f.* radiculectomy, excision of the root of a nerve, esp. a spinal nerve.

radiculitis *f.* radiculitis, infl. of a nerve root.

radiculomielopatía *f.* radiculomyelopathy, a disease affecting the spinal cord and the roots of the spinal nerves.

radiculoneuritis *f.* radiculoneuritis, Guillain-Barré syndrome, infl. of the roots of a spinal nerve.

radiculoneuropatía *f.* radiculoneuropathy, disease of the nerves and nerve roots.

radiculopatía *f.* radiculopathy, disease of the roots of the spinal nerves.

radio *m.* 1. radium, metallic, radioactive, fluorescent element used in some of its variations in the treatment of malignant tumors; **agujas de ___** / ___ needles, needle-shaped, radium-containing device used in radiotherapy; 2. radius, the outer bone of the forearm; 3. radio.

radiobiología *f.* radiobiology, the study of the effect of radiation on living tissue.

radiocardiografía *f.* radiocardiography, graphic recording of a radioactive substance as it travels through the heart.

radiocurable *a.* radiocurable, curable using radiotherapy.

radiodiagnosis *f.* radiagnosis, diagnosis by means of x-rays.

radiofármaco *m.* radiopharmaceutical, radioactive drug used for diagnosis and treatment of diseases.

radiografía *f.* radiography. roentgenograma.

radioisótopo *m.* radioisotope, radioactive isotope.

radiología *f.* radiology, the study of x-rays and rays emanating from radioactive substances, esp. for medical use.

radiológico-a *a.* radiologic, rel. to radiology.

radiólogo-a *m., f.* radiologist, specialist in radiology.

radiolúcido-a *a.* radiolucent, that allows the passage of most x-rays.

radionecrosis *f.* radionecrosis, disintegration of tissue by means of radiation.

radiopaco-a *a.* radioopaque, that does not allow the passage of x-rays or any other form of radiation; **colorante** ___ / ___ dye.

radiorresistente *a.* radioresistant, having the quality of being resistant to the effects of radiation.

radioscopía *f.* radioscopy, exam of the internal structures of the body by means of x-rays and rays emitted by electrons and positrons known as *roentgen.*

radiosensitivo-a *a.* radiosensitive, that is affected by or responds to radiation treatment.

radioterapia *f.* radiotherapy, radiation therapy.

radón *m.* radon, colorless, gaseous radioactive element.

rafe *m.* raphe, joining line of two symmetrical halves of a structure such as the tongue.

raíz *f.* root.

rajadura *f.* crack, slit.

rama *f.* ramus, branch.

ramificación *f.* ramification, separation into branches.

ramificarse *vr., vi.* to ramify.

rancio-a *a.* rancid, stale, having an unpleasant smell, gen. due to decomposition.

ránula *f.* ranula, cystic tumor under the tongue caused by an obstruction of a gland duct.

ranura *f.* groove, slit.

rapidez *f.* speed, velocity.

rápido-a *a.* quick, fast; swift; **-mente** *adv.* quickly.

raptus *L.* raptus, sudden, violent attack such as of a maniacal or nervous nature.

raquídeo-a *a.* rachial, rel. to the rachis or the spine.

raquis *m.* rachis, the vertebral column, backbone.

raquítico-a *a.* rachitic. 1. rel. to rachitism; 2. stunted, feeble.

raquitis *f.* rickets.raquitismo.

raquitismo *m.* rachitism, rachitis, a deficiency disease that affects skeletal growth in the young, usu. caused by lack of calcium, phosphorus, and vitamin D; *pop.* rickets.

raro-a *a.* rare, different, unusual; **-mente** *adv.* rarely, seldom.

rascar *vi.* to scratch; **rascarse** *vr.* to scratch oneself.

rasgo *m.* trait, feature, strain; ___ **adquirido** / acquired ___; ___ **heredado** / inherited ___ .

rasguño, rascuño *m.* scratch.

raspado *m.* curettage, scraping of the interior of a cavity; ___ **uterino** / ___dilation and curettage.

raspador *m.* scraper.

raspadura, rasponazo *f., m.* scrape.

raspante *a.* abrasive.

raspar *v.* to scrape.

rastrear *v.* to scan, trace, and record with a sensitive detecting device.

rastreo *m.* scan.escán.

rastro *m.* trace. 1. small quantity; 2. a visible sign or mark.

rasura *f.* rasura, scrapings or filings.

rata *f.* rat.

ratio *L.* ratio, quantity of one substance in relation to another.

rato *m.* while, a short time.

Rauwolfia serpentina *f.* Rauwolfia serpentina, a plant species that is the source of reserpine, an extract used in the treatment of hypertension and some mental disorders.

raya *f.* streak.

Raynaud, enfermedad de *f.* Raynaud's disease. acrocianosis.

Raynaud, fenómeno de *m.* Raynaud's phenomenon, the symptoms associated with Raynaud's disease.

rayo *m.* ray.___ **láser** / laser beam; ___ **alfa** / alpha ___; **infrarrojo** / infrared ___; ___ **ultravioleta** / ultraviolet ___ .

rayos gamma *m., pl.* gamma rays, high-energy rays emitted by radioactive substances.

rayos-x *m., pl.* 1. x-rays, high-energy electromagnetic short waves used to penetrate tissues and record densities on film; 2. films obtained through the use of x-rays.

raza *f.* race, a distinctive ethnic group with common inherited characteristics.

razón *f.* the faculty of reason; **a ___ de** / at the rate of; ___ **de ingreso** / ___ for admission; *v.* **tener** ___ / to be right.

razón fundamental *f.* rationale.

razonable *a.* reasonable.

razonamiento *m.* reasoning.

razonar *v.* to reason.

reabsorber *v.* to reabsorb.

reacción *f.* reaction, response; ___ **alérgica** / allergic ___; ___ **anafiláctica** / anaphylactic ___; ___ **de ansiedad** / anxiety ___; ___ **de conversión** / conversion ___; ___ **depresiva psicótica** / psychotic depressive ___; ___ **en cadena** / chain ___; ___ **inmune** / immune ___ .

reaccionar *v.* to react, to respond to a stimulus.

reactivación *f.* reactivation; the act of activating again; ___ **de una vacuna** / booster shot.

reactivar *v.* to stimulate or activate again.

reactividad *f.* reactivity, manifestation of a reaction.

reactivo *m.* reagent, agent that stimulates a reaction; **-a** *a.* reactive, that has the property of reacting or causing a reaction.

readmisión *f.* readmission.

reagina *f.* reagin, antibody used in the treatment of allergies that causes the production of histamine.

reajustar *v.* to adjust, [*de pago, de precio*] to readjust.

real *a.* real, actual; **-mente** *adv.* really.

realidad *f.* reality.

realimentación, retroalimentación *f.* feedback, regeneration of energy, action of taking the energy or the effects of the process back to its original source.

realizar *v.* to perform, to execute, to carry out; **se decidió ___ la operación** / it was decided to ___ the operation.

realzar *vi.* to enhance, to intensify, to increase; to highlight.

reanimar *v.* to reanimate, to bring back to life.

reanudable *a.* renewable.

rebajar *v.* to lower, to reduce, [*a liquid*] to dilute.

rebelde *a.* rebellious.

reblandecimiento *m.* ripening, softening, dilation, such as of the cervix during childbirth.

reborde *m.* ridge, elongated elevation.

rebote *m.* rebound, a return to a previous condition after the removal of a stimulus; **fenómeno de ___** / ___ phenomenon, intensified onward movement of a part when the initial resistance is removed.

rebuscado-a *a.* farfetched.

recado *m.* message.

recaer *vi.* to relapse.

recaída *f.* relapse, setback, the recurrence of a disease after a period of recovery.

recalcificación *f.* recalcification, restoration of calcium compounds to tissues.

recámara *f. Mex.* bedroom.

recapacitar *v.* to reconsider.

receptáculo *m.* receptacle, vessel for liquids.

receptaculum *n., L. (pl. receptacula)* receptaculum, container, receptacle.

receptivo-a *a.* receptive.

receptor *m.* 1. recipient of an organ; 2. receptor, a nerve end that receives a nervous stimulus and passes it on to other nerves; ___ **auditivo** / auditory ___; ___ **de contacto** / contact ___; ___ **de estiramiento** / stretch ___; ___ **de temperature** / temperature ___; ___ **gustativo** / taste ___; ___ **propioceptivo** / proprioceptive ___; ___ **sensorial** / sensory ___ .

recesión *f.* recession, pathological withdrawal of tissue such as gums receding.

recesivo-a *a.* recessive. 1. tending to withdraw; 2. in genetics, rel. to nondominant genes.

receta *f.* prescription; recipe.

recetar *v.* to prescribe medication, to medicate.

recetario *m.* 1. prescription pad; 2. recipe book, cookbook.

rechazar *vi.* to reject, to drive back.

rechazo *m.* rejection. 1. immune reaction of incompatibility to transplanted tissue cells; ___ **agudo** / acute ___; ___ **crónico** / chronic ___; ___ **hiperagudo** / hyperacute ___; 2. denial, refusal.

rechinamiento *m.* [*los dientes*] gnashing.

rechinar *v.* [*los dientes*] to chatter; to squeak; to gnash

recibir *v.* to receive.

recibo *m.* receipt.

recidiva *f.* recidivation, recidivism, the recurrence of a disease or symptom.

recién *adv.* recently.

recién nacido-a *m., f.* newborn; **sala de ___ -s** / nursery.

reciente *a.* recent; **-mente** *adv.* recently.

recipiente *m.* 1. recipient, individual who receives blood, or an implant of tissue or organ from a donor; 2. container.

recipiente universal *m.* universal recipient, person belonging to blood group AB.

reciprocidad *f.* reciprocity.

recíproco-a *a.* reciprocal.

reclamación *f.* claim; [process] complaint.

reclinado-a *a.* reclined, reclining, recumbent.

reclinarse *vr.* to recline, to lean back.

recluido-a *a.* confined.

recluir *vi.* to confine.

reclutamiento *m.* recruitment, gradual intensification of a reflex action by an unaltered prolonged stimulus.

recobrar *v.* to regain; ___ **el conocimiento** / ___ consciousness; to regain; to retrieve.

recoger *vi.* to gather; to pick up.

recomendable *a.* advisable.

recomendación *f.* recommendation; referral.

recomendar *vi.* to recommend, to advise.

recompresión *f.* recompression, the return to normal environmental pressure.

reconocer *vi.* 1. to examine physically; 2. to recognize; to admit; to acknowledge.

reconocimiento *m.* 1. physical examination; 2. recognition.

reconstitución *f.* reconstitution, restitution of tissue to its initial form.

reconstituir *vi.* to reconstitute; ___ la salud / to build up one's health.

reconstituyente *m.* tonic.

reconstruir *vi.* to reconstruct.

récord *m.* record, chart.

recordar *vi.* to recall; to recollect; to remind.

recordarse *vr.* to remember.

recostado-a *a.* lying down, recumbent.

recostarse *vr., vi.* to lie down.

recreo *f.* recreation.

recrudescencia *f.* recrudescence, relapse, return of symptoms.

rectal *a.* rectal, rel. to the rectum; absceso ___ / ___ abscess; biopsia ___ / ___ biopsy; **inflamación** ___ / ___ inflammation; proctitis **protuberancia, bulto** ___ / ___ lump; **prolapso** ___ / ___ prolapse.

rectificación *f.* rectification, correction.

rectificar *vi.* to rectify, to correct.

recto *m.* rectum, the distal portion of the long intestine that connects the sigmoid and the anus; **-a** *a.* straight.

rectocele *m.* rectocele, herniation of part of the rectum into the vagina.

rectosigmoide *a.* rectosigmoid, rel. to the sigmoid and the rectum.

rectovaginal *a.* rectovaginal, rel. to the rectum and the vagina.

rectovesical *a.* rectovesical, rel. to the rectum and the bladder.

rectus *L.* rectus. 1. straight; 2. rel. to any of a group of straight muscles such as the ones in the eye and the abdominal wall.

recuento sanguíneo completo *m.* complete blood count.

recumbente *a.* recumbent, lying down position.

recuperación *f.* recuperation, recovery, restoration to health.

recuperado-a *a., pp.* de **recuperar**, recovered; improved.

recuperar *v.* to recover; ___ el conocimiento / to regain consciousness; **recuperarse** *vr.* to get well, *pop.* to pull through, to recoup.

recurrencia *f.* recurrence. 1. the return of symptoms after a period of remission; 2. relapse; repetition.

recurrente *a.* recurrent, that reappears temporarily; **cistitis** ___ / ___ cystitis; **dolor** ___ / ___ pain.

recurso *m.* recourse; resource; ___ -s **económicos** / source of income.

red *f.* web, network, netlike arrangement of nerve fibers and blood vessels; ___ de membranas arteriopulmonares / pulmonary arterial ___ .

redondo-a *a.* round, circular.

reducción *f.* reduction, lowering of, diminishing.

reducción del seno *f.* reduction mammaplasty, plastic surgery that reduces the breast and improves its position and appearance.

reducible *a.* reducible, able to be reduced.

reducido-a *a.* reduced, diminished.

reducir *vi.* to reduce, to cut down. 1. to restore to its normal position, such as a fragmented or dislocated bone; 2. to weaken the potency of a compound by adding hydrogen or suppressing oxygen; 3. to lose weight.

reductasa *f.* reductase, enzyme that acts as a catalyst in reduction.

reductor *m.* reducer, agent that causes reduction.

reeducación *f.* reeducation, training to regain motor and mental functions.

reemplazar *vi.* to replace, to substitute; to supplant.

reemplazo *m.* replacement, substitution.

reevaluación *f.* reevaluation; reassessment.

referencia *f.* reference; **valores de** ___ / ___ values.

referir *vi.* to refer; to direct; **referirse** *vr.* to refer to, to cite.

refinar *v.* to refine, to purify.

reflejar *v.* to reflect.

reflejo *m.* reflex, a conscious or unconscious motor response to a stimulus; **acto, acción** ___ / ___ action; **arco** ___ / ___ arc. V. cuadro en la página 221.

reflejo hepatoyugular *a.* hepatojugular reflex, ingurgitation of the jugular veins, produced by pressure on the liver in cases of right cardiac failure.

reflexión *f.* reflection. 1. the throwing off or bending back of light or another form of radiant energy from a surface; 2. turning or bending back, as of a membrane lining a body wall, that passes over the surface of an organ and returns to the body wall; 3. introspection.

reflexógeno-a *a.* reflexogenic, that causes a reflex action.

Reflejo	Reflex
adquirido	behavior
condicionado	conditioned
de estiramiento	stretch
del tendón de Aquiles	Achilles tendon
en cadena	chain
instintivo	instinctive
no condicionado, natural	unconditioned
patelar o rotuliano	patellar
radial	radial
rectal	rectal

reflujo *m.* reflux, backflow of a fluid substance;___ **abdominoyugular /** abdominojugular ___; ___ **esofágico /** esophageal ___; ___ **hepatoyugular /** hepatojugular ___; ___ **intrarenal /** intrarenal ___; ___ **ureterorenal /** ureterorenal ___ .

reflujo gastroesofágico *m.* gastroesophageal reflux, reflux concerning the stomach and the esophagus.

reforzar *vi.* to reinforce, to strengthen.

refracción *f.* refraction, the act of refracting; ___ **ocular /** ocular ___ .

refractar *v.* to refract. 1. to change the direction from a straight path, such as of a ray of light when it passes from one medium to another of different density; 2. to detect abnormalities of refraction in the eyes and correct them.

refractario-a *a.* refractory. 1. resistant to treatment; 2. nonresponsive to a stimulus.

refractividad *f.* refractivity, the ability to refract.

refrescante *a.* refreshing, cooling.

refrescar *vi.* to refresh, to revive; **refrescarse** *vr.* to cool off.

refresco *m.* refreshment, soft drink.

refrigeración *f.* refrigeration, reduction of heat by external means.

refrigerante *m.* refrigerant; antipyretic.

refrigerar *v.* to refrigerate.

refringente *a.* refringent, rel. to or that causes refraction.

refugiado-a *m., f.* refugee.

refugiar *v.* to shelter; **refugiarse** *vr.* to seek refuge, to seek shelter.

refugio *m.* shelter, refuge; asylum.

regalo *m.* present, gift.

regazo *m.* lap.

regeneración *f.* regeneration, restoration, renewal; feedback.

regenerar *v.* to regenerate.

régimen *m.* regimen, structured plan, such as a regulated diet.

región *f.* region, a part of the body with more or less definite boundaries.

regional *a.* regional.

registrar *v.* to register, to record.

registro *m.* recording, [*cinta magnética*] taping.

regla *f.* 1. menstruation; 2. rule; 3. ruler, device for measuring.

reglamento *m.* set of rules, policy.

regresar *v.* to return to a place.

regresión *f.* regression. 1. return to an earlier condition; 2. abatement of the symptoms or process of a disease.

regeldo *m.* belch.

regulación *f.* regulation.

regular *a.* regular, normal; *v.* to regulate; **-mente** *adv.* regularly.

regurgitación *f.* regurgitation. 1. the act of expelling swallowed food; 2. the backflow of blood through a defective valve of the heart; ___ **de la válvula aórtica** ___ / aortic valve ___; ___ **de la válvula mitral /** mitral valve ___; ___ **valvular /** valvular ___ .

regurgitante *a.* regurgitant, rel. to regurgitation.

regurgitar *v.* to regurgitate.

rehabilitación *f.* rehabilitation, the act of rehabilitating.

rehabilitado-a *a.* rehabilitated.

rehabilitar *v.* to rehabilitate, to help regain normal functions through therapy.

rehén *m., f.* hostage.

rehidratación *f.* rehydration, establishment of normal liquid balance in the body.

rehuir *vi.* to evade, to shun.

rehusar *v.* to refuse, deny; ___ **la medicina /** ___ taking the medication;

reimplantación *f.* reimplantation. 1. restoration of a tissue or part; 2. restitution into the uterus of an ovum removed from the body and fertilized *in vitro*.

reinervación *f.* reinnervation, grafting of a nerve to restore the function of a muscle.

reinfección *f.* reinfection, subsequent infection caused by the same microorganism.

reinfusión *f.* reinfusion, reinjection of blood serum or cerebrospinal fluid.

reinoculación *f.* reinoculation, subsequent inoculation with the same microorganisms.

r

reírse *vr., vi.* to laugh.

rejuvenecer *vi.* to rejuvenate; **rejuvenecerse** *vr.* to become rejuvenated.

rejuvenecimieno *m.* rejuvenescence.

relación *f.* relation; relationship; ___ **armoniosa** / rapport.

relacionado-a *a.* rel. to, related.

relacionar *v.* to relate, to establish a relationship; **relacionarse** *vr.* to become acquainted.

relajación *f.* relaxation, act of relaxing or becoming relaxed.

relajado-a *a.* relaxed.

relajante *m.* relaxant, agent that reduces tension.

relajar *v.* to relax, to reduce tension; **relajarse** *vr.* to become less tense, *pop.* to loosen up.

relativo-a *a.* relative; **-mente** *adv.* relatively.

religión *f.* religion.

religioso-a *a.* religious.

rellenar *v.* to refill.

relleno *m.* padding; stuffing.

reloj *m.* watch; clock.

remediador-a *a.* remedial, rel. to remedy.

remediar *v.* to remedy, to help, to alleviate.

remedio *m.* remedy, relief.

remineralización *f.* remineralization, replacement of lost minerals from the body.

reminiscencia *f.* reminiscence. 1. something remembered; a memory; 2. a vague or imprecise memory; 3. act to bring back images of past memories.

remisión *f.* remission. 1. diminution or cessation of the symptoms of a disease; 2. period of time during which the symptoms of a disease diminish.

remitente *a.* remittent, occurring at intervals.

remojar *v.* to soak; to wet again.

remolacha *f.* beet.

remordimiento *m.* remorse.

remoto-a *a.* remote, distant.

removible *a.* removable; that can be removed surgically.

renal *a.* renal, rel. to or resembling the kidney; **aclaración** ___ , **aclaramiento** ___ / ___ clearance; **cólico nefrítico, cólico** ___ / ___ colic; **fallo** ___ / ___ failure; **hipertensión de origen** / ___ hypertension; **intervención** ___ / ___ intervention; **pelvis** ___ / ___ pelvis; **prueba de aclaramiento o depuración** ___ / ___ clearance test; **prueba funcional** ___ / ___ function test; **diálisis, terapia de reemplazo** ___ / ___ dialisis, replacement therapy.

rendido-a *a.* tired out, exhausted.

rendimiento *m.* output, yield; **fallo en el** ___ / ___ failure.

renina *f.* renin, an enzyme released by the kidney that is a factor in the regulation of blood pressure.

renograma *m.* renogram, monitoring of the rate at which the kidney eliminates from the blood a radioactive substance previously injected intravenously.

renovar *vi.* to renew, to renovate.

renuente *a.* reluctant.

reñir *vi.* to quarrel, to fight.

reparación *f.* repair, restoration.

reparar *v.* to repair, to restore.

repartir *v.* to distribute, to divide.

repasar *v.* to review, to look over.

repaso *m.* review; ___ **del caso** / case ___ ; ___ **por sistemas, aparatos** / ___ of systems.

repelente *m.* repellent.

repentino-a *a.* sudden; **-mente** *adv.* suddenly.

repercusión *f.* repercussion. 1. penetration or spreading of a swelling, tumor, or eruption; 2. ballottement.

repetir *vi.* to repeat, to reiterate.

repleto-a *a.* replete, full.

repliegue *m.* replication, reproduction, duplication.

reporte *m.* report, account.

reposar *v.* to repose, to rest.

reposo *m.* rest, repose; **cura de** ___ / ___ cure; **en** ___ / resting.

represión *f.* repression. 1. inhibition of an action; 2. exclusion from consciousness of unacceptable desires or impulses.

reprimir *v.* to repress, to hold back.

reproducción *f.* reproduction.

reproducir *vi.* to reproduce.

reproductivo-a *a.* reproductive, rel. to reproduction.

reprovisión *f.* feedback. 1. [*información*] regeneration of information; 2. regeneration of energy *v.* realimentación.

repugnante *a.* repugnant, disgusting.

repulsión *f.* repulsion, the act of driving back or away; aversion.

repulsivo-a *a.* repulsive, repugnant.

reputación *f.* reputation.

requerido-a *a.* required, mandatory, necessary.

requerimiento *m.* requirement.

requerir *vi.* to require.

requisito *m.* requirement, condition. ___ **de ingreso** / admission ___ ; ___ **necesario** / mandatory ___ .

resbaladizo-a, resbaloso-a *a.* slippery.
resbalar *v.* to slip; to slide.
rescatar *v.* to rescue, to save.
rescate *m.* rescue; **método de ___ , método de salvamento / ___ method.**
resecar *v.* to resect. 1. to perform a resection; 2. to cut a portion of tissue or organ; 3. to dry thoroughly.
resección *f.* resection, the act of cutting a portion of tissue or organ; **___ en cuña /** wedge ___; **___ gástrica / gastric ___; ___ transuretral / transurethral ___ .**
reseco-a *a.* dried up; parched.
resectoscopía *f.* resectoscopy, resection of the prostate with a resectoscope.
resectoscopio *m.* resectoscope, instrument provided with a cutting electrode used in surgery within cavities, such as the one used for the resection of the prostate through the urethra.
resentimiento *m.* resentment, rancor, hard feelings.
reserpina *f.* reserpine, derivative of *Rauwolfia serpentina* used primarily in the treatment of hypertension and emotional disorders.
reserva *f.* reserve, that which is kept in store for future use.
reservar *v.* to reserve.
resfriado *m.* a cold.
resfriarse *vr.* to catch a cold.
residencia *f.* residency, period of specialized training in a hospital following completion of medical school.
residente *m.* resident, physician completing a residency.
residir *v.* to reside, to live.
residual *a.* residual, remainder; **función ___ / ___ function; orina ___ / ___** urine.
residuo *m.* residue; **dieta de bajo ___ / low- ___** diet; **dieta de ___ alto / high- ___ diet.**
resiliente *a.* resilient, elastic.
resina *f.* resin, resina, organic substance of vegetable origin, insoluble in water but readily soluble in alcohol and ether, that has a variety of uses in medicine and dentistry.
res ipsa loquitor *L.* res ipsa loquitor, evident, that which speaks for itself.
resistencia *f.* resistance, endurance, capacity of an organism to resist harmful effects; **___ adquirida / acquired ___; ___ a un colorante /** fast resistant; **___ inicial / initial ___; ___ periférica / peripheral ___ .**
resistente *a.* resistant.

resolución *f.* resolution. 1. termination of an inflammatory process; 2. the ability to distinguish fine and subtle details as through a microscope.
resolver *vi.* to resolve. 1. to cause resolution; 2. to become separated into components.
resonancia *f.* resonance, capacity to increase the intensity of a sound; **___ normal /** normal ___; **___ vesicular / vesicular ___; ___ vocal / vocal ___ .**
resonante *a.* resonant, ringing, that gives out a vibrant sound on percussion.
resorcinol *m.* resorcinol, agent used in the treatment of acne and other forms of dermatosis.
resorción *f.* resorption, partial or total loss of a process, tissue, or exudate by means of biochemical reactions such as lysis and absorption.
respetar *v.* to respect.
respeto *m.* respect.
respiración *f.* breathing, respiration; **aguantar o sostener la ___ / to hold one's breath; ___ abdominal / abdominal ___; ___ acelerada /** accelerated ___; **___ aeróbica / aerobic ___; ___ anaeróbica / anaerobic ___; ___ diafragmática / diaphragmatic ___; ___ gruesa / coarse ___; ___ laboriosa /** labored ___; **___ profunda / deep ___ .**
respiración sibilante *f.* wheezing.
respirador *m.* respirator, breather, device used to purify the air reaching the lungs or to administer artificial respiration; **___ torácico / chest ___ .**
respirar *v.* to breathe; **___ por la boca /** ___ through the mouth; **___ por la nariz / ___** through the nose.
respiratorio-a *a.* respiratory, rel. to respiration; **alkalosis ___ / ___ alkalosis; aparato ___ superior / upper ___ tract; arritmia ___ / ___** arrhythmia; **ataxia ___ / ___ ataxia; bronquíolos ___ -s / ___ bronchioles; capacidad ___ / ___ capacity; cociente ___ / ___ quotient; conducto, pasaje ___ / ___ airway; ejercicios ___ -s /** breathing exercises; **enzima ___ / ___ enzyme; índice ___ / ___ rate; infección del tracto ___ superior / upper ___ tract infection; infecciones y enfermedades de las vías ___ -s / ___ tract** infections and diseases; **inhibidor ___ / ___** inhibitor; **insuficiencia o fallo ___ / ___ failure,** insufficiency; **lóbulo ___ / ___ lobule; metabolismo ___ / ___ metabolism; mucosa ___ / ___ mucosa; pruebas de función ___ / ___ function tests;**

r

ruidos ___ / ___ sounds; **unidad de cuidado** ___ / ___ care unit.

respiratorio, centro *m.* respiratory center, region in the medulla oblongata that regulates respiratory movements.

responsabilidad *f.* responsibility.

responsable *a.* responsible; **persona** ___ / responsible party.

respuesta *f.* response; answer. 1. reaction of an organ or tissue to a stimulus; 2. reaction of a patient to a treatment; ___ **evocada** / evoked ___ , sensorial test; ___ **no condicionada** / unconditioned ___ , nonrestricted reaction.

restablecer *vi.* to restore; **restablecerse** *vr.* to recover.

restablecido-a *a.* [*de una enfermedad*] recovered.

restablecimiento *m.* recuperation.

restauración *f.* restoration; remodeling.

restaurativo-a *a.* restorative, that stimulates recuperation.

restenosis *f.* restenosis, recurrence of stenosis after corrective surgery.

restitutio ad integrum *L.* restitutio ad integrum, total restitution of health.

resto *m.* rest, remainder.

restricción *f.* restraint, confinement; ___ **de movimiento** / limitation of motion; ___ **en cama** / bed confinement.

restringido-a *a.* restricted.

restringir *vi.* to restrict, to confine.

resucitación *f.* resuscitation. 1. return to life; 2. artificial respiration; ___ **cardiaca** / cardiac ___ .

resucitador *m.* resuscitator, an apparatus to provide artificial respiration; **cardiac** ___ / ___ cardiasis.

resucitar *v.* to resuscitate, to revive.

resultado *m.* result, outcome.

resumen *m.* summary.

resurgencia *f.* resurgence.

retardo *m.* retraso.

rete *L.* (*pl. retia*) *retia*rete. network; plexus. red.

retención *f.* retention; **enema de** ___ / ___ enema; ___ **de líquido** / fluid ___ ; ___ **gástrica** / gastric ___ ; ___ **urinaria** / urinary ___ .

retener *vi.* to retain; to keep.

reticulación *f.* reticulation, reticular formation.

reticular, retiforme *a.* reticular, resembling a network.

retículo *m.* reticulum, a network, esp. of nerve fibers and blood vessels.

retículo endoplásmico *m.* endoplasmic reticulum, a network of canals in a cell in which

the functions of anabolism and catabolism take place.

reticulocito *m.* reticulocyte, an immature red blood cell with a network of threads and granules that appears primarily during blood regeneration.

reticulocitopenia *f.* reticulocytopenia, an abnormal decrease in the number of reticulocytes in the blood.

reticulocitosis, reticulosis *f.* reticulocytosis, abnormal increase in the nmber of reticulocytes in the bloodstream, as a result of active blood regeneration by means of bone marrow stimulation, or as a symptom of anemia.

reticuloendotelial, sistema *m.* reticuloendothelial system, network of phagocytic cells (except circulating leukocytes) throughout the body, involving processes such as blood cell formation, elimination of worn-out cells, and immune responses to infection.

reticuloendotelio *m.* reticuloendothelium, tissue of the reticuloendothelial system.

reticuloendotelioma *m.* reticuloendothelioma, tumor of the reticuloendothelial system.

reticulohistiocitoma *m.* reticulohistiocytoma, a large aggregate of granular and giant cells.

reticulopenia *f.* reticulopenia. reticulocitopenia.

retina *f.* retina, the innermost layer of the eyeball that receives images and transmits visual impulses to the brain; **conmoción de la** ___ / commotio retinae, traumatic condition of the retina that produces temporary blindness; **desprendimiento de la** ___ / retinal detachment, separation of all or part of the retina from the choroid; **deterioración de la** ___ / retinal degeneration.

retináculo *m.* retinaculum, structure that supports an organ or tissue in its place.

retiniano-a *a.* retinal, rel. to the retina; **perforación** ___ / ___ perforation.

retinitis *f.* retinitis, infl. of the retina.

retinoblastoma *m.* retinoblastoma, gen. inherited malignant tumor of the retina genetic in origin.

retinol *m.* retinol, vitamin A_1.

retinopatía *f.* retinopathy, any abnormal condition of the retina. ___ **diabética** / diabetic ___ .

retinoscopía *f.* retinoscopy, method of determination and evaluation of refractive errors of the eye.

retirado-a *a.* retired; isolated.

retoque *m.* touch-up.

retorno *m.* return.

retortijón *m.* brief and acute intestinal cramp.

retracción *f.* retraction, the act of drawing or pulling back; ___ **del coágulo** / clot ___ .

retractable, retráctil *a.* retractile, capable of being retracted.

retractar *v.* to retract, to draw back, to withdraw.

retractor *m.* retractor. 1. instrument for holding back the edges of a wound; 2. retractile muscle.

retraído-a *a.* withdrawn, introverted, that keeps to himself or herself.

retrasado-a, retardado-a *a.* retarded; ___ **mental** / mentally ___ .

retraso *m.* retardation, abnormal slowness of a motor or a mental process.

retroacción *f.* retroaction, retroactive action.

retroactivo-a *a.* retroactive, that acts upon or affects a past event.

retroauricular *a.* retroauricular, rel. to or situated behind the ear.

retrocecal *a.* retrocecal, rel. to or situated behind the cecum.

retroceder *v.* [*water*] recede, diminish; to go back.

retroceso *m.* retrocession, throwback.

retrofaríngeo-a *a.* retropharyngeal, rel. to or situated behind the pharynx.

retroflexión *f.* retroflexion, the flexing back of an organ.

retrógrado-a *a.* retrograde, that moves backward or returns to the past; **amnesia** ___ / ___ amnesia; **aortografía** ___ / ___ aortography; **pielografía** ___ / ___ pyelography.

retrogresión *f.* 1. retrogression, return to a simpler level of development; 2. flashback, sudden vivid memory of images from the past.

retrolental *a.* retrolental, rel. to or situated behind the lens of the eye; **fibroplasia** ___ / ___ fibroplasia.

retroperitoneal *a.* retroperitoneal, rel. to or situated behind the peritoneum.

retroplasia *f.* anaplasia.

retroprovisión *f.* feedback.

retrospectivo-a *a.* retrospective; **estudio** ___ / ___ study.

retroversión *f.* retroversion, turning backward, such as an organ.

retroversión uterina *f.* retroversion of the uterus, condition of the uterus in which it is tipped backward.

retrovirus *m.* retrovirus, a virus belonging to a group of RNA viruses, some of which are oncogenic; ___ **endógeno humano** / human endogenous ___ .

Retzius, espacio de *m.* Retzius' space, space between the bladder and the pubic bones.

reuma *f.* rheum. 1. aqueous secretion; 2. rheumatism.

reumático-a *a.* rheumatic, rel. to or afflicted by rheumatism.

reumatide *f.* rheumatid, any dermatosis associated with rheumatic fever.

reumatismo *m.* rheumatism, painful chronic or acute disease marked by infl. and pain in the joints.

reumatoide *a.* rheumatoid, rel. to or resembling rheumatism; **artritis** ___ / ___ arthritis.

reunión *f.* meeting; attachment 1. meeting parts such as those of a fractured bone on the edge of a wound; 2. meeting of a group of persons.

revacunación *f.* booster shot.

revascularización *f.* revascularization. 1. restoration of blood supply to a part following a lesion or a bypass; 2. bypass.

reventar *vi.* to burst; **reventarse** *vr.* to burst open.

reversión *f.* reversal, reversion, restitution to a previously existing condition.

revestimiento *m.* covering.

revisar *v.* to review; to revise.

revisión *f.* revision, review. ___ **del caso** / case ___ ; ___ **ingreso** / ___ review.

revista *f.* magazine.

revivificación *f.* revivification, recovery of life and strength after an illness.

revivir *v.* to revive, to bring back to life.

revólver *m.* revolver, handgun.

revulsión *f.* revulsion. contrairritación.

revulsivo-a *a.* revulsive, rel. to or causing revulsion.

Reye, síndrome de *m.* Reye's syndrome, acute disease in children and adolescents manifested by severe edema that can affect the brain and other major organs of the body such as the liver.

rezar *vi.* to pray.

riboflavina *f.* riboflavin, component of vitamin B_2 complex, essential to nutrition.

ribonucleasa *f.* ribonuclease, enzyme that catalyzes the hydrolysis of ribonucleic acid.

ribonucleoproteína *f.* ribonucleoprotein, a substance containing both protein and ribonucleic acid.

ricino *m.* castor oil plant; **aceite de** ___ / castor oil.

rickettsia *f.* rickettsia, any of the gram-negative microorganisms of the group *Rickettsiaceae* that multiply only in host cells of fleas, lice, ticks, and mice, and are transmitted to humans via the bite of these vectors.

rico-a *a.* rich; affluent; *pop.* very tasty.

riego *m.* flow; ___ **sanguíneo** / blood ___ .

r

riesgo *m.* risk; hazard; **grupos de alto** ___ / high ___ groups ___; **posible** ___ / potential ___; ___ **de contaminación** / ___ of contamination; ___ **de infección** / ___ of infection; ___ **de una lesión** / ___ of injury; ___ **de violencia** / ___ of violence; ___ **-s** / ___ factors.

riesgoso-a *a.* risky.

rigidez *f.* rigidity, stiffness, inflexibility; ___ **cadavérica** / cadaveric ___ , rigor mortis.

rígido-a *a.* rigid, stiff.

rigor *m.* rigor. 1. inflexibility of a muscle; 2. chill with high temperature; ___ **mortis** / ___ mortis.

rinal *a.* rhinal, rel. to the nose.

rinitis *f.* rhinitis, infl. of the nasal mucosa.

rinofaringitis *f.* rhinopharyngitis, infl. of the nasopharynx.

rinofima *f.* rhinophyma, severe form of acne rosacea in the area of the nose.

rinolaringitis *f.* rhinolaryngitis, simultaneous infl. of the mucous membranes of the nose and the larynx.

rinoplastia *f.* rhinoplasty, plastic surgery of the nose.

rinorrea *f.* rhinorrhea, liquid mucous discharge from the nose.

rinoscopia *f.* rhinoscopy, examination of the nasal cavities.

riñón *m.* kidney, organ situated in the back of each side of the abdominal cavity; **fallo del** ___ / ___ failure; **necrosis papilar del** ___ / renal papillary necrosis; **piedras en el** ___ / ___ stones; ___ **artificial** / hemodyalizer; ___ **poliquístico** / polycystic ___; **transplante del** ___ / renal transplant. *V.* ilustración en la página 227.

risa *f.* laugh, laughter; ___ **histerica** / hysteric ___; ___ **sardónica** / sardonic ___ , contraction of facial muscles that gives the appearance of a smile.

risorio *m.* risorius, muscle inserted at the corners of the mouth.

ristocetina *f.* ristocetin, antibiotic substance used in the treatment of infections by gram-positive cocci.

risueño-a *a.* smiling, affable.

Ritalin, clorhidrato de *m.* Ritalin hydrochloride, stimulant and antidepressant.

ritidectomía *f.* rhytidectomy, face-lift, removal of wrinkles through plastic surgery.

ritidosis *f.* rytidosis, contraction of the cornea before death.

rítmico-a *a.* rhythmical.

ritmo *m.* rhythm, regularity in the action or function of an organ of the body such as the heart; ___

acoplado / coupled ___; ___ **alfa** / alpha ___; ___ **atrioventricular** / atrioventricular ___; ___ **bigeminal** / bigeminal ___; ___ **circadiano** / circadian ___; ___ **de galope** / gallop ___; ___ **de tic-tac** / tic-tac ___; ___ **ectópico** / ectopic ___; ___ **idioventricular** / idioventricular ___; ___ **nodal** / nodal ___; ___ **pendular** / pendulum ___; ___ **sinusal** / sinus ___

ritmo circadiano *m.* circadian rhythm, rhythmic biological variations in a 24-hour cycle.

ritual *m.* ritual.

rizotomia *f.* rhizotomy, transection of the root of a nerve.

Robitussin *m.* Robitussin, expectorant.

robustecer *vi.* to strengthen.

robusto-a *a.* robust, stout.

rociar *v.* to spray.

rodar *vi.* to roll; to wheel.

rodeado-a *a.* surrounded.

rodenticida *m.* rodenticide, agent that destroys rodents.

rodilla *f.* knee; **dislocación de la** ___ / ___ dislocation.

rodillera *f.* knee protector.

rodopsina *f.* rhodopsin, purple-red pigment found in the retinal rods that enhances vision in dim light.

roedor *m.* rodent.

roentgen *m.* roentgen, the international unit of x- or gamma radiation; **rayos de** ___ / ___ rays, x-rays.

roentgenograma *m.* roentgenogram, radiograph, photograph made with x-rays on a fluorescent surface.

rojizo-a *a.* reddish.

rojo-a *a.* red; ___ **Congo** / Congo ___; ___ **escarlata** / scarlet ___ .

Romberg, signo de *m.* Romberg's sign, swaying of the body when in an erect position with eyes closed and feet close together as a sign of an inability to maintain balance.

romero *m.* rosemary.

romper *v.* to break; **romperse** *vr.* to break into pieces.

roncar *vi.* to snore.

roncha *f.* blotch; wheal; hives.

ronco-a *a.* hoarse, with a husky voice.

rongeur *Fr.* rongeur, forceps to remove minute bone chips.

ronquera *f.* hoarseness.

ronquido *m.* snore.

ropa *f.* clothing; ___ **de cama** / bed clothes, bed linens; ___ **interior** / underclothing.

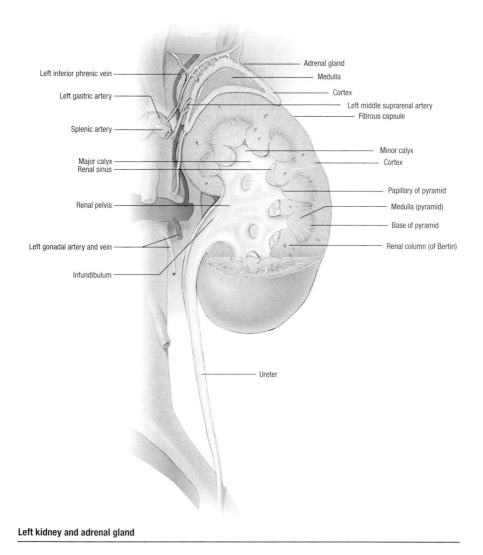

Left inferior phrenic vein

Left gastric artery

Splenic artery

Major calyx
Renal sinus

Renal pelvis

Left gonadal artery and vein

Infundibulum

Adrenal gland
Medulla
Cortex
Left middle suprarenal artery
Fibrous capsule

Minor calyx
Cortex

Papillary of pyramid
Medulla (pyramid)
Base of pyramid
Renal column (of Bertin)

Ureter

Left kidney and adrenal gland

Rorschach, prueba de *f.* Rorschach test, psychological test by which personality traits are revealed through the subject's interpretation of a series of ink blots.

rosáceo-a *a.* pinkish, rosy.

rosado-a *a.* pink.

rosario *m.* rosary, structure that resembles a string of beads.

rosbif *m.* roast beef.

roséola *f.* roséola, rose-colored skin eruption.

rosette *Fr.* rosette, a rose-shaped cluster of cells.

rostral *a.* rostral, rel. to or resembling a rostrum.

rostro *m.* rostrum. 1. human face; 2. beak or projection.

rotación *f.* rotation.

rotador-a *a.* rotator.

rotar *v.* to rotate, to turn around.

rotatorio-a *a.* rotatory, that rotates.

roto-a *a. pp.* de **romper,** broken.

rotula *f.* patella, kneecap; ball-and-socket joint.

rotura *f.* breakage; fracture.

rubefaciente *a.* rubefacient, that causes redness of the skin.

rubeola *f.* rubella, German measles, highly contagious benign viral infection manifested by fever, rose-colored eruption, and sore throat. It can have serious effects on the development of the fetus if acquired by the mother during early pregnancy.

rubio-a *a.* fair, blond, of light coloring.

rubor *m.* rubor, redness of the skin; blush.

ruborizado-a *a.* rubescent, that blushes.

ruborizarse *vr., vi.* to blush.

rudimento *m.* rudiment. 1. a partially developed organ; 2. an organ or part with a partial or total loss of function.

rueda de andar *f.* [*acondicionamiento físico*] treadmill.

ruga *L.* ruga, (*pl. rugae*); wrinkle or fold.

ruido *m.* noise, sound; [*corazón*] bruit, murmur; ___ **sordo** / rumble.

ruptura *f.* rupture.

ruta *f.* route, direction.

rutina *f.* routine.

rutinario-a *a.* routine, done habitually.

S

S *abr.* **sulfuro** / sulphur;

s *abr.* **sacral** / sacral; **sección** / section; **segundo** / second.

sábana *f.* sheet.

sabañón *m.* chilblain, a hand or foot sore produced by cold.

saber *vi.* to know; **hacer** ___ / to make known; ___ **cómo** / ___ how; ___ **de** / ___ of, about.

Sabin, vacuna de *f.* Sabin vaccine, oral poliomyelitis vaccine.

sabor *m.* taste; flavor, aftertaste;*v.* **tener** ___ **a,** ___ **de** / to taste like.

sabroso-a *a.* tasteful, pleasurable to the taste.

sacabocados *m.* punch, surgical instrument used to perforate or cut a resistant tissue.

sacar *vi.* to take out; to draw out.

sacárido *m.* saccharide, chemical compound, one of a series of carbohydrates that includes sugars.

sacarina *f.* saccharin, crystalline substance used as an artificial sweetener.

sacerdote *m.* priest, clergyman.

saciado-a *a.* satiated.

saciar*v.* to quench; to satiate; ___ **la sed** / ___ the thirst.

saciedad *f.* satiety, the state of being fully satisfied.

saco *m.* sac, pocket, pouchlike structure; jacket.

sacral *a.* sacral, rel. to or near the sacrum; **nervios** ___ **-es** / ___ nerves; **plexo** ___ / ___ plexus.

sacralización *f.* sacralization, fusion of the fifth lumbar vertebra and the sacrum.

sacrificar *vi.* to sacrifice.

sacro *m.* sacrum, the large triangular bone formed by five fused vertebrae that lies at the base of the spine between the two hip bones.

sacroilitis *f.* sacroilitis, infl. of the sacroiliac joint.

sacrolumbar *a.* sacrolumbar, rel. to the sacral and the lumbar regions.

sacudida *f.* jerk, jolt.

sacudir*v.* to shake; to jerk.

sáculo *m.* saccule, small sac.

sádico-a *a.* sadistic, rel. to sadism.

sadismo *m.* sadism, perverted sexual pleasure derived from inflicting physical or psychological pain on others.

sadista *m., f.* sadist, person who practices sadism.

sadomasoquismo *m.* sadomasochism, perverted sexual pleasure derived from inflicting pain on oneself or on others.

sadomasoquista *m., f.* person who practices sadomasochism; *a.* sadomasochistic, rel. to the practice of sadomasochism.

safeno-a *a.* saphenous, rel. to or associated with the saphenous veins or nerves; **venas** ___ **-s** / ___ veins, the veins of the leg.

safismo *m.* sapphism, lesbianism.

sagital *a.* sagittal, resembling an arrow; **plano** ___ / ___ plane, parallel to the long axis of the body.

sal *f.* salt, sodium chloride; ___ **-es aromáticas** / smelling ___ -s; ___ **corriente** / noniodized ___; ___ **yodada** / iodized ___; *v.* **echar o poner** ___ / to salt or add salt; **sin** ___ / unsalted.

sala *f.* room; living room; [*hospital*] ward; ___ **de aislamiento** / isolation ward; ___ **de cuidado cardíaco** / cardiac care unit; ___ **de cuidados intensivos** / intensive care unit; ___ **de emergencia** / emergency ___; ___ **de espera** / waiting ___; ___ **de operaciones** / operating ___; ___ **de parto** / delivery ___; ___ **de recuperación** / recovery ___ .

salado-a *a.* salty.

salario *m.* salary, wages.

salchicha *f.* sausage.

salcochar, sancochar *v.* to parboil.

salicilato *m.* salicylate, any salt of salicylic acid.

salicilismo *m.* salicylism, toxic condition produced by excess intake of salicylic acid.

salida *f.* outlet; exit, way out.

saliente *m.* protrusion; *a.* salient, projecting, protruding.

salino-a *a.* saline; **solución** ___ / ___ solution, distilled water and salt.

salir *vi.* to go out; to leave; to come out.

saliva *f.* saliva, spit, secretion of the salivary glands that moistens and softens foods in the mouth.

salivación *f.* salivation, excessive discharge of saliva.

salival *a.* salivary, rel. to saliva.

Salk, vacuna de *f.* Salk vaccine, poliomyelitis vaccine.

salmón *m.* salmon.

Salmonela *f.* Salmonella, a genus of gram-negative bacteria of the *Enterobacteriaceae* family that causes enteric fever, gastrointestinal disorders, and septicemia.

salmonelosis *f.* salmonellosis, infectious condition caused by ingestion of food contaminated by bacteria of the genus *Salmonella.*

salón *m.* large hall or room.

salpingectomía *f.* salpingectomy, removal of one or both fallopian tubes.

salpingitis *f.* salpingitis, infl. of a fallopian tube.

salpingooforectomía *f.* salpingo-oophorectomy, removal of a fallopian tube and an ovary.

salpingoplastia *f.* salpingoplasty, plastic surgery of the fallopian tubes.

salpinx *Gr.* salpinx, *pl.* salpinges, a tube, such as the fallopian tube.

salpullido, sarpullido *m.* heat rash.

salsa *f.* sauce; gravy.

saltar *v.* to jump; to skip; ___ **un turno** / to skip an appointment or turn.

saltear *v.* to stagger; to alternate.

salto *m.* jump; skip; omission, [*del corazón*] palpitation.

saltón, saltona *a.* jumpy.

salubre *a.* salubrious, healthy.

salubridad *f.* the state of public health.

salud *f.* health **atención a la** ___ / ___ care; **centros de** ___ / ___ care facilities; **certificado de** ___ / ___ certificate; **cuidado de la** ___ / ___ care; **cuidado de** ___ **en el hogar** / home ___ care; ___ **de las personas de mayor edad** / senior ___; **estado de** ___ / ___ status; **instituciones de** ___ **pública** / public ___ facilities; ___ **mental** / mental ___; ___ **precaria** / uncertain ___; **profesional de atención de la** ___ / ___ care provider; **servicios de** ___ / ___ services; **servicios de** ___ **para los ancianos** / ___ services for the aged; ___ **pública** / public ___; ___ **rural** / rural ___; ___ **urbana** / urban ___ .

saludable *a.* healthy; **conducta** ___ / ___ behavior ___ .

saludar *v.* to greet.

saludo *m.* greeting.

salvado *m.* bran, a by-product of the milling of grain.

salvamento *m.* salvage, rescue.

salvar *v.* to save.

sanar *v.* to cure, to heal.

sanatorio *m.* sanatorium, sanitarium, health establishment for physical and mental rehabilitation.

saneamiento *m.* sanitation.

sangrado, sangramiento *m.* bleeding; ___ **por la nariz** / nosebleed.

sangrar *v.* to bleed.

sangre *f.* blood; ___ **autóloga** / autologous ___; **coágulo de** ___ / ___ clot; **conteo de** ___ / ___ count; **donante de** ___ / ___ donor; ___ **periférica** / peripheral ___; **prueba selecta de** ___ / ___ screening; **transfusión de** ___ / ___ transfusion; ___ **vital** / lifeblood; **a** ___ **fría** / in cold ___; **banco de** ___ / ___ bank.

sangre oculta *f.* occult blood, blood that is present in such a minute amount that it cannot be seen with the naked eye.

sangría *f.* bloodletting.

sangriento-a *a.* bloody.

sanguíneo-a *a.* 1. sanguineous, rel. to blood or that contains it; **derivados** ___ **-s, hemoderivados** / blood derivatives; **determinación de grupos** ___ **-s** / blood grouping; **gases** ___ **-s** / blood gases; **plasma** ___ / blood plasma; **producto** ___ / blood product; **proteína** ___ / blood protein; **sustitutos** ___ **-s** / blood substitutes; **tipo** ___ / blood group; **tiempo de coagulación** ___ / blood coagulation time; 2. sanguine, of a cheerful nature.

sanguinolento-a *a.* sanguinolent, containing blood; **esputo** ___ / bloody sputum.

sanitario-a *m., f.* sanitarian, person trained in matters of sanitation and public health; *a.* sanitary, hygienic; **toalla, servilleta** ___ / ___ napkin.

sano-a *a.* healthy; sound; wholesome.

saprófito *m.* saprophyte, vegetable organism that lives on decaying or dead organic matter.

sarampión *m.* measles, highly contagious disease esp. in school age children, caused by the rubeola virus; **suero de globulina preventivo al** ___ / ___ immune serum globulin administered within five days after exposure to the disease.

sarcoidosis *f.* sarcoidosis. Schaumann, enfermedad-de.

sarcoma *m.* sarcoma, malignant neoplasm of the connective tissue. ___ **condroblástico** / chondroblastic ___; ___ **de tejido blando** / soft tissue ___; ___ **fibroblástico** / fibropastic ___; ___ **gástrico** / gastric ___; ___ **linfático** / lymphatic ___; ___ **medular** / medullary ___; ___ **mielógeno** / myelogenic ___; ___ **óseo** / osteogenic ___; ___ **prostático** / prostatic ___; ___ **pulmonar** / pulmonary ___; ___ **renal** / renal ___ .

sardina *f.* sardine.

sarna *f.* scabies, mange, parasitic cutaneous infection that produces itching.

satélite *m.* satellite, a small structure accompanying a larger one.

satisfacer *vi.* to satisfy.

satisfecho-a *a., pp.* desatisfacer, satisfied.

saturación *f.* saturation.

saturado-a *a.* saturated, unable to absorb or receive any given substance beyond a given limit; **no** ___ / unsaturated;

saturar *v.* to saturate.

savia *f.* sap, natural juice.

saya *f.* skirt.

sazonado-a *a.* seasoned.

sazonar *v.* to season.

Schaumann, enfermedad de *f.* Schaumann's disease, chronic disease of unknown cause manifested by the presence of small tubercles, esp. in the lymph nodes, lungs, bones, and skin.

Schilling, prueba de *f.* Schilling test, use of radioactive Vitamin B_{12} for the purpose of diagnosing primary pernicious anemia.

sebáceo-a *a.* sebaceous, rel. to or containing sebum; **glándulas** ___ **-s** / ___ glands, glands of the skin; **quiste** ___ / ___ cyst.

sebo *m.* sebum, fatty thick substance secreted by the sebaceous glands.

seborrea *f.* seborrhea, malfunction of the sebaceous glands characterized by an excessive discharge of sebum from the glands.

seborréico-a *a.* seborrheic, rel to seborrhea; **blefaritis** ___ / ___ blepharitis; **dermatitis** ___ / ___ dermatitis; **queratosis** ___ / ___ keratosis.

secar *vi.* to dry; **secarse** *vr.* to dry oneself.

sección *f.* section, portion, part; ___ **media** / midsection.

seccionar *v.* to divide, to cut.

seco-a *a.* dry.

secreción *f.* secretion.1. the production of a given substance as a result of glandular activity; 2. substance produced by secretion; ___ **apocrina** / apocrine ___; ___ **externa** / external ___; ___ **interna** / internal ___; ___ **purulenta** / purulent ___ .

secretagogo *m.* secretagogue, secretogogue, agent that stimulates glandular secretion.

secretar *v.* to secrete.

secretario-a *m., f.* secretary.

secretor-a *a.* secretory, that has the property of secreting; **capilares** ___ **-es** / ___ capillaries; **carcinoma** ___ / ___ carcinoma; **fibra** ___ / ___ fiber; **nervio** ___ / ___ nerve.

secuela *f.* sequela, aftereffects, condition following or resulting from a disease or treatment.

secuencia *f.* sequence, succession, order.

secuestración *f.* sequestration. 1. the act of isolating; 2. the formation of sequestrum.

secuestrar *v.* to sequester, to isolate.

secuestro *m.* sequestrum, fragment of dead bone that has become separated from adjoining bone.

secundario-a *a.* secondary.

secundinas *f., pl.* afterbirth, placenta and membranes expelled at the time of delivery.

sed *f.* thirst; *v.* **tener** ___ / to be thirsty.

seda *f.* silk.

sedación *f.* sedation, the act and effect of inducing calm through medication.

sedante, sedativo *m.* sedative, agent with a quieting and tranquilizing effect.

sedentario-a *a.* sedentary. 1. having little or no physical activity; 2. rel. to a sitting position.

sediento-a *a.* thirsty.

sedimentación *f.* sedimentation, the process of depositing sediment; **índice de** ___ / ___ rate.

sedimento *m.* sediment, matter that settles at the bottom of a solution.

segmentación *f.* segmentation, the act of dividing into parts.

segmento *m.* segment, section or part.

seguido-a *a.* continuous, unbroken; following.

seguimiento *m.* follow-up.

Seguin, síntoma de *m.* Seguin's signal symptom, involuntary contraction of the muscles before an epileptic seizure.

seguir *vi.* to follow; to continue.

según *prep.* according to; in accordance with.

segundo *m.* second, unit of time; **-a** *a.* [*ordinal number*] second, ordinal form of the number two.

seguridad *f.* safety, security; assurance; **medidas de** ___ / ___ measures.

seguro *m.* insurance; ___ **de incapacidad** / disability ___; ___ **de vida** / life ___; ___ **médico** / health ___; ___ **social** / social security; *seguro-a* *a.* safe; certain; **-mente** *adv.* surely.

selección *f.* selection, choice; sampling.

selenio *m.* selenium, a nonmetallic chemical element resembling sulfur, used in electronic devices.

sellar *v.* to seal, to close tightly.

semana *f.* week; **la** ___ **pasada** / last ___; **la** ___ **próxima, la** ___ **que viene** / next ___ .

semanal *a.* weekly;**-mente** *adv.* weekly.

semántica *f.* semantics, the study of the meaning of words.

semblante *m.* appearance of the face.

semejante *a.* resembling, similar.

semejar *v.* to resemble.

semen *m.* semen, sperm, thick whitish secretion of the male reproductive organs.

semicoma *m.* semicoma, slight comatose state.

semilla *f.* seed; pit.

seminal *a.* seminal, concerning the semen or seed; **conducto** ___ / ___ duct; **emision** ___ / ___ emission.

seminífero-a *a.* seminiferous, that produces or bears seeds or semen; **conductos** ___ -s / ___ tubules.

seminuria *f.* seminuria, presence of semen in the urine.

semiótica *f.* semiotics, the branch of medicine concerned with signs and symptoms of diseases.

semiótico-a *a.* semiotic, rel. to the signs and symptoms of a disease.

sencillo-a *a.* simple, plain.

senescencia *f.* senescence, the process of becoming old.

senil *a.* senile, rel. to old age esp. as it affects mental and physical functions.

senilidad *f.* senility, the state of being senile.

seno *m.* breast, bust, bosom; **autoexamen de los** ___ -s / ___ self-examination.

senos paranasales *m., pl.* paranasal sinuses, any of the air cavities in the adjacent bones of the nasal cavity.

sensación *f.* sensation, feeling, perception through the senses.

sensato-a *a.* sensible, reasonable.

sensibilidad *f.* sensitivity, the condition of being sensitive to touch or palpation; tenderness; ___ **cruzada** / cross ___; **entrenamiento de la** ___ / ___ training; ___ **profunda** / deep ___; ___ **táctil** / touch sensation; ___ **térmica** / thermal ___ .

sensibilización *f.* sensitization, the act of making sensible.

sensibilizar *vi.* to sensitize, to make sensitive.

sensible *a.* sensitive, sensible; wise, prudent.

sensífero-a *a.* sensiferous, that causes, transmits, or conducts sensations.

sensitivo-a *a.* 1. sensorial, that is perceived through the senses; 2. tender, sensitive to touch or palpation.

sensitivomotor *a.* sensorimotor, rel. to sensory and motor activities of the body.

sensorial, sensorio-a *a.* sensory, rel. to sensation or to the senses; **afasia** ___ / ___ aphasia; **epilepsia** ___ / ___ epilepsy; **ganglio** ___ / ___ ganglion; **imagen** ___ / ___ image; **integración** ___ / ___ integration; **nervio** ___ / ___ nerve; **nivel de agudeza** ___ / ___ acuity level; **privación** ___ / ___ deprivation; **procesamiento** ___ / ___ processing; **sobrecarga** ___ / ___ overload; **umbral** ___ / ___ threshold.

sensual *a.* sensual, sensuous; carnal.

sentado-a *a.* seated.

sentarse *vr., vi.* to sit down.

sentido *m.* sense; a perception or impression received through the senses; ___ **de la vista** / ___ of sight; ___ **del oído** / ___ of hearing; ___ **del olfato** / ___ of smell; ___ **del sabor** / ___ of taste; ___ **del tacto** / ___ of touch; ___ **común** / common ___; ___ **del humor** / ___ of humor.

sentimiento *m.* feeling; sentiment.

sentir *vi.* to feel, to perceive through the senses; **sentirse** *vr.* [*estado corporal*] to feel, general state of the body or mind; ___ **bien** / to ___ good; ___ **mal** / to ___ sick.

señal *f.* sign, indication.

señalado-a *a.* conspicuous, pronounced.

señalar *v.* to point out, to indicate; to mark.

señor *m.* mister; *abr.* Mr.

señora *f.* married woman; *abr.* Mrs.

señorita *f.* miss, young lady; *abr.* Miss.

separación *f.* separation; in obstetrics, disengagement.

separado-a *a.* separate; **-mente** *adv.* separately.

separar *v.* to separate, to sever.

sepsis *L.* sepsis, toxic condition caused by bacterial contamination.

septal *a.* septal, rel. to a septum; **desviación** ___ / ___ deviation.

septectomía *f.* septectomy, partial or total excision of the septum.

septicemia *f.* septicemia, blood poisoning, invasion of the blood by virulent microorganisms.

séptico-a *a.* septic, rel. to sepsis; **choque** ___ / ___ shock.

septimetritis *f.* septimetritis, infl. of the uterus due to sepsis.

septostomía *f.* septostomy, surgical opening of a septum.

septum *L.* septum, (*pl. septa*) partition between two cavities.

sequedad *f.* dryness.

sequía *f.* drought.

ser *vi.* to be.

sereno-a *a.* serene, calm; *pop.* cool.

serie *f.* distribution, set, succession; series, a group of specimens or types arranged in sequence; **en** ___ / serial; ___ **selectiva bioquímica** / biochemical screening.

serio-a *a.* serious; [*caso médico*] complicated; **en** ___ / seriously; **-mente** *adv.* seriously.

seroconversión *f.* seroconversion, development of antibodies as a response to an infection or to the administration of a vaccine.

serología *f.* serology, the science that studies sera.

serológico-a *a.* serologic, serological, rel. to serum.

seroma *m.* seroma, accumulation of blood serum that produces a tumorlike swelling, gen. subcutaneous.

seronegativo-a *a.* seronegative, presenting a negative reaction in serological tests.

seropositivo-a *a.* seropositive, presenting a positive reaction in serological tests.

serosa *f.* serosa, serous membrane.

serosanguíneo-a *a.* serosanguineous, of the nature of serum and blood.

serositis *f.* serositis, infl. of a serous membrane, an important sign in diseases of the connective tissue such as systemic erythematous lupus.

seroso-a *a.* serous.1. of the nature of serum; 2. producing or containing serum.

serotipo *m.* serotype, type of microorganism determined by the class and combination of antigens present in the cell; **determinación del** ___ / serotyping.

serpiente *f.* snake, serpent; ___ **de cascabel** / rattlesnake; **mordida de** ___ / ___ bite; ___ **venenosa** / poisonous ___ .

serpiginoso-a *a.* serpiginous, that crawls from one place to another.

servible *a.* usable.

servicio *m.* service; ___ **-s de cuidado exterior** / extended care facility; ___ **-s de emergencia** / emergency ___ ; ___ **-s de salud preventiva** / preventive health ___ .

servilleta *f.* napkin.

servir *vi.* to serve; to be of help or service.

sesamoideo-a *a.* sesamoid, rel. to or resembling a small mass in a joint or cartilage.

sésil *a.* sessile, attached by a broad base with no peduncle.

sesión *f.* session.

seso *m.* brain.

seudogota *f.* pseudogout, recurrent arthritic condition with symptoms similar to gout.

severo-a *a.* severe; **síndrome respiratorio** ___ / ___ acute respiratory syndrome; **inmunodeficiencia combinada** ___ / ___ combined immunodeficiency.

sexo *m.* sex; **relacionado con el** ___ / ___ -linked, transmitted by genes located in the sex chromosome.

sexual *a.* sexual, rel. to sex; **agresión** ___ / ___ assault; **características** ___ **-es** / ___ characteristics; **conducta** ___ / ___ behavior; **desarrollo** ___ / ___ development; **educación** ___ / ___ education; **madurez** ___ / ___ maturity; **relaciones** ___ **-es** / ___ intercourse; **salud** ___ / ___ health; **trastorno** ___ / ___ disorder; **vida** ___ / ___ life; **-mente** *adv.* sexually; **enfermedad** ___ **transmitida, enfermedad venérea** / ___ transmitted disease. *V.* cuadro en la página XX.

sexualidad *f.* sexuality, collective characteristics of each sex.

shigelosis *f.* shigellosis, bacillary dysentery.

shock *m.* shock, abnormal state generated by insufficient blood circulation that can cause disorders such as low blood pressure, rapid pulse, pallor, abnormally low body temperature, and general weakness; ___ **anafiláctico** / anaphylactic ___ ; ___ **endotóxico** / endotoxic ___ ; ___ **insulínico** / insulin ___ ; ___ **séptico** / septic ___ .

Shy-Drager, síndrome de *m.* Shy-Drager syndrome, neurodegenerative disease of middle-aged or older persons that affects the autonomous nervous system and is characterized by chronic orthostatic hypotension and cardiac arrhythmia.

si *conj.* if, in case.

sí *adv.* yes; **diga** ___ **o no, di** ___ **o no** / say ___ or no.

sialadenitis *f.* sialadenitis, sialoadenitis, infl. of a salivary gland.

sialogogo *m.* sialogogue, agent that stimulates secretion of saliva.

sialograma *m.* sialogram, x-ray of the salivary tract.

SIDA *abr.* AIDS, acquired immunodeficiency syndrome, characterized by immunodeficiency, infections (such as pneumonia, tuberculosis, and chronic diarrhea), and tumors esp. lymphoma and Kaposi's sarcoma.

siempre *adv.* always; **para** ___ / forever.

sien *f.* temple, the flattened lateral region on either side of the head.

siesta *f.* nap; break of activities at midday.

sietemesino-a *a.* born at seven months' gestation.

sífilis *f.* syphilis, contagious venereal disease usu. transmitted by direct contact and manifested by structural and cutaneous lesions; ___ **terciaria** / tertiary ___ , the third and most advanced stage of syphilis.

sifilítico-a *m., f.* syphylitic, person infected with syphilis; *a.* rel. to or caused by syphilis. **mácula** ___ / ___ macule;

sifilología *f.* syphilology, branch of medicine that studies the diagnosis and treatment of syphilis.

sifón *m.* syphon.

sigmoide, sigmoideo-a *a.* sigmoid. 1. shaped like the letter *s*; 2. rel. to the sigmoid colon.

sigmoidoscopía *f.* sigmoidoscopy, examination of the sigmoid flexure with a sigmoidoscope.

sigmoidoscopio *m.* sigmoidoscope, long hollow tubular instrument used for the examination of the sigmoid flexure.

significado *m.* meaning, significance.

significar *vi.* to signify, to mean.

significativo-a *a.* significant; meaningful, important.

signo *m.* sign; mark, objective manifestation of a disease; ___ **-s vitales** / vital ___ -s.

siguiente *a.* following, next.

sílaba *f., gr.* syllable.

silbar *v.* to whistle.

silbido *m.* whistle, the sound of a.

silencio *m.* silence.

silencioso-a *a.* silent.

silicio *m.* silicon, nonmetallic element found in the soil.

silicón *m.* silicone, organic silicon compound used in lubricants, synthetics and also in plastic surgery and prostheses.

silicosis *f.* silicosis, dust inhalation; a pathological condition of the lungs resulting from long term inhalation of silica dust.

Silvio, acueducto de *m.* aqueduct of Silvius, narrow channel connecting the third and fourth ventricles of the brain.

silla *f.* chair; ___ **de ruedas** / wheelchair;

silla turca *f.* sella turcica, depression on the superior surface of the sphenoid bone that contains the hypophysis.

sillón *m.* armchair; *Cu.* rocking chair.

simbiosis *f.* symbiosis, close association of two dissimilar organisms.

simbiótico-a *a.* symbiotic, rel. to symbiosis.

simbolismo *m.* symbolism. 1. mental abnormality by which the patient conceives occurrences as symbols of his or her own thoughts; 2. in psychoanalysis, symbolic representation of repressed thoughts and emotions.

símbolo *m.* symbol.

simetría *f.* symmetry, perfect correspondence of parts situated on opposite sides of an axis or plane of a body.

simétrico-a *a.* symmetrical.

similar *a.* similar.

simpatectomía *f.* sympathectomy, interruption of the sympathetic nerve pathways.

simpatía *f.* sympathy, relationship, affinity. 1. affinity between mind and body whereby one is affected by the other; 2. relationship between two organs in which an anomaly in one affects the other.

simpático-a *a.* sympathetic, rel. to the sympathetic nervous system.

simpatolítico-a *a.* sympatholytic, resistant to the activity produced by the stimulation of the sympathetic nervous system.

simpatomimético-a *a.* sympathomimetic, having the capacity to cause physiological changes similar to those produced by the action of the sympathetic nervous system.

simple *a.* simple; **-mente** *adv.* merely.

simplificar *vi.* to simplify.

simulación *f.* simulation, imitation; feigning an illness or symptom.

simulador-a *m., f.* malingerer, person who deliberately feigns or exaggerates the symptoms of an illness.

sin *prep.* without; ___ **embargo** / nevertheless;

sinapsis *f.* 1. synapse, the point of contact between two neurons, where the impulse traveling through the first neuron originates an impulse in the second one; 2. synapsis, the pairing of homologous chromosomes at the start of meiosis.

sináptico-a *a.* synaptic, rel. to synapse or synapsis.

sinartrosis *f.* synarthrosis, an immovable joint in which the bony elements are fused.

sincanto *m.* syncanthus, adhesion of the eye to the orbital tissues.

sincitial *a.* syncytial, rel. to or constituting syncytium.

sincitio *m.* syncytium, mass of protoplasm resulting from cell fusion.

sinclono *m.* synclonus, spasm or tremor of various muscles at one time.

sincondrosis *f.* synchondrosis, an immovable joint in which the surfaces are joined by cartilaginous tissue.

sincopal *a.* syncopal, rel. to a syncope.

síncope *m.* syncope, temporary loss of consciousness due to inadequate supply of blood to the brain.___ **anginoso** / anginal ___; ___ **de deglución** / deglutition ___; ___ **cardíaco** / cardiac ___; ___ **convulsivo** / convulsive ___; ___ **histérico** / hysterical ___; ___ **laríngeo** / laryngeal ___ .

sincrónico-a *a.* synchronous, occurring at the same time.

sindactilia *f.* syndactylism, syndactyly, congenital anomaly consisting of the fusion of two or more fingers or toes.

sindesmitis *f.* syndesmitis. 1. infl. of one or more ligaments; 2. infl. of the conjunctiva.

sindesmona *f.* syndesmona, connective tissue tumor.

síndrome *m.* syndrome, the totality of the symptoms and signs of a disease; ___ **adiposo** / adipose ___; ___ **de choque tóxico** / toxic shock ___ , blood poisoning due to *Staphylococci*; ___ **de dificultad respiratoria** / respiratory distress ___; ___ **de escaldadura** / scalded skin ___ , burns of the epidermis that gen. do not harm the underlying dermis; ___ **de intestino irritado** / irritable bowel ___; ___ **de malabsorción** / malabsorption ___ , gastro-intestinal disorder caused by poor absorption of food; ___ **de niños maltratados** / battered children ___; ___ **de privación** / withdrawal ___ , resulting from discontinued use of alcohol or a drug; ___ **de transfusión múltiple** / multiple transfusion ___ ; ___ **de vaciamiento gástrico rápido** / dumping ___ , rapid dumping of the stomach contents into the small intestine; ___ **del lóbulo medio del pulmón** / middle lobe ___ of the lung; ___ **del secuestro subclavicular** / subclavian steal ___; ___ **nefrótico** / nephrotic ___ , excessive loss of protein; ___ **premenstrual** / premenstrual ___; ___ **suprarrenogenital** / adrenogenital ___ .

síndrome de inmunodeficiencia adquirida *m.* acquired immunodeficiency syndrome. SIDA.

síndrome de muerte infantil súbita *m.* sudden infant death syndrome, sudden unexplained death of an apparently healthy infant during sleep the cause of which remains unknown. sis.

síndrome del mentón entumecido *m.* numb chin syndrome, loss of sensation and cramps in part of the cheek and lower lip that can result from disorders such as multiple myeloma, or mammary or prostrate carcinoma.

síndrome hemolítico urémico *m.* hemolytic uremic syndrome, hemolytic anemia and thrombocytopenia presenting acute renal failure; during infancy it is accompanied by symptoms of gastrointestinal bleeding, hematuria, oliguria, and hemolytic anemia.

síndrome neuroléptico maligno *m.* neuroleptic malignant syndrome, due to the use of neuroleptic agents and characterized by symptoms of hyperthermia, loss of consciousness, and serious reactions related to the central nervous system that could be fatal.

sinequia *f.* synechia, union or abnormal adherence of tissue or organs, esp. in reference to the iris, the lens, and the cornea.

sinérgico-a *a.* synergistic, synergic, the capacity to act together.

sinergismo *m.* synergism, correlated or harmonious action between two or more structures or drugs.

sínfisis *f.* symphysis, a joint in which adjacent bony surfaces are united by fibrocartilage.

singular *m., gr.* singular, only one. *a.* singular, not common, unique.

singulto *m.* singultus, hiccup, hiccough.

sinoauricular o sinusal, nódulo *m.* sinoauricular, sinoatrial node located at the meeting point of the vena cava and the right cardiac atrium, point of origin of the impulses that stimulate the heartbeat.

sinograma *m.* sinogram, x-ray of a sinus by means of a contrasting dye.

sinostosis *f.* synostosis, osseous joining of two adjacent bones; ___ **senil** / senile ___; ___ **tribacilar** / tribacilar ___.

sinovia *f.* synovia, synovial fluid, transparent and viscid liquid secreted by synovial membranes that lubricates joints and connective tissue.

sinovial *a.* synovial, rel. to or producing synovia; **bursa, saco** ___ / ___ bursa; **membrana** ___ / ___ membrane; **quiste** ___ / ___ cyst.

sinovioma *m.* synovioma, tumor that originates in the synovial membrane.

sinovitis *f.* synovitis, an infl. of the synovial membrane; ___ **purulenta** / purulent ___; ___ **seca** / dry ___; ___ **serosa** / serous ___ .

sinquiria *f.* synchiria, condition by which a stimulus applied to one part of the body is referred to another part.

sinquisis *f.* synchysis, state of fluidity of the vitreous humor.

síntesis *f.* synthesis, the composition of a whole by union of the parts.

sintético-a *a.* synthetic, rel. to or produced by synthesis.

sintetizar *vi.* to synthesize, to produce synthesis.

síntoma *m.* symptom, any manifestation of a disease as perceived by the patient; ___ **constitucional** / constitutional ___ ; ___ **demorado** / delayed ___ ; ___ **de supresión** / withdrawal ___ ; ___ **objetivo** / objective ___ ; ___ **patognomónico** / pathognomonic ___ ; ___ **presente** / presenting ___ ; ___ **prodrómico** / prodromal ___ ; ___ **-s premonitorios** / warning ___ -s.

sintomático-a *a.* symptomatic; *-mente adv.* symptomatically.

sintomatolítico-a *a.* symptomatolytic, that takes away the symptoms.

sintomatología *f.* symptomatology, symptoms pertaining to a given condition or case.

sintónico-a *m., f.* syntonic, a type of personality that responds and adjusts normally to his or her environment.

sinuoso-a *a.* sinuous, winding, wavy.

sinus *L.* sinus, cavity or hollow passage.

sinusitis *f.* sinusitis, infl. of a sinus, esp. a paranasal sinus.

sinusoide *m.* sinusoid, a minute passage that carries blood to the tissues of an organ, such as the liver; *a.* resembling a sinus.

siringobulbia *f.* syringobulbia, the presence of abnormal cavities in the medulla oblongata.

siringocele *m.* syringocele. 1. the central canal of the spinal cord; 2. a meningomyelocele containing a cavity in the ectopic spinal cord.

siringomielia *f.* syringomyelia, chronic, progressive disease of the spinal cord manifested by formation of liquid-filled cavities, gen. in the cervical region and sometimes extending into the medulla oblongata.

sirope *m.* syrup, concentrated sugar solution.

sistáltico-a *a.* systaltic, that alternates dilations and contractions.

sistema *m.* system, a group of correlated parts or organs constituting a whole that performs one or more vital functions. *V.* cuadro en esta página.

sistema de circulación cardiopulmonar *m.* application of a heart-lung machine.

sistema sensorio nervioso *m.* sensory nervous system.

Sistema	System
cardiovascular	cardiovascular
digestivo	digestive
endocrino	endocrine
genitourinario	genitourinary
hematopoyético	hematopoietic
inmunológico	immune
linfático	lymphatic
nervioso	nervous
óseo	osseous
portal	portal
reproductivo	reproductive
respiratorio	respiratory
reticuloendotelial	reticuloendothelial

sistemático-a *a.* systematic, that follows a system; *-mente adv.* systematically.

sistematización *f.* systematization, the act of arranging thoughts or objects in a systematic and orderly manner.

sistémico-a *a.* systemic, that affects the body as a whole; **circulación** ___ / ___ circulation;

sístole *f.* systole, the contractive cycle of the heartbeat, esp. of the ventricles; ___ **auricular** / atrial ___ ; ___ **prematura** / premature ___ ; ___ **ventricular** / ventricular ___ .

sistólico-a *a.* systolic, rel. to the systole; **murmullo** ___ / ___ murmur; **presión** ___ / ___ pressure.

situación *f.* situation.

situado-a *a.* situated, placed, located.

situs *L.* situs, position or place.

Sjogren, síndrome de *m.* Sjogren's syndrome, autoimmune disorder that results in diminished salivary and lacrimal secretion, causing dryness of the eyes and the lips.

Snellen, prueba de ojo de *f.* Snellen's eye test, a chart of black letters that gradually diminish in size, used in testing visual acuity.

sobra *f.* excess, surplus; **hay de** ___ / there is more than enough.

sobrante *m.* surplus, leftover, excess.

sobrar *v.* to be or have in excess.

sobre *prep.* above, over; ___ **todo** / above all;

sobrealimentación *f.* hyperalimentation; ___ **intravenosa** / parenteral ___ .

sobrecierre *m.* overclosure, condition caused when the mandible closes before the upper and lower teeth meet.

sobrecompensación *f.* overcompensation; an exaggerated attempt to conceal feelings of guilt or inferiority.

sobrecorrección *f.* overcorrection, use of too powerful a lens to correct an eye defect.

sobredosis *f.* overdose, excessive dose of a drug.

sobreextensión *f.* overextension.

sobrellevar *v.* to endure.

sobremordida *f.* overbite.

sobrenombre *m.* surname, family name.

sobrepeso *m.* overweight.

sobreponerse *vr., vi.* to overcome.

sobreproducción *f.* overproduction.

sobrerrespuesta *f.* overresponse, excessive reaction to a stimulus.

sobresalir *vi.* to protrude; to be conspicuous.

sobresaltado-a *a.* frightened, startled.

sobretodo *m.* overcoat, coat.

sobrevivir *v.* to survive.

sobrino-a *m., f.* nephew; niece.

sobrio-a *a.* sober.

socavar *v.* to undermine.

sociable *a.* sociable.

social *a.* social; **seguro ___ / ___** security; **asistencia ___ / ___** work; **trabajador-a ___ / ___** worker.

socialización *f.* socialization, social adaptation.

socializado-a *a.* socialized; **medicina ___ / ___** medicine.

sociedad *f.* society; corporation; fellowship.

socio-a *m., f.* member; partner; fellow.

sociobiología *f.* sociobiology, the science that studies genetic factors as determinants of social behavior.

sociología *f.* sociology, the science that studies social relations and phenomena.

sociólogo-a *m., f.* sociologist, specialist in sociology.

sociópata *m., f.* sociopath, an individual that manifests antisocial behavior.

socorrer *v.* to help, to assist, to aid.

soda *f.* soda, sodium carbonate.

sodio *m.* sodium, soft alkaline metallic element found in the fluids of the body; **bicarbonato de ___ /** baking soda; **carbonato de ___ /** soda.

sodomía *f.* sodomy, term used in reference to dual intercourse most often between males.

sodomita *m., f.* sodomite, one who commits sodomy.

sofisticación *f.* sophistication; the adulteration of a substance.

sofocación *f.* suffocation, asphyxia, shortness of breath.

sofocar *vi.* to suffocate, to smother; to choke.

sofoco *m.* hot flash; suffocation.

soja, soya *f.* soy, soybean.

sol *m.* sun; **baño de ___ /** sunbathing; **bloqueador del ___ /** sunscreen; **estar expuesto al ___ / ___** exposure; **mancha del ___ /** sunspot; **quemadura de ___ /** sunburn; **tomar el ___ /** to sunbathe.

solar *a.* solar, rel. to the sun; **bloqueador ___ /** sunscreen.

solaz *m.* solace, comfort, rest from work.

sólido-a *a.* solid; firm; sound.

solo-a *a.* alone, only; **-mente** *adv.* only.

soltar *vi.* to release; to loosen.

soltero-a *a.* single, unmarried.

soluble *a.* soluble.

solución *f.* solution.

solvente *m.* solvent, liquid that dissolves or is capable of producing a solution; thinner; *a.* financially responsible; having financial assets.

sollozar *vi.* to sob; to cry.

somático-a *a.* somatic, rel. to the body.

somatización *f.* somatization; the process of converting mental experiences into bodily manifestations.

sombra *f.* shadow; opacity; shade; **a la ___ /** in the shade.

sombrero *m.* hat.

someter *v.* to submit; **someterse** *vr.* to undergo; to submit oneself.

somnífero *m.* sleeping pill.

somniloquia *f.* somniloquism, the act of talking while asleep. *Syn.* sleeptalking.

somnolencia *f.* sleepiness, drowsiness.

sonambulismo *m.* somnambulance, somnambulism, sleepwalking.

sonámbulo-a *m., f.* somnambule, person who walks in his or her sleep.

sonar *vi.* to sound, to ring.

sonda *f.* probe, thin, smooth, and flexible instrument used to explore cavities and body passages or to measure the depth and direction of a wound; **___ acanalada /** hollow **___**; **___ intestinal /** intestinal decompression tube; **___ uretral /** urethral catheter.

sonido *m.* sound.

sonografía *f.* sonography. ultrasonografía.

sonograma *m.* sonogram, image obtained by ultrasonography.

sonoluciente *a.* sonolucent, in ultrasonography, having the quality of permitting the passage of ultrasound waves without remitting them back to their source.

sonoro-a *a.* sonorous, resonant, having a deep or full sound.

sonreír *vi.* to smile.

sonrisa *f.* smile.

soñar *vi.* to dream; ___ **despierto -a** / to daydream.

sopa *f.* soup.

soplar *v.* to blow.

soplo *m.* murmur, bruit, flutter; short, raspy, or fluttering sound, esp. an abnormal beat of the heart; ___ **aórtico, regurgitante** / aortic, regurgitant in value; ___ **cardíaco** / cardiac ___; ___ **continuo** / continuous ___; ___ **creciente, en crescendo** / crescendo ___; ___ **diastólico** / diastolic ___; ___ **endocardial** / endocardial ___; ___ **en vaivén** / to-and-fro ___; ___ **exocardial** / exocardial ___; ___ **funcional** / functional ___; ___ **inocente** / innocent ___; ___ **mitral** / mitral ___; ___ **pansistólico** / pansystolic ___; ___ **presistólico** / presystolic ___; ___ **sistólico** / systolic ___ . *V.* cuadro en la página 456.

sopor *m.* drowsiness, sleepiness.

soporífero, soporífico *m.* soporific, agent that produces sleep.

soporoso-a *a.* soporose, soporous, in a state of stupor.

soportable *a.* bearable, tolerable.

soportar *v.* to endure, to bear, to sustain.

soporte *m.* support.

sorber *v.* to sip; to suck; to absorb.

sorbo *m.* sip.

sordera *f.* deafness.

sordo-a *m., f.* a deaf person; *a.* deaf.

sordomudo-a *m., f.* deaf-mute person.

soso-a *a.* tasteless.

sostén *m.* support, backing; buttress; brassiere.

sostener *vi.* to sustain; to maintain.

sostenido-a *a.* sustained; maintained.

Still, enfermedad de *f.* Still's disease, juvenile rheumatoid arthritis.

stratum *L.* stratum, (*pl. strata*) layer.

Streptococcus *Gr.* Streptococcus, a genus of gram-positive bacteria of the tribe *Streptococceae* that occur in pairs or chains, many of which are causal agents of serious infection.

suave *a.* soft, smooth; **-mente** *adv.* softly.

suavizar *vi.* to soften.

subacromial *a.* subacromial, below the acromion.

subagudo-a *a.* subacute, rel. to a condition that is neither acute nor chronic.

subaracnoideo-a *a.* subarachnoid, situated or occurring below the arachnoid membrane; **espacio** ___ / ___ space.

subatómico-a *a.* subatomic, smaller than an atom.

subcapsular *a.* subcapsular, located below a capsule.

subclavicular *a.* subclavian, subclavicular, located beneath the clavicle; **arteria** ___ / ___ artery; **vena** ___ / ___ vein.

subclínico-a *a.* subclinical, without clinical manifestations.

subconsciencia, subconsciente *f., m.* subconscious, state during which mental processes affecting thought, feeling, and behavior occur without the individual's awareness.

subconsciente *a.* subconscious, rel. to the part of the mind of which one is not fully aware.

subcostal *a.* subcostal, below the ribs.

subcultivo *m.* subculture, a culture of bacteria derived from another culture.

subcutáneo-a *a.* subcutaneous, under the skin.

subdesarrollado-a *a.* underdeveloped.

subdesarrollo *m.* underdevelopment.

subdural *a.* subdural, under the dura mater. **espacio** ___ / ___ space.

subependimario-a *a.* subependymal, situated under the ependyma.

subescapular *a.* subscapular, below the scapula.

subesternal *a.* substernal, below the sternum.

subestructura *f.* substructure, supporting structure.

subfrénico-a *a.* subphrenic, situated below the diaphragm; **absceso** ___ / ___ abscess.

subhepático-a *a.* subhepatic, situated under the liver.

subintimal *a.* subintimal, situated below the intima.

subinvolución *f.* subinvolution, incomplete involution; ___ **del útero** / ___ of the uterus.

subir *v.* to go up; to lift up; to climb; ___ **las escaleras** / to climb the stairs.

súbito-a *a.* sudden; **muerte** ___ / ___ death; **-mente** *adv.* suddenly.

subjetivo-a *a.* subjective; **síntomas** ___**-s** / ___ symptoms.

sublimación *f.* sublimation. 1. the change from a solid state to vapor; 2. a Freudian term indicating a process by which instinctual drives and impulses are modified into socially acceptable behavior.

sublimado *m.* sublimate, substance obtained by sublimation.

sublingual *a.* sublingual, under the tongue; **glandula** ___ / ___ gland.

subluxación *f.* subluxation, an incomplete dislocation.

submandibular *a.* submandibular, under the mandible.

submental *a.* submental, under the chin.

submucosa *f.* submucosa, layer of cellular tissue situated under a mucous membrane.

subnormal *a.* subnormal, below normal or below average.

subóptimo-a *a.* suboptimal, less than optimum.

subproducto *m.* by-product.

subrogado-a *a.* surrogate, that takes the place of someone or something.

subscripción *f.* subscription, part of the prescription that contains instructions for its preparation.

subsistir *v.* to subsist, to survive.

substantivo, sustantivo *m., gr.* substantive, noun.

subtotal *m.* subtotal.

subungueal *a.* subungual, beneath a nail.

succión *f.* suction; **dispositivo de** ___ / ___ device.

suceder *v.* to happen.

sucesivo-a *a.* successive, consecutive.

suceso *m.* happening, event.

suciedad *f.* filth.

sucio-a *a.* dirty, filthy.

suco *m.* succus, juice; sap.

sucrosa *f.* sucrose, natural saccharose obtained mostly from sugarcane and sugar beets.

sudado-a *a.* sweaty, moist with perspiration; perspiring.

sudamina *f.* sudamina, non-inflammatory cutaneous eruption that presents whitish vesicles filled with aqueous liquid and that gen. occurs after profuse sweating or accompanying some febrile disorder.

sudar *v.* to sweat, to perspire.

sudatorio, sudorífico *m.* sudorific, an agent promoting sweat.

sudor *m.* sweat, perspiration, secretion of the sweat glands; ___ **-es nocturnos** / night ___-s.

sudores fríos *m., pl.* cold sweat.

sudoriento-a *a.* sweaty, covered with sweat.

sudorífico-a *a.* sudorific, that produces sweat.

sudoroso-a *a.* perspiring, sweaty.

suegro-a *m., f.* father-in-law; mother-in-law.

sueldo *m.* salary, wages.

suelo *m.* ground; floor.

suelto-a *a.* , *pp.* de **soltar**, loose, unattached.

sueño *m.* sleep; dream; **ciclos del** ___ / ___ cycles; ___ **crepuscular** / twilight ___ ; **estadíos del** ___ / ___ stages; ___ **profundo** / deep ___ ; ___ **reparador** / balmy ___ ; **trastornos del** ___ / sleep disorders; *v.* **tener** ___ / to be sleepy;

sueño, enfermedad del *f.* sleeping sickness, endemic, acute disease of Africa caused by a protozoon transmitted by the tsetse fly and characterized by a state of lethargy, chills, loss of weight, and general weakness.

suero *m.* serum.1. clear, watery portion of the plasma that remains fluid after clotting of blood; 2. any serous fluid;3. immune serum of an animal that is inoculated to produce passive immunization;___ **antitóxico** / immune ___; ___ **de globulina** / globulin ___; ___ **de la verdad** / truth ___ .

suerte *f.* luck;*v.* **tener** ___ / to be lucky;

suficiente *a.* sufficient, enough;*-mente adv.* sufficiently.

sufijo *m., gr.* suffix.

sufrible *a.* sufferable, bearable.

sufrimiento *m.* suffering.

sufrir *v.* to suffer; [*herida*] to sustain; [*operación*] to undergo.

sufusión *f.* suffusion, infiltration of a bodily fluid into the surrounding tissues.

sugerencia, sugestión *f.* suggestion, intimation, indication.

sugerir *vi.* to suggest, to indicate, to hint.

sugestivo-a *a.* suggestive, rel. to suggestion or that suggests.

suicida *a.* suicidal, prone to commit suicide.

suicidarse *vr.* to commit suicide.

suicidio *m.* suicide; **intento de** ___ / attempted ___ .

sujeto *m.* subject.1. term used in reference to the patient; 2. topic; 3. *gr.* subject of the verb.

sulciforme *a.* sulciform, in the shape of a furrow.

sulcus *L. sulci*sulcus, slight depression, fissure.

sulfa, medicamentos de *m., pl.* sulfa drugs, *sulfonamides,* antibacterial drugs of the sulfonamide group.

sulfato *m.* sulfate, a salt of sulfuric acid.

sulfonamidas *f. pl.* sulfonamides, a group of bacteriostatic sulfur organic compounds.

sulfúrico-a *a.* sulfuric, rel. to sulfur.

sulfuro *m.* sulphur.

suma *f.* summation, total amount.

sumamente *adv.* extremely, very.

sumar *v.* to add.

sumario *m.* summary, clinical history of the patient.

sumergir *vi.* to submerge, to immerse.

superar *v.* to overcome.

superfecundación *f.* superfecundation, successive fertilization of two or more ova from the same menstrual cycle in two separate instances of sexual intercourse.

superfetación *f.* superfetation, fecundation of two ova in the same uterus corresponding to two different menstrual cycles but occurring within a short period of time from each other.

superficial *a.* superficial, rel. to a surface; **tensión** ___ / surface tension; shallow; *-mente adv.* superficially, shallowly.

superficie *f.* surface, outer portion or limit of a structure.

superhembra *f.* superfemale, a female organism that contains more than the normal number of sex-determining chromosomes.

superinfección *f.* superinfection, new infection that occurs while a previous one is still present, gen. caused by a different organism.

superior *a.* superior; upper; higher; greater.

supernumerario-a *a.* supernumerary, that exceeds the normal number.

superolateral *a.* superolateral, situated above and to the side.

supersaturado-a *a.* supersaturated, beyond saturation.

supersaturar *v.* to supersaturate, to add a substance in an amount greater than that which can be dissolved normally by a liquid.

supersensibilidad *f.* supersensitiveness, hypersensibility.

supersónico-a *a.* supersonic, rel. to vibrations of sound waves at speeds above the capacity of human hearing.

superstición *f.* superstition.

supersticioso-a *a.* superstitious.

supervisar *v.* to supervise.

supervisor-a *m., f.* supervisor.

supervivencia *f.* survivorship; annuity.

superyó *m.* superego, in psychoanalysis the part of the psyche concerned with social standards, ethics, and conscience.

supinación *f.* supination, turning the hand with the palm facing forward and upward.

supino-a *a.* supine, rel. to the position of lying on the back, face up, with palms of the hands turned upward.

suplemental *a.* supplemental, additional.

suplemento *m.* supplement, supply.

suplicio *m.* torture, punishment, extreme suffering.

suponer *vi.* to suppose, to surmise.

suposición *f.* supposition, guess.

supositorio *m.* suppository, a semisolid, soluble, medicated mass that is introduced in a body passage such as the vagina or the rectum.

supraclavicular *a.* supraclavicular, situated above the clavicle.

supraglótico-a *a.* supraglottic, situated above the glottis.

suprap?bico-a *a.* suprapubic, above the pubis; **catéter** ___ / ___ catheter; **cistotomia** ___ / ___ cystotomy.

suprarrenal *a.* suprarenal, above the kidney; **glandula** ___ / ___ gland.

suprasillar *a.* suprasellar, above the sella turcica.

supratentorial *a.* supratentorial, above the dura mater.

supresión *f.* suppression; withdrawal; 1. arrest in the production of a secretion, excretion, or any normal discharge; 2. in psychoanalysis, inhibition of an idea or desire.

suprimir *v.* to discontinue, to withdraw.

supuración *f.* suppuration, formation or discharge of pus.

supurar *v.* to suppurate, to fester, to ooze.

supurativo-a *a.* suppurative, rel. to suppuration.

sur *m.* south.

sural *a.* sural, rel. to the calf of the leg.

surco *m.* furrow, line, wrinkle; groove, track; ___ **atrioventricular** / atrioventricular ___; ___ **bicipital** / bicipital ___; ___ **costal** / costal ___; ___ **digital** / digital ___; ___ **glúteo** / gluteal ___ .

surfactante *m.* surfactant, active agent that modifies the surface tension of a liquid.

susceptibilidad *f.* susceptibility.

susceptible *a.* susceptible.

suscitar *v.* to rouse, to stir up.

suspender *v.* to suspend, to cancel, to halt.

suspensión *f.* suspension. 1. temporary stoppage of a vital process; 2. treatment that consists of immobilizing and suspending a patient in a desired position; 3. the state of a substance when its particles are not dissolved in a fluid or solid; 4. detention, stoppage.

suspenso-a *a.* pending.

suspensorio-a *a.* suspensory, sustaining or providing support; **ligamento** ___ / ___ ligament.

sustancia *f.* substance, matter; ___ **blanca** / white matter, neural tissue formed mainly by myelinated fibers that constitute the conducting portion of the brain and the spinal cord; ___ **fundamental** / ground ___ , gelatinous matter of connective tissue, cartilage, and bone that fills the space between cells and fibers.

sustancioso-a *a.* nutritious.

sustantivo *m., gr.* substantive, noun.

sustentacular *a.* sustentacular, sustaining or supporting.

sustentaculum *L.* sustentaculum, support.

sustento *m.* sustenance.

sustitución *f.* substitution, the act of replacing one thing for another; **terapéutica por** ___ / ___ therapy.

sustituir *vi.* to substitute.

sustituto *m.* substitute.

susto *m.* fright, sudden fear.

sustrato *m.* 1. substrate, a substance acted upon by an enzyme; 2. substratum, an underlying foundation.

susurro *m.* whisper, murmur.

sutil *a.* subtile, subtle, fine, delicate; inadvertent.

sutura *f.* suture, line of union; ___ **absorbable** / absorbable surgical ___; ___**compuesta** / bolster ___; ___ **continua, de peletero** / continuous, uninterrupted ___; ___ **de aposición y aproximación** / near and far ___; ___**de catgut** / catgut ___; ___**de colchonero** / vertical mattress ___; ___ **de herida** / wound ___; ___ **de seda** / silk ___; ___ **en bolsa de tabaco** / pursestring ___; ___ **facial** / fascial ___; ___ **implantada** / implanted ___; ___ **interrumpida** / interrupted ___; ___ **no absorbible** / nonabsorbable ___; ___ **plana** / flat ___ .

Swan-Ganz, catéter de *m.* Swan-Ganz catheter, soft, flexible catheter with a balloon near the tip used to measure the blood pressure in the pulmonary artery.

Sydenham, corea de *f.* Sydenham's chorea, rare type of chorea with relatively moderate movements that is gen. accompanied by symptoms and manifestations of rheumatic fever.

t

T *abr.* **temperatura absoluta** / absolute temperature; **T +, tensión aumentada** / T +, increased tension; **T +, tensión disminuida** / T +, diminished tension.

tabaco *m.* 1. tobacco, the dried and prepared leaves of *Nicotiana tabacum* that contain nicotine; 2. cigar; **contaminación por humo de ___** / ___ smoke pollution.

tabaquismo *m.* tabacism, tabacosis, acute or chronic intoxication due to excessive intake of tobacco dust.

tabardillo *m. pop.* name given to typhus, or typhoid fever in certain regions of Mexico and Latin America.

tabes *L.* tabes, progressive deterioration of the body or any part of it caused by a chronic illness.

tabético-a *a.* tabetic, rel. to or suffering from tabes.

tabicado-a *a.* septate, that has a dividing wall.

tabique *m.* thin wall; ___ **nasal, o de la nariz** / nose ridge.

tabla *f.* table. 1. a flat osseous plate or lamina; 2. an arranged collection of many particulars that have a common standard.

tableta *f.* tablet, a solid dosage of medication; ___ **de capa entérica** / enteric-coated ___ .

tabú *m.* taboo, tabu, a forbidden thing or behavior; *a.* forbidden.

tabular *a.* tabular, resembling a table or square; *v.* to tabulate, to make lists or tables.

tacha *f.* defect, blemish, imperfection.

tacón *m.* heel of a shoe.

táctica *f.* tactic.

táctil *a.* tactile, rel. to touch or to the sense of touch; **discriminación ___** / ___ discrimination; **sistema ___** / ___ system.

tacto *m.* the sense of touch.

taenia *L.* taenia. tenia.

tajada *f.* slice, cut.

tal, tales *a.* such, as, so, so much; **¿qué ___ ?** / how goes it?; ___ **cual,** ___ **como** / ___ as; *adv.* thus, in such a way, in such manner.

talámico-a *a.* thalamic, rel. to the thalamus.

tálamo *m.* thalamus, one of the two large, oval-shaped masses of gray matter situated at the base of the cerebrum that are the main relay centers of sensory impulses to the cerebral cortex.

talar *a.* talar, rel. to the ankle.

talasemia *f.* thalassemia, group of different types of hereditary hemolytic anemia found in populations of the Mediterranean region and Southeast Asia; ___ **mayor** / major ___; ___ **menor** / minor ___.

talasofobia *f.* thalassophobia, morbid fear of the sea.

talasoterapia *f.* thalassotherapy, the treatment of disease by sea bathing or by exposure to the sea.

talco *m.* talc, talcum powder.

talidomida *f.* thalidomide, hypnotic sedative known to cause severe malformation in developing fetuses.

talitoxicosis *f.* thallitoxicosis, incidental poisoning by ingestion of thallium sulfate used in pesticides.

talla *f.* size, height or length of the body taken from head to toe.

taller *m.* workshop.

tallo *m.* stalk; stem, an elongated, slender structure resembling the stalk or stem of a plant.

talon *m.* talon, posterior part of a molar tooth.

talón *m.* talus, astragalus, heel, ankle bone.

talotibial *a.* talotibial, rel. to the talus and the tibia.

tamaño *m.* size.

tambalearse *vr.* to stagger, to waver.

también *adv.* also, as well, too.

tampoco *adv.* neither, not either.

tan *adv.* so, as well, as much.

tanatología *f.* thanatology, branch of medicine that deals with death in all its aspects.

tanatomania *f.* thanatomania, suicidal or homicidal mania.

tanatómetro *m.* thanatometer, instrument used to determine when a death took place by taking an internal measurement of the temperature of the body.

tangible *a.* tangible.

tanto-a *a.* so much, as much, so many, as many; *adv.* so much, as much; **estar al ___ de** / to be alerted to; **por lo ___** / therefore; ___ **mejor** / ___ the better; ___ **peor** / ___ the worse.

tapa *f.* cover; lid.

tapado-a *a.* covered; clogged.

tapar *v.* to cover.

tapón *m.* 1. pledget, pack of absorbent material applied to a part of the body or inserted in a cavity to stop hemorrhage or absorb secretions; 2. plug, tampon, buffer.

taponamiento *m.* tamponade, packing.1. the process of filling a cavity with cotton, gauze or some other material; 2. wrapping.

taponamiento cardíaco *m.* cardiac tamponade, acute compression of the heart due to excess fluid in the pericardium.

taquiarritmia *f.* tachyarrhythmia, arrhythmia combined with a rapid pulse.

taquiarritmia paroxística *f.* paroxismal taquicardia, palpitation episodes that begin and end abruptly or may last hours or days and can be recurrent.

taquicardia *n.* tachycardia, acceleration of the heart activity, gen. at a frequency of more than one hundred beats per minute in adults; ___ **auricular** / atrial ___; ___ **auricular paroxística** / paroxysmal atrial ___; ___ **ectópica** / ectopic ___; ___ **en salves** / ___ en salves; ___ **exoftálmica** / exophthalmica; ___ **fetal** / fetal ___; ___ **paroximal** / paroxysmal ___; ___ **refleja** / reflex ___; ___ **sinusal** / sinus ___; ___ **supraventricular** / supraventricular ___; ___ **ventricular** / ventricular ___ .

taquifagia *f.* tachyphagia, an acquired habit of eating too fast.

taquifasia *f.* tachyphasia, characteristic of rapid speech. *Sin.* tachyphrasia.

taquipnea *f.* tachypnea, rapid breathing.

tara *f.* 1. weight of a container deducted from the total weight of a load; 2. physical or mental inherited disorder of importance; 3. defect or imperfection that devalues an object.

tarado-a *a.* defective, damaged; [*person*] handicapped; idiot; nitwit.

tarántula *f.* tarantula, large, black, venomous spider.

tardar *v.* to delay; to take time; **a más** ___ / at the latest; **¿cuánto tarda la operación?** / the operation, how long does the operation take?; **tarda menos de una hora** / It takes less than an hour; *fam.* **no tardes mucho** / do not be long ___; **tardarse** *vr.* to be delayed.

tarde *f.* afternoon; *adv.* late; **más** ___ **o más temprano** / sooner or later.

tardío-a *a.* late; delayed.

tardive *Fr.* tardive, late in appearing.

tarea *f.* task.

tarjeta *f.* card; ___ **de crédito** / credit ___; ___ **de visita** / calling ___ .

tarsal, tarsiano-a *a.* tarsal, rel. to the connective tissue that supports the eyelid or the tarsus.

tarso *m.* tarsus, posterior part of the foot located between the bones of the lower leg and the metatarsus; **huesos del** ___ / tarsal bones.

tarsometatarsiano-a *a.* tarsometatarsal, rel. to the tarsus and the metatarsus.

tartamudear *v.* to stammer, to stutter.

tartamudo-a *m., f.* stutter, a person that stutters.

tartamudeo, tartamudez *m., f.* stammering, stuttering.

tatuaje *m.* tattooing, the act of puncturing the skin for the purpose of creating designs with permanent colors.

tatuar *v.* to tatoo; **tatuarse** *vr.* to have a tatoo.

taxis *L.* taxis. 1. manipulation or reduction of a part or an organ to restore it to its normal position; 2. directional reaction of an organism to a stimulus.

taza *f.* cup.

té *m.* tea; ___ **de jazmín** / jasmine ___ .

tebaína *f.* thebaine, toxic alkaloid obtained from opium.

teca *f.* theca, covering or sheath of an organ.

techo *m.* roof; ceiling.

tecnecio 99m *m.* technetium 99m, a radioisotope that emits gamma rays and that is the most frequently used radioisotope in nuclear medicine.

técnica *f.* technic, technique, method, or procedure.

técnico-a *m., f.* technician, an individual who has the necessary knowledge and skill to carry out specialized procedures and treatments, gen. under the supervision of a health care professional; ___ **dental** / dental ___; ___ **de rayos-x** / x-ray ___; ___ **de terapia respiratoria** / respiratory therapy ___ .

tecnología *f.* technology, the science of applying technical knowledge for practical purposes.

tecnológico-a *a.* technological.

tecnólogo-a *m., f.* technologist, an expert in technology.

tecoma *m.* thecoma, tumor of an ovary, gen. benign.

tectorium *L.* tectorium, membrane that covers Corti's organ.

tectum *L.* tectum, rooflike structure.

tedioso-a *a.* tedious; tiresome.

tegumento *m.* tegument, the skin.

tejido *m.* tissue, a group of similar cells and their intercellular substance that act together in the performance of a particular function; ___ **adiposo** / adipose ___; ___ **cartilaginoso** /

cartilaginous ___; ___ **cicatrizante** / scar ___; ___ **conectivo** / connective ___; ___ **de granulación** / granulation ___; ___ **elástico** / elastic ___; ___ **endotelial** / endothelial ___; ___ **epitelial** / epithelial; ___ **eréctil** / erectile ___; ___ **fibroso** / fibrous ___; ___ **glandular** / glandular ___; ___ **interstitial** / ___ fluid; ___ **linfoide** / lymphoid ___; ___ **mesenquimatoso** / mesenchymal ___; ___ **mucoso** / mucous ___; ___ **muscular** / muscular ___; ___ **nervioso** / nerve, nervous ___; ___ **óseo** / bony, bone ___; ___ **subcutáneo** / subcutaneous ___ .

tela *f.* fabric, cloth.

telangiectasia *f.* telangiectasia, telangiectasis, condition caused by an abnormal dilation of the capillary vessels and arterioles that sometimes can produce angioma.

telecardiófono *m.* telecardiophone, an instrument that allows to hear the heart sounds.

teledirigido *a. pp.* de **teledirigir**; *a.* remote controlled.

teléfono *m.* telephone; **llamar por** ___ , **telefonear** / to telephone.

telemetría *f.* telemetry, electronically transmitted data.

telencéfalo *m.* telencephalon, anterior portion of the prosencephalon.

teleopsia *f.* teleopsy, visual disorder by which close objects seem farther than they really are.

telepatia *f.* telepathy, apparent communication of thought by extrasensory means.

telerradiografía *f.* teleradiography, x-ray taken with the radiation source at a distance of about two meters or more from the subject to minimize distortion.

televisión *f.* television.

televisor *m.* television set.

telofase *f.* telophase, last phase of a process.

tembladera *f. pop.* the shakes.

temblar *v.* to quiver, to shiver.

temblor *m.* tremor, an involuntary quivering or trembling; ___ **alcohólico** / alcoholic ___; ___ **continuo** / continuous ___; ___ **de aleteo** / flapping ___; ___ **de reposo** / rest ___; ___ **de variaciones rápidas** / fine ___; ___ **esencial** / essential ___; ___ **fisiológico** / physiologic ___; ___ **intencional** / intentional ___; ___ **intermitente** / intermittent ___; ___ **lento y acentuado** / coarse ___; ___ **muscular** / muscular ___ .

temblores *m., pl. pop.* the shakes.

temer *v.* to fear, to dread.

temor *m.* fear, dread.

temperamento *m.* temperament, the combined physical, emotional, and mental constitution of an individual that distinguishes him or her from others.

temperatura *f.* temperature. 1. degree of heat or cold as measured on a specific scale; ___ **absoluta** / absolute ___; ___ **ambiente** / room ___; ___ **axilar** / axillary ___; ___ **crítica** / critical ___; ___ **del cuerpo** / body ___; ___ **máxima** / maximum ___; ___ **mínima** / minimum ___; ___ **normal** / normal ___; ___ **oral** / oral ___; ___ **rectal** / rectal ___; ___ **subnormal** / subnormal ___; 2. the natural degree of heat of a living body.

temple *m.* temper; character.

temporal *a.* 1. temporal, rel. to the temple; **huesos** ___ -es / ___ bones; **lóbulo** ___ / ___ lobe; **músculo** ___ / ___ muscle; 2. temporary, limited in time.

temporomandibular *a.* temporomandibular, rel. to or affecting the joint between the temporal bone and the mandible; **articulaciones** ___ -es / ___ joints.

temprano-a *a.* early.

tenáculo *m.* tenaculum, type of hook used in surg. to grasp or hold a part.

tenar *a.* thenar, rel. to the palm of the hand; **eminencia** ___ / ___ eminence; **músculos** ___ -es / ___ muscles.

tenaz *a.* tenacious, persistent, determined.

tenaza *f.* clamp, pincers.

tendencia *f.* tendency, propensity; trend.

tendinitis *f.* tendinitis, tendonitis, infl. of a tendon.

tendinoso-a *a.* tendinous, rel. to or resembling a tendon; **reflejo** ___ / tendon reflex; **reflejo profundo** / deep tendon reflex; **tirón** ___ / tendon jerk.

tendón *m.* tendon, sinew, highly resistant, fibrous tissue that attaches the muscles to the bones or to other parts; ___ -es de la corva / hamstring; ___ **de Aquiles** / Achilles ___ .

tenedor *m.* fork.

tener *vi.* to have, to possess; ___ **diez años** / to be ten years old; ___ **dolor** / to be in pain; ___ **ganas de** / to want to; ___ **hambre** / to be hungry; ___ **miedo** / to be afraid; ___ **que** / to have to; ___ **razón** / to be right; ___ **sed** / to be thirsty.

tenesmo *m.* tenesmus, continuously painful, ineffectual, and straining efforts to urinate or defecate.

tenia *f.* flatworm of the class *Cestoda* that in the adult stage lives in the intestines of vertebrates; *pop.* tapeworm.

teniasis *f.* taeniasis, infestation by taenia.

tenosinovitis *f.* tenosynovitis, infl. of a tendon sheath.

tensión *f.* tension, tenseness; 1. the act or effect of stretching or being extended; 2. the degree of stretching; 3. physical, emotional, or mental stress; ___ **premenstrual** / premenstrual ___; ___ **superficial** / surface ___; 4. the expansive pressure of a gas or vapor.

tenso-a *a.* tense, in a state of tension; rigid, stiff.

tensoactivo *m.* surfactant, an agent that modifies the surface tension of a liquid.

tensor *a.* tensor, term applied to any muscle that stretches or produces tension.

tentativo-a *a.* tentative, experimental, or subject to change.

tentorial *a.* tentorial, rel. to a tentorium.

tentorium *L.* tentorium, tentlike structure.

tenue *a.* tenuous, slight.

teñir *vi.* to dye; to color.

teoría *f.* theory. 1. an exposition of the principles of any science; 2. hypothesis that lacks scientific proof.

teórico-a *a.* theoretical, rel. to a theory.

terapeuta, terapista *m., f.* therapist, person skilled in giving or applying therapy in a given health field; ___ **fisico** / physical ___; ___ **patólogo-a del habla y del lenguage** / speech ___ .

terapéutica *f.* therapeutics, the branch of medicine that deals with treatments and remedies. ___ **electroconvulsiva** / electroconvulsive ___; ___ **endocrina** / endocrine ___; ___ **específica** / specific ___; ___ **experimental** / experimental ___; ___ **farmacológica** / pharmacological ___; ___ **hidrológica** / hydrologic ___; ___ **ocupacional** / occupational ___; ___ **química** / chemical ___; ___ **quirúrgica** / surgical ___; ___ **sustitutiva** / substitution ___ .

terapia, terapéutica *f.* therapy, the treatment of a disease. V. cuadro en esta pagina.

terapéutica por realidad *f.* reality therapy, method by which the patient is confronted with his or her real-life situation and helped to accept it as such.

terapéutico-a *a.* therapeutic. 1. rel. to therapy; **indicaciones** ___ **-s** / therapeutic ___-s; 2. that has healing properties.

Terapia, terapéutica	Therapy
anticoagulante	anticoagulant
biológica	biological
de conducta	behavioral
de grupo	group
de oxígeno	oxygen
diatérmica	diathermic
inespecífica	nonspecific
inmunosupresiva	immunosuppressive
ocupacional	occupational
por choque	shock
por inhalación	inhalation
por radiación	radiation
por sugestión	suggestion
respiratoria	respiratory
sustitutiva	substitutive

teratogénesis *f.* teratogenesis, the production of gross fetal abnormalities.

teratógeno *m.* teratogen, agent that causes teratogenesis.

teratoide *a.* teratoid, resembling a monster; **tumor** ___ / ___ tumor.

teratología *f.* teratology, the study of malformations in fetuses.

teratoma *m.* teratoma, neoplasm derived from more than one embryonic layer and therefore constituted by different types of tissues.

terciano-a *a.* tertian, that repeats itself every three days.

terco-a *a.* stubborn, obstinate; *pop.* hardheaded.

teres *L.* teres, term applied to describe some elongated, cylindrical muscles and ligaments.

termal *a.* thermal, thermic, rel. to heat or produced by it.

terminación *f.* ending; [*de un nervio*] twig.

terminal *a.* terminal, final.

terminar *v.* to terminate, to rescind.

término *m.* term. 1. a definite period of time or its completion, such as a pregnancy; 2. word.

terminología *f.* terminology, nomenclature.

termistor *m.* thermistor, a type of thermometer used for measuring minute changes of temperature.

termo *m.* thermos.

termocoagulación *f.* thermocoagulation, coagulation of tissue with high-frequency currents.

termodinámica *f.* thermodynamics, the science that studies the relationship between heat and other forms of energy.

termoesterilización *f.* thermosterilization, sterilization by heat.

termografía *f.* thermography, recording obtained by the use of a thermograph.

termógrafo *m.* thermograph, infrared detector that registers variations in temperature by reaction to the blood flow.

termómetro *m.* thermometer; device that measures heat or cold; ___ **clínico** / clinical ___; ___ **de Celsius** / Celsius ___ , centrigrade; ___ **de Fahrenheit** / Fahrenheit ___; ___ **de registro automático** / self-recording ___; ___ **rectal** / rectal ___ .

termonuclear *a.* thermonuclear.

termorregulación *f.* thermoregulation, regulation by heat and temperature.

termostato *m.* thermostat, instrument used for regulating temperature.

termotaxis *f.* thermotaxis. 1. regulation of the temperature of the body; 2. the reaction of an organism to heat.

termoterapia *f.* thermotherapy, therapeutic use of heat.

ternario-a *a.* ternary, triple, made up of three elements.

ternura *f.* tenderness, sensitivity.

Terramicina *f.* Terramycin, trade name for a tetracycline antibiotic.

terremoto *m.* earthquake.

terrible *a.* terrible.

terror *m.* terror; panic.

tesis *f.* thesis.

testamento *m.* testament, last will.

testarudo-a *a.* hardheaded, stubborn, headstrong.

testicular *m.* testicular, rel. to a testicle; **tumores** ___ **-es** / ___ tumors.

testículo *m.* testicle, the male gonad, one of the two male reproductive glands that produce spermatozoa and the hormone testosterone; ___ **ectópico** / ectopic ___ ; ___ **no descendido** / undescended testis.

testificar *vi.* to testify.

testigo *m., f.* to witness; ___ **experto especializado** / expert witness.

testis *L.* testis, (*pl. testes*) testicle.

testosterona *f.* testosterone, male hormone produced chiefly by the testicle and responsible for the development of male secondary characteristics such as facial hair and a deep voice; **implante de** ___ / ___ implant.

teta *f.* teat. 1. mammary gland; 2. nipple.

tetania *f.* tetany, a neuromuscular affliction associated with parathyroid deficiencies and diminished mineral balance, esp. calcium, and manifested by intermittent tonic spasms of the voluntary muscles.

tetánico-a *a.* tetanic, rel. to tetanus; **antitoxina** ___ / tetanus antitoxin; **convulsión** ___ / ___ convulsion; **toxoide** ___ / ___ toxoid;

tétano *m.* tetanus, an acute infectious disease caused by the toxin of the tetanus bacillus, gen. introduced in the body through a wound and manifested by muscular spasms and rigidity of the jaw, neck, and abdomen; *pop.* lockjaw; **globulina inmune para el** ___ / ___ immune globulin.

tetera, teto *f., m.* pacifier; nipple of a nursing bottle.

tetilla *f.* male nipple.

tetraciclina *f.* tetracycline, a type of broad-spectrum antibiotic effective against gram-positive and gram-negative bacteria, rickettsia, and a variety of viruses.

tétrada *f.* tetrad, a group of four similar elements.

tetralogía *f.* tetralogy, term applied to the combination of four factors or elements.

tetraplejía *f.* tetraplegia, paralysis of the four extremities.

tetraploide *a.* tetraploid, having four sets of chromosomes.

tetravalente *m.* tetravalent, element that has a chemical valance of four.

textura *f.* texture, the composition of a tissue or structure.

tez *f.* complexion.

thrill *m.* thrill, a vibration felt on palpation; ___ **aneurismal** / aneurysmal ___; ___ **aórtico** / aortic ___; ___ **arterial** / arterial ___; ___ **diastólico** / diastolic ___ .

tibia *f.* tibia, the inner and larger bone of the leg below the knee.

tibial *a.* tibial, rel. to or situated close to the tibia.

tibio-a *a.* tepid, lukewarm.

tic *Fr.* tic, spasmodic, involuntary movement or twitching of a muscle; ___ **convulsivo** / convulsive ___; ___ **coordinado** / coordinated ___; ___ **doloroso** / ___ douleureux; ___ **facial** / facial ___ .

tiempo *m.* 1. time, the duration of an event; **a** ___ / in ___; **a su debido** ___ / in due ___; **¿cuánto** ___ **?** / how long?; **espacio**

de ___ / ___ frame; **medir el** ___ / to ___ , to set the ___; **pérdida de** ___ / waste of ___; **por algún** ___ / for some ___; **regulador de** ___ / timer; ___ **de coagulación** / coagulation ___; ___ **de exposición** / exposure ___; ___ **de latencia** / ___ lag; ___ **de percepción** / perception ___; ___ **de protrombina** / prothrombin ___; ___ **de sangramiento** / bleeding ___; ___ **limitado** / a limited ___; ___ **medido** / timed; ___ **suplementario** / overtime; 2. weather; **hace buen** ___ / the ___ is good; **hace mal** ___ / the ___ is bad; **pronóstico del** ___ / ___ forecasting.

tiempo de trombina *m.* thrombin time, necessary length of time to form a fibrin clot after adding thrombin to the citrated plasma.

tienda *f.* tent, a cover or shelter made of fabric, gen. used to enclose the patient within a given area; ___ **de oxígeno** / oxygen ___ .;

tierno-a *a.* tender, sensitive.

tierra *f.* soil; earth.

tieso-a *a.* stiff, rigid.

tífico-a *a.* typhoid, rel. to typhus.

tiflitis *f.* typhlitis, infl. of the cecum.

tifoidea, fiebre *f.* typhoid fever, acute intestinal infection caused by a bacterium of the genus *Salmonella,* characterized by fever, prostration, headache, and abdominal pain.

tifus *m.* typhus, acute infectious disease caused by *rickettsia* with manifestations of high fever, delirium, prostration, and severe headache, gen. transmitted by lice, fleas, ticks, and mites.

tijeras *f., pl.* scissors.

tila, tilo *m.* tea made with linden flowers.

timectomía *f.* thymectomy, excision of the thymus.

tímico-a *a.* thymic, rel. to the thymus gland.

tímido-a *a.* timid, bashful, shy.

timo *m.* thymus, glandular organ situated in the inferior portion of the neck and the antero-superior portion of the thoracic cavity. It plays an important part in the immunological process of the body.

timocito *m.* thymocyte, a lymphocyte arising in the thymus.

timoma *m.* thymoma, tumor derived from the thymus.

timpanectomía *f.* tympanectomy, excision of the tympanic membrane.

timpánico-a *a.* tympanic, resonant or rel. to the tympanum; **membrana** ___ / ___ membrane.

timpanismo *m.* tympanites, distension of the abdomen caused by accumulation of gas in the intestine.

timpanítico-a *a.* tympanitic, rel. to or affected with tympanites; **resonancia** ___ / ___ resonance.

timpanitis *f.* tympanitis, infl. of the middle ear.

tímpano *m.* tympanum, the eardrum, middle ear.

timpanoplastia *f.* tympanoplasty, surgical correction of a damaged middle ear.

timpanotomía *f.* tympanotomy, incision of the tympanic membrane.

tina *f.* tub.

tinea *L.* tinea, cutaneous fungal infection in the form of a ring; ___ **capitis** / ___ capitis; ___ **corporis** / ___ corporis; ___ **pedis** / ___ pedis, athlete's foot; ___ **versicolor** ___ / versicolor.

tinnitus *L.* tinnitus, buzzing or ringing sound in the ears.

tinta *f.* ink.

tinte *m.* dye.

tintura *f.* tincture, an alcoholic extract of animal or vegetable origin.

tiña *f.* tinea, ringworm. tinea.

tío-a *m., f.* uncle; aunt.

típico-a *a.* typical; characteristic.

tipificación *f.* typing, determination by types; ___ **de tejido** / tissue ___; ___ **inmunológica** / immunotyping.

tipo *m.* type; kind, the general character of a given entity.

tira *f.* strap.

tirante *a.* tense, extended; pulling; stretched; [*relación*] strained.

tirar *v.* 1. to throw, to toss; to throw out; 2. to pull, to tug, as in tracheal tugging.

tiritar *v.* to shiver.

tiro *m.* shot from a firearm.

tiroadenitis *f.* thyroadenitis, inf. of the thyroid gland.

tiroglobulina *f.* thyroglobulin. 1. a glycoprotein secreted by the thyroid gland; 2. a substance obtained by the fractioning of the thyroid gland of the hog, used in the treatment of hyperthyroidism.

tirogloso-a *a.* thyroglossal, rel. to the thyroid and the tongue; **conducto** ___ / ___ duct.

tiroidea *a.* thyroid related; **hormona estimulante** ___ / thyroid stimulating hormone.

tiroidectomía *f.* thyroidectomy, excision of the thyroid gland.

tiroideo-a *a.* thyroid, rel. to the thyroid gland; **cartílago** ___ / ___ cartilage; **crisis** ___ / ___ storm; **hormonas** ___ -s / ___ hormones.

tiroides, glándula *f.* thyroid gland, one of the endocrine glands situated in the front part of the trachea and made up of two lateral lobules that connect in the middle; **prueba del funcionamiento de la** ___ / thyroid function test.

tiroiditis *f.* thyroiditis, infl. of the thyroid gland.

tiromegalia *f.* thyromegaly, enlargement of the thyroid gland.

tirón *m.* forceful pull; tugging.

tiroparatiroidectomía *f.* thyroparathyroidectomy, excision of the thyroid and parathyroid glands.

tirotóxico-a *a.* thyrotoxic, rel. to or affected by toxic activity of the thyroid gland.

tirotoxicosis *f.* thyrotoxicosis, disorder caused by hyperthyroidism and marked by an enlargement of the thyroid gland, increased metabolic rate, tachycardia, rapid pulse, and hypertension.

tirotropina *f.* thyrotropin, thyroid-stimulating hormone produced in the anterior lobe of the pituitary gland; **hormona estimulante de la** ___ / ___ -releasing hormone.

tiroxina *f.* thyroxine, iodine containing hormone produced by the thyroid gland, also obtained synthetically for use in the treatment of hypothyroidism.

titulación *f.* titration, determination of volume using standard solutions of known strength.

titular *v.* to titrate, to determine by titration.

título *m.* titer, titre, the required amount of a substance to produce a reaction with a given volume of another substance.

toalla *f.* towel.

tobillera *f.* ankle brace.

tobillo *m.* ankle.

tocar *vi.* to touch, to palpate.

tocino *m.* bacon.

tocógrafo *m.* tocograph, device used to estimate and record the force of uterine contractions.

tocómetro *m.* tocometer.

todavía *adv.* still, yet.

todo-a *a.* all, entire; **ante** ___ / above all; ___ **el día** / the whole day; ___ **-s los días** / every day; ___ **-s los meses** / every month.

tofáceo-a *a.* tophaceous, rel. to a tophus or of a gritty nature.

tofo *m.* tophus. 1. deposits of urates in tissues as seen in gout; 2. dental calculus.

toilette *Fr.* toilette, cleansing, as related to a medical procedure.

tolerable *a.* tolerable, bearable.

tolerancia *f.* tolerance, the ability to endure the use of a medication or performance of a given amount of physical activity without ill effects.

tolerante *a.* tolerant.

tolerar *v.* to tolerate, to endure.

tomar *v.* to take; to eat or drink.

tomate *m.* tomato.

tomografía *f.* tomography, scan, diagnostic technique by which a series of x-ray pictures taken at different depths of an organ are obtained; ___ **axial computada** / computed ___; ___ **axial computarizada** / computerized axial ___; ___ **computada** / computed ___; ___ **computada de alta resolución** / high-resolution computed ___; ___ **computada dinámica auricular** / atrial bolus dynamic computerized ___; ___ **con rayos de electrón** / electron beam ___; ___ **convencional** / conventional ___; ___ **de emisión de positron** / positron emission ___; ___ **dinámica computada** / dynamic computed ___; ___ **magnética nuclear de resonancia** / nuclear magnetic resonance ___ .

tomógrafo *m.* tomograph, x-ray machine used in tomography.

tomograma *m.* tomogram, sectional x-ray of a part of the body.

tonicidad *f.* tonicity, normal quality of tone or tension.

tónico *m.* tonic, medication for restoring tone and vitality; **-a** *a.* 1. that restores the normal tone; 2. characterized by continuous tension.

tono *m.* tone; pitch. 1. the quality of the body with its organs and parts in a normal and balanced state; ___ **muscular** / muscle ___; 2. a particular quality of sound or voice.

tonoclónico-a *a.* tonoclonic, rel. to muscular spasms that are both tonic and clonic.

tonometría *f.* tonometry, the measurement of tension or pressure.

tonómetro *m.* tonometer, instrument that measures tone, esp. intraocular tension.

tonsila *f.* tonsil; ___ **cerebelosa** / cerebellar ___; ___ **faríngea** / pharyngeal ___; ___ **lingual** / lingual ___; ___ **palatina** / palatine ___ .

tonsilar *a.* tonsillar, rel. to a tonsil; **cripta**___ **o amigdalina** / ___ crypt ; **fosa** ___ / ___ fossa.

tonsilectomía *f.* tonsillectomy. amigdalotomía.

tonsilitis *f.* tonsillitis. amigdalitis.

tonsiloadenoidectomía *f.* tonsilloadenoidectomy, excision of the tonsils and adenoids.

tonto-a *a.* foolish, fatuous.

tonus *L.* tonus, tone.

tópico-a *a.* topical, rel. to a specific area.

toracentesis *f.* thoracentesis, surgical puncture and drainage of the thoracic cavity.

torácico-a *a.* thoracic, rel. to the thorax; **cavidad** ___ / ___ cavity; **conducto** ___ / ___ duct; **pared** ___ / ___ cage, chest wall, osseous structure enclosing the thorax.**traumatismos** ___ -s / ___ injuries.

toracicoabdominal *a.* thoracicoabdominal, rel. to the thorax and the abdomen.

Toracina *f.* Thorazine, antiemetic sedative.

toracolumbar *a.* thoracolumbar, rel. to the thoracic and lumbar vertebrae.

toracoplastia *f.* thoracoplasty, plastic surgery of the thorax that consists in removing a portion of the ribs to allow the collapse of a diseased lung.

toracostomía *f.* thoracostomy, incision of the chest wall to allow for drainage.

toracotomía *f.* thoracotomy, incision of the thoracic wall.

tórax *m.* thorax, the chest; ___ **inestable** / flail chest, condition of the wall of the thorax caused by multiple fracture of the ribs.

torcedura *f.* strain, sprain, warp, twisting of a joint with distension and laceration of its ligaments, usu. accompanied by pain and swelling.

torcer *vi.* to twist, to strain, to curve, to warp; **torcerse** *vr.* to sprain.

torcido-a *a.* twisted, sprained.

tormenta *f.* storm, abrupt and temporary intensification of the symptoms of a disease.

tormento *a.* torment.

tornillo *m.* screw.

torniquete *m.* tourniquet, tourniquette, device used to apply pressure over an artery to stop the flow of blood.

toronja *f.* grapefruit.

torpe *a.* dull, clumsy, slow.

torpeza *f.* dullness; clumsiness.

tórpido-a *a.* torpid, sluggish, slow.

torpor *m.* sluggishness, cloudiness; ___ **mental** / clouding of consciousness.

torque *m.* torque, a force that produces rotation.

torsión *f.* torsion, twisting or rotating of a part on its long axis; ___ **ovárica** / ovarian ___; ___ **testicular** / testicular ___ .

torso *m.* torso, trunk of the body.

tortícolis *f.* torticollis, toniclonic spasm of the muscles of the neck that causes cervical torsion and immobility of the head.

tortuoso-a *a.* tortuous, twisted.

tortura *f.* torture.

torus *L.* torus, (*pl. tori*) prominence, swelling.

tos *f.* cough; **ataque de** ___ / coughing spell; **calmante para la** ___ / ___ suppressant; **jarabe para la** ___ / ___ syrup; **pastillas para la** ___ / lozenges; ___ **metálica, bronca** / brassy ___; ___ **seca recurrente** / hacking ___ .

tos ferina *f.* pertussis, whooping cough, infectious children's disease that gen. begins with a cold followed by a persistent dry cough.

tosecilla *f.* slight cough.

toser *v.* to cough.

tostada *f.* toast.

tostado-a *a.* toasted; **pan** ___ / toast.

total *a.* total, whole; **mente** *adv.* totally.

totipotencia *f.* totipotency, ability of a cell to regenerate or develop into another type of cell.

totipotente *a.* totipotent, that can generate totipotency.

toxemia *f.* toxemia, generalized intoxication due to absorption of toxins formed at a local source of infection.

toxicidad *f.* toxicity, the quality of being poisonous.

tóxico-a *a.* toxic, rel. to a poison or of a poisonous nature.

toxicología *f.* toxicology, the study of poisons and their effects and treatment.

toxicológico-a *a.* toxicological, rel. to toxicology; **protocolo** ___ / toxicology screen.

toxicólogo-a *m., f.* toxicologist, a specialist in toxicology.

toxicosis *f.* toxicosis, morbid state caused by a poison.

toxina *f.* toxin, a noxious substance produced by a plant or animal microorganism; ___ **bacteriana** / bacterial ___ .

toxina antitoxina *f.* toxin-antitoxin, a nearly neutral mixture of a toxin and its antitoxin used for immunization against the specific disease caused by the toxin.

toxoide *m.* toxoid, a toxin void of toxicity that causes antibody formation and produces immunity to the specific disease caused by the toxin; ___ **diftérico** / diphtheria ___; ___ **tetánico** / tetanus ___ .

Toxoplasma *m. Toxoplasma,* a genus of parasitic protozoa; **anticuerpo del** ___ / ___ antibody; ___ **serológico** / serologic ___ .

toxoplasmosis *f.* toxoplasmosis, infection with organisms of the genus Toxoplasma that can cause minimal symptoms of malaise or swelling of the lymph glands, or serious damage to the central nervous system.

trabajador-a *m., f.* worker; ___ **social** / social ___ .

trabajar *v.* to work, to labor.

trabajo *m.* work, job, occupation; ___ **de beneficencia social** / welfare ___; ___ **de casa** / housework; ___ **excesivo** / overwork.

trabajoso-a *a.* laborious, hard.

trabécula *f.* trabecula, term used to designate a supporting structure of connective tissue that divides or secures an organ.

trabeculado-a *a.* trabeculate, having trabeculae.

tracción *f.* traction. 1. the action of drawing or pulling; 2. a pulling force; ___ **cervical** / cervical ___; ___ **lumbar** / lumbar ___ .

tracoma *f.* trachoma, a viral contagious disease of the conjunctiva and the cornea, manifested by photophobia, pain, tearing, and, in severe cases, blindness.

tracto *m.* tract, an elongated system of tissue or organs that acts to carry out a common function; ___ **alimenticio** / alimentary ___; ___ **dorsolateral** / dorsolateral ___; ___ **genitourinario** / genitourinary ___; ___ **intestinal** / intestinal ___; ___ **respiratorio** / respiratory ___ .

tractor *m.* tractor, any instrument or machine used to apply traction.

traducción *f.* translation.

traer *vi.* to bring; to fetch.

tragar *vi.* to swallow; ___ **apresuradamente** / to gulp down.

trago *m.* tragus, triangular cartilaginous eminence in the outer part of the ear.

traicionero-a *a.* deceitful, treacherous; **enfermedad** ___ / ___ disease.

trance *m.* trance, hypnotic-like state characterized by detachment from the surroundings and diminished motor activity.

tranquilidad *f.* tranquility, rest; ___ **de espíritu** / peace of mind.

tranquilizante *m.* tranquilizer, sedative.

tranquilizar *vi.* to tranquilize, to calm; **tranquilizarse** *vr.* to quiet down; to ease one's mind.

tranquilo-a *a.* tranquil, calm, restful.

transabdominal *a.* transabdominal, through or across the abdominal wall.

transaminasa glutámica oxalacética *f.* glutamic-oxaloacetic transaminase, enzyme present in several tissues, such as the heart, liver, and brain, that presents a high concentration of serum when there is cardiac or hepatic damage.

transaminasa glutámica pirúvica *f.* glutamicpyruvic transaminase, enzyme that presents an elevated serum content when there is an injury or acute damage to liver cells.

transaxial *a.* transaxial, through or across the long axis of a structure.

transcapilar *a.* transcapillary, existing or taking place across the capillary walls.

transcurrir *v.* to elapse; [*tiempo*] to go by.

transcutáneo-a *a.* transcutaneous, through the skin; **neuroestimulación eléctrica** ___ / ___ electrical nerve stimulation.

transductor *a.* transducer, device that transforms one form of energy to another.

transección *f.* transection, cross section, cutting across the long axis of an organ.

transexual *a.* transexual. 1. individual with a psychological urge to be of the opposite sex; 2. person who has undergone a ical sex change.

transferencia *f.* transfer, transference.1. in psychoanalysis, shifting feelings and behavior towards a new object, gen. the psychoanalyst;2. transmission of symptoms from one part of the body to another.

transferir *vi.* to transfer.

transferrina *f.* transferrin, a type of beta globulin in blood plasma that fixes and transports iron.

transfixión *f.* transfixion, the act of cutting through soft tissues from the inside outwards, such as in amputations and excision of tumors.

transformación *f.* transformation, change of form or appearance.

transformar *v.* to transform, to change the appearance, character, or structure of something or someone.

transfusión *f.* transfusion, the process of transferring fluid into a vein or artery; ___ **directa** / direct ___; ___ **indirecta** / indirect ___ .

transición *f.* transition.

transicional *a.* transitional, rel. to or subject to change.

transiluminación *f.* transillumination, passage of light through a body part.

transitorio-a *a.* transitory, of a temporal nature.

translocación *f.* translocation, displacement of all or part of a chromosome to another chromosome.

translúcido-a *a.* translucent.

transmigración *f.* transmigration, the passing from one place to another such as of blood cells in diapedesis.

transmisible *a.* transmissible, that can be transmitted.

transmisión *f.* transmission, the act of transmitting, such as an infectious disease or a hereditary condition; ___ **patógena /** pathogen ___; ___ **placentaria /** placental ___; ___ **por contacto /** ___ by contact; ___ **por instilación /** droplet ___ .

transmisor *m.* transmitter.

transmural *a.* transmural, that occurs or is administered through a wall.

transmutación *f.* transmutation. 1. transformation, evolutionary change; 2. change of one chemical into another.

transocular *a.* transocular, occurring or passing through the orbit of the eye.

transonancia *f.* transonance, transmitted resonance.

transorbitorio-a *a.* transorbital, occurring or passing through the orbit of the eye.

transparencia *f.* transparency; [*diapositiva*] slide.

transparente *a.* transparent, clear.

transplacentario-a *a.* transplacental, occurring through the placenta.

transpleural *a.* transpleural, occurring or administered through the pleura.

transporte *m.* transport, the movement of materials within the body, esp. across the cellular membrane.

transposición *f.* transposition. 1. displacement of an organ to the opposite side; 2. displacement of genetic material from one chromosome to another resulting at times in congenital defects.

transposición de los grandes vasos *f.* transposition of great vessels, congenital defect by which the aorta rises from the right ventricle and the pulmonary artery from the left ventricle.

transuretral *a.* transurethral, occurring or administered through the urethra.

transvaginal *a.* transvaginal, occurring or done through the vagina.

transversal *a.* transverse, across; **plano** ___ / ___ plane.

transverso-a *a.* transverse; **colon** ___ / ___ colon.

transvestido-a, transvestita *m., f.* transvestite, person who practices transvestism.

transvestismo *m.* transvestism, adoption of modalities of the opposite sex, esp. dress; cross-dressing.

trapecio *m.* trapezius, flat, triangular muscle essential in the rotation of the scapula.

tráquea *f.* trachea, respiratory conduit between the inferior extremity of the larynx and the beginning of the bronchi;*pop.* windpipe.

traqueal *a.* tracheal, rel. to the trachea.

traqueítis *f.* tracheitis, infl. of the trachea.

traqueoesofágico-a *a.* tracheoesophageal, rel. to the trachea and the esophagus.

traqueomalacia *f.* tracheomalacia, softening of the cartilages of the trachea.

traqueostenosis *f.* tracheostenosis, narrowing of the trachea.

traqueostomía *f.* tracheostomy, incision into the trachea through the neck to allow the passage of air in cases of obstruction.

traqueotomía *f.* tracheotomy, incision into the trachea through the skin and muscles of the neck.

tras *prep.* after, behind.

trasero *m. pop.* buttocks, rear.

trasmitir *v.* to transmit.

trasplantación *f.* transplantation, the act of transplanting; ___ **autoplástica /** autoplastic ___; ___ **heteroplastíca /** heteroplastic ___; ___ **homotópica /** homotopic ___ .

trasplantar *v.* to transplant.

trasplante *m.* transplant, the transfer of an organ or tissue from a donor to a recipient, or from one part of the body to another in order to replace a diseased organ or to restitute impaired function.

trasplante de médula ósea *m.* bone marrow transplantation, grafting of bone marrow tissue to cancer patients after an extenuating degree of chemotherapy, or to patients suffering from aplastic anemia or severe leukemia.

trasplante de órgano *m.* organ transplantation.

trasplante cardíaco *m.* heart transplantation.

trasplante hepático *m.* liver transplantation

trastornado-a *a.* deranged, mentally disturbed.

trastorno *m.* disturbance, disorder, derangement; ___ **del procesor metabólico /** deranged metabolic process; ___ **mental /** mental disorder. V. cuadro en la pagina 252.

trasudado *m.* transudate, fluid that has passed through a membrane or that has been forced out from a tissue as a result of infl.

tratado-a *a.* treated; **no** ___ / untreated;

tratamiento *m.* treatment, method, or procedure used in curing illnesses, lesions, or malformations; **método o plan de** ___ / ___ plan; **sujeto a** ___ / **under** ___ **de desintoxicación /** withdrawal ___ .

tratar *v.* [a un paciente] to treat; to try.

trato *m.* care; treatment; **buen** ___ / good ___; **mal** ___ / bad ___ .

Trastornos de la personalidad ejemplos	Personality disorders examples
trastorno de:	**disorder:**
__ ansiedad depresión aguda	anxiety __ acute depression
__ dependencia de adicción: dependencia en las drogas	addiction dependency__ drug dependence
__ de ajuste personalidad antisocial	adjustment__ antisocial personality
__ ciclotímico de cambios emocionales cíclicos	cyclothymic__ cyclic mood swings
__ de deglución bulimia, deglución excesiva	eating __ bulimia, binge eating
__de fobias miedo a las alturas	phobias __ fear of heights
__de cambios emocionales ataques de llanto	mood change __ crying attacks
__ de pánico miedo anormal a la oscuridad	panic__ abnormal fear of darkness
__ de falta de atención impulsividad, falta de concentración	attention deficit __ impulsivity, lack of concentration

trauma, traumatismo *m.* 1. trauma, a psychological state; **Una muerte en la familia es un trauma familiar.** / A death in the family is a trauma; 2. traumatismo, refering to a physiological condition; **Un golpe en la cabeza es un traumatismo cerebral ___** / A blow to the head is cerebral trauma;

traumático-a *a.* traumatic, rel. to, resulting from, or causing trauma.

traumatizado-a *a.* traumatized.

traumatizante *a.* traumatising, rel. to a phychological situation.

traumatizar *vi.* to traumatize, to injure.

traumatología *f.* traumatology, the branch of surg. that deals with injuries and wounds and their treatment.

travestido *m.* transvestite.

trazador *m.* tracer, a radioisotope that when introduced into the body leaves a trace that can be detected and followed.

trazar *vi.* to trace.

trazo *m.* tracing, the graphic record of movement or change made by an instrument.

trefinación *f.* trephination, the act of removing a circular disk of bone, gen. from the skull, or of removing tissue from the cornea or sclera.

Trematoda *Gr. Trematoda*, a class of parasitic worms that includes the flatworms and the flukes, both pathogenic to humans.

tremendo-a *a.* tremendous.

tremor *m.* tremor, trembling.

trémulo-a *a.* tremulous, rel. to or affected by a tremor.

Trendelenburg, posición de *f.* Trendelenburg position, slanted position used in abdominal surgery in which the body and lower extremities are placed higher than the head.

trepanación *f.* trepanation, perforation of the skull with a special instrument to relieve increased pressure caused by fracture or accumulation of intracranial blood or pus.

trepanar *v.* to trepan, to perforate with a trepan.

trépano *m.* trepan, bur, burr, type of drill used for trepanation.

Treponema *Gr. Treponema*, microorganisms of the genus Spirochaetales, some of which are pathogenic to humans and other animals; ___ **pallidum** / ___ pallidum, causing agent of syphilis.

treponema *m.* treponema, any organism of the genus Treponema.

treponemiasis *f.* treponemiasis, infection with organisms of the genus Treponema.

tríada *f.* triad, a group of three related elements, objects, or symptoms.

triage *Fr.* triage, screening and classification of injured persons during a battle or disaster for the purpose of establishing priority of treatment in order to maximize the number who will survive.

triangular *a.* triangular

triángulo *m.* triangle.

tribu *f.* tribe.

tríceps *m.* triceps, a three-headed muscle; **reflejo del** ___ / ___ reflex.

Trichinella *Gr. Trichinella* a genus of nematode worms parasitic in carnivorous mammals.

Trichomonas *Gr.tricomonas m. Trichomonas*, a genus of parasitic protozoa that lodge in the alimentary and genitourinary tracts of vertebrates; ___ **vaginal** / ___ vaginalis.

tricobezoar *m.* trichobezoar, concretion or bezoar of hair found in the intestine or stomach.

tricomonas *m. Trichomonas*

tricomoniasis *f.* trichomoniasis, infestation with *Trichomonas.*

tricromático-a *a.* trichromatic, rel. to or consisting of three colors.

tricúspide *a.* tricuspid.1. having three points;2. rel. to the tricuspid valve of the heart; **atresia** ___ / ___ atresia; **soplo** ___ / ___ murmur; **válvula** ___ / ___ valve.

trifásico-a *a.* triphasic, occurring in three stages, esp. in relation to electric currents.

trifocal *a.* trifocal.

trigémino-a *a.* trigeminal, rel. to the trigeminus nerve; **neuralgia** ___ / ___ neuralgia.

trigeminus *L.* trigeminus, trigeminus nerve. craneales, nervios.

triglicéridos *m. triglycerides* combination resulting from one molecule of glycerol and three molecules of fatty acids; elevated triglycerides are considered an important factor in heart disease.

trigo *m.* wheat; **germen de** ___ / ___ germ.

trigonitis *f.* trigonitis, infl. of the trigone of the urinary bladder.

trígono *m.* trigone, space or area in a triangular shape.

trigueño-a *a.* dark-complexioned, brunet, brunette.

trimestre *m.* trimester, three-month period.

trinchera *f.* trench, ditch, moat; **fiebre de** ___ / ___ fever; **pie de** ___ / ___ foot, infection caused by exposure to severe cold;

tripa *f.* tripe, gut.

tripanosomiasis *f.* trypanosomiasis, infection caused by a flagellated organism of the genus Trypanosoma.

tripanosómico-a *a.* trypanosomal, caused by or belonging to the genus Trypanosoma.

triple *a.* triple, consisting of three components.

triplopia *f.* triplopia, eye disorder in which three images of the same object are seen at one time.

tripsina *f.* trypsin, an enzyme present in the pancreatic juice formed by trypsinogen.

tripsinógeno *m.* trypsinogen, inactive substance released by the pancreas into the duodenum to form trypsin.

triptófano *m.* tryptophan, crystalline amino acid present in proteins essential to animal life.

triquina *f.* trichina, a worm that lives as a parasite in the muscles in the larval stage, and in the intestines when mature.

triquinosis *f.* trichinosis, disease acquired by ingestion of raw or inadequately cooked meat, esp. pork, that contains the larvae of Trichinella spiralis.

triquitis *f.* trichitis, infl. of hair bulbs.

trismo *m.* trismus, a spasm of the mastication muscles.

trisomía *f.* trisomy, genetic disorder in which there are three homologous chromosomes per cell instead of the usual two (diploid), causing severe fetal malformation.

triste *a.* sad, sorrowful.

tristeza *f.* sadness; sorrow.

trituración *f.* trituration; pulverization.

triturar *v.* to triturate, to crush, to grind; to shatter in many small fragments.

triunfar *v.* to succeed.

triunfo *m.* success, triumph.

trocánter *m.* trochanter, each of the two outer prominences below the neck of the femur; ___ **mayor** / major ___; ___ **menor** / lesser ___ .

tróclea *f.* trochlea, structure that functions as a pulley.

trófico-a *a.* trophic, rel. to nutrition.

trombectomía *f.* thrombectomy, removal of a thrombus.

trombina *f.* thrombin, an enzyme present in extravasated blood which catalyzes the conversion of fibrinogen to fibrin.

trombinógeno *m.* thrombinogen.protrombina.

trombo *m.* thrombus, a blood clot that causes a total or partial vascular obstruction; ___ **blanco** / white ___ , pale; ___ **estratificado** / stratified ___ , layered; ___ **mural** / mural ___ , attached to the wall of the endocardium; ___ **oclusivo** / occluding ___ , that closes the vessel completely.

tromboangiítis *f.* thromboangiitis, thrombosis of a blood vessel.

trombocito *m.* thrombocyte, platelet.

trombocitopenia *f.* thrombocytopenia, abnormal decrease in the number of blood platelets.

trombocitopénico-a *a.* thrombocytopenic, rel. to thrombocytopenia.

trombocitosis *f.* thrombocytosis, abnormal increase in the number of blood platelets.

tromboembolia *f.* thromboembolism, obstruction of a blood vessel by a blood clot that has broken away from its site of origin.

tromboflebitis *f.* thrombophlebitis, dilation of a vein wall associated with thrombosis.

tromboflebitis migratoria *f.* thrombophlebitis migrans, slowly progressing thrombophlebitis moving from one vein to another.

trombogénesis *f.* thrombogenesis, formation of blood clots.

trombólisis *f.* thrombolysis, dissolution of a thrombus.

trombolítico-a *a.* thrombolytic, rel. to or causing the dissolution of a thrombus.

trombosado-a *a.* thrombosed, rel. to a blood vessel containing a thrombus.

trombosis *f.* thrombosis, formation, development, or presence of a thrombus; ___ **biliar** / biliary ___; ___ **cardíaca** / cardiac ___; ___ **coronaria** / coronary ___; ___ **embólica** / embolic ___; ___ **traumática** / traumatic ___; ___ **venosa** / venous ___ .

trombótico-a *a.* thrombotic, rel. to or affected by thrombosis.

trompa *f.* tube, conduit; **ligadura de las** ___ **-s** / tubal ligation;

troncal *a.* truncal, rel. to the trunk of the body.

tronco *m.* trunk, the human body exclusive of the head and the extremities.

tropezar *vi.* to bump or stumble into something or somebody.

tropical *a.* tropical, rel. to the tropics.

tropismo *m.* tropism, the reaction of a cell or living organism toward or away from the source of an external stimulus.

truncado-a *a.* truncate, having the end squarely cut off; amputated.

truncar *vi.* to truncate, to cut off, to shorten; to amputate.

truncus *L.* truncus, trunk.

Trypanosoma *m.* *Trypanosoma*, a genus of parasitic protozoa found in the blood of many vertebrates, transmitted to them by insect vectors.

tsetsé *m.* tsetse fly, bloodsucking fly of southern Africa that transmits sleeping sickness.

tuba *L.* tuba, tube; ___ **acústica** / eustachian tube.

tubárico-a *a.* tubal, rel. to a tube; **embarazo** ___ / ___ pregnancy occurring in the fallopian tube.

tuber *L.* *tuber*tuber, enlargement.

tubercular *a.* tubercular, rel. to or marked by tubercles.

tuberculicida *a.* tuberculocidal, that destroys the tubercle bacilli.

tuberculina *f.* tuberculin, compound prepared from the tubercle bacillus and used in the diagnosis of tuberculosis infection; **prueba de la** ___ / ___ test.

tubérculo *m.* tubercle.1. small nodule;2. small knobby prominence of a bone;3. the characteristic lesion produced by the tuberculosis bacilli.

tuberculosis *f.* tuberculosis, an acute or chronic bacterial infection caused by the germ *Mycobacterium tuberculosis* that gen. affects the lungs, although it can affect other organs as well; ___ **espinal** / spinal ___; ___ **infantil** / childhood ___; ___ **meníngea** / meningeal ___; ___ **pulmonar** / pulmonary ___; ___ **urogenital** / urogenital ___ .

tuberculosis miliar *f.* miliary tuberculosis, disease that invades the organism through the bloodstream and is characterized by the formation of minute tubercles in the different organs affected by it.

tuberculoso-a *a.* tuberculous, rel. to or affected by tuberculosis.

tuberculum *L.* tuberculum, tubercle.

tuberosidad *f.* tuber, a swelling or enlargement.

tuberoso-a *a.* tuberous, rel. to or resembling a tuber.

tubo *m.* tube, elongated, cylindrical, hollow structure; ___ **colector** / collecting tubule; ___ **contorneado del riñón** / convoluted tubule of the kidney; ___ **de drenaje** / drainage ___; ___ **de ensayo** / test ___; ___ **de inhalación** / inhalation ___; ___ **de toracostomía** / thoracostomy ___; ___ **de traqueotomía** / tracheotomy ___; ___ **endotraqueal** / endotracheal ___; ___ **en T** / T- ___; ___ **nasogástrico** / nasogastric ___; ___ **urinífero** / uriniferous tubule.

tubo-ovaritis *f.* tubo-ovaritis, infl. of the ovary and the Fallopian tube.

tuboovárico-a *a.* tubo-ovarian, rel. to the fallopian tube and the ovary; **absceso** ___ / ___ abscess.

tuboplastia *f.* tuboplasty, plastic surgery of a tube, esp. the fallopian tube.

túbulo *m.* tubule, a small anatomical tube; ___
  colector / collecting ___; ___ **renal** / renal ___ .
tuerto-a *a.* one-eyed or blind in one eye.
tularemia *f.* tularemia, rabbit fever, infection
  transmitted to humans by the bite of a vector
  insect or by handling of infected meat.
tumefacción, tumescencia *f.* tumefaction,
  the process of swelling.
tumor *m.* tumor, swelling, new spontaneous
  growth of mass or tissue of no physiological
  use; ___ **desdiferenciado** /
  undifferentiated ___; ___ **difundido o difuso** /
  diffuse ___; ___ **escirroso** / scirrhous ___; ___
  inflamatorio / inflammatory ___; ___ **medular** /
  medullary ___; ___ **necrótico** /
  necrotic ___; ___ **no solido** / nonsolid ___; ___
  radiocurable / radiocurable ___; ___
  radiorresistente / radioresistant ___; ___
  radiosensitivo / radiosensitive ___; ___ **sin**
  diferenciación / undifferentiated ___ .
tumoral *a.* tumorous, rel. to a tumor.
tumorectomía *f.* lumpectomy, excision of a
  breast tumor excluding lymph nodes and
  adjacent tissue.
tumoricida *a.* tumoricidal, that destroys
  tumorous cells.
tumorigénesis *f.* tumorigenesis, production of
  tumors.

túnel *m.* tunnel, a bodily channel; ___ **del carpo** /
  carpal ___; ___ **flexor** / flexor ___; ___ **torsal,**
  tarsiano / torsal ___ .
túnica *L.* tunica, tunic, protective membrane; ___
  adventicia / ___ adventitia; ___ **albugínea** / ___
  albuginea; ___ **dartos** / ___ dartos; ___
  mucosa / ___ mucosa; ___ **muscular** / ___
  muscularis; ___ **serosa** / ___ serosa; ___
  vaginal / ___ vaginalis.
túnica *f.* tunic, covering, outer layer of an organ
  or part.
tupido-a *a.* plugged, obstructed; **oídos** ___ / ___
  ears.
turbinado-a *a.* turbinate. 1. rel. to the nasal
  concha; 2. shaped like a dome.
turbio-a *a.* turbid, cloudy, not translucent.
turgido-a *a.* turgid, distended, swollen.
turgor *m.* turgor. 1. swelling, distension; 2.
  normal cellular tension.
Turner, sindrome de *m.* Turner's syndrome,
  congenital endocrine abnormality manifested by
  amenorrhea, failure of sexual maturation, short
  stature and neck, and the presence of only forty-
  five chromosomes.
turno *m.* turn; [*cita*] appointment; shift.
tusivo-a *a.* tussive, rel. to cough or caused by it.
tussis *L.* tussis, cough.
tympanum *L.* tympanum, the middle ear.
  tímpano.

u

U *abr.* **unidad** / unit; **uranio** / uranium; **urología** / urology.

u *conj.* or, used instead of *o* before words beginning with *o* or *ho*.

ubre *f.* udder, mammary gland of female animals, such as cows.

úlcera *f.* ulcer, sore, or lesion of the skin or mucous membrane with gradual disintegration of tissue; ___ **chancroide** / chancroidal; ___ **crónica** / chronic ___; ___ **duodenal** / duodenal ___; ___ **fagedénica** / phagedenic ___; ___ **gástrica** / gastric ___; ___ **hemorrágica** / hemorrhagic ___; ___ **indolente** / indolent ___; ___ **marginal** / marginal ___; ___ **micótica** / mycotic ___; ___ **péptica** / peptic ___ ; ___ **perforante** / perforating ___; ___ **por decúbito** / decubitus ___ , bedsore; ___ **roedora** / rodent ___ , that destroys gradually; ___ **sifilítica** / syphilitic ___; ___ **varicosa crónica de la pierna** / chronic varicose leg ___; ___ **vesical** / vesical ___ .

úlcera péptica *f.* peptic ulcer, ulceration of the mucous membranes of the esophagus, stomach, or duodenum caused by excessive acidity of the gastric juice, gen. produced by acute or chronic stress.

ulceración *f.* ulceration, the formation process of an ulcer; **-es genitales** / genital ___ -s.

ulcerado-a *a.* ulcerated, rel. to or of the nature of an ulcer.

ulcerar *v.* to ulcerate.

ulcerativo *a.* ulcerative, rel. to or causing an ulcer.

ulceroso-a *a.* ulcerous, rel. to or affected by an ulcer.

uleritema *m.* ulerythema, erythematous dermatitis characterized by formation of scars.

ulitis *f.* ulitis. gingivitis.

ulnar *a.* ulnar, rel. to the ulna or to the arteries and nerves related to it; **disfunción del nervio** ___ / ___ nerve dysfunction.

ulocarcinoma *m.* ulocarcinoma, cancer of the gums.

último-a *a.* last, ultimate, final; **-mente** *adv.* lately; **por** ___ / finally.

ultracentrífuga *f.* ultracentrifuge, machine with a centrifugal force capable of separating and sedimenting the molecules of a substance.

ultraestructura *f.* ultrastructure, structure of the smallest elements of a body, visible only through an electron microscope.

ultrafiltración *f.* ultrafiltration, a filtration process that allows the passage of small molecules, holding back larger ones.

ultramicroscopio *m.* ultramicroscope, a microscope that makes visible objects that cannot be seen under a common light microscope.

ultrasónico-a *a.* ultrasonic.supersónico-a.

ultrasonido *m.* ultrasound, a sound wave with a frequency above the range of human hearing used in ultrasonography for diagnostic and therapeutic purposes;**diagnóstico por** ___ / ultrasonic diagnosis; ___ **abdominal** / abdominal ___; ___ **de la mama** / breast ___; ___ **de la tiroides** / thyroid ___; ___ **del embarazo** / pregnancy ___ .

ultrasonografía *f.* ultrasonography, diagnostic technique that uses ultrasound waves to develop the image of a structure or tissue of the body.

ultrasonograma *m.* ultrasonogram, the image produced by ultrasonography.

ultravioleta *a.* ultraviolet, beyond the visible, violet end of the spectrum; **rayos** ___ / ___ rays; **terapia de radiación** ___ / ___ therapy.

ululación *f.* ululation, the act of screaming hysterically as seen in mental patients.

umbilical *a.* umbilical, rel. to the umbilicus.

umbral *m.* threshold, the minimum degree of stimulus needed to produce an effect or response; ___ **absoluto** / absolute ___; ___ **auditivo** / auditory ___; ___ **de la conciencia** / ___ of consciousness; ___ **renal** / renal ___; ___ **sensorio** / sensory ___ .

unánime *a.* unanimous.

unción *f.* unction; ointment.

ungueal *a.* ungual, rel. to the nails.

ungüento *m.* unguent, liniment, salve, medicated preparation for external use.

uniarticular *a.* uniarticular, rel. to a single joint.

unibásico-a *a.* unibasal, rel. to a single base.

unicelular *a.* unicellular, having only one cell.

único-a *a.* only, sole; **-mente** *adv.* only, solely.

unidad *f.* unit. 1. one of a kind; ___ **motora** / motor ___ , that provides motor activity; 2. standard of measurement; 3. unity

unidad internacional *f.* international unit, standard measurement of a given substance as adopted by the International Conference for Unification of Formulae.

unido-a *a.* joined; close.

uniforme *m.* uniform; *a.* uniform, even.

unigrávida *f.* unigravida, woman who is pregnant for the first time.

unilateral *a.* unilateral, rel. to one side only.

unión *f.* union. 1. the action or effect of joining two things into one; 2. the growing together of severed parts of a bone or of the lips of a wound.

unípara *f.* uniparous, woman who gives birth to only one child.

unipolar *a.* unipolar, having one pole, such as the nerve cells.

unir *v.* to join; to unite, to merge.

unitario-a *a.* unitary, rel. to a single unit.

universal *a.* universal, general.

universidad *f.* university.

universo *m.* universe.

Unna, bota de pasta de *f.* Unna's paste boot, compression dressing applied to the lower part of the leg in the treatment of varicose ulcers consisting of layers of gauze applied with and covered with Unna's paste.

unsinaria *f.* hookworm, intestinal parasite; **enfermedad de la ___ / ___** disease.

untadura *f.* application; ointment.

untar *v.* to apply ointment; to rub, to smear.

untuoso-a *a.* unctuous, greasy, oily.

uña *f.* nail; **___ del dedo del pie** / toenail; **___ encarnada** / ingrown **___;** *vr.* **comerse las ___ -s** / to bite one's **___ -s.**

uñero *m.* ingrown nail.

uránico-a *a.* uranic, rel. to uremia.

uranio *m.* uranium, heavy metallic element.

urato *m.* urate, uric acid salt.

urea *f.* urea, crystalline substance found in the blood, lymph, and urine that is the final product of the metabolism of proteins and is excreted through the urine as nitrogen.

ureico-a *a.* ureal, rel. to urea; **ciclo ___ hereditario anormal** / hereditary urea cycle abnormality.

urelcosis *f.* urelcosis, formation of ulcers in the urinary tract.

uremia *f.* uremia, toxic condition caused by renal insufficiency that produces retention of nitrogen substances, phosphates, and sulfates in the blood; **___ eclámptica** / eclamptic **___ .**

urémico-a *a.* uremic, rel. to or affected by uremia.

uréter *m.* ureter, one of the ducts by which urine passes from the kidney to the urinary bladder.

ureteral, uretérico-a *a.* ureteral, rel. to a ureter; **lesión ___ / ___**

injury.**obstrucción ___ / ___** obstruction; **reflejo ___ / ___** reflex.

ureterectasis *f.* ureterectasis, abnormal dilation of the ureter.

ureterectomía *f.* ureterectomy, partial or total excision of the ureter.

ureteritis *f.* ureteritis, infl. of the ureter.

ureterocele *m.* ureterocele, cystic dilation of the distal intravesical portion of the ureter due to stenosis of the ureteral orifice.

ureterocistoneostomía *f.* uretercystoneostomy. ureteroneocistomía.

ureterocistostomía *f.* ureterocystostomy. ureteroneocistostomía.

ureterografía *f.* ureterography, x-ray of the ureter with the use of a radiopaque substance.

ureteroheminefrectomía *f.* ureteroheminephrectomy, resection of a portion of the kidney and its ureter in cases of duplication of the upper urinary tract.

ureterohidronefrosis *f.* ureterohydronephrosis, distension of the ureter and the kidney due to obstruction.

ureteroileostomía *f.* ureteroileostomy, anastomosis of a ureter to an isolated segment of the ileum.

ureterolitiasis *f.* ureterolithiasis, formation of a ureteral calculus.

ureterolitotomía *f.* ureterolithotomy, incision into a ureter for removal of a calculus.

ureteronefrectomía *f.* ureteronephrectomy, excision of the kidney and its ureter.

ureteroneocistomía *f.* ureteroneocystostomy, reimplantation of the ureter into the bladder.

ureteropélvico-a *a.* ureteropelvic, rel. to the ureter and the pelvis.

ureteropieloplastia *f.* ureteropyeloplasty, plastic surgery of a ureter and the renal pelvis.

ureteroplastia *f.* ureteroplasty, plastic surgery of the ureter.

ureterosigmoidostomía *f.* ureterosigmoidostomy, implantation of a ureter in the sigmoid colon.

ureterostomía *f.* ureterostomy, formation of a permanent fistula for drainage of a ureter.

ureterotomía *f.* ureterotomy, incision into a ureter.

ureteroureterostomía *f.* ureteroureterostomy, anastomosis of two ureters or of extreme parts of the same ureter.

ureterovesical *a.* ureterovesical, rel. to the ureter and the urinary bladder.

uretra *f.* urethra, urinary canal.

uretral *a.* urethral, rel. to the urethra;
catéter ___ / ___ catheter;
obstrucción ___ / ___ obstruction;
procedimiento ___ / ___ process;
secreción ___ / ___ discharge;
síndrome ___ / ___ syndrome;
suspensión ___ / ___ suspension.

uretralgia *f.* urethralgia, pain in the urethra.

uretrectomía *f.* urethrectomy, partial or total excision of the urethra.

uretritis *f.* urethritis, chronic or acute infl. of the urethra.

uretrografía *f.* urethrography, x-ray of the urethra after injection of a radiopaque substance.

uretroscopio *m.* urethroscope, instrument for viewing the interior of the urethra.

uretrotomía *f.* urethrotomy, incision of the urethra, usu. to alleviate a stricture.

uretrótomo *m.* urethrotome, instrument used in urethrotomy.

urgente *a.* urgent, pressing; **-mente** *adv.* urgently.

uricemia *f.* uricemia, excess uric acid in the blood.

úrico-a *a.* uric, rel. to the urine.

uricosuria *f.* uricosuria, presence of an excessive amount of uric acid in the urine.

urinación *f.* urination, the act of urinating.

urinálisis *m.* urinalysis, analysis of the urine.

urinario-a *a.* urinary, rel. to the urine;
infección ___ / ___ infection; **órganos** ___
-s / ___ organs; **sedimento** ___ / ___ sediment.

urinario, sistema *m.* urinary system, the group of organs and conduits that participate in the production and excretion of urine.

urinífero-a *a.* uriniferous, containing or carrying urine.

urinogenital, urogenital *a.* urinogenital, urogenital, rel. to the urinary and the genital tracts.

urinoma *m.* urinoma, urine containing cyst or tumor.

urobilinógeno *m.* urobilinogen, pigment derived from the reduction of bilirubin by action of intestinal bacteria.

urocinasa *f.* urokinase, enzyme present in human urine used to dissolve blood clots.

urodinámica *f.* urodynamics, the study of the active process and pathophysiology of urination.

urodinia *f.* urodynia, painful urination.

urogenital *a.* urogenital, rel. to the urinary and the genital tracts; **diafragma** ___ / ___ diaphragm.

urografía *f.* urography, x-ray of a part of the urinary tract by injection of a radiopaque substance; ___ **descendente o excretora** / descending or excretory ___; ___ **retrógrada** / retrograde ___ .

urograma *m.* urogram, x-ray record of a urography.

urohematonefrosis *f.* urohematonephrosis, pathological condition of the kidney by which the pelvis distends with blood and urine.

urolitiasis *f.* urolithiasis, formation of urinary calculi and disorders associated with their presence.

urolítico-a *a.* urolithic, rel. to urinary calculi.

urología *f.* urology, the branch of medicine that studies the diagnosis and treatment of diseases of the genitourinary tract in men and the urinary tract in women.

urologico-a *a.* urologic, rel. to urology.

urologo-a *m., f.* urologist, specialist in urology.

uropatía *f.* uropathy, any disease that affects the urinary tract.

urosquesis *f.* uroschesis, suspension or retention of urine.

urticaria *f.* urticaria, hives, eruptive skin disease characterized by pink patches accompanied by intense itching, gen. allergic in nature and caused by an internal or external agent; ___
papulosa / papular ___; ___ **pigmentosa** / ___
pigmentosa; ___ **térmica** / heat rash.

usado-a *a.* used.

usar *v.* to use; [*ropa*] to wear.

uso *m.* use; function; usage; **de poco** ___ /
under ___; ___ **no aprobado** / off-label ___ .

usual *a.* usual, customary; **-mente** *adv.* usually.

uterino-a *a.* uterine, rel. to the uterus;
prolapso ___ / ___ prolapse; **ruptura** ___ / ___
rupture; **sangramiento** ___ / ___ bleeding
unrelated to menstruation.

útero *m.* uterus, womb, hollow, muscular organ of the female reproductive system that contains and nourishes the embryo and fetus during the period of gestation; **cáncer del** ___ **o de la matriz** / uterine cancer; ___ **didelfo** / didelphys ___ , double uterus.

uterosalpingografía *f.* uterosalpingography, x-ray examination of the uterus and the fallopian tubes following injection of a radiopaque substance.

uterovaginal *a.* uterovaginal, rel. to the uterus and the vagina.

uterovesical *a.* uterovesical, rel. to the uterus and the urinary bladder.

útil *a.* useful, practical.

utrículo *m.* utriculus, small bag; ___ **del oído o del vestíbulo** / ___ of the ear or of vestibule; ___ **prostático o uretral** / ___ prostaticus or urethral.

uva *f.* grape.

uvea *f.* uvea, the vascular layer of the eye formed by the iris and the ciliary body together with the choroid coat.

uveitis *f.* uveitis, infl. of the uvea.

úvula *f.* uvula, small, fleshy structure hanging in the middle of the posterior border of the soft palate; ___ **hundida** / cleft ___; ___ **vesical** / vesical ___ .

uvulitis *f.* uvulitis, infl. of the uvula.

uvulotomía *f.* uvulotomy, partial or total cutting of the uvula.

V

V *abr.* **válvula** / valve; **vena** / vein; **visión** / vision; **volumen** / volume.

vaca *f.* cow.

vacaciones *f., pl.* vacations.

vaccinia *L.* vaccinia, cowpox, a virus that causes disease in cattle and when inoculated in humans gives a degree of immunity against smallpox.

vaciar *v.* to empty; to flush out, to void; **vaciarse** *vr.* to become empty.

vacilante *a.* vacillating, fluctuating; shaky.

vacilar *v.* to vacillate; to fluctuate; to hesitate.

vacío-a *a.* empty; **envasado al ___** / vacuum packed.

vacuna *f.* vaccine, a preparation of attenuated or killed microorganisms that when introduced in the body establishes immunity to the specific disease caused by microorganisms; **reacción a la ___** / ___ reaction; **___ antipolio oral, trivalente atenuada de Sabin** / poliovirus, live oral trivalent ___ , Sabin; **___ antirrábica** / rabies ___; **___ antisarampión de virus, vivo** / measles virus ___ , live; **___ antisarampión, inactivada** / measles virus ___ , inactivated; **___ antitífica** / typhoid fever ___; **___ antivariólica, antivariolosa** / smallpox ___; **___ contra la tuberculosis** / BCG ___ against tuberculosis; **___ contra el tétano** / tetanus ___; **___ contra la hepatitis A** / hepatitis A. ___; **___ contra la hepatitis B** / hepatitis B ___; **___ contra la influenza** / influenza ___; **___ contra la varicela** / chickenpox ___; **___ de Salk, contra la poliomielitis** / Salk ___ , antipolio; **___ de virus vivo contra la rubéola** / rubella virus ___ , live; **___ neumocócica polisacárida** / pneumovax ___; **___ neumocócica polivalente** / pneumococcal polyvalent virus ___; **___ triple contra la difteria, el tétano y la tos ferina** / ___ , against diphtheria, pertussis, and tetanus.

vacunación *f.* vaccination, inoculation of vaccine.

vacunar *v.* to vaccinate.

vacuola *f.* vacuole, small cavity or space filled with fluid or air in the cellular protoplasm.

vacuolización *f.* vacuolization, formation of vacuoles.

vacuum *L.* vacuum, emptiness, a space devoid of air or matter.

vagal *a.* vagal, rel. to the pneumogastric or vagus nerve.

vagante *a.* vagrant, wandering; loose, free.

vagar *vi.* to wander.

vagina *f.* vagina. 1. female canal extending from the uterus to the vulva; 2. structure resembling a sheath.

vaginal *a.* vaginal, rel. to the vagina or to a sheathlike structure; **candidiasis ___** / ___ candidiasis; **cultivo ___** / ___ culture ; **flujo ___** / ___ discharge; **hemorragia, sangrado ___** / ___ bleeding; **picazón ___** / ___ itching; **quistes ___** / ___ cysts; **reparación de la pared ___** / ___ wall repair; **tratamiento de secamiento ___** / ___ drying treatment; **tumor ___** / ___ tumor.

vaginismus *L.* vaginismus, sudden and painful spasm of the vagina.

vaginitis *f.* vaginitis, infl. of the vagina; **___ bacteriana** / bacterial ___ .

vago-a *a.* vague, indistinct; **-mente** *adv.* vaguely.

vago, nervio *m.* vagus nerve.nervios craneales.

vagolítico-a *a.* vagolytic, inhibiting the function of the vagus nerve.

vagotomía *f.* vagotomy, interruption of the vagus nerve.

vahído *m.* dizziness, fainting spell.

vaina *f.* sheath, a protective covering structure.

vainilla *f.* vanilla.

vaivén *m.* swaying;*pop.* to and fro.

valencia *f.* valence, valency.

valer *vi.* to cost; to be worth; to be valid, good, or acceptable; **valerse** *vr.* **___ por sí mismo** / to be self-sufficient.

valgus *L.* valgus, bent or twisted outward.

validez *f.* validity.

válido-a *a.* valid, acceptable.

valiente *a.* valiant, brave, courageous.

valioso-a *a.* valuable, of worth.

valor *m.* value, worth.

valorización *f.* valorization, evaluation.

Valsalva, maniobra de *f.* Valsalva's maneuver, procedure to test the patency of the eustachian tubes or to adjust the pressure of the middle ear by forcibly exhaling while holding the nostrils and mouth closed.

válvula *f.* valve, a membranous structure in a canal or orifice that closes temporarily to prevent the backward flow of the contents passing through it; **___ aórtica** / aortic ___ , between the left ventricle and the aorta; **___**

atrioventricular derecha, tricúspide / atrioventricular ___ right, tricuspid; ___
atrioventricular izquierda, bicúspide, mitral / atrioventricular ___ left, bicuspid, mitral; ___ **ileocecal /** ileocecal ___ ; ___ **pilórica /** pyloric ___; ___ **pulmonar /** pulmonary ___ .

válvula mitral *f.* mitral valve, the left atrioventricular valve of the heart; **insuficiencia de la** ___ / insufficiency of the ___; **prolapso de la** ___ / prolapse of the ___ .

valvular *a.* valvular, rel. to a valve or of its nature;**estenosis pulmonar** ___ / ___ pulmonary stenosis.

válvulas conniventes *f., pl.* valvulae conniventes, circular membranous folds found in the small intestine that slow the passage of food along the bowels.

valvuloplastia *f.* valvuloplasty, plastic surgery of a heart valve.

valvulótomo *m.* valvulotome, instrument to incise a valve.

vano-a *a.* vain; **en** ___ / in vain, needlessly.

vapor *m.* vapor, gas, fume.

vaporización *f.* vaporization. 1. action and effect of vaporizing; 2. therapeutic use of vapors.

vaporizador *m.* vaporizer, device used to convert a substance into a vapor for therapeutic purposes.

vaporizar *vi.* to vaporize, to change a substance into vapor.

variabilidad *f.* variability.

variable *f.* variable, a changing factor; *a.* that can change.

variación *f.* variation, diversity in the characteristic of related elements.

variado-a *a.* varied.

variante *f.* variant, that which is essentially the same as another but different in form; *a.* different, changing.

variar *v.* to change, to vary.

várice, variz *f.* varix, an enlarged and tortuous vein, artery or lymphatic vessel.

varicella *L.* varicella, chicken pox, viral contagious disease, gen. manifested during childhood, characterized by an eruption that evolves into small vesicles.

varicocele *m.* varicocele, varicose condition of the veins of the spermatic cord that produces a soft mass in the scrotum.

varicoide *a.* varicoid, resembling a varix.

varicoso-a *a.* varicose, resembling or related to varices; **venas** ___ **-s /** ___ veins.

varicotomía *f.* varicotomy, excision of a varicose vein.

variedad *f.* variety.

varilla *f.* thin, short rod; wand; ___ **de aceite /** dipstick.

variola *L.* variola. viruela.

variólico-a, varioloso-a *a.* variolous, rel. to smallpox or affected by it.

varioliforme *a.* varioliform, resembling smallpox.

varios-as *a.* several.

varón *m.* male.

varonil *a.* manly.

varus *L.* varus, twisted or turned inward.

vas *L.* vas, (*pl. vasa*) vessel; ___ **recta /** ___ recta; ___ **vasorum /** ___ vasorum.

vas deferens *L.* vas deferens, the excretory duct of the spermatozoa.

vascular *a.* vascular, rel. to the blood vessels; **cambio cutáneo** ___ / ___ skin change; **ectasia** ___ **del colon /** ___ ectasia of the colon; **espasmo** ___ / ___ spasm; **púrpura** ___ / ___ purpura; **sistema** ___ / ___ system, all the vessels of the body, esp. the blood vessels; **túnica** ___ / ___ tunic.

vascularización *f.* vascularization, formation of new blood vessels.

vascularizar *vi.* to vascularize, to develop new blood vessels.

vasculatura *f.* vasculature, arrangement of blood vessels in an organ or part.

vasculitis *f.* vasculitis. angiitis.

vasculopatía *f.* vasculopathy, any disease of a blood vessel.

vasectomía *f.* vasectomy, partial excision and ligation of the vas deferens to prevent the passage of spermatozoa into the semen, usu. done as a means of birth control.

vaselina *f.* vaseline, petroleum jelly.

vasija *f.* receptacle, vessel.

vaso *m.* vessel; conduit.1. any channel or tube that carries fluid such as blood or lymph; **grandes** ___ **-s /** great ___ -s; ___ **colateral /** collateral ___; ___ **linfático /** lymphatic ___; ___ **sanguíneo /** blood ___; 2. a drinking glass.

vasoactivo *m.* vasoactive, agent that affects the blood vessels.

vasoconstricción *f.* vasoconstriction, decrease in the caliber of the blood vessels.

vasoconstrictor *m.* vasoconstrictor, that which causes vasoconstriction; **-a** *a.* vasoconstrictive, rel. to constriction of the blood vessels.

vasodilatación *f.* vasodilation, increase in the caliber of the blood vessels.

vasodilatador *m.* vasodilator, that which causes vasodilation; **-a** *a.* that causes vasodilation.

vasoespasmo *m.* vasospasm. angioespasmo; ___ **coronario** / coronary ___ .

vasomotor *m.* vasomotor, that which regulates the contraction and dilation of blood vessels; **rinitis** ___ / ___ rhinitis; **-a** *a.* rel. to dilation or contraction of blood vessels.

vasopresina *f.* vasopressin, hormone secreted by the posterior pituitary gland that increases the reabsorption of water by the kidneys, raising the blood pressure.

vasopresor *m.* vasopressor, that which has a vasoconstrictive effect; **-a** *a.* having a vasoconstrictive effect.

vasotónico-a *a.* vasotonic, rel. to a vessel tone.

vasovagal *a.* vasovagal, rel. to the vessels and the vagus nerve; **síncope** ___ / ___ syncope, brief fainting spell caused by vascular and vagal disturbances.

vasto-a *a.* vastus.

vastus *L.* vastus, dilated, large, extensive.

Vater, ámpula de *f.* Vater's ampulla or papilla, the point where the biliar and pancreatic excretory systems enter the duodenum.

vecino-a *m., f.* neighbor.

vector *m.* vector, a carrier that transmits infectious agents.

vegetación *f.* vegetation, a wartlike, abnormal growth on a body part as seen in endocarditis.

vegetal *m.* vegetable; *a.* vegetal, rel. to plants.

vegetarianismo *m.* vegetarianism, the practice of eating only vegetables and fruits. Dairy products may not be excluded.

vegetariano-a *m., f.* individual who eats mainly vegetables; *a.* rel. to vegetables.

vegetativo-a *a.* vegetative. 1. rel. to functions of growth and nutrition; 2. rel. to involuntary or unconscious bodily movements; 3. pertaining to plants.

vehículo *m.* vehicle. 1. agent without therapeutic action that carries the active ingredient of a medication; 2. an agent of transmission.

vejez *f.* old age.

vejiga *f.* bladder; **cálculos de la** ___ / ___ calculi; **irrigación de la** ___ / ___ irrigation; ___ **llena de aire** / air ___; ___ **neurogénica** / neurogenic ___ .

vejiga urinaria *f.* urinary bladder, sac-shaped organ that serves as a receptacle to urine secreted by the kidneys.

vela *f.* candle.

velar *v.* to watch over, to take care of someone.

velo *m.* veil. 1. thin membrane or covering of a body part; 2. a piece of amniotic sac seen sometimes covering the face of a newborn; 3. slight alteration in the voice.

velocidad *f.* speed, velocity; ___ **de desplazamiento** / movement of travel.

vello *m.* body hair; ___ **axilar** / axillary ___ ; ___ **púbico** / pubic hair.

vellosidad *f.* villus, short, filiform projection from a membranous surface; ___ **aracnoidea** / arachnoid ___; ___ **coriónica** / chorionic ___; ___ **-es intestinales** / intestinal ___; ___ **-es sinoviales** / synovial ___ .

velloso-a, velludo-a *a.* villous, hairy.

vena *f.* vein, fibromuscular vessel that carries blood from the capillaries toward the heart; ___ **-s varicosas** / ___ veins, *pop.* spider ___ .

vena cava *f.* vena cava, either of two large veins returning deoxygenated blood to the right atrium of the heart; ___ **inferior** / inferior ___; ___ **superior** / superior ___ .

vencimiento *m.* expiration; **fecha de** ___ / ___ date.

venda *f.* bandage.

vendaje *m.* bandage, dressing, curative, protective covering; ___ **abdominal** / abdominal binder; ___ **de yeso** / plaster cast; ___ **protector** / surgical dressing.

vendar *v.* to bandage.

vender *v.* to sell.

veneno *m.* poison, venom, toxic substance; **centro de control de** ___ **-s** / ___ control center.

venenoso-a *a.* poisonous, venomous, toxic; **hiedra** ___ / poison ivy.

venéreo-a *a.* venereal, resulting from or transmitted by sexual intercourse; **enfermedad** ___ / ___ disease; **verruga** ___ / ___ wart.

venina *f.* venin, toxic substance present in snake venom.

veninantivenina *f.* venin-antivenin, vaccine to counteract the effect of snake poison.

venipuntura *a.* venepuncture, venipuncture, surgical puncture of a vein.

venir *vi.* to come; ___ **al caso** / to be relevant.

venisección *f.* venisection.flebotomía.

venoclusivo-a *a.* veno-occlusive, rel. to the obstruction of veins.

venoconstricción *f.* venoconstriction, constriction of the muscular walls of the veins.

venografía *f.* venography, recording of a venogram.

venografía radionuclear *f.* radionuclear tomography, study of the veins by means of gamma rays.

venograma *m.* venogram, x-ray of a vein with the use of a contrasting medium; ___ **renal** / renal ___ .

venoso-a *a.* venous, rel. to the veins; **congestión** ___ / ___ congestion; **insuficiencia** ___ / ___ insufficiency; **retorno** ___ / ___ return; **sangre** ___ / ___ blood; **seno** ___ / ___ sinus; **tromboembolismo** ___ / ___ thromboembolism; **trombosis** ___ / ___ thrombosis.

venotomía *f.* venotomy. flebotomía.

vent *Fr.* vent, opening.

ventaja *f.* advantage.

ventajoso-a *a.* advantageous.

ventana *f.* window; ___ **oval** / oval ___ , aperture in the middle ear.

ventilación *f.* ventilation; ___ **pulmonar** / pulmonary ___; 1. the act of circulating fresh air in a given area; 2. oxygenation of blood; 3. open discussion and airing of grievances.

ventilador *m.* ventilator, artificial respirator; fan.

ventilar *v.* to ventilate, to air.

ventolera *f.* strong gust of wind.

ventral *a.* ventral, abdominal, rel. to the belly or to the front side of the body; **hernia** ___ / ___ hernia.

ventricular *a.* ventricular, rel. to a ventricle; **defecto del tabique** ___ / ___ septal defect; **defecto septal** ___ / ___ septal defect; **fibrilación** ___ / ___ fibrillation; **punción** ___ / ___ puncture; **taquicardia** ___ / ___ tachycardia.

ventriculitis *f.* ventriculitis, infl. of a ventricle.

ventrículo *m.* ventricle, a small cavity, esp. in reference to such structures as seen in the heart, the brain, or the larynx; **cuarto** ___ **del cerebro** / fourth ___ of the brain; **tercer** ___ **del cerebro** / third ___ of the brain; ___ **de la laringe** / ___ of the larynx; ___ **derecho del corazón** / right ___ of the heart; ___ **izquierdo del corazón** / left ___ of the heart; ___ **lateral del cerebro** / lateral ___ of the brain.

ventriculografía *f.* ventriculography.neumoencefalografía.

ventriculotomía *f.* ventriculotomy, incision of a ventricle.

ventrodorsal *a.* ventrodorsal, rel. to the ventral and the dorsal surfaces.

vénula *f.* venule, minute vein that connects the capillaries with larger veins.

ver *vi.* to see; **está por** ___ / it remains to be seen; **tener que** ___ **con** / to have to do with; **verse** *vr.* to see oneself; to see each other.

verano *m.* summer

verbatim *L.* verbatim, exactly as stated.

verbo *m. gr.* verb.

verdad *f.* truth; **decir la** ___ / to tell the ___; **de** ___ / truly, really; **¿no es** ___ ? / isn't it so?

verdadero-a *a.* true, real; **pelvis** ___ / ___ pelvis; **-mente** *adv.* truly.

verde *a.* green; not ripe.

verdugón *m.* welt.

verdura *f.* [*vegetales*] greens.

veredicto *m.* verdict.

vergonzoso-a *a.* shameful.

vergenza *f.* shame; bashfulness; *v.* **tener** ___ / to be ashamed.

verificación *f.* verification, proof.

verificar *vi.* to verify, to prove true.

vermicida, vermífugo *m.* vermicide, agent that destroys worms.

vermiforme *a.* vermiform, wormlike, resembling worm; **apéndice** ___ / ___ appendix.

vermis *L.* vermis. 1. parasitic worm; 2. wormlike structure.

vernix *L.* vernix, varnish; ___ **caseosa** / ___ caseosa, sebaceous secretion protecting the skin of a fetus;

verruca *L.* verruca, (*pl. verrucae*) wart; ___ **filiformis** / ___ filiformis; ___ **plantaris** / ___ plantaris; ___ **vulgaris** / ___ vulgaris.

verruga *f.* verruca; ___ **planas juveniles** / ___ planae juveniles; ___ **seborreica** / seborrheic ___; ___ **simple** / simple ___ .

verrugoso-a *a.* verrucose, warty, or rel. to warts.

versátil *a.* versatile, having multiple applications.

versión *f.* version. 1. change of direction of an organ, such as the uterus; 2. change of position of the fetus in utero to facilitate delivery; ___ **bimanual** / bimanual ___ ; ___ **bipolar** / bipolar ___; ___ **cefálica** / cephalic ___; ___ **combinada** / combined ___; ___ **externa** / external ___; ___ **espontánea** / spontaneous ___ .

vértebra *f.* vertebra, any of the thirty-three bones of the vertebral column; ___ **cervical** / cervical ___; ___ **coccígea** / coccygeal ___; ___ **lumbar** / lumbar ___; ___ **sacra** / sacral ___; ___ **torácica** / thoracic ___ .

vertebrado-a *a.* vertebrate, having or resembling a vertebral column.

vertebral *a.* vertebral, rel. to the vertebrae; **arteria** ___ / ___ artery; **conducto** ___ / ___ canal; **costillas** ___ **-es** / ___ ribs.

vertebrobasilar *a.* vertebrobasilar, rel. to the basilar and vertebral arteries;

insuficiencia ___ / ___ insufficiency; **trastornos** ___ **es de la circulación** / ___ circulatory disorders.

verter *vi.* to spill; to pour.

vertex *n.* vertex, pl. vértices 1. the highest point of a structure, such as the top of the head; 2. convergence point of the two sides of an angle.

vertical *a.* vertical. 1. upright; 2. rel. to the vertex.

vértice *m.* vertex.

vertiginoso-a *a.* vertiginous, rel. to, affected by, or producing vertigo.

vértigo *m.* vertigo, sensation of whirling motion either of oneself (subjective vertigo), or of surrounding objects (objective vertigo) gen. caused by a disease of the inner ear or by gastric or cardiac disorders; ___ **laberíntico** / labyrinthine ___ .

verumontanitis *f.* verumontanitis, infl. of the verumontanum.

verumontanum *L.* verumontanum, an elevation in the urethra at the point of entry of the seminal ducts.

vesicación *f.* vesication. 1. the formation of blisters; 2. a blister.

vesical *a.* vesical, rel. to or resembling a bladder.

vesicouretral *a.* vesicoureteral, rel. to the urinary bladder and the ureters.

vesicovaginal *a.* vesicovaginal, rel. to the urinary bladder and the vagina.

vesícula *f.* vesicle, vesicula, small sac or elevation of the skin containing serous fluid.

vesícula biliar *f.* gallbladder, pear-shaped receptacle on the lower part of the liver that stores bile.

vesicular *a.* vesicular, rel. to a vesicle.

vesiculoso-a *a.* vesiculate, of the nature of a vesicle.

vestibular *a.* vestibular, rel. to a vestibule; **bulbo** ___ / ___ bulb; **nervio** ___ / ___ nerve.

vestíbulo *m.* vestibule. 1. space or cavity that gives acccss to a duct or canal; 2. lobby, waiting room.

vestigial *a.* vestigial, rudimentary, rel. to a vestige.

vestigio *m.* vestige, remains of a structure that was fully developed in a previous stage of the species or of the individual.

vestimenta *f.* clothing; garment.

vestir *vi.* to dress; **vestirse** *vr.* to dress oneself.

veterano-a *m., f.* veteran.

veterinaria *f.* veterinary medicine, the science that deals with prevention and cure of animal diseases, esp. domestic animals.

veterinario-a *m., f.* veterinarian, specialist in veterinary medicine; *a.* rel. to veterinary medicine.

vez *f.* time, occasion; **a la** ___ / at the same ___; **alguna** ___ / sometime; **cada** ___ / each ___; **de una** ___ / all at once; **de** ___ **en cuando** / once in a while; **en** ___ **de** / instead of; **otra** ___ / again; **rara** ___ / rarely; **tal** ___ / perhaps; **una** ___ / once.

vía *f.* tract, via, passage, conduit; ___ **olfatoria** / olfactory ___; ___ **piramidal** / pyramidal ___; ___ **-s biliares** / biliary ___; ___ **-s digestivas** / gastrointestinal ___; ___ **-s respiratorias** / respiratory ___; ___ **-s urinarias** / urinary ___ .

vías descendientes *f., pl.* descending tracts, tracts of nerves in the dorsal spine that carry impulses from the brain to the rest of the body.

viabilidad *f.* viability, the quality of being viable.

viable *a.* viable, capable of surviving, gen. in reference to a newborn; **no** ___ / nonviable.

viajar *v.* to travel.

viaje *m.* trip.

vianda *f.* starchy vegetables such as potatoes.

víbora *f.* viper.

vibración *f.* vibration, oscillation.

vibrante *a.* vibrant.

vibrar *vi.* to vibrate.

vibratorio-a *a.* vibratory, vibratile, vibrating or producing vibration; **sentido** ___ / ___ sense.

vicario-a *a.* vicarious, acting or assuming the place of another.

vicio *m.* vice, bad habit.

vicioso-a *a.* given to vice.

víctima *f.* victim; ___ **de accidente** / casualty.

vida *f.* life; vitality; **medidas para el sostenimiento de la** ___ / ___ saving measures; **promedio de duración de** ___ / ___ expectancy; **que pone la** ___ **en peligro** / ___ -threatening; ___ **cotidiana** / daily ___ .

vida media *f.* half-life. 1. the time required for half the nuclei of a radioactive substance to disintegrate; 2. the time required for half the amount of a substance taken in by the body to dissolve by natural means.

video *m.* video.

videocinta *f.* videotape.

vidrio *m.* glass; ___ **de fibra** / fiberglass.

viejo-a *a.* old, aged; stale.

viento *m.* wind; **hace** ___ / it is windy.

vientre *m.* belly; abdomen.

vigente *a.* in force, in effect.

vigilancia *f.* 1. vigilance, state of alertness or responsiveness; 2. surveillance.

vigilar *v.* to watch, to guard; to survey.

vigilia *f.* vigil. 1. the state of being consciously responsive to a stimulus; 2. insomnia.

vigor *m.* vigor, strength; fortitude; stamina.

vigorizar *vi.* to invigorate, to strengthen, to energize.

vigoroso-a *a.* vigorous, strong; having fortitude; **-mente** *adv.* vigorously.

VIH *m.* HIV, human immunodeficiency virus-1, a retrovirus considered to be the cause of AIDS that can be transmitted by sexual relations or by blood transfusion from someone who is infected with HIV. The virus can be transmitted to children of mothers with HIV in utero, at birth, or, likely, through breast-feeding.

vinagre *m.* vinegar, solution of acetic acid.

vínculo *m.* link.

vino *m.* wine.

violáceo-a *a.* purplish.

violación *f.* rape; violation; ___ **estatutaria** / statutory ___ .

violar *a.* to rape; to harm or injure.

violencia *f.* violence; ___ **doméstica** / domestic ___ .

violento-a *a.* violent.

violeta *a.* [*color*] violet.

violeta de genciana *f.* gentian violet, coloring agent used to dye tissues and microorganisms in their microscopic study; used also as anti-infective.

viral *a.* viral, rel. to a virus; **artritis** ___ / ___ arthritis; **crup** ___ / ___ croup; **fiebre hemorrágica** ___ / ___ hemorrhagic fever; **gastroenteritis** ___ / ___ gastroenteritis; **hepatitis** ___ / ___ hepatitis; **infección** ___ **del sistema respiratorio superior** / ___ upper respiratory infection; **neumonía** ___ / ___ pneumonia; **replicación** ___ / ___ replication.

virar *a.* to turn; *virarse* *vr.* to turn oneself around.

viremia *f.* viremia, the presence of virus in the blood.

virgen *f.* virgin. 1. uncontaminated, pure; 2. having had no sexual intercourse.

virginal *a.* virginal, pure.

virginidad *f.* virginity.

viril *a.* virile, rel. to the male.

virilidad *f.* virility. 1. sexual potency; 2. the quality of being virile.

virilización *f.* virilization, the process by which secondary male characteristics develop in the female, gen. due to adrenal malfunction or to intake of hormones.

virión *m.* virion, mature viral particle that constitutes the extracellular, infectious form of a virus.

virolento-a *a.* 1. rel. to or afflicted with smallpox; 2. pockmarked.

virología *f.* virology, the study of viruses.

virtual *a.* virtual, existing in appearance and effect, but not in reality.

viruela *f.* smallpox, highly contagious viral disease characterized by high temperature and generalized blisters and pustules; ___ -s **locas** / chickenpox.

virulencia *f.* virulence. 1. the power of an organism to produce disease in the host; 2. the quality of being virulent.

virulento-a *a.* virulent, highly poisonous or infectious.

virus *m.* virus, ultramicroscopic microorganisms capable of causing infectious diseases; ___ **atenuado** / attenuated ___ ; ___ **citomegálico** / cytomegalic ___ ; ___ **Coxsackie** / Coxsackie ___ ; ___ **de la parainfluenza** / parainfluenza ___ ; ___ **ECHO** / ECHO ___ ; ___ **entérico** / enteric ___ ; ___ **herpético** / herpes ___ ; ___ **oncogénico, tumoral** / tumor ___ ; ___ **sincitial respiratorio** / respiratory syncytial ___ ; ___ **variólico** / pox ___ .

visceral *a.* visceral, rel. to viscera.

vísceras *f., pl.* viscera, large internal organs of the body, esp. the abdomen.

visceromegalia *f.* visceromegaly, abnormal enlargement of a viscus.

viscosidad *f.* viscosity, the quality of being viscous, esp. the property of fluids to offer resistance due to molecular friction.

viscoso-a *a.* viscous, gummy, sticky; slimy.

visibilidad *f.* visibility.

visible *a.* visible; evident; **-mente** *adv.* visibly.

visión *f.* vision, the sense of sight. 1. the ability to see, to perceive things through the action of light on the eyes and on related centers in the brain; ___ **acromática** / achromatic ___ ; ___ **a la distancia** / distance ___ ; ___ **binocular** / binocular ___ ; ___ **central** / central ___ ; ___ **cromática** / chromatic ___ ; ___ **diurna, fotoscópica** / day ___ , photoscopic; ___ **doble, diplopía** / double ___ , diplopia; ___ **en túnel** / in tunnel field; ___ **estocópica** / stocopic ___ ; ___ **monocular** / monocular ___ ; ___ **nocturna** / night ___ ; 2. imaginary apparition.

visión en tunel *f.* tunnel vision, eye anomaly manifested by a great reduction in the visual field, as if looking through a tunnel, such as occurs in cases of glaucoma.

visita *f.* visit; call; **horas de** ___ / visiting hours; ___ **médica** / house call.

visitar *v.* to visit.

vista *f.* sight; eyesight; view; **corto de** ___ / nearsighted; **enfermedades de la** ___ / eye diseases; ___ **cansada** / eyestrain; ___ **nublada** / bleary-eyed; *v.* **a primera** ___ / at first ___ ; **en** ___ **de** / in view of; **tener buena** ___ / to have good eyesight.

vistazo *m.* glance, glimpse; *v.* **dar un** ___ / to take a look.

visto-a *a. pp.* de **ver**, seen.

visual *a.* visual, rel. to vision; **campo** ___ / ___ field, field of vision; **contacto** ___ / eye contact; **memoria** ___ / eye memory.

visualización *f.* visualization, 1. the act of viewing an image or picture, as in the study of an x-ray, when a body part is examined in detail; 2. mental conception of health created for the purpose of aiding the healing process.

visualizar *vi.* to visualize. 1. to form a mental image; 2. to make visible, such as through x-rays.

vital *a.* vital, rel. to life or essential to maintaining it; **capacidad** ___ / ___ capacity; **signos** ___ -**es** / ___ signs.

vitalicio-a *a.* for life.

vitalidad *f.* vitality. 1. the quality of having life; 2. physical or mental vigor.

vitalizar *vi.* to vitalize, to give life; to reanimate.

vitamina *f.* vitamin, any one of a group of organic compounds found in small amounts in foods and essential to the growth and development of the body and its functions; **pérdida de** ___ -**s** / loss of ___ -s.

vitamínico-a *a.* vitaminic, rel. to vitamins.

vitiligo *m.* vitiligo, benign skin disease characterized by smooth white spots, gen. in exposed areas.

vitrectomía *f.* vitrectomy, partial or total extirpation of the vitreous humor of the eye. It is sometimes recommended in cases of advanced proliferative diabetic retinopathy.

vítreo-a *a.* vitreous, glassy, hyaline; **camara** ___ / ___ chamber; **cuerpo** ___ / ___ body; **humor** ___ / ___ humor.

viudo-a *m., f.* widower; widow.

vivificante *a.* vivifying.

vivir *v.* to live.

vivisección *f.* vivisection, the cutting or operating upon living animals for research purposes.

vivo-a *a.* alive; living; *pop.* ingenuous.

vocabulario *m.* vocabulary.

vocación *f.* vocation, profession.

vocal *f. gr.* vowel; *a.* rel. to the voice or produced by it; **ligamentos** ___ -**es** / ___ ligaments.

vocalización *f.* vocalization.

volar *vi.* to fly; to travel by airplane.

volátil *a.* volatile, readily vaporized.

volición *f.* volition, will, the power to determine.

Volkmann, contractura de *f.* Volkmann contracture, ischemic contracture as a result of irreversible necrosis of the muscular tissue, gen. seen in the forearm and hands.

volumen *m.* volume, space occupied by a body or substance; ___ **cardíaco** / heart ___; ___ **de reserva espiratoria o aire de reserva** / expiratory air reserve ___; ___ **de ventilación pulmonar** / tidal ___; ___ **residual** / residual ___; ___ **sanguíneo** / blood ___; ___ **sistólico** / stroke ___ .

volumétrico-a *a.* volumetric, rel. to the measurement of volume.

voluntad *f.* will, determination; **fuerza de** ___ / ___ power.

voluntario-a *m., f.* volunteer; *a.* voluntary; **músculo** ___ / ___ muscle.

voluptuoso-a *a.* voluptuous, sensually provocative.

volver *vi.* to return; to turn; ___ **en sí** / to come to; **volverse** *vr.* to turn over; to return to.

vólvulo *m.* volvulus, intestinal obstruction caused by torsion of the intestine on its mesentery.

vómer *m.* vomer, the impaired flat bone that forms part of the nasal septum.

vomitar *v.* to vomit.

vomitivo *m.* vomitive, emetic.

vómito *m.* vomit, vomiting.

Von Gierke, enfermedad de *f.* Von Gierke disease, abnormal storage of glycogen.

von Recklinghausen, enfermedad de *f.* von Recklinghausen's disease.neurofibromatosis.

Von Willenbrand, enfermedad de *f.* Von Willenbrand's disease, hereditary blood disorder characterized by bleeding episodes gen. from the mucous membranes.

voraz *a.* voracious, having an excessive appetite.

vórtice *m.* vortex, spiral-shaped structure.

voyeur *Fr.* voyeur, one who practices voyeurism.

voyeurismo *m.* voyeurism, sexual perversion by which erotic gratification is derived from watching sexual organs or activity.

voz *f.* voice.

vozarrón *m.* strong, deep voice.

vuelo *m.* flight; trajectory.

vuelta *f.* turning; turn; rotation; **media** ___ / about-face; *v.* **dar una** ___ / to take a stroll, ride, or walk; *v.* **estar de** ___ / to be back.

vulnerable *a.* vulnerable, prone to injury or disease.

vulva *f.* vulva, external female organ.

vulvar *a.* vulval, vulvar, rel. to the vulva.

vulvectomía *f.* vulvectomy, excision of the vulva.

vulvitis *f.* vulvitis, infl. of the vulva.

vulvovaginal *a.* vulvovaginal, rel. to the vulva and the vagina.

vulvovaginitis *f.* vulvovaginitis, infl. of the vulva and the vagina.

Waldenstrom, macroglobulinemia de *f.*
Waldenstrom's macroglobulinemia, sickness of
elderly persons, hemorrhagic syndrome with
anemia and symptoms of enlarged lymph nodes,
liver and spleen, with frequent manifestations of
bleeding and purpura.

Waldeyer, anillo de *m.* Waldeyer's ring, the
ring of lymphatic tissue that consists of the
palatine, lingual, and pharyngeal tonsils.

Waller, degeneración de *f.* Wallerian
degeneration, degeneration of nerve fibers that
have been separated from their center of
nutrition.

warfarina *f.* warfarin, generic name for
Coumadine, anticoagulant used in the prevention
of thrombosis and infarcts.

Wasserman, reacción de *f.* Wasserman
reaction, serological test for syphilis.

Waterhouse-Friderichsen, síndrome de
m. Waterhouse-Friderichsen syndrome, acute
hemorrhage of the glands with skin hemorrhage
associated to a sudden acute bacteriogenic shock.

Weneger, granulomatosis de *f.* Weneger's
granulomatosis, disease characterized by the
formation of granulomas in the artery affecting
the nasal cavity, the lungs, and the kidneys.

Western Blot *m.* Western Blot, immunoblot,
test to confirm HIV infection in patients with
evidence of exposure to HIV by a previous
enzyme-linked immunosorbent assay.

Wharton, conducto de *m.* Wharton's duct,
excretory duct of the submandibular gland.

Whipple, enfermedad de *f.* Whipple's
disease, rare disease caused by deposit of lipids
in the lymphatic and intestinal tissues.

Wilms, tumor de *m.* Wilms tumor, rapidly
developing neoplasm of the kidney, seen esp. in
children.

Wilson, enfermedad de *f.* Wilson's disease,
hereditary disease manifested by severe hepatic
and cerebral disorders.

X

X *abbr.* **xantina** / xanthine.

xantelasma *f.* xanthelasma, yellow plaques or spots that appear gen. around the eyelids.

xantina *f.* xanthine, one of a group of stimulants of the central nervous system and the heart, such as caffeine.

xantocromía *f.* xanthochromia, yellowish discoloration as it is seen in skin patches or in the cerebrospinal fluid.

xantocrómico-a *a.* xanthochromic, having a yellowish appearance or rel. to xanthochromia.

xantoderma *m.* xanthoderma, yellowish coloration of the skin.

xantoma *m.* xanthoma, condition characterized by the presence of yellowish plaques or nodules in the skin, gen. due to deposit of lipids; ___ **diabético** / diabetic ___; ___ **diseminado** / disseminatum ___; ___ **eruptivo** / eruptive ___; ___ **plano** / planar ___; ___ **tendinoso** / tendinous ___; ___ **tuberoso** / tuberosum ___ .

xantomatosis *f.* xanthomatosis, presence of multiple xanthomas on the skin.

xantosis *f.* xanthosis, yellowing of the skin due to excessive ingestion of foods such as carrots and egg yolks.

xenofobia *f.* xenophobia, morbid fear or aversion to anything foreign.

xenoinjerto *m.* xenograft; **rechazo de**___ / ___ rejection.

xenón *m.* xenon, a dense, colorless element found in small amounts in the atmosphere.

xenotransplante *m.* xenotransplant, the act of transplanting an organ, tissue, or part from one species to another.

xerodermia *f.* xeroderma, xerosis, excessively dry skin.

xeroftalmìa *f.* xerophthalmia, dryness of the conjunctiva due to lack of vitamin A.

xerografía *f.* xerography. xerorradiografía.

xeromamografía *f.* xeromammography, xeroradiography of the breast.

xerorradiografía *f.* xeroradiography, dry process of registering electrostatic images by the use of metal plates covered with a substance such as selenium.

xerosis *f.* xerosis, abnormal dryness as seen in the skin, eyes, and mucous membranes.

xerostomía *f.* xerostomia, abnormal dryness of the mouth due to deficiency of salivary secretion.

xifoide, xifoideo-a *a.* xiphoid, shaped like a sword, as the xiphoid process.

xifoides, apéndice *m.* xiphoid process, cartilaginous, sword-shaped formation joined to the lowest portion of the sternum.

X

y

y *conj.* and.

ya *adv.* already; ___ **que** / as long as.

yarda *f.* yard.

yatrogénico-a, yatrógeno-a *a.* iatrogenic, rel. to the adverse condition of a patient resulting from an erroneous medical treatment or procedure.

yaws *m.* yaws.frambesia.

yema *f.* yolk. 1. the yolk of the egg of a bird; 2. contents of the ovum that supply the embryo.

yerbabuena, hierbabuena *f.* peppermint.

yerno *m.* son-in-law.

yersinia *f.* yersinia, genus of the species *Yersinia pestis*, parasitic bacteria in humans that does not form spores and that contains rods of ovoid, gamma negative cells.

yeso *m.* plaster, plaster cast.

yeyunal *a.* jejunal, rel. to the jejunum.

yeyunectomía *f.* jejunectomy, excision of part or all of the jejunum.

yeyuno *m.* jejunum, portion of the small intestine that extends from the duodenum to the ileum.

yeyunostomía *f.* jejunostomy, permanent opening in the jejunum through the abdominal wall.

yo *m.* self, [*el yo*] the ego, Freudian term that refers to the part of the psyche that mediates between the person and reality; *gr. pron.* I.

yodismo *m.* iodism, poisoning by iodine.

yodo *m.* iodine, nonmetallic element used in medications, esp. those that stimulate the function and development of the thyroid gland and the prevention of goiter; **prueba radiactiva del** ___ / radioactive ___ excretion test, used for evaluating the function of the thyroid gland.

yododerma, yododermia *f.* iododerma, skin rash caused by allergy to the ingestion of iodites.

yodofilia *f.* iodophilia, affinity for iodine.

yodurar *v.* to iodize, to treat with iodine.

yoga *m.* yoga, Hindu system of beliefs and practices by which the individual tries to reach the union of self with a universal self through contemplation, meditation, and self-control.

yogurt *m.* yogurt, milk that is fermented by the action of *Lactobacillus bulgaricus* and credited with nutritious and therapeutic value.

yugular *a.* jugular, rel. to the throat; **foramen** ___ / ___foramen; **fosa** ___ / ___ fossa; **glándula** ___ / ___ gland; **glomo** ___ / ___ glomus; **nervio** ___ / ___ nerve; **pulso** ___ / ___ pulse; **venas**___-es / ___ veins, veins that carry blood from the cranium, the face, and the neck to the heart.

yuxtaglomerular *a.* juxtaglomerular, close to a glomerulus; **aparato** ___ / ___ apparatus; group of cells that participate in the production of renin and in the metabolism of sodium situated around arterioles leading to a glomerulus of the kidney.

yuxtaponer *vi.* to juxtapose, to put next to.

yuxtaposición *f.* juxtaposition, a position that is adjacent to or side by side to another.

Z

z *abr.* **zona** / zone.

zambo-a *a.* bandy-legged; bow-legged.

zanahoria *f.* carrot.

zapato *m.* shoe; ___ortopédico / orthopedic ___; ___ **para escayola** / cast ___ .

zinc, cinc *m.* zinc, crystalline metallic chemical element with astringent properties; **pomada de**___ / ___ ointment.

Zollinger-Ellison, síndrome de *m.* Zollinger-Ellison syndrome, manifested by gastric hypersecretion and hyperacidity and by peptic ulceration of the stomach and small intestine.

zona *f.* 1. zona, a specific area or layer; 2. zoster; 3. zone, a belt-like anatomical structure; ___ **de apoyo** / rest area; ___ **de bienestar** / comfort ___; ___ **de deslizamiento** / gliding ___; ___ **de equivalencia** / equivalence ___; ___ **de transición** / transition ___; ___ **radiada** / radiated ___; ___ **respiratoria** / respiratory ___ .

zona desencadenante *f.* trigger zone, a sensitive area of the body whose stimulation triggers a reaction in a different part of the body.

zoofilia *f.* zoophilia. 1. love to animals; 2. bestiality.

zoofobia *f.* zoophobia, anxiety and irrational fear of animals.

zoógeno-a *a.* zoogenous, acquired from animals or derived from them.

zooinjerto *m.* zoograft, graft taken from an animal.

zootoxina *f.* zootoxin, poisonous substance produced from an animal such as the snake venom.

zóster *f.* zoster, *pop.* shingles. herpes.

zoster oftálmico *m.* zoster ophthalmicus, herpetic infection of the eye, esp. affecting the optical nerve.

zumbar *v.* to hum, to buzz, to ring.

zumbido *m.* hum, buzz, ring.

Gramática inglesa simplificada

Simplified English Grammar

EL NOMBRE O SUSTANTIVO / THE NOUN
GÉNERO / GENDER

Los nombres o sustantivos en inglés se clasifican en masculinos, femeninos y neutros. El género de cosas inanimadas es generalmente neutro.

Femenino	nombre de mujer o animal hembra
	la mujer / **the woman**
Masculino	nombre de hombre o animal varón
	el hombre / **the man**
Neutro	nombres de cosas, concretas o abstractas
	la inyección / **the shot**; el dolor / **the pain**

En ciertos nombres se distingue el género por medio de las palabras: hembra / **female,** varón / **male,** o por niño / **boy** y niña / **girl.**

enfermera / **female nurse**   enfermero / **male nurse**
bebita / **baby girl**   bebito / **baby boy**

Note: En este diccionario se ha incorporado la palabra **person** / persona a palabras como **chairman,** cambiada a **chairperson,** para evitar el uso exclusivo del masculino en nombres que pueden referirse al sexo masculino o femenino.

NÚMERO / NUMBER

El plural de los nombres

Añada **-s** para formar el plural de la mayor parte de los nombres.

síntoma / **symptom**   síntomas / **symptoms**

Añada **-es** si la palabra termina en **ch, h, sh, ss, x,** u **o.**

punto quirúrgico / **stitch**   puntos quirúrgicos / **stitches**
fogaje / **hot flash**   fogajes / **hot flashes**
absceso / **abscess**   abscesos / **abscesses**
reflejo / **reflex**   reflejos / **reflexes**
mosquito / **mosquito**   mosquitos / **mosquitoes**

Añada **-es** si la palabra termina en **y;** cambie la **y** por **i.**

deformidad / **deformity**   deformidades / **deformities**

Añada **-es** si la palabra termina en **f** o **fe;** cambie la **f** por **v.**

vida / **life**   vidas / **lives**
hoja / **leaf**   hojas / **leaves**

PLURALES IRREGULARES MÁS COMUNES EN INGLÉS / MOST COMMON IRREGULAR PLURALS IN ENGLISH

Singular	Plural	Singular	Plural
diente / **tooth**	dientes / **teeth**	hombre / **man**	hombres / **men**
mujer / **woman**	mujeres / **women**	niño / **child**	niños / **children**
pie / **foot**	pies / **feet**	piojo / **louse**	piojos / **lice**
ratón / **mouse**	ratones / **mice**		

EL CASO POSESIVO DE LOS NOMBRES

El caso posesivo de los nombres en inglés se forma invirtiendo el orden del caso posesivo en español.

Poseedor + ' (apóstrofe) + **s** + nombre de lo que posee

la enfermedad de la mujer / **the woman's illness**

Los nombres que terminan en **-s** y los nombres plurales añaden solamente un apóstrofe al final de la palabra.

Poseedor + ' (apóstrofe) + nombre de lo que posee

la opinión de los doctores / **the doctors' opinion**

Comparativo de igualdad de los nombres

Singular: **as much** + nombre + **as**

Ella tiene tanta fiebre hoy como ayer. / **She has as much fever today as yesterday.**

Plural: **as many** + nombre + **as**

Ella tiene tantos síntomas hoy como ayer. / **She has as many symptoms today as yesterday.**

EL ARTÍCULO / THE ARTICLE

Los artículos en inglés son invariables en género y número.

EL ARTÍCULO DEFINIDO / THE DEFINITE ARTICLE

el, la, los, las / **the**

el hospital / **the hospital**
la medicina / **the medicine**
los riñones / **the kidneys**
las recetas / **the prescriptions**

El artículo definido se omite en inglés cuando:

1. el sustantivo es un nombre común que expresa una idea general.

   una vacuna contra la difteria / **a vaccine against diptheria**
2. precede a los títulos de Sr., Sra. y Srta., o a cargos dignatarios o profesionales.

   El Sr. Jones / **Mr. Jones**; el Dr. Jones / **Dr. Jones**

EL ARTÍCULO INDEFINIDO / THE INDEFINITE ARTICLE

un, una / **a**

un, una / **an**

una píldora / **a pill**
un laboratorio / **a laboratory**
una unión / **a union**
un eufemismo / **a euphemism**
una hora / **an hour**
un accidente / **an accident**

1. **a:** Se emplea delante de las palabras que empiezan con consonante **o** con la vocal **u,** o el diptongo **eu** cuando éste se pronuncia como la letra **y.**
2. **an:** Se emplea delante de palabras que empiezan con una vocal o una **h** muda.

USOS DEL ARTÍCULO INDEFINIDO

1. Con nombres que designan el empleo o la profesión después del verbo **to be.**

   Ella es enfermera. / **She is a nurse.**

2. En generalizaciones sobre especies o clases precediendo a un nombre en singular; si el nombre está en plural el artículo se omite.

   El mosquito puede transmitir enfermedades. / **A mosquito can transmit disease.**
   Los antibióticos son indispensables. / **Antibiotics are indispensable.**

Nota: El plural del artículo indefinido **unos, unas,** se traduce al inglés como **some:**

   unas indicaciones preventivas / **some preventive indications**
   unos procedimientos quirúrgicos / **some surgical procedures**

EL ADJETIVO Y EL ADVERBIO / THE ADJECTIVE AND THE ADVERB

Los adjetivos en inglés generalmente preceden al nombre y son invariables en género y número. Los adjetivos demostrativos son una excepción a esta regla, ya que cambian del singular al plural de acuerdo con el nombre que modifican.

La mesa pequeña / **the small table**
Las mesas pequeñas / **the small tables**
esta mesa / **this table**
estas mesas / **these tables**

FORMACIÓN DEL ADVERBIO / HOW ADVERBS ARE FORMED

1. Los adverbios de modo que en español terminan generalmente en **-mente,** se forman en inglés añadiendo la terminación **-ly** al adjetivo.

>   frecuente / **frequent**   frecuentemente / **frequently**

2. Si el adjetivo en inglés termina en **-ble**, la **e** se convierte en **y.**

>   posible / **possible**   posiblemente / **possibly**

3. Si el adjetivo en inglés termina en **-ic,** el adverbio se forma añadiendo la terminación **-ally:**

>   crónico / **chronic**   crónicamente / **chronically**

COMPARACIÓN DE LOS ADJETIVOS Y ADVERBIOS / COMPARATIVE FORMS OF ADJECTIVES AND ADVERBS

Tanto los adjetivos como los adverbios admiten grados de comparación.

1. Los monosílabos y algunos bisílabos cortos añaden la terminación **-er** y **-est** a la forma positiva:

a.	frío / **cold**	más frío / **colder**	(el)(la) más frío-a / **the coldest**
adv.	despacio / **slow**	más despacio / **slower**	(el)(la) más despacio / **the slowest**

2. Palabras que terminan en **-y** cambian la **-y** en **i** y añaden **-er** y **-est** para formar el comparativo y el superlativo, respectivamente:

a.	contento-a / **happy**	más contento-a / **happier**	(el)(la) más contento-a / **the happiest**
adv.	temprano / **early**	más temprano / **earlier**	(el)(la) más temprano-a / **the earliest**

3. El resto de los adjetivos y adverbios forman el comparativo de superioridad y el superlativo anteponiendo las palabras **more** y **most.**

a.	doloroso-a / **painful**	más doloroso-a / **more painful**	(el)(la) más doloroso-a / **the most painful**
adv.	frecuentemente / **frequently**	más frecuentemente / **more frequently**	(el)(la) más frecuentemente / **the most frequently**

4. El comparativo y el superlativo de inferioridad se forma anteponiendo las palabras **less** y **least.**

a.	contagioso-a / **contagious**	menos contagioso-a / **less contagious**	(el)(la) menos contagioso-a / **the least contagious**
adv.	frecuentemente / **frequently**	menos frecuentemente / **less frequently**	(el)(la) menos frecuentemente / **the least frequently**

5. El comparativo de igualdad se forma usando la palabra **as** antes y después del adjetivo y del adverbio.

as+adjetivo+**as**	tan infeccioso como / **as infectious as**
as+adverbio+**as**	tan temprano como / **as early as**

Adjetivos comunes con comparativos y superlativos irregulares

malo / **bad**	peor / **worse**	(el)(la) peor / **the worst**
bueno / **good**	mejor / **better**	(el)(la) mejor / **the best**
poco / **little**	menos / **less**	(el)(la) menos / **the least**
mucho / **much, many**	más / **more**	(el)(la) más / **the most**

Adverbios comunes con comparativos y superlativos irregulares

lejos / **far**	más lejos / **farther**	(el)(la) más lejos / **the farthest**
poco / **little**	menos / **less**	menor / **the least**
much / **mucho**	más / **more**	mayor / **the most**
bien / **well**	mejor / **better**	(el)(la) mejor / **the best**

PRONOMBRES Y ADJETIVOS / PRONOUNS AND ADJECTIVES

PRONOMBRES PERSONALES / SUBJECT PRONOUNS

1. Los pronombres personales nominativos, es decir, los que sirven de sujeto, nunca se omiten en inglés:

> (Yo) Tengo dolor / **I have a pain; I am in pain.**

El pronombre **I** (yo) siempre se escribe con mayúscula en inglés.

Pronombres personales / Subject Pronouns

PERSONAL	SINGULAR	*PLURAL*
1a.	I	we
2a.	you	you
3a. (*m.*)	he	they
3a. (*f.*)	she	they
3a. (*neut.*)	it	they

2. El pronombre (objeto directo) siempre precede al pronombre (objeto indirecto). El pronombre que actúa de objeto indirecto va precedido por un preposición (**to, from, for, of**).

> Me las dio. / She gave **them to me.**

Cuando el objeto directo es un nombre y el objeto indirecto es un pronombre, el pronombre precede al objeto directo.

> La enfermera me dio las instrucciones / **The nurse gave me the instructions.**

Pronombres como complemento

PERSONA	SINGULAR	*PLURAL*
1a.	me	us
2a.	you	you
3a. (*m.*)	him	them
3a. (*f.*)	her	them
3a. (*neut.*)	it	them

3. Además de actuar como sujeto o complemento, el pronombre personal en inglés puede también ser reflexivo cuando el complemento es la misma persona que el sujeto:

Él **se** curó a **si** mismo. / He cured **himself.**

Pronombres reflexivos

PERSONA	SINGULAR	PLURAL
1a.	myself	ourselves
2a.	yourself	yourselves
3a. (*m.*)	himself	themselves
3a. (*f.*)	herself	themselves
3a. (*neut.*)	itself	themselves

PRONOMBRES Y ADJETIVOS DEMOSTRATIVOS / DEMONSTRATIVE PRONOUNS AND ADJECTIVES

Los demostrativos son los únicos adjetivos que cambian del singular al plural de acuerdo con el número del nombre que modifican.

ADJETIVOS DEMOSTRATIVOS

este	esta	**this**
estos	estas	**these**
ese	esa	**that**
aquel	aquella	**that**
esos	esas	**those**
aquellos	aquellas	**those**

esta enfermedad / **this disease**
estas enfermedades / **these diseases**
esa pastilla / **that pill**.

PRONOMBRES DEMOSTRATIVOS

éste, ésta, esto	**this one, this**
éstos, éstas	**these**
ése, ésa, eso	**that one, that**
aquél, aquélla, aquello	**that one, that**
ésos, ésas	**those**
aquéllos, aquéllas	**those**

Tome ésta. / **Take this one.**
Tome éstas. / **Take these.**

Ése es mejor. / **That one is better.**
Es aquélla. / **It is that one.**

PRONOMBRES Y ADJETIVOS POSESIVOS / POSSESSIVE ADJECTIVES AND PRONOUNS

PERSONA	ADJETIVO	PRONOMBRE
Sing. 1a.	my	mine
2a.	your	yours
3a. (*m.*)	his	his
3a. (*f.*)	her	hers
3a. (*neut.*)	its	its
Plur. 1a.	our	ours
2a.	your	yours
3a.	their	theirs

mi paciente / **my patient**
sus síntomas / **her symptoms**
La medicina es mía. / **The medicine is mine.**
El problema es nuestro. / **The problem is ours.**

Nota: En inglés el adjetivo posesivo se emplea con las partes del cuerpo:
Me lastimé el brazo. / **I hurt my arm.**

PRONOMBRES Y ADJETIVOS INTERROGATIVOS / INTERROGATIVE ADJECTIVES AND PRONOUNS

INTERROGATIVOS / INTERROGATIVES

¿quién?, ¿quiénes?	who?
¿de quién?, ¿de quiénes?	whose?
¿a quién?, ¿a quiénes?	whom?
¿qué?, ¿cuál?, ¿cuáles?	what, which?

¿Quién está enfermo? / **Who is ill?**
¿De quién es la receta? / **Whose is the prescription?**
¿A quién vio ella? / **Whom did she see?**
¿Qué medicina prefiere? / **Which medicine do you prefer?**
¿Qué recomendó el doctor? / **What did the doctor recommend?**
¿Cuál recomendó el doctor? / **Which did the doctor recommend?**
De esos antibióticos, ¿cuáles prefiere? / **Of those antibiotics, which do you prefer?**

PRONOMBRES RELATIVOS / RELATIVE PRONOUNS

que, el cual, la cual, el que, la que, lo que, los que, las que	**that**
que, quien, el cual, la cual, el que, etc.	**which**
quien, que, el cual, la cual, etc.	**who**
que, quien, el cual, la cual, etc.	**whom**
de quien, cuyo, del cual, de la cual, etc.	**whose**

el jarabe que (ella) tomó / **the cough syrup that she took**

la medicina que se recetó / **the medicine which was prescribed**

el paciente que está esperando / **the patient who is waiting**

el paciente que (a quién) la enfermera atiende / **the patient whom the nurse is helping**

el paciente cuya radiografía necesita el doctor / **the patient whose x-rays the doctor needs**

Nota: Las terminaciones **-ever** y **-soever** se añaden a **who, which,** y **what** para formar los pronombres relativos compuestos **whoever** / quienquiera, **whichever** / cualquiera y **whatever** / quienquiera o cualquiera.

PRONOMBRES Y ADJETIVOS INDEFINIDOS MÁS COMUNES / MOST COMMON INDEFINITE ADJECTIVES AND PRONOUNS

all	todo	many	muchos
another	otro	nobody	nadie
any	cualquiera	none	ninguno, ninguna
anybody	cualquiera	no one	nadie
anyone	cualquiera	nothing	nada
anything	cualquier cosa, algo	one	uno-a
both	ambos, ambas	other	otro-a
each (one)	cada (uno), cada cual	some	algunos, algunas
everybody	todos	somebody	alguien
everyone	todos	someone	alguien
everything	todo	something	algo
few	pocos		
a few	unos pocos		

EL VERBO / THE VERB
FORMAS DEL VERBO / FORMS OF THE VERB

Infinitivo	Pasado	Participio	Gerundio
curar / to heal	healed	healed	healing
comer / to eat	ate	ate	eating
Infinitivo / Infinitive		El verbo precedido de la preposición to: examina / **to examine**	
Presente / Present		La misma forma verbal del infinitivo sin la preposición **to** precedida del pronombre correspondiente: yo examino / **I examine** nosotros examinamos / **we examine**	
Pasado / Past		El infinitivo + la terminación **-d** o **-ed** yo examiné / **I examined** nosotros examinamos / **we examined**	
Participio pasado / Past Participle		La misma forma verbal que el pasado: examinado / **examined**	
Participio de presente / Present Participle		El infinitivo + **-ing**: examinando / **examining**	

Nota: Para formar el pasado o el participio de verbos regulares se añade la terminación **-ed** al infinitivo. Las variaciones a esta regla son las siguientes.

a. Si el infinitivo termina en **e**, se añade **-d** (die, di**ed**).
b. Si el infinitivo termina en la letra **y** precedida de una consonante, se cambia la **y** por **i** antes de añadir **-ed** (try, tri**ed**).
c. Si el infinitivo termina en consonante precedida de una vocal y la sílaba final lleva el énfasis, se dobla la consonante antes de añadir **-ed** (permit, permit**ted**).

Nota: Para formar el gerundio se añade la terminación **-ing** al infinitivo; **to drink** / beber; **drink-ing** / bebiendo. Las variaciones a esta regla son las siguientes:

a. Si el infinitivo termina en **-e** precedida de una consonante, la **e** se pierde antes de añadir la terminación **-ing** (arise, arising).
b. Si el infinitivo termina en **ie**, la **ie** se sustituye por la letra **y** antes de añadir **-ing** (l**ie**, l**y**ing).
c. En algunos verbos se dobla la consonante antes de añadir -ing si la sílaba final del infinitivo lleva el énfasis (spit, spit**ting**), excepto en verbos terminados en **h**, **w**, **e y**, los cuales no doblan la consonante al formar el gerundio **to chew** / masticar; **chewing** / masticando.

TIEMPOS DEL VERBO / TENSES OF THE VERB
TIEMPOS SIMPLES / SIMPLE TENSES

to cough / toser

Presente / Present	yo toso / **I cough**
Pasado (pretérito e imperfecto) / Past	yo tosí, tosía / **I coughed**
Futuro / Future	yo toseré / **I will, shall cough**

El imperfecto se traduce al inglés con las formas **used to** o **would** para indicar una acción repetida indefinidamente o habitualmente en el pasado.

Yo tomaba la medicina todos los días. / **I used to take the medicine every day.**

El futuro de todas las personas se forma con el verbo auxiliar **will** o **shall,** que precede a la forma del verbo en todos los tiempos.

Tomaré la medicina. / **I will take the medicine.**

TIEMPOS COMPUESTOS / COMPOUND TENSES

Los tiempos compuestos se forman con el verbo auxiliar haber / **to have.** (Véase la conjugación del verbo **to have** al final de la explicación del verbo.)

Perfecto / Present perfect	yo he tosido / **I have coughed**
Pluscuamperfecto / Past perfect	yo había, hube tosido / **I had coughed**
Futuro anterior / Future perfect	yo habré tosido / **I will, I shall have coughed**

Nota: Además de los seis tiempos indicados, todos los verbos tienen una forma progresiva que indica una acción continuada dentro de la configuración del tiempo a que se refieren. Se forma con el verbo auxiliar estar / **to be,** seguido del participio presente (gerundio). (Véase la conjugación del verbo **to be** al final de la explicación del verbo.)

Presente	yo estoy tosiendo / **I am coughing**
Pasado	yo estaba, estuve tosiendo / **I was coughing**
Futuro	yo estaré tosiendo / **I will, shall be coughing**
Perfecto	yo he estado tosiendo / **I have been coughing**
Pluscuamperfecto	yo había, hube estado tosiendo / **I had been coughing**
Futuro anterior	yo habré estado tosiendo / **I will, shall have been coughing**

MODOS DEL VERBO / MOODS OF THE VERB
INDICATIVO / INDICATIVE

Yo toso / **I cough.**

La oración interrogativa, negativa y enfática se forma con el verbo auxiliar **to do.** (Véase la conjugación del verbo al final de la explicación del verbo.)

285

Interrogación	¿Tose usted por las mañanas? / **Do you cough in the morning?**
Negación	No toso durante el día. / **I do not cough during the day.**
Énfasis	Toso mucho por las noches. / **I do cough a lot at night.**

Nota: El verbo **to do** también se emplea para dar énfasis a la respuesta de sí o no a una pregunta:

¿Tose mucho? / **Do you cough much?**   **Yes, I do.**
                                                         No, I do not.

IMPERATIVO / IMPERATIVE

Tosa, por favor. / **Cough please.**

CONJUGACIÓN DE UN VERBO REGULAR / CONJUGATION OF A REGULAR VERB

preparar / to prepare

INFINITIVO	PARTICIPIO	GERUNDIO
preparar / **to prepare**	preparado / **prepared**	preparando / **preparing**

Indicativo

PRESENTE / PRESENT

yo preparo / **I prepare**	nosotros preparamos / **we prepare**
Ud. prepara, tú preparas / **you prepare**	vosotros preparáis, ustedes preparan / **you prepare**
él, ella prepara / **he, she, it prepares**	ellos, ellas preparan / **they prepare**

PRETÉRITO / IMPERFECTO / PAST

preparé, preparaba / **I prepared**	preparamos, preparábamos / **we prepared**
preparó, preparaba, preparaste, preparabas / **you prepared**	prepararon, preparaban, preparasteis, preparabais / **you prepared**
preparó, preparaba / **he, she, it, prepared**	prepararon, preparaban / **they prepared**

FUTURO / FUTURE

prepararé / **I will, shall prepare**	prepararemos / **we will, shall prepare**
preparará, prepararás / **you will prepare**	prepararéis, prepararán / **you will prepare**
preparará / **he, she, it will prepare**	prepararán / **they will prepare**

PERFECTO / PERFECT

he preparado / **I have prepared**	hemos preparado / **we have prepared**
ha preparado, has preparado / **you have prepared**	habéis, han preparado / **you have prepared**
ha preparado / **he, she, it has prepared**	han preparado / **they have prepared**

PLUSCUAMPERFECTO / PAST PERFECT

había preparado / **I had prepared**	habíamos preparado / **we had prepared**
había, habías preparado / **you had prepared**	habíais, habían preparado / **you had prepared**
había preparado / **he, she, it had prepared**	habían preparado / **they had prepared**

FUTURO ANTERIOR / FUTURE PERFECT

habré preparado / **I will, shall have prepared**	habremos preparado / **we will, shall have prepared**
habrá, habrás preparado / **you will have prepared**	habréis, habrán preparado / **you will have prepared**
habrá preparado / **he, she, it will have prepared**	habrán preparado / **they will have prepared**

Imperativo / Imperative

prepara (tú), prepare (usted), preparad (vosotros), preparen (ustedes, ellos)	**prepare**
preparemos (nosotros)	let's prepare

En inglés no existe la distinción entre el **tú** familiar y el **usted** formal. La segunda persona del singular es siempre **you.** La segunda persona del plural (**vosotros** y **ustedes**) tiene igualmente una sola forma, que se traduce también como **you.**

La tercera persona singular del presente es la única forma verbal que difiere de las demás al tomar la terminación **-s.** Las excepciones a esta regla son las siguientes:

a. Si el verbo en el infinitivo termina en **-s, -x, -z, -ch,** o **-sh,** se añade **-es;** alcanzar / **to reach;** he, she, it **reaches.**

b. Si el verbo termina en **-z,** precedida por una sola vocal, la **z** se dobla y se añade **-es;** preguntar / **to quiz;** he, she, it **quizzes.**

c. Si el verbo termina en **y,** precedida de consonante, la **y** cambia a **i** y se añade **-es;** llevar / **to carry;** he, she, it **carries.**

CONJUGACIÓN DE LOS VERBOS AUXILIARES / CONJUGATION OF AUXILIARY VERBS

haber / to have

INFINITIVO	PARTICIPIO	GERUNDIO
haber / **to have**	habido / **had**	habiendo / **having**

Indicativo / Indicative

PRESENTE / PRESENT

yo he / **I have**	nosotros hemos / **we have**
Ud. ha, tú has / **you have**	vosotros habéis, ustedes han / **you have**
él, ella ha / **he, she, it has**	ellos han / **they have**

PRETÉRITO / IMPERFECTO / PAST

hube, había / **I had**	hubimos, habíamos / **we had**
hubo, había, hubiste, habías/ **you had**	hubisteis, habíais, hubieron, habían / **you had**
hubo, había / **he, she, it had**	hubieron, habían / **they had**

FUTURO / FUTURE

habré / **I will, shall have**	habremos / **we will, shall have**
habrá, habrás / **you will have**	habréis, habrán / **you will have**
habrá / **he, she, it will have**	habrán / **they will have**

Nota: Para formar los tiempos compuestos se añade el participio de pasado **had** a las formas simples: **I have had, I had had, I will, shall have had.**

ser, estar / to be

INFINITIVO	PARTICIPIO	GERUNDIO
ser / **to be**	sido / **been**	siendo / **being**

PRESENTE / PRESENT

yo soy / **I am**	nosotros somos / **we are**
Ud. es, tú eres / **you are**	vosotros sois, ustedes son / **you are**
él, ella es / **he, she, it is**	ellos, ellas son / **they are**

PRETÉRITO / IMPERFECTO / PAST

fui, era / **I was**	fuimos, éramos / **we were**
fue, era, fuiste, eras / **you were**	fuisteis, erais, fueron, eran / **you were**
fue, era / **he, she, it was**	fueron, eran / **they were**

seré / **I will, shall be**	seremos / **we will, shall be**
será, serás / **you will be**	seréis, serán / **you will be**
será / **he, she, it will be**	serán / **they will be**

Nota: Para formar los tiempos compuestos se usan las formas simples del verbo auxiliar **to have** y el participio de **to be: been. I have been; I had been; I will, shall have been.**

hacer / to do

El verbo **to do** no existe como verbo auxiliar en español; por lo tanto, las formas **do, does** y **did** en oraciones interrogativas, negativas y enfáticas no tienen traducción al español.

INFINITIVO	PARTICIPIO	GERUNDIO
hacer / **to do**	hecho / **done**	haciendo / **doing**

PRESENTE / PRESENT

yo hago / **I do**	nosotros hacemos / **we do**
Ud. hace, tú haces / **you do**	vosotros hacéis, ustedes hacen / **you do**
él, ella hace / **he, she, it does**	ellos, ellas hacen / **they do**

PRETÉRITO / IMPERFECTO / PAST

hice, hacía / **I did**	hicimos, hacíamos / **we did**
hiciste, hacías / **you did**	hicisteis, hacíais, hicieron, hacían / **you did**
hizo, hacía / **he, she, it did**	hicieron, hacían / **they did**

FUTURO / FUTURE

haré / **I will, shall do**	haremos / **we will, shall do**
hará, harás / **you will do**	haréis, harán / **you will do**
hará / **he, she, it will do**	harán / **they will do**

Nota: Para formar los tiempos compuestos se usan las formas simples del verbo auxiliar **to have** y el participio de **to do, done: I have done, I had done, I will, shall have done.**

Imperativo / Imperative

haz (tú), haga (usted), haced (vosotros), hagan (ustedes, ellos)	**do**
hagamos (nosotros)	**let us do**

Subjuntivo / Subjunctive

El modo subjuntivo se emplea en inglés con mucha menos frecuencia que en español, y para los efectos de este diccionario, no lo hemos incluído.

PARTICIPIOS Y PRETÉRITOS IRREGULARES / IRREGULAR PAST PARTICIPLES AND PRETERITES

Infinitivo / Infinitive	Pretérito / Preterit	Participio pasado / Past Participle
to arise / levantarse, surgir	arose	arisen
to awake / despertarse	awoke	awoke, awoken
to be / ser, estar	was, were	been
to become / volverse, hacerse	became	become
to begin / empezar	began	begun
to bend / inclinarse, doblarse	bent	bent
to bite / morder	bit	bit, bitten
to bleed / sangrar	bled	bled
to blow / soplar	blew	blown
to break / romper; quebrar	broke	broken
to bring / traer	brought	brought
to build / construir	built	built
to burn / quemar	burnt, burned	burnt, burned
to burst / reventar	burst	burst
to buy / comprar	bought	bought
can (defectivo, aux.) / poder	could	—
to catch / agarrar, coger	caught	caught
to choose / escoger, elegir	chose	chosen
to come / venir	came	come
to cost / costar	cost	cost
to cut / cortar	cut	cut
to deal out / repartir, alocar	dealt out	dealt out
to deal with / tratar de, resolver	dealt with	dealt with
to dig / cavar, extraer	dug	dug
to draw / dibujar	drew	drawn
to dream / soñar	dreamt, dreamed	dreamt, dreamed
to drink / beber, tomar	drank	drunk
to drive / manejar, conducir	drove	driven
to eat / comer	ate	eaten
to fall / caerse; desprenderse	fell	fallen
to feed / alimentar, dar de comer	fed	fed
to feel / sentir; palpar	felt	felt
to fight / pelear	fought	fought
to find / encontrar, hallar	found	found
to fly / volar	flew	flown
to foresee / prever	foresaw	foreseen

Infinitivo / Infinitive	Pretérito / Preterit	Participio pasado / Past Participle
to forget / olvidar	forgot	forgot, forgotten
to forgive / perdonar	forgave	forgiven
to freeze / congelar	froze	frozen
to get / conseguir, obtener	got	got, gotten
to give / dar	gave	given
to grind / moler; pulverizar	ground	ground
to grow / crecer; madurar	grew	grown
to hang / colgar; suspender	hung	hung
to have / tener, haber	had	had
to hear / oír, escuchar	heard	heard
to hide / esconder (se)	hid	hid, hidden
to hit / pegar	hit	hit
to hold / aguantar	held	held
to hurt / lastimar, doler	hurt	hurt
to keep / guardar	kept	kept
to kneel / arrodillarse	knelt	knelt
to knit / tejer	knit, knitted	knit, knitted
to know / saber, conocer	knew	known
to lay / poner, colocar	laid	laid
to lead / dirigir	led	led
to leap / saltar	leapt, leaped	leapt, leaped
to leave / irse, dejar	left	left
to lend / prestar	lent	lent
to let / permitir, dejar	let	let
to lie / echarse, acostarse	lay	lain
to light / encender	lit, lighted	lit, lighted
to lose / perder	lost	lost
to make / hacer	made	made
may / poder	might	—
to meet / conocer	met	met
to melt / derretir	melted	melted, molten
to mistake / equivocarse	mistook	mistaken
must (*defectivo; aux.*) / deber de; tener que	—	—
ought (*defectivo; aux.*) / deber de	—	—
to pay / pagar	paid	paid
to put / poner	put	put
to quit / renunciar, dejar	quit	quit
to read / leer	read	read

Infinitivo / Infinitive	Pretérito / Preterit	Participio pasado / Past Participle
to rid / librar, deshacerse	rid, ridded	rid, ridded
to ride / montar, pasear	rode	ridden
to ring / sonar	rang, rung	rung
to rise / alzarse, levantarse	rose	risen
to run / correr	ran	run
to say / decir	said	said
to see / ver	saw	seen
to seek / buscar	sought	sought
to sell / vender	sold	sold
to send / enviar	sent	sent
to set / colocar, poner	set	set
to sew / coser	sewed	sewn
to shake / batir, temblar	shook	shaken
to shine / brillar	shone	shone
to shoot / disparar	shot	shot
to show / mostrar	showed	shown, showed
to shrink / encogerse	shrank, shrunk	shrunk, shrunken
to shut / cerrar	shut	shut
to sit / sentarse	sat	sat
to sleep / dormir (se)	slept	slept
to slide / deslizar (se)	slid	slid
to slit / rajar	slit	slit
to speak / hablar	spoke	spoken
to speed / acelerar	sped	sped
to spend / gastar	spent	spent
to spill / botar, derramar	spilled, spilt	spilled, spilt
to spin / dar vueltas	spun	spun
to spit / escupir	spit, spat	spit, spat
to split / partir	split	split
to spread / regar, esparcir	spread	spread
to stand / pararse	stood	stood
to steal / robar	stole	stolen
to stick / punzar, picar	stuck	stuck
to sting / picar, pinchar	stung	stung
to stink / apestar	stank, stunk	stunk
to strike / golpear, herir	struck	struck, stricken
to swear / jurar	swore	sworn
to sweep / barrer	swept	swept
to swell / hincharse	swelled	swollen, swelled

Infinitivo / Infinitive	Pretérito / Preterit	Participio pasado / Past Participle
to swim / nadar	swam	swum
to swing / mecer (se)	swung	swung
to take / tomar	took	taken
to teach / enseñar	taught	taught
to tear / rasgar, desgarrar	tore	torn
to tell / decir, contar	told	told
to think / pensar	thought	thought
to throw / tirar	threw	thrown
to understand / comprender, entender	understood	understood
to undo / deshacer	undid	undone
to upset / indisponer (se)	upset	upset
to visualize / visualizar, visualizado	visualized	visualized
to wake / despertar	woke, waked	waked, woken
to wear / usar, llevar	wore	worn
to weep / llorar	wept	wept
to wet / mojar, humedecer	wet, wetted	wet, wetted
will / (*v. aux.*)	would	—
to win / ganar	won	won
to withstand / soportar, resistir	withstood	withstood
to write / escribir	wrote	written

Glosario inglés-español
English-Spanish Glossary

a

a *abbr.* **absolute** / absoluto; **accommodation** / acomodación; **acidity** / acidez; **allergy** / alergia; **anterior** / anterior; **aqua** / agua; **artery** / arteria.

a *art. indef.* un, una; **a contagious disease** / una enfermedad contagiosa; **a good doctor** / un buen médico; (antes de vocal o *h* muda); **an; an abdominal pain** / un dolor abdominal; *a.* algún, alguna; **Is there a doctor on duty?** / ¿Hay algún médico de guardia? *prep.* a; **three times a day** / tres veces al (a+el) día.

abandon *v.* abandonar, dejar; desamparar.
abandoned *a.* abandonado-a; irresponsable.
abasia *n.* abasia, movimiento incierto.
abbreviate *v.* abreviar, acortar, reducir, resumir.
abbreviation *n.* abreviación, abreviatura.
abdomen *n.* abdomen, vientre. *pop.* barriga, panza; **pendulous** ___ / ___ colgante, pendular; **scaphoid** ___ / ___ escafoideo. See illustration on this page.

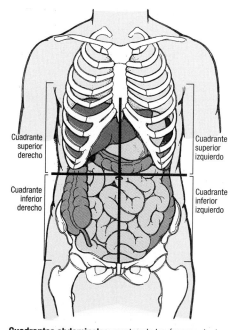

Cuadrante superior derecho
Cuadrante superior izquierdo
Cuadrante inferior derecho
Cuadrante inferior izquierdo

Cuadrantes abdominales: mostrando los órganos dentro de cada cuadrante

abdominal *a.* abdominal, rel. al abdomen; ___ **bandage** / vendaje ___; ___ **breathing** / respiración ___; ___ **cavity** / cavidad ___; ___ **cramps** / retortijón, torzón; ___ **dyspnea** / disnea ___; ___ **distention** / distensión ___; ___ **fistula** / fístula ___; ___ **injuries** / traumatismos ___-es; ___ **puncture** / punción ___; ___ **rigidity** / rigidez ___; ___ **tumor** / tumor ___.

abdominocentesis *n.* abdominocentesis, punción abdominal.

abdominohysterectomy *n.* abdominohisterectomía, excisión del útero por medio de una incisión abdominal.

abdominoplasty *n.* abdominoplastia, reparación de la pared abdominal.

abdominovaginal *a.* abdominovaginal, rel. al abdomen y la vagina.

abduce *v.* abducir, desviar, separar.
abducent *a.* abducente; abductor.
abduction *n.* abducción, separación.
aberrant *a.* aberrante, desviado del curso normal; anómalo.

aberration *n.* aberración. 1. visión defectuosa o imperfecta; **chromatic** ___ / ___ cromática; 2. desviación de lo normal; 3. trastorno mental; **mental** ___ / ___ mental.

abhor *v.* aborrecer; tener aversión a algo o a alguien.

ability *n.* habilidad, aptitud; talento, capacidad.

abiotrophy *n.* abiotrofia, pérdida prematura de la vitalidad.

ablatio *n.* ablación, separación, desprendimiento; ___ **placentae** / desprendimiento de la placenta; ___ **retinae** / desprendimiento de la retina.

ablation *n.* ablación.

able *a.* hábil, capaz, apto-a; *v.* **to be** ___ / [*to be or do something*] ser capaz de; poder.

abnormal *a.* anormal, anómalo-a; disforme, irregular.

abnormality *n.* anormalidad, anomalía; irregularidad; deformidad.

abort *v.* abortar; hacer abortar, interrumpir el curso de una gestación o de una enfermedad antes del término natural.

abortifacient *n.* abortivo, estimulante para inducir un aborto.

abortion *n.* aborto, interrupción prematura del embarazo. See chart on page 298.

abortionist *n.* abortista, persona que interrumpe un embarazo.

about *prep.* cerca de; junto a; alrededor de; a eso de, sobre; **it is** ___ **a block from here** / está

Abortion	Aborto
accidental	accidental
afebrile	afebril
ampullar	ampollar
artificial	artifical
cervical	cervical
complete	completo
contagious	contagioso
criminal	criminal
elective	electivo
epizootic	epizoótico
incomplete	incompleto
induced	provocado o inducido
infectious	infeccioso
in progress	en curso
natural	natural
recurrent	recurrente
septic	séptico
spontaneous	espontáneo
therapeutic	terapéutico
tubal	tubárico

cerca de una cuadra de aquí; *adv.* [*time*]; **it is ___ one thirty** / es alrededor de la una y media; *v.* **to speak ___** / hablar de.

above *n.* antecedente, precedente; *a.* antedicho-a, anterior; *prep.* sobre, por encima de; **___ the heart** / encima del corazón; *adv.* arriba; la parte alta; más de o más que; **___ all** / sobre todo; **from ___** / desde lo alto, desde arriba.

abrasion *n.* abrasión, excoriación, irritación o raspadura de las mucosas o de una superficie a causa de una fricción o de un trauma; **___ collar** / círculo de ___ , marca circular de pólvora que deja en la piel el disparo de un arma de fuego.

abrasive *a.* abrasivo-a, irritante, raspante, rel. a una abrasión o que la causa.

abreast *adv.* de frente; en frente.

abrupt *a.* abrupto-a, precipitado-a, repentino-a.

abruptio *n. L.* abruptio, abrupción, acción violenta de separación, desprendimiento; **___ placentae, placental abruption** / desprendimiento prematuro de la placenta.

abruption *n.* abrupción.

abscess *n.* absceso, acumulación de pus gen. debido a una desintegración del tejido; **acute ___** / **___** agudo; **alveolar ___** / **___** alveolar; **chronic ___** / **___** crónico; **cutaneous ___** / **___** cutáneo; **dental ___** / **___** dental; **drainage ___** / **___** de drenaje; **encysted ___** / **___** enquistado; **facial ___** / **___** facial; **fecal ___** / **___** fecal; **follicular ___** / **___** folicular; **gingival ___** / **___** de las encías; **hepatic ___** / **___** hepático; **mammary ___** / **___** mamario; **mastoid ___** / **___** mastoideo; **osseous ___** / **___** óseo; **pancreatic ___** / **___** pancreático; **paronchial ___** / **___** de la uña; **pelvic ___** / **___** de la pelvis; **peritonsicular ___** / **___** de las amígdalas; **pulmonary ___** / **___** pulmonar o en un pulmón; **radicular ___** / absceso de la raíz; **tubo-ovarian ___** / **___** tubárico. See chart on page 40.

absence *n.* ausencia, falta; pérdida momentánea del conocimiento.

absent *a.* ausente; distraído-a, absorto-a.

absentia epileptica *n.* absencia epiléptica (epilepsia menor), pérdida momentánea del conocimiento en ciertos casos de ataques epilépticos.

absentminded *a.* distraído-a; absorto-a.

absolute *a.* absoluto-a, incondicional; **___ alcohol (ethyl)** / alcohol **___** (alcohol etílico).

absorb *v.* absorber, sorber, chupar.

absorbency *n.* absorbencia.

absorbent *a.* absorbente; que puede absorber.

absorption *n.* absorción.1. acto de ingerir o introducir líquidos u otras sustancias en el organismo; **cutaneous ___** / **___** cutánea; **mouth ___** / **___** bucal; **parenteral ___** / **___** parenteral; **intestinal ___** / **___** entérica; **stomach ___** / **___** estomacal; 2. ensimismación.

abstain *v.* abstenerse, privarse de; **___ from sexual intercourse** / **___** de relaciones sexuales; *Mex.* cuidarse.

abstainer, abstemious *a.* abstemio-a; persona sobria.

abstention *n.* abstinencia, abstención, privación.

abstinence *n.* abstinencia, privación voluntaria, templanza, moderación.

abstract *n.* extracto, cantidad pequeña; resumen; *a.* abstracto-a; *v.* separar, alejar; extractar; resumir.

abstracted *a.* pensativo-a, abstraído-a; puro-a, sin mezcla alguna.

absurd *a.* absurdo-a; ridículo-a.

abulia *n.* abulia, pérdida de la voluntad; **cyclic** ___ / ___ cíclica.

abundance *n.* abundancia.

abundant *a.* abundante, copioso-a.

abuse *n.* abuso, uso exagerado; maltrato; ___ of medication / uso exagerado de medicamentos o drogas; **spouse** ___ / ___ conyugal; **verbal** ___ / maltrato de palabra, insulto; *v.* [*to take advantage of*] abusar de; maltratar; seducir.

abutment *n.* refuerzo, remate; [*dentistry*] soporte.

acanthoid *n.* acantoide, espinoso-a, en forma de espina.

acanthosis *n.* acantosis, enfermedad que causa una condición áspera y verrugosa en la piel.

acapnia *n.* acapnia, estado producido por una disminución de ácido carbónico en la sangre.

acariasis *n.* acariasis, infección causada por ácaros; comezón; sarna.

acarid *n.* ácaro, parásito; *a.* acárido-a.

accelerate *v.* acelerar, apresurar, aumentar la velocidad; **to** ___ **the healing process** / ___ la cura.

acceleration *n.* aceleración, aceleramiento.

accelerator *n.* acelerador, sustancia o agente que tiene la propiedad de acelerar un proceso.

accent *n.* acento, énfasis, intensificación; *v.* acentuar, hacer énfasis; recalcar.

accented *a.* acentuado-a.

accept *v.* aceptar, admitir, acoger, aprobar.

acceptable *a.* aceptable, permitido-a; admitido-a.

access *n.* 1. ataque, acceso; paroxismo; 2. [*entrance*] entrada.

accessible *a.* accesivo-a, asequible, accesible.

accessory *a.* accesorio-a, adicional, adjunto-a.

accident *n.* accidente; **by** ___ / por casualidad, sin querer; **car** ___ / ___ automovilístico; **occupational** ___ / ___ del trabajo, ocupacional; **traffic** ___ / ___ de tráfico.

accidental *a.* accidental, inesperado-a, casual.

acclimate *v.* aclimatar.

acclimatization *n.* aclimatación.

accommodate *v.* acomodar, ajustar, cuadrar; [*to lodge*] alojar, hospedar.

accommodation *n.* acomodación, ajustamiento; [*lodging*] alojamiento; **amplitude of** ___ / amplitud de ___; **histologic** ___ / ___ histológica; **negative** ___ / ___ negativa; **nerve** ___ / ___ del nervio; **positive** ___ / ___ positiva; **range of** ___ / jerarquía de ___ .

accompany *v.* acompañar.

accomplish *v.* acabar, realizar, lograr, cumplir, finalizar.

accomplishment *n.* realización, éxito, logro.

accord *n.* acuerdo, convenio, arreglo, transacción; *v.* acordar, poner de acuerdo; **of one's own** ___ / espontáneamente, voluntariamente; **of mutual** ___ / de acuerdo mutuo.

accordingly *adv.* de acuerdo con, por consiguiente; conformemente, en conformidad.

account *n.* cuenta, cálculo; nota, relación; **bank** ___ / ___ bancaria; **current** ___ / ___ corriente; **on** ___ **of** / por motivo de; *v.* **to pay the** ___ / pagar la ___; **to settle the** ___ / arreglar la ___; **to take into** ___ / tener en ___ , tener en consideración.

accountable *a.* responsable, contable.

accredit *v.* dar crédito, acreditar; certificar; dar credenciales.

accreditation *n.* crédito; credencial; capacitación.

accredited *a.* acreditado-a.

accretion *n.* aumento, acrecentamiento; acumulación.

accumulate *v.* acumular, añadir, aumentar.

accumulation *n.* acumulación, amontonamiento; hacinamiento.

accuracy *n.* exactitud, precisión, cuidado.

accurate *a.* exacto-a, preciso-a, correcto-a.

accurateness *n.* precisión, exactitud, esmero.

accusation *n.* acusación, imputación.

accuse *v.* acusar, denunciar, culpar.

accustom *v.* acostumbrar, hacer algo de costumbre.

accustomed *a.* acostumbrado-a; *v.* **to be** ___ **to** / estar acostumbrado-a a.

acellular *a.* acelular, que no contiene células.

acentric *a.* acéntrico, fuera del centro.

acerbic *a.* agrio-a, ácido-a, áspero-a.

acetabulum *n.* acetábulo, hueso cóncavo de la cadera.

acetate *n.* acetato, sal o éster de ácido acítico.

acetic *a.* acético, agrio, relacionado con el vinagre; ___ **acid** / ácido ___ .

acetone *n.* acetona, sustancia fragante que se usa como solvente y se observa en cantidad excesiva en casos de diabetes.

acetonemia *n.* acetonemia, exceso de acetona en la sangre.

acetonuria *n.* acetonuria, exceso de acetona en la orina, característico de la diabetes.

acetylsalicylic acid *n.* ácido acetilsalicílico, aspirina.

achalasia *n.* acalasia, falta de capacidad de relajación esp. de una abertura o esfínter.

ache *n.* dolor constante, padecimiento, *pop.* achaque.

achieve *v.* llevar a cabo, realizar, lograr un éxito.

achievement quotient *n.* cociente de inteligencia.

Achilles tendon *n.* tendón de Aquiles, tendón mayor que se une a los músculos posteriores de la pierna y se inserta en el talón del pie.

achilloburfitis *n.* aquilobursitis, infl. de la bursa situada en la parte anterior del tendón de Aquiles.

achillodynia *n.* aquilodinia, dolor en la región del tendón de Aquiles.

aching *a.* doloroso-a, doliente; mortificante.

achlorhydria *n.* aclorhidria, ausencia de ácido hipoclorhídrico en las secreciones estomacales.

achloropsia *n.* acloropsia, inhabilidad de distinguir el color verde.

acholia *n.* acolia, ausencia de bilis.

achondroplasia *n.* acondroplasia, deformidad ósea de nacimiento; enanismo.

achromasia *n.* acromasia, falta o pérdida de la pigmentación de la piel, característica de los albinos.

achromatic *a.* acromático-a, sin color.

achromatopsia *n.* acromatopsia, ceguera cromática.

achromocyte *n.* acromocito, tipo de eritrocito con escasa hemoglobina y en forma de semiluna.

achylia *n.* aquilia, deficiencia de jugos estomacales.

acid *n.* ácido;**acetic** ___ / ___ acético; ___ **-fast** / acidorresistente; ___ **-proof** / a prueba de ___; **aminoacetic** ___ / ___ aminoacético (suplemento dietético); **ascorbic** ___ / ___ ascórbico; **aspartic** ___ / ___ aspártico; **boric** ___ / ___ bórico; **butyric** ___ / ___ butírico; **chlorogenic** ___ / ___ clorogénico; **cholic** ___ / ___ cólico o coleico; **citric** ___ / ___ cítrico; **deoxyribonucleic** ___ / ___ desoxirribonucleico; **fatty** ___ / ___ graso; **folic** ___ / ___ fólico; **gastric** ___ / ___ gástrico; **glucuramic** ___ / ___ glucurámico; **glutamic** ___ / ___ glutámico; **glycolic** ___ / ___ glicólico; **lactic** ___ / ___ láctico; **nicotinic** ___ / ___ nicotínico; **nitric** ___ / ___ nítrico; **nucleic** ___ / ___ nucleico; **phenic** ___ / ___ fenílico; **ribonucleic** ___ / ___ ribonucleico; **salicylic** ___ / ___ salicílico; **sulfonic** ___ / ___ sulfónico; **sulfuric** ___ / ___ sulfúrico; **uric** ___ / ___ úrico.

acidemia *n.* acidemia, exceso de ácido en la sangre.

acidify *v.* acedar, agriar, acidular.

acidity *n.* acidez, exceso de ácido, acedia, agrura.

acidosis *n.* acidosis, exceso de acidez en la sangre y los tejidos del cuerpo; **diabetic** ___ / ___ diabética; **metabolic** ___ / ___ metabólica.

acknowledge *v.* reconocer, agradecer; [*correspondence*] acusar recibo.

acne *n.* acné, condición inflamatoria de la piel; ___ **rosacea** / ___ rosácea; ___ **vulgaris** / ___vulgar o común.

acoustic *a.* acústico-a, rel. al sonido o la audición.___ **neuroma** / neuroma ___; ___ **radiation** / radiación ___; ___ **reflex** / reflejo ___ .

acoustics *n.* acústica, la ciencia de los sonidos, su producción, transmisión y efectos.

acquaint *v.* dar a conocer, enterar, informar.

acquaintance *n.* conocimiento; trato; [*person*] un conocido, una conocida.

acquainted *a.* conocido-a, informado-a; **to be** ___ **with a case** / tener conocimiento del caso.

acquire *v.* adquirir, obtener, conseguir.

acquired *a.* adquirido-a; contraído-a.

acquired immunodeficiency syndrome *n.* síndrome de inmunodeficiencia adquirida, colapso del sistema inmune del organismo que lo incapacita a responder a la invasión de infecciones.

acquisition *n.* adquisición.

acrid *a.* amargo-a, agrio-a, acre, irritante.

acridity *n.* acritud, amargura.

acroarthritis *n.* acroartritis, infl. de las articulaciones de las extremidades.

acrocyanosis, Raynaud's disease *n.* acrocianosis, Raynaud, enfermedad de, cianosis y frialdad en las extremidades a causa de un trastorno circulatorio asociado con tensión emocional o por exposición al frío.

acrodermatitis *n.* acrodermatitis, infl. de la piel de las manos y los pies; **chronic** ___ / ___ crónica atrófica.

acromegaly *n.* acromegalia, enfermedad crónica de la edad madura manifestada por un agrandamiento progresivo de las extremidades óseas y los huesos de la cabeza debido a un malfuncionamiento de la pituitaria.

acromial *a.* acromial, rel. al acromion; ___ **bone** / hueso ___; ___ **process** / proceso ___; ___**reflex** / reflejo ___ .

acromion *n.* acromión, parte del hueso escapular del hombro.

acrophobia *n.* acrofobia, mal de altura; temor excesivo a la altitud.

acropustulosis *n.* acropustulosis, erupciones pustulares de las manos y de los pies; forma de psoriasis; **infantile** ___ / ___ infantil.

across *adv.* a través, de una parte a otra, al otro lado de; *prep.* a través de, por, sobre, contra; *v.* **to come** ___ / encontrarse con.

acrotic *a.* acrótico-a, rel. a acrotismo.

acrotism *n.* acrotismo, falta o deficiencia del pulso.

acrylamide *n.* acrilamida, agente causante potencial de cáncer.

act *n.* acto; ___ **of God** / fuerza mayor; *v.* actuar, obrar, ejecutar, hacer algo; portarse; **do not** ___ **like that** / no se porte así, no te portes así.

actine *n.* actina, proteína del tejido muscular que, unida a la miosina, hace posible la contracción muscular.

actinic *a.* actínico-a, rel. a rayos químicamente activos tal como los rayos-x, la luz ultravioleta y particularmente el sol; ___ **dermatitis** / dermatitis ___; ___ **granuloma** / granuloma ___; ___ **keratosis** / queratosis ___ .

action *n.* acción, actuación.

activate *v.* activar.

active *a.* activo-a; diligente, hábil, enérgico-a.

activities of daily living *n.* actividades de la vida diaria.

activity *n.* actividad, ejercicio, ocupación.

actual *a.* actual, real, verdadero-a; **-ly** *adv.* en realidad, actualmente; **the** ___ **symptom** / el síntoma verdadero.

acuity *n.* agudeza; precisión; **visual** ___ / ___ visual.

acupuncture *n.* acupuntura, método de cura por inserción de agujas en áreas determinadas del cuerpo con el propósito de reducir o suprimir un dolor.

acute *a.* agudo-a punzante; ___ **-care-center** / centro-de-emergencia; ___ **care facility** / centro de cuidado crítico; **an** ___ **pain** / un dolor ___ .

Adam's apple *n.* nuez de Adán.

adapt *v.* adaptar; *vr.* adaptarse, ajustarse.

adaptation *n.* adaptación, ajuste.

adaptometer *n.* adaptómetro, instrumento que determina el tiempo requerido para la adaptación de la retina.

add *v.* añadir, sumar, agregar.

addict *n.* adicto-a; vicioso-a, *a.* adicto-a, entregado-a, dependiente física o psicológicamente de una sustancia esp. referente a una persona alcohólica o narcómana.

addicted *a.* enviciado-a; entregado-a, habituado-a a una sustancia, esp. alcohol o narcóticos; *v.* **to become** ___ / enviciarse, entregarse a una droga.

addiction *n.* adicción, propensión, dependencia.

Addison's disease *n.* enfermedad de Addison, hipofunción de las glándulas suprarrenales.

additive *n.* aditivo, sustancia que se agrega.

address *n.* dirección, señas; *v.* [*to speak or write to*] dirigirse a; hablar con; [*to write*] escribir a; [*to speak to an audience*] hablar en público.

adduct *v.* aducir, mover hacia la línea media.

adduction *n.* aducción.1. movimiento hacia la línea media del cuerpo o hacia adentro de un miembro o parte del cuerpo; 2. movimiento hacia un centro común.

adductor *n.* músculo aductor, músculo que tira hacia una línea media o hacia el centro.

adenectomy *n.* adenectomía, extirpación de una glándula.

adenitis *n.* adenitis, infl. de una glándula.

adenoacanthoma *n.* adenoacantoma, cáncer en el útero que crece lentamente.

adenocarcinoma *n.* adenocarcinoma, cáncer maligno que se origina en una glándula.

adenocystoma *n.* adenocistoma, tumor benigno de una glándula formado por quistes.

adenofibroma *n.* adenofibroma, tumor benigno formado por tejido fibroso y glandular, visto en el útero y en los pechos.

adenoid *a.* adenoideo, semejante a una glándula.

adenoidectomy *n.* adenoidectomía, extirpación de la adenoide.

adenoiditis *n.* adenoiditis, infl. de la adenoide.

adenoids *n., pl.* adenoides, acumulación de tejido linfático en la nasofaringe durante la niñez.

adenoma *n.* adenoma, tumor de una consistencia parecida a la del tejido glandular; **acidophil** ___ / ___ acidófilo; ___ **of nipple** / ___ de la mama; **adrenocortical** ___ / ___ adrenocortical; **basal cell** ___ / ___ de células basales; **basophil** ___ / ___ basófilo; **bronquial** ___ / ___ bronquial; **embryonal** ___ / ___ embriónico; **follicular** ___ / ___ folicular; **hepatic** ___ / ___ hepático; **renal cortical** ___ / ___ corticorenal; **sebaceous** ___ / ___ sebáceo; **toxic** ___ / ___ tóxico.

adenomyoma *n.* adenomioma, tumor benigno visto con frecuencia en el útero.

adenopathy, adenopalia *n.* adenopatía, adenopalia, enfermedad de una glándula linfática.

adenosarcoma *n.* adenosarcoma, tumor maligno.

adenosis *n.* adenosis, engrosamiento de una glándula.

adequate *a.* adecuado-a, proporcionado-a.

adherent lens *n.* lente de contacto.

adhesion *n.* adhesión, adherencia.

adhesive *n.* adhesivo, tela adhesiva; ___ **strips** / esparadrapo.

adipocyte *n.* adipocito, célula adiposa.

adipose tissue *n.* tejido adiposo, grasa.

adiposogenital *a.* adiposogenital.

adjacent *a.* adyacente, contiguo, al lado de.

adjective *n.* adjetivo.

adjoin *v.* juntar, asociar, unir.

adjunct *a.* adjunto-a, unido-a, asociado-a, arrimado-a.

adjust *v.* ajustar, arreglar, acomodar.

adjustment *n.* ajuste, adaptación; **occlusal** ___ / ___ de oclusión, ___ oclusal.

adjuvant *n.* adjutor, agente o sustancia que acentúa la potencia de un medicamento.

administer *v.* administrar, proveer, dar algo necesario.

administration *n.* administración.

admirable *a.* admirable, digno-a.

admission *n.* [*to a hospital*] ingreso; internación, admisión.

admit *v.* admitir, dar entrada o ingreso a una institución.

admittance *n.* entrada, admisión.

admix *v.* mezclar, juntar.

admonish *v.* advertir, amonestar.

admonition *n.* advertencia, admonición, consejo.

adnexa *n., pl.* anejos, anexos, apéndices tales como las trompas de Falopio.

adolescence *n.* adolescencia, pubertad.

adolescent *n.* adolescente; pubescente.

adopt *v.* adoptar, prohijar.

adoption *n.* adopción.

adoptive *a.* adoptivo-a.

adrenal *a.* suprarrenal, adrenal; ___ **congenital hyperplasia** / hiperplasia ___ congenital; ___ **crisis** / crisis ___; ___ **cortex hormones** / corticosteroides ___-es; **gland diseases** / enfermedades de la glándula ___; ___ **glands** / glándulas ___-es; ___ **gland neoplasms** / neoplasmas de las glándulas ___-es; ___ **hypertension** / hipertensión ___.

adrenalectomy *n.* adrenalectomía, extirpación de las glándulas suprarrenales.

adrenaline *n.* adrenalina, marca registrada de la epinefrina, hormona usada como vasoconstrictor secretada por la médula suprarrenal.

adrenalism *n.* adrenalismo, disfunción de la glándula suprarrenal que ocasiona síntomas de debilidad y decaimiento.

adrenergic blocking agents *n., pl.* agentes bloqueadores adrenérgicos. 1. tipo de drogas que copian las acciones del sistema nervioso simpático; 2. drogas que aumentan el flujo sanguíneo y reducen la tensión arterial.

adrenocorticotropin *n.* adrenocorticotropina, hormona secretada por la pituitaria, estimulante de la corteza suprarrenal.

adrenogenic *a.* adrenogénico, que proviene de las glándulas suprarrenales.

adsorbent *a.* adsorbente.

adsorption *n.* adsorción, adherencia de un gas o líquido a una superficie sólida.

adult *n., a.* adulto-a.

adulterate *v.* adulterar, cambiar el original, viciar; falsificar.

adultery *n.* adulterio.

advance *v.* avanzar, adelantar, pasar adelante; **in** ___ / por adelantado.

advancement *n.* [*improvement*] mejora, mejoría, progreso; promoción, ascenso.

advantage *n.* ventaja, ganancia, beneficio; *v.* **to take** ___ / aprovecharse, valerse de.

advantageous *a.* provechoso-a, ventajoso-a, favorable, propicio-a.

adverb *n.* adverbio.

adverbial *a.* adverbial.

adverse *a.* desfavorable, adverso-a, contrario-a, opuesto-a; ___ **effects** / efectos ___; ___ **reaction** / reacción ___.

advisable *a.* recomendable, conveniente.

advise *n.* advertencia, consejo; opinión, parecer; *v.* advertir; aconsejar, recomendar.

aerate *v.* airear, ventilar. 1. saturar un líquido de aire; 2. cambiar la sangre venosa en sangre arterial en los pulmones.

aerobe *n.* aerobio, organismo que requiere oxígeno para vivir.

aerobic *a.* aeróbico-a. 1. rel. a un aerobio; 2. rel. a un ejercicio coordinado como una actividad física; ___ **dance** / baile ___; ___ **exercises** / ejercicios ___-s; 3. que ocurre o vive en la presencia de oxígeno.

aerobics *n.* aeróbic, técnica gimnástica que consiste en ejercicios y calistenia combinados con una rutina de baile.

aerocele *n.* aerocele, hernia de la tráquea.

a

aeroembolism *n.* aeroembolismo, ''enfermedad de los buzos'', condición causada por burbujas de nitrógeno liberadas en la sangre debido a un cambio brusco de presión atmosférica; *pop.* **the bends**.

aeroemphysema *n.* aeroenfisema, ''enfermedad de los aviadores'', condición causada por un ascenso súbito en el espacio sin decompresión adecuada; *pop.* **the chokes**.

aerogenic *a.* aerógeno-a, que produce gas.

aerophagia *n.* aerofagia, tragar aire en exceso.

afebrile *a.* afebril, sin fiebre, sin calentura.

affair *n.* asunto, cuestión.

affect *v.* afectar, causar un cambio en la salud; conmover, excitar.

affectation *n.* artificio, afectación.

affected *a.* afectado-a, que padece de una enfermedad física o de un sufrimiento emocional; ___ **by** / ___ por.

affection *n.* [*sickness*] afección, dolencia, enfermedad; [*feeling*] expresión de cariño, afecto o afección.

affectionate *a.* afectuoso-a, cariñoso-a.

affective *a.* afectivo-a; ___ **disorders** / trastornos ___ -s; ___ **symptoms** / síntomas ___ -s.

afferent *a.* aferente, que se dirige hacia el centro o hacia adentro; ___ **fibers** / fibras ___ -s; ___ **glomerular arteriole** / arteriola glomerular ___; ___ **lymphatic vessel** / vaso linfático ___; ___ **nerve** / nervio ___; ___ **vessel** / vaso ___ .

affinity *n.* afinidad, conformidad; conexión.

affirm *v.* afirmar, asegurar.

affirmation *n.* afirmación, confirmación, ratificación de una medida.

affirmed *a.* afirmado-a, confirmado-a, ratificado-a.

affix *v.* aplicar, colocar, adaptar; ligar, unir.

affixture *n.* ligadura, adición.

afflict *v.* afligir, causar dolor o sufrimiento; [*lament*] afligirse, inquietarse.

afflicted *a.* afligido-a, sufrido-a.

affliction *n.* aflicción, padecimiento, sufrimiento.

afflux *n.* flujo.

afford *v.* poder costear, tener solvencia; soportar.

affront *v.* hacer frente, confrontar; encararse.

afibrinogenemia *n.* afibrinogenemia, deficiencia de fibrinógeno en la sangre.

afire *a.* encendido-a; *adv.* en llamas.

afraid *a.* temeroso-a, miedoso-a, intimidado-a, *v.* **to be** ___ / tener miedo.

after *prep.* después; *adv.* después, más tarde; ___ **effects** / consecuencias, secuelas; acción

retardada de una droga; ___ **treatment** / tratamiento de recuperación.

afterbirth *n.* secundinas, placenta y membranas que se expelen en el parto.

aftercare *n.* convalecencia, restablecimiento; tratamiento post-operatorio.

afterimage *n.* impresión mantenida por la retina.

aftermath *n.* secuela, consecuencias de una enfermedad.

afterpains *n., pl.* entuertos, dolores siguientes al parto.

aftersleep *n.* sueño secundario.

aftersound *n.* impresión auditiva que persiste después de cesar el estímulo.

aftertaste *n.* permanencia de la sensación del gusto.

afterwards *adv.* después, luego, más tarde.

again *adv.* otra vez; ___ **and** ___ / una y otra vez, muchas veces; **do it** ___ / hágalo, hazlo___ .

against *prep.* contra, enfrente; *v.* **to be** ___ / oponerse; enfrentarse a, con.

agalorrhea *n.* agalorrea, cesación o falta de leche en los pechos.

agamic *a.* agámico-a, rel. a la reproducción sin unión sexual.

agammaglobulinemia *n.* agammaglobulinemia, deficiencia de gamma globulina en la sangre.

age *n.* edad; ___ **of consent** / mayor de ___ , mayoría de ___; **full** ___ / mayor de edad; **legal** ___ / ___ legal; **tender** ___ / infancia, primera edad.

agenesis, agenesia *n.* agénesis, agenesia.1. defecto congénito en el desarrollo de un órgano o parte del cuerpo; 2. esterilidad; impotencia.

agent *n.* agente, factor.

Agent Orange *n.* Agente Naranja, causante de defoliación que contiene el elemento químico-tóxico dioxina.

agglomeration *n.* aglomeración, acumulación.

agglutinants *n., pl.* aglutinantes, agentes o factores que unen partes separadas en un proceso de curación.

agglutinate *v.* aglutinar; causar unión.

agglutination *n.* aglutinación, acción de aglutinar o causar unión.

aggravate *v.* agravar, empeorar, irritar.

aggression *n.* agresión, actitud y acción hostil.

aggressive *a.* agresivo-a, hostil.

agile *a.* ágil, ligero-a, expedito-a.

aging *n.* envejecimiento.

agitate *v.* [*to shake*] agitar, sacudir; [*to upset*] inquietar, perturbar.

agitation *n.* agitación, perturbación; alboroto.

agnosia *n.* agnosia, desorden o incapacidad debido a una lesión cerebral por la cual una persona pierde total o parcialmente el uso de los sentidos y no reconoce a personas u objetos familiares; **visual** ___ / ___visual.

ago *adv.* atrás; [*with time*] hace; **ten years** ___ / [*hace + length of time*] hace diez años.

agonize *v.* agonizar, estar en agonía; sufrir en extremo.

agony *n.* agonía.1. sufrimiento extremo; 2. estado que precede a la muerte.

agoraphobia *n.* agorafobia, temor excesivo a los espacios abiertos.

agranulocytosis *n.* agranulocitosis, condición aguda causada por la disminución excesiva de leucocitos en la sangre.

agraphia *n.* agrafia, pérdida de la habilidad de escribir causada por un trastorno cerebral.

agree *v.* acordar; estar de acuerdo; sentar bien, caer bien; **we** ___ / estamos de acuerdo; **coffee does not** ___ **with me** / el café no me sienta bien; el café no me cae bien.

agreeable *a.* agradable, ameno-a, placentero-a, grato-a.

agreement *n.* acuerdo, pacto, consolidación, ajustamiento; **to come to an** ___ / llegar a un acuerdo; acordar.

ahead *adv.* adelante, enfrente, hacia adelante; *v.* **look** ___ / mire, mira ___ .

aid *n.* ayuda, asistencia; **government** ___ / subsidio del gobierno; **nurse** ___ / enfermero, enfermera asistente.

AIDS *abbr.* acquired immunodeficiency syndrome; *n.* SIDA; síndrome de inmunodeficiencia adquirida, estado avanzado de infección por el virus VIH, caracterizado por inmunodeficiencia, infecciones (tales como neumonía, tuberculosis y diarrea crónica) y tumores (esp. linfoma y sarcoma de Kaposi).

ailing *a.* achacoso-a, enfermizo-a.

ailment *n.* dolencia, achaque, indisposición.

air *n.* aire;___ **bladder** / vejiga llena de ___; ___ **blast injury** / lesión por una explosión; ___ **bubbles** / burbujas de ___; ___ **chamber** / cámara de ___; ___ **-conditioned** / ___ acondicionado; ___ **contamination** / ___ contaminado; contaminación del ___ , polución; ___ **dressing** / vendaje; ___ **embolism** / embolia gaseosa; ___ **hole** / respiradero; ___ **hunger** / falta de ___; ___ **mattress** / colchón neumático; ___ **passages** / conductos de ___; ___ **pocket** / bolsa de ___; ___ **pollution** / polución atmosférica; ___ **sac [lung]** / alvéolo pulmonar; **cool** ___ / ___ fresco; **tidal** ___ / ___ respiratorio; **ventilated** ___ / ___ de ventilación; *v.* [*to ventilate*] airear, ventilar.

airborne *a.* en vuelo; [*transported*] llevado-a por el aire;___**spores** / esporas transmitidas por el aire.

airing *n.* aéreo, ventilación.

airless *a.* falto de respiración, sin aire.

airmail *n.* correo aéreo.

airplane *n.* avión, aeroplano.

airsickness *n.* mareo de altura.

airtight *a.* hermético-a.

airway *n.* 1. conducto de aire; 2. vías respiratorias; **lower** ___ / vía respiratoria inferior; **oclussive** ___ / conducto de aire; vía respiratoria oclusiva; **respiratory** ___ / vías respiratorias; **upper** ___ / vía respiratoria superior.

akin *a.* consanguíneo, de cualidades uniformes.

akinesthesia *n.* aquinestesia, falta del sentido de movimiento.

alalia *n.* pérdida del habla.

alar *a.* alar, rel. a o semejante a una ala;___ **artery** / arteria ___; ___ **cartilage** / cartílago ___ .

alarm *n.* alarma, peligro; **fire** ___ / ___ de fuego; *v.* alarmar, inquietar, impacientar; turbar.

alarming *a.* alarmante, inquietante, desesperante; sorprendente.

albinism *n.* albinismo, falta de pigmentación en la piel, el cabello y los ojos.

albino *n.* albino-a, persona afectada por albinismo.

albumin *n.* albúmina, componente proteínico.

albuminuria *n.* albuminuria, presencia de proteína en la orina, esp. albúmina o globulina.

alcohol *n.* alcohol; ___ **detoxification** / detoxificación alcohólica; ___ **withdrawal syndrome** / síndrome de privación alcohólica;

alcoholic *n., a.* alcohólico-a.

alcoholism *n.* alcoholismo, uso excesivo de bebidas alcohólicas.

aldosterone *n.* aldosterona, hormona producida por la corteza suprarrenal.

aldosteronism *n.* aldosteronismo, trastorno causado por una secreción excesiva de aldosterona.

alert *a.* alerta, dispuesto-a.

alertness *n.* estado de alerta.

aleukemia *n.* aleucemia, falta o deficiencia de leucocitos en la sangre.

alexia *n.* alexia, inhabilidad de comprender la palabra escrita.

algesia *n.* algesia, hipertesia.
algid *a.* álgido-a, frío-a.
algor *n.* escalofrío, algor.
algorithm *n.* algoritmo, método aritmético y algebraico que se usa en el diagnóstico y tratamiento de una enfermedad.
alien *a.* incompatible; extranjero-a, forastero-a.
alienation *n.* separación; ofuscación.
alimentary *a.* alimenticio-a, rel. a los alimentos; ___ **tract** / tubo digestivo, tracto ___ .
alimentation *n.* alimentación, nutrición; **forced** ___ / ___ forzada; **rectal** ___ / ___ por el recto.
alimony *n.* manutención, pensión alimenticia, apoyo monetario.
alive *a.* vivo-a, con vida; *v.* **to be** ___ / estar ___ .
alkaloid *n.* alcaloide, grupo de sustancias orgánicas básicas de origen vegetal.
alkalosis *n.* alcalosis, trastorno patológico en el balance acidobásico del organismo.
all *n.* el todo, compuesto de partes iguales; *a.* todo-a, todos-as; [*everyone*] todo el mundo;___ **day** / todo el día; ___ **night** / toda la noche; **at** ___ **risks** / a todo riesgo; **before** ___ / ante todo; *adv.* todo, del todo, completamente; enteramente; ___ **along** / todo el tiempo; ___**of a sudden** / de pronto, de golpe, de repente; ___ **the better** / tanto mejor; ___ **the worse** / tanto peor; **by** ___ **means** / sin duda, por supuesto; ___**right** / está bien.
allele *n.* alelo, alelomorfo, uno de dos o más genes de una serie que ocupa la misma posición en cromosomas homólogos y que determina características alternantes en los descendientes.
allergen *n.* alérgeno, antígeno que induce una respuesta alérgica o hipersensitiva. See chart on this page.
allergens *n., pl.* alérgenos, agentes causantes de alergias.
allergic *a.* alérgico-a; ___ **reaction** / reacción alérgica; ___ **rhinitis** / rinitis ___ .
allergist *n.* alergista, especialista en alergias.
allergy *n.* alergia; **delayed** ___ / reacción alérgica retardada;
alleviate *v.* aliviar, calmar, mejorar, atenuar.
alliance *n.* alianza, unión; acuerdo.
allogeneic, allogenic *a.* alogénico-a, de constitución genética distinta dentro de una misma especie; ___ **cells** / células ___ s; ___ **system** / sistema ___;
allograft *n.* aloinjerto. homograft.
allow *v.* admitir, aceptar, consentir.

Allergens	Alérgenos
acarus	ácaros de polvo
alcoholic beverages	bebidas alcohólicas
aspirin	aspirina
birds (feathers, droppings)	pájaros (pluma, excremento)
cat (urine, hair)	gato (orina, pelo)
colorants (food)	colorantes (comidas)
cosmetics	cosméticos
chocolate	chocolate
detergents	detergentes
glue	pegamentos
horse (sweat, hair)	caballo (sudor, pelo)
insecticide	insecticida
medicines	medicinas
milk	leche
mushrooms	hongos
nuts	nueces
paints	pinturas
plants	plantas
pollen	polen

allowance *n.* 1. asignación, regalía; 2. dieta alimenticia.
almanac *n.* almanaque, calendario.
Almighty *n.* Dios; **almighty** *a.* todopoderoso-a, omnipotente.
almond *n.* almendra.
almost *adv.* casi, cerca de, alrededor de.
alone *a.* solo-a, solitario-a.
along *adv.* a lo largo de, próximo a, junto a; *v.* **come** ___ / venga; ven; **to get** ___ / llevarse bien.
alongside *adv.* al costado de, junto a.
aloof *a.* apartado-a, aislado-a, lejos de todo o de todos.
alopecia *n.* alopecia, pérdida del cabello.
aloud *adv.* en voz alta; **to speak** ___ / hablar recio.
already *adv.* ya.
also *adv.* del mismo modo, también.
alter *v.* cambiar, variar; reformar.
alteration *n.* alteración, modificación, reforma, cambio.
alternate *v.* alternar, turnar.
alternative *n.* alternativa, opción.
although *conj.* aunque, si bien, bien que.

altitude *n.* altitud, altura, elevación.

alveolalgia *n.* alveolalgia, complicación postoperativa de una extracción dental.

alveolar *a.* alveolar, rel. a un alvéolo.

alveolitis *n.* alveolitis. 1. infl. de los alveolos pulmonares; 2. infl. de la fosa de un diente; **allergic** ___ / ___ alérgica; **acute pulmonary** ___ / ___ pulmonar aguda; **chronic fibrotic** ___ / ___ fibrosa crónica; **cryptogenic fibrotic** ___ / ___ fibrosa criptogénica; **extrinsic allergic** ___ / ___ alérgica extrínseca;

alveolus *n.* alvéolo, cavidad.

always *adv.* siempre, para siempre.

alymphocytosis *n.* alinfocitosis, reducción anormal de linfocitos.

Alzheimer's disease *n.* enfermedad de Alzheimer, deteriorización cerebral progresiva con características de demencia senil.

am *v.* soy, estoy, primera persona pres. ind. *v.* **to be** / ser; estar.

amalgamate *v.* amalgamar, mezclar, juntar.

amastia *n.* amastia, ausencia de los pechos.

amateur *a.* aficionado-a; principiante.

amaurosis *n.* amaurosis, ceguera sin aparente cambio en los ojos, posiblemente causada por una lesión cerebral.

amaurotic *a.* amaurótico-a, rel. a amaurosis.

amaze *v.* asombrar, maravillar, pasmar.

amazement *n.* asombro, pasmo, admiración.

amber *n.* ámbar; *a.* ambarino-a.

ambiance *n.* ambiente.

ambidextrous *a.* ambidextro-a.

ambisexual *a.* ambisexual, bisexual.

ambition *n.* ambición, aspiración; *v.* ambicionar, aspirar.

ambivalence *n.* ambivalencia.

amblyopia *n.* ambliopía, visión reducida.

ambulance *n.* ambulancia.

ambulant *a.* ambulante.

ambulatory *a.* ambulatorio-a; ambulante.

amebiasis *n.* amebiasis, amibiasis, estado infeccioso causado por amebas.

amebic *a.* amebiano-a, rel. a la ameba o causado por ésta.

ameliorate *v.* mejorar; adelantar; mejorarse.

amend *v.* enmendar, corregir.

amenorrhea *n.* amenorrea, ausencia del período menstrual.

American *n., a.* americano-a.

ametropia *n.* ametropía, falta de visión causada por una anomalía de los poderes refractores del ojo.

amine *n.* amina, uno de los compuestos básicos derivados del amoníaco.

amino acid *n.* aminoácido, compuesto orgánico metabólico necesario en el desarrollo y crecimiento humano esencial en la digestión e hidrólisis de proteínas.

amitosis *n.* amitosis, división nuclear directa.

ammonia *n.* amoníaco, gas alcalino que se forma por la descomposición de sustancias nitrogenadas y por aminoácidos.

ammoniuria *n.* amoniuria, excreción de orina con un alto grado de amoníaco.

amnesia *n.* amnesia, pérdida de la memoria.

amniocentesis *n.* amniocentesis, punción del útero para obtener líquido amniótico.

amnion *n.* amnios, saco membranoso que envuelve el embrión.

amnioscope *n.* amnioscopio, endoscopio que se usa para el estudio del líquido amniótico.

amnioscopy *n.* amnioscopía, visualización directa del feto y del líquido amniótico por medio de un endoscopio.

amniotic *n.* amniótico, en relación con el amnios; ___ **fluid** / fluido ___; ___ **sac** / saco ___ .

amniotomy *n.* amniotomía, ruptura artificial de las membranas fetales para estimular el parto.

amoeba, ameba *n.* ameba, organismo de una sola célula.

amorphous *a.* amorfo-a, sin forma.

amphetamine *n.* anfetamina, tipo de droga usada como estimulante del sistema nervioso.

ampicillin *n.* ampicilina, penicilina semisintética.

ample *a.* amplio-a, ancho-a; abundante, copioso-a.

amplification *n.* amplificación, ampliación, extensión.

amplify *v.* ampliar, extender, dilatar.

ampoule, ampule *n.* ámpula, ampolla, tubo de jeringuilla.

amputate *v.* amputar, desmembrar.

amputation *n.* amputación, desmembración.

Amsler Grid *n.* Amsler, gráfico de, gráfico que sirve de ayuda para revelar signos de degeneración macular aguda.

amygdala *n.* amígdala. V. **tonsil**.

amyloid *n.* amiloide, proteína que se asemeja a los almidones; ___ **degeneration** / degeneración ___; ___ **disease** / enfermedad ___; ___ **kidney** / riñón ___; ___ **nephrosis** / nefrosis ___.

amyloidosis *n.* amiloidosis, acumulación de amiloide en los tejidos.

anabolic *a.* anabólico-a, rel. al anabolismo; ___ **steroid** / esteroide ___ .

anabolism *n.* anabolismo, proceso celular por el cual sustancias simples se convierten en complejas, fase constructiva del metabolismo.

anacidity *n.* anacidez, sin ácido.

anacusia *n.* anacusia, sordera total.

anaerobe *n.* anaerobio, microorganismo que se multiplica en ausencia de aire u oxígeno.

anaerobic *a.* anaeróbico, rel. a los anaerobios o de la naturaleza de éstos.

anal *a.* anal, rel. al ano; ___ **fistula** / fístula ___ .

analgesic *n.* analgésico, calmante.

analogy *n.* analogía, semejanza.

analphabet *n.* analfabeto-a.

analysis *n.* análisis, prueba; **accumulation** ___ / ___ de acumulación; **amino acid** ___ / ___ de aminoácido; **bite** ___ / ___ de la mordida; **breath** ___ / ___ del aliento; **cephalometric** ___ / ___ cefalométrico; **character** ___ / ___ del carácter; **cost** ___ / ___ de costos; **data** ___ / ___ de datos; **dream** ___ / ___ de los sueños; **gastric** ___ / ___ gástrico; **hair** ___ / ___ del pelo; **qualitative** ___ / ___ cualitativo; **quantitative** ___ / ___ cuantitativo. See chart on page 48.

analyze *v.* analizar, hacer análisis.

anaphase *n.* anafase, etapa de la división celular.

anaphylactic *a.* anafiláctico-a, rel. a la anafilaxis.

anaphylaxis *n.* anafilaxis, hipersensibilidad, reacción alérgica extrema.

anaplasia *n.* anaplasia, falta de diferenciación en las células.

anaplastic *a.* anaplástico-a, rel. a la anaplasia.

anasarca *n.* anasarca, edema generalizado, hidropesía.

anastomosis *n.* anastomosis, pasaje o comunicación entre dos o más órganos.

anatomic, anatomical *a.* anatómico-a, rel. a la anatomía.

anatomy *n.* anatomía, ciencia que estudia la estructura del cuerpo humano y de sus órganos; **macroscopic** ___ / ___ macroscópica, estudio de estructuras que se distinguen a simple vista; **topographic** ___ / ___ topográfica, estudio de estructuras y partes de las mismas en las distintas regiones del cuerpo.

ancestors *n., pl.* antepasados, padres o abuelos; *pop.* los mayores.

ancestry *n.* ascendencia; extracción étnica, raza; alcurnia.

anconal *a.* anconal, referente al codo.

and *conj.* y; e (gr. used instead of y before words beginning with i or hi; **father and son** / padre *e* hijo; **two thirty** / las dos *y* media.

androgen *n.* andrógeno, hormona masculina.

androgenic *a.* androgénico-a, rel. a las características sexuales masculinas.

androgynous *a.* androginoide, que tiene las características de ambos sexos.

androtomy *n.* androtomía, disección de un cadáver.

anemia *n.* anemia, insuficiencia hemática o de glóbulos rojos en calidad, cantidad o en hemoglobina; **aplastic** ___ / ___ aplástica, falta anormal de producción de glóbulos rojos; **hemorrhagic, hemolytic** ___ / ___ hemorrágica, hemolítica, destrucción progresiva de glóbulos rojos; **hyperchromic** ___ / ___ hipercrómica, aumento anormal en la hemoglobina; **hypochromic microcytic** ___ / ___ hipocrómica microcítica, (células pequeñas), deficiencia de glóbulos rojos en menor cantidad que de hemoglobina; **macrocytic** ___ / ___ macrocítica, glóbulos rojos de un tamaño exagerado (anemia perniciosa); **sickle cell** ___ / ___ de glóbulos falciformes; **iron deficiency** ___ / ___ por deficiencia de hierro.

anergy *n.* anergia.1. astenia, falta de energía; 2. reducción o falta de respuesta a un antígeno específico.

anesthesia *n.* anestesia;**endotracheal** ___ / ___ endotraqueal; **epidural** ___ / ___ epidural; **general** ___ / ___ general; **general** ___ **by inhalation** / general por ___ inhalación; **general** ___ **by intubation** / general por ___ intubación; **hypnosis** ___ / ___ por hipnosis; **hypotensive** ___ / ___ con hipotensión controlada; **intercostal** ___ / ___ intercostal; **intravenous general** ___ / ___ general intravenosa; **local** ___ / ___ local; **regional** ___ / ___ regional; **saddle block** ___ / ___ en silla de montar; **spinal** ___ / ___ raquídea; **topical** ___ / ___ tópica; **thermal** ___ / ___ térmica. See chart on page 49.

anesthesiologist *n.* anestesista, anestesiólogo-a.

anesthesiology *n.* anestesiología.

anesthetic *n.* anestésico.

anesthetize *v.* anestesiar.

aneurysm *n.* aneurisma, dilatación de una porción de la pared de una arteria; **aortic** ___ / ___ aórtico; **berry** ___ / ___ cerebral saculado; **cerebral** ___ / ___ cerebral; **dissecting** ___ / ___ disecante; **false** ___ / ___ falso; **fusiform** ___ / ___ fusiforme; **true** ___ / ___verdadero.

aneurysmal *a.* aneurismal, rel. a un aneurisma.

aneurysmectomy *n.* aneurismectomía, extirpación de un aneurisma.

anger *n.* ira, cólera.

angiitis *n.* angiitis, infl. de un vaso linfático o de un vaso sanguíneo.

angina *n.* angina, sensación de dolor constrictivo o ahogo; ___ **pectoris, angor pectoris** / ___ de pecho, dolor en el pecho causado por insuficiencia de flujo sanguíneo al músculo cardíaco; **intestinal** ___ / ___ intestinal, dolor abdominal agudo debido a insuficiencia de flujo sanguíneo a los intestinos; **laryngeal** ___ / ___ laríngea, infl. de la garganta; **unstable** ___ / ___ inestable.

angiocardiography *n.* angiocardiografía, visión radiográfica de las aurículas y los ventrículos del corazón.

angiodysplasia *n.* angiodisplasia, trastorno del desarollo vascular.

angioedema *n.* edema angioneurótico, infl. alérgica localizada gen. en la cara.

angiogenesis *n.* angiogénesis, desarrollo del sistema vascular.

angiogram *n.* angiograma, visualización radiográfica de un vaso sanguíneo mediante inyección de una sustancia radioopaca; **coronary** ___ / ___ coronario; **lymph** ___ / ___ linfático.

angiography *n.* angiografía, proceso de obtener una radiografía de los vasos sanguíneos haciendo resaltar su contorno.

angioma *n.* angioma, tumor vascular benigno.

angioplasty *n.* angioplastia, intervención quirúrgica para la reconstrucción de vasos sanguíneos enfermos o traumatizados; **percutaneous coronary** ___ / ___ coronaria percutánea; **peripheral percutaneous** ___ / ___ periférica percutánea.

angiosarcoma *n.* angiosarcoma, neoplasma maligno que ocurre mayormente en tejidos blandos; se cree que se origina en las células endoteliales de los vasos sanguíneos.

angiospasm *n.* angioespasmo, contracción prolongada y fuerte de un vaso sanguíneo.

angiostenosis *n.* angioestenosis, estrechamiento de un vaso, esp. un vaso sanguíneo.

angiotensin *n.* angiotensina, agente presor en los trastornos hipotensivos, estimulante de la aldosterona.

angle *n.* ángulo, abertura formada por dos líneas que salen separadamente de un mismo punto.

anguish *n.* agonía, angustia. *v.* angustiarse.

anhidrosis *n.* anhidrosis, deficiencia o falta de secreción sudoral.

animal *n.* animal.

animate *v.* animar, dar vida.

animosity *n.* animosidad, rencor, aversión, mala voluntad; *v.* **to have** ___ / tener ___ .

anisocoria *n.* anisocoria, condición por la cual ambas pupilas de los ojos son desiguales; **central simple** ___ / ___ central simple; **essential** ___ / ___ esencial; **physiologic** ___ / ___ fisiológica; **simple** ___ / ___ simple.

anisocytosis *n.* anisocitosis, tamaño desigual de los glóbulos rojos.

ankle *n.* tobillo; ___ **bone** / hueso del ___ .

ankylosis *n.* anquilosis, inflexibilidad o falta de movimiento de una articulación.

ankylotic *a.* anquiloso-a, anquilosado-a.

annexive *a.* anexo, contiguo.

annihilation *n.* aniquilación, destrucción total.

annotate *v.* anotar, hacer un comentario.

annotation *n.* anotación, nota.

announce *v.* anunciar, publicar.

announcement *n.* anuncio, aviso, declaración pública.

annoy *v.* importunar, fastidiar, molestar.

annual *a.* anual; *-ly adv.* anualmente, cada año.

annul *v.* anular, cancelar, revocar.

annular *a.* anular, en forma de anillo; ___ **eruption** / erupción ___ .

anodyne *n.* anodino, agente mitigador del dolor; *a.* insípido-a.

anoint *v.* untar, administrar la extremaunción.

anomalous *a.* anómalo-a, irregular, disforme.

anomaly *n.* trastorno, anomalía, irregularidad contraída o congénita.

anorexia *n.* anorexia, trastorno causado por falta de apetito; ___ **nervosa** / ___ nerviosa, aversión histérica a la comida.

anosmia *n.* anosmia, falta de olfato.

another *a.* otro-a, otros-as; *pron.* el otro, la otra.

anovulation *n.* anovulación, cese de ovulación.

anovulatory drugs *n., pl.* drogas anticonceptivas, drogas para evitar la ovulación.

anoxemia *n.* anoxemia, insuficiencia de oxígeno en la sangre.

anoxia *n.* anoxia, ausencia de oxígeno en los tejidos; **altitude** ___ / ___ de altitud; **anemic** ___ / ___ anémica; **neonatorum** ___ / ___ del nenonato; **stagnant** ___ / ___ de estancamiento.

anoxic *a.* anóxico-a, rel. o causado por falta de oxígeno.

answer *n.* contestación, respuesta.

ant *n.* hormiga.

antacid *n.* antiácido, neutralizador de acidez.

antagonist *a.* antagonista, droga que neutraliza los efectos de otra.

antecubital *a.* antecubital, en posición anterior al codo.

anteflexion *n.* anteflexión, acto de doblarse hacia adelante.

antemetic *n.* antiemético, medicamento para controlar las naúseas.

anterior *a.* anterior, precedente; [*body position*] anterior o ventral; [*time*] previo-a.

anteversion *n.* anteversión, vuelta hacia el frente.

anthracosis *n.* antracosis, condición pulmonar causada por la inhalación prolongada de polvo de carbón.

anthrax *n.* ántrax, infección estafilocócica causada por el *Bacillus anthracis* que da lugar a abscesos cutáneos profundos que pueden formar grandes pústulas. *V.* **Appendix C**.

anthropomorphic *a.* antropomórfico-a, de forma humana.

antiallergic *a.* antialérgico-a, rel. a los medicamentos que se usan para combatir alergias.

antiarrhythmic *a.* antiarrítmico-a, que previene la arritmia cardíaca o es efectivo en tratamientos contra ésta; ___ **agents** / agentes ___-s.

antiarthritics *n., pl.* antiartríticos, medicamentos para combatir la artritis o aliviarla.

antibiotic *n., pl.* antibióticos, drogas antibacterianas; **antineoplastic** ___ / ___ antineoplástico; **bactericidal** ___ / ___ bactericida; **broad spectrum** ___ / ___ de amplio espectro.

antibody *n.* anticuerpo, sustancia de proteína que actúa como respuesta a la presencia de antígenos; ___ **formation** / formación de ___-s; **cross-reacting** ___ / ___ de reacción cruzada; **monoclonal** ___ / ___ monoclónico, derivado de células de hibridoma.

anticancer drug, anticarcinogen *n.* anticarcinógeno, droga usada en el tratamiento del cáncer.

anticholinergic *a.* anticolinérgico-a, rel. al bloqueo de los impulsos transmitidos a través de los nervios parasimpáticos.

anticipate *v.* anticipar, prevenir.

anticoagulant *n.* anticoagulante, medicamento usado para evitar coágulos.

anticonvulsant *n.* anticonvulsivo, medicamento usado en la prevención de convulsiones o ataques.

antidepressant *n.* antidepresivo, medicamento o proceso curativo usado para evitar estados de depresión.

antidiabetic *n.* antidiabético, medicamento usado en el tratamiento de la diabetes.

antidiarrheal *a.* antidiarreico.

antidiuretic *n.* antidiurético, sustancia que evita la emisión excesiva de orina.

antidote *n.* antídoto, contraveneno.

antiemetic *n.* antiemético, medicamento usado en el tratamiento de la náusea.

antiestrogen *n.* antiestrógeno, sustancia que detiene o modifica la acción del estrógeno.

antigen *n.* antígeno, sustancia tóxica que estimula la formación de anticuerpos; **carcinoembriogenic** ___ / ___ carcinoembriogénico.

antigenic *a.* antigénico-a, que tiene las propiedades de un antígeno; ___ **determinant** / determinante ___; ___ **drift** / variaciones antigénicas menores; ___ **shift** / variación ___ mayor; ___ **specificity** / especificidad ___ .

antigenicity *n.* antigenicidad, el estado o propiedad de producir una reacción inmune a un anticuerpo. *Syn.* **immunogenicity.**

antiglobulin test *n.* prueba de la antiglobulina.

antihistamine *n.* antihistamina, medicamento usado en el tratamiento de reacciones alérgicas.

antihypertensive *n.* antihipertensivo, medicamento para bajar la presión arterial.

anti-inflammatory agents *n., pl.* agentes anti-inflamatorios.

antineoplastic *a.* antineoplástico-a, droga que controla o mata células cancerosas.

antioncotic *n.* antioncótico, agente reductor de la tumefacción.

antipathy *n.* antipatía, adversión.

antipruritic *a.* antipruriginoso-a, sustancia que trata o alivia la picazón.

antipyretic *n.* antipirético-a, agente reductor de la fiebre.

antiseptic *n.* antiséptico, agente desinfectante que destruye bacterias.

antiserum anaphylaxis *n.* antisuero anafiláctico.

antisocial *a.* antisocial, opuesto-a a los derechos humanos o a las normas legales de la sociedad.

antispasmodic *n.* antiespasmódico, medicamento usado para aliviar o prevenir espasmos.

antitoxic *n.* antitóxico, neutralizador de los efectos de las toxinas.

antitoxin *n.* antitoxina, anticuerpo que actúa como neutralizante de la sustancia tóxica introducida por un microorganismo; **bovine** ___ / ___ bovina; **diphtheria** ___ / ___ diftérica; **scarlet fever** ___ / ___ de la escarlatina; **tetanus** ___ / ___ tetánica.

antivenum *n.* antiveneno. V. **antitoxin**.

antiviral *a.* antivirósico-a, antiviral, que detiene la acción de un virus.

antrectomy *n.* antrectomía, excisión de la pared de un antro.

antrum *n.* antro, cavidad o cámara casi cerrada; **auris** ___ / cavidad del oído; **cardiaum** ___ / ___ cardial; **follicular** ___ / ___ folicular; **mastoid** ___ / ___ mastoideo; **maxillary** ___ / ___ maxilar o seno maxilar; **pyloricum** ___ / ___ pilórico; **tympanic** ___ / ___ timpánico.

anuria *n.* anuria, escasez o ausencia de orina.

anus *n.* ano, orificio del recto.

anxiety *n.* ansiedad, angustia; estado de preocupación excesiva; aprehensión, abatimiento de ánimo, desasosiego; ___ **attack** / crisis de ___; ___ **disorders** / trastornos ___; ___ **neurosis** / neurosis de ___ .

anxious *a.* ansioso-a, anheloso-a, abatido-a, perturbado-a.

any *a.* algún, alguna, cualquier, cualquiera; **are you taking any medicine ?** / ¿toma, tomas alguna medicina?; ¿toma, tomas algún medicamento?; ___ **further** / más lejos; ___ **more** / no más; **don't go** ___ **further** / no vaya, no vayas más lejos; **don't take** ___ **of those pills** / no tome, no tomes ninguna de esas pastillas; **you don't need** ___ **more pills** / no necesita, no necesitas más pastillas; [*after negation*] ningún, ninguno-a.

anybody *pron.* alguien, alguno-a; cualquiera; **did** ___ **call ?** / ¿llamó alguien?; [*negative*] nada, nadie, ninguno-a; **no one called** / no llamó nadie.

anything *pron.* algo, alguna cosa, cualquier cosa; [*negative*] nada; **do you feel** ___? / ¿siente, sientes algo?; **don't you feel** ___? / ¿no siente, no sientes nada?

anyway *adv.* de todas maneras, de cualquier modo, sea lo que fuera.

anywhere *adv.* dondequiera, en cualquier parte.

aorta *n.* aorta, arteria mayor que se origina en el ventrículo izquierdo del corazón; **ascending** ___ / ___ ascendiente; **arch of the** ___ / cayado de la ___; **coarctation of the** ___ / coartación o compresión de la ___; **descending** ___ / ___ descendiente, descendente.

aortic *a.* aórtico-a, rel. a la aorta; ___ **murmur** / soplo, ruido ___; ___ **stenosis** / estenosis o estrechamiento ___ .

aortocoronary *n.* aortocoronaria, rel. a las arterias aorta y coronaria.

aortogram *n.* aortograma, rayos-x de la aorta.

aortography *n.* aortografía, técnica empleada con rayos-x para ver el contorno de la aorta.

aortoiliac *a.* aortoilíaca, rel. a las arterias aorta e ilíaca.

aortoplasty *n.* aortoplastia, procedimiento quirúrgico para reparar la aorta.

apart *adv.* aparte, separadamente; hacia un lado.

apathetic *a.* apático-a, indolente, insensible.

apathy *n.* apatía, insensibilidad.

apepsia *n.* apepsia, mala digestión.

aperitive *n.* aperitivo. 1. purgante suave; 2. estimulante del apetito.

aperture *n.* apertura, abertura, paso, boquete.

apex *n.* apex. 1. ápice, extremo superior o punta de un órgano; 2. extremidad puntiaguda de una estructura.

aphasia *n.* afasia, incapacidad de coordinar el pensamiento y la palabra; **amnestic** ___ / ___ amnéstica; **ataxic** ___ / ___ atáxica.

aphemia *n.* afemia, pérdida del habla, gen. debido a una hemorragia cerebral, coágulo o tumor.

aphonia *n.* afonía, pérdida de la voz debido a una afección localizada en la laringe.

aphonic *a.* afónico-a, sin sonido, sin voz.

aphrodisiac *a.* afrodisíaco-a, que estimula deseos sexuales.

aphtha *n.* afta, úlcera pequeña que aparece como señal de infección en la mucosa oral.

aphthous stomatitis *n.* estomatitis aftosa, dolor de garganta acompañado de pequeñas aftas en la boca.

apicoectomy *n.* apicoectomía, resección de la raíz de un diente.

aplasia *n.* aplasia, falta de desarrollo normal en un órgano.

apnea *n.* apnea, falta de respiración.

aponeurosis *n.* aponeurosis, membrana que cubre los músculos.

apophysis *n.* apófisis, parte saliente de un hueso.

apoplexy *n.* apoplejía, hemorragia cerebral.

appalling *a.* espantoso-a, aterrador-a, atemorizante.

a

apparent *a.* aparente, evidente, preciso-a; claro-a; patente; *-ly adv.* aparentemente, evidentemente, precisamente.

appeal *n.* apelación, recurso, súplica; *v.* apelar, recurrir, suplicar.

appear *v.* aparecer, parecer, responder; manifestarse.

appearance *n.* apariencia, aspecto.

appendage *n.* apéndice; dependencia; accesorio.

appendectomy *n.* apendectomía, extirpación del apéndice.

appendicitis *n.* apendicitis, infl. del apéndice.

appendicular *a.* apendicular, rel. al apéndice.

appendix *n.* apéndice.

appetite *n.* apetito, deseos de, ganas de comer; **altered** ___ / ___ alterado; **excessive** ___ / ___ excesivo; **poor** ___ , **loss of** ___ / falta de ___ , pérdida del ___ .

appetizing *a.* grato-a, gustoso-a.

apple *n.* manzana.

appliance *n.* aplicación; accesorio, instrumento, aparato eléctico.

applicable *a.* aplicable, adecuado-a, apropiado-a para utilizarse.

application *n.* aplicación, solicitud; ___ **blank** / formulario; [*ointment*] untadura.

applicator *n.* aplicador; **cotton** ___ / ___ de algodón.

apply *v.* aplicar, solicitar, requerir.

appointment *n.* cita, consulta, turno; [*job related*] nombramiento, cargo.

appraise *v.* apreciar, estimar, evaluar, ponderar.

appreciate *v.* apreciar, agradecer, reconocer.

approach *n.* [*avenue*] acceso, entrada; [*words*] las palabras acertadas; método; [*decision*] las medidas necesarias; *v.* abordar; *vr.* acercarse, aproximarse.

appropriate *a.* apropiado-a, adecuado-a, apto-a.

approval *n.* aprobación, aceptación, consentimiento, admisión.

approve *v.* aprobar, aceptar, dar estimación.

approximate *a.* aproximado-a.

apraxia *n.* apraxia, falta de coordinación muscular en los movimientos causada por una afección cerebral.

apricot *n.* albaricoque; *Mex.* chabacano.

apron *n.* delantal.

aptitude *n.* aptitud, capacidad, destreza para hacer algo; ___ **test** / prueba de ___ .

aqua *n.* *L.* agua; **aq. abbr.** / aq. *abr.*; ___ **bull,** ___ **bulliens** / ___ hirviendo; ___ **dest.,** ___ **destillata,** / ___ destilada; ___ **pur.,** ___ **pura** / ___ pura; ___ **tep.,** ___ **tepid** / ___ tépida, tibia; water.

aqueous *a.* acuoso-a, aguado-a; ___ **humor** / humor ___ .

aquiline *a.* aquilino-a; ___ **nose** / nariz aguileña.

arachnoid *n.* aracnoides, membrana media cerebral que cubre el cerebro y la médula espinal.

arch *n.* arco, estructura de forma circular o en curva; ___ **like** / arqueado-a; **carotid** ___ / ___ carotideo; **maxillary** ___ / ___ del paladar; **plantar** ___ / ___ plantar.

archetype *n.* arquetipo, tipo original ideal del que se derivan versiones modificadas.

archiblastoma *n.* arquiblastoma, tumor cerebral compuesto principalmente de células no diferenciadas.

arching *n.* arqueamiento.

ardor *n.* ardor, sensación quemante.

areflexia *n.* arreflexia, ausencia de reflejos.

areola *n.* aréola, areola, área circular alrededor de un centro.

argue *v.* razonar, discutir, sostener.

Argyll Robertson symptom *n.* signo de Argyll Robertson, condición de la pupila de acomodarse a una distancia, pero no a refracciones de la luz.

arise *vi.* subir, levantarse, surgir.

arm *n.* brazo, una de las extremidades superiores; ___ **sling** / cabestrillo; ___ **span** / de mano a mano, distancia de la mano derecha a la izquierda con los ___-s extendidos; **open arms** / ___-s abiertos.

armless *a.* sin brazos.

armpit *n.* axila, *pop.* sobaco.

aroma *n.* aroma, olor agradable.

aromatic *a.* aromático-a, rel. al aroma.

around *prep.* en, cerca de; *adv.* alrededor, cerca, a la vuelta; más o menos; ___ **here** / por aquí, en los alrededores; *v.* **to look** ___ / buscar; **to turn** ___ / voltear, dar la vuelta; virarse.

arrange *v.* arreglar, colocar, poner en su sitio.

arrest *n.* paro, arresto; detención; **cardiac** ___ / ___ del corazón, ___ cardíaco.

arrhenoblastoma *n.* arrenoblastoma, tumor ovárico.

arrhythmia *n.* arritmia, falta de ritmo, esp. latidos irregulares del corazón.

arrival *n.* arribo, llegada; **dead on** ___ / paciente que llega sin vida, que llega muerto-a; [*newborn*] **new** ___ / neonato-a, recién nacido-a.

arsenic *n.* arsénico; ___ **poisoning** / envenenamiento por ___ .

arterial *a.* arterial, referente a las arterias; ___ **blood gases** / gases ___-es ; ___ **occlusive**

diseases / enfermedades oclusivas ___-es; ___
system / sistema ___ .

arteriogram *n.* arteriograma, angiograma de las
arterias; **cerebral or carotid** / ___ cerebral o
carotinoide; **mesenteric** ___ / ___ mesentérico;
peripheral ___ / ___ periférico;
renal ___ / ___ renal.

arteriography *n.* arteriografía, proceso de
obtener una radiografía de las arterias.

arteriole *n.* arteriola, arteria diminuta que
termina en un capilar.

arteriosclerosis *n.* arterioesclerosis,
endurecimiento de las paredes de las arterias.

arteriotomy *n.* arteriotomía, apertura de una
arteria.

arteriovenous *a.* arteriovenoso-a, relacionado
con una arteria y una vena; ___ **fistula** /
fístula ___; ___ **malformations** /
malformaciones ___-s; ___ **shunt, surgical** /
anastomosis ___ quirúrgica.

arteritis *n.* arteritis, infl. de una arteria.

artery *n.* arteria, uno de los vasos mayores que
llevan la sangre del corazón a otras partes del
cuerpo; **innominate** ___ / ___ innominada.

arthritic *a.* artrítico-a, que padece de artritis.

arthritis *n.* artritis, infl. de una articulación o
coyuntura; **acute** ___ / ___ aguda;
chronic ___ / ___ crónica;
degenerative ___ / ___ degenerativa;
hemophilic ___ / ___ hemofílica;
rheumatoid ___ / ___ reumatoidea; **juvenile**
rheumatoid ___ / ___ reumatoidea juvenil;
rheumatoid coronary ___ / ___ coronaria
reumatoide; **septic** ___ / ___ séptica;
traumatic ___ / ___ traumática.

arthrodesis *n.* artrodesis.1. fusión de los huesos
que hacen una articulación; 2. anquilosis
artificial.

arthrogram *n.* artrograma, radiografía de una
articulación por medio de un tinte opaco.

arthropathy *n.* artropatía, enfermedad de las
articulaciones.

arthroplasty *n.* artroplastia, reparación
quirúrgica plástica de una articulación.

arthroscope *n.* artroscopio, instrumento que se
usa para el diagnóstico y tratamiento de ciertas
condiciones en las articulaciones.

arthroscopy *n.* artroscopia, examen del interior
de una articulación.

arthrotomy *n.* artrotomía, incisión en una
articulación con fines terapéuticos.

articular *a.* articular, rel. a las articulaciones.

articulate *a.* articulado-a, que se pronuncia con
precisión; ___ **person** / persona que tiene

facilidad de palabra, que puede expresarse bien;
v. articular, pronunciar las palabras claramente.

articulation *n.* articulación.1. unión de dos o
más huesos; 2. pronunciación clara y distinta de
los sonidos de las palabras; ___ **disorders** /
trastornos de la ___ .

artificial *a.* artificial, artificioso-a; ___
impregnation / impregnación,
fecundación ___; ___ **insemination** /
inseminación ___; ___ **limb** / extremidad o
parte ___; ___ **respiration** / respiración ___ .

artificial heart *n.* corazón artificial, aparato
que bombea la sangre con la capacidad funcional
de un corazón normal.

as *conj.* como, del mismo modo; ___ **a child** / de
niño; *comp.* ___ **much** / tanto ___; ___ **as**
much ___ **possible** / lo más posible; ___
soon ___ **you can** / tan pronto como pueda,
puedas; ___ **usual** / como de costumbre; ___
you please / como Ud. quiera, como tú quieras;
not ___ **yet** / todavía no.

asbestos *n.* asbesto, amianto.

asbestosis *n.* asbestosis, infección crónica de
los pulmones causada por el polvo del asbesto.

ascariasis *n.* ascariasis, infección causada por
parásitos del género *Ascaris.*

ascaris *n. Ascaris,* género de parásitos que se
aloja en el intestino de animales vertebrados.

ascend *v.* ascender, subir, escalar.

ascendent *a.* ascendiente, ascendente.

ascites *n.* ascitis, acumulación de líquido en la
cavidad abdominal.

ascorbic acid *n.* ácido ascórbico, vitamina C.

asepsia *n.* asepsia, ausencia total de gérmenes.

aseptic *a.* aséptico-a, estéril.

asexual *a.* asexual, sin género; ___
reproduction / reproducción sin unión sexual.

ash *n.* ceniza; ___ **-colored** / ceniciento-a.

ashamed *a.* avergonzado-a, apenado-a; *v.* **to**
be ___ / tener vergenza, tener pena.

Asiatic flu *n.* gripe asiática.

aside *adv.* aparte, a un lado; *v.* **to lay** ___ / dejar
de lado.

ask *v.* preguntar, interrogar, hacer preguntas;
[*about someone*] preguntar por; **to** ___ **for** / [*to*
request] pedir.

asking *n.* súplica, petición, demanda.

asleep *a.* dormido-a; *v.* **to fall** ___ / dormirse,
quedarse ___ .

aspartame *n.* aspartamo, dulcificante artificial
de baja caloría.

aspartate transaminasa *n.* aspartato
transaminasa, agente diagnóstico en casos de
hepatitis viral e infarto de miocardio.

aspect *n.* aspecto, apariencia.

Asperger's disorder *n.* Asperger, síndrome de, trastorno de la personalidad que en casos extremos se caracteriza por retraimiento social, falta de habilidad ocupacional, habla de estilo pedante y excesivo interés en asuntos banales.

aspergilloma *n.* aspergiloma, masa redonda de *Aspergillus hyphae* que coloniza una cavidad existente en el pulmón.

aspergillosis *n.* aspergilosis, infección producida por el hongo *Aspergillus* que suele afectar el oído; **acute invasive** ___ / ___ invasiva aguda; **disseminated** ___ / ___ diseminada.

aspermia *n.* aspermia, fallo en la emisión de semen.

asphyxia *n.* asfixia, sofocación, falta de respiración; ___ **fetalis** / ___ del feto.

asphyxiate *v.* asfixiarse.

aspirate *v.* aspirar.

aspiration *n.* aspiración, inhalación, succión, extracción de un líquido sin dejar entrar el aire; ___ **biopsy** / biopsia con aguja.

aspirin *n.* aspirina, ácido acetilsalicílico.

assay *n.* ensayo; análisis.

assert *v.* afirmar, sostener.

assessment *n.* evaluación; **clinical** ___ / ___ clínica; **health** ___ / ___ del estado de salud.

assets *n.* capital existente, fondos.

assign *v.* asignar, indicar, señalar.

assignment *n.* asignación, tarea, misión.

assimilate *v.* asimilar, convertir los alimentos en sustancias.

assimilation *n.* asimilación, transformación y absorción por el organismo de los alimentos digeridos.

assist *v.* ayudar, asistir, socorrer.

assistance *n.* asistencia, ayuda.

assistant *n., a.* asistente, ayudante.

associate *a.* asociado-a, socio-a.

association *n.* asociación, sociedad, unión.

assurance *n.* seguridad, confianza, certeza.

assure *v.* asegurar, dar confianza.

astasia *n.* astasia, condición histérica.

asthenia *n.* astenia, pérdida de vigor.

asthma *n.* asma, condición alégica con ataques de coriza y falta de respiración a causa de la infl. de las membranas mucosas; **cardiac** ___ / ___ cardíaca.

asthmatic *a.* asmático-a, rel. al asma.

astigmatism *n.* astigmatismo, defecto de la visión a causa de una irregularidad en la curvatura del ojo.

astragalus *n.* astrágalo, calus, hueso del tobillo.

astringent *a.* astringente, agente con poder de constricción de los tejidos y las membranas mucosas.

astrocytoma *n.* astrocitoma, tumor cerebral.

asylum *n.* asilo.

asymmetry *n.* asimetría, falta de simetría.

asymptomatic *a.* asintomático-a, sin síntoma alguno.

asynclitism *n.* asinclitismo, presentacion del neonato y de los planos pélvicos en el parto.

asynergy *n.* asinergia, falta de coordinación entre órganos gen. armónicos.

asystole, asystolia *n.* asístole, asistolia, paro del corazón, ausencia de contracciones cardíacas.

ataraxia *n.* ataraxia; impasividad.

atavism *n.* atavismo, reproducción de rasgos y características ancestrales.

ataxia *n.* ataxia, deficiencia de coordinación muscular.

atelectasis *n.* atelectasis, colapso parcial o total de un pulmón.

athermic *a.* atérmico-a, sin fiebre.

atheroma *n.* ateroma, depósito graso o lípido en la capa íntima de una arteria que causa endurecimiento de la misma.

atherosclerosis *n.* aterosclerosis, condición causada por la deposición de grasa en las capas interiores de las arterias y fibrosis de las mismas.

athetosis *n.* atetosis, condición con síntomas de contracciones involuntarias en las manos y los dedos y movimientos sin coordinación de las extremidades, esp. los brazos.

athlete's foot *n.* pie de atleta. V. **dermatophytosis.**

atmosphere *n.* atmósfera.

atmospheric *a.* atmosférico-a.

atom *n.* átomo.

atomic *a.* atómico-a.

atomizer *n.* atomizador.

atonia, atony *n.* atonía, falta de tono, esp. en los músculos.

atopic *a.* atópico-a, rel. a la atopía.

atopy *n.* atopía, tipo de alergia considerada de carácter hereditario.

atresia *n.* atresia, cierre congénito anormal de una abertura o conducto del cuerpo.

atrial *a.* auricular, atrial, rel. al atrio o la aurícula; ___ **septal defect** / defecto septal ___ .

atrioventricular *a.* atrioventricular, rel. a la aurícula y ventrículo del corazón; ___ **node** / nudo aurículoventricular; ___ **orifice** / orificio ___ .

atrium *n.* (*pl.* **atria**) atrio-a.1. cavidad que tiene comunicación con otra estructura; 2. cavidad superior del corazón.

atrophy *n.* atrofia, deteriorización de las células, tejidos y órganos del cuerpo; **acute yellow** ___ **of the liver** / ___ amarilla hepática aguda; **alveolar** ___ / ___ alveolar; **arthritic** ___ / ___ artrítica; **artificial** ___ / ___ artificial; **cerebellar** ___ / ___ cerebelosa; **epileptic absence** ___ / ___ por ausencia epiléptica; **infantile progressive spinal muscular** ___ / ___ músculo-espinal infantil progresiva; **ischemic muscular** ___ / ___ isquémica muscular; **juvenile muscular** ___ / ___ muscular juvenil; **macular** ___ / ___ macular; **multiple system** ___ / ___ de sistema múltiple; **neurogenic** ___ / ___ neurogénica; **nutritional type cerebellar** ___ / ___ cerebelar de tipo nutricional; **ocular** ___ / ___ ocular; **periodontal** ___ / ___ periodontal; **postmenopausal** ___ / ___ postmenopausia; **primary macular** ___ **of the skin** / ___ macular primaria de la piel; **primary vascular** ___ **of the skin** / ___ primaria vascular de la piel; **progressive cerebral** ___ / ___ progresiva cerebral.

atropine sulfate *n.* atropina, agente usado como relajador muscular, esp. aplicado para dilatar la pupila y paralizar el músculo ciliar durante un examen de la vista.

attach *v.* añadir, juntar, pegar, unir.

attached *a.* añadido-a, pegado-a, unido-a.

attack *n.* ataque, acceso; **heart** ___ / ataque al corazón; *v.* atacar, combatir.

attempt *v.* intentar, tratar de obtener algo; hacer un esfuerzo; esforzarse, arriesgarse.

attend *v.* atender, asistir, cuidar, tener cuidado; **to** ___ **the sick** / asistir, cuidar a los enfermos.

attendant *n.* auxiliar, asistente.

attending physician *n.* médico-a de cabecera.

attention *n.* atención, cuidado; **lack of** ___ / falta de ___; *v.* **to pay** ___ / atender, prestar atención.

attentive *a.* atento-a; *-ly adv.* atentamente, con cuidado.

attenuation *n.* atenuación, acto de disminución, esp. de una virulencia.

attitude *n.* actitud; ___ **of health personnel** / ___ del personal de salud; ___ **toward death** / ___ frente a la muerte.

attorney *n.* abogado-a, agente legal.

attract *v.* atraer.

attraction *n.* atracción.

attribute *n.* atributo, característica.

atypical *a.* atípico-a, que no es común; fuera de lo corriente.

audiogram *n.* audiograma, instrumento para anotar la agudeza de la audición.

audiovisual *a.* audiovisual, rel. a la vista y a la audición.

auditory *a.* auditivo-a, rel. a la audición; ___ **canal** / conducto ___; ___ **nerve** / nervio ___ .

augment *n.* aumento, crecimiento; *v.* aumentar, crecer; agrandarse.

aunt *n.* tía.

aura *n.* aura, síntoma premonitorio de un ataque epiléptico.

aural, auricular *a.* aural, auricular.1. rel. al sentido del oído; 2. rel. a una aurícula del corazón.

auricle, auricula *n.* aurícula. 1. oreja, la parte externa del oído; 2. cada una de las dos cavidades superiores del corazón; 3. orejuela.

auscultate *v.* auscultar, examinar, detectar sonidos de órganos tales como el corazón y los pulmones con el propósito de hacer un diagnóstico.

auscultation *n.* auscultación, acto de auscultar, detección de sonidos en un examen directo o por medio del estetoscopio.

authority *n.* autoridad, facultad.

authorization *n.* autorización.

authorize *v.* autorizar, permitir.

autism *n.* autismo, trastorno de la conducta que se manifiesta en un egocentrismo extremo; **infantile** ___ / ___ infantil.

autistic *a.* autístico-a, rel. al autismo o que padece de éste.

autoclave *n.* autoclave, aparato de esterilización al vapor.

autodiagnosis *n.* autodiagnosis, diagnóstico propio, de si mismo-a.

autodigestion *n.* autodigestión, digestión de tejidos por las mismas sustancias que los producen.

autogenous *n.* autógeno-a, que se produce en el mismo organismo.

autogenous vaccine *n.* vacuna autógena, inoculación que proviene del cultivo de bacterias del mismo paciente y se hace para crear anticuerpos.

autograft *n.* autoinjerto, injerto que se transfiere de una parte a otra del cuerpo del mismo paciente.

autohypnosis *n.* autohipnosis, hipnotismo propio, de si mismo-a.

autoimmunization *n.* autoinmunización, inmunidad producida por una sustancia desarrollada dentro del organismo de la persona afectada.

autoinfection *n.* autoinfección, infección causada por un agente del propio organismo.

autoinoculable *a.* autoinoculable, suceptible a organismos que provienen del propio cuerpo.

autologous *a.* autólogo-a, que indica algo que proviene del propio individuo.

automatic *a.* automático, de movimiento propio.

automatism *n.* automatismo, conducta que no está bajo control voluntario.

automobile *n.* automóvil, carro, *Cuba* máquina, *Spain* coche.

autonomic, autonomous *a.* autonómico-a, autónomo-a, que funciona independientemente; ___ **division of nervous system** / división ___ del sistema nervioso; ___ **dysreflexia** / disrreflexia ___; ___**hypereflexia** / hiperreflexia ___; ___**imbalance** / desequilibrio ___; ___ **nervous system** / sistema nervioso ___; ___ **neurogenic bladder** / vejiga neurogénica ___; ___ **plexus** / plexo ___; ___ **seizure** / convulsión ___; ___**visceral motor nuclei** / núcleos viscerales motores autonómicos.

autonomy *n.* autonomía, de funcionamiento propio.

autoplastic *a.* autoplástico-a, rel. a la autoplastia.

autoplasty *n.* autoplastia, cirugía plástica con el uso de un injerto que se obtiene de la misma persona que lo recibe.

autopsy *n.* autopsia, examen de un cadáver.

autosuggestion *n.* autosugestión, acto de sugestionarse.

autotransplant *n.* autotransplante, autoinjerto, autograft.

auxiliary *a.* auxiliar; ayudante.

availability *n.* disponibilidad, facilidad.

available *a.* disponible, servicial; a la mano; **to be** ___ / estar a la disposición, estar ___ .

avaricious *a.* avaricioso-a, ruin, miserable.

average *n.* promedio, término medio; de mediana proporción.

aversion *n.* aversión, aborrecimiento, odio.

avitaminosis *n.* avitaminosis, trastorno o enfermedad causada por una deficiencia vitamínica.

avoid *v.* evitar.

avulsion *n.* avulsión, extracción o remoción de una estructura o parte de ésta.

awake *a.* despierto-a.

aware *a.* enterado-a; conocedor-a; *v.* **to be** ___ / estar al tanto.

away *adv.* lejos; *a.* distante, ausente; *v.* **to go** ___ / irse, ausentarse; *interj.* **get** ___ ! / quítese, quítate; váyase, vete.

awful *a.* terrible, desagradable; tremendo-a.

awhile *adv.* por un rato, por algún tiempo.

awkward *a.* [*movement*] torpe; desmañado-a; [*appearance*] extraño-a; ___ **feeling** / sentimiento extraño.

axial *a.* axil, axial, rel. al axis o a un eje.

axilla *n.* (*pl.* **axillae**) axila, *pop.* sobaco.

axillary *a.* axilar, rel. a la axila.

axis *n.* axis, eje, línea central imaginaria que pasa a través del cuerpo o de un órgano.

axon *n.* axon, fibra nerviosa, proyección que va desde el cuerpo celular de una neurona y transporta impulsos nerviosos lejos de ésta.

ay, aye *adv.* sí, claro, desde luego, seguramente.

Ayerza's syndrome *n.* síndrome de Ayersa, síndrome caracterizado por multiples síntomas, esp. dispnea y cianosis, gen. como resultado de insuficiencia pulmonar.

azoospermia *n.* azoospermia, falta de espermatozoos en el esperma.

azotemia *n.* azotemia, exceso de urea en la sangre.

azure *n.* azul celeste.

b

b *abbr.* **bacillus** / bacilo; **behavior** / conducta; **buccal** / bucal.

babble *n.* balbuceo; *v.* balbucear.

Babinski's sign *n.* reflejo de Babinski, dorsiflexión del dedo gordo al estimularse la planta del pie.

baby, babe *n.* bebé, *dim.* bebito-a; nene, nena.

bachelor *n.* soltero-a, célibe; [*degree*] bachiller.

bacillar, bacillary *a.* bacilar, rel. a un bacilo.

bacillemia *n.* bacilemia, presencia de bacilos en la sangre.

bacillicarrier *n.* portador de bacilos.

bacillosis *n.* bacilosis, infección provocada por bacilos.

bacilluria *n.* baciluria, presencia de bacilos en la orina.

bacillus *n.* (*pl.* **bacilli**) bacilo, microbio, bacteria en forma de bastoncillo; **Calmette-Guérin, bacille bilié** ___ / ___ de Calmette Guérin, bacille bilié; **Koch's** ___ , **Mycobacterium tuberculosis** / ___ de Koch, micobacteria de la tuberculosis; **typhoid** ___ , **Salmonella typhi** / ___ de la fiebre tifoidea, Salmonela tifoidea.

bacitracin *n.* bacitracin, antibiótico efectivo en contra de ciertos estafilococos.

back *n.* espalda; ___ **tooth** / muela; **low** ___ **pain** / lumbalgia; *adv.* atrás, detrás.

backache *n.* dolor de espalda.

backboard *n.* respaldar.

backbone *n.* columna vertebral, espina dorsal.

background *n.* fondo; [*knowledge*] preparación, experiencia.

backing *n.* apoyo, sostén.

backlash *n.* contragolpe.

backside *n.* nalgas, *pop.* sentaderas, posaderas, trasero.

backslide *v.* resbalar o caer hacia atrás.

backward *a.* atrasado-a, tardío-a, lento-a, retraído-a; *adv.* atrás, hacia atrás, al revés; [*direction*] en sentido contrario.

backwardness *n.* atraso, retraso, ignorancia, torpeza.

bacon *n.* tocino.

bacteria *n., pl.* bacterias, gérmenes.

bacterial *a.* bacteriano-a; ___ **infections** / infecciones ___ -s; ___ **endocarditis** / endocarditis ___ ; ___ **sensitivity tests** / pruebas de sensibilidad ___ .

bactericidal *n.* bactericida, exterminador de bacterias.

bacteriogenic *a.* bacteriogénico-a. 1. de origen bacteriano; 2. que produce bacterias.

bacteriological *a.* bacteriológico-a, rel. a las bacterias.

bacteriologist *n.* bacteriólogo-a, especialista en bacteriología.

bacteriology *n.* bacteriología, ciencia que estudia las bacterias.

bacteriolysin *n.* bacteriolisina, anticuerpo antibacteriano que destruye bacterias.

bacteriolysis *n.* bacteriolisis, destrucción de bacterias.

bacteriosis *n.* bacteriosis, toda infección causada por gérmenes o bacterias.

bacteriostatic *a.* bacteriostático-a, que detiene el desarrollo o multiplicación de bacterias.

bacterium *n.* (*pl.* **bacteria**) bacteria, germen.

bacteriuria *n.* bacteriuria, presencia de bacterias en la orina.

bactermia *n.* bacteremia, presencia de bacterias en la sangre.

bacteroides *n.* bacteroides, tipo de bacterias anaeróbicas, sin formación de esporas, con bastoncillos de gramnegativo, que constituyen parte de la flora normal del tracto intestinal y se encuentran en menor cantidad en las cavidades respiratoria y urinaria.

bad *a.* malo-a mal, nocivo-a, [*harmful*] dañino-a; **from** ___ **to worse** / de mal en peor; **it is** ___ **for your health** / es dañino a la salud; ___ **breath** / mal aliento; ___ **looking** / mal parecido; ___ **mood** / mal humor; ___ **taste in the mouth** / mal sabor en la boca; *slang* ___ **trip** / mala experiencia con una droga; **to look** ___ / tener mal aspecto, tener mala cara; *adv.* mal; *v.* **to feel** ___ / ___ sentirse mal; -ly *adv.* mal, malamente; **to need** ___ / necesitar con urgencia.

bag *n.* bolsa, bolso; saco; ___ **of waters** / saco amniótico, *pop.* ___ de aguas; **colostomy** ___ / bolso de colostomía; **ice** ___ / ___ de hielo.

baked *a.* asado-a, guisado-a al horno, horneado-a.

baking soda *n.* bicarbonato de sodio.

balance *n.* balance.1. pesa, balanza, instrumento para medir pesos; **acid-base** ___ / ___ acidobásico; **fluid** ___ / ___ hídrico; 2. balance, estado de las cantidades y concentraciones de las partes y fluidos que en forma normal constituyen el cuerpo humano; 3. estado normal del equilibrio físico o emocional.

balanced *a.* balanceado-a; en control; ___ **diet** / dieta ___ .

balanitis *n.* balanitis, infl. del glande gen. acompañada de infl. del prepucio.

balanoposthitis *n.* balanopostitis, infl. del glande y del prepucio.

bald *a.* calvo-a, sin pelo; franco-a, espontáneo-a, escueto-a.

baldness *n.* calvicie.

ball *n.* bola; asiento del pie; ___ **forceps** / pinzas sacabalas; ___ **of the foot** / antepié.

ball-and-socket joint *n.* enartrosis, articulación multiaxial sinovial en la cual la cabeza del hueso hace cabida dentro de la cavidad redondeada del otro hueso, *p. ej.* la articulación de la cadera.

ballistocardiogram *n.* balistocardiograma, registro fotográfico del volumen sistólico para calcular el volumen por minuto.

balloon *n.* globo, balón; slang [*heroin*] globo; **angioplasty** ___ / ___ de angioplastia; **detachable** ___ / ___ desmontable; **intraaortic** ___ / ___ para uso intraaórtico.

ballottement *n., Fr.* peloteo, movimiento manual de rebote por palpación usado en el examen abdominal y pélvico para determinar la presencia de un tumor o el agrandamiento de un órgano.

balm *n.* bálsamo, ungento, calmante de uso externo.

balmy *a.* balsámico; suave, reparador; ___ **sleep** / sueño reparador.

balsam *n.* bálsamo, agente suavizante.

ban *v.* prohibir, suspender, suprimir.

banana *n.* banana, plátano.

Band-Aid *n. pop.* curita; parche.

bandage *n.* venda, vendaje, faja; *v.* vendar, ligar, atar.

bandy-legged *n.* zambo-a, patizambo-a.

bane *n.* veneno; ruina.

baneful *a.* venenoso-a, dañino-a, destructivo-a.

bang *n.* golpe; detonación.

bank *n.* banco; **blood** ___ / ___ de sangre.

B antigens *n.* antígenos B, proteínas presentes en las membranas de los eritrocitos que pueden causar una reacción seria en una transfusión.

baragnosis *n.* baragnosis, pérdida de la capacidad de reconocer pesos y presiones.

barbiturate *n.* barbitúrico, hipnótico, sedante.

bare *a.* desnudo-a, descubierto-a; ___ **-legged** / sin medias; **-ly** *adv.* apenas.

barefoot *a.* descalzo-a, sin zapatos.

baresthesia *n.* barestesia, sensación de presión o peso.

barium *n.* bario, metal alcalino de número atómico 56; ___ **enema** / enema de ___; ___ **swallow** / trago de ___ .

barium sulfato *n.* sulfato de bario, suspensión lechosa de sulfato de bario que se da a los pacientes como medio de contraste antes de hacer una radiografía del tubo digestivo.

barley *n.* cebada.

barometer *n.* barómetro, instrumento para medir la presión atmosférica.

baroreceptor *n.* barorreceptor, terminación nerviosa sensorial que reacciona a los cambios de presión.

barotrauma *n.* barotrauma, lesión física debida a una falta de balance de la presión ambiental y la presión dentro de una cavidad afectada del organismo, tal como sucede a los buzos con la dolencia de descompresión; **otic** ___ / ___ ótico; **sinus** ___ / ___ sinusal.

barrel *n.* [*part of a syringe*] cilindro; barril.

barren *a.* estéril, infecundo-a.

barrier *n.* obstrucción, barrera.

bartholinitis *n.* bartolinitis, infl. de la glándula de Bartolino o glándula vulvovaginal.

baryphonia *n.* barifonía, tipo de voz gruesa.

basal, basilar *a.* basal, basilar, rel. a una base; ___ **ganglia diseases** / enfermedades de los ganglios ___ -es; ___ **metabolic rate** / índice del metabolismo ___ .

basal ganglia *n.* ganglios basales, masas grises localizadas debajo de la corteza cerebral que toman parte en la coordinación muscular.

base, basis *n.* base, fundación.

bashful *a.* tímido-a, *pop.* corto-a.

basic *a.* básico-a, fundamental.

basil *n.* albahaca.

basilar *a.* basilar, rel. a la base o parte basal.

basiloma *n.* basiloma, carcinoma compuesto por células basales.

basin *n.* 1. vasija redonda tal como una palangana; 2. cavidad de la pelvis.

basophobia *n.* basofobia, temor excesivo de caminar.

bassinet *n.* bacinete, cuna.

bastard *n.* bastardo-a; hijo o hija ilegítimo-a.

bath *n.* baño; **alcohol** ___ / fricción de alcohol; **antipyretic** ___ / ___ antipirético, para reducir la fiebre; **aromatic** ___ / ___ aromático; **cold** ___ / ___ de agua fría; **hot** ___ / ___ caliente; **full** ___ / ___ completo; **kinetotherapeutic** ___ / ___ cinetoterapéutico; **immersion** ___ / ___ con inmersión; **oil** ___ / ___ aceitado; **Sitz** ___ / ___ de asiento caliente; **sponge** ___ / ___ con esponja; **warm** ___ / ___ tibio.

bathe *v.* bañar, lavar; bañarse, lavarse.

bathrobe *n.* bata de baño.
bathroom *n.* baño, cuarto de baño.
bathtub *n.* tina, bañadera.
battered *a.* abatido-a, maltratado-a.
battle *n.* batalla, lucha; *v.* batallar, combatir, luchar.
bay leaves *n., pl.* hojas de laurel.
bay-salt *n.* sal marina.
B cell receptor *n., pl.* receptor de células tipo B.
B cells *n., pl.* células tipo B, linfocitos que proceden de la médula ósea y producen anticuerpos, por lo que representan una ayuda importante en la respuesta inmune.
be *vi.* ser, estar; **there is, there are** / hay; **there was** / hubo, había; **there will be** / será,estará, habrá; [*pp.*] **been** / sido, estado; [*pp.*] **being** / siendo, estando; **to ___ afraid** / tener miedo; **to ___ at a loss** / estar confundido-a; **to ___ calm** / calmarse; **to ___ careful** / tener cuidado; **to ___ cold** / tener frío; **to ___ hot** / tener calor; **to ___ hungry** / tener hambre; **to ___ quiet** / callarse; estar tranquilo-a; **to ___ right** / tener razón; **to ___ all right** / estar bien; **to ___ ... years old** / tener ... años; **to ___ sick** / estar enfermo-a; **to ___ sleepy** / tener sueño; **to ___ successful** / tener éxito; **to ___ thirsty** / tener sed; **to ___ warm** [*with a temperature*] / tener fiebre, tener calentura; tener calor; **to want to ___** / querer ser; **to want to ___** [*somewhere*] / querer estar.
bean *n.* frijol; **___ -shaped** / en forma de riñon o frijol.
bear *vi.* soportar; aguantar; **___ down** / pujar, empujar hacia afuera con fuerza.
bearable *a.* soportable, tolerable.
beard *n.* barba.
bearded *a.* barbudo.
bearer *n.* soporte, apoyo.
bearing *n.* gestación; conexión; [*in obstetrics*]; **___ down** / [*second stage of labor*] pujo, expulsión hacia afuera.
beat *n.* [*heart*] latido, pulsación; **heart ___ / ___** del corazón; *vi.* pulsar; [*heart*] palpitar; pegar, golpear.
beaten *a. pp.* de to beat, maltratado-a; golpeado-a; vencido-a, derrotado-a.
beating *n.* pulsación, latido; paliza, zurra.
beautiful *a.* hermoso-a, bello-a.
beauty *n.* belleza, hermosura, beldad.
become *vi.* hacerse, convertirse; **___ a** / convertirse en; **___ accustomed** / acostumbrarse; **___ a doctor** / hacerse médico-a; [*conversion*] **___ crazy** / volverse loco-a; **___**

frightened / asustarse; **___ ill** / ponerse enfermo-a; enfermarse; **___ inflamed** / inflamarse; **___ swollen** / hincharse.
becoming *a.* apropiado-a, conveniente, que sienta o cae bien.
bed *n.* cama, lecho; **___ occupancy** / ocupación de ___ -s; **___ rest** / reclusión en ___ .
bedbug *n.* chinche.
bedclothes *n., pl.* ropa de cama.
bedding *n.* ropa de cama; colchón y almohada.
bedfast *a.* recluido-a en cama.
bedpan *n.* bacín, chata, cuña.
bedridden *a.* postrado-a en cama.
bedroom *n.* cuarto de dormir, alcoba, dormitorio; *Mex.* recámara.
bedside *a.* al lado de la cama.
bedsore *n.* úlcera por decúbito.
bedspread *n.* colcha, sobrecama, cubrecama.
bedtime *n.* hora de acostarse.
bed-wetting *n.* enuresis; orinarse en la cama, mojar la cama.
bee *n.* abeja; **___ venom** / veneno de ___ .
beef *n.* carne de res, carne de vaca; **___ broth** / caldo de carne; **___ steak** / biftec; **roast ___** / carne asada, rosbif.
beer *n.* cerveza.
beet *n.* remolacha.
before *adv.* delante; enfrente de; antes de; anterior a; *conj.* antes que; antes de que.
beforehand *adv.* con anterioridad, con anticipación; de antemano.
beg *v.* pedir, rogar, mendigar.
begin *vi.* comenzar, empezar, principiar.
beginner *n.* principiante, novicio-a; autor-a, iniciador-a.
beginning *n.* principio, origen, génesis.
behalf *n.* en beneficio, a favor; **on your ___** / a su favor, por usted.
behavior *n.* conducta, comportamiento; **___ reflex** / reflejo adquirido; **___ therapy** / terapia de la ___; **high-risk ___** / comportamiento arriesgado.
behind *adv., prep.,* detras, trás, atrás, hacia atrás.
bel *n.* bel, belio, unidad que expresa la intensidad relativa de un sonido.
belch *n.* eructo, regeldo; *v.* eructar.
belief *n.* creencia, opinión.
belittle *n.* dar poca importancia, humillar.
belladonna *n.* belladona, yerba medicinal cuyas hojas y raíces contienen atropina y alcaloides.
bellied *a.* panzudo-a, barrigón-a, con barriga.
belligerent *a.* beligerante.
Bell's palsy *n.* parálisis de Bell, parálisis de un lado de la cara causada por una afección del nervio facial.

belly *n.* abdomen, barriga, vientre, *pop.* panza; ___ **button** / ombligo; ___ **worm** / lombriz intestinal.

bellyache *n.* dolor de estómago, de barriga.

below *prep.* después de, debajo de; *adv.* abajo, bajo, debajo; **down** ___ / en la parte baja; más abajo.

belt *n.* cinturón, cinto.

bend *vi.* doblarse, inclinarse; ___ **back** / ___ hacia atrás; ___ **forward** / ___ hacia adelante.

beneath *prep., adv.* abajo, debajo, bajo.

Benedict test *n.* prueba de Benedict, análisis químico para encontrar la presencia de azúcar en la orina.

beneficial *a.* beneficioso-a, favorable, provechoso-a.

beneficiary *n., a.* beneficiado-a, favorecido-a.

benefit *n.* beneficio, favor; servicio, provecho; **allocation of** ___ **-s** / asignación de ___ -s.

benign *a.* benigno-a, que no es de naturaleza maligna.

bent *n.* inclinación, curvatura; *a.* encorvado-a; inclinado-a.

Benzedrine *n.* Bencedrina, nombre comercial del sulfato de anfetamina.

benzoin *n.* benjuí, resina usada como expectorante.

beriberi *n.* beriberi, tipo de neuritis múltiple causada por deficiencia de vitamina B1 (tiamina).

beside *adv.* además, *prep.* al lado de, cerca de, junto a; ___ **oneself** / fuera de sí, loco-a.

best *a., sup.* mejor, superior, óptimo; *v.* **to do one's** ___ / hacer lo ___ posible.

bestial *a.* bestial, irracional, brutal.

bestiality *n.* bestialidad, relaciones sexuales con animales.

beta blocker *n.* beta bloqueador, agente que bloquea la acción de la epinefrina.

better *a. comp.* mejor, superior; [*better than*] mejor que; **so much the** ___ / tanto mejor; *v.* **to be** ___ / estar mejor, ponerse mejor; **to be** ___ **than** / ser mejor que; **to be** ___ **than before** / estar, ser mejor que antes; **to change for the** ___ / recuperarse, restablecerse; **to like** ___ / preferir; **to make** ___ / mejorar, aliviar.

between *adv.* en medio; *prep.* entre, en medio de.

beverage *n.* bebida; **alcoholic** ___ **-s** / bebidas alcoholicas; **nonalcoholic** ___ / ___ no alcoholica.

beware of *vi.* cuidarse de.

bewilder *v.* confundir, perturbar, turbar.

bewildered *a.* perplejo-a, confundido-a; atolondrado-a.

beyond *adv.* más allá, más lejos.

bezoar *n.* bezoar, concreción formada de distintas materias como fibras vegetales y pelo, presente en el estómago y en el intestino humano así como en el de los animales.

bias *n.* parcialidad, prejuicio, tendencia.

biaxial *a.* biaxial, que tiene dos ejes.

bib *n.* babero; pechera.

bibliography *n.* bibliografía.

bicarbonate *n.* bicarbonato, sal de ácido carbónico.

biceps *n.* músculo bíceps.

bicipital *a.* bicipital. 1. rel. al músculo bíceps; 2. bicípite, que tiene dos cabezas.

biconcave *a.* bicóncavo-a, de dos superficies cóncavas.

biconvex *a.* biconvexo-a, de dos caras convexas, tal como los lentes para la presbicia.

bicuspid *a.* bicúspide, que presenta dos puntas.

bicycle *n.* bicicleta; **stationary** ___ / ___ estacionaria.

bicycling *n.* ciclismo.

bifid *a.* bífido-a, partido en dos.

bifocal *a.* bifocal, referente a dos focos o enfoques.

bifurcation *n.* bifurcación, división en dos ramas o derecciones.

big *a.* grande, enorme; mayor; ___ **bellied** / barrigón-a, panzudo-a; ___ **head** / cabezón-a; ___ **sister, brother** / hermana mayor, hermano mayor; ___ **toe** / dedo gordo; ___ **with child** / encinta, en estado.

bigeminy *n.* bigeminia, pulsación duplicada en sucesión rápida.

bigger *a. comp.* mayor, más grande.

bilabial *a.* bilabial.

bilateral *a.* bilateral, de dos lados.

bile *n.* bilis, hiel, producto de la secreción del hígado; ___ **acids and salts** / ácidos y sales biliares; ___ **ducts** / conductos biliares; ___ **pigments** / pigmentos biliares.

bilharziasis *n.* bilharziasis. V. **schistosomiasis.**

biliary *a.* biliar, rel. a la bilis, los conductos biliares o la vesícula; ___ **duct obstruction** / obstrucción del conducto ___; ___ **stasis** / colestasis; ___ **tract diseases** / enfermedades de las vías ___-es; ___ **tract hemorrhage** / hemobilia.

bilingual *a.* bilingüe.

bilious *a.* bilioso-a, con exceso de bilis.

biliousness *n.* biliosidad, trastorno con síntomas de estreñimiento, dolor de cabeza e indigestión atribuídos a un exceso de secreción biliar.

bilirubin *n.* bilirrubina, pigmento rojo de la bilis.

bilirubinemia *n.* bilirrubinemia, presencia de bilirrubina en la sangre.

bilirubinuria *n.* bilirrubinuria, presencia de bilirrubina en la orina.

bill *n.* [*statement*] cuenta; [*currency*] billete.

bimanual *a.* bimanual, rel. a las dos manos.

binary *a.* binario, doble.

bind *vi.* unir, ligar, vendar.

binding *n.* enlace; ligazón; venda; vendaje.

binocular *n.* binocular, lentes, gemelos.

bioassay *n.* bioensayo, prueba de determinación de la potencia de una droga en animales.

biochemical *a.* bioquímico-a, rel. a la bioquímica.

biochemistry *n.* bioquímica, ciencia que estudia los organismos vivos.

biologic, biological *a.* biológico-a, rel. a la biología; ___ **assay** / análisis ___; ___ **control** / control ___; ___ **evolution** / evolución ___; ___ **half-life** / semivida ___; ___ **immunotherapy** / inmunoterapia ___; ___ **indicator** / indicador ___; ___ **psychiatry** / siquiatría ___; ___ **warfare** / guerra ___ .

biologist *n.* biólogo-a.

biology *n.* biología, ciencia que estudia los organismos vivos; **cellular** ___ / ___ celular; **molecular** ___ / ___ molecular.

biomedical *a.* biomédico-a, rel. a la aplicación de las ciencias naturales, esp. los campos de las ciencias biológicas y fisiológicas que se relacionan con el estudio de la medicina.

biometrics *n.* biométrica, rama de la biología que estudia los fenómenos biológicos y sus observaciones por medio de análisis de estadística.

biopsy *n.* biopsia, proceso para obtener un espécimen de tejido con fines de diagnóstico; **aspiration** ___ / por aspiración; ___ **by ablation** / ___ por ablación; ___ **by frozen section** / ___ en frío; ___ **of the bone marrow** / ___ de la medula ósea; ___ **of the breast** / ___ de la mama, del seno; ___ **of the cervix** / ___ del cuello uterino; ___ **of the lymph nodes** / ___ de los ganglios linfáticos; **brush** ___ / ___ con cepillo; **endoscopic** ___ / ___ endoscópica; **excision** ___ / ___ por excisión; **fine needle** ___ / ___ de aguja fina; **incision** ___ / ___por incisión; **muscle** ___ / ___ muscular; **needle** ___ / ___ por aspiración; **sentinel** ___ / ___ del ganglio vigilante; **specimen wedge** ___ / ___ de espécimen cuneiforme; **temporal artery** ___ / ___ de la arteria temporal.

bioscience *n.* biociencia, cualquiera de las ciencias naturales relacionadas con el estudio de la conducta y la estructura de organismos vivos.

biosynthesis *n.* biosíntesis, formación de sustancias químicas en los procesos fisiológicos de los organismos.

bioterrorism *n.* terrorismo biológico, bioterrorismo. V. Appendix C.

biotype *n.* biotipo, grupo de individuos con igual genotipo.

biped *n.* bípedo, animal de dos pies.

birefringent *a.* birrefringente, de refracción doble.

birth *n.* nacimiento, parto, alumbramiento;___ **canal** / canal del parto; ___ **certificate** / certificado de ___; ___ **control** / control de la natalidad, planeamiento familiar; ___ **-death ratio** / índice de mortalidad; ___ **rate** / natalidad; ___ **right** / derechos naturales; ___ **weight** / peso al nacer; **post-term** ___ / ___ tardío; **premature** ___ / ___ prematuro; *v.* **to give** ___ / dar a luz, estar de parto.

birth date *n.* fecha de nacimiento.

birthday *n.* cumpleaños, natalicio.

birthplace *n.* lugar de nacimiento.

bisect *v.* bisecar, dividir en dos partes.

bisexual *a.* bisexual, con gónadas de los dos sexos.

bite *n.* mordida, picadura; [*snake*] mordida de serpiente; [*insect*] picadura; ___ **block** / bloque de ___; ___ **rim** / reborde de la ___; ___ **testing** / análisis de la ___; *vi.* morder, picar.

biting *a.* penetrante, picante.

Bitot spots *n., pl.* Bitot, manchas de, pequeñas manchas grises triangulares que aparecen en la conjuntiva y se asocian a la deficiencia de vitamina A.

bitter *a.* agrio-a, amargo-a; [*person*] amargado-a.

black *a.* negro-a; ___ **and blue** / amoratado; ___ **eye** / ojo amoratado; ___ **death** / peste bubónica; ___ **urine** / melanuria.

blackhead *n.* barro, espinilla, comedón.

blackout *n.* desmayo, vértigo, condición caracterizada por la falta de visión y pérdida momentánea del conocimiento.

bladder *n.* vejiga; saco musculomembranoso situado en la cavidad pélvica; ___ **calculi** / cálculos, piedras de la ___; ___ **infection** / infección de la ___; ___ **irrigation** / irrigación de la ___, **neurogenic** / ___ neurogénica.

blain *n.* llaga, ampolla, pústula.

Blalock-Tausig operation *n.* Blalock-Tausig, operación de, cirugía para reparar una malformación congénita del corazón.

blame *n.* culpa; *v.* **to blame** / echar la culpa; **to blame someone** / echarle la culpa.

bland *a.* blando-a, suave; ___ **diet** / dieta ___ .

blanket *n.* manta, frazada, cobija.

blastema *n.* blastema, sustancia primaria de la que se originan las células.

blastomycosis *n.* blastomicosis, infección causada por hongos que se inicia gen. en los pulmones.

blastula *n.* blástula, etapa primitiva del óvulo.

bleach *n.* blanqueador, lejía; *v.* blanquear.

bleariness *n.* lagaña, secreción pegajosa del ojo; vista nublada.

bleary-eyed *a.* [*eye*] legañosos; [*sight*] vista nublada; vista cansada.

bleed *vi.* sangrar, derramar, perder sangre; [*profusely*] desangrarse.

bleeder's disease *n. pop.* hemofilia.

bleeding *n.* sangrado, hemorragia; ___ **disorders** / trastornos hemorrágicos; ___ **from an artery** / hemorragia arterial; ___ **from the vagina** / ___ vaginal; ___ **from the nose** / ___ por la nariz, epistaxis; ___ **piles** / hemorroides; ___ **tendency** / diátesis hemorrágica; ___ **rectal** / rectorrhagia; **life threatening** ___ / hemorragia con peligro mortal.

blemish *n.* mancha, imperfección, defecto.

blend *n.* mezcla; *v.* mezclar, combinar.

blennorrhagia *n.* blenorragia, flujo de mucus.

blepharectomy *n.* blefarectomía, excisión de una parte o de todo el párpado.

blepharitis *n.* blefaritis, infl. de los párpados.

blepharochalasis *n.* blefarocalasis, relajación o caída del párpado superior por pérdida de elasticidad del tejido intersticial.

blepharoplasty *n.* blefaroplastia, operación plástica de los párpados.

blepharoplegia *n.* blefaroplejía, parálisis del párpado.

blind *a.* ciego-a, sin vista, ofuscado-a; *v.* cegar, deslumbrar; ___ **in one eye** / tuerto-a; ___ **spot** / punto ___ .

blindness *n.* ceguera; **color** ___ / acromatopsia, ___ al color; **night** ___ / nictalopía, ___ nocturna; **red** ___ / ___ roja; **total** ___ / pérdida completa de la visión.

blinds *n., pl.* cortinas.

blink *v.* parpadear.

blinking *n.* parpadeo.

blister *n.* ampolla, vesícula, flictena.

bloat *n.* aventación; *v.* entumecerse, hincharse.

bloated *a.* aventado-a, hinchado-a, inflado-a.

block *n.* bloqueo, obstrucción; *v.* obstruir, bloquear.

blocked *a.* bloqueado-a, obstruído-a; ___ **bowel** / obstrucción intestinal; ___ **ureter** / obstrucción ureteral.

blocker *n.* bloqueador; **calcium channel** ___ / ___ del canal cálcico.

blond *a.* rubio-a, *Mex.* gero-a.

blood *n.* sangre; **autologous** ___ / ___ autóloga; ___ **alcohol concentration** / concentración de alcohol en la ___ ; ___ **alcohol test** / prueba de alcoholemia; ___ **bank** / banco de ___ ; ___ **cell count** / conteo globular, conteo de células sanguíneas; ___ **clotting ability** / propiedad de coagulación; ___ **count** / conteo sanguíneo; ___ **culture** / hemocultivo; ___ **clot** / coágulo de ___ ; ___ **coagulation time** / tiempo de coagulación sanguínea; ___ **derivatives** / derivados sanguíneos, hemoderivados; ___ **donor** / donante de ___ ; ___ **gases** / gases sanguíneos; ___ **groups** / grupos sanguíneos; ___ **grouping** / determinación de grupos sanguíneos; ___ **oxygen analysis** / análisis del oxígeno contenido en la ___ ; ___ **plasma** / plasma sanguíneo; ___ **pressure** / presión arterial; ___ **products** / productos sanguíneos; ___ **proteins** / proteínas sanguíneas; ___ **relation** / consanguíneo-a; ___ **screening** / prueba selecta de ___ ; ___ **sputum** / esputo sanguinolento; ___ **substitutes** / substitutos sanguíneos; ___ **sugar** / glucemia; ___ **transfusion** / transfusión sanguínea; ___ **type** / grupo sanguíneo; ___ **typing** / determinación del grupo sanguíneo; ___ **vessel** / vaso sanguíneo; **packed** ___ **cells** / células paquete, células sanguíneas compactadas; **peripheral** ___ / ___ periférica.

bloodless *a.* exange, debilitado-a.

bloodletting *n.* efusión de sangre; *pop.* sangría.

blood pressure *n.* presión sanguínea, tensión de la sangre en las arterias producida por la contracción del ventrículo izquierdo, la resistencia de las arteriolas y capilares, la elasticidad de las paredes arteriales y la viscosidad y volumen de la sangre, expresada en relación con la presión atmosférica; **high** ___ / ___ alta; **low** ___ / ___ baja; **normal** ___ / ___ normal.

bloodshot *a.* [*eye*] inyectado de sangre.

bloody *a.* ensangrentado-a, con sangre, sanguinolento-a, cruento.

bloody sputum *n.* expectoración sanguínea; expectoración hemorrágica.

blotch *n.* marca, roncha.

blouse *n.* blusa, corpiño.

blow *n.* golpe; *vi.* soplar, **to __ one's nose** / soplarse, sonarse la nariz; **to give a __** / golpear.

blown *a., pp.* de to blow, soplado-a; **__ up** / hinchado-a.

blue *n.* color azul; *a.* triste, malancólico-a; **__ baby syndrome** / cianosis congénita, *pop.* mal azul.

blunder *n.* disparate, desatino.

blunt *a.* despuntado-a; embotado-a; **__ injuries** / heridas contusas.

blur *v.* empañar, nublar los ojos.

blurred *a., pp.* de **to blur**, borroso-a, nublado-a, empañado-a.

blush *vr.* sonrojarse, ruborizarse.

blushing *n.* rubor.

board *n.* tabla.

body *n.* cuerpo; [*dead*] cadáver; tronco; materia, sustancia; **__ fluid** / líquido corporal; **__ height** / estatura; **__ temperature** / temperatura corporal; **__ weight** / peso corporal; **__ wall** / tronco. See illustration on this page.

body-building *n.* esculturismo, restauración del cuerpo con ejercicios.

bogus *a.* falso-a; podrido-a.

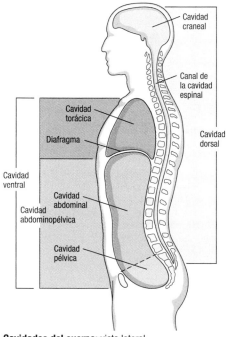

Cavidades del cuerpo: vista lateral

boil *n.* forúnculo, *Cuba* nacido; *Mex.* elacote; *v.* hervir, cocer.

boiled *a.* hervido-a; **__ water** / agua **__** .

boiling point *n.* punto de ebullición.

bolster *n.* cabezal; sostén, refuerzo; **__ suture** / sutura compuesta.

bolus *n.* bolo. 1. cantidad de una sustancia que se administra en determinado tiempo por vía oral o intravenosa para obtener una respuesta inmediata; 2. masa de consistencia suave lista para ser ingerida; **alimentary __** / **__** alimenticio.

bond *n.* vínculo, unión.

bonding *n.* vínculo afectivo.

bone *n.* 1. hueso. 2. [*fish*] espina; **__ cell** / osteoblasto; **__ chips** / astillas de **__**; **__ density** / densidad ósea; **__ development** / desarrollo óseo; **__ fracture** / fractura, **__** quebrado; **__ fragility** / fragilidad ósea; **__ graft** / injerto óseo; **__ hook** / gancho óseo; **__ lesions** / lesiones en los **__** -s; **__ loss** / osteopenia; **__ marrow** / médula ósea, *pop.* tuétano; **__ marrow failure** / fallo de la médula ósea; **__ plate** / placa ósea; **__ splinter** / esquirla, astilla ósea; **hard __** / **__** compacto; **he swallowed a fish __** / se tragó una espina de **__**; **spongy __** / **__** esponjoso; *v.* **to make no __ -s about it** / hablar sin rodeos; **skin and __ -s** / piel y **__** -s, muy delgado *pop.* estar en el hueso; *v.* deshuesar / sacar los **__** -s.

bonelet *n. dim.* huesecillo.

bonesetter *n.* componedor de huesos; curandero-a.

book *n.* libro.

boost *v.* estimular, aumentar, [*electricity*] elevar.

booster shot *n.* búster, inyección de refuerzo; dosis suplementaria; reactivación de una vacuna o agente inmunizador.

boot *n.* bota.

booze *n.* bebida alcohólica.

borax *n.* bórax, borato de sodio.

border *n.* borde, margen; frontera.

bordering *a.* cercano-a, fronterizo-a, adyacente.

border-line case *n.* caso indeciso, precario, difícil de pronosticar.

bored *a.* aburrido-a.

boredom *n.* fastidio, aburrimiento.

boric acid *n.* ácido bórico.

born *a.* nacido-a; **__ alive** / **__** vivo; **new __** / recién nacido-a; *v.* **to be __** / nacer.

borne *a.* acarreado-a; transmitido-a; llevado-a.

bosom *n.* seno, pecho.

both *a., pron.* ambos, los dos.

bothersome *a.* incómodo-a, molesto-a.

botox *n.* bótox, proteína purificada por la bacteria de botulismo *clostridium* que se emplea en aplicaciones cosméticas.

bottle *n.* botella, frasco, [*infant*] biberón, mamadera; *Mex.* pote, tele; ___ **feeding** / alimentación por biberón; ___ **propping** / suplemento con biberón;

bottle-feeding *n.* alimentación con biberón.

bottled water *n.* agua embotellada.

bottom *n.* fondo, parte inferior; asiento; *pop.* posaderas, asentaderas; *Cuba* fondillo.

botulin *n.* botulina, toxina causante del botulismo.

botulism *n.* botulismo, intoxicación ocasionada por la ingestión de alimentos contaminados por *Clostridium botulinum* que se desarrolla en alimentos que no han sido propiamente conservados.

bougie *n.* bujía; candelilla, instrumento usado en la dilatación de la uretra.

bouillon *n.* caldo, líquido alimenticio.

bounding pulse *n.* pulso saltón.

bounding pupil *n.* pupila saltona.

bouquet *n. Fr.* bouquet, grupo de estructuras en forma de racimo similares a la letra b.

bout *n.* acceso, ataque, episodio.

bovine *n.* bovino, referente al ganado.

bowel *n.* intestino. ___ **movement** / evacuación, deposición; ___ **obstruction** / obstrucción intestinal.

bowels *n., pl.* intestinos.

bowl *n.* bacín, taza.

bowleg *n.* V. **genu varum**.

box *n.* caja, estuche.

boy *n.* niño, muchacho.

boyfriend *n.* amigo, novio.

brace *n.* braguero, corsée, vendaje; abrazadera; **ankle** ___ / tobillera; **neck** ___ / ___ de cuello; abrazadera; *n., pl.* [*dentristy*] ganchos, aros.

brachial *a.* braquial, rel. al brazo; ___ **artery** / arteria braquial; ___ **plexus** / plexo ___; ___ **veins** / venas ___ -es o del brazo;

brachiocephalic *a.* braquiocefálico, rel. a la cabeza y al brazo.

brachydactyly *n.* braquidactilia, condición de manos y pies anormalmente pequeños.

bracing *n.* aplicación de una abrazadera.

bradycardia *n.* bradicardia, espanocardia, lentitud anormal en los latidos del corazón.

bradypnea *n.* bradipnea, movimientos respiratorios lentos.

bradytachycardia *n.* braditaquicardia, frecuencia cardíaca que alterna entre frecuencias cardíacas muy elevadas a frecuencias muy bajas.

Braille, reading system *n.* Braille, sistema de lectura, método de escritura e impreso de puntos alzados que identifican letras, números y puntuación y permite a los ciegos leer por medio del tacto.

b

brain *n.* cerebro, parte del sistema nervioso central que se localiza en el cráneo y actúa como regulador principal de las funciones del cuerpo; **blood** ___ **barrier** / barrera hematoencefálica; ___ **abscess** / asbceso cerebral; ___ **center** / centro cerebral; ___ **death** / muerte cerebral; ___ **edema** / edema cerebral; ___ **injuries** / traumatismo cerebral; ___ **or cerebral concussion** / concusión o conmoción cerebral; ___ **puncture** / punción cerebral; ___ **scan** / escán del ___; ___ **tumor** / tumor cerebral. See illustration on page 324.

brain stem *n.* cuello encefálico, parte que conecta el encéfalo con la espina dorsal.

brain stimulator surgery *n.* cirugía estimuladora del cerebro, tipo nuevo de cirugía cerebral que ayuda a controlar los temblores en los pacientes de Parkinson.

braincase *n.* cráneo, parte que encierra el cerebro.

brainless *a.* tonto-a, insensato-a.

brainwashing *n.* lavado de cerebro.

brainy *a.* inteligente, listo-a, talentoso-a.

braise *v.* asar al fuego; a la brasa.

bran *n.* salvado, producto procesado del trigo.

branch *n.* rama, bifurcación; sección, dependencia.

brassiere *n.* sostén, ajustador, corpiño.

brassy cough *n.* tos metálica, tos bronca.

BRCA 1 breast cancer *n.* cáncer del seno, cáncer de la mama, acrónimo que identifica al gene del cáncer de la mama, que se encuentra en un porciento bajo de pacientes descendientes de familiares que han sufrido de cáncer de la mama.

BRCA 2 uterine cancer *n.* acrónimo del gene del cáncer uterino que se encuentra en un porciento bajo de pacientes descendientes de familiares que padecieron del mismo tipo de cáncer.

bread *n.* pan; ___ **and butter** / ___ y mantequilla.

break *n.* fractura, rotura; quebradura; *vi.* romper, quebrar, fracturar; *v.* fracturarse, romperse, quebrarse; **to** ___ **down** / [*health*] perder la salud; **to** ___ **in** / forzar, abrir; **to** ___ **loose** / separarse, desprenderse; **to** ___ **through** / avanzar; **to** ___ **up** / fraccionar.

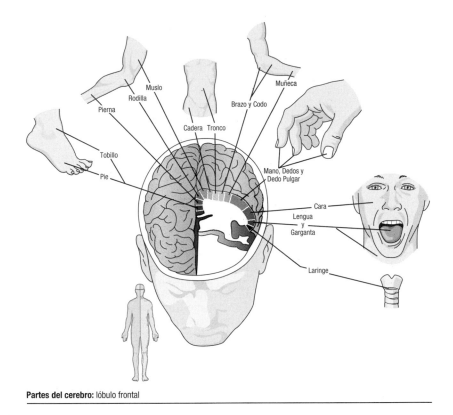

Partes del cerebro: lóbulo frontal

breakable *a.* frágil, quebradizo.

breakage *n.* rotura, quebradura.

breakdown *n.* distribución detallada; descomposición; colapso; **nervous ___** / crisis nerviosa.

breakfast *n.* desayuno.

breakout *n.* erupción.

breast *n.* pecho, seno, busto, mama, *slang* teta; **benign ___ disease** / enfermedad benigna de la mama; **caked ___** / mastitis por estasis; *v.* to **___ -feed** / dar el pecho, dar de mamar, dar la teta, *Mex. A.* criar con pecho; **___ pump** / sacaleche, mamadera; **___ self-examination** / autoexamen de los senos.

breastbone *n.* esternón.

breastfeeding *n.* lactancia materna.

breath *n.* respiración, aliento, soplo; *pop.* resuello; **___ sounds** / ruidos respiratorios; **coarse ___** / **___ gruesa**; **short of ___** / corto de **___** , falto de aliento; **out of ___** / falto de **___** , sin aliento; *v.* to **be out of ___** / faltar la **___** , estar sofacado-a; to **gasp for ___** / jadear; **to take a deep ___** / respirar

profundamente; **to hold one's ___** / sostener, aguantar la **___** .

breathanalyzer *n.* instrumento que analiza el aliento de una persona para indicar el grado de consunción de alcohol.

breathe *v.* respirar; [*to exhale*] exhalar; [*to inhale*] aspirar; **to ___ through the mouth** / **___** por la boca; **to ___ through the nose** / **___** por la nariz.

breather *n.* respirador; tregua, reposo.

breathing *n.* respiración, aliento, respiro; inhalación, aspiración; **___ exercises** / ejercicios respiratorios; **___ space, ___ time** / descanso, parada, reposo.

breathless *a.* sofocado-a, sin aliento; falto de respiración.

breathlessness *n.* sofocación.

breathtaking *a.* impresionante, asombroso-a.

breech *n.* trasero, posaderas, nalgas; [*in obstetrics*] **___ birth** / presentación de nalgas, presentación trasera.

breed *vi.* criar, producir, engendrar.

breeding *n.* cria, crianza.

breeze *n.* brisa, aire suave.

bregma *n. Gr.* bregma, intersección de las suturas coronal y sagital del cráneo.

bridge *n.* puente; [*dental*]; ___ **abutment** / pilar de ___ anclaje.

brief *n.* sumario, resumen; *a.* breve, corto-a, conciso-a; **-ly** *adv.* brevemente, concisamente; en pocas palabras.

bright *a.* brillante, lustroso-a, luminoso-a.

Bright's disease *n.* enfermedad de Bright. glomerulonephritis.

brim *n.* borde.

bring *vi.* traer; inducir; **to** ___ **down** / bajar; **to** ___ **down the fever** / bajar la fiebre; [*raise children*] **to** ___ **up** / educar, criar.

brochure *n.* folleto, panfleto.

broken *a. pp.* of **to break,** [*bone*] fracturado-a, quebrado-a; **broken arm** / brazo fracturado, quebrado; [*home, person*] **broken home** / hogar deshecho, destrozado; **broken hearted** / descorazonado.

bromhidrosis *n.* bromhidrosis, perspiración fétida; sudor fétido.

bromide *n.* bromuro, bromo, elemento no metálico, miembro del grupo de halógenos, muy irritante a las membranas mucosas. Se emplea como oxidante y antiséptico.

bronchial *a.* bronquial, rel. a los bronquios;___ **adenoma** / adenoma ___; ___ **arch** / arco ___; ___ **asthma** / asma ___; ___ **blockade** / bloqueo ___; ___ **breathing** / murmullo vesicular; ___ **cleft** / fisura ___; ___ **glands** / glándulas bronquiales; ___ **plexus injury** / lesión del plexo ___; ___ **spasm** / espasmo ___; ___ **stenosis** / estenosis ___; ___ **tree** / árbol ___; ___ **veins** / venas bronquiales; ___ **washing** / lavado ___ .

bronchiectasis *n.* bronquiectasia, dilatación crónica de los bronquios debida a una obstrucción o a una condición inflamatoria.

bronchiocele *n.* bronquiocele, dilatación localizada de un bronquiolo.

bronchiole *n.* bronquiolo, una de las ramas menores del árbol bronquial.

bronchiolitis *n.* bronquiolitis, infl. de los bronquiolos.

bronchitis *n.* bronquitis, infl. de los tubos bronquiales.

bronchoconstriction *n.* broncoconstricción, reducción de calibre bronquial.

bronchodilation *n.* broncodilatación, dilatación bronquial.

bronchodilator *n.* broncodilatador, medicamento que dilata el calibre de un bronquio; ___ **agents** / agentes ___ -es.

bronchogenic *a.* broncogénico-a, broncógeno-a, que se origina en los bronquios; ___ **carcinoma** / carcinoma ___; ___ **cyst** / quiste ___ .

bronchography *n.* broncografía, radiografía del árbol bronquial usando un medio de contraste.

broncholith *n.* broncolito, cálculo bronquial.

bronchopneumonia *n.* bronconeumonía, infl. aguda de los bronquiolos y de los lóbulos pulmonares que afecta gen. ambos pulmones.

bronchopulmonary *a.* broncopulmonar, rel. a los bronquios y los pulmones; ___ **lavage** / lavado ___; ___ **lymph nodes** / ganglios linfáticos ___ -es.

bronchoscopy *n.* broncoscopía, examen del árbol bronquial por medio del broncoscopio.

bronchospasm *n.* broncoespasmo, contracción espasmódica de los bronquios y los bronquiolos.

bronchospirometry *n.* broncoespirometría, proceso de medir la función de ventilación de cada pulmón separadamente por medio de un broncoespirómetro.

bronchostomy *n.* broncostomía, incisión de un bronquio.

bronchotomogram *n.* broncotomograma, escán o barrido de imágenes tomadas del sistema respiratorio superior, comprendiendo desde la tráquea a los bronquios inferiores.

bronchovesicular *a.* broncovesicular, rel. a los bronquios y alvéolos pulmonares esp. durante la auscultación. *Syn.* **broncoalveolar.**

bronchus *n.* (*pl.* **bronchia**) bronquio, uno de los tubos por los cuales el aire pasa a los pulmones; **eparterial** ___ / ___ superior a una arteria; **intermediate** ___ / ___ intermedio; **left main** ___ / ___ principal izquierdo; **lobar bronchi** / broncolobares; **main** ___ / ___ principal; **mucoid impaction of** ___ / impacto mucoso del ___; **right main** ___ / ___ principal derecho.

bronzed *a. pp.* of **to bronze,** bronceado-a.

brother *n.* hermano; ___ **-in-law** / cuñado; **half-** ___ / medio ___ .

brow *n.* ceño; frente.

brown *n.* castaño, café, carmelita; [*skin*] moreno-a.

Brown-Séquard syndrome *n.* síndrome de Brown Séquard, hemisección de la médula espinal que causa hiperestesia en el lado lesionado y pérdida de la sensibilidad en el lado opuesto.

brow presentation *n.* [*delivery*] presentación frontal del feto.

brucellosis *n.* brucelosis, fiebre ondulante o fiebre mediterránea, condición infecciosa bacteriana que se contrae por contacto con ganado vacuno o sus productos.

bruise *n.* magulladura, *Lat. Am.* magullón, cardenal; *vr.* magullarse, hacerse una magulladura, un morado o cardenal.

brunet, brunette *a.* trigueño-a, de piel oscura.

brush *n.* cepillo; *v.* cepillar; cepillarse.

brutal *a.* brutal, bruto-a.

bubble *n.* burbuja, ampolla; **to ___ over with joy** / rebozar de gozo.

bubo *n.* bubón, infl. linfática de la ingle.

bubonic plague *n.* peste bubónica.

bucca *n.* boca.

buccal *a.* bucal.

buccogingival *a.* bucogingival, rel. a la boca y encías.

buccolabial *a.* bucolabial, rel. a los labios y las mejillas.

bucket *n.* cubeta, cubo, balde.

buckle *n.* hebilla; *v.* **to ___ together** / unir, atar, juntar.

bud *n.* brote, retoño.

budget *n.* presupuesto.

buffer *n.* tampón, tope; *v.* neutralizar, tamponar; **___ system** / sistema amortiguador.

build *vi.* construir; **___ -up phase** / fase de ascenso; **to ___ up one's health** / reconstituir la salud.

bulb *n.* bulbo, pera; bombillo; 1. [*syringe*] pera de goma; 2. expansión oval o circular de un conducto o cilindro.

bulbocavernosus *n.* bulbocavernoso, localizado siguiendo la espina dorsal.

bulbourethral *a.* bulbouretral, uretrobulbar, rel. al bulbo del pene y la uretra.

bulbus cordis *n. L.* bulbo del corazón.

bulge *n.* hinchazón, protuberancia.

bulging *n.* protuberancia; **___ abdomen** / abdomen prominente, vientre abombado; **___ eyes** / ojos saltones.

bulimia *n.* bulimia, apetito exagerado.

bulk *n.* volumen.

bulla *n.* ampolla.

bullet *n.* bala; **___ wound** / balazo, herida de ___ .

bulletin *n.* boletín, aviso.

bump *n.* golpe, [*on the head*] chichón; *v.* tropezar; golpearse, darse un golpe.

bundle *n.* manojo, haz; bulto; **___ -branch block** / bloque de rama.

bunion *n.* bunio, juanete, infl. de la bursa en la primera coyuntura del dedo pulgar del pie. V. **Hallux valgus**.

bunionectomy *n.* extirpación de un juanete.

burden *v.* agobiar.

burn *n.* quemadura; **___ , dry heat** / ___ por calor seco; **___ -s, chemical** / ___ -s por sustancias químicas; **first-, second-, and third-degree ___ -s** / ___ -s de primer, segundo y tercer grado; **minor ___** / ___ leve; **sun ___** / insolación, eritema solar; **thermal ___** / ___ térmica; *n.* arder, quemar, incendiar.

burning *n.* ardor, quemadura; irritación; **a ___ feeling** / sensación de ___ , quemazón; **___ on urination** / al orinar.

burnt-out *a.* [*persona*]. extenuado-a. quemado-a; [*worn-out*] *a.* extenuado-a.

burp *n.* eructo, eructación; *v.* eructar, sacar el aire.

burr *n.* taladro; [*dentistry*] fresa; **fissure ___** / ___ de fisura; **diamond point ___** / ___ diamantada.

bursa *n. L.* bursa, bolsa o saco en forma de cavidad que contiene líquido sinovial en áreas de los tejidos donde puede ocurrir una fricción.

bursitis *n.* bursitis, infl. de una bursa.

burst *n.* [*a sudden outbreak*] reventón; *v.* reventar, reventarse, abrirse; **___ into laughter** / echarse a reír; **___ into tears** / deshacerse en lágrimas; **to ___ out** / brotar, reventar; **to ___ open** / abrirse, reventarse; echarse a llorar.

bushed *a. pop.* [*exhausted*] hecho polvo; agotado-a, molido-a, exhausto-a.

butter *n.* mantequilla.

butter milk *n.* 1. suero de leche; 2. leche agria.

buttocks *n., pl.* nalgas, *pop. Mex.* asentaderas, *Cuba* fondillo.

button *n.* botón.

buttress *n.* contrafuerte, resfuerzo, sostén.

buy *vi.* comprar.

buzz *n.* murmullo, zumbido.

by *prep.* por, cerca de, al lado de, según; **___ day** / de día, por el día; **___ night** / de noche, por la noche;

bypass *n. pop.* baipás, derivación. 1. conducto auxiliar, comunicación, derivación; *v.* 2. cambiar el curso de fluidos de un órgano o parte a otro a través de una nueva vía quirúrgica; **aortocoronary ___** / ___ aortocoronario o derivación aortocoronaria; **aortoiliac ___** / ___ aortoilíaco; **aortorenal ___** / ___ aortorenal; **cardiopulmonary ___** / ___ cardiopulmonar; **coronary ___** / ___ derivación coronaria; **extracraneal-intracraneal ___** / ___ extracranial-intracranial; **internal mammary artery ___** / ___ derivación de la arteria mamaria interna.

by-product *n.* subproducto.

C

C *abbr.* **carbon** / carbono; **celsius** / Celsius; **centigrade** / centígrado; **Kilocalorie** / kilocaloría.

c *abbr.* **calorie** / caloría; **cobalt** / cobalto; **cocaine** / cocaína; **contraction** / contracción.

cabbage *n.* col, repollo.

cacao *n.* cacao, planta de la cual se deriva el chocolate, alcaloide diurético.

cachexia *n.* caquexia, condición grave que se caracteriza por pérdida excesiva de peso y debilidad general progresiva.

cacosmia *n.* cacosmia, percepción de olores imaginarios, esp. olores fétidos.

cadaver *n.* cadáver.

cadaveric *a.* rel. a cadáver.

cadaverous *a.* cadavérico-a.

cafeteria *n.* cafetería.

caffeine *n.* cafeína, alcaloide presente esp. en el café y el té, estimulante y diurético.

calamine *n.* calamina, antiséptico astringente secante que se usa en afecciones de la piel.

calcaneus *n.* calcáneo, hueso del talón; *pop.* calcañal, calcañar.

calcareous *n.* calcáreo, que contiene calcio o cal.

calcemia *n.* calcemia, presencia de calcio en la sangre.

calcic *a.* cálcico, rel. a la cal.

calciferol *n.* calciferol, producto derivado de ergosterol, vitamina D2.

calcification *n.* calcificación, endurecimiento de tejidos orgánicos por depósitos de sales de calcio.

calcified *a.* calcificado-a.

calcinosis *n.* calcinosis, presencia de sales cálcicas en la piel, los tejidos subcutáneos y los órganos.

calcitonin *n.* calcitonina, hormona segregada por la tiroides que estimula el transporte del calcio de la sangre a los huesos.

calcium *n.* calcio, sustancia mineral necesaria en el desarrollo de los huesos y tejidos.

calciuria *n.* calciuria, presencia de calcio en la orina.

calculate *v.* calcular.

calculation *n.* calculación.

calculus *n.* (*pl.* **calculi**) cálculo, concreción o pequeña piedra que puede formarse en las secreciones y fluidos del organismo; **biliary** ___ / ___ biliar; **calcium oxalate** ___ / ___ de oxalato de calcio; **cystine** ___ / ___ de cistina; **fibrin** ___ / ___ de fibrina; **urinary** ___ / ___ urinario.

calendar *n.* calendario, almanaque.

calf *n.* pantorrilla; [*animal*] ternero-a.

caliber *n.* calibre, diámetro de un conducto o canal.

calibrator *n.* calibrador, instrumento para medir el diámetro de un conducto o canal.

caliceal *n.* caliceal, rel. a un cáliz.

call *n.* llamada; *v.* llamar; **to be on** ___ / estar de guardia; **to** ___ **for** / pedir.

callosity *n.* callosidad.

callous *a.* calloso-a.

callus *n.* callo, callosidad.

calm *n.* calma, serenidad; *v.* calmar, tranquilizar; calmarse, serenarse, tranquilizarse.

calmative *a.* calmante, sedante.

calmodulin *n.* calmodulina, proteína que se fija o se une a los iones de calcio interviniendo en todos los procesos celulares en los cuales los iones intervienen.

calomel *n.* calomel, cloruro mercurioso usado como agente local antibacteriano.

caloric *n.* calórico-a, rel. al calor o las calorías; ___ **intake** / ingestión ___ .

calorie *n.* caloría, unidad de calor a la que se refiere al evaluar la energía alimenticia; **kilocalorie, large** ___ / gran ___; **small** ___ / pequeña ___ .

calorific *n.* calorífico.

calvaria, skullcap *n.* calvaria, bóveda craneal.

calyx *n.* cáliz, colector en forma de copa.

camera *n.* cámara.1. espacio abierto o ventrículo; 2. cámara fotográfica.

camphor *n.* alcanfor; ___ **julep** / aqua alcanforada.

can *n.* lata, bote, envase; *vi.* poder.

canal *n.* canal, pasaje, estructura tubular; **birth** ___ / ___ del parto; **femoral** ___ / ___ femoral; **inguinalis** ___ / ___ inguinal; **root** ___ / ___ radicular.

canaliculus *n.* canalículo, canal o pasaje diminuto; **bilary** ___ / ___ biliar, entre las células del hígado; **lacrimal** ___ / ___ lacrimal, lagrimal.

cancel *v.* cancelar, suprimir.

cancellation *n.* cancelación.

cancellous *a.* canceloso-a, esponjoso-a, reticulado-a; ___ **bone** / hueso ___ .

cancer *n.* cáncer, tumor maligno; **breast** ___ / ___ de la mama; ___ **grading /**

determinacíon del grado patológico del ___; ___
staging / estado o extensión del tumor
canceroso; ___ **survivors** / supervivientes de
cáncer; **chemoprevention of** ___ / prevención
química de ___; **early** ___ / ___ incipiente.

cancerophobia *n.* cancerofobia, fobia a
contraer cáncer.

cancerous *a.* canceroso-a.

candid *a.* cándido-a; sincero-a.

candida albicans susceptibility *n.*
susceptibilidad a candida albicans.

candidiasis *n.* candidiasis, infección de la piel
producida por un hongo semejante a la levadura.

candy *n.* dulce, confite, caramelo.

cane *n.* bastón; caña; ___ **sugar** / azúcar de caña,
sucrosa, sacarosa.

canine *n.* canino; cúspide; diente; *a.* rel. a los
perros.

canker *n.* ulceración de la boca o los labios; ___
sore / afta, llaga ulcerosa.

cannabis, marijuana *n.* canabis, marijuana,
mariguana, marihuana, planta de hojas que
producen un efecto narcótico y halucinógeno al
fumarse; *slang* **grass; bomber** / cigarrillo de
marijuana; *v. slang;* **to blast, to blow weed** /
fumar marijuana.

cannula *n.* (*pl.* **cannulae**) cánula, sonda, tubo
que insertado en el cuerpo conduce o saca
líquidos.

cannulation *n.* canulación, acto de introducir
una cánula a través de un vaso o conducto;
aortic ___ / ___ aórtica.

canthus *n.* 1. canto, borde; 2. ángulo formado
por el párpado externo y el interno al unirse en
ambas partes del ojo.

cap *n.* gorra; tapa.

capable *a.* capaz.

capacity *n.* a capacidad; **vital** ___ / ___ vital.

capillary *n.* capilar; vaso capilar; *a.* semejante a
un cabello; **arterial** ___ / ___ arterial;
lymph ___ / ___ linfático; **venous** ___ / ___
venoso.

capitellum *n.* capitelum.1. bulbo de un pelo; 2.
parte del húmero.

capsula, capsule *n.* cápsula.1. envoltura
membranosa; 2. pastilla; **articular** ___ / ___
articular, que envuelve una articulación sinovial;
enclosed in a ___ / encapsulado.

capsulation *n.* encapsulación, acto de envolver
en una cápsula o envoltura.

car *n.* automóvil, carro; *Sp.* coche; ___ **accident** /
accidente automovilístico.

carbohydrase *n.* carbohidrasa.

carbohydrate *n.* carbohidrato, grupo de
compuestos de carbono, hidrógeno y oxígeno

entre los que se encuentran los almidones,
azúcares y celulosas.

carbolic *a.* carbólico-a, rel. al fenol o ácido
fenílico.

carbon *n.* carbono; ___ **dioxide** / dióxido
de ___; ___ **monoxide** / monóxido de ___ .

carbonated *a.* carbonatado-a.

carbonic *a.* carbónico-a.

carbonization *n.* carbonización.

carboxyhemoglobin *n.* carboxihemoglobina,
combinación de monóxido de carbono y
hemoglobina que desplaza el oxígeno e
interrumpe la función oxidante de la sangre.

carbuncle *n.* carbunco, furúnculo, infl. con
pus,*pop.* avispero.

carcinogen *n.* carcinógeno, cualquier sustancia
que puede producir cáncer.

carcinogenesis *n.* carcinogénesis, origen del
cáncer.

carcinogenic *n.* carcinógeno-a, de origen
canceroso.

carcinoma *n.* carcinoma, tumor canceroso. See
chart on page 329.

carcinoma in situ *n.* carcinoma in situ, células
tumorales localizadas en estado de desarrollo
quo no han invadido aún estructuras adyacentes.

carcinomatosis *n.* carcinomatosis, invasión de
cáncer diseminado en varias partes del cuerpo.

carcinosarcoma *n.* carcinosarcoma, neoplasma
maligno formado por células carcinogénicas y de
sarcoma. Este tipo de neoplasma se observa en
la tiroides, la garganta y los ovarios.

cardiac *a.* cardíaco-a, referente al corazón. See
chart on page 329.

cardiac ultrasonography *n.* V.
echocardiography.

cardias *n.* cardias, desembocadura del esófago en
el estómago.

cardiataxia *n.* cardiataxia, falta de coordinación
de los movimientos cardíacos.

cardiectomy *n.* cardiectomía, extirpación de la
región superior extrema del estómago.

cardioangiogram *n.* cardioangiograma, imagen
por rayos-x de los vasos sanguíneos y las
cámaras del corazón usando un medio de
contraste.

cardiocentesis *n.* cardiocentesis,
cardiopuntura, punción de una cavidad del
corazón.

cardiodynamics *n.* cardiodinámica; la
dinámica de la acción cardíaca.

cardiogram *n.* cardiograma, trazado que
representa los impulsos del corazón.

Carcinoma	Carcinoma
adenocystic	adenoquístico
adenosquamous	adenoescamoso
adrenocortical	corticosuprarrenal
alveolar cells of the lung	de células alveolares del pulmón
apocrine	de apocrinocitos
basal cells of the face	de células basales de la cara
basal squamous cells	de células basales escamosas
borderline	de límite
bronchogenic	broncógeno, de broncocitos
bronchial	bronquiolar
colloid	coloide
cuboidal	cuboide
cutaneous	cutáneo
cylindromatous	cilindromatoso
cystic	quístico
duodenal	duodenal
ductal	ductal, de conducto
early cancer	precoz
embryonal	embrional
endometrial	endometrial
follicular	folicular
giant cell	de célula gigante
glandular	glandular
in situ	localizado
latent	latente
lipomatous	lipomatoso
liver cell	de hepatocitos
lobular non invasive	lobular no invasivo
medullary	medular
metastatic	metastásico
occult	escondido
of anaplastic cells	de células anaplásticas
of cervix	del cuello uterino
of salivary glands	de glándulas salivares
of the bladder	de la vejiga
of the breast	de la mama
ovarian	ovárico
papillar	papilar
pharyngeal	faríngeo
prostatic	de la próstata
uterine	del útero
verrugous	verrugoso

Cardiac	Cardíaco
apex	ápex
arrest, standstill	paro
asthma	asma
catheterization	cateterización
chambers	cavidades
depressants	agentes antiarrítmicos
edema	edema
examination	auscultación
failure	insuficiencia
massage	masaje
output	gasto, rendimiento
pacing, artificial	estimulación ___ artificial
pulse generator	generador del impulso
resuscitation	reanimación
rupture	ruptura
sounds	ruidos
sphincter	esfínter
stimulants	estimulantes
tamponade	taponamiento

cardiograph *n.* cardiógrafo, instrumento que traza gráficamente los movimientos del corazón.
cardiography *n.* cardiografía, uso del cardiógrafo para registrar los movimientos del corazón.
cardiologist *n.* cardiólogo-a, especialista del corazón.
cardiology *n.* cardiología, ciencia que estudia el corazón, sus funciones y enfermedades.
cardiomegaly *n.* cardiomegalia, hipertrofia cardíaca.
cardiomyopathy *n.* cardiomiopatía, alteración del músculo del corazón; **alcoholic** ___ / ___ alcohólica; **congestive** ___ / ___ congestiva; **dilated** ___ / ___ dilatada; **hypertrophic** ___ / ___ hipertrófica familiar; **hypertrophic** ___ / ___ hipertrófica; **idiopathic** ___ / ___ idiopática; **puerperal** ___ / ___ puerperal.
cardiopathy *n.* cardiopatía, enfermedad cardíaca.
cardioplegia *n.* cardioplegia, paro o traumatismo cardíaco.
cardiopulmonary *a.* cardiopulmonar, rel. al corazón y los pulmones; ___ **bypass /**

puente ___; ___ **resuscitation** /
resucitación ___; ___ **resuscitator** / resucitador,
reanimador ___ .

cardiospasm *n.* cardiospasmo, espasmo o
contracción del cardias.

cardiotomy *n.* cardiotomía, incisión en el
corazón.

cardiotonic *a.* cardiotónico-a, de efecto tónico o
favorable al corazón.

cardiovascular *a.* cardiovascular, rel. al
corazón y los vasos sanguíneos; ___ **failure** /
insuficiencia ___ .

cardioversion *n.* cardioversión, restauración del
ritmo sinusal normal del corazón por medio de
una corriente directa.

carditis *n.* carditis, infl. del pericardio, miocardio
y endocardio; **rheumatic** ___ / ___ reumática.

care *n.* cuidado, asistencia, atención; **cardiac**___
unit / sala de ___ cardíaco; **comprehensive
medical** ___ / médico-comprensiva;
delivery ___ / asistencia obstétrica; **end-of-
life** ___ / ___ terminal; **free of** ___ / libre
de ___; **health** ___ **system** / sistema de
asistencia sanitaria; **inpatient** ___ / asistencia
hospitalaria; **intensive** ___ **unit** / sala de ___
intensivo; **managed** ___ / atención
administrativa; **postnatal** ___ / ___ después del
parto; **prenatal** ___ / ___ y atención prenatal;
primary___ / ___ primario; **proper** ___ / ___
apropiado; **quality** ___ / calidad asistencial;
refusal of ___ / negación de ___; **self-care** /
atención o cuidado personal; *v.* **to be under
the** ___ **of** / estar bajo el ___ de.

career *n.* profesión.

careful *a.* cuidadoso-a; esmerado-a; atento-a.

caregiver *n.* asistente de salud, facilitador de
atención sanitaria.

careless *a.* descuidado-a; desatento-a.

carelessness *n.* descuido; negligencia.

caries *n., pl.* caries. 1. destrucción progresiva de
tejido óseo; 2. caries dentales, *pop.* dientes
picados; **dental carie** / ___ dental;
distal ___ / ___ distal; **fissure** ___ / ___ de
fisura.

carmine *n.* carmín, carmesí.

carnivorous *a.* carnívoro-a.

carnosity *n.* carnosidad, excrecencia carnosa.

carotene *n.* caroteno, pigmento amarillo rojizo
presente en vegetales que se convierte en
vitamina A en el cuerpo.

carotid *n.* carótida, arteria principal del
cuello; ___ **arteries** / arterias ___ -s; ___ **sinus** /
seno de la ___; ___ **sinus syncope** / síncope del
seno de la ___ .

carotodynia *n.* carotodinia, dolor causado por
presión de la arteria carótida.

carotid sinus *n.* sinus (seno) de la carótida,
pequeña dilatación de la arteria carótida y su
bifurcación; ___ **sinus syncope** / *n.* síncope del
seno de la carótida .

carpal *a.* carpal, rel. al carpo.

carpus *n.* (*pl.* **carpi**) carpo, muñeca de la mano,
porción de la extremidad superior situada entre
el antebrazo y la mano.

carrier *n.* portador, agente transmisor. 1. una
persona o animal que lleva oculto temporalmente
un agente patógeno específico al que es inmune,
y se convierte en un foco potencial de esa
infección a otros; 2. un agente genético que
puede convertirse en un foco de infección; ___
state / estado portador; **latent** ___ / ___ latente;
manifesting ___ / ___ manifestado;
passive ___ / ___ pasivo.

carrot *n.* zanahoria.

carry *v.* llevar; cargar; **to** ___ **out** / /llevar a cabo.

carrying capacity *n.* capacidad de
sustención; ___ **fatality rate** / índice de
letalidad; ___ **management** / administración de
casos.

car sickness *n.* mareo.

cartilage *n.* cartílago, tejido semiduro que cubre
los huesos.

caruncle *n.* carúncula, pequeña irritación de la
piel; **urethral** ___ / uretral.

cascara sagrada *n.* cáscara sagrada, corteza
de la planta *Rhamnus purshiana*, comúnmente
usada como medicamento en casos de
estreñimiento crónico.

case *n.* caso; ___ **fatality rate** / índice de
mortalidad por ___-s; ___ **history** / historia
clínica; ___ **reporting** / presentación
del ___; ___ **control study** / estudio
comparativo de ___ -s.

casein *n.* caseína, proteína principal de la leche.

caseous *a.* caseoso, de queso o parecido al
queso.

cash *n.* dinero al contado; ___ **payment** / ___ ,
pago al contado; *v.* **to pay** ___ / pagar al
contado.

casket *n.* ataúd, caja.

cast *n.* 1. molde, vaciado; **bronchial** ___ / ___
bronquial; 2. escayola; **plaster** ___ / ___ de
yeso; 3. cilindro; **blood** ___ / cilindro hemático;
v. **to put in a** ___ / enyesar, moldear; **to** ___
aside / desechar. V. **granular cast**.

castor oil *n.* aceite de ricino, palmacristi.

castrate *v.* castrar.

casual *a.* casual, accidental.

casualty *n.* víctima de accidente, herido, muerto; [*war*] bajas.[*wounded*] herido-a; ___ **list** / lista de accidentados.

casualty report *n.* informe de urgencias.

cat *n.* gato-a.

catabolism *n.* catabolismo, proceso por el cual sustancias complejas se reducen a compuestos más simples.

catalepsy *n.* catalepsia, condición caracterizada por la pérdida de la capacidad de movimiento muscular voluntario y disminución acentuada de la habilidad de reaccionar a estímulos, gen. asociada con transtornos psicológicos.

catalysis *n.* catálisis, alteración de la velocidad de una reacción química por la presencia de un catalítico.

catalyst, catalytic *a.* catalítico-a, agente estimulante de una reacción química sin afectarla.

cataplexy *n.* cataplejía, pérdida repentina del tono muscular causada por un estado emocional intenso.

cataract *n.* catarata, opacidad del cristalino; **anular** ___ / ___ anular; **black** ___ / ___ negra; **blue** ___ / ___ cerúlea; **complete** ___ / ___ completa; **congenital** ___ / ___ congénita; **green** ___ / ___ verde; **mature** ___ / ___ madura; **senile** ___ / ___ senil; **soft** ___ / ___ blanda.

cataractogenic *a.* cataratogénico, causante de catarata.

catarrh *n.* catarro, resfriado, constipado.

catarrhal *a.* catarral, referente a un catarro.

catatonia *n.* catatonía, esquizofrenia caracterizada por mutismo, postura rígida y resistencia a cooperar para activar los movimientos o el habla. Los mismos síntomas se asocian con otras enfermedades mentales.

catch *vi.* contraer; agarrar; coger; ___ **an illness** / ___ una enfermedad.

catecholamines *n., pl.* catecolaminas, aminas de acción simpatomimética producidas en las glándulas suprarrenales (incluyen la dopamina, la epinefrina y la norepinefrina).

category *n.* categoría, clase.

catgut *n.* catgut, tipo de ligadura que se hace con la tripa del intestino de algunos animales.

catharsis *n.* catarsis. 1. acción purgativa; 2. análisis con el fin terapéutico de liberar al paciente de un estado de ansiedad.

cathartic *n.* catártico, medicamento con efectos laxativos o purgativos; *a.* catártico-a, rel. a la catarsis.

catheter *n.* catéter, sonda, tubo usado para drenar o introducir líquidos; ___ **holder** / portacatéter.

catheterization *n.* cateterización, inserción de un catéter.

catheterize *v.* cateterizar, insertar un catéter.

cat-scratch disease *n.* enfermedad causada por rasguño de gato.

cauda *n.* cauda, apéndice similar a una cola.

caudal *a.* caudal, rel. a la cola.

cauliflower *n.* coliflor.

causal *a.* causal.

causalgia *n.* causalgia, dolor con ardor en la piel.

causative *a.* causal, etiológico-a.

cause *n.* causa, lo que produce un efecto o condición, un cambio mórbido o enfermedad; **constitutional** ___ / ___ constitucional; **existing** ___ / ___ actual, presente; **necessary** ___ / ___ necesaria; **precipitating** ___ / factor desencadenante; **predisposing** ___ / factor predisponente; **proximate** ___ / ___ inmediata; **specific** ___ / ___ específica; **without** ___ / sin ___; *v.* causar, ocasionar.

caustic *a.* cáustico-a.

cauterization *n.* cauterización, quemadura producida por medio de un agente cauterizante tal como el calor, la corriente eléctrica, o un cáustico.

cauterize *v.* cauterizar, quemar por medio de un agente cauterizante.

cautery-assisted uvulopalatoplasty *n.* cauterización asistida por uvulopalatoplastía.

caution *n.* advertencia, precaución, cautela.

cautious *a.* precavido-a, prudente; **to make a** ___ **decision** / hacer una decisión precavida.

cava *n., pl.* de cavum, cavidad, hueco. V. **vein, cava**.

cave *n.* depresión.

cavern *n.* caverna, cavidad patológica.

cavernous *a.* cavernoso-a, que contiene espacios huecos.

cavity *n.* cavidad, lugar hueco; **abdominal** ___ / ___ abdominal; **cranial** ___ / ___ craneal; **pelvic** ___ / ___ pelviana; **thoracic** ___ / ___ torácica.

cease *v.* cesar, parar, detener.

cecostomy *n.* cecostomía, creación de una apertura artificial en el ciego.

cecum *n.* ciego, bolsa que forma la primera parte del intestino grueso.

celery *n.* apio.

celiac *a.* celíaco, abdominal, rel. al abdomen.

celiotomy *n.* celiotomía. V. **laparotomy**.

cell *n.* célula, unidad estructural de todo organismo viviente. See illustration and chart on this page.

cellular *a.* celular, de naturaleza semejante o referente a la célula; ___ **compartmentation** / compartimentos ___ -es; ___ **counting device** / cuenta células; ___ **growth** / crecimiento ___; ___ **-like** / en forma ___; ___ **tissue** / tejido ___; ___ **water** / agua ___ .

cellularity *n.* celularidad, condición y calidad de las células presentes en un tejido o masa.

cellulitis *n.* celulitis, infl. del tejido conectivo celular.

cellulose *n.* celulosa.

cement *n.* cemento.

cemetery *n.* cementerio, camposanto.

census *n.* censo.

center *n.* centro.

Center for Disease Control *n.* Centro para Control de Enfermedades.

centigrade *n.* centígrado.

Cell	Célula
adipose	adiposa
anaplastic	anaplástica
accesory	accesoria
acoustic	acústica
B lymphocyte	linfocito B, tipo de
basal	basal
columnar	columnar
giant	gigante
goblet	calciforme
ependymal	ependimaria
epidermal	epidérmica
interstitial	intersticial
mononuclear	mononuclear
phagocyte	fagocitaria
pyramidal	piramidal
red blood	sanguíneas
reproductive	reproductiva
scavenger	basurera
sickle	falciforme

centimeter *n.* centímetro.

central *a.* central; céntrico-a; ___ **nervous system** / sistema nervioso ___ .

central deafness *n.* sordera central.

centrifugal *a.* centrífugo-a, rel. al movimiento de repulsión, del centro hacia afuera.

centripetal *a.* centrípeto-a, con movimiento de atracción hacia el centro.

cephalalgia *n.* cefalalgia, dolor de cabeza,*pop.* jaqueca.

cephalic *a.* cefálico-a, rel. a la cabeza.

cephalosporin *n.* cefalosporina, antibiótico de espectro amplio.

cerclage *n.* cerclaje, en ortopedia procedimiento usado en ciertas fracturas por el cual se unen partes rodeándolas con un hilo metálico o con catgut.

cereal *n.* cereal.

cerebellum *n.* cerebelo, parte posterior del cerebro, centro de coordinación de los movimientos musculares voluntarios.

cerebral *a.* cerebral, rel. al cerebro; ___ **edema** / edema ___; ___ **embolism and thrombosis** / embolia y trombosis ___; ___ **hemorrhage** / hemorragia ___; ___ **palsy** / parálisis ___; ___ **tumor** / tumor ___ .

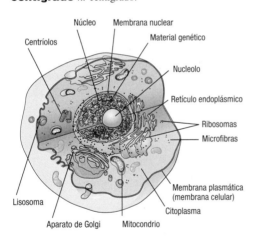

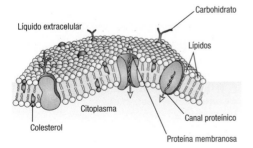

La célula: (A) La célula y los organillos; (B) Célula típica de un animal y membrana plasmática

cerebral paralysis *n.* parálisis cerebral, falta de coordinación muscular debido a una lesión cerebral congénita.

cerebrospinal *a.* cefalorraquídeo, cerebroespinal; ___ **axis** / eje ___; ___ **fluid** / líquido ___; ___ **meningitis** / meningitis ___; ___ **pressure** / presión ___ .

cerebrovascular *a.* cerebrovascular; ___ **accident** / apoplegía, hemorragia cerebral.

cerebrum *n.* cerebro, encéfalo, centro de coordinación de actividades sensoriales e intelectuales.

certain *a.* cierto-a; seguro-a; *v.* **to be** ___ / estar seguro-a; **-ly** *adv.* ciertamente, seguramente.

certainty *n.* certeza.

certificate *n.* certificado; **death** ___ / ___ de defunción.

cerumen *n.* cerumen, segregación cerosa que lubrica y protege el óido.

cervical *a.* cervical. 1. referente al área del cuello; 2. rel. al cuello uterino; ___ **dilator** / dilatador ___; ___ **dysplasia** / displasia ___; ___ **incompetence** / incompetencia del cuello uterino; ___ **erosion** / erosión ___; ___ **polyp** / pólipo ___ .

cervical cap *n.* capa o cubierta del cuello uterino.

cervical dystonia *n.* distonia cervical, trastorno de tonicidad en los tejidos de la nuca que resulta en incapacitación de movimiento voluntario del cuello.

cervical range of motion *n.* alcance del movimiento cervical.

cervical traction vest *n.* chaleco de tracción cervical.

cervicovesical *a.* cervicovesical, rel. al cuello uterino y a la vejiga.

cervix *n.* cuello uterino, parte baja del útero en forma de cuello; **dilation of the** ___ / dilatación del ___ .

cesarean *n.* cesárea; ___ **section** / cirugía de parto.

cesium *n.* cesio, elemento metálico perteneciente al grupo de metales alcalinos.

chain *n.* cadena; ___ **reaction** / reacción en ___; ___ **suture** / sutura en ___ .

chair *n.* silla.

chalazion *n.* chalazión, quiste del párpado, quiste meiboniano.

chalk *n.* yeso.

chamber *n.* cámara, cavidad; **anterior** ___ / ___ anterior, situada entre la córnea y el iris; **aqueous** ___ / ___ acuosa; ___ **-s of the**

eye / ___ -s oculares; ___ **-s of the heart** / cavidades del corazón: aurículas y ventrículos del corazón; **hyperbaric** ___ / ___ hiperbárica.

chamomile *n.* manzanilla, té, sedante gastrointestinal.

chancre *n.* chancro; lesión primaria de la sífilis.

chancroid *n.* chancroide, úlcera venérea no sifilítica.

change *n.* cambio, alteración; ___ **of life** / menopausia; *v.* cambiar, mudar.

changeless *a.* invariable, inmutable.

channel *n.* canal; estructura tubular; **birth** ___ / ___ del parto.

chaos *n.* caos, desorden.

chaotic *n.* caótico-a, desordenado-a.

chap *n.* hendidura, raja, grieta.

chapel *n.* capilla.

chapped *a.* agrietado-a, cuarteado-a; rajado-a; ___ **hands** / manos ___ -s; ___ **lips** / labios ___ -s.

chapter *n.* capítulo.

character *n.* 1. carácter; 2. calidad, naturaleza; 3. [*actor, actress in a play or movie*] personaje.

characteristic *n.* característica, peculiaridad; *a.* característico-a; peculiar; **it is a symptom** ___ **of this illness** / es un síntoma ___ de esta enfermedad.

charcoal *n.* carbón vegetal.

charge *n.* costo; *v.* cobrar.

charitable *a.* caritativo-a.

charity *n.* caridad; beneficencia.

charity institution *n.* institución benéfica.

charlatan *n.* charlatán-a; dícese de una persona que pretende tener cualidades o conocimientos para curar enfermedades.

charley horse *n.* dolor y sensibilidad en un músculo; *pop.* calambre.

charred *a.* carbonizado-a.

chart *n.* plano, gráfico; **medical** ___ / hoja clínica.

chat *n.* charla, plática; *v.* charlar, platicar.

chatter *v.* [*teeth*] rechinar los dientes.

cheap *a.* barato-a.

check *n.* control; acción o efecto de regular; [*bank*] cheque; *v.* controlar; chequear, verificar.

checkbook *n.* chequera; talonario.

checkup *n.* *Am.* chequeo, examen físico completo.

cheek *n.* mejilla.

cheekbone *n.* carrillo, pómulo, hueso malar.

cheer up *v.* animarse, alegrarse.

cheese *n.* queso.

cheilectomy *n.* queilectomía, excisión parcial del labio.

cheilitis, chilitis *n.* queilitis, infl. de los labios.

cheiloplasty *n.* queiloplastia, reparación del labio.

cheiloschisis *n.* queilosquisis V. **harelip**.

cheilosis *n.* queilosis, manifestación con marcas y fisuras en la comisura de los labios debida a deficiencia de vitamina B$_2$ (riboflavina).

cheilotomy *n.* queilotomía

cheirology *n.* quirología. 1. estudio de la mano; 2. uso del lenguaje por señas como medio de comunicación con los sordomudos.

chemical *a.* químico-a; ___ **peel** / peladura ___ .

chemist *n.* químico-a; farmacéutico-a, boticario-a.

chemistry *n.* química, ciencia que estudia los elementos, estructura y propiedades de las sustancias y las transformaciones que éstas sufren.

chemocoagulation *n.* quimiocoagulación, co-agulación por medio de agentes químicos.

chemonucleolysis *n.* quimionucleólisis, disolución por inyección de una enzima proteolítica del núcleo pulposo de una hernia.

chemoprophylaxis *n.* quimioprofilaxis, uso de una droga o de una sustancia química que contiene preventivos.

chemoreceptor *n.* quimiorreceptor-a, célula suceptible a cambios químicos o que puede ser afectada por éstos.

chemosurgery *n.* quimiocirugía, extirpación o remoción de tejidos por medio de sustancias químicas.

chemotaxis *n.* quimiotaxis, movimiento de un organismo o célula como reacción a un estímulo químico.

chemotherapy *n.* quimioterapia, tratamiento de una enfermedad por medio de agentes químicos.

cherubism *n.* querubismo, condición fibroósea infantil que causa agrandamiento de los huesos de la mandíbula.

chest *n.* tórax, pecho; ___ **cold** / catarro bronquial; *pop.* catarro al pecho; ___ **respirator** / respirador torácico; ___ **surgery** / cirugía torácica; ___ **wall** / pared torácica;

chew *v.* masticar, mascar.

Cheyne-Stokes respiration syndrome *n.* síndrome de respiración de Cheyne-Stokes, respiración cíclica con períodos de apnea y aumento rápido y profundo de la respiración gen. asociada con trastornos del centro neurológico respiratorio.

chiasm, chiasma *n.* quiasma. 1. cruzamiento de dos vías o conductos; 2. punto de cruzamiento de las fibras de los nervios ópticos.

chiasma opticum *n.* quiasma óptico.

chicken *n.* pollo; ___ **breast** / pechuga.

chickenpox, varicella *n.* varicela, enfermedad viral contagiosa que se manifiesta gen. en la infancia y se caracteriza por una erupción que se convierte en pequeñas vesículas; *pop.* viruelas locas.

chief *n.* jefe-a; ___ **complaint** / queja principal.

chilblain *n.* sabañón, eritema debido a frío intenso que gen. se manifiesta en las manos y los pies.

child *n.* niño-a; ___ **nurse** / niñera; ___ **nursery** / guardería infantil, jardín de la infancia; ___ **support** / manutención, pensión alimenticia; ___ **welfare** / asistencia social a la infancia.

childbearing *n.* gestación, embarazo.

childbirth *n.* parto, nacimiento, alumbramiento.

childhood *n.* infancia, niñez.

chill *n.* enfriamiento, escalofrío.

chin *n.* barba, mentón, barbilla.

chiropodist *n.* quiropodista. V. **podiatrist**.

chiropractic *n.* quiropráctica, sistema terapéutico que recurre a la manipulación y ajustamiento de las estructuras del cuerpo esp. la columna vertebral en relación con el sistema nervioso.

chisel *n.* cincel.

chloasma *n.* cloasma, hiperpigmentación facial que puede ocurrir en algunas mujeres durante el embarazo.

chlorambucil *n.* clorambucil, forma de mostaza nitrogenada usada para combatir algunas formas de cáncer.

chloramphenicol, chloromycetin *n.* cloranfenicol, cloromicetina, antibiótico esp. efectivo en el tratamiento de la fiebre tifoidea.

chlorhydria *n.* clorhidria, exceso de ácido clorhídrico en el estómago.

chloride *n.* cloruro.

chlorine *n.* cloro, agente desinfectante y blanqueador.

chloroform *n.* cloroformo, anestésico.

chloroma *n.* cloroma, tumor de color verde que puede manifestarse en distintas partes del cuerpo.

chlorophyll *n.* clorofila, pigmento verde de las plantas esencial en la producción de carbohidratos por fotosíntesis.

chloroquine *n.* cloroquina, compuesto usado en el tratamiento de la malaria.

chlorosis *n.* clorosis, tipo de anemia vista esp. en la mujer y usu. relacionada con deficiencia de hierro.

chlorpromazine *n.* cloropromacina, antiemético y tranquilizante.

chlortetracycline *n.* clorotetraciclina, antibiótico antimicrobiano de espectro amplio.

chocolate *n.* chocolate.

choice *n.* opción, alternative; elección.

choke *v.* ahogar, sofocar, estrangular; [*choke on something*] atragantarse.

cholangiectasis *n.* colangiectasis, dilatación de los conductos biliares.

cholangiogram *n.* colangiograma, radiografía de las vías biliares usando un medio de contraste.

cholangiography *n.* colangiografía, rayos-x de las vías biliares.

cholangitis *n.* colangitis, infl. de los conductos biliares.

cholecystectomy *n.* colecistectomía, extirpación de la vesícula biliar.

cholecystitis *n.* colecistitis, infl. de la vesícula biliar.

cholecystoduodenostomy *n.* colecistoduodenostomía, anastomosis de la vesícula y el duodeno.

cholecystogastrostomy *n.* colecistogastrostomía, anastomosis de la vesícula y el estómago.

cholecystogram *n.* colecistograma, radiografía de la vesícula biliar.

cholecystography *n.* colecistografía, rayos-x de la vesícula biliar usando un medio radiopaco.

cholecystopathy *n.* colecistopatía, enfermedad de la vesícula biliar.

choledochojejunostomy *n.* coledocoyeyunostomía, anastomosis del coledóco y el yeyuno.

choledocholithiasis *n.* coledocolitiasis, cálculos en el coledóco.

choledochus *n.* coledóco, conducto biliar formado por la unión de los conductos hepático y cístico.

cholelithiasis *n.* colelitiasis, litiasis biliar, presencia de cálculos en la vesícula biliar o en un conducto biliar.

cholemia *n.* colemia, presencia de bilis en la sangre.

cholera *n.* cólera, enfermedad infecciosa grave caracterizada por diarrea severa y vómitos; ___ **fulminans** / ___ fulminante.

choleric *a.* colérico-a.

cholestasis *n.* colestasis, estasis biliar.

cholesteatoma *n.* colesteatoma, tumor que contiene colesterol, situado comúnmente en el oído medio.

cholesteremia, cholesterolemia *n.* colesteremia, colesterolemia, exceso de colesterol en la sangre.

cholesterol *n.* colesterol, lípido precursor de las hormonas sexuales y corticoides adrenales, componente de las grasas y aceites animales, del tejido nervioso y de la sangre; ___ **reducer** / reductor de ___; **high** ___ / ___ alto.

cholic acid *n.* ácido cólico, uno de los ácidos no conjugados de la bilis.

cholinesterase *n.* colinesterasa, familia de enzimas.

choluria *n.* coluria, presencia de bilis en la orina.

chondritis *n.* condritis, infl. de un cartílago.

chondrocalcinosis *n.* condrocalcinosis, condición semejante a la gota, con manifestaciones de cicatrización por calcificación y deteriorización o alteraciones degenerativas de los cartílagos.

chondrocostal *a.* condrocostal, rel. a los cartílagos costales y las costillas.

chondrodynia *n.* condrodinia, dolor en un cartílago.

chondromalacia *n.* condromalacia, reblandecimiento anormal de los cartílagos.

choose *vi.* escoger, elegir.

chord *n.* cuerda; **vocal** ___ / ___ vocal.

chorea, Huntington's disease *n.* corea; enfermedad de Huntington, padecimiento nervioso que se manifiesta en movimientos abruptos coordinados aunque involuntarios de las extremidades y los músculos faciales; *pop.* baile se San Vito.

choriocarcinoma *n.* coriocarcinoma, tumor maligno visto gen. en el útero y en los testículos.

chorion *n.* corión, una de las dos membranas que rodean al feto.

chorionic *a.* coriónico-a, rel. al corión.

choroid *n.* coroides, membrana situada en el ojo al que nutre con la sangre.

choroiditis *n.* coroiditis, infl. de la coroides.

chromatic *a.* cromático-a, rel. al color.

chromatin *n.* cromatina, parte del núcleo de la célula más propensa a absorber color.

chromocyte *n.* cromocito, célula pigmentada.

chromogen *n.* cromógeno, sustancia que produce color.

chromophobe *n.* cromófobo, tipo de célula que ofrece resistencia al color.

chromophobia *n.* cromofobia, aversión anormal a ciertos colores.

chromosomal *a.* cromosómico-a, rel. al cromosoma; ___ **aberrations** / aberraciones ___ -s.

chromosome *n.* cromosoma, la parte dentro del núcleo de la célula que contiene los genes.

chronic *a.* crónico-a, de larga duración, de efecto prolongado.

chronological *a.* cronológico-a, rel. a la secuencia del tiempo.

chronotropism *n.* cronotropismo, modificación de funciones regulares tales como los latidos del corazón.

chubby *a.* regordete-a, macizo-a.

chyle *n.* quilo, sustancia lechosa que resulta de la absorción y emulsión de las grasas, presente en el intestino delgado.

chylemia *n.* quilemia, presencia de quilo en la sangre.

chylomicron *n.* quilomicrón, pequeña partícula de lípido vista en la sangre después de la ingestión de grasas.

chylorrhea *n.* quilorrea, derrame de quilo debido a una ruptura del conducto torácico.

chylous *a.* quiloso-a, que contiene quilo o de la naturaleza de éste.

chyluria *n.* quiluria. V. **galacturia.**

chyme *n.* quimo, sustancia o materia semilíquida que proviene de la digestión gástrica.

chymotrypsin *n.* quimotripsina, tripsina, enzima de la secreción pancreática.

chymotrypsinogen *n.* quimotripsinógeno, enzima pancreática precursora de la quimotripsina.

cicatrix *n.* (*pl.* **cicatrices**) *L.* cicatriz.

cicatrizant *n.* cicatrizante, agente que contribuye a la cicatrización.

cicatrization *n.* cicatrización.

cigar *n.* puro, *H.A.* tabaco.

cigarette *n.* cigarro, cigarrillo.

ciliary *n.* ciliar, rel. a las pestañas o al párpado.

cilium *n.* (*pl.* **cilial**) *L.* párpado.

cineradiography *n.* cinerradiografía, película radiográfica de un órgano en movimiento.

cinerea *n.* cinérea, la sustancia gris del sistema nervioso.

cinnamon *n.* canela.

circadian rhythm *n.* ritmo circadiano, ref. a variaciones rítmicas biológicas en un ciclo de 24 horas.

circinate *a.* circinado-a, semejante a un anillo o círculo.

circle *n.* círculo, circunferencia.

circuit *n.* circuito, vuelta, rotación.

circulation *n.* circulación; ___ **rate** / volumen circulatorio por minuto; **peripheral** ___ / ___ periférica; **poor** ___ / mala ___ .

circulatory *a.* circulatorio-a.

circumcise *v.* circuncidar.

circumcision *n.* circuncisión, excisión del prepucio.

circumduction *n.* circunducción, movimiento circular de una parte del cuerpo tal como el ojo o alguna extremidad.

circumference *n.* circunferencia; círculo.

cirrhosis *n.* cirrosis, enfermedad asociada con infl. intersticial, fallo en la función de hepatocitos y trastornos en la circulación de la sangre en el hígado; **alcoholic** ___ / ___ alcohólica; **biliary** ___ / ___ biliar.

cistern *n.* cisterna, receptáculo de agua, aljibe.

cite *v.* citar, referirse a.

citizen *n.* ciudadano-a.

citizenship *n.* ciudadanía.

citric, citrous *a.* cítrico-a; ___ **acid** / ácido ___ .

city *n.* ciudad.

claim *n.* reclamación; petición; ___ **review procedure** / proceso para revisión de peticiones (reclamaciones); *v.* reclamar, demandar.

clam *n.* almeja.

clammy *a.* frío y húmedo.

clamp *n.* pinza; presilla.

clamping *n.* pinzado.

clap *n. pop.* gonorrea, blenorragia; [*hand*] palmada.

clarification *n.* aclaración, clarificación.

clarify *v.* aclarar, clarificar.

clarity *n.* claridad.

clasp *n.* gancho.

class *n.* clase; tipo.

classification *n.* clasificación; distribución.

classify *v.* clasificar, distribuir.

claudication *n.* claudicación; **intermittent** ___ / ___ intermitente.

claustrophobia *n.* claustrofobia, miedo o fobia a espacios cerrados.

clavicle *n.* clavícula, hueso de la faja pectoral que conecta al esternón con la escápula.

clavicular *a.* clavicular, rel. a las clavículas.

claw *n.* garra; ___ **foot** / pie en ___; ___ **hand** / mano en ___ .

clean *a.* limpio-a, aseado-a; *v.* limpiar, asear.

clear *a.* claro-a.

clearance *n.* aclaramiento, eliminación renal de una sustancia en el plasma sanguíneo.

cleft *n.* fisura, abertura alargada.

cleft lip *n.* labio leporino. V. **harelip.**

cleft palate *n.* paladar hendido, defecto congénito del velo del paladar por falta de fusión en la línea media.

cleidocostal *a.* cleidocostal, rel. a la clavícula y las costillas.

clergyman *n.* clérigo.

climacteric *a.* climatérico-a.

climacterium *n. L.* climaterio, menopausia, cese de actividad reproductiva.

climate *n.* clima.

climax *n. L.* climax. 1. crisis de una enfermedad; 2. orgasmo sexual.

climb *v.* subir; trepar; subirse, treparse.

clinic *n.* clínica; **small ___ /** dispensario.

clinical *a.* clínico-a. 1. rel. a una clínica; 2. rel. a la observacíon directa de pacientes; **___ history /** historia **___ ,** expediente; **___ picture /** cuadro **___; ___ procedure /** procedimiento **___; ___ trials /** ensayos **___ -s.**

clip *n.* pinza; *v.* sujetar con pinzas.

clitoridectomy *n.* clitoridectomía, excisión del clítoris.

clitoris *n.* clítoris, pequeña protuberancia situada en la parte anterior de la vulva.

cloaca *n.* cloaca, abertura común del intestino y de las vías urinarias en la fase de desarrollo primario del embrión.

clock *n.* reloj; **around the ___ /** durante las veinticuatro horas, de día y de noche.

clone *n.* clon, reproducción o copia idéntica.

clonic *a.* clónico-a, rel. a un clono.

cloning *n.* clonación.

clonorchiasis *n.* clonorquiasis, infección parasitaria que afecta los conductos biliares distales.

clonus *n. Gr.* clono, serie de contracciones rápidas y rítmicas de un músculo.

close *v.* cerrar.

closed *a.* cerrado-a; **___ -circuit television /** televisión en circuito **___; ___ ecological system /** sistema ecológico **___ .**

closure *n.* acto de cerrar o sellar; encierro.

clot *n.* cóagulo, cuajo, grumo, *pop.* cuajarón.

clothes, clothing *n.* ropa.

clotting *n.* coagulación; **___ factor /** factor de **___; ___ time /** tiempo de **___ .**

cloudiness *n.* nebulosidad, enturbamiento.

cloudy *a.* turbio-a, nebuloso-a, oscuro-a.

clove *n.* clavo de especia.

clubbing *n.* dedo en palillo de tambor.

club foot *n.* pie torcido, *pop.* patizambo, *slang* chueco.

club hand *n.* mano zamba, *pop.* mano de gancho.

cluster *n.* racimo, grupo.

cluster headache, Horton's syndrome *n.* cefalalgia de Horton, dolor de cabeza producido por histaminas.

clysis *n.* clisis, administración de líquidos por cualquier vía excepto la oral.

coagglutination *n.* coaglutinación, aglutinación de grupos.

coagglutinine *n.* coaglutinina, aglutinante que afecta a dos o más organismos.

coagulant *n.* coagulante, agente que causa o acelera la coagulación. *Syn.* **coagulative**.

coagulate *v.* coagular, coagularse.

coagulation *n.* coagulación, coágulo; **disseminated intravascular ___ / ___** intravascular diseminada.

coagulopathy *n.* coagulopatía, enfermedad o condición que afecta el mecanismo de la coagulación de la sangre.

coalescense *n.* coalescencia, fusión de dos o más partes.

coal miners' disease *n.* enfermedad de los mineros. V. **anthracosis**.

coarctation *n.* coartación, estrechez.

coarse *a.* grueso-a; rudo-a, tosco-a, burdo-a, ordinario-a.

coat *n.* membrana, cubierta; [*clothing*] abrigo.

coated *a.* cubierto-a, pintado-a; **___ with adhesive tape / ___** con esparadrapo.

cobalt *n.* cobalto.

coca *n.* coca, planta de cuyas hojas se extrae la cocaína.

cocaine *n.* cocaína, narcótico alcaloide adictivo complejo obtenido de las hojas de coca; *slang* nieve.

coccidioidin *n.* coccidioidina, solución estéril suministrada por medio intercutáneo en la prueba de la coccidioidomicosis (fiebre del valle).

coccidioidomycosis, valley fever *n.* coccidioidomicosis, fiebre del valle, infección respiratoria endémica en el suroeste de los Estados Unidos, México y algunas partes de América del Sur.

coccus *n. L.* (*pl.* **cocci**) coco, bacteria de forma esférica.

coccygeal *a.* coccígeo, rel. al cóccix.

coccygodynia *n.* coccigodinia, dolor en la región coccígea.

coccyx *n.* cóccix; último hueso de la columna vertebral; *pop.* rabadilla.

cochlea *n.* cóclea, parte del oído interior en forma de caracol.

cochleare *n. L.* cucharada; **___ magnum / ___** de sopa; **___ medium / ___** de postre; **___ parvum /** cucharita de café.

cockroach *n.* cucaracha.

cod *n.* bacalao; **___ liver oil /** aceite de hígado de **___ .**

codeine *n.* codeína, narcótico analgésico.

coefficient *n.* coeficiente, indicación de cambios físicos o químicos producidos por variantes de ciertos factores.

coenzyme *n.* coenzima, sustancia que activa la acción de una enzima.

coffee *n.* café.

coffin *n.* ataúd, caja.

cognac *n.* coñac, aguardiente.

cognate *n.* cognado, palabra que proviene del mismo tronco o raíz; *a.* cognado-a, de la misma naturaleza o calidad.

cognition *n.* cognición, conocimiento, acción y efecto de conocer.

cognitive *a.* cognitivo-a. 1. rel. al conocimiento; 2. rel. al proceso mental de comprensión.

cognitive development *n.* desarrollo cognitivo, cambio en el desarrollo infantil de las funciones intelectuales.

cohabit *v.* cohabitar, vivir en unión sin matrimonio legal.

coherence *n.* 1. coherencia, cohesión; 2. coherencia, referencia a cualquier grupo designado, seguido o copiado por un período de tiempo, tal como en un estudio epidemiológico.

coherent *a.* coherente.

cohesion *n.* cohesión, unión, fuerza que une a las moléculas.

coil *n.* espiral, serpentina, dispositivo intrauterino.

coincide *v.* coincidir.

coincidence *n.* coincidencia; **by** ___ / por casualidad.

coitus *n. L.* coito, acto sexual.

cold *n.* catarro; resfriado; [*weather*] frío; *a* [*temperature*] frío-a; ___ **-blooded** / de sangre fría o de temperatura muy baja; ___ **cream** / crema, pomada facial; ___ **pack** / compresa fría; ___ **sore** / úlcera de herpes simple; ___ **sweat** / sudor frío; *v.* **to be** ___ / tener frío; **it is** ___ / hace frío.

coldness *n.* frialdad.

colectomy *n.* colectomía, extirpación de una parte o de todo el colon.

colic *n.* cólico, dolor espasmódico abdominal agudo.

colicky *a.* rel. al cólico.

colitis *n.* colitis, infl. del colon; **chronic** ___ / ___ crónica; **pseudomembranous** ___ / ___ mucomembranosa; **spasmodic** ___ / ___ espasmódica; **ulcerative** ___ / ___ ulcerativa.

collaborate *v.* colaborar, cooperar.

collagen *n.* colágeno, principal proteína de sostén del tejido conectivo de la piel, huesos, tendones y cartílagos.

collapse *n.* colapso; postración; desplome; **circulatory** ___ / ___ circulatorio; ___ **therapy** / terapia de ___; *v.* sufrir un ___.

collapsed *a.* desplomado-a; derrumbado-a; estado de vacuidad.

collar *n.* cuello.

collarbone *n.* clavícula.

collateral *n.* colateral. 1. indirecto, subsidiario o accesorio a la cuestión principal; 2. una rama subsidiaria del axon de un nervio o vaso sanguíneo; *a.* accesorio-a; *adv.* al lado.

collateral vessel *n.* vaso colateral. 1. rama de una arteria que sigue el curso paralela al tronco protector; 2. un vaso que sigue su curso paralelo a otro vaso, nervio u otra estructura mayor. *Syn.* **vas collaterale.**

collaterization *n.* colaterización.

colleague *n.* colega; compañero-a.

collect *v.* coleccionar, recoger, juntar; acumular.

collodion *n.* colodión, sustancia usada para proteger heridas en la piel.

colloid *n.* coloide, sustancia gelatinosa producida por ciertas formas de degeneración de los tejidos.

collyrium *n.* colirio, medicamento aplicado a los ojos.

coloboma *n.* coloboma, defecto congénito, patológico, o artificial especialmente manifestado en el ojo debido a un cierre incompleto de la fisura óptica; ___ **iridis** / ___ del iris; ___ **lentis** / ___ del lente; ___ **of choroid** / ___ de la coroides; ___ **of optic nerve** / ___ del nervio óptico; ___ **of vitreous** / ___ del vítreo; **macular** ___ / ___ macular.

colon *n.* colon, porción del intestino grueso entre el ciego y el recto; **ascending** ___ / ___ ascendente; **descending** ___ / ___ descendente.

colonic *a.* colónico, referente al colon; ___ **neoplasms** / neoplasmas del colon.

colonoscopy *n.* colonoscopía, examen de la superficie interna del colon a través del colonoscopio.

colony *n.* colonia, cultivo de bacterias derivadas del mismo organismo.

coloproctitis *n.* coloproctitis, infl. del colon y del recto.

color *n.* color; ___ **index** / guía colorimétrica; *v.* colorar; teñir o dar color; ___ **confusion** / confusión de colores; ___ **perception** / percepción del ___; **complementary colors** / colores complementarios; **extrinsic colors** / colores extrínsecos; **intrinsic colors** / colores intrínsecos; **primary colors** / colores primarios;

pure ___ / ___ puro; **reflected** ___ / ___
reflejado; **saturated** ___ / ___ saturado;
simple ___ / ___ simple; **structural** ___ / ___
estructural; **tone** ___ / tono de ___ . See chart
on page 77.

coloration *n.* coloración.

colorectal cancer *n.* cáncer colorectal,
carcinoma colónico rectal.

colostomy *n.* colostomía, creación de un ano
artificial.

colostrum *n.* colostro, secreción de la glándula
mamaria anterior a la leche.

colpitis *n.* colpitis, vaginitis, infl. de la vagina.

colpocele *n.* colpocele, hernia vaginal.

colporrhagia *n.* colporragia, hemorragia
vaginal.

colporrhaphy *n.* colporrafia, sutura de la
vagina.

colposcope *n.* colposcopio, instrumento que se
usa para examinar visualmente la vagina y el
cuello uterino.

colposcopy *n.* colposcopía, examen de la
vagina y del cuello uterino a través de un
colposcopio.

colpotomy *n.* colpotomía, incisión de la vagina.

column *n.* columna.

coma *n.* coma, en estado de coma; sueño
profundo o estado inconsciente.

comatose *a.* comatoso-a; **in a** ___ **state** / en
estado de coma.

comb *n.* peine; *v.* peinar, peinarse.

combat *n.* combate, lucha; *v.* combatir.

combatting *v. p.p.* of **to combat**, combatiendo.

combine *v.* combinar, unir.

come *vi* venir; ___ **in!** / pase, pasa; entre, entra;
to ___ **to terms** / ponerse de acuerdo.

comfort *n.* comodidad, alivio, bienestar; *v.*
confortar, alentar.

comfortable *a.* cómodo-a; a gusto.

comfortless *a.* incómodo-a.

command *n.* orden, mandato.

commensal *n.* comensal, organismo que vive a
expensas de otro sin beneficiarlo ni perjudicarlo.

comment *n.* comentario; *v.* comentar; hacer un
comentario.

comminute *v.* pulverizar, triturar.

comminuted *a.* conminuto-a, roto-a en
fragmentos tal como en una fractura.

commiserate *v.* tener compasión, tener lástima;
apiadarse, compadecerse; tenerse lástima.

commission *n.* comisión, encargo.

commissure *n.* comisura, punto de unión de
estructuras tal como la unión de los labios.

commisurotomy *n.* comisurotomía, incisión de
las bandas fibrosas de una comisura tal como la
de los labios o la de los bordes de válvulas
cardíacas.

commit *v.* cometer; [*intern*] internar, encerrar.

commitment *n.* obligación, compromiso.

commode *n.* inodoro, servicio.

common *a.* común, corriente; ___ **name** /
nombre ___; ___ **place** / lugar ___; ___ **sense** /
sentido ___ .

commotion *n.* conmoción; agitación.

commotio retinae *n. L.* conmoción retinal,
condición traumática que produce ceguera
momentánea.

communicable *a.* contagioso-a;
comunicable; ___ **disease control** / control de
enfermedades ___ .

communicate *v.* comunicar; [*to get in touch*]
comunicarse.

communication *n.* comunicación; acceso;
entrada.

community *n.* comunidad, sociedad, barrio; ___
health center / centro de servicio de la
salud; ___ **medicine** / medicina comunitaria.

companion *n.* compañero-a; acompañante; ___
disease / enfermedad concomitante.

company *n.* compañía, establecimiento.

comparative *a.* comparativo-a.

compare *v.* comparar.

compassion *n.* compasión, lástima.

compatible *a.* compatible.

compensate *v.* compensar, recompensar.

compensation *n.* compensación. 1. cualidad de
compensar o equilibrar un defecto; 2. mecanismo
de defensa; 3. remuneración.

competent *a.* competente, capaz.

complain *v.* quejarse, lamentarse.

complainer *a.* persona que se queja en exceso.

complaint *n.* queja, síntoma; trastorno, molestia;
chief ___ / ___ principal.

complement *n.* complemento, sustancia
proteínica presente en el plasma que destruye las
bacterias y las células con que se pone en
contacto.

complex *n.* complejo, serie de procesos mentales
interrelacionados que afectan la conducta y la
personalidad; **castration** ___ / ___ de castración;
guilt ___ / ___ de culpa; **inferiority** ___ / ___
de inferioridad; **Electra's** ___ / ___ de Electra;
Oedipus ___ / ___ de Edipo; *a.* complejo-a;
complicado-a.

complexion *n.* cutis, complexión, tez.

compliance *n.* adaptabilidad, conformidad,
grado de elasticidad de un órgano para

distenderse o de una estructura para perder la forma; ___ **with standards** / ___ a las normas.

complicate *v.* complicar.

complication *n.* complicación.

component *n.* componente.

composition *n.* composición, mezcla, compuesto.

composure *n.* compostura, serenidad.

compote *n.* compota.

compound *n.* compuesto.

comprehension *n.* comprensión.

compress *n.* compresa, apósito; **cold** ___ / ___ fría; **hot** ___ / fomento; *v.* comprimir, apretar.

compromise *v.* comprometerse, obligarse.

compulsion *n.* compulsión.

compulsive *a.* compulsorio-a, compulsivo-a; obsesivo-a.

computer diagnosis *n.* diagnóstico computado.

concave *a.* cóncavo-a.

conceive *v.* concebir.

concentrate *v.* concentrar.

concentration *n.* concentración.

concept *n.* concepto, opinión, noción, idea.

conception *n.* concepción, acto de concebir.

concern *n.* preocupación, cuidado.

concise *a.* conciso-a; definido-a.

conclusion *n.* conclusión.

concoction *n.* cocimiento, mezcla, concocción.

concrete *a.* concreto-a; definido-a.

concretio cordis *n., L.* concretio cordis, obliteración parcial o total de la cavidad del pericardio debido a una pericarditis constrictiva.

concretion *n.* concreción, bezoar o masa inorgánica que se acumula en partes del cuerpo.

concubitus *n., L.* concúbito.

concussion *n.* concusión, conmoción, traumatismo esp. del cerebro causado por una lesión en la cabeza que puede presentar síntomas de náusea y mareos; **cerebral** ___ / ___ cerebral.

condemn *v.* condenar.

condense *v.* condensar, hacer más denso o compacto.

condition *n.* condición, cualidad; **guarded** ___ / en estado de gravedad; **preexisting** ___ / ___ preexistente; **undiagnosed** ___ / ___ sin diagnosticar.

conditioning *n.* acondicionamiento, condicionamiento.

condole *v.* condolerse; dar el pésame.

condolence *n.* condolencia, pésame.

condom *n.* condón, contraceptivo masculino.

conduct *v.* dirigir, conducir.

conduit *n.* conducto; **airway** ___ / ___ para aire; **tear** ___ / ___ lagrimal.

condyle *n.* cóndilo, porción redondeada de un hueso, usu. en la articulación.

condyloma *n.* condiloma, tipo de verruga vista alrededor de los genitales y el perineo.

cone *n.* cono, uno de los órganos sensoriales que, con los bastoncillos de la retina, facilitan la visión del color; ___ **cells** / ___ -s de la retina.

confabulation *n.* confabulación, condición en la que el individuo imagina situaciones que olvida fácilmente.

confer *v.* consultar; conferenciar.

confess *v.* admitir, reconocer; confesar.

confidential *a.* confidencial; en secreto.

confidentiality *n.* confidencialidad.

confine *v.* recluir, internar, confinar; **to** ___ **in bed** / ___ en la cama.

confined *a.* recluido-a, confinado-a.

confinement *n.* confinación, reclusión, internación.

confirm *v.* confirmar.

conflict *n.* conflicto, problema.

confluence *n.* confluencia, punto de reunión de varios canales.

confront *v.* confrontar.

confuse *v.* confundir, trastornar, aturdir.

confused *a.* confuso-a, confundido-a, distraído-a; *v.* **to be** ___ / estar ___ , confundirse.

confusion *n.* confusión; atolondramiento; aturdimiento.

congenital *a.* congénito-a; engendrado-a, rel. a una característica que se hereda y existe desde el nacimiento.

congenital cataract *n.* catarata congénita, no común, usualmente bilateral, producida a causa de una infección intrauterina, a toxicidad, a una lesión, o a trastornos metabólicos o cromosomáticos.

congested *a.* congestionado-a; en estado de congestión.

congestion *n.* congestión, aglomeración; acumulación excesiva de sangre en un órgano; **active** ___ / ___ activa; **functional** ___ / ___ funcional; **passive** ___ / ___ pasiva; **venous** ___ / ___ venosa.

congestive *a.* congestivo-a, rel. a la congestión; ___ **heart failure** / insuficiencia cardíaca ___ .

conical, conic *a.* cónico-a, semejante a un cono.

conization *n.* conización, extirpación de tejido que tiene forma cónica, semejante al de la mucosa del cuello uterino.

conjunctiva *n.* conjuntiva, membrana mucosa protectora del ojo; **bulbar** ___ / ___ bulbar; **palpebral** ___ / ___ palpebral.

conjunctival *a.* conjuntivo-a, rel. a la conjuntiva; ___ **diseases** / enfermedades de la conjuntiva.

conjunctivitis *n.* conjuntivitis, infl. de la conjuntiva; **allergic** ___ / ___ alérgica; **catarrhal** ___ / ___ catarral; **chronic** ___ / ___ crónica; ___ **acute, contagious** / ___ aguda contagiosa; **epidemic** ___ / ___ epidémica; **follicular** ___ / ___ folicular; **hemorrhagic** ___ / ___ hemorrágica; **infantile purulent** ___ / ___ infantil purulenta; **vernal** ___ / ___ vernal; **viral** ___ / ___ viral.

consanguineous *a.* consanguíneo-a, de la misma sangre u origen.

conscious *a.* consciente, en posesión de las facultades mentales.

consciousness *n.* consciencia, conocimiento, sentido; estado consciente; **clouding of** ___ / torpor, confusión, entorpecimiento mental; *v.* **to lose** ___ / perder el conocimiento; perder el sentido.

consensus *n.* consenso.

consent *n.* consentimiento, autorización; *v.* permitir, consentir; **informed** ___ / ___ autorizado.

consequences *n., pl.* consecuencias, secuelas.

conservation *n.* conservación, preservación.

conservative *a.* conservador-a; preservativo-a.

conserve *v.* conservar, mantener.

consider *v.* considerar, ponderar.

considerate *a.* considerado-a; moderado-a.

consideration *n.* consideración.

consist *v.* consistir; estar formado de; constar de.

consistency *n.* consistencia; solidez.

consistent *a.* consistente, firme, estable.

console *v.* consolar, confortar; dar aliento.

consomme *n.* consomé, caldo.

conspicuous *a.* sobresaliente, señalado-a, conspicuo-a.

constant *a.* constante, persistente.

constipate *v.* estreñir, constipar.

constipated *a.* estreñido-a; constipado-a; *v.* **to be** ___ / estar ___ .

constipation *n.* estreñimiento, trastorno intestinal caracterizado por la imposibilidad de evacuar con facilidad.

constituent *n.* constituyente.

constitute *v.* constituir, componer, formar.

constitution *n.* constitución, fortaleza.

constrain *v.* restringir; impedir.

constrict *v.* apretar, estrangular.

constriction *n.* constricción.

consult *v.* consultar.

consultant *n.* consultor-a, consejero-a.

consultation *n.* consulta.

consulting room *n.* consultorio médico.

consume *v.* consumir.

consummation *n.* consumación.

consumption *n.* consunción; desgaste progresivo; tisis, tuberculosis.

contact *n.* contacto; **close** ___ / ___ íntimo; ___ **lenses** / lentes de ___; **initial** ___ / ___ inicial.

contagion *n.* contagio, transmisión de una enfermedad por contacto.

contagious *a.* contagioso-a; infeccioso-a; que se comunica por contagio.

contain *v.* contener; reprimir.

container *n.* recipiente, envase.

contaminate *v.* contaminar, infectar.

contamination *n.* contaminación; infección.

content *n.* contenido.

contented *a.* satisfecho-a.

contiguous *a.* contiguo-a, adyacente.

continence *n.* continencia, control o automoderación en relación con actividades sexuales o físicas.

continuation *n.* continuación.

continue *v.* continuar.

continuity *n.* continuidad.

continuous *a.* continuo-a, seguido-a.

contour *n.* contorno.

contraception *n.* contracepción, anticoncepción.

contraceptive *n.* contraceptivo, anticonceptivo, agente o método para impedir la concepción; ___ **agents** / agentes anticonceptivos; ___ **implant** / implante de ___; ___ **methods** / métodos ___ -s, métodos anticonceptivos; **oral** ___ / ___ oral.

contract *v.* [*a disease*] contraer.

contracted *n.* contraído-a; retenido-a.

contractile *a.* contráctil, que tiene la capacidad de contraerse.

contractility *n.* contractilidad, capacidad de contraerse.

contraction *n.* contracción; **after -** ___ / ___ ulterior; **deep** ___ / ___ de fondo; **hunger** ___ / ___ de hambre; **muscular** ___ / ___ muscular; **spasmodic** ___ / ___ espasmódica.

contracture *n.* contractura, contracción prolongada involuntaria.

contradict *v.* contradecir, negar.

contradiction *n.* contradicción, oposición.

contraindicated *a.* contraindicado-a.

contraindication *n.* contraindicación.

contralateral *a.* contralateral, rel. al lado opuesto.

contrary *a.* contrario-a, adverso-a, opuesto-a.

contrast *n.* contraste; ___ **medium** / medio de ___; *v.* contrastar, resaltar.

contribute *v.* contribuir.

control *n.* control, regulación; *v.* controlar, regular, dominar; **to ___ oneself** / controlarse, dominarse.

contuse *v.* magullar.

contusion *n.* contusión, magulladura.

convalesce *v.* convalecer, reponerse.

convalescence *n.* convalecencia, proceso de restablecimiento, estado de recuperación.

convalescent *a.* convaleciente.

convalescent carrier *n.* portador convaleciente, aún capaz de transmitir un agente infeccioso.

convergence *n.* convergencia, inclinación de dos o más elementos hacia un punto común.

conversion *n.* conversión. 1. cambio, transformación; 2. transformación de una emoción en una manifestación física; ___ **disorder** / enajenamiento.

convex *a.* convexo-a.

convict *n.* preso-a, detenido-a, presidiario-a.

convulsion *n.* convulsión, contracción involuntaria de un músculo; **febrile** ___ / ___ febril; **Jacksonian** ___ / ___ Jacksoniana; **tonic-clonic** ___ / ___ tonicoclónica.

convulsive, convulsant *a.* convulsivo-a, rel. a la convulsión; ___ **activity** / actividad ___ .

cook *n.* cocinero-a; *v.* cocinar.

cooked *a.* cocinado-a; guisado-a; **well ___** / bien ___ .

cool *a.* fresco-a; refrescado-a; ___ **headed** / sereno-a, calmado-a; [*weather*] **it is ___** / hace fresco; [*body temperature*] **he, she, it is ___** / está fresco-a.

cool-down *n.* [*physical fitness*] enfriamiento.

cooler *n.* refrigerante, refresco.

coolness *n.* frialdad; serenidad.

cooperate *v.* cooperar, ayudar.

coordinate *v.* coordinar.

coordination *n.* coordinación; **lack of ___** / falta de ___ .

copayment *n.* pago compartido.

copious *a.* abundante, copioso-a.

coprolith *n.* coprolito, pequeña masa fecal de consistencia dura.

coprophagy *n.* coprofagia, trastorno mental manifestado en la ingestión de heces fecales.

copulation *n.* copulación, relaciones sexuales.

copy *n.* copia; imitación; *v.* copiar; imitar.

cor *n.* L. cor, corazón.

coracoclavicular *a.* coracoclavicular, referente a la escápula y la clavícula.

coracoid *n.* coracoides, apófisis del omóplato.

Coramine *n.* Coramina, nombre comercial de la niquetamida.

cord *n.* cordón, cuerda, cordel; **umbilical ___** / ___ umbilical.

cordectomy *n.* cordectomía, excisión de una cuerda vocal o parte de ésta.

core *n.* centro, corazón, núcleo.

corium *n.* L. corion, dermis o piel.

corn *n.* callo, callosidad; [*grain*] maíz.

cornea *n.* córnea, parte anterior transparente del globo del ojo.

corneal grafting *n.* injerto de la córnea.

corneous *a.* córneo, rel. a la córnea; calloso-a.

coronary *a.* coronario-a, que circunda tal como una corona; ___ **artery** / arteria ___ ; ___ **bypass** / desviación ___ ; ___ **care unit** / unidad de cuidado ___ ; ___ **thrombosis** / trombosis ___ ; ___ **vasospasm** / vasoepasmo ___ .

coronary angiography *n.* angiografía coronaria, imágenes tomadas por medio de un medio de contraste de la circulación del miocardio, hecha gen. por caterización selectiva de cada una de las arterias coronarias.

coronary artery aneurysm *n.* aneurisma de la arteria coronaria, gen. debido a aterosclerosis, a procesos inflamatorios o a una fístula coronaria.

coronary artery bypass *n.* conducto o derivación aortocoronaria, intervención usualmente con uso de una vena como injerto, o de una arteria mamaria interna interpuesta entre la aorta y una rama de la arteria coronaria, y puesta como derivación sanguínea mas allá de la obstrucción formada. *Syn.* **aortocoronary bypass.**

coronary atherectomy *n.* aterectomía coronaria, excisión de obstrucciones en la arteria coronaria con un instrumento cortante que se inserta usando un catéter coronario.

coronary care unit *n.* unidad de atención coronaria; sala de hospital reservada para el cuidado de pacientes que requieren atención relacionada con infarto coronario.

coronary collaterization *n.* colaterización coronaria, desarrollo espontáneo de nuevos vasos sanguíneos alrededor de las regiones cardíacas bajo un restringido fluido sanguíneo.

coronary failure *n.* insuficiencia coronaria aguda.

coronary insufficiency *n.* insuficiencia coronaria, deficiencia en la circulación coronaria con riesgo de sufrir un dolor provocado por angina, trombosis o ateroma, que puede dar como resultado un infarto del miocardio. *Syn.* **coronarism.**

coronary occlusion *n.* oclusión coronaria, bloqueo de un vaso coronario.

coronary-prone behavior *n.* conducta hostil que puede ocasionar el padecimiento de una enfermedad cardíaca.

coronary thrombosis *n.* trombosis coronaria debido a formación de un trombo, gen. como resultado de cambios ateromatosos en la pared de la arteria, posible causa de infarto de miocardio.

coroner *n.* médico-a forense.

corporeal *a.* corporal, físico-a, rel. al cuerpo.

corpse *n.* cadáver, muerto-a.

corpus *n.* (*pl.* **corpora**) *L.* corpus, el cuerpo humano.

corpus callosum *n. L.* corpus callosum, comisura mayor del cerebro.

corpuscle *n.* corpúsculo, cuerpo diminuto.

corpuscular *a.* corpuscular, diminuto-a.

corpus luteum *n. L.* corpus luteum, cuerpo lúteo, cuerpo amarillo, masa glandular amarillenta que se forma en el ovario por la ruptura de un folículo y produce progesterona.

correct *a.* correcto-a, exacto-a; *v.* corregir, enmendar.

correction *n.* corrección.

corrective *a.* correctivo-a.

corrective lenses *n.* lentes correctoras.

correspondence *n.* correspondencia; reciprocidad.

corroded *a.* corroído-a, desgastado-a.

corrosion *n.* corrosión, desgaste.

corset *n.* corsé.

cortex *n.* corteza, córtex, la capa más exterior de un órgano; **adrenal ___ / ___ suprarrenal; cerebral ___ / ___** cerebral.

cortical *a.* cortical, rel. a la corteza.

corticoid, corticosteroid *n.* corticoide, corticoesteroide, esteroide producido por la corteza suprarrenal.

corticosteroid-binding globulin *n.* globulina de enlace corticoesteroide.

corticotropin *n.* corticotropina, sustancia hormonal de actividad adrenocorticotrópica.

cortisol *n.* cortisol, hormona secretada por la corteza suprarrenal.

cortisone *n.* cortisona, esteroide glucogénico derivado del cortisol o sintéticamente.

Corti's organ *n.* órgano de Corti, órgano terminal de la audición a través del cual se perciben directamente los sonidos.

cosmetic *n.* cosmético; *a.* cósmetico-a.

cosmetic surgery *n.* cirugía plástica con fines estéticos.

cost *n.* coste, costo, precio; *v.* costar.

costal *a.* costal, rel. a las costillas.

costalgia *n.* costalgia, neuralgia, dolor en las costillas.

costly *a.* costoso-a, caro-a; *adv.* costosamente.

costochondritis *n.* costocondritis, infl. de uno o más cartílagos costales.

costoclavicular *a.* costoclavicular, rel. a las costillas y la clavícula.

costovertebral *a.* costovertebral, rel. a las costillas y vértebras torácicas.

cotton *n.* algodón.

cough *n.* tos; **___ lozenges** / pastillas para la; **___ suppressant** / calmante para la **___**; **___ syrup** / jarabe para la **___**; **hacking ___ / ___** seca recurrente; *v.* toser; **coughing spell** / ataque de **___**; **to ___ up phlegm** / expectorar la flema.

count *v.* contar.

counter *n.* contador.

counteract *v.* contrarrestar, oponerse a; contraatacar.

counterattack *n.* contraataque.

countercoup *n.* contragolpe.

counterpoison *n.* antídoto, contraveneno.

counterreaction *n.* reacción opuesta; reacción en contra de.

countershock *n.* contrachoque, corriente eléctrica aplicada al corazón para normalizar el ritmo cardíaco.

courage *n.* coraje, valor, firmeza.

courageous *a.* valiente, valeroso-a.

course *n.* curso, dirección.

cousin *n.* primo-a.

cover *n.* cobertor, manta, cobija; *v.* cubrir, proteger; tapar; abrigar.

covered *a.* cubierto-a; protegido-a.

cow *n.* vaca.

coward *a.* cobarde.

cowperitis *n.* cowperitis, infl. de las glándulas de Cowper (bulbouretrales).

Cowper's glands *n.* glándulas de Cowper (bulbouretrales), pequeñas glándulas adyacentes al bulbo de la uretra masculina en la que vacían una secreción mucosa.

cowpox *n.* vacuna, cowpox.

coxa *L.* (*pl.* **coxae**) coxa, cadera.

coxa magna *n.* coxa magna, ensanchamiento anormal de la cabeza y del cuello del fémur.

coxa valga *n.* coxa valga, deformidad de la cadera por desplazamiento lateral angular del fémur.

coxa vara *n.* coxa vara, deformidad de la cadera por desplazamiento angular interno del fémur

coxalgia *n.* coxalgia, dolor en la cadera.

coxitis *n.* coxitis, infl. de la articulación coxofemoral, (articulación de la cadera).

crab *n.* cangrejo, cámbaro.

crack *n.* rajadura, quebradura; *v.* rajar, quebrar.

cracker *n.* galleta.

cradle *n.* cuna; ____ **cap** / costra láctea.

cramp *n.* calambre, entumecimiento; contracción dolorosa de un músculo.

cranial *a.* craneal, craneano-a, del cráneo o rel. al mismo.

cranial nerves *n.* nervios craneales, cada uno de los doce pares de nervios que salen de la región inferior del cerebro. See chart on this page.

craniopharingioma *n.* craneofaringioma, tipo de tumor cerebral maligno visto esp. en los niños.

cranioplasty *n.* craneoplastia, operación para reparar un defecto del cráneo, tal como un injerto óseo.

craniotomy *n.* craneotomía. trepanación del cráneo.

Cranial nerves	Nervios craneales
olfactory	olfatorio
optic	óptico
oculomotor	motor ocular común
trochlear	patético
trigeminal	trigémino
abducens	motor ocular externo, abducente
facial	facial
auditory	auditivo
glossopharyngeal	glosofaríngeo
vagus	neumogástrico
spinal accesory	espinal
hypoglossal	hipoglosal

cranium *n.* cráneo, parte ósea de la cabeza que cubre el cerebro.

cranky *a.* majadero-a; inquieto-a.

crash *n.* choque violento; accidente de tráfico.

crater *n.* cráter. V. **niche.**

crave *v.* apetecer; ansiar; desear algo excesivamente.

craving *n.* deseo exagerado.

crawl *v.* arrastrarse; andar a gatas, gatear.

craze *n.* manía, locura.

crazy *a.* loco-a, demente.

cream *n.* crema, nata.

create *v.* crear.

creatine *n.* creatina, componente del tejido muscular, esencial en la fase anaeróbica de la contracción muscular.

creatinine *n.* creatinina, sustancia presente en la orina que representa el producto final del metabolismo de la creatina; ____ **clearance** / depuración de ____ , volumen de plasma libre de ____ .

creation *n.* creación, obra; universo.

credit *n.* crédito; *v.* acreditar, dar crédito.

cremasteric *a.* cremastérico, referente al músculo cremastérico del escroto.

cremate *v.* incinerar.

cremation *n.* incineración.

creosote *n.* creosota, líquido aceitoso gen. usado como desinfectante y como expectorante catarral.

crepitation *n.* crepitación, chasquido, crujido; **pleural** ____ / ____ pleural.

crest *n.* cresta, prominencia; copete. 1. reborde o prominencia de un hueso; 2. la elevación máxima de una línea en un gráfico.

crestfallen *a.* decaído-a, alicaído-a; acobardado-a.

cretin *n.* cretino-a, persona con manifestaciones de cretinismo.

cretinism *n.* cretinismo, hipotiroidismo congénito debido a una deficiencia acentuada de la hormona tiroidea.

cretinoid *a.* cretinoide, con características similares a un cretino.

crib *n.* cuna, camita.

crib death *n.* muerte de cuna, síndrome de muerte infantil súbita.

cribriform *a.* cribriforme, perforado-a.

cricoid *a.* cricoide, de forma anular.

crime *n.* crimen, delito.

criminal *n.* criminal.

cripple *a.* lisiado-a, paralítico-a, inválido-a, tullido-a; *v.* lisiar, baldar, paralizar; tullir.

crisis *n.* crisis. 1. El punto culminante del estado severo del paciente en el curso de una enfermedad que puede resultar en el cambio a una condición favorable o drástica; 2. ataque convulsivo; **adolescent** ___ / ___ de maduración; **adrenal** ___ / ___ adrenal; **anaphylactoid** ___ / ___ anafiláctica; **febrile** ___ / ___ febril; **gastric** ___ / ___ gástrica; **hypertensive** ___ / ___ hipertensiva; **identity** ___ / ___ de identidad; **midlife** ___ / ___ de la edad madura; **myasthenic** ___ / ___ miasténica; **tabetic** ___ / ___ tabética; **thyrotoxic** ___ / ___ tiroidea tóxica.

crisscross *a.* cruzado-a, entrelazado-a; *adv.* en cruz.

crista *n.* cresta, proyección.

critical *a.* crítico-a; ___ **condition** / estado ___ , gravedad extrema.

cross-cultural *a.* intercultural.

cross-dressed *n.* travestismo.

cross-eyed *n.* bizco-a.

cross-legged *a.* patizambo-a; cruzado-a de piernas.

cross matching *n.* pruebas sanguíneas cruzadas que comprueban la compatibilidad de la sangre antes de una tranfusión.

cross-section *n.* sección transversal.

cross studies *n., pl.* estudios cruzados.

crossing-over, crossover *n.* acción de cruzar a través.

crossed eyes, strabismus *n.* estrabismo, *pop.* bizquera, debilidad de los músculos que controlan la posición del ojo impidiendo la coordinación visual.

crossway *adv.* transversalmente.

crotch *n.* bifurcación, horquilla.

croup *n.* crup, *pop.* garrotillo, síndrome respiratorio visto en los niños, causado gen. por una infección o una reacción alérgica; **spasmodic** ___ / ___ espasmódico.

crown *n.* corona; **artificial** ___ / ___ artificial; **bell shaped** ___ / ___ en forma de campana.

crowning *n.* coronamiento, coronación. 1. etapa del parto cuando la cabeza se localiza en la salida pélvica; 2. preparación de un diente natural para recubrirlo usando el material dental elegido.

crucial *a.* crucial, definitivo-a.

crude *a.* rudo-a, crudo-a.

cruel *a.* cruel, inhumano-a.

crus *n. L.* crus. 1. pierna o parte semejante a una pierna; 2. parte de la pierna entre la rodilla y el tobillo.

crush *v.* triturar, moler, aplastar.

crust *n.* costra.

crutches *n., pl.* muletas.

cry *v.* llorar.

cryoanesthesia *n.* crioanestesia. 1. anestesia producida por aplicación de frío localizado; 2. pérdida de la sensibilidad al frío.

cryogenic *n.* criogénico, que produce temperaturas bajas.

cryoglobulin *n.* crioglobulina, globulina que se precipita del suero por acción del frío.

cryoprecipitate *n.* crioprecipitado, precipitado producido por enfriamiento.

cryosurgery *n.* criocirugía, destrucción de tejidos por aplicación de temperatura fría local o general.

cryotherapy *n.* crioterapia, tratamiento terapéutico por aplicación de frío local o general.

crypt *n.* cripta, pequeño receso tubular.

cryptic *a.* críptico-a, escondido-a.

cryptococcosis *n.* criptococosis, infección que afecta distintos órganos del cuerpo, esp. el cerebro y sus meninges.

cryptogenic *a.* criptogénico, de causa desconocida.

cryptorchism *n.* criptorquismo, falta de descenso testicular al escroto.

crystal *n.* cristal, vidrio.

crystalline *a.* cristalino-a, transparente.

crystalline lens *n.* cristalino, lente del ojo.

cubiform *a.* cúbico-a, rel. a la forma cúbica.

cubital *a.* cubital, codal.

cubitus, ulna *n., L.* cubitus, cúbito, hueso interno del antebrazo.

cucumber *n.* pepino, pepinillo.

cuff *n.* manguito, tejido fibroso que rodea una articulación; **rotator** ___ / ___ rotador, músculo tendinoso; **rotator** ___ **tear** / ruptura del ___ rotador.

cul-de-sac *n., Fr.* 1. cul-de-sac, fondo de saco, bolsa sin boquete de salida; 2. saco rectouterino.

culdoscope *n.* culdoscopio, instrumento endoscópico que se inserta en la vagina para examinar visualmente la pelvis y la cavidad abdominal.

culdoscopy *n.* culdoscopía, examen de la pelvis y la cavidad abdominal por medio del culdoscopio.

cultivate *v.* cultivar; estudiar.

culture *n.* cultivo, crecimiento artificial de microorganismos o células de tejido vivo en el

C

laboratorio; **blood** ___ / ___ de sangre; ___; ___ **medium** / medio de ___; **tissue** ___ / ___ de tejido.

cunnilingus *a.* cunnilinguo-a, rel. a la práctica de estimulación oral del pene o del clítoris.

cup *n.* copa; ventosa; **optic** ___ / ___ de ojo, ___ ocular; **measuring** ___ / taza de medir.

cupful *n.* una taza llena.

curable *a.* curable, sanable.

curare *n.* curare, veneno extraído de varios tipos de plantas y usado como relajante muscular y anestésico.

curative *n.* curativo, remedio, agente que tiene propiedades curativas.

curd *n.* cuajo, cuajarón, coágulo sanguíneo grande; [*milk*] leche cuajada.

curdle *v.* cuajarse, coagularse, engrumecerse.

cure *n.* curación, remedio; *v.* curar, sanar, remediar.

cureless *a.* incurable.

curettage *n.* curetaje, raspado de una superficie o cavidad con uso de la cureta.

curette *n.* cureta, instrumento quirúrgico en forma de cuchara o pala usado para raspar los tejidos de una superficie o cavidad.

curious *a.* curioso-a, extraño-a.

current *n.* corriente, trasmisión de fluido o electricidad que pasa por un conductor; *a.* corriente, actual; **-ly** *adv.* actualmente.

curvature *n.* curvatura.

curve *n.* curva; *v.* torcer, encorvar.

Cushing's syndrome *n.* síndrome de Cushing, síndrome adrenogenital asociado con una producción excesiva de cortisol, caracterizado por obesidad y debilitamiento muscular.

cushion *n.* cojinete, cojín.

cusp *n.* cúspide, punta.

cuspid *n.* [*tooth*] colmillo.

cuspidal *a.* cuspídeo, puntiagudo.

custard *n.* flan, natilla.

custodial care *n.* cuidado bajo custodia.

custom *n.* costumbre, hábito.

cut *n.* cortada, cortadura; *v.* cortar; **to ___ down** / rebajar, reducir; **to ___ off** / extirpar, amputar; [*oneself*] cortarse.

cutaneous *a.* cutáneo-a; ___ **absorption** / absorción ___; ___ **glands** / glándulas ___ -s o sebáceas.

cuticle *n.* cutícula, capa exterior de la piel.

cutis *n.* cutis; piel de la cara.

cyanide *n.* cianuro, compuesto extremadamente venenoso.

cyanocobalamin *n.* cianocobalamina, vitamina B$_{12}$ usada en el tratamiento de la anemia perniciosa.

cyanosis *n.* cianosis, condición azulada o amoratada de la piel y las mucosas a causa de anomalías cardíacas o funcionales.

cyanotic *a.* cianótico-a, rel. a la cianosis o causado por ésta.

cybernetics *n.* cibernética, estudio del uso de medios electrónicos y mecanismos de comunicación aplicados a sistemas biológicos tales como los sistemas nervioso y cerebral.

cyclamate *n.* ciclamato, agente artificial dulcificante.

cycle *n.* ciclo, período; **pregnancy** ___ / ___ gravídico.

cyclectomy *n.* cicletomía, excisión de una parte del músculo ciliar.

cyclic *a.* cíclico-a, que ocurre en períodos o ciclos.

cyclical chemotherapy *n.* quimoterapia cíclica.

cyclitis *n.* ciclitis, infl. del músculo ciliar.

cyclophoria *n.* cicloforia, rotación del globo ocular debido a debilidad muscular.

cyclophosphamide *n.* ciclofosfamida, droga antineoplástica usada también como inmunosupresor en trasplantes.

cyclophotocoagulation *n.* ciclofotocoagulación, fotocoagulación a través de la pupila con un laser, procedimiento usado en el tratamiento de glaucoma.

cycloplegia *n.* cicloplejía, parálisis del músculo ciliar.

cyclosporine *n.* ciclosporina, agente inmunosupresivo usado en tranplantes de órganos.

cyclothymia *n.* ciclotimia, personalidad cíclica con trastornos de agitación y depresión.

cyclotomy *n.* ciclotomía, incisión a través del músculo ciliar.

cyclotropia *n.* ciclotropia, desviación del ojo alrededor del eje anteroposterior.

cylinder *n.* cilindro. 1. émbolo de una jeringa; 2. forma geométrica semejante a una columna.

cylindrical *a.* cilíndrico-a.

cylindrical lens *n.* lente cilíndrico

cylindrical renal cast *n.* molde renal cilíndrico

cylindroma *n.* cilindroma, tumor generalmente maligno visto en la cara o en la órbita del ojo.

cylindruria *n.* cilindruria, presencia de cilindros en la orina.

cynic *a.* cínico-a.

cyst *n.* quiste, saco o bolsa que contiene líquido o materia semilíquida; **pilonidal** ___ / ___

pilonidal, que contiene pelo, gen. localizado en al área sacrococcígea; **sebaceous** ___ / ___ sebáceo, gen. localizado en el cuero cabelludo.

cystadenocarcinoma *n.* cistadenocarcinoma, carcinoma y cistadenoma combinados.

cystadenoma *n.* cistadenoma, adenoma que contiene uno o various quistes.

cystectomy *n.* cistectomía, extirpación o resección de la vejiga.

cysteine *n.* cisteína, aminoácido derivado de la cistina, presente en la mayor parte de las proteínas.

cystic *a.* cístico-a, rel. a la vesícula biliar o la vejiga urinaria; ___ **duct** / conducto ___ .

cystic fibrosis *n.* fibrosis cística del páncreas, fibroquiste.

cystine *n.* cistina, aminoácido producido durante la digestión de las proteínas, presente a veces en la orina.

cystinuria *n.* cistinuria, exceso de cistina en la orina.

cystitis *n.* cistitis, infl. de la vejiga urinaria caracterizada por ardor, dolor y micción frecuente.

cystocele *n.* cistocele, hernia de la vejiga.

cystofibroma *n.* cistofibroma, tipo de fibroma en el cual se han formado quistes o formaciones semejantes a quistes.

cystofibroscope *n.* cistofibroscopio.

cystogram *n.* cistograma, rayos-x de la vejiga.

cystography *n.* cistografia, rayos-x de la vejiga urinaria usando un medio de contraste.

cystolithotomy *n.* cistolitotomía, extracción de una piedra o cálculo por medio de una incisión en la vejiga.

cystometer *n.* cistómetro, instrumento usado para estudiar la patofisiología de la vejiga que mide la capacidad y las reacciones de ésta a presiones aplicadas.

cystometry *n.* cistometría, estudio de las funciones de la vejiga con uso del cistómetro.

cystopexy *n.* cistopexia, fijación de la vejiga urinaria a la pared abdominal.

cystoscope *n.* cistoscopio, instrumento en forma de tubo usado para examinar y tratar trastornos de la vejiga, los uréteres y los riñones.

cystoscopy *n.* cistoscopía, examen por medio del cistoscopio.

cystostomy *n.* cistostomía, creación de un boquete o fistula en la vejiga para permitir el drenaje urinario.

cystotomy *n.* cistotomía, incisión en la vejiga.

cystourethrography *n.* cistouretrografía, radiografía de la vejiga y la uretra.

cystourethroscope *n.* cistouretroscopio, instrumento usado en la exploración de la vejiga y la uretra.

cytochrome *n.* citocromo, hemocromógeno importante en el proceso de oxidación.

cytology *n.* citología, ciencia que estudia la estructura, forma y función de las células.

cytolytic *a.* citolítico-a, que tiene la cualidad de disolver o destruir células.

cytomegalic *a.* citomegálico-a, caracterizado-a por células agrandadas.

cytomegalovirus *n.* citomegalovirus, grupo de virus pertenecientes a la familia *Herpesviridae* que infectan humanos y otros animales, y son causantes de la enfermedad de inclusión citomegálica.

cytometer *n.* citómetro, dispositivo usado en el conteo y medida de los hematíes.

cytopenia *n.* citopenia, deficiencia de elementos celulares en la sangre.

cytoplasm *n.* citoplasma, protoplasma de una célula con exclusión del núcleo.

cytotoxic agents *n., pl.* agentes citotóxicos, compuestos químicos usados en quimioterapia con el propósito de destruir células cancerosas.

cytotoxicity *n.* citotoxicidad, la capacidad de un agente de destruir ciertas células.

cytotoxin *n.* citotoxina, agente tóxico que afecta a las células de ciertos órganos.

cytula *n.* cítula, término que define al óvulo o pequeña célula impregnada.

d

d *abbr.* **death** / muerte; **deceased** / difunto-a;
degree / grado; **density** / densidad; **dose** / dosis.

dacryadenitis *n.* dacriadenitis, infl. de una
glándula lagrimal.

dacryagogue *n.* dacriagogo, agente estimulante
de las glándulas lagrimales.

dacrycystalgia *n.* dacricistalgia, dolor en el
saco lagrimal.

dacryoadenectomy *n.* dacrioadenectomía,
extirpación de una glándula lagrimal.

dacryocyst *n.* dacriocisto, saco lacrimal interno.

dacryocystectomy *n.* dacriocistectomía,
cirugía para restaurar el drenaje del saco lacrimal
cuando ocurre obstrucción en el conducto
nasolacrimal.

dacryocystitis *n.* dacriocistitis, infl. del saco
lagrimal.

dacryocystotomy *n.* dacriocistotomía, incisión
del saco lagrimal.

dacryolithiasis *n.* dacriolitiasis, formación de
cálculos lacrimales.

dacryopyorrhea *n.* dacriopiorrea, excreción de
lágrimas que contienen leucocitos.

dacryostenosis *n.* dacriostenosis, estenosis del
conducto lacrimal.

dactyl *n.* dáctilo, dedo de la mano o del pie.

dactylogram *n.* dactilograma, proceso de
determinación de las huellas digitales.

dactylography *n.* dactilografía, estudio de las
huellas digitales.

dactylology *n.* dactilología, lenguaje mímico o
por señas.

dactylomegaly *n.* dactilomegalia, dedos de los
pies o las manos de tamaño demasiado grande.

dad *n.* papá; **daddy** / *H.A.* papi, papacito, tata.

dagger *n.* puñal.

daily *a.* diario-a, cotidiano-a; ___ **life** / vida
cotidiana; *adv.* diariamente, todos los días, cada
día, cotidianamente.

dairy products *n., pl.* productos lácteos.

daltonism *n.* daltonismo, dificultad para percibir
colores.

dam *v.* acción de detener, estancar, tapar.

damage *n.* daño, deterioro, lesión. *v.* dañar,
perjudicar; dañarse, perjudicarse.

damages *n., pl.* daños y perjuicios.

damaging *a.* perjudicial.

damiana *n.* damiana, planta originaria de Mex.
cuyas hojas tienen acción diurética.

damp *a.* húmedo-a.

dampen *v.* humedecer, mojar.

danazol *n.* danazol, hormona sintética que
suprime la acción de la pituitaria anterior.

dance *n.* baile; **St. Vitus'** ___ / ___ de San Vito;
chorea; *v.* bailar, danzar.

dandruff *n.* caspa.

danger *n.* peligro, riesgo; *v.* **to be in** ___ /
correr ___ .

dangerous *a.* peligroso-a, arriesgado-a.

dapsone *n.* dapsona, sulfonildianilina, droga
usada en el tratamiento de la lepra.

dare *v.* atreverse, arriesgarse.

dark *a.* oscuro-a; ___ **adaptation** / adaptación a
la oscuridad; ___ **field illumination** /
iluminación del campo ___, iluminación lateral u
oblicua.

darken *v.* oscurecer.

darkness *n.* oscuridad.

Darwinian reflex *n.* reflejo de Darwin, la
tendencia en los niños pequeñitos de suspenderse
agarrados de una barra.

Darwinian theory *n.* Darwin, teoría de, teoría
de selección y de evolución.

data *n., pl.* datos.

date *n.* fecha; **effective** ___ / ___ de vigencia;
expiration ___ / ___ de vencimiento;
specimen ___ / ___ del espécimen o muestra;
up-to- ___ / hasta la fecha; [*current*] al
corriente.

daughter *n.* hija; ___ **-in-law** / nuera.

Daviel's operation *n.* Daviel, operación de,
extracción extracapsular de una catarata.

dawn *n.* amanecer.

day *n.* día, **all** ___ / todo el ___; **by** ___ / por
el ___, de___; ___ **after tomorrow** / pasado
mañana; ___ **before yesterday** / anteayer; ___
in ___ **out** / ___ tras ___; **each** ___ / cada ___;
every ___ / todos los ___ -s; **every other** ___ /
un ___ sí y un ___ no; **three times a** ___ / tres
veces al ___; **twice a** ___ / dos veces al ___ .

daybreak *n.* amanecer, alba.

daydream *n.* ilusión, ensueño; *v.* **to**___ / soñar
despierto-a.

daylight *n.* luz del día.

daytime *a.* de día.

daze *n.* ofuscación, desorientación.

deacidify *v.* neutralizar un ácido.

deactivation *n.* desactivación, proceso de
transformar lo activo en inactivo.

dead *a.* difunto-a; muerto-a.
dead weight *n.* carga innecesaria; estorbo.
deaden *v.* [*sound*] amortigar; [*nerve*] adormecer; anestesiar.
deadly *a.* mortífero-a; mortal, que puede causar la muerte; ___ **poison** / veneno ___; ___ **wound** / herida ___ .
deaf *n. a.* sordo-a.
deaf-mute *n.* sordomudo-a.
deaf-muteness, deafmutism *n.* sordomudez.
deafen *v.* ensordecer.
deafness *n.* sordera.
deal *n.* cantidad, porción; **a good** ___ / bastante; **a great** ___ **of time** / mucho tiempo; *v.* repartir, distribuir; **to** ___ **with** / tratar con.
deambulatory *a.* ambulatorio-a; móvil.
dear *a.* querido-a; estimado-a.
death *n.* muerte, fallecimiento; **apparent** ___ / ___ aparente; ___ **certificate** / certificado de defunción; ___ **instinct** / instinto mortal; ___ **rate** / mortalidad; ___ **rattle** / estertor agónico; **fetal** ___ / ___ del feto.
debanding *n.* acción de remover.
debilitate *v.* debilitar; debilitarse.
debilitated *a.* debilitado-a.
debilitating *a.* debilitante, rel. a una enfermedad o agente que debilita.
debility *n.* debilidad; atonía.
debridement *n.* desbridamiento, proceso quirúrgico de limpieza de una herida o quemadura para prevenir una infección.
debris *n.* detrito, partículas, [*building*] escombros.
debt *n.* deuda.
debulking operation *n.* extirpación de la mayor parte de un tumor.
decalcification *n.* descalcificación, pérdida o disminución de sales de calcio en los huesos o dientes.
decapacitation *n.* decapacitación, proceso que previene que la espermatozoa pase por el proceso de capacitación.
decapsulation *n.* decapsulación, incisión y extirpación de una cápsula.
decay *n.* deteriorización, deterioro, descomposición gradual; [*teeth*] caries; **dental** ___ / carie dental, *pop.* dientes picados; ___ **rate** / índice de descomposición gradual; *v.* deteriorar, descomponer, decaer, declinar; deteriorarse, descomponerse, [*teeth*] cariarse; [*wood*] carcomerse; [*matter*] podrirse, pudrirse.
decayed *a.* deteriorado-a, decaído-a; empeorado-a; cariado-a; carcomido-a; podrido-a; putrefacto-a.

deceased *n.* difunto-a, persona muerta.
deceit *n.* engaño, fraude.
deceitful *a.* traicionero-a, engañador-a; ___ **sickness** / enfermedad ___ .
deceive *v.* engañar, defraudar, embaucar.
deceleration *n.* desaceleración, disminución de la velocidad tal como en la frecuencia cardíaca.
decency *n.* decencia.
decent *a.* decente.
decentered *a.* descentrado-a, fuera del centro.
decholesterolization *n.* decolesterolización, reducción terapéutica de la concentración de colesterol en la sangre.
decide *v.* decidir, determinar.
decided *a.* decidido-a.
decidua *n.* decidua, tejido membranoso formado por la mucosa uterina durante la gestación y expulsado después del parto.
decidua menstrualis *n., L.* decidua menstrual, también llamada membrana caduca, es la capa mucosa del útero que se desprende durante la menstruación.
deciduous *a.* deciduo-a, de permanencia temporal; ___ **dentition** / primera dentición; ___ **teeth** / dientes ___ -s, dientes de leche.
decimate *v.* diezmar.
decimation *n.* gran mortalidad, diezma.
decipher *v.* descifrar, resolver un problema.
decision *n.* decisión, resolución.
decisive *a.* decisivo-a, terminante.
declination *n.* declinación. 1. rotación del ojo; 2. declive, descenso.
decline *n.* declinación; decadencia, decaimiento. *v.* declinar, decaer; [*invitation, offer*] declinar, rehusar, rechazar; [*health*] desmejorarse.
decoction *n.* cocimiento, té de yerbas medicinales.
decompensation *n.* descompensación, inhabilidad del corazón para mantener una circulación adecuada.
decompose *v.* descomponerse, corromperse; [*food*] podrirse, pudrirse.
decomposed *a.* descompuesto-a; [*food*] podrido-a, putrefacto-a.
decomposition *n.* descomposición, disolución de una sustancia en elementos químicos.
decompression *n.* descompresión, reducción de presión; ___ **chamber** / cámara de ___; ___ **sickness** / condición por ___; **surgical** ___ / ___ quirúrgica.
decongest *v.* descongestionar.
decongestant *n.* descongestionador, descongestionante.

decontaminate *v.* descontaminar, librar de contaminación.

decontamination *n.* descontaminación, proceso de librar el ambiente, objetos o personas de sustancias o agentes contaminados o nocivos tales como sustancias radiactivas.

decortication *n.* decorticación, excisión del tejido cortical de un órgano o estructura.

decrease *n.* disminución; reducción v. decrecer, disminuir, reducir; ___ **saliva** / ___ de saliva o reducción de saliva; ___ **tears** / ___ de lágrimas o reducción de lágrimas; ___ **urine output** / ___ o reducción del rendimiento urinario.

decreased *a., pp.* of **to decrease**, decrecido-a, disminuido-a, reducido-a.

decreasing *a.* decreciente, disminuyendo.

decrepit *a.* decrépito-a, senil.

decrepitude *n.* decrepitud.

decrudescence *n.* decrudescencia, disminución de la gravedad de los síntomas.

decubitus *n.* decúbito, posición acostada; ___ **ventral** / ___ prono; **dorsal** ___ / ___ supino; **lateral** ___ **x-ray** / radiografía ___ lateral.

decussation *n.* decusación, cruzamiento de estructuras en forma de X; ___ **of pyramids** / ___ de las pirámides, cruzamiento de fibras nerviosas de una pirámide a otra en la médula oblongata; **optic** ___ / ___ óptica, cruzamiento de las fibras del nervio óptico.

dedicate *v.* dedicar.

deduce *v.* deducir, inferir.

deduct *v.* descontar; rebajar.

deductible *a.* deducible.

deduction *n.* deducción.

deep *a.* profundo-a, hondo-a; ___ **artery of arm** / arteria ___ del brazo; ___ **artery of clitoris** / arteria ___ del clítoris; ___ **artery of penis** / arteria ___ del pene; ___ **breathing** / respiración ___; ___ **cerebral veins** / venas cerebrales ___; ___ **cervical veins** / venas cervicales ___ -as; ___ **contractions** / contracciones ___ -s, de fondo; ___ **-chested** / ancho-a de pecho; ___ **dredging** / dragado; ___ **facial vein** / vena facial ___; ___ **inguinal ring** / anillo inguinal ___; ___ **-rooted** / arraigado-a; ___ **sensibility** / sensibilidad ___; ___ **sleep** / sueño ___, sopor; ___ **tendon reflex** / reflejos tendónicos ___ -s; ___ **venous thrombosis** / trombosis venosa ___; ___ **x-ray therapy** / terapia ___ .

deer fly disease *n.* V. **tularemia.**

deface *v.* mutilar, deformar, desfigurar.

defacement *n.* deformación; deterioro; mutilación.

defecate *v.* defecar, evacuar; *Mex.* obrar.

defecation *n.* defecación, evacuación intestinal.

defect *n.* defecto; insuficiencia; fallo.

defective *a.* defectuoso-a; incompleto-a.

defend *v.* defender.

defense *n.* defensa; protección; resistencia; ___ **mechanism** / mecanismo de ___; [*organic*] antitoxina; autoprotección.

defenseless *a.* indefenso-a, inerme.

defensive medicine *n.* medicina defensiva, medidas terapéuticas o de diagnóstico que se toman con el propósito de evitar un posible riesgo de negligencia médica.

defer *v.* diferir, aplazar.

deferent *a.* deferente, hacia afuera.

deferred *a.* aplazado-a, diferido-a.

defibrillation *n.* desfibrilación, acción de cambiar latidos irregulares del corazón a su ritmo normal.

defibrillator *n.* desfibrilador, dispositivo eléctrico usado para restaurar el ritmo normal del corazón.

deficiency *n.* deficiencia, falta de algún elemento esencial al organismo; ___ **disease** / enfermedad por deficiencia; **galactokinasa** ___ / ___ de galactocinasa; **lactase** ___ / ___ de lactasa; **mineral** ___ / ___ mineral; **mental** ___ / ___ mental; **oxygen** ___ / falta de oxígeno.

deficient *a.* deficiente, careciente.

deficit *n.* déficit, deuda; falta; deficiencia.

definition *n.* definición.

definitive *a.* definitivo; determinado; ___ **diagnosis** / diagnóstico ___ .

definitive host *n.* huésped definitivo, aquél en el cual el parásito se desarrolla hasta alcanzar la madurez sexual.

deflate *v.* desinflar, deshinchar.

deflect *v.* desviar, apartar.

deflection, deflexion *n.* deflexión, desviación, desvío; diversión inconsciente de ideas.

deform *v.* deformar.

deformed *a.* deformado-a, irregular.

deformity *n.* deformidad, irregularidad, defecto congénito o adquirido.

defurfuration *n.* defurfuración, acto de soltar escamas de la piel semejantes a hojuelas.

degenerate *a.* degenerado-a; anómalo-a.

degeneration *n.* degeneración, deteriorización.

degenerative joint disease *n.* enfermedad degenerativa de una articulación o coyuntura.

deglutition *n.* deglución, acto de ingerir.

degree *n.* grado. 1. unidad de medida de la temperatura; 2. intensidad.

dehiscence *n.* dehiscencia, abertura espontánea de una herida.

dehumidifier *n.* deshumectante, aparato para disminuir la humedad.

dehydrate *v.* deshidratar, eliminar el agua de una sustancia; deshidratarse, perder líquido del cuerpo o de los tejidos.

dehydrated *a.* deshidratado-a.

dehydrocholesterol *n.* dehidrocolesterol, esterol presente en la piel que se convierte en vitamina D por la acción de rayos solares.

déjà vu *n. Fr.* déjà vu, impresión ilusoria de haber experimentado antes una situación que es totalmente nueva.

dejection *n.* deyección. 1. estado de abatimiento, depresión; 2. expulsión de excremento.

delay *n.* demora; *v.* demorar, atrasar; postergar.

delayed *a.* tardío-a, demorado-a; ___ **delivery** / parto ___ .

deleterious *a.* deletéreo-a, nocivo-a, dañino-a.

delicate *a.* delicado-a.

delicious *a.* delicioso-a; exquisito-a.

delight *n.* deleite; delicia; *v.* agradar, deleitar.

delighted *a.* encantado-a; *v.* **to be** ___ / tener mucho gusto.

delinquency *n.* delincuencia; **juvenile** ___ / ___ juvenil.

delirious *a.* delirante, en estado de delirio.

delirium *n.* delirium, estado de confusión mental acompañado gen. de alucinaciones y sensaciones distorsionadas; ___ **tremens** / ___ tremens, tipo de psicosis alcohólica.

deliver *v.* extraer; partear; [*in childbirth*] **to be delivered** / dar a luz, estar de parto,; *Mex. A.* aliviarse.

delivery *n.* parto, alumbramiento; **after** ___ / ___ después del ___; **before** ___ / antes del ___; ___ **of the placenta** / expulsión de la placenta; ___ **room** / sala de ___ -s; sala de maternidad; **false** ___ / ___ falso; **hard** ___ / ___ laborioso; **induction of** ___ / ___ inducido; **normal** ___ / ___ normal; **premature** ___ / ___ prematuro; **prolonged** ___ / ___ prolongado; **stages of** ___ / etapas del ___ .

deltoid *a.* deltoideo-a. 1. en forma de delta; 2. rel. al músculo deltoides.

delusion *n.* delirio, decepción, engaño; creencias falsas; ___ **of control** / ___ de control; ___ **of grandeur** / ___ de grandeza; ___ **of negation** / ___ de negación; ___ **of persecution** / ___ de persecución.

demand *n.* petición, demanda; ___ **feeding** / alimentación por demanda.

demand oxygen delivery device *n.* servicio de entrega de oxígeno por demanda de un dispositivo eléctrico que conserve oxígeno.

demented *a.* demente, enajenado-a; que sufre de demencia.

dementia *n.* demencia, locura; declinación de las funciones mentales; ___ **paralytica** / ___ paralítica; ___ **praecox** / ___ precoz, esquizofrenia; **organic** ___ / ___ orgánica; **senile** ___ / ___ senil.

demineralization *n.* desmineralización, pérdida de sales minerales del organismo.

demoplastic *a.* desmoplásico-a, causante de adherencias.

demulcent *n.* emoliente, demulcente, aceite u otro agente que suaviza y alivia molestias de la piel.

demyelination *n.* desmielinización, pérdida de la capa de mielina de un nervio.

dendrite *n.* dendrita, prolongación protoplasmática de la célula de un nervio que recibe los impulsos nerviosos.

denervated *a.* desnervado, enervado, rel. a la pérdida de energía nerviosa.

dengue fever *n.* dengue, fiebre endémica producida por un virus, transmitida por el mosquito *Aedes*.

denomination *n.* denominación, nombre.

dense *a.* denso-a, espeso-a.

density *n.* densidad; **bone** ___ / ___ ósea; **optic** ___ / ___ óptica; **urinary** ___ / ___ urinaria; **vapor** ___ / ___ del vapor;

dental *a.* dental, dentario-a, rel. a los dientes;___ **abscess** / absceso ___; ___ **ankylosis** / anquilosis ___; ___ **arch** / arco ___; ___ **bulb** / bulbo ___; ___ **care** / cuidado ___; ___ **caries** / caries ___ -es; ___ **drill** / taladro, torno; ___ **enamel** / esmalte dentario; ___ **floss** / hilo ___, hilo de seda encerada; ___ **flossing system** / sistema para aplicar hilo ___; ___ **follicle** / folículo ___; ___ **health services** / servicios de salud ___; ___ **hygienist** / técnico-a en profiláctica ___; ___ **implants** / implantes ___ -es; ___ **impression** / impresión, mordisco; ___ **impactation** / inclusión dentaria; ___ **plaque** / placa dentaria; ___ **public health** / salud pública ___; ___ **school** / escuela de odontología; ___ **surgeon** / cirujano; ___ **tartar** / sarro ___; ___ **technician** / mecánico ___ .

dentiform *a.* odontoide, dentado-a, de proyección similar a un diente.

dentifrice *n.* dentífrico, pasta dental.
dentilabial *a.* dentilabial, rel. a los dientes y los labios.
dentin *n.* dentina, marfil dentario, tejido calcificado de un diente.
dentinogenesis *n.* dentinogénesis, formación de la dentina.
dentinoma *n.* dentinoma, tumor benigno que consiste mayormente de dentina.
dentist *n.* dentista.
dentistry *n.* arte o profesión de dentistas.
dentition *n.* dentición, brote de los dientes; ___ **primary** / ___ primaria [*first teeth*] o dientes de leche; ___ , **secondary** / ___ secundaria o dientes permanentes.
denture *n.* dentadura, prótesis; [*artificial*] dentadura postiza; ___ **plates** / ___ parcial, *pop.* plancha dental.
denudation *n.* denudación, privación de la cubierta de una superficie de una manera traumática, sea por cirugía, trauma, o por un cambio patológico.
denutrition *n.* desnutrición, malnutrición, deficiencia alimenticia; **protein-calorie** ___ / ___ proteinocalórica.
deny *v.* negar, rehusar.
deodorant *n.* desodorante.
deodorize *v.* desodorizar, destruir olores fétidos o desagradables.
deoxycorticosterone *n.* desoxicorticosterona, hormona producida en la corteza de las glándulas suprarrenales de efecto marcado en el metabolismo del agua y los electrólitos.
deoxygenated *a.* desoxigenado-a.
deoxyhemoglobin *n.* desoxihemoglobina, forma reducida de hemoglobina que ocurre cuando la oxihemoglobina pierde el oxígeno.
depart *v.* partir, salir.
departed *a.* difunto-a; ausente.
depend *v.* depender.
dependence, dependency *n.* dependencia, subordinación; ___ **producing drugs** / drogas adictivas, de dependencia.
dependent *n.* depediente *a.* depediente; ___ **drainage** / drenaje ___; ___ **edema** / edema ___; ___ **personality** / personalidad ___ .
depersonalization *n.* despersonalización, pérdida de la personalidad.
depigmentation *n.* despigmentación, pérdida parcial o completa de pigmento.
depilate *v.* depilar, acción de quitar o extirpar pelo.
depilation *n.* depilación, procedimiento de extirpación del pelo y la raíz.

depilatory *n.* depilatorio.
deplete *v.* agotar, vaciar; depauperarse.
depleted *a.* agotado-a, vaciado-a, depauperado-a.
depletion *n.* deplección. 1. acción de vaciar; 2. pérdida o remoción de los líquidos del cuerpo; ___ **of body liquids** / pérdida de líquidos del cuerpo; **fluid** ___ , **dehydration** / pérdida de fluido, deshidratación; **potassium** ___ / pérdida de potasio, hipopotasemia; **saline** ___ / pérdida salina.
deposit *n.* depósito; *v.* depositar.
depravation *n.* depravación.
depress *v.* deprimir; desalentar, desanimar.
depressant *n.* depresor; tranquilizante; ___ **drug** / medicamento tranquilizante;
depressed *a.* deprimido-a, abatido-a; *v.* **to become** ___ / deprimirse.
depression *n.* depresión. 1. sensación de tristeza o melancolía acompañada de apatía y estados de abatimiento; 2. cavidad.
depressive *a.* depresivo-a, deprimente; ___ **disorder** / trastorno ___ .
depressor *n.* depresor. 1. agente usado para reducir un nivel establecido de una función o actividad del organismo; 2. tranquilizante que produce depresión.
depurate *v.* depurar.
depurated *a.* depurado-a.
depuration *n.* depuración, purificación.
derange *v.* perturbar, desordenar, causar trastorno.
deranged *a.* perturbado-a; trastornado-a; ___ **metabolic process** / trastorno del proceso metabólico.
derangement *n. Fr.* trastorno, desequilibrio, irregularidad de una función del cuerpo.
derivation *n.* derivación. 1. desviación, curso alterado o lateral que tiene lugar por anastomosis o por una característica anatómica natural; 2. descendencia.
derive *v.* derivar, inferir, deducir; descender, proceder.
dermabrasion *n.* dermabrasión, abrasión cutánea, proceso empleado para eliminar los nevos y cicatrices de la acné.
dermatitis *n.* dermatitis, dermitis, cualquier infl. de la piel;**atopic** ___ / ___ atópica; ___ **by contact** / ___ por contacto; ___ **medicamentosa** / ___ medicamentosa; ___ **papillaris capillitii** / ___ papillaris capillitii; **erythematic** ___ / ___ eritematosa; **gangrenous** ___ / ___ gangrenosa; **occupational** ___ / ___ ocupacional, industrial; **seborrheic** ___ / ___ seborréica.

dermatological *a.* dermatológico-a, rel. a la dermis.

dermatologist *n.* dermatólogo-a, especialista en dermatología.

dermatology *n.* dermatología, parte de la medicina que estudia la piel, su estructura, sus funciones y el tratamiento de la misma.

dermatolysis *n.* dermatolisis, exfoliación de la epidermis causada por una enfermedad.

dermatoma *n.* dermatoma, neoplasma de la piel.

dermatome *n.* dermátomo, instrumento quirúrgico empleado para cortar capas o tejidos finos de la piel.

dermatomere *n.* dermatomera, segmento del tegumento embrionario.

dermatomycosis *n.* dermatomicosis, infl. de la piel producida por hongos.

dermatomyositis *n.* dermatomiositis, enfermedad del tejido conectivo con manifestaciones de dermatitis, edema e infl. de los músculos.

dermatoneurosis *n.* dermatoneurosis, erupción cutánea causada por un estímulo emocional.

dermatopathy, dermatosis *n.* dermatopatía, dermatosis, cualquier enfermedad de la piel.

dermatophiliasis *n.* dermatofiliasis, infección de la piel producida por pulgas o niguas.

dermatophyte *n.* dermatófito, hongo parásito que ataca la piel.

dermatophytosis *n.* dermatofitosis, pie de atleta, infección fungosa producida por dermatófilos.

dermatoplasty *n.* dermatoplastia, cirugía plástica de la piel.

dermatosyphilis *n.* dermatosífilis, manifestación sifilítica en la piel.

dermic *a.* dermal, dermático-a, cutáneo-a.

dermis, derma *n.* dermis, piel.

dermoid *a.* dermoideo-a, semejante o rel. a la piel; ___ **cyst** / quiste ___, de origen congénito, gen. benigno.

descend *v.* descender, bajar; derivarse.

descendant *n. a.* descendiente.

descending *a.* descendente, descendiente; ___ **aorta** / aorta ___, parte mayor de la aorta; ___ **colon** / colon ___ .

descending tracts *n., pl.* ramas descendentes de nervios en la espina dorsal que llevan impulsos del cerebro al resto del cuerpo.

descent *n.* descenso, bajada; descendencia, sucesión.

describe *v.* describir.

described *a.* descrito-a, narrado-a.

desensitize *v.* desensibilizar, reducir o eliminar una sensibilidad de origen físico o emocional.

desert *n.* desierto, yermo, páramo.

deserve *v.* merecer.

desexualizing *n.* desexualización. 1. eliminación de un impulso sexual; 2. castración.

desiccant *a.* desecante, que tiene la propiedad de secar.

desiccate *v.* desecar, secar, quitar la humedad.

desiccated *a. pp.* of **to desiccate**, desecado-a.

design *n.* diseño.

desirable *a.* deseado-a; conveniente.

desire *n.* deseo, ansia; *v.* desear, ansiar.

desk *n.* enscritorio; **front** ___ / mesa de admisión.

desmoid *a.* desmoide, en forma de ligamento.

desmoma *n.* desmoma, tumor del tejido conjuntivo.

desmoplastic *a.* desmoplásico-a, causante de adherencias.

despair *n.* desesperación; *v.* [*to lose hope*] perder la esperanza; desesperarse.

despondency *n.* desaliento; desesperación.

despondent *a.* desesperado-a, desalentado-a; *v.* **to be** ___ / estar ___ .

desquamation *n.* descamación, exfoliación, desprendimiento de la piel en forma de escamas.

destroy *v.* destruir, aniquilar; arruinar.

detach *v.* separar, desprender, despegar; desprenderse; soltarse.

detachment *n.* desprendimiento, separación; ___ **of the retina** / ___ de la retina.

detail *n.* detalle; **in** ___ / con detalle, detalladamente; *v.* detallar, destacar; **to go into** ___ / explicar todo detalladamente.

detain *v.* detener, parar.

detect *v.* detectar, descubrir.

detector *n.* detector, revelador, descubridor.

detergent *n.* detergente, agente limpiador, *a.* detergente, limpiador-a.

deteriorate *v.* deteriorar, desmejorar; deteriorarse; desmejorarse.

deterioration *n.* deterioración, deterioro, desmejoramiento.

determinant *n.* determinante, elemento que predomina o causa una determinación.

determination *n.* determinación, decisión, resolución.

determine *v.* determinar, decidir; resolver; concluir.

determined *a.* decidido-a; [*in tests*] comprobado-a.

determinism *n.* determinismo, teoría que establece que todo fenómeno influido físico o psíquico está predeterminado y no es influido por la voluntad individual.

detorsion *n.* destorsión. 1. corrección de la curvatura o malformación de una estructura; 2. corrección quirúrgica de la torsión de un testículo o del intestino.

detoxicate *v.* desintoxicar.

detoxification *n.* destoxificación, reducción de las propiedades tóxicas de una sustancia.

detoxify *v.* destoxificar, desintoxicar, extraer sustancias tóxicas.

detrimental *a.* perjudicial, nocivo-a.

detritus *n., pl.* desechos.

detrusor *n.* detrusor, músculo que expulsa o echa hacia afuera.

deuteranopia *n.* deuteranopía, ceguera al color verde.

develop *v.* [*to expand, to grow*] desarrollar, crecer, progresar; evolucionar; avanzar; [*film*] revelar; [*symptom*] surgir; manifestarse.

developed *a.* desarrollado-a; revelado-a, manifestado-a.

development *n.* desarrollo; adelanto; progreso, crecimiento; [*germs*] proliferación; **child** ___ / ___ infantil; **physical** ___ / ___ físico; **psychomotor and physical** ___ / ___ psicomotor y físico.

developmental disability *n.* inhabilidades de desarrollo o pérdida de una función adquirida debido a causas congénitas o post natales, tales como la adquisición del lenguaje o la habilidad motora o social.

developmental psychology *n.* sicología del desarrollo mental.

deviation *n.* desviación, desvío. 1. alejamiento de una pauta establecida; 2. aberración mental; mala conducta, mal comportamiento.

device *n.* dispositivo; mecanismo.

devious *a.* desviado-a; descaminado-a; extraviado a.

devise *v.* idear, inventar, considerar.

devitalize *v.* devitalizar, debilitar, privar de la fuerza vital.

devolution *n.* devolución. V. **catabolism**.

dexter *a.* diestro-a; a la derecha.

dextrality *n.* dextrismo, preferencia de uso de la mano derecha.

dextrocardia *n.* dextrocardia, dislocación del corazón hacia la derecha.

dextromanual *a.* dextromanual, preferencia por el uso de la mano derecha.

dextroposition *n.* dextroposición, desplazamiento hacia la derecha.

dextrose *n.* dextrosa, glucosa, forma de azúcar simple, *pop.* azúcar de uva.

diabetes *n.* diabetes, enfermedad que se manifiesta por excesiva emisión de orina.

diabetes insipidus *n.* diabetes insípida nefrógena, causada por una deficiencia en el gasto de hormona antidiurética.

diabetes mellitus *n.* diabetes mellitus, diabetes causada por una deficiencia en la producción de insulina que resulta en hiperglucemia y glucosuria; ___ **noninsulin-dependent** / ___ sin dependencia de insulina.

diabetic *a.* diabético-a; rel. a la diabetes o que padece de ella; **brittle** ___ / ___ inestable; ___ **angiopathies** / angiopatías ___ -s; ___ **coma** / coma ___, por falta de insulina; ___ **diet** / dieta ___; ___ **neuropathy** / neuropatía ___; ___ **retinopathy** / retinopatía ___ .

diabetogenic *a.* diabetogénico-a, que produce diabetes.

diabetograph *n.* diabetógrafo, aparato para medir la proporción de glucosa en la orina.

diacetemia *n.* diacetemia, presencia de ácido diacético en la sangre.

diacetic acid *n.* ácido diacético.

diacetylmorphine *n.* diacetilmorfina, heroína.

diagnose *v.* diagnosticar, dar un diagnóstico, hacer un diagnóstico o diagnosis.

diagnosis *n.* diagnóstico, diagnosis, determinación de la enfermedad del paciente; **computer** ___ / ___ por computadora; ___ **error** / errores de ___; **differential** ___ / ___ diferencial, por comparación; **physical** ___ / ___ físico, por medio de un examen físico completo.

diagnostic *n.* diagnóstico; ___ **chart** / ficha de ___; ___ **imaging** / ___ de imágenes por medios radioactivos.

diagonal *a.* diagonal, sección transversal.

diagram *n.* diagrama.

dialysate *n.* dializado, líquido que pasa por la membrana separadora o dializadora.

dialysis *n.* diálisis, procedimiento para filtrar y eliminar toxinas presentes en la sangre de pacientes con insuficiencia renal; ___ **machine** / aparato de ___ (riñón artificial); **peritoneal** ___ / ___ peritoneal; **renal** ___ / ___ renal.

dialyze *v.* dializar, hacer una diálisis.

dialyzer *n.* dializador, instrumento usado en el proceso de diálisis.

diameter *n.* diámetro.

Diana, complex of *n.* complejo de Diana, la adopción de características y conducta masculina por parte de una mujer.

diapedesis *n.* diapédesis, paso de células sanguíneas, esp. leucocitos, a través de la pared intacta de un vaso capilar.

diaper *n.* pañal; culero; *Mex.* pavico; zapeta; ___ **rash** / eritema de los pañales, erupción.

diaphoretic *n.* diaforético, agente que estimula la transpiración.

diaphragm *n.* diafragma. 1. músculo que separa el tórax del abdomen; 2. anticonceptivo uterino.

diaphragmatic *a.* diafragmático-a, rel. al diafragma.

diaphysis *n.* diáfisis, porción media de un hueso largo tal como se presenta en el húmero.

diaplasis *n.* diaplasis, reducción de una luxación o fractura.

diarrhea *n.* diarrea; **acute** ___ / ___ severa; ___ **infantile** / ___ infantil; ___ **of the newborn** / ___ epidémica del recién nacido; **dysenteric** ___ / ___ disentérica; **emotional** ___ / ___ emocional; **lienteric** ___ / ___ lientérica; **mucous** ___ / ___ mucosa; **nervous** ___ / ___ nerviosa; **pancreatic** ___ / ___ pancreática; **purulent** ___ / ___ purulenta; **summer** ___ / ___ estival o de verano; **travelers'** ___ / ___ del viajero. See chart on page 95.

diarrheal *a.* diarreico-a, rel. a la diarrea.

diarthrosis *n.* diartrosis, tipo de articulación que permite movimiento amplio, tal como la de la cadera.

diastase *n.* diastasa, enzima que actúa en la digestión de almidones y azúcares.

diastasis *n.* diastasis. 1. separación anormal de partes unidas esp. huesos; 2. tiempo de descanso del ciclo cardíaco inmediatamente anterior a la sístole.

diastole *n.* diástole, fase de dilatación del corazón durante la cual se llenan de sangre las cavidades cardíacas.

diastolic *a.* diastólico-a, rel. a la diástole del corazón; ___ **pressure** / presión ___ .

diathermy *n.* diatermia, aplicación de calor a los tejidos del cuerpo por medio de una corriente eléctrica.

diathesis *n.* diátesis, propensión constitucional u orgánica a contraer ciertas enfermedades; **hemorrhagic** ___ / ___ hemorrágica; **rheumatic** ___ / ___ reumática.

diatrizoate meglumine *n.* diatrizoate de meglumina, sustancia radiopaca que se usa para hacer visibles las arterias y venas del corazón y del cerebro así como la vesícula, los riñones y la vejiga.

dichorionic *n.* dicoriónico, que tiene dos coriones.

dichotomy, dichotomization *n.* dicotomía, dicotomización, división en dos partes; bifurcación.

dichroism *n.* dicroísmo, propiedad de algunas soluciones o cristales de diferenciar colores a través de la luz reflejada o transmitida.

dichromic *a.* dicrómico-a, rel. a dos colores.

dichromophil *a.* dicromófilo-a, que permite la coloración básica y ácida.

dictate *v.* dictar, ordenar.

dictyoma *n.* dictioma, tumor del epitelio que protege el cuerpo ciliar del ojo.

didactic *a.* didáctico-a, instructivo-a, que se enseña por medio de libros de texto y conferencias a diferencia de un planteamiento clínico.

didelphic *a.* didélfico-a, rel. a un útero doble.

didymitis *n.* didimitis. V. **orchitis**.

die *n.* molde, troquel; *v.* morir, fallecer, dejar de existir; morirse.

diembryony *n.* diembrionismo, producción de dos embriones de un solo óvulo.

diencephalon *n.* diencéfalo, parte del cerebro.

dienestrol *n.* dienestrol, estrógeno sintético.

diet *n.* dieta, régimen; **balanced** ___ / ___ balanceada, equilibrada; **bland** ___ / ___ blanda; **diabetic** ___ / ___ diabética; **gluten-free** ___ / ___ libre de gluten; **high fiber** ___ / ___ alta en fibria; **liquid** ___ / ___ líquida; **low in fat** ___ / ___ baja en grasa; **low-salt** ___ / ___ baja de sal; **salt-free** ___ / ___ sin sal; **weight reduction** ___ / ___ para bajar de peso.

dietary *a.* dietético-a; alimenticio-a; ___ **vitamins** / vitaminas ___ -s.

dietetic *a.* dietético-a, rel. a la dieta o aplicado a ésta.

dietetics *n.* dietética, ciencia que regula el régimen alimenticio para preservar o recuperar la salud.

dietitian *n.* dietista, especialista en nutrición.

difamation *n.* difamación.

different *a.* diferente, distinto-a.

differential *a.* diferencial, rel. a la diferenciación; ___ **diagnosis** / diagnóstico ___ .

differentiate *v.* diferenciar.

differentiation *n.* diferenciación, comparación y distinción de una sustancia, enfermedad o entidad con otra o de otra.

difficult *a.* difícil.

difficulty *n.* dificultad; penalidad; obstáculo.

diffraction *n.* difracción. 1. desviación de dirección; 2. la descomposición de un rayo de luz y sus componentes al atravesar un cristal o prisma; ___ **pattern** / patrón de ___ .

diffuse *v.* difundir, extender.

diffused *a.* difuso-a; ___ **abscess** / absceso ___ ; ___ **cutaneous mastocystosis** / mastocitosis cutánea ___ ; ___ **injury** / lesión extensa; ___ **obstructive enphysema** / enfisema obstructivo ___ .

diffusion *n.* difusión. 1. proceso de difundir; 2. diálisis a través de una membrana.

diffusion respiration *n.* proceso de difusión de respiración en apnea.

dig *vi.* excavar, extraer.

digest *v.* digerir.

digestant *n.* digestivo, agente que facilita la digestión.

digestion *n.* digestión, transformación de líquidos y sólidos en sustancias más simples para ser asimiladas por el organismo; **gastric** ___ / ___ gástrica; **intestinal** ___ / ___ intestinal, del intestino; **pancreatic** ___ / ___ pancreática.

digestive *a.* digestivo-a; rel. a la digestión; ___ **system** / sistema ___ .

digit *n.* dedo.

digital *a.* digital, rel. a los dedos.

digitalis *n.* digitalis, agente cardiotónico que se obtiene de las hojas secas de la *Digitalis purpurea;* ___ **intoxication** / intoxicación por ___ .

digitalization *n.* digitalización, uso terapéutico de digitalis.

digital radiography *n.* radiografía de imagen digital, transmisión de una imagen directa de rayos-x por medio de una computadora (ordenador).

digitation *n.* digitación, proceso en forma de dedos.

digitoxin *n.* digitoxina, glucósido cardiotónico obtenido de digitalis y usado en el tratamiento de la congestión pasiva del corazón.

digitus *n.* dígito, dedo; ___ **malleus, mallet finger** / dedo en martillo; ___ **valgus, varus** / desviación de un dedo.

digoxin *n.* digoxina, un derivado de digitalis que se emplea en el tratamiento de arritmias cardíacas.

dihydrostreptomycin *n.* dihidroestreptomicina, antibiótico derivado de la estreptomicina más usado que ésta por causar menos neurotoxicidad.

Dilantin *n.* Dilantin, droga antiespasmódica.

dilatation, dilation *n.* dilatación, aumento o expansión anormal de un órgano u orificio.

dilate *v.* dilatar, expandir.

dilation and curettage *n.* dilatación y curetaje; *pop.* raspado.

dilator *n.* dilatador. 1. músculo que dilata un órgano al contraerse; 2. instrumento quirúrgico para expandir o dilatar un orificio o paredes; **Hegar's** ___ / ___ de Hegar, instrumento usado para dilatar el canal uterino.

diluent *a.* diluente, diluyente, agente o medicamento que tiene la propiedad de diluir.

dim *a.* débil, mortecino-a; confuso-a; opaco-a.

dimension *n.* dimensión, medida de un cuerpo.

dimercaprol *n.* dimercaprol, antídoto usado en el envenenamiento producido por metales tales como oro y mercurio.

dimethylsulfoxide *n.* dimetilsulfóxido, medicamento antiinflamatorio y analgésico.

dimetria *n.* dimetría, útero o matriz doble.

diminish *v.* disminuir, reducir; amortiguar.

diminution *n.* disminución, proceso de disminuir o reducir.

diminutive *n.* diminutivo; *a.* diminuto-a, pequeño-a.

dimness *n.* opacidad; obscurecimiento de la vista.

dimorphism *n.* dimorfismo, caracterización de dos formas diferentes; **sexual** ___ / ___ sexual, hermafrodismo.

dimple *n.* hoyuelo o hendidura en la piel, esp. en la mejilla o la barbilla.

dinner *n.* cena.

diopter, dioptre *n.* dioptría, unidad de medida de refracción de un lente.

dioptometer *n.* dioptómetro, instrumento usado para medir la refracción ocular.

dioptric *a.* dióptrico, referente a la refración de la luz.

dioptrics *n.* dióptrica, ciencia que trata de la formación de imágenes y lentes.

diphallus *n.* difalo, duplicación parcial o completa del pene.

diphasic *a.* difásico-a, que tiene lugar en dos etapas diferentes.

diphenhydramine *n.* difenhidramina, nombre comercial Benadryl, antihistamínico.

diphonia *n.* difonía, producción de dos tonos diferentes.

diphtheria *n.* difteria, enfermedad contagiosa e infecciosa aguda, causada por el bacilo *Corynebacterium diphtheriae* (Klebs-Löffler), caracterizada por la formación de membranas falsas esp. en la garganta; ___ **antitoxin** / antitoxina contra la ___ .

diphtherotoxin *n.* difterotoxina, toxina derivada del cultivo de bacilos de la difteria.

diplacusis *n.* diplacusia, desorden auditivo caracterizado por la percepción de dos tonos por cada sonido producido.

diplegia *n.* diplejía, parálisis bilateral; **facial** ___ / ___ facial, parálisis de ambos lados de la cara; **spastic** ___ / ___ espástica.

diplocoria *n.* diplocoria, pupila doble.

diploe *n.* diploe, tejido esponjoso localizado entre las dos capas compactas de los huesos craneales.

diploid *a.* diploide, que posee dos combinaciones de cromosomas.

diplopagus *n.* diplópagos, mellizos unidos, cada uno de cuerpo casi completo, pero que comparten algunos órganos.

diplopia *n.* diplopía, visión doble.

dipsesis, dipsosis *n.* dipsesis, dipsosis, sed insaciable.

dipsomania *n.* dipsomanía, tipo de alcoholismo en el cual el paciente sufre una urgencia incontrolable por consumir sustancias alcohólicas.

direct *a.* directo-a; *v.* dirigir, ordenar; instruir.

direction *n.* dirección; instrucción.

directory *n.* directorio; junta; **telephone** ___ / guía telefónica.

dirty *a.* sucio-a, mugriento-a; *pop.* cochino-a.

disability *n.* incapacidad, inhabilidad; invalidez, impedimento; disminución de una capacidad física o mental.

disabled *a.* inválido-a; impedido-a; incapacitado-a.

disadvantage *n.* desventaja; alguna capacidad disminuida.

disagree *v.* no estar de acuerdo; disentir; altercar, argumentar.

disagreeable *a.* desagradable; ofensivo-a.

disappoint *v.* contrariar, desengañar.

disappointment *n.* contrariedad; desengaño, desilusión.

disarticulated *a.* desarticulado-a, dislocado-a, rel. a un hueso separado de la articulación.

disarticulation *n.* desarticulación, separación o amputación de dos o más huesos articulados entre sí.

disassimilation *n.* disasimilación, proceso destructivo.

disaster *n.* desastre; desdicha, infortunio.

disbelief *n.* incredulidad, escepticismo.

disbelieve *v.* desconfiar, dudar.

discard *n.* desecho, descarte; *v.* descartar, desechar.

discharge *n.* flujo; supuración; excreción; descarga; derrame; ___ **summary** / sumario o nota de egreso; *v.* [*fluid, pus*] secretar, supurar; [*from the hospital*] dar de alta; librar; soltar; [*electricity*] descargar.

discipline *n.* disciplina, comportamiento estricto.

discitis *n.* discitis, infl. de un disco.

disclose *v.* revelar, descubrir; destapar, abrir.

discogenic *a.* discogénico, rel. a un disco intervertebral.

discography *n.* discografía, radiografía de un disco vertebral usando un medio de contraste.

discolor *v.* cambiar de color, quitar el color.

discolored *a.* descolorido-a, [*skin*] ensombrecido-a, sin color, empañado-a.

discomfort *n.* incomodidad, malestar, aflicción.

discomposed *a.* descompuesto-a; desordenado-a.

disconnect *v.* desconectar, desunir, quitar la conexión; separar.

disconnected *a.* desconectado-a, separado-a, sin conexión, desunido-a.

discontented *a.* descontento-a; insatisfecho-a; disgustado-a.

discontinue *v.* suspender, interrumpir, descontinuar; **to** ___ **the medication** / ___ la medicina.

discontinued *a.* suspendido-a, interrumpido-a, descontinuado-a.

discourage *v.* desanimar, desalentar; **to** ___ **from** / disuadir.

discouraged *a.* desanimado-a, desalentado-a.

discovery *n.* descubrimiento, revelación.

discredit *v.* desacreditar.

discreet *a.* discreto-a, prudente.

discrepancy *n.* desacuerdo, discrepancia, diferencia.

discretion *n.* discreción, prudencia; acuerdo.

discriminate *v.* discriminar; mostrar prejuicio; hacer notar diferencias.

discrimination *n.* discriminación; diferenciación de raza o cualidad.

discuss *v.* discutir, argumentar.

discussion *n.* discusión, debate, argumento.

disease *n.* enfermedad, dolencia, anomalía; indisposición; **a crippling** ___ / ___ que causa invalidez; **blood** ___ / ___ sanguínea; **bone** ___ / ___ ósea; **cardiac** ___ / ___ cardíaca; **chronic obstructive pulmonary** ___ / ___ pulmonar crónica obstructiva; **coal miner's** ___ / ___ de los mineros; **communicable** ___ / ___ contagiosa;

communicable ___ **control** / control de ___ -es contagiosas; **companion** ___ / ___ concomitante; **functional** ___ / ___ funcional; **gallbladder** ___ / colecistopatía; **heavy chain** ___ / ___ de red o de cadena; **kidney** ___ / nefropatía; **liver** ___ / ___ hepática, renal; **venereal** ___ / ___ venérea; *v.* causar una enfermedad, contagiar, enfermar, dañar, hacer daño.

disease related *n.* relacionado a una enfermedad.

diseased *a.* enfermo-a.

disengage *v.* librar, separar, desplazar.

disengagement *n.* desencajamiento, separación, desunión; [*in obstetrics*] desplazamiento de la cabeza del feto de la vulva.

disfiguration *n.* desfiguración, desfiguramiento.

disfigure *v.* desfigurar, afear.

disillusion *n.* desencanto, desilusión; *v.* perder la ilusión; desilusionarse.

disinfect *v.* desinfectar, esterilizar.

disinfectant *n.* desinfectante, antiséptico, esterilizante.

disinfection *n.* desinfección. 1. proceso de limpieza extensa y eliminación de organismos patógenos; 2. limpieza de control de eliminación diaria de materiales contaminados y destrucción de microorganismos, tal como se hace en hospitales.

disinfestation *n.* desinfestación, limpieza extensa y eliminación de parásitos, rumiantes e insectos causantes de infección.

disintegrate *v.* desintegrar, reducir a fragmentos o partículas; desintegrarse; separarse.

disintegration *n.* desintegración, descomposición, separación.

disjoint *v.* desunir, separar, desarticular.

disjointed *a.* desarticulado-a, descoyuntado-a, dislocado-a.

disjunction *n.* disyunción, desunión, separación de cromosomas en la anafase de la división celular.

disk, disc *n.* disco; **herniated** ___ / ___ herniado; **ruptured** ___ / ruptura del ___ .

dislike *n.* aversión, antipatía; *v.* aborrecer, desagradar, repugnar; **I** ___ **this medicine** / no me gusta, me desagrada, me repugna esta medicina.

dislocate *v.* dislocar, descoyuntar, desencajar.

dislocated *a. pp.* of **to dislocate**; dislocado-a; ___ **shoulder** / luxación del hombro.

dislocation *n.* dislocación, luxación, desviación, desplazamiento de una articulación;

cervical ___ / luxación cervical; **closed** ___ / ___ cerrada; **complicated** ___ / ___ complicada; **congenital** ___ / ___ congénita; **congenital** ___ **of the hip** / ___ congénita de la cadera; **habitual** ___ / ___ recidivante.

dislocation of the lens *n.* desplazamiento del cristalino.

dismember *v.* desmembrar, amputar; [*to break apart*] despedazar.

dismemberment *n.* desmembración, amputación.

dismiss *v.* rechazar; descartar; [*an employee*] despedir.

disobedience *n.* desobediencia.

disobedient *a.* desobediente.

disorder *n.* desorden, desarreglo, trastorno; **mental** ___ / desarreglo emocional, trastorno mental.

disorganized *a.* desorganizado-a.

disorient *v.* desorientar.

disorientation *n.* desorientación, incapacidad de encontrar una dirección o local, de reconocer a otras personas, y de establecer una relación temporal lógica.

disoriented *a.* desorientado-a; confundido-a, confuso-a.

dispensary *n.* dispensario, clínica, establecimiento que proporciona asistencia médica y dispensa medicamentos.

dispense *v.* dispensar; distribuir.

disperse *v.* dispersar, disipar.

dispirited *a.* descorazonado-a, desalentado-a.

displace *v.* desplazar; poner fuera de lugar.

displaced *a.* desplazado-a; dislocado-a; *v.* **to be** ___ / estar fuera de lugar, estar ___ [*bone, joint*] estar dislocado-a.

displacement *n.* desplazamiento; dislocación; transferencia de una emoción a otra distinta de la inicial; ___ **of pelvic bone** / ___ del hueso pélvico.

display *n.* muestra, exhibición, *v.* mostrar, exhibir, extender.

displease *v.* desagradar; incomodar.

displeased *a.* descontento-a; insatisfecho-a.

disposable *a.* desechable.

dispose *v.* disponer; desechar; **to** ___ **of** / deshacerse de.

disposition *n.* disposición; tendencia.

disproportion *n.* desproporción; desproporcionamiento.

disproportionate *a.* desproporcionado-a, desigual, sin simetría.

disprove *v.* refutar.

disregard *v.* ignorar; no prestar atención, descuidar.

disrespect *n.* falta de respeto, irreverencia; *v.* desatender; dejar de respetar, faltar el respeto.

dissect *v.* disecar, acto de dividir y cortar; hacer una disección.

dissecting hook *n.* erina.

dissecting knife *n.* escalpelo, bisturí.

dissection *n.* disección.

disseminated *a.* diseminado-a, difundido-a; ___ **intravascular coagulation** / coagulación intravascular ___ .

dissemination *n.* diseminación, esparcimiento.

dissipation *n.* disipación, vida disipada; dispersión.

dissociation *n.* disociación. 1. acción y efecto de separar; 2. descomposición de un agregado molecular en otros más sencillos; 3. separación inconsciente de la personalidad propia de la esquizofrenia, con efectos que resultan en un trastorno de las asociaciones del pensamiento; **atrial** ___ / ___ atrial; **atrioventricular** ___ / ___ atrioventricular; **pupillary light-near** ___ / ___ pupilar por cercanía de luz; **sleep** ___ / ___ del sueño; **visual-kinetic** ___ / ___ visual quinética.

dissolution *n.* disolución; descomposición; muerte.

dissolve *v.* disolver, diluir, deshacer; destruir.

dissolved *a. pp.* of **to dissolve**, disuelto-a, diluído-a.

dissolvent *a.* disolvente, capaz de disolver.

distal *a.* distal, distante, rel. a la parte más lejana; ___ **end** / extremo ___ .

distance *n.* distancia, lejanía; **at a** ___ / a lo lejos; *v.* **to keep at a** ___ / mantener a ___ .

distaste *n.* aversión, disgusto.

distemper *n.* destemplanza, cualquier trastorno físico o mental.

distend *v.* distender, dilatar; distenderse, dilatarse.

distensibility *n.* distensibilidad, capacidad de una estructura de ser extendida, dilatada o agrandada en tamaño.

distension, distention *n.* distensión, condición de dilatación o expansión.

distill *v.* destilar, crear vapor por medio de calor.

distillation *n.* destilación.

distinct *a.* diferente; definido-a; **-ly** *adv.* definidamente; con diferencia, con precisión.

distinguish *v.* distinguir; diferenciar, clasificar.

distinguished *a.* [*person*] distinguido-a; [*characteristics*] señalado-a, marcado-a.

distobuccal *a.* distobucal, rel. a la superficie distal y bucal de un diente.

distoclusion *n.* distoclusión, mordida irregular.

distort *v.* torcer, deformar, desfigurar.

distorted *a.* torcido-a; deformado-a; desfigurado-a.

distortion *n.* distorsión, deformación, desfiguración.

distract *v.* distraer, interrumpir.

distracted *a.* distraído-a, [*madness*] trastornado-a.

distraction *n.* distracción. 1. inhabilidad para concentrarse en una experiencia determinada; 2. separación de articulaciones sin dislocación.

distraught *a.* atolondrado-a, confundido-a, desconcertado-a; [*irrational*] demente.

distress *n.* angustia, apuro, preocupación, aflicción. *v.* **to be in** ___ / estar angustiado-a, estar afligido-a.

distressed *a.* adolorido-a, angustiado-a, afligido-a.

distribute *v.* distribuir, dispensar, repartir.

distribution *n.* distribución.

distrust *n.* desconfianza, falta de confianza; *v.* desconfiar.

disturb *v.* perturbar, incomodar, molestar, inquietar.

disturbance *n.* confusión, disturbio.

diuresis *n.* diuresis, aumento en la secreción de orina.

diuretic *a.* diurético, rel. a agentes que provocan aumento en la secreción de orina.

diuria *n.* diuria, frecuencia de excreción de orina durante el día.

diver *n.* buzo-a; ___ **'s paralysis** / parálisis de los ___ -s.

divergence *n.* divergencia, separación de un centro común.

divergent *a.* divergente, movimiento en sentido opuesto; ___ **reactor** / reactor de potencia ___ .

diverticulitis *n.* diverticulosis, diverticulitis, infl. de un divertículo, esp. de pequeños sacos que se forman en el colon.

diverticulosis *n.* diverticulosis, formación de divertículos en las paredes del intestino grueso o colon; **degenerative** ___ / ___ degenerativa; **electrolyte** ___ / ___ hidroeléctrica.

diverticulum *n.* (*pl.* **diverticula**) divertículo, saco o bolsa que se origina en la cavidad de un órgano o estructura.

divide *v.* dividir, repartir.

divided *a.* dividido-a, separado-a.

division *n.* división, desunión; separación.

divorce *n.* divorcio, disolución.

divulsion *n.* divulsión, separación o desprendimiento.

dizygotic twins *n., pl.* gemelos dicigóticos, mellizos de embriones producidos por dos óvulos.

dizziness *n.* mareo, sensación de desvanecimiento, vahído.

dizzy *a.* mareado-a.

do *vi. aux.* hacer; ___ **it!** / ,hágalo!,,hazlo!; ___ **not** ___ **it!** / ,No lo haga!, ,no lo hagas!; ___ **you cough a lot?** / ¿Tose mucho?, ¿toses mucho?; **he, she does** / él, ella hace. (Do is not translated in Spanish when used as an auxiliary verb.); **How do you** ___ **?** / ¿cómo está usted?, ¿cómo estás tú? **that will** ___ / eso es suficiente; **to** ___ **away with** / deshacerse de; **to** ___ **harm** / hacer daño; **to** ___ **one's best** / hacer lo mejor posible; **to** ___ **someone good** / mejorar, ayudar a alguien; **to** ___ **without** / pasar sin, prescindir de; **What do you** ___ **?** / ¿Qué hace usted?, ¿qué haces tú?; **whatever you** ___ / cualquier cosa que haga, hagas.

doctor *n.* doctor-a, médico-a; ___ **'s discretion** / al criterio del ___; según opinión facultativa.

document *n.* documento.

documentation *n.* documentación.

doer *n.* hacedor-a, agente, ejecutor-a.

dog *n.* perro-a; ___ **bite** / mordida de ___ .

dolichocephalic *a.* dolicocefálico-a, de cráneo alargado y estrecho.

domestic *a.* doméstico-a.

domiciliary *a.* domiciliario-a, rel. a lo que se trata en el domicilio.

dominance *n.* dominancia, predominio.

dominant *a.* dominante, característica primordial; ___ **characteristics** / características ___ -s, con tendencia a heredarse; ___ **factor** / factor ___ .

donate *v.* donar, regalar.

donation *n.* donativo, donación.

done *a., pp.* of **to do**, hecho, terminado; ___ **for** / gastado-a, destruido-a.

donor *n.* donante, donador; persona contribuyente; ___ **card** / tarjeta de ___ .

Donovania granulomatosis, Donovan's body *n.* Donovania granulomatosis, cuerpos de Donovan, infección bacteriana que afecta la piel y las membranas mucosas de los genitales y el ano.

door *n.* puerta; [*entrance*] ___ de entrada; **back** ___ / ___ de atrás.

dopamine *n.* dopamina, neurotransmisor, sustancia sintetizada por la glándula suprarrenal que aumenta la presión arterial; gen. usada en el tratamiento de choque.

dope *n.* narcótico; ___ **addict** / drogadicto-a; ___ **fiend** / narcómano-a; *v.* dopar, estimar la potencia de la dosis de una droga.

Doppler technique *n.* Doppler, técnica de, técnica de diagnóstico basada en el hecho de que la frecuencia de las ondas ultrasónicas cambia cuando éstas se reflejan en una superficie en movimiento; ___ **echocardiography** / ecocardiografía de ___; ___ **effect** / efecto de ___; ___ **ultrasonography** / ultrasonografía de ___ .

dormancy *n.* sueño pesado, estupor, letargo.

dorsal *a.* dorsal, situado-a en la parte posterior del cuerpo o rel. a ésta; ___ **recumbent position** / posición recumbente; ___ **slit** / fisura o corte ___ .

dorsalgia *n.* dorsalgia, dolor de espalda.

dorsiflexion *n.* dorsiflexión, movimiento de doblar o de doblarse hacia atrás.

dorsocephalad *a.* dorsocefálico-a, situado-a en la parte posterior de la cabeza.

dorsodynia *n.* dorsodinia, dolor en los músculos de la parte superior de la espalda.

dorsolateral *a.* dorsolateral, rel. a la espalda y un costado.

dorsolumbar *a.* dorsolumbar, lumbodorsal, rel. a la espalda y la región lumbar de la columna.

dorsospinal *a.* dorsoespinal, rel. a la espalda y la espina dorsal.

dorsum *n.* (*pl.* **dorsa**) dorso. 1. porción posterior, tal como el dorso de la mano o el pie; 2. espalda.

dose, dosage *n.* dosis, dosificación. 1. cantidad prescrita de medicina u otro agente terapéutico; 2. en medicina nuclear, una cantidad farmacéutica determinada; **absorbed** ___ / ___ de absorción; **average** ___ / ___ promedio, media; **bone marrow** ___ / ___ de la médula ósea; **booster** ___ / ___ de refuerzo; **cumulative** ___ / ___ acumulada; **curative** ___ / ___ curativa; **daily** ___ / ___ diaria; **divided** ___ / ___ dividida; **effective** ___ / ___ efectiva; **equivalent** ___ / ___ equivalente; **exposure** ___ / ___ de exposición; **initial** ___ / ___ inicial; **integral** ___ / ___ integral; **lethal** ___ / ___ letal; **maximal** ___ / ___ máxima; **maximal permissible** ___ / máxima ___ permitida; **maximum tolerated** ___ / ___ máxima tolerable; **minimal** ___ / ___ mínima; **minimal lethal** ___ / ___ letal mínima; **minimal reacting** ___ / ___ reactiva mínima;

optimum __ / __ óptima; **preventive** __ / __ preventiva; **radiation** __ / __ de radiación; **reduction** __ / __ de reducción; **skin** __ / __ dermal; **therapeutic** __ / __ terapéutica; **tolerated** __ / __ tolerada; **unit** __ / __ individual; **volume** __ / __ de volumen.

dosimeter *n.* dosímetro, instrumento usado para detectar y medir la exposición a radiaciones.

dosimetry *n.* dosimetría, determinación precisa y sistemática de las dosis de radiación.

dossier *n.* expediente.

dot *n.* cúmulo, mancha.

dotage *n.* senilidad, chochera, chochez.

double *a.* doble; __ **-edged** / con dos bordes; __ **personality** / desdoblamiento de la personalidad; __ **uterus** / útero didelfo, útero o matriz doble; *v.* duplicar.

doubt *n.* duda, incertidumbre.

douche *n.* 1. ducha, regadera; 2. lavado vaginal; irrigación. *v.* tomar una ducha; ducharse.

Douglas cul-de-sac *n.* saco de Douglas, pliegue del peritoneo que se introduce entre el recto y el útero.

down *adv.* abajo, hacia abajo; __ **below** / más abajo; *v.* **to cut** __ / recortar; reducir; **to lie** __ / acostarse, recostarse.

downcast *a.* deprimido-a, alicaído-a, abatido-a.

downstairs *v.* **to go** __ / bajar las escaleras; *adv.* abajo.

Down syndrome *n.* síndrome de Down, anormalidad citogenética del cromosoma 21 caracterizada por retraso mental y facciones mongoloides.

downtown *n.* centro (de la ciudad).

doze *v.* dormitar, quedarse medio dormido.

dozen *n.* docena.

draft *n.* 1. líquido prescrito para ser tomado en una sola dosis; 2. [*air*] corriente de aire; 3. [*art design*] diseño, bosquejo.

drain *n.* desage, escurridor. *v.* drenar, desaguar, eliminar una secreción o pus de una parte infectada.

drainage *n.* drenaje; **open** __ / __ abierto; **continuous** __ / __ continuo; __ **tube** / tubo de __; **postural** __ / __ postural, por gravedad; **tidal** __ / __ periódico.

Dramamine, dimenhydrinate *n.* Dramamina, dimenhidrinato, anthistamínico usado en el tratamiento de náusea.

dramatism *n.* dramatismo, conducta espectacular y lenguaje dramatizado manifestados en ciertos trastornos mentales.

drape *v.* cubrir el campo operatorio con paños esterilizados.

drastic *a.* drástico-a; __ **therapy** / tratamiento __ .

draw *vi.* extraer, sacar; [*air*] aspirar; [*art*] dibujar, trazar; **to** __ **back** / retroceder; **to** __ **in** / atraer; incitar; **to** __ **near** / acercarse, arrimarse.

drawer *n.* gaveta, cajón.

dream *n.* sueño, ilusión. *v.* soñar, imaginar, hacerse ilusiones.

dreary *a.* monótono-a, escabroso-a, pesado-a.

drenched *a.* empapado-a, mojado-a.

drepanocyte *n.* drepanocito, glóbulo rojo de células falciformes.

dress *n.* vestido. *v.* [*a wound*] vendar, curar; [*a corpse*] amortajar; [*put on clothes*] vestirse.

dressing *n.* apósito o vendaje, venda de gasa u otro material para cubrir una herida; **adhesive, absorbent** __ / __ adhesivo, absorbente; **antiseptic** __ / __ antiséptico; **dry** __ / __ seco; **fixed** __ / __ fijo; **occlusive** __ / __ oclusivo; **pressured** __ / __ presionado; **removable** __ / __ desechable; **tie-over** __ / __ amarrado; **wet** __ / __ humedecido.

dribble *n.* goteo.

drill *n.* taladro; [*dentistry*] fresa.

drink *n.* bebida, trago. *v.* beber, tomar.

drinker *a.* bebedor, tomador.

drip *n.* gota, goteo; gotera; **postnasal** __ / __ postnasal; *v.* gotear.

drive *n.* paseo, vuelta; impulso; [*haste*] exigencia; [*energy*] energía, vigor; *v.* **to go for a** __ / dar un paseo; *vi.* [*vehicles*] conducir, manejar, guiar; **to** __ **someone crazy** / enloquecer, volver loco-a.

drivel *n.* baba o saliva que sale por los extremos de la boca.

dromotropic *a.* dromotrópico-a, que afecta la conductividad de una fibra muscular o nerviosa.

drop *n.* gota; caída; __ **by** __ / gota a gota; *v.* dejar caer; [*from school*] dejar la escuela; caerse.

droplet *n.* partícula, gotica; __ **infection** / infección trasmitida por goticas o partículas.

dropper *n.* gotero.

dropsy *n.* hidropesía, acumulación excesiva de fluido seroso en una cavidad o tejido celular.

drought *n.* sequía.

drown *v.* ahogar; anegar; sumergir; sofocar; ahogarse.

drowning *n.* ahogamiento, acción de ahogar o ahogarse.

drowse *v.* adormecerse, adormitarse.

drowsiness *n.* sopor, somnolencia, abotagamiento, pesadez.

drug *n.* droga, medicamento, narcótico, barbitúrico; ___ **abuse** / uso excesivo de una ___ por adicción; ___ **addict** / narcómano-a, drogadicto-a; ___ **-induced abnormality** / anomalía causada por el uso de ___ -s; ___ **interactions** / interacciones de medicamentos; ___ **resistance, microbial** / resistencia microbiana a las ___ -s; **long acting** ___ / ___ de acción prolongada.

drugged *a.* endrogado-a, drogado-a.

drunk *n.* borracho-a, ebrio-a.

drunkenness *n.* borrachera, embriaguez.

dry *a.* seco-a; árido-a; *v.* secar; ___ **abscess** / absceso ___; ___ **cough** / tos ___; ___ **gangrene** / gangrena ___; **to** ___ **out** / secarse.

dryness *n.* sequedad; aridez.

duck *n.* ánade, pato.

duct *n.* conducto, canal; **biliary** ___ / ___ biliar; **common bile** / colédoco; **cystic** ___ / ___ cístico; **deferent** ___ / ___ defrente; **ejaculatory** ___ / ___ eyaculatorio; **excretory** ___ / ___ excretorio; **hepatic** ___ / ___ hepático; **lacrimal** ___ / ___ lacrimal; **lactiferous** ___ / ___ lactífero; **lymphatic** ___ / ___ linfático; **mullerian** ___ / ___ mullerian; **nasolacrimal** ___ / ___ nasolagrimal; **lacrimal** ___ / ___ lacrimal; **mammary** ___ / ___ mamario; **seminal** ___ / ___ seminal; **seminiferous tubule** ___ / ___ seminífero. See chart on page 80.

ductal *a.* rel. a un conducto o canal.

ductile *a.* dúctil, que tiene la propiedad de admitir deformaciones sin romperse.

ductule *n.* túbulo, conducto pequeño.

dues *n., pl.* deuda; obligación.

dull *a.* aburrido-a; [*pain*] dolor sordo; [*blade*] mellado-a.

dullness *n.* 1. matidez, resonancia disminuída en la palpación; 2. estado de aburrimiento, torpeza, estupidez; 3. [*instrument's edge*] melladura.

dumb *a.* mudo-a; torpe, estúpido-a.

dumping syndrome *n.* síndrome de vaciamiento gástrico demasiado rápido del contenido estomacal en el intestino delgado.

duodenal *a.* duodenal, rel. al duodeno.

duodenal ulcer *n.* úlcera duodenal.

duodenectomy *n.* duodenectomía, excisión del duodeno o una parte de éste.

duodenitis *n.* duodenitis, infl. del duodeno.

duodenoenterostomy *n.* duodenoenterostomía, anastomosis entre el duodeno y el intestino delgado.

duodenography *n.* duodenografía, radiografía del duodeno.

duodenojejunostomy *n.* duodenoyeyunostomía, operación para construir un pasaje artificial entre el yeyuno y el duodeno.

duodenoplasty *n.* duodenoplastia, operación para reparar el duodeno.

duodenostomy *n.* duodenostomía, creación de una salida en el duodeno, para aliviar la estenosis del píloro.

duodenum *n.* duodeno, parte esencial del canal alimenticio y del intestino delgado situado entre el píloro y el yeyuno.

duplication *n.* doblez, pliegue; duplicación.

dura mater *n.* duramadre, membrana externa que cubre el encéfalo y la médula espinal.

durability *n.* durabilidad, duración.

durable *a.* durable, duradero-a; estable.

duration *n.* duración, continuación.

duress *n.* coerción; coacción, **under** ___ / bajo ___ .

during *prep.* durante; mientras, entre tanto.

dust *n.* polvo; [*mortal remains*] cenizas, restos mortales; ___ **count** / conteo de partículas de ___ en el aire.

duty *n.* deber, obligación; [*tax*] impuesto; **on** ___ / de guardia.

dwarf *n.* enano-a, persona de estatura inferior a la normal; **achondroplastic** ___ / ___ acondroplástico-a; **asexual** ___ / ___ asexual; **infantile** ___ / ___ infantil; **micrometic** ___ / ___ micromético-a.

dwarfism *n.* enanismo, insuficiencia del desarrollo en el crecimiento de una persona.

dye *n.* tinte, color saturado; colorante.

dying *a.* moribundo-a, agonizante, mortal.

dynamic cardiomyoplastia *n.* cardiomioplastia dinámica, intervención que se lleva a cabo en pacientes clasificados bajo cardiopatía clase III que han sufrido fallo cardíaco o que padecen de isquemia cardíaca.

dynamics *n.* dinámica, estudio de órganos o partes del cuerpo en movimiento.

dyne *n.* unidad de fuerza necesaria para acelerar un gramo de masa un centímetro por segundo.

dysacousia, dysacusia *n.* disacusis, disacusia, trastorno o dificultad para oír.

dysaphia *n.* disafia, entorpecimiento del sentido del tacto.

dysarthria *n.* disartria, dificultad del habla a causa de una afección de la lengua u otro músculo esencial al lenguaje.

dysautonomy, dysautonomia *n.*
disautonomía, trastorno del sistema nervioso autónomo.

dysbarism *n.* disbarismo, condición causada por descompresión.

dyscalculia *n.* discalculia, incapacidad de resolver problemas matemáticos debido a una anomalía cerebral.

dyscephalia *n.* discefalia, malformación de la cabeza y los huesos de la cara.

dyschiria *n.* disquiria, incapacidad de percibir sensaciones táctiles en ciertas áreas.

dyscoria *n.* discoria, pupila deformada.

dyscrasia *n.* discrasia, sinónimo de enfermedad.

dyscrinism *n.* discrinismo, funcionamiento anormal en la producción de secreciones, esp. de las glándulas endocrinas.

dysdiadochokinesia *n.* disdiadocoquinesia, alteración de la función de detener un impulso motor y substituirlo por otro diametralmente opuesto.

dysentery *n.* disentería, condición inflamatoria del intestino grueso causada por bacilos o parásitos con síntomas de diarrea y dolor abdominal; **amebic___ / ___** amebiana; **bacillar___ / ___** bacilar.

dysergia *n.* disergia, falta de coordinación en los movimientos musculares voluntarios.

dysesthesia *n.* disestesia, reacción excesiva de molestia a algunas sensaciones que por lo común no producen dolor.

dysfunction *n.* desorden, trastorno, malfuncionamiento de un órgano o parte.

dysgenesis *n.* disgénesis, defecto, malformación hereditaria.

dysgerminoma *n.* disgerminoma, tumor maligno del ovario.

dysgnosia *n.* disgnosia, cualquier impedimento relacionado con el intelecto.

dyshidrosis *n.* dishidrosis. 1. trastorno transpiratorio; 2. erupción recurrente de vesículas y picazón tal como en el pie de atleta.

dyskinesia *n.* discinesia, disquinesia, inhabilidad de realizar movimientos voluntarios tal como sucede en la enfermedad de Parkinson.

dyslalia *n.* dislalia, impedimento en el habla debido a trastornos vocálicos funcionales.

dyslexia *n.* dislexia, impedimento en la lectura, dificultad que puede ser una condición hereditaria o causada por una lesión cerebral.

dysmenorrhea, dysmenorrhoea *n.* dismenorrea, menstruación difícil, acompañada de dolor y trastornos.

dysmetria *n.* dismetría, afección del cerebelo que incapacita el control de la distancia en movimientos musculares.

dysmetropsia *n.* dismetropsia, defecto en la apreciación visual del tamaño y forma de objetos.

dysmnesia *n.* dismnesia, trastorno de la memoria.

dysmorphism *n.* dismorfismo, malformación anatómica.

dysmyotonia *n.* dismiotonía, distonía muscular con tonicidad muscular anormal.

dysosmia *n.* disosmia, malfuncionamiento de la función olfatoria.

dysostosis *n.* disostosis, desarrollo deficiente de los huesos y dientes.

dyspareunia *n.* dispareunia, relaciones sexuales dolorosas.

dyspepsia *n.* dispepsia, indigestión caracterizada por irregularidades digestivas tales como eructos, náuseas, acidez, flatulencia y pérdida del apetito.

dyspermia *n.* dispermia, dolor durante la eyaculación.

dysphagia *n.* disfagia, dificultad al tragar a causa de una obstrucción; **esophageal ___ / ___** esofágica; **oropharyngeal ___ / ___** orofaríngea.

dysphasia *n.* disfasia, defecto del habla causado por una lesión cerebral.

dysphonia *n.* disfonía, ronquera.

dysphoria *n.* disforia, excesiva depresión o angustia.

dyspigmentation *n.* despigmentación, decoloración anormal de la piel y del pelo.

dysplasia *n.* displasia, cambio o desarrollo anormal de los tejidos.

dysplastic *a.* displásico-a, pertaining to dysplasia.

dyspnea, dyspnoea *n.* disnea, dificultad en la respiración; **exertional ___ / ___** por esfuerzo.

dyspneic *a.* disneico-a, rel. a o que padece de disnea.

dyspraxia *n.* dispraxia, impedimento o dolor al realizar cualquier movimiento coordinado.

dysreflexia *n.* disrreflexia, condición por la cual las reacciones a estímulos son inapropiadas o fuera de orden.

dysrhythmia *n.* disritmia, sin coordinación o ritmo.

dysstasia *n.* distasia, dificultad de mantenerse en pie.

dyssynergia *n.* disinergia. V. **ataxia.**

dystocia *n.* distocia, parto difícil, laborioso.

dystonia *n.* distonía, tonicidad alterada, esp. muscular.

dystrophy *n.* distrofia. 1. anomalía causada por desnutrición; 2. desarrollo defectuoso o de malformación.

dysuria *n.* disuria, dificultad o dolor al orinar.

d

e

E *abbr.* **emmetropia** / emetropía; **enema** / enema; **enzyme** / enzima; **eye** / ojo.

each *a.* cada; todo; cualquier-a; *pron.* cada uno, cada una; cada cual.

eager *a.* ansioso-a, deseoso-a; impaciente.

ear *n.* oreja; oído, órgano de la audición formado por el oído interior, el medio, y el externo;___ **ache** / dolor de oídos, otalgia; ___ **canal** / conducto auditivo; ___ **cup** / audífono; ___ **discharge** / otorrea; ___ **drops** / gotas para los oídos; ___ **infection** / infección auditiva; ___ **injury** / oído lastimado, lesión auditiva; ___ **lap** / pabellón de la oreja; ___ **lobe** / lóbulo de la oreja; ___ **lobe crease** / pliegue del lóbulo del oído; ___ **plug** / tapón auditivo; ___ **protector** / orejera; ___ **specialist** / otólogo, audiólogo; ___ **wax** / cerumen; *a.* ___ **deafening** / ensordecedor-a. See illustration on this page.

earache *n.* dolor de oído.

eardrum *n.* tímpano del oído.

early *adv.* temprano, pronto; **as** ___ **as possible** / lo más ___ posible; **at the earliest** / lo más ___; ___ **age** / infancia; ___ **cancer** / cáncer incipiente; ___ **childhood** / primera infancia; ___ **death** / muerte prematura; ___ **morning** / madrugada; ___ **pregnancy** / principio del embarazo; ___ **stage of** / la primera fase de, al principio de.

earn *v.* ganar, merecer.

earphone *n.* auricular, audífono.

earthquake *n.* terremoto, temblor de tierra, sismo.

earthworm *n.* lombriz de tierra; gusano.

ease *n.* alivio; descanso; facilidad; *v.* aliviar, facilitar; **to** ___ **one's mind** / tranquilizarse.

easily *adv.* fácilmente, sin dificultad.

east *n.* este, oriente; **to the** ___ / al ___ .

easy *a.* fácil; **within** ___ **reach** / al alcance de la mano.

easygoing *a.* sereno-a, tranquilo-a, de buena disposición.

eat *vi.* comer, sustentarse, ingerir alimentos; **to** ___ **breakfast** / desayunarse, tomar el

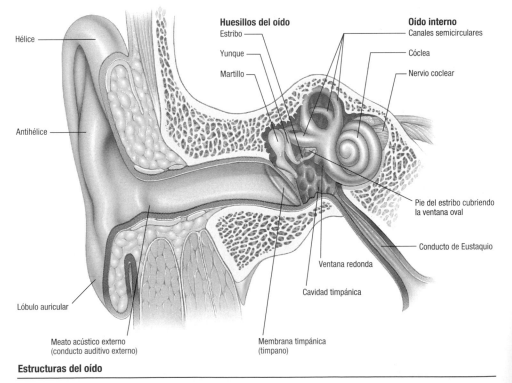

Hélice

Antihélice

Lóbulo auricular

Meato acústico externo
(conducto auditivo externo)

Huesillos del oído
Estribo
Yunque
Martillo

Membrana timpánica
(timpano)

Ventana redonda

Cavidad timpánica

Oído interno
Canales semicirculares
Cóclea
Nervio coclear

Pie del estribo cubriendo la ventana oval

Conducto de Eustaquio

Estructuras del oído

desayuno; **to ___ lunch** / almorzar; tomar el almuerzo; **to ___ supper** / cenar;

eating *n.* acto de comer; *a.* rel. a comer o para comer.

ebullient *a.* hirviente; **___ water** / agua ___ .

ebullition *n.* ebullición, acto de hervir.

eccentric *a.* excéntrico-a; extravagante.

ecchymosis *n.* equimosis, *pop.* morado, moratón. 1. cambio de color de la piel de azulado a verde debido a extravasación de sangre en el tejido subcutáneo celular; 2. hematoma.

eccrine sweat glands *n.* glándulas sudoríparas ecrinas, secretoras de la transpiración.

echinococcosis *n.* equinococosis, infestación de equinococos; **hepatic ___** / ___ hepática;

Echinococcus *n.* Equinococo, especie de tenia o trematodo.

echo *n.* eco, repercusión del sonido; *v.* **to ___** / hacer eco.

echocardiogram *n.* ecocardiograma, gráfico producido por una ecocardiografía.

echocardiography *n.* ecocardiografía, método de diagnóstico por sonido ultrasónico para hacer visuales estructuras internas del corazón.

echoencephalography *n.* ecoencefalografía, técnica de diagnóstico por medio de ultrasonido para examinar estructuras intracraneales.

echogram *n.* ecograma, registro de una ecografía.

echography *n.* ecografía. V. **ultrasonography**.

echolalia *n.* ecolalia, trastorno de repetición involuntaria de sonidos y palabras después de oírlas.

Echo virus *n.* Echo virus, virus presente en el tracto gastrointestinal asociado con la meningitis, enteritis e infecciones respiratorias agudas.

eclampsia *n.* eclampsia, desorden convulsivo tóxico que se presenta gen. al final del embarazo o pocos días después del parto.

eclamptic *a.* eclámptico-a, rel. a la eclampsia.

ecology *n.* ecología, estudio de plantas y animales en relación con el ambiente.

economic *a.* económico-a; módico-a, moderado-a.

ecosystem *n.* ecosistema, microcosmo ecológico.

ecstasy *n.* éxtasis, trance acompañado de un sentimiento de placer.

ectopic pregnancy *n.* embarazo ectópico, gestación fuera del útero.

ectoplasm *n.* ectoplasma, capa externa del citoplasma en una célula viva.

ectopy *n.* ectopia, desplazamiento de un órgano, condición gen. congénita.

ectropion *n.* ectropión, anomalía de eversión congénita o adquirida, gen. vista en la comisura del párpado.

eczema *n.* eczema, infección cutánea inflamatoria no contagiosa.

edema *n.* edema, acumulación anormal de líquido en los tejidos intracelulares; **angioneurotic ___** / ___ angioneurótico; **brain ___** / ___ cerebral; **cardiac ___** / ___ cardíaco; **dependent ___** / ___ dependiente; **pitting ___** / ___ de fóvea; **pulmonary ___** / ___ pulmonar.

edematous *a.* edematoso-a, rel. a un edema o afectado por éste.

edentulous *n.* desdentado, sin dientes.

edetate, calcium disodium *n.* disodio de calcio, agente usado en el tratamiento de envenenamiento por plomo.

edge *n.* borde, orilla, canto; [*of cutting instruments*] filo; **on ___** / irritable, impaciente, nervioso-a.

edible *a.* comestible; edible.

educate *v.* educar, enseñar, instruir.

education *n.* educación, enseñanza; **medical ___** / ___ médica.

effacement *n.* borradura, deformación de las características de un órgano tal como la del cuello uterino durante el parto.

effect *n.* efecto, impresión, resultado; *v.* **to carry into ___** / llevar a cabo; **to this ___** / en este sentido; **in ___** / en ___ , en realidad; **no ___** / sin ___ .

effective *a.* efectivo-a.

effectiveness *n.* eficacia, efectividad.

effector *n.* efector, terminación nerviosa que produce un efecto eferente en una glándula de secreción o en una célula muscular.

effeminate *a.* afeminado, *pop.* invertido-a.

efferent *a.* eferente, de fuerza centrífuga; **___ arterioles** / arteriolas ___; **___ nerves** / nervios ___; **___ neurons** / neuronas ___ -es.

effervescence *n.* efervescencia, producción de burbujas.

effervescent *a.* efervescente, que produce efervescencia.

efficacious, efficient *a.* eficaz, eficiente, competente.

efficiency *n.* eficiencia, competencia.

efficient *a.* eficiente; **-ly** *adv.* eficientemente.

effluent *a.* efluente, que tiene salida de dentro hacia afuera.

effort *n.* esfuerzo, empeño; *v.* **to make every** —— **to** / hacer todo lo posible por.

effortless *a.* fácil, sin esfuerzo.

effusion *n.* efusión, derrame, escape de líquido a una cavidad o tejido; **pericardial** —— / —— pericardial; **pleural** —— / —— pleural.

egg *n.* huevo; *Mex.* blanquillos; —— **cell** / óvulo; —— **-shaped** / ovoide; —— **white** / clara de ——; —— **yolk** / yema de ——; **fried** —— / huevo frito; **hard-boiled** —— / huevo duro; **soft-boiled** —— / —— pasado por agua.

eggplant *n.* berenjena.

eggshell *n.* cáscara de huevo.

ego *n.* ego, el yo; la conciencia humana; término freudiano que se refiere a la parte de la psique mediadora entre la persona y la realidad.

egocentric *a.* egocéntrico-a, concentrado-a en si mismo-a.

egoism *n.* egoísmo.

egomania *n.* egomanía, concentración excesiva en sí mismo-a.

ego-syntonic *a.* egosintónico-a, en armonía o correspondencia con el ego.

either *a., pron.* uno-a u otro-a; *conj.* o; *adv.* también; [*after negation*] tampoco.

ejaculate *v.* eyacular, expeler.

ejaculation *n.* eyaculación, expulsión rápida y súbita tal como la emisión del semen.

ejaculatory duct *n.* conducto eyaculatorio.

ejection *n.* eyección, acto de expulsar con fuerza.

elaborate *a.* elaborado-a, complejo-a, detallado-a; *a.* relacionado con un método complejo de hacer algo; **an elaborate operation** / una operación compleja, elaborada; *v.* elaborar, explicar en detalle.

elastase *n.* elastasa, enzima que cataliza la digestión de las fibras elásticas, esp. en el jugo pancreático.

elastic *n.* elástico, cinta de goma; *a.* elástico-a, capaz de extenderse y de volver luego a la forma inicial; —— **tissue** / tejido —— .

elasticity *n.* elasticidad, habilidad de expandirse.

elastinase *n.* elastinasa. V. **elastase**.

elation *n.* estado de exaltación o euforia, caracterizado por excitación física y mental.

elbow *n.* codo; —— **joint** / coyuntura del ——; —— **room** / espacio suficiente; **tennis** —— / —— de tenista.

elder *a.* mayor, de más edad; anciano-a; antepasados, los mayores.

elderly *adv.* de avanzada edad.

eldest *a. sup.* el mayor, la mayor.

elect *v.* elegir, escoger.

elective *a.* electivo-a, elegido-a; —— **surgery** / cirugía —— , planeada; —— **therapy** / terapia —— .

electric *a.* eléctrico-a; —— **current** / corriente ——; —— **eye** / ojo mágico, ojo —— .

electrical *a.* eléctrico-a.

electricity *n.* electricidad.

electrocardiogram *n.* electrocardiograma, gráfico de cambios eléctricos que se producen durante las contracciones del músculo cardíaco.

electrocardiograph *n.* electrocardiógrafo, instrumento para registrar las variaciones eléctricas del músculo cardíaco en acción.

electrocauterization *n.* electrocauterización, destrucción de tejidos por medio de una corriente eléctrica.

electroconvulsive therapy *n.* terapéutica de choque, electrochoque, tratamiento de ciertos desórdenes mentales con aplicación de corriente eléctrica al cerebro.

electrodiagnosis *n.* electrodiagnosis, el uso de instrumentos electrónicos para uso de diagnóstico.

electroencephalogram *n.* electroencefalograma, registro obtenido de una encefalografía.

electroencephalography *n.* electroencefalografía, gráfico descriptivo de la actividad eléctrica desarrollada en el cerebro.

electrolysis *n.* electrolisis, descomposición de una sustancia por medio de una corriente eléctrica.

electrolyte *n.* electrolito, ion que conduce una carga eléctrica.

electrolyzation *n.* electrolización, descomposición por electricidad.

electromagnetic *a.* electromagnético-a; —— **spectrum** / espectro —— .

electromyogram *n.* electromiograma, reporte gráfico por medio de una electromiografía.

electromyography *n.* electromiografía. 1. grabación de la actividad eléctrica generada en un músculo para uso de diagnóstico; 2. estudio de laboratorio sobre electrodiagnóstico que incluye no sólo la electromiografía sino también estudios sobre la conducción de los nervios.

electronic *a.* electrónico-a.

electron microscope *n.* microscopio electrónico, microscopio visual y fotográfico en el cual los rayos electrónicos poseen la longitud de onda miles de veces más corta que la luz visible. La capacidad de resolución y magnificación de este microscopio permite la ampliación máxima de objetos muy pequeños.

electrophoresis *n.* electroforesis, movimiento de partículas coloidales en un medio que, al someterse a una corriente eléctrica, las separa, tal como ocurre con la separación de proteínas en el plasma.

electrophysiology *n.* electrofisiología, estudio de la relación entre procesos fisiológicos afectados por fenómenos eléctricos.

electrosurgery *n.* electrocirugía, uso de electricidad en procesos quirúrgicos.

electrosurgical *a.* electroquirúrgico-a; ___ **destruction of lesions** / destrucción ___ de lesiones.

electroversion *n.* electroversión, cesación de una disrritmia cardíaca por un medio eléctrico.

element *n.* elemento, componente.

elementary *a.* elemental; rudimentario-a.

elephantiasis *n.* elefantiasis, enfermedad crónica caracterizada por obstrucción de los vasos linfáticos e hipertrofia de la piel y tejido celular subcutáneo que afecta gen. las extremidades inferiores y los órganos genitales externos.

elevate *v.* elevar, levantar, alzar.

elevation *n.* elevación; altura.

elevator *n.* elevador. 1. instrumento quirúrgico que se usa para levantar partes hendidas o para extirpar tejido óseo; 2. ascensor.

eligible *a.* elegible, electivo-a.

eliminate *v.* eliminar, expeler del organismo; suprimir.

elimination *n.* eliminación; exclusión.

elimination diet *n.* dieta de eliminación, una dieta reguladora del tipo de alimentos que el paciente debe ingerir después de detectar los ingredientes que pueden producirle una reacción alérgica y retirarlos de la dieta habitual.

elixir *n.* elixir, licor dulce y aromático que contiene un ingrediente medicinal activo.

elliptocyte *n.* eliptocito, eritrocito, célula roja ovalada.

elongated *a.* alargado-a, estirado-a, como el sistema de las vías digestivas.

else *a.* otro-a; más; **anyone** ___ / alguien más; **anything** ___ / algo más; **nothing** ___ / nada más; **Who** ___ **needs help?** / ¿Quién más necesita ayuda?

elsewhere *adv.* en otra parte, a otra parte.

emaciated *a.* enflaquecido-a; excesivamente delgado-a.

emasculation *n.* emasculación; castración; mutilación.

embalm *v.* embalsamar.

embalming *n.* embalsamamiento, preservación del cuerpo después de la muerte por medio de sustancias químicas.

embarrass *v.* avergonzar, trastornar, turbar, interferir, desconcertar.

embolism *n.* embolismo, embolia, oclusión súbita de un vaso por un coágulo, placa o aire; **cerebral** ___ / ___ cerebral; **pulmonary** ___ / ___ pulmonar.

embolus *n.* émbolo, coágulo u otro tipo de materia que, al circular a través de la corriente sanguínea, se aloja en un vaso de menor diámetro.

embrace *n.* abrazo; *v.* abrazar; [*each other*] abrazarse.

embryo *n.* embrión. 1. fase primitiva de desarrollo del ser humano desde la concepción hasta la séptima semana; 2. organismo en la fase primitiva de desarrollo.

embryology *n.* embriología, estudio del embrión y su desarrollo hasta el momento del nacimiento.

embryonic *a.* embriónico-a, embrional.

emerge *v.* brotar, emerger, surgir.

emergency *n.* emergencia, urgencia; **an** ___ **case** / un caso de ___; ___ **care** / servicio de ___; ___ **childbirth** / nacimiento repentino; ___ **medical identification bracelets** / brazaletes para identificación médica de ___; ___ **operation** / intervención quirúrgica de urgencia; ___ **room** / sala de ___; ___ **tracheostomy** / traqueotomía de urgencia.

emetic *a.* emético-a, que estimula el vómito.

emetine *n.* emetina, droga emética y antiamébica.

emigration *n.* emigración o migración, escape tal como el de leucocitos a través de las paredes de los capilares y las venas.

eminence *n.* eminencia o prominencia, forma de elevación semejante a la de la superficie de un hueso.

emission *n.* emisión, salida de líquido; derrame; **nocturnal** ___ / ___ nocturna, escape involuntario de semen durante el sueño.

emit *v.* emitir, descargar; manifestar una opinión.

emollient *a.* emoliente, que suaviza la piel o mucosas interiores.

emotion *n.* emoción, sentimiento intenso.

emotional *a.* emocional, rel. a las emociones; ___ **disturbances** / síntomas afectivos; ___ **life** / vida afectiva.

emotive *a.* emotivo-a.

empathy *n.* empatía, comprensión y apreciación de los sentimientos de otra persona.

emphasis *n.* énfasis; acentuación.

emphatic *a.* enfático-a, acentuado-a, marcado-a.

emphysema *n.* enfisema, enfermedad crónica pulmonar en la cual los alvéolos pulmonares se distienden y los tejidos localizados entre los mismos se atrofian y dificultan el proceso respiratorio.

emphysematous *a.* enfisematoso-a, rel. al enfisema.

empiric *a.* empírico-a, que se basa en observaciones prácticas.

emplacement *n.* colocación, ubicación.

employ *v.* emplear, ocupar.

employee *n.* empleado-a.

employment *n.* empleo, ocupación.

empty *a.* vacío-a, desocupado-a; *v.* vaciar, desocupar; **to ___ itself** / vaciarse, desocuparse.

empyema *n., L. (pl.* **empyemato)** empiema, acumulación de pus en una cavidad, esp. la cavidad torácica.

emulsifier *n.* emulsionador.

emulsify *v.* emulsionar, convertir en emulsión.

emulsion *n.* emulsión, mezcla de dos líquidos, uno de los cuales permanece suspendido.

enamel *n.* esmalte, sustancia dura que protege la dentina del diente.

enarthrosis *n.* enartrosis, forma ósea en la que la cabeza del hueso hace cabida dentro de la cavidad redondeada del otro hueso, como en la articulación de la cadera.

encephalalgia *n.* encefalalgia, dolor de cabeza intenso.

encephalic *a.* encefálico-a, rel. al encéfalo o cerebro.

encephalitis *n.* encefalitis, infl. del encéfalo; **acute hemorrhagic ___** / **___** aguda hemorrágica; **acute necrotizing ___** / **___** aguda necrotizante; **bacterial ___** / **___** bacteriana; **epidemic ___** / **___** epidémica; **experimental allergic ___** / **___** experimental alérgica; **herpes ___** / **___** herpética; **lethargic ___** / **___** letárgica; **neonatorum ___** / **___** del recién nacido; **purulent ___** / **___** purulenta; **pyogenic ___** / **___** piogénica; **suppurative ___** / **___** supurativa.

encephalocele *n.* encefalocele, hernia del encéfalo, protrusión del encéfalo a través de una abertura congénita o traumática en el cráneo.

encephalography *n.* encefalografía, examen radiográfico del cerebro.

encephaloma *n.* encefaloma, tumor del encéfalo.

encephalomalacia *n.* encefalomalacia, reblandecimiento del encéfalo.

encephalomyelitis *n.* encefalomielitis, infl. del encéfalo y de la médula espinal.

encephalon *n.* encéfalo, porción del sistema nervioso contenido en el cráneo.

encephalopathy *n.* encefalopatía, cualquier enfermedad cerebral.

enchondroma *n.* encondroma, tumor que se desarrolla en un hueso.

encircle *v.* rodear, circundar.

enclose *v.* encerrar, cercar; [*in a letter*] incluir, adjuntar.

enclosed *a. pp.* of **to enclose**, [*in a letter*] incluido-a, adjunto-a.

encopresis *n.* encopresis, incontinencia de heces fecales.

encounter *n.* encuentro; *v.* encontrar, salir al encuentro.

encourage *v.* alentar, animar.

encouragement *n.* aliento, incentivo.

encysted *a.* enquistado-a, que se encuentra envuelto en un saco o quiste.

end *n.* fin, término, extremidad; extremo; [*aim*] objetivo; **at the ___ of** / al extremo de; [*date*] a fines de; **To what ? ___** / ¿Con qué ___ ?; *a.* terminal, final; **___ artery** / arteria terminal; **___ organ** / órgano terminal.

endanger *v.* poner en peligro. *v.* arriesgarse.

endangered *a. pp.* of **to endanger.** 1. puesto en peligro; 2. en peligro de extinción.

endarterectomy *n.* endarterectomía, extirpación de la túnica interna (íntima) engrosada de una arteria.

endarteritis *n.* endarteritis, infl. de la túnica (íntima) de una arteria.

endbrain *n.* telencéfalo, porción o parte del sistema nervioso que comprende la corteza cerebral, el cuerpo calloso, el cuerpo estriado y el rinencéfalo.

endeavor *n.* empeño, esfuerzo.

endemic *a.* endémico-a, rel. a una enfermedad que permanece por un tiempo indefinido en una comunidad o región; **___ area** / área ___; **___ disease** / enfermedad ___ .

endemoepidemic *n.* endemoepidemia, término que indica un aumento de casos de una enfermedad endémica.

ending *n.* final; terminación, conclusión.

endless *a.* interminable, inacabable, sin fin.

endocarditis *n.* endocarditis, infl. aguda o crónica del endocardio; **acute bacterial ___** / **___** aguda bacteriana; **bacterial ___** / **___** bacteriana; **chronic ___** / **___** crónica; **constrictive ___** / **___** constrictiva;

infectious ___ / ___ infecciosa;
malignant ___ / ___ maligna;
mucomembranous ___ / ___ mucomembranosa;
rheumatic ___ / ___ reumática; **subacute
bacterial**___ / ___ subaguda bacteriana;
tuberculous ___ / ___ tuberculosa;
valvular___ / ___ valvular;
vegetative ___ / ___ vegetativa.

endocardium *n.* (*pl.* **endocardia**) endocardio, membrana serosa interior del corazón.

endocervix *n.* endocérvix, mucosa glandular del cuello uterino.

endocrine *a.* endocrino-a, rel. a secreciones internas y a las glándulas que las producen.

endocrine glands *n.* glándulas endocrinas, glándulas que segregan hormonas directamente en la corriente sanguínea (gónadas, pituitaria y suprarrenales).

endocrinologist *n.* endocrinólogo, especialista en endocrinología.

endocrinology *n.* endocrinología, estudio de las glándulas endocrinas y las hormonas segregadas por éstas.

endoderm *n.* endodermo, la más interna de las tres membranas del embrión.

endogenous *a.* endógeno-a, que ocurre debido a factores internos del organismo.

endolymph *n.* endolinfa, fluido contenido en el laberinto membranoso del oído.

endolymphatic duct *n.* conducto endolinfático localizado en el oído.

endometrial *a.* endometrial, rel. al endometrio; ___ **biopsy** / biopsia ___ .

endometrioma *n.* endometrioma, tumor constituído por tejido endometrial.

endometriosis *n.* endometriosis, trastorno por el cual tejido similar al del endometrio se manifiesta en otras partes fuera del útero.

endometritis *n.* endometritis, infl. de la mucosa uterina.

endometrium *n.* endometrio, membrana mucosa interior del útero.

endomorph *a.* endomorfo-a, de torso más pronunciado que las extremidades.

endophlebitis *n.* endoflebitis, infl. de la íntima de una vena.

endophthalmitis, endophthalmia *n.* endoftalmitis, infl. de los tejidos interiores del globo ocular, la cual puede ser causada por una reacción alérgica, la reacción a una droga o una reacción bacteriológica. El ojo se enrojece, se infecta, y a veces tiene pus. Otros síntomas que pueden manifestarse son vómito, fiebre

(calentura) y dolor de cabeza; ___ **ophthalmia
nodose** / ___ oftalmia nodular; ___
phacoanaphylactica / ___ facoanafiláctica;
granulomatous ___ / ___ granulomatosa.

endoplasmic *a.* endoplásmico-a. rel. al endoplasma.

endoplasmic reticulum *n.* retículo endoplásmico, sistema de canales en los cuales se llevan a cabo las funciones de anabolismo y catabolismo de la célula.

end organ *n.* órgano terminal.

endorphins *n., pl.* endorfinas, sustancias químicas naturales del cerebro a las que se le atribuye la propiedad de aliviar el dolor.

endorse *v.* apoyar, endosar.

endoscope *n.* endoscopio, instrumento usado para examinar un órgano o una cavidad interior hueca.

endoscopic *a.* endoscópico-a, rel. a la endoscopía.

endoscopy *n.* endoscopía, examen interior hecho con el endoscopio.

endostatin assay *n.* análisis endostático, un método para confirmar la diagnosis de ántrax por medio de una reacción de precipitación que indica la presencia del antígeno de calor-estable del *Bacillus antraxis* en el tejido extraído.

endosteum *n.* (*pl.* **endostea**) endostio, células localizadas en la cavidad medular central de los huesos y sirven de cobertura a la superficie interior del hueso.

endothelial *a.* endotelial, rel. al endotelio.

endothelium *n.* (*pl.* **endothelia**) endotelio, capa celular interna que reviste los vasos sanguíneos, los canales linfáticos, el corazón y otras cavidades.

endothermic *a.* endotérmico-a, rel. a la absorción de calor.

endotoxemia *n.* endotoxemia, presencia en la sangre de endotoxinas.

endotoxic shock *n.* choque endotóxico.

endotoxin *n.* endotoxina, toxina venenosa excretada después que el organismo venenoso muere; es menos potente que la exotoxina. La persona infectada puede tener síntomas de fiebre, escalofríos y choque.

endotracheal *a.* endotraqueal, dentro de la tráquea; ___ **tube, cuffed** / tubo ___ con manguito.

endotracheal anesthesia *n.* anestesia endotraqueal, el anestésico y los gases respiratorios pasan por vía bucal y nasal a través de un tubo a la tráquea.

end-stage *n.* fase final.

endurable *a.* soportable, aguantable, tolerable.

endurance *n.* resistencia; tolerancia;
beyond ___ / más allá de lo que puede
soportarse, intolerable.

endure *v.* soportar, sobrellevar, resistir, aguantar.

enema *n.* enema, lavado, lavativa;
barium ___ / ___ de bario; **cleansing** ___ /
lavativa, lavado; **double contrast** ___ / ___ de
contraste doble; **retention** ___ / ___ de
retención.

energetic *a.* enérgico-a, vigoroso-a, lleno-a de
energía.

energize *v.* desplegar energía; vigorizar.

energy *n.* energía, la capacidad de trabajar, de
moverse y hacer ejercicio con vigor;
chemical ___ / ___ química; ___ **of**
activation / ___ de activación; **free** ___ / ___
libre; **fusion** ___ / ___ de fusión;
internal ___ / ___ interna; **kinetic** ___ / ___
cinética; **latent** ___ / ___ latente;
nuclear ___ / ___ nuclear; **nutritional** ___ / ___
nutritiva; **potential** ___ / ___ potencial;
psychic ___ / ___ síquica; **solar** ___ / ___ solar;
total ___ / ___ total.

enervate *v.* 1. extirpar un nervio; 2. debilitar,
enervar.

enforce *v.* [*rules, law*] hacer cumplir.

engage *v.* encajar, ajustar, conectar; [*in a*
relationship] comprometerse.

engaged *a.* encajado-a, ajustado-a, conectado-a;
[*undertaken*] comprometido-a.

engagement *n.* [*birth*] encajamiento de la
cabeza fetal.

engender *v.* engendrar, procrear.

English *n.* [*language*] inglés; [*native*] *a.* inglés,
inglesa.

engorged *a.* ingurgitado-a. 1. distendido por
exceso de líquidos; 2. congestionado de sangre.

engram *n.* engrama. 1. marca permanente hecha
en el protoplasma por un estímulo pasajero; 2.
vestigio o visión imborrable producida por una
experiencia sensorial.

enhance *v.* aumentar el valor, intensificar;
[*beautify*] realzar.

enhancement *n.* aumento de un efecto tal
como el de radiaciones por oxígeno u otro
elemento químico.

enjoy *v.* disfrutar, gozar de.

enkephalins *n., pl.* encefalinas, sustancias
químicas (polipéptidos) producidas en el cerebro.

enlarge *v.* ampliar, expandir, agrandar;
ensanchar.

enlarged *pp.* dilatado, agrandado,
aumentado; ___ **liver** / hígado agrandado; ___
prostate / próstata aumentada.

enophthalmos *n.* enoftalmia, hundimiento del
globo ocular.

enormous *a.* enorme, muy grande.

enough *a. adv.* bastante, suficiente; **fair** ___ / de
acuerdo; **large** ___ / bastante grande; **sure** ___ /
sin duda; *int.* basta!; no más!

enrich *v.* enriquecer.

enriched *a.* [*added qualities*] enriquecido-a, de
valor aumentado.

enrichment *n.* enriquecimento.

enter *v.* entrar, introducir, penetrar.

enteral, enteric *a.* entérico-a, rel. al intestino.

enteric coated *n.* cubierta entérica,
revestimiento de ciertas tabletas y cápsulas para
evitar que se disuelvan antes de llegar al
intestino.

enteritis *n.* enteritis, infl. del intestino delgado.

enterocholecystostomy *n.*
enterocolecistotomía, abertura entre la vesícula
biliar y el intestino delgado.

enteroclysis *n.* enteroclisis. 1. irrigación del
colon; 2. enema intenso.

enterococcus *n.* (*pl.* **enterococci**) enterococo,
clase de estreptococo que se aloja en el intestino
humano.

enterocolitis *n.* enterocolitis, infl. del intestino
grueso y delgado.

enterocutaneous *a.* enterocutáneo-a, que
comunica la piel y el intestino.

enteropathogen *n.* enteropatógeno,
microorganismo causante de una enfermedad
intestinal.

enteropathy *n.* enteropatía, cualquier anomalía
o enfermedad del intestino.

enterostomy *n.* enterostomía, apertura o
comunicación entre el intestino y la piel de la
pared abdominal.

enterotoxin *n.* enterotoxina, toxina producida
en el intestino.

enterovirus *n.* enterovirus, grupo de virus que
infecta el tubo digestivo y que puede ocasionar
enfermedades respiratorias y trastornos
neurológicos.

enthusiasm *n.* entusiasmo.

entire *a.* entero-a, completo-a, íntegro-a; **-ly** *adv.*
completamente, del todo, totalmente.

entity *n.* entidad, integridad, esencia o cualidad
de algo.

entrance *n.* [*local*] entrada; [*acceptance*]
ingreso; acceso a una cavidad.

entropion *n.* entropión, inversión del párpado.

entropy *n.* entropía, disminución de la capacidad de convertir la energía en trabajo.

entry *n.* entrada, acceso.

enucleate *v.* enuclear. 1. extirpar un tumor sin causar ruptura; 2. destruir o separar el núcleo de una célula; 3. extirpar el globo ocular.

enucleation *n.* enucleación, extirpación de un tumor o estructura.

enumerate *v.* enumerar, contar.

enuresis *n.* enuresis, incontinencia de orina; **nocturnal** ___ / ___ nocturna.

envelope *n.* sobre 1. objeto de papel de uso postal; 2. cubierta; 3. cápsula.

enveloping membrane *n.* membrana cubridora.

envenomation *n.* 1. envenenamiento por picadura de un miembro de la clase *Artropoda*: cangrejos, langostas, arañas, etc; 2. acto de introducir un agente venenoso por medio de una mordida, picazo, u otra forma inyectable.

environment *n.* ambiente, medio ambiente, entorno.

environmental *a.* rel. al medio ambiente; ___ **hazards** / peligros del medio ambiente.

envy *v.* envidia.

enzygotic *a.* encigótico-a, que se deriva del mismo óvulo fecundado.

enzyme *n.* enzima, proteína que actúa como catalítico en reacciones químicas vitales; **mucomembranous** ___ / ___ mucomembranosa; **tuberculous** ___ / ___ tuberculosa.

enzymology *n.* enzimología, estudio de las enzimas.

eosin *n.* eosina, sustancia insoluble usada como colorante rojo en algunos tejidos que se estudian bajo el microscopio.

eosinopenia *n.* eosinopenia, número reducido de células eosinófilas en la sangre.

eosinopenic *a.* eosinopénico-a, rel. a la eosinopenia.

eosinophil *n.* eosinófilo, célula granulocítica que acepta fácilmente la acción colorante de la eosina.

eosinophilia *n.* eosinofilia, aumento en exceso de eosinófilos en la sangre por unidad de volumen.

eosinophilic *a.* eosinófilo-a, que tiene afinidad con o por la eosina.

eosinophilic leukocytes *n.* leucocitos eosinofílicos, leucocitos con abundante granulación ácida que con los colorantes básicos se tiñen de color violeta.

ependyma *n.* epéndimo, membrana que cubre los ventrículos del cerebro y el canal central de la médula espinal.

ependymal *a.* ependimario-a, rel. al epéndimo: ___ **cells** / células ___ -as; ___ **layer** / membrana ___ .

ependymitis *n.* ependimitis, infl. del epéndimo.

ependymoma *n.* ependimoma, tumor del sistema nervioso central que se origina de inclusiones fetales ependimarias.

ephedrine *n.* efedrina, alcaloide, tipo de adrenalina de efecto broncodilatador.

ephemeral *a.* efímero-a, pasajero-a.

epicardium *n.* (*pl.* **epicardia**) epicardio, cara visceral del pericardio.

epicondyle *n.* epicóndilo, eminencia sobre el cóndilo de un hueso.

epidemic *n.* epidemia, enfermedad que se manifiesta con alta frecuencia y que afecta a un número considerable de personas en una región o comunidad; *a.* epidémico-a; ___ **outbreak** / brote ___ .

epidemiologist *n.* epidemiólogo-a, especialista en el estudio de enfermedades epidémicas.

epidemiology *n.* epidemiología, estudio de las enfermedades epidémicas.

epidermic *a.* epidérmico-a, rel. a la epidermis.

epidermis *n.* epidermis, cubierta externa epitelial de la piel.

epidermoid *a.* epidermoide. 1. semejante a la piel; 2. rel. a un tumor que contiene células epidérmicas.

epidermolysis *n.* epidermólisis, descamación de la piel.

epididymis *n.* epidídimo, conducto situado en la parte posterior del testículo que recoge el esperma que es transportado por el conducto deferente a la vesícula seminal.

epididymitis *n.* epididimitis, infección e infl. del epidídimo.

epidural *a.* epidural, situado-a sobre o fuera de la duramadre.

epigastric *a.* epigástrico-a, rel. al epigastrio; ___ **reflex** / reflejo ___ .

epigastrium *n.* (*pl.* **epigastria**) epigastrio, región superior media del abdomen.

epiglottis *n.* epiglotis, cartílago que cubre la laringe e impide la entrada de alimentos en la misma durante la deglución.

epiglottitis *n.* epiglotitis, infl. de la epiglotis.

epilation *n.* epilación, depilación por medio de electrólisis.

epilepsy, grand mal *n.* epilepsia, desorden neurológico gen. crónico y con frecuencia hereditario que se manifiesta con ataques o convulsiones y a veces con pérdida del conocimiento.

epileptic *n.* epiléptico-a, persona que padece de epilepsia; *a.* epiléptico-a, rel. a la epilepsia o que sufre de ella; ___ **seizure** / ataque ___ , crisis ___ .

epileptogenic, epileptogenous *a.* epileptógeno-a, causante de crisis epilépticas.

epinephrine *n.* epinefrina. V. **adrenaline**.

epiphora *n.* epifora, lagrimeo.

epiphysial *a.* epifisiario-a, rel. a la epífisis.

epiphysis *n.* epífisis, extremo de un hueso largo, gen. parte más ancha que la diáfisis.

epiphysitis *n.* epifisitis, infl. de una epífisis.

epiploic *a.* epiploico-a, rel. al epiplón.

epiploic foramen *n.* foramen epiploico, abertura que comunica la cavidad mayor peritoneal con la menor.

epiploon *n.* epiplón, repliegue de grasa que cubre el intestino.

episiotomy *n.* episiotomía, incisión del perineo durante el parto para evitar desgarros.

episode *n.* episodio, evento no regulado, en serie o independiente que puede formar parte de una condición física o de un estado mental, o de ambos, y se manifiestan en ciertas enfermedades tal como la epilepsia.

epispadias *n.* epispadias, abertura congénita anormal de la uretra en la parte superior del pene.

epistaxis *n.* epistaxis, sangramiento por la nariz.

epithalamus *n.* epitálamo, porción extrema superior del diencéfalo.

epithelial *a.* epitelial, rel. al epitelio.

epithelial casts *n.* cilindro epitelial, cilindro urinario constituido por células epiteliales renales y células redondas.

epithelialization *n.* epitelialización, crecimiento del epitelio sobre una superficie expuesta tal como en la cicatrización de una herida.

epithelioma *n.* epitelioma, carcinoma compuesto mayormente de células epiteliales.

epithelium *n., L.* (*pl.* **epitelia**) epitelio, tejido que cubre las superficies expuestas e interiores del cuerpo; **ciliated** ___ / ___ ciliado; **columnar** ___ / ___ columnar; **cuboidal** ___ / ___ cuboidal; **squamous** ___ / ___ escamoso; **stratified** ___ / ___ estratificado; **transitional** ___ / ___ de transición, transicional.

epitympanum *n.* epitímpano, porción superior del tímpano.

eponym *n.* epónimo, uso del nombre propio de una persona para nombrar instrumentos médicos, anomalías o síndromes tal como el síndrome de Down.

epoxy *n.* epoxia, adhesivo.

epsilon-amino caproic acid *n.* ácido epsilónamino caproico; ácido sulfúrico.

Epsom salt *n.* sal de Epsom, sal de higuera; sulfato de magnesio; medicamento usado como catártico.

Epstein-Barr virus *n.* virus de Epstein-Barr, virus del herpes que causa mononucleosis.

epulis gravidarum *n.* epúlide grávida, granuloma piogénico de la encía que puede surgir durante el embarazo.

equal *a.* igual; parejo-a; uniforme; ___ **rights** / igualdad de derechos; **-ly** *adv.* igualmente.

equality *n.* igualdad, uniformidad.

equalize *v.* igualar, emparejar, uniformar.

equanimity *n.* ecuanimidad; entereza.

equator *n.* ecuador, línea imaginaria que divide un cuerpo en dos partes iguales.

equilibrate *v.* equilibrar, balancear.

equilibration *n.* equilibración, mantenimiento del equilibrio.

equilibrium *n.* equilibrio, balance.

equinovarus *n.* equinovarus, deformidad congénita del pie.

equipment *n.* equipo, provisión; accesorios.

equitable *a.* equitativo-a; justo-a.

equivalence *n.* equivalencia.

equivalent *a.* equivalente, del mismo valor.

equivocal *a.* equívoco-a; ___ **symptom** / síntoma equívoco.

eradicate *v.* erradicar, extirpar; desarraigar.

erase *v.* borrar; raspar.

erectile *a.* eréctil, capaz de ponerse en erección o de dilatarse; ___ **tissue** / tejido ___ .

erection *n.* erección, estado de rigidez, endurecimiento o dilatación de un tejido eréctil cuando se llena de sangre, tal como el pene.

erector *n.* erector, con propiedad de erección.

ergonomics *n.* ergonomía, rama de la ecología que estudia la creación y diseño de maquinarias en su ambiente físico y la relación de las mismas con el bienestar humano.

ergot *n.* cornezuelo de centeno, hongo que en forma seca o en extracto se usa como medicamento para detener hemorragias o para inducir contracciones uterinas.

ergotamine *n.* ergotamina, alcaloide usado en el tratamiento de migraña.

ergotism *n.* ergotismo, intoxicación crónica producida por el uso excesivo de alcaloides del cornezuelo de centeno.

erode *v.* desgastar.

erogenous *a.* erógeno-a, que produce sensaciones eróticas; ___ **zone** / zona erótica.

erosion *n.* erosión, desgaste.

erosive *a.* erosivo-a, que causa erosión.

erotic *a.* erótico-a, rel. al erotismo o capaz de despertar impulsos sexuales.

eroticism, erotism *n.* erotismo, exaltación sexual.

erratic *a.* errático-a, que no sigue un curso o ritmo estable.

error *n.* error, falta, equivocación.

eructation *n.* eructación, eructo.

erupt *v.* brotar, salir con fuerza, hacer erupción.

eruption *n.* erupción, brote; salpullido.

erysipelas *n* erisipelas, infección de celulitis cutánea por el estreptococo β-hemolítico que se caracteriza por una erupción enrojecida, o carmelita, con tamaño definido; **ambulant** ___ / ___ ambulante; ___ **internum** / ___ interna; ___ **migrans** / ___ migrante; ___ **pustulosum** / ___ pustulosa; **surgical** ___ / ___ quirúrgica.

erythema *n.* eritema, enrojecimiento de la piel debido a una congestión de los capilares.

erythematic, erithematous *a.* eritematoso-a, rel. al eritema.

erythremia *n.* eritremia. V. **polycythemia**.

erythroblast *n.* eritroblasto, hematíe, glóbulo rojo primitivo.

erythroblastosis *n.* eritroblastosis, número excesivo de eritoblastos en la sangre.

erythrocyte *n.* eritrocito, célula roja producida en la médula ósea que actúa como transportadora de oxígeno a los tejidos; ___ **sedimentation rate** / índice de sedimentación de ___ -s.

erythrocytopenia *n.* eritrocitopenia, deficiencia en la cantidad de glóbulos rojos circulantes.

erythrocytosis *n.* eritrocitosis, aumento de eritrocitos en la sangre.

erythroid *n.* eritroide, de color semejante al rojo.

erythroleukemia *n.* eritroleucemia, enfermedad sanguínea maligna caracterizada por el crecimiento anormal de glóbulos rojos y blancos.

erythromelia *n.* eritromelia, trastorno cutáneo de las extremidades inferiores que se manifiesta en eritema de origen desconocido y dermis atrofiada.

erythromycin *n.* eritromicina, antibiótico usado en el tratamiento de bacterias gram-positivas.

erythron *n.* eritrón, concepto de la sangre como un sistema compuesto por los eritrocitos y sus precursores, así como también los órganos de los que provienen.

erythropoiesis *n.* eritropoyesis, producción de eritrocitos.

erythropoietic hormone *n.* hormona eritropoyética, cualquier tipo de hormona de proteína que toma parte en la formación de eritrocitos.

erythropoietin *n.* eritropoyetina, proteína no dializable que estimula la producción de eritrocitos.

erytromelalgia *n.* eritromelalgia, trastorno de las extremidades caracterizado por ataques de paroxismo con dolores severos, hinchazón, y que gen. ocurre en la edad madura.

eschar *n.* escara, costra de color oscuro que se forma en la piel después de una quemadura.

esophageal *a.* esofágico-a, rel. al esófago; ___ **dilatation** / dilatación ___; ___ **dysphagia** / disfagia esofágica; ___ **obstruction** / obstrucción ___; ___ **scintigraphy** / cintigrafía ___; ___ **spasm** / espasmo ___ .

esophagectomy *n.* esofagectomía, excisión de una porción del esófago.

esophagitis *n.* esofagitis, infl. del esófago.

esophagodynia *n.* esofagodinia, dolor en el esófago.

esophagogastritis *n.* esofagogastritis, infl. del estómago y del esófago.

esophagogastroduodenoscopy *n.* esofagogastroduodenoscopía, examen del estómago, esófago y duodeno por medio de un endoscopio.

esophagogastroscopy *n.* esofagogastroscopía, examen del esófago y del estómago por medio de un endoscopio.

esophagus *n.* esófago, porción del tubo digestivo situado entre la faringe y el estómago.

esophoria *n.* esoforia, movimiento del ojo hacia adentro; *pop.* bizquera.

esotropia *n.* esotropia. V. **esophoria**.

essence *n.* esencia, cualidad indispensable.

essential *a.* esencial, indispensable.

establish *v.* establecer, determinar.

estate *n.* estado, condición de una persona, animal o cosa.

ester *n.* éster, compuesto formado por la combinación de un ácido orgánico con alcohol.

esterification *n.* esterificación, transformación de un ácido en un éster.

e

esthesia *n.* estesia. 1. percepción, sensación; 2. cualquier anomalía que afecte las sensaciones.

esthetics *n.* estética, rama de la filosofía que se refiere a la belleza y el arte.

estradiol *n.* estradiol, esteroide producido por los ovarios.

estrinization *n.* estrinización, cambios epiteliales de la vagina producidos por estimulación de estrógeno.

estrogen *n.* estrógeno, hormona sexual femenina producida por los ovarios; ___ **receptor** / receptor de ___ .

estrogenic *a.* estrogénico-a, rel. al estrógeno.

estrone *n.* estrona, hormona estrogénica.

eternal *a.* eterno-a.

ethanol *n.* alcohol etílico.

ether *n.* éter, fluido químico cuyo vapor es usado en anestesia general.

ethics *n.* ética, normas y principios que gobiernan la conducta profesional.

ethmoid *n.* etmoides, hueso esponjoso situado en la base del cráneo.

ethmoidectomy *n.* etmoidectomía, extirpación de las células etmoideas o de parte del hueso etmoide.

ethmoid sinus *n.* seno etmoideo, cavidad aérea situada dentro del etmoide.

ethylene *n.* etileno, anestésico.

etiologic *a.* etiológico-a, rel. a la etiología.

etiology *n.* etiología, rama de la medicina que estudia la causa de las enfermedades.

eubolism *n.* eubolismo, metabolismo normal.

eucalyptus *n.* eucalipto.

eugenics *n.* eugenesia, ciencia que estudia el mejoramiento de la especie humana de acuerdo con las leyes biológicas de la herencia.

eunuch *n.* eunuco, hombre castrado.

euphoria *n.* estado exagerado de sensación de bienestar.

euploidy *n.* euploidia, grupos completos de cromosomas.

Eustachian tube *n.* trompa de Eustaquio, parte del conducto auditivo.

Eustaquian catheter *n.* Eustaquio, catéter de, catéter usado a través del tubo eustaquiano en el oído medio.

euthanasia *n.* eutanasia, muerte infringida sin sufrimiento en casos de una enfermedad incurable.

euthyroid *a.* eutiroideo-a, rel. a la función normal de la glándula tiroides.

evacuant *a.* evacuante, catártico, estimulante de la evacuación.

evacuate *v.* evacuar, eliminar; defecar; vaciar, *Mex.* obrar.

evacuation *n.* evacuación. 1. acción de vaciar esp. los intestinos; 2. acción de hacer un vacío.

evagination *n.* evaginación, salida o protuberancia de un órgano o parte de éste de su propia localización.

evaluate *v.* evaluar, estimar.

evaluation *n.* evaluación, consideración del estado de salud mental y físico de una persona enferma o sana.

evanescent *a.* evanescente, que se desvanece, efímero-a.

evaporation *n.* evaporación, conversión de un estado líquido a vapor.

even *a.* igual, uniforme; [*same*] mismo-a, parejo-a; *adv.* ___ **so** / aun cuando; ___ **though** / aun cuando.

evening *n.* tardecita, anochecer, por la noche; **last** ___ / ayer por la noche; **this** ___ / esta noche.

ever *adv.* siempre; **for** ___ **and** ___ / por ___ jamás; **hardly** ___ / casi nunca; ___ **since** / desde entonces, desde que.

eversion *n.* eversión, versión hacia afuera, esp. la de una mucosa que rodea un orificio natural.

every *a.* todo; cada; ___ **day** / ___-s los días; ___ **once in a while** / a veces, de vez en cuando; ___ **other day** / día por medio, cada dos días, un día sí y otro no.

everybody *pron.* todos, todo el mundo.

everything *pron.* todo.

evidence *n.* evidencia, manifestación; [*legal*] evidencia, testimonio.

evil *n.* maldad; *a.* malo-a, maligno-a.

evisceration *n.* evisceración, extirpación del contenido de una víscera o de una cavidad.

evoke *v.* evocar.

evoked response *n.* respuesta evocada.

evolution *n.* evolución, cambio gradual.

evulsion *n.* evulsión, acción de sacar hacia afuera, arranque.

exacerbation *n.* exacerbación, agravamiento de un síntoma o enfermedad.

exact *a.* exacto-a; **-ly** *adv.* exactamente.

exaggerate *v.* exagerar.

exaggeration *n.* exageración, alarde.

exam *n.* examen, evaluación, investigación.

examination *n.* examen, exploración, reconocimiento, auscultación; **abdominal** ___ / exploración abdominal; **bladder** ___ / cistoscopia; **cardiac** ___ / auscultación cardíaca; ___ **table** / mesa de exploración;

medical ___ / reconocimiento médico;
neurological ___ / exploración neurológica;
vaginal ___ / examen vaginal.
examine *v.* examinar, evaluar, investigar, indagar.
example *n.* ejemplo, muestra.
exanthem, exanthema *n.* exantema, erupción cutánea secundaria a un síntoma de un virus o enfermedad cócica, por ejemplo, la escarlatina o el sarampión; **epidemic** ___ / ___ epidémico; ___ **subitum** / ___ súbito; **keratoid** ___ / ___ queratoideo.
exasperate *v.* exasperar, agravar.
exasperated *a.* exasperado-a.
excellent *a.* excelente, óptimo-a.
excementosis *n.* excementosis, una excrecencia nodular en el cemento de la superficie de la raíz de un diente.
except *prep.* excepto, menos.
exception *n.* excepción; **with the** ___ **of** / a ___ de.
excess *n.* exceso, sobrante.
excessive *a.* excesivo-a.
exchange *v.* cambiar, trocar.
exchange transfusion *n.* ex-sanguinotransfusión, transfusión gradual y simultánea de sangre al recipiente mientras se saca la sangre del donante.
excise *v.* extirpar, cortar, dividir.
excision *n.* excisión, extirpación, ablación.
excitability *n.* excitabilidad.
excitation *n.* excitación, reacción a un estímulo.
excite *v.* excitar, estimular; provocar.
excited *a.* excitado-a; acalorado-a.
exclude *v.* excluir, suprimir.
exclusive *a.* exclusivo-a.
excoriation *n.* excoriación, abrasión de la epidermis.
excrement *n.* excremento, heces fecales, *pop.* [*infant's*] caca.
excrescence *n.* excrecencia, tumor saliente en la superficie de un órgano o parte.
excreta *n.* excreta, todo lo excretado por el cuerpo.
excrete *v.* excretar, eliminar desechos del cuerpo.
excretion *n.* excreción, expulsión de lo secretado.
excretory *a.* excretorio-a, rel. a la excreción.
excuse *v.* excusar, perdonar, dispensar; ___ **me** / con permiso.
exenteration *n.* exenteración. V. **evisceration**.
exercise *n.* ejercicio, esfuerzo saludable moderado con el propósito de restaurar la

vitalidad máxima a los órganos y funciones del cuerpo;**active** ___ / ___ activo;
aerobic ___ / ___ aeróbico;
corrective ___ / ___ correctivo; **deep-breathing** ___ / ___ de respiración profunda; ___ **electrocardiogram, stress test** / prueba de esfuerzo máximo; ___ **-induced amenorrea** / amenorrea inducida por ___ excesivo; ___ **test** / prueba de esfuerzo; ___ **tolerance test** / prueba física de ___ tolerado; **isometric** ___ / ___ isométrico; **isotonic** ___ / ___ isotónico; **passive** ___ / ___ pasivo; **physical** ___ / ___ físico.
exertional dyspnea *n.* disnea por esfuerzo excesivo.
exfoliation *n.* exfoliación, descamación del tejido.
exhalation *n.* exhalación, proceso de salida del aire hacia afuera.
exhale *v.* espirar, exhalar.
exhaust *v.* agotar; extraer; vaciar; **to** ___ **all means** / agotar todos los recursos.
exhausted *a.* agotado-a, exhausto-a, extenuado-a.
exhaustion *n.* agotamiento, postración, fatiga extrema.
exhaustive *a.* completo, minucioso, extenso; **to do an** ___ **evaluation of the case** / hacer una evaluación completa del caso.
exhibition *n.* exhibición, exposición.
exhibitionism *n.* exhibicionismo, deseo obsesivo de exhibir partes del cuerpo esp. los genitales.
exhibitionist *n.* exhibicionista, persona que practica el exhibicionismo.
exhumation *n.* exhumación, desenterramiento.
exist *v.* existir, ser, vivir.
existent *a.* existente.
exit *n.* salida.
exocrine *a.* exocrino-a, rel. a la secreción externa de una glándula.
exocrine glands *n.* glándulas exocrinas, glándulas que secretan hormonas a través de un conducto o tubo tal como las mamarias y las sudoríparas.
exogenous *a.* exógeno-a, externo-a, que se origina fuera del organismo.
exomphalos *n.* exónfalo. V. **omphalocele**.
exophthalmia, exophthalmos *n.* exoftalmia, protrusión anormal del globo del ojo.
exophthalmic *a.* exoftálmico-a, rel. a la exoftalmia.
exophthalmic goiter *n.* bocio exoftálmico.

exostosis *n.* exóstosis, hipertrofia ósea cartilaginosa que sobresale hacia afuera de un hueso o de la raíz de un diente.

exotic *a.* exótico-a, raro-a, extraño-a.

exotoxin *n.* exotoxina, veneno excretado por una bacteria que es un organismo vivo, contraria a la endotoxina, que no es liberada hasta que el organismo bacteria muere.

exotropia *n.* exotropía, tipo de estrabismo divergente, rotación anormal de un ojo o de ambos hacia afuera por falta de balance muscular.

expand *v.* ensanchar, expandir, dilatar; expandirse.

expansion *n.* expansión, extensión.

expect *v.* esperar; suponer.

expectancy *n.* esperanza, expectativa, anhelo.

expecting *n.* anticipación, esperanza, anhelo; ___ **mother** / mujer embarazada.

expectorant *n.* expectorante, agente que estimula la expectoración.

expectoration *n.* expectoración, esputo, expulsión de mucosidades o flema de los pulmones, tráquea y bronquios.

expel *v.* expulsar.

expense, expenditure *n.* gasto; **covered** ___ **-s** / ___ -s cubiertos.

experience *n.* experiencia, práctica.

experiment *n.* experimento; *v.* experimentar.

expert *a.* experto-a, perito-a.

expiration *n.* expiración, terminación; espiración. 1. acto de dar salida al aire aspirado por los pulmones; 2. acto de fallecer o morir.

expire *v.* 1. espirar, expeler el aire aspirado; 2. expirar, morir, dejar de existir.

explain *v.* explicar, aclarar.

explanation *n.* explicación, interpretación.

explanatory *a.* explicativo, aclaratorio; **self-explanatory** / que no necesita explicación o aclaración.

exploration *n.* exploración, investigación, búsqueda.

exploratory *a.* exploratorio-a, rel. a una exploración.

expose *v.* exponer, mostrar; expulsar bajo presión.

exposition *n.* exposición, demostración, exhibición.

expression *n.* expresión, aspecto o apariencia que se registra en la cara; medio de expresar algo.

expressivity *n.* expresividad, apreciación de un rasgo heredado según se manifiesta en el descendiente portador del gene.

expulsion *n.* expulsión; ___ **of the placenta** / ___ de la placenta; ___ **of the infant** / ___ del recién nacido.

extended care facility *n.* centro de atención médica externa.

extension *n.* 1. prolongación, extensión; 2. acto de enderezar un dedo o alinear un miembro o hueso dislocado.

extensor *a.* extensor-a, que tiene la propiedad de extender.

extenuate *v.* mitigar, atenuar, disminuir.

extenuating cases *n., pl.* casos atenuantes.

exterior *a.* exterior, externo-a; visible.

exteriorize *v.* exteriorizar, exponer un órgano o una parte temporalmente.

externalia *n., pl.* genitales externos.

externalize *v.* externalizar. V. **exteriorize**.

extinction *n.* extinción; supresión; cesación.

extinguish *v.* extinguir, apagar.

extirpation *n.* extirpación, ablación de una parte u órgano.

extra *a.* extraordinario-a; adicional.

extracellular *a.* extracelular, fuera de la célula.

extracorporeal *a.* extracorporal, fuera del cuerpo.

extract *n.* extracto, producto concentrado.

extraction *n.* extracción, proceso de extraer, separar o sacar afuera.

extradural *a.* extradural. V. **epidural**.

extraneous *a.* extraño-a, sin relación con un organismo o fuera del mismo.

extraocular *a.* extraocular, fuera del ojo.

extrasensory perception *n.* percepción extrasensorial, percepción o conocimiento de las acciones o pensamientos de otras personas adquirido sin participación sensorial.

extrasystole *n.* extrasístole, latido arrítmico del corazón.

extravasated *a.* extravasado-a, rel. al escape de fluido de un vaso a tejidos circundantes.

extravascular *a.* extravascular, que ocurre fuera de un vaso o vasos.

extreme *a.* extremo-a, excesivo-a; último-a; **-ly** *adv.* extremadamente, excesivamente; sumamente.

extremity *n.* extremidad, la parte terminal de algo.

extrinsic *a.* extrínseco-a ___ **muscle** / músculo ___ .

extrophy *n.* extrofia. V. **eversion**.

extrovert *a.* extrovertido-a, tipo de personalidad que dirige la atención a sucesos u objetos fuera de sí mismo-a.

extrude *v.* exprimir, forzar hacia afuera.

extrusion *n.* extrusión, expulsión.

extubation *n.* extubación, extracción de un tubo.

exuberant *a.* exuberante, de proliferación excesiva.

exudate *n.* exudado, fluido inflamatorio tal como el de secreciones y supuraciones.

exudation *n.* exudación.

exude *v.* exudar, sudar, supurar a través de los tejidos.

eye *n.* ojo; **amaurotic** ___ / ___ amaurótico; **artificial** ___ / ___ postizo; **black** ___ / ___ amoratado, contusión ocular; **bleary** ___ / ___ nublado; ___ legañoso; **bloodshot** ___ / ___ inyectado; **chemical burns in** ___ / quemaduras químicas oculares; **crossed-eyed** / bizco; **cyclopian** ___ / ___ de cíclope; ___ **bank** / banco de ojos; ___ **contact** / contacto visual; ___ **diseases** / enfermedades de los ojos, enfermedades de la vista; ___ **drops** / gotas para

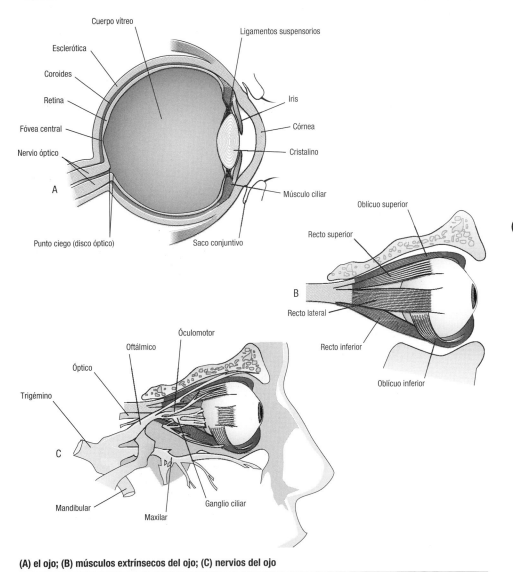

(A) el ojo; (B) músculos extrínsecos del ojo; (C) nervios del ojo

los ojos; ___ **injuries** / traumatismos oculares; ___ **injury** / lesión ocular; ___ **memory** / memoria visual; ___**strain** / fatiga ocular; **foreign body in the** ___ / cuerpo extraño en el ___; **glass** ___ / ___ de cristal, ___ de vidrio; **lazy** ___ / ambliopía; **light-adapted** ___ / ___ adaptado a la luz; **master** ___ / ___ maestro; **squinting** ___ / ___ estrábico; **to keep an** ___ **on** / cuidar, vigilar; **watery** ___ / ___ lacrimoso. See illustration on page 377.

eyeball *n.* globo del ojo, globo ocular.

eyeband *n.* venda para los ojos.

eyebrow *n.* ceja.

eyecup *n.* copita para los ojos.

eyeglasses *n. pl.* espejuelos, gafas, lentes, anteojos; **bifocal** ___ / ___ bifocales; **trifocal** ___ / ___ trifocales.

eyeground *n.* fondo del ojo.

eyelash *n.* pestaña.

eyelid *n.* párpado.

eye memory *n.* memoria visual.

eyepiece *n.* ocular.

eyesight *n.* vista; *v.* **to have good** ___ / tener buena ___ .

eye socket *n.* órbita ocular; cuenca del ojo.

eyestrain *n.* vista cansada.

eyewash *n.* solución ocular, colirio, solución para los ojos.

eyewitness *n.* testigo ocular o visual.

f

F *abbr.* **Fahrenheit** / Fahrenheit.

f *abbr.* **failure** / fallo; **feminine** / femenino; **formula** / fórmula; **function** / función.

fabella *n.* fabela, fibrocartílago sesamoideo que puede desarrollarse en la cabeza del músculo gastronecmio.

face *n.* cara, rostro, faz; ___ **-down** / boca abajo; ___ **-lift** / estire de la cara, ritidectomía; ___ **peeling** / peladura de la ___; ___ **to face** / frente a frente; ___ **-up** / boca arriba.

facet *n.* faceta, pequeña parte lisa en la superficie de una estructura dura semejante a la de los huesos.

facetectomy *n.* extirpación de la faceta auricular.

facial *a.* facial, rel. a la cara; ___ **artery** / arteria ___; ___ **axis** / axis ___; ___ **bone defects** / defectos óseos ___ -es; ___ **bones** / huesos de la cara, huesos ___ -es; ___ **canal** / canal ___; ___ **hemiplegia** / hemiplejía ___; ___ **injuries** / traumatismos ___ -es; ___**nerve** / nervio ___; ___ **nerves** / nervios ___ -es; ___ **palsy** / parálisis ___; ___ **paralysis** / parálisis ___; ___ **reconstruction** / reconstrucción ___; ___**spasm** / espasmo ___; ___**tic** / tic ___; ___**vein** / vena ___.

facies *n.* (*pl.* **facies**) facies, expresión o apariencia de la cara; **leontina** ___ / ___ leontina; **masklike** ___ / ___ inexpresiva.

facilitate *v.* facilitar; proporcionar.

facility *n.* facilidad; instalación; [*conveniences*] *pl.* comodidades; servicios en general.

facing *n.* [*dental*] revestimiento.

facioplegia *n.* facioplejía, parálisis facial.

fact *n.* de hecho, hecho, realidad; **in** ___ / en efecto, en realidad.

factitious *a.* facticio-a, artificial, no natural.

factor *n.* factor, elemento que contribuye a producir una acción; **antihemophilic** ___ / ___ antihemofílico; **clotting, coagulation** ___ / ___ de coagulación; **fibroblast growth** ___ / ___ de crecimiento fibroplástico; **releasing** ___ / ___ liberador; **Rh** ___ / ___ Rh [*erre ache*]; **rheumatoid** ___ / ___ reumatoideo; **tumor angiogenesis** ___ / ___ angiogenético tumoral.

factual *a.* objetivo-a, real.

facultative *a.* facultativo-a. 1. voluntario, no obligatorio; 2. de naturaleza profesional.

faculty *n.* facultad. 1. cuerpo facultativo; 2. aptitud o habilidad para llevar a cabo funciones normales.

fade *v.* descolorar; perder el color, atenuar la imagen o el color, desteñirse.

Faget, sign of *n.* signo de Faget, un pulso bajo en relación a la alta temperatura presente.

Fahrenheit scale *n.* escala de Fahrenheit, escala de temperatura que usa el punto de congelación a 32 y el de ebullición a 212.

fail *v.* [*to be deficient*] fallar, faltar; dejar de; **without** ___ / sin falta.

failing *n.* debilidad; deterioro; flaqueza; falla, falta.

failure *n.* insuficiencia, fallo; omisión; fracaso; ___ **neurosis** / neurosis de fracaso; **gross** ___ / fiasco; **heart** ___ / ___ cardíaca, fallo cardíaco; **renal** ___ / ___ renal; **respiratory** ___ / ___ respiratoria.

faint *n.* desmayo, desvanecimiento, vahído; *v.* dar un vahído; desmayarse, desvanecerse; **-ly** *adv.* débilmente, lánguidamente; escasamente.

fainting *n.* desmayo; desfallecimiento; ___ **spell** / desmayo.

faintness *n.* desaliento, [*weakness*] debilidad.

fair *a.* [*blonde*] rubio-a; [*light skin*] de tez blanca; [*average*] regular; ___ **complexion** / rubio-a, de tez clara; [*weather*] claro, despejado, favorable; [*decision*] imparcial, razonable, justa.

faith *n.* fe; **in good** ___ / de buena ___.

faithful *a.* exacto-a, veraz; **-ly** *adv.* fielmente, exactamente.

faith healer *n.* curandero-a.

faith healing *n.* curanderismo.

fake *v.* fingir; falsificar, simular.

falciform *a.* falciforme, en forma de hoz; ___ **ligament** / ligamento ___; ___ **ligament of liver** / ligamento ___ del hígado; ___**process** / proceso ___.

fall *n.* caída; [*season*] otoño; *vi.* caer; caerse; **to** ___ **asleep** / quedarse dormido-a; **to** ___ **back** / echarse atrás; **to** ___ **behind** / atrasarse, quedarse atrás; **to** ___ **short** / faltar, ser deficiente.

fallen *a. pp.* of **to fall**, caído-a.

falling *n.* caída; [*temperature*] descenso.

Fallopian tubes *n.* trompas de Falopio, conductos que se extienden del útero a los ovarios.

Fallot, tetralogy of *n.* tetralogía de Fallot, deformación cardíaca congénita que comprende cuatro defectos de los grandes vasos sanguíneos y de las paredes de las aurículas y ventrículos.

fallout *n.* cenizas radioactivas.

false *a.* falso-a, incorrecto-a. no real; ___ **anemia** / anemia ___; ___ **aneurysm** / aneurisma ___; ___ **ankylosis** / anquilosis ___; ___ **blepharoptosis** / blefaroptosis ___; ___ **diverticulum** / divertículo ___; ___ **hematuria** / hematuria ___; ___ **hermaphroditism** / hermafroditismo ___; ___ **image** / imagen ___; ___ **joint** / articulación ___; ___ **lumen** / lúmen ___; ___ **membrane** / membrana ___; ___ **memory syndrome** / síndrome ___ de la memoria; ___ **negative** / ___ negativo; ___ **neuroma** / neuroma ___; ___ **positive** / ___ positivo; ___ **pregnancy** / embarazo ___; ___ **rib** / costilla ___; ___ **suture** / sutura ___; ___ **vocal chords** / cuerdas vocales ___ -s.

falsification *n.* falsificación, distorsión o alteración de un suceso u objeto.

fame *n.* fama, nombre.

familial, familiar *a.* familiar, rel. a la familia; frecuente; ___ **adenomatous polyposis** / poliposis adenomatosa ___; ___ **amyloid neuropathy** / neuropatía amiloide ___; ___ **dysautonomia** / disautonomía ___; ___ **goiter** / bocio ___; ___ **hypercholesteremia** / hipercolesteremia ___; ___ **jaundice** / icteria ___; ___ **Mediterranean fever** / fiebre ___ del Mediterráneo; ___ **periodic paralysis** / parálisis periódica ___; ___ **pseudoinflammatory macular degeneration** / degeneración macular pseudo-inflamatoria ___; ___ **screening** / escrutinio ___ .

family *n.* familia; ___ **man** / padre de familia; ___ **name** / apellido; ___ **practice** / práctica de ___; ___ **therapy** / terapia de ___ .

family planning *n.* planificación familiar, planeamiento de la concepción de los hijos gen. con el uso de métodos contraceptivos.

family practice *n.* medicina familiar, atención médica especial de la familia como unidad.

famine *n.* hambre, carestía.

famished *a.* famélico-a, hambriento-a.

fanatic, fanatical *a.* fanático-a.

Fanconi's syndrome *n.* síndrome de Fanconi, anemia hipoplástica congénita.

fancy *v.* imaginar, fantasear.

fantasy, phantasy *n.* fantasía, uso de la imaginación para transformar una realidad desagradable en una experiencia satisfactoria.

far *adv.* lejos; distante; ___ **apart** / infrecuente; ___ **better** / mucho mejor; ___ **cry** / gran diferencia; ___ **off** / a lo lejos, distante; **from** ___ **away** / de lejos, a lo lejos; **so** ___ / hasta ahora, hasta aquí.

farfetched *a.* rebuscado-a; inconcebible.

farina *n.* farina, harina, combinación de harina de trigo con otro cereal.

farmer *n.* campesino-a, granjero-a.

farmer's lung *n.* pulmón de granjero, hipersensibilidad de los alvéolos pulmonares causada por exposición a heno fermentado.

farsighted *a.* hiperópico-a, que sufre de hipermetropía.

farsightedness *n.* presbiopía, hiperopía, hipermetropía, defecto visual en el cual los rayos de luz hacen foco detrás de la retina y los objetos lejanos se ven mejor que los que están a corta distancia.

fascia *n.* fascia, tejido fibroso conectivo que envuelve el cuerpo bajo la piel y protege los músculos, los nervios y los vasos sanguíneos; ___ , **aponeurotic** / ___ aponeurótica, tejido fibroso que sirve de soporte a los músculos; ___ , **Buck's** / ___ de Buck, tejido fibroso que cubre el pene; ___ , **Colles'** / ___ de Colles, cubierta interna de la fascia perineal; ___ **graft** / injerto de una ___; ___ , **lata** / ___ lata, protectora de los músculos del muslo; ___ , **tranversalis** / tranversal, localizada entre el peritoneo y el músculo transverso del abdomen.

fascial *a.* fascial, rel a una fascia; ___ **sheath of eye-ball** / cubierta ___ del globo del ojo.

fascicle, fasciculum *n.* (*pl.* **fascicula**) fascículo, haz de fibras musculares y nerviosas.

fascicular *a.* fascicular, rel a un fascículo; ___ **degeneration** / degeneración ___; ___ **graft** / injerto ___.

fasciculation *n.* fasciculación. 1. formación de fascículos; 2. contracción involuntaria breve de fibras musculares.

fascietomy *n.* fascietomía, excisión parcial o total de una fascia.

fasciitis *n.* fascitis, infl. de una fascia.

fasciodesis *n.* fasciodesis, operación de adherir un tendón a una fascia.

fasciola *n., L.* (*pl.* **fasciolae**) fasciola, grupo pequeño de fibras.

fascioplasty *n.* fascioplastía, cirugía plástica de una fascia.

fasciorrhaphy *n.* fasciorrafía, sutura de una fascia.

fasciotomy _n._ fasciotomía, incisión de una fascia.

fast _n._ ayuno; _a._ [_speed_] rápido-a, ligero-a; [_of a color_] que tiene resistencia a un colorante: ___ **asleep** / profundamente dormido-a; ___ **day** / día de ayuno; _v._ ayunar, estar en ayunas.

fasten _v._ sujetar; amarrar; abrochar; abotonar.

fastening _n._ amarre.

fastidious _a._ fastidioso-a, en bacteriología rel. a demandas nutricionales complejas.

fasting _n._ ayuno.

fastness _n._ resistencia.

fat _n._ [_grease_] grasa; _a._ gordo-a, grueso-a, obeso-a; [_greasy_] grasoso-a; ___ **embolism** / embolia grasosa; _v._ **to get** ___ / engordar.

fatal _a._ fatal.

fatality _n._ fatalidad, desgracia; muerte.

fatality rate _n._ índice de mortalidad.

fate _n._ destino.

father _n._ padre; papá; _pop._ tata.

father-in-law _n._ suegro.

fatherless _n._ huérfano-a de padre.

fatigability _n._ fatigabilidad, predisposición a la fatiga.

fatigue _n._ cansancio; sensación de agotamiento; _v._ fatigarse, cansarse.

fatness _n._ gordura.

fatty _a._ adiposo-a, grasoso-a; ___ **acids** / ácidos grasos; ___ **cirrhosis** / cirrosis ___; ___ **degeneration** / degeneración ___; ___ **heart** / corazón ___; ___ **hernia** / hernia ___; ___ **infiltration** / infiltración ___; ___ **kidney** / riñón ___; ___ **liver** / hígado ___; ___ **oil** / aceite ___; ___ **tumor** / lipoma; ___ **tissue** / tejido ___.

fauces _n., L._ fauces, región intermedia entre la boca y la faringe.

faucet _n._ pila, llave de agua.

fault _n._ falta, defecto, culpa; _v._ **to be at** ___ / ser culpable.

faultless _a._ perfecto-a; intachable.

faulty _a._ defectuoso-a, imperfecto-a.

favor _n._ favor.

favorable _a._ favorable; propicio-a.

fear _n._ temor, miedo, aprehensión. _v._ temer, tener miedo.

fearful _a._ temeroso-a, miedoso-a.

fearless _a._ sin temor, intrépido-a.

feasible _a._ posible, factible.

feast _n._ banquete.

feather _n._ pluma.

feature _n._ rasgo, característica.

febrile _a._ febril, calenturiento-a; ___ **convulsion** / convulsión ___.

fecal _a._ fecal, que contiene heces fecales; ___ **abscess** / absceso ___; ___ **examination** / examen ___; ___ **fistula** / fístula ___.

fecalith _n._ fecalito, concreción intestinal formada alrededor de materia fecal.

fecaloid _a._ fecaloide, semejante a materia fecal.

fecaloma _n._ fecaloma, acumulación de heces fecales en el recto con apariencia de tumor abdominal.

fecaluria _n._ presencia de materia fecal en la orina.

feces _n., pl._ heces, excremento.

feculent _a._ feculento, lleno de heces fecales.

fecund _a._ fecundo-a; fértil.

fecundation _n._ fecundación, el acto de hacer fértil.

fecundity _n._ fecundidad, fertilidad.

fed _a. pp._ of **to feed**; **to be** ___ **up** / estar harto-a, _pop._ estar hasta la coronilla.

fee _n._ honorario, cuota.

feeble _a._ débil, endeble.

feed _vi._ alimentar, dar de comer; proveer materiales o asistencia.

feedback _n._ 1. [_information_] reprovisión de material informativo distribuido; 2. retroalimentación, retorno parcial del rendimiento o efectos de un proceso a su fuente de origen o a una fase anterior; _v._ proveer de nuevo material informativo; regenerar la energía.

feeding _n._ alimentación; **breast-** ___ / lactancia materna; **enteral** ___ / ___ enteral; ___ **time** / horario de ___; **forced** ___ / ___ forzada; **intravenous** ___ / ___ intravenosa; **rectal** ___ / ___ por el recto; **tube** ___ / ___ por sonda.

feel _vi._ sentir, percibir, sentirse; **Do you** ___ **the effects of the medication?** / ¿Siente, sientes los efectos de la medicina?; **to** ___ **hungry** / tener hambre; **to** ___ **the effects of** / sentir los efectos de; **to** ___ **like** / tener ganas de; **to** ___ **sleepy** / tener sueño; **to** ___ **sorry for** / compadecerse de; tener lástima de; **to** ___ **the pulse** / tomar el pulso; **to** ___ **thirsty** / tener sed; **to** ___ **bad** / sentirse mal; **to** ___ **better** / ___ mejor; **to** ___ **good, fine** / ___ bien; **to** ___ **uncomfortable** / ___ incómodo-a.

feeling _n._ sensación; [_emotion_] sentimiento, emoción, sensibilidad.

feet _n., pl._ de **foot**; pies.

feline _a._ felino-a, rel. a la familia de los gatos o con características semejantes a éstos.

fellatio _n._ felación. V. **cunnilingus.**

felon _n._ 1. panadizo, absceso doloroso de la falange distal de un dedo; 2. felón, criminal.

female *n.* hembra; *a.* femenino-a, rel. a la mujer; ___ **catheter** / catéter para mujer; ___ **circumcision** / circuncisión de la mujer; ___ **pseudohermaphrotidism** / pseudohermafrotidismo femenino.

feminine *a.* femenino-a; afeminado.

femininity *n.* feminidad; ___ **complex** / complejo de ___.

feminist *a.* feminista.

feminization *n.* feminización, desarrollo de características femeninas.

femoral *a.* femoral, rel. al fémur; **deep** ___ **arch** / arco ___ profundo; ___ **artery** / arteria ___; ___ **canal** / canal ___; ___ **hernia** / hernia ___; ___ **nerve** / nervio ___; ___ **nutrient artery** / arteria nutricional ___; ___ **sheath** / capa ___; ___ **triangle** / triángulo ___; ___ **vein** / vena ___.

femorotibial *a.* femorotibial, rel. al fémur y a la tibia; ___ **capillary** / capilar ___; ___ **membrane** / membrana ___.

femur *n.* fémur, hueso del muslo.

fenestrated *a.* fenestrado-a; que tiene orificios o aperturas.

fenestration *n.* fenestración. 1. creación de una abertura en el laberinto del oído para restaurar la audición; 2. acto de perforar.

ferment *n.* fermento. 1. sustancia o agente que activa la fermentación; 2. producto de fermentación; *v.* fermentar, hacer fermentar.

fermentation *n.* fermentación, descomposición de sustancias complejas por la acción de enzimas o fermentos.

fermentative *a.* fermentativo, que tiene la propiedad de hacer fermentar.

ferritin *n.* ferritina, una de las formas en que el hierro se almacena en el organismo.

ferroprotein *n.* ferroproteína, proteína compuesta de un radical ferruginoso.

ferruginous *a.* ferruginoso-a, ferrugíneo-a. 1. que contiene hierro; 2. que tiene el color de hierro oxidado.

fertile *a.* fértil, fecundo-a, productivo-a.

fertility *n.* fertilidad.

fertilization *n.* fertilización, fecundación.

fertilize *v.* fecundar, hacer fértil.

fertilizer *n.* fertilizante.

fester *v.* enconarse; supurar superficialmente.

festinant *a.* festinante, acelerado, rápido.

fetal *a.* fetal, rel. al feto; ___ **alcohol syndrome** / síndrome alcohólico ___; ___ **aspiration syndrome** / síndrome de aspiración ___; ___ **circulation** / circulación ___; ___ **death** / muerte ___; ___ **drug syndrome** / síndrome ___ del abuso de droga; ___ **dystocia** / distocia ___; ___ **growth retardation** / retardo del crecimiento ___; ___ **heart tone** / latido del corazón ___; ___ **hydrops** / hidropesía ___; ___ **maturity, chronologic** / edad gestacional; ___ **medicine** / medicina ___; ___ **membrane** / membrana ___; ___ **monitoring** / monitorización ___; ___ **placenta** / placenta ___; ___ **pulse oximeter** / oxímetro de pulso ___; ___ **transfusion** / transfusión de sangre *in utero*; ___ **viability** / viabilidad ___; ___ **wastage** / desperdicio ___.

feticide *n.* feticidio, destrucción del feto en el útero.

fetid *a.* fétido-a, hediondo-a, de mal olor.

fetish *n.* fetiche.

fetometry *n.* fetometría, estimación del tamaño del feto, esp. la cabeza antes del nacimiento

fetoplacental *a.* fetoplacental, rel. al feto y a la placenta.

fetoprotein *n.* fetoproteína, antígeno presente en el feto humano.

fetor *n.* fetor, mal olor, hedor.

fetoscope *n.* fetoscopio, endoscopio que se usa en la fetoscopía.

fetoscopy *n.* fetoscopía, inspección antenatal fetal transabdominal de la placenta y el feto con el propósito de diagnosticar posibles trastornos fetales.

fetotoxic *a.* fetotóxico-a, que puede toxificar al feto.

fetus *n.* feto, embrión en desarrollo, fase de la gestación desde los tres meses hasta el parto.

fever *n.* fiebre, calentura; **enteric** ___ / ___ entérica, intestinal; ___ **blister** / herpes febril; ___ **of unknown origin** / ___ de origen desconocido; **intermittent** ___ / ___ intermitente; **rabbit** ___ / ___ de conejo, tularemia; **rheumatoid** ___ / ___ reumatoidea; **remittent** ___ / ___ remitente; **Rocky Mountain** ___ / ___ manchada de las Montañas Rocosas; **scarlet** ___ / escarlatina; **yellow** ___ / ___ amarilla, paludismo, malaria; **typhoid** ___ / ___ tifoidea; **undulant** ___ / brucelosis.

fiber *n.* fibra, filamento en forma de hilo.

fiberoptic *a.* fibróptico, rel. a las fibras ópticas.

fiberoptics *n., pl.* fibras ópticas, filamentos flexibles de cristal o plástico que conducen una imagen transmitida.

fibril *n.* filamento, fibrilla, fibra pequeña.

fibrillar, fibrillary *a.* fibrilar, rel. a una fibra; ___ **astrocyte** / astrocito ___; ___ **contractions** / contracciones ___ -es.

fibrillation *n.* fibrilación. 1. contracción muscular involuntaria que afecta fibras musculares individuales; 2. formación de fibrillas; **atrial** ___ / ___ auricular; **flutter** ___ / ___ de aleteo; **ventricular** ___ / ___ ventricular.

fibrin *n.* fibrina, proteína insoluble indispensable en la coagulación de la sangre.

fibrinogen *n.* fibrinógeno. 1. proteína presente en el plasma sanguíneo que se convierte en fibrina en el proceso de coagulación; 2. el Factor I.

fibrinogenemia *n.* fibrinogenemia, presencia de fibrógeno en la sangre.

fibrinogenic, fibrinogenous *a.* fibrinogénico-a, que produce fibrina.

fibrinogenolysis *n.* fibrinogenólisis, disolución o inactivación del fibrinógeno en la corriente sanguínea.

fibrinoid *a.* fibrinoide, semejante a la fibrina;___ **degeneration** / degeneración ___.

fibrinolysis *n.* fibrinólisis, disolución de fibrina por la acción de enzimas; **primary** ___ / ___ primaria; **therapeutic** ___ / ___ terapéutica.

fibrinolytic *a.* fibrinolítico-a, rel. a la desintegración de fibrina.

fibrinous, fibrous *a.* fibrinoso-a, fibroso-a. 1. rel. a la naturaleza de una fibra; 2. semejante a un hilo; ___ **bronchitis** / bronquitis ___; ___ **inflammation** / inflamación ___; ___ **pericarditis** / pericarditis ___; ___ **pleurisy** / pleuresía ___; ___ **polyp** / pólipo ___.

fibrinuria *n.* fibrinuria, presencia de fibrina en la orina.

fibroadenoma *n.* fibroadenoma, tumor benigno formado por tejido fibroso y glandular.

fibroadipose *a.* fibroadiposo, constituido por tejido fibroso y adiposo.

fibroblast *n.* fibroblasto, células de soporte de las que proviene el tejido conectivo.

fibrocartilage *n.* fibrocartílago, tipo de cartílago en el que la matriz contiene abundante tejido fibroso.

fibrocellular *a.* fibrocelular, que es de constitución fibrosa y celular.

fibrochondritis *n.* fibrocondritis, infl. de un fibrocartílago.

fibrochondroma *n.* fibrocondroma, tumor benigno compuesto por tejido conjuntivo fibroso y cartilaginoso.

fibrocyst *n.* fibroquiste. 1. fibroma formado por quistes; 2. neoplasma de degeneración cística.

fibrocystic *a.* fibrocístico-a, fibroquístico-a, de naturaleza fibrosa con degeneración cística; ___

disease of the breast / enfermedad ___ de la mama.

fibrocystoma *n.* fibrocistoma, tumor benigno con elementos císticos.

fibroid *a.* fibroide, de naturaleza fibrosa; ___ **adenoma** / adenoma ___; ___ **cataract** / catarata ___.

fibroidectomy *n.* fibroidectomía, excisión de un tumor fibroide.

fibrolabile *n.* fibrolábil, que puede ser destruído fácilmente por el frío.

fibrolipoma *n.* fibrolipoma, tumor que contiene tejido fibroso y adiposo en exceso.

fibroma *n.* fibroma, tumor benigno compuesto de tejido fibroso.

fibromatosis *n.* fibromatosis, producción de fibromas múltiples en la piel o en el útero.

fibromuscular *a.* fibromuscular, de naturaleza muscular y fibrosa; ___ **dysplasia** / displasia ___ .

fibromyalgia *n.* fibromialgia, condición crónica generalizada que resulta en dolor y rigidez en los músculos y los tejidos blandos.

fibromyoma *n.* fibromioma, tumor benigno formado por tejido muscular y fibroso.

fibroneuroma *n.* fibroneuroma, tumor del tejido conjuntivo de los nervios.

fibroplasia *n.* fibroplasia, producción de tejido fibroso tal como en la cicatrización de una herida.

fibrosarcoma *n.* fibrosarcoma, tumor maligno constituído por células fusiformes, colágeno y fibras de reticulina.

fibrosis *n.* fibrosis, formación anormal de tejido fibroso; **diffuse interstitial pulmonary** ___ / ___ intersticial del pulmón; **proliferative** ___ / ___ proliferativa; **retroperineal** ___ / ___ retroperineal.

fibrositis *n.* fibrositis, infl. de tejido blanco conjuntivo esp. en el área de las articulaciones.

fibrotic *a.* fibrótico-a, rel. a la fibrosis.

fibrous *a.* fibroso-a. 1. rel. a la fibrina; 2. estructura en forma de hilo; ___ **ankylosis** / anquilosis ___; ___ **cortical defect** / defecto cortical ___; ___ **degeneration** / degeneración ___; ___ **goiter** / bocio ___; ___ **joint** / articulación ___; ___ **tissue** / tejido ___; ___ **tubercule** / tubérculo ___.

fibula *a.* peroné, el hueso más externo y más delgado de la pierna.

fibular *a.* fibular, rel. al peroné; ___ **artery** / arteria ___; ___ **veins** / venas ___ .

fictitious *a.* ficticio-a, falso-a.

fidelity *n.* fidelidad, lealtad; precisión.

field *n.* campo. 1. área o espacio abierto; ___ **of vision** / ___ visual; 2. área de especialización.

fight *n.* pelea, lucha; *vi.* pelear, combatir, luchar con.

figure *n.* figura; cifra, número.

filament *n.* filamento, fibra o hilo fino.

file *n.* [*instrument*] lima; [*record*] expediente, ficha; *v.* limar; registrar.

fill *v.* llenar; rellenar; llenarse.

filling *n.* [*dental*] empaste; obturación; restauración.

film *n.* 1. película; radiografía; 2. telilla, membrana o capa fina.

filter *n.* filtro; *v.* filtrar; **to ___ through** / filtrarse.

filtering *n.* filtración, el acto de filtrar a través de un filtro que impide el paso de ciertas moléculas; ___ **operation** / operación de ___.

filth *n.* suciedad, immundicias, mugre; *H. A.* cochinada.

filthy *a.* sucio-a, mugriento-a, mugroso-a.

filtration *n.* filtración, colación, acción de pasar a través de un filtro.

fimbria *n.* (*pl.* **fimbriae**) fimbria, borde o canto; apéndice de ciertas bacterias; ___ **hippocampi** / ___ del hipocampo; ___ **of uterine tube** / ___ del tubo uterino; ___ **ovaricae** / ___ ovárica.

final *a.* final, último-a; conclusivo-a; definitivo-a.

financial *a.* financiero-a, monetario-a; ___ **expenses** / gastos ___ -s; ___ **income** / ingresos, honorarios; ___ **responsibility** / solvencia, capacidad ___; **-ly** *adv.* ___ **responsible** / persona solvente, persona responsable de los gastos.

find *vi.* hallar, encontrar, descubrir.

findings *n., pl.* hallazgos, resultados de una investigación o indagación.

fine *a.* fino-a, delicado-a; *v.* **to feel ___** / sentirse bien.

finger *n.* dedo de la mano; ___ **agnosia** / agnosia del ___; ___ **nose test** / prueba de la nariz y el ___; ___ **-shaped** / digitiforme; **first ___** / dedo índice; **little ___** / dedo meñique; **mallet ___** / dedo en martillo.

fingernail *n.* uña.

fingerprint *n.* impresión, huella digital; *v.* tomar las impresiones digitales; ___ **expert** / dactiloscopista.

finish *n.* final, terminación; *v.* acabar, terminar.

finished *a.* acabado-a, terminado-a.

finite *a.* finito-a, que tiene límites.

Finney operation *n.* operación de Finney, gastroduodenostomía que crea una apertura grande para asegurar el vaciamiento total del estómago.

fire *n.* fuego; [*conflagration*] incendio; ___ **alarm** / alarma de ___; ___ **department** / cuerpo de bomberos; ___ **escape** / escalera de ___; *v.* **to catch ___** / encenderse, prenderse; **to set ___ to** / encender, quemar.

firearm *n.* arma de fuego.

firm *a.* firme, fijo-a, consistente.

first *n.* primero-a; *a.* primero-a, primer (before a *m.* singular *n.*) ___ **degree** / de primer grado; ___ **name** / nombre de pila.

first aid *n.* primeros auxilios; ___ **kit** / botiquín de ___.

firstborn *n.* primogénito-a.

fish *n.* pez; [*fish caught*] pescado.

fish poisoning *n.* intoxicación de pescado.

fission *n.* fisión. 1. división en partes; 2. división de un átomo para ser descompuesto y desplazar energía y neutrones.

fissure *n.* fisura. V. **cleft.**

fist *n.* puño *v.* **to make a ___** / cerrar el ___.

fistula *n.* fístula, canal o pasaje anormal que permite el paso de secreciones de una cavidad a otra o a la superficie exterior; **anal ___** / ___ anal; **arteriovenous ___** / ___ arteriovenosa; **biliary ___** / ___ biliar.

fistulization *n.* fistulización, formación de una fístula por un medio quirúrgico o patológico súbito.

fistulous *a.* fistuloso-a, rel. a una fístula.

fit *n.* ataque súbito; convulsión; *a.* [*suitable*] adecuado-a; *vi.* [*glasses*] ajustar, encajar, montar.

fitness *n.* aptitud, vigor físico, acondicionamiento físico; **physical ___** / ___ física.

fix *v.* [*fasten*] fijar, asegurar; **to fix up** / arreglar; convenir.

fixation *n.* fijación. 1. inmovilización de una parte; 2. acción de fijar la vista en un objeto; 3. interrupción del desarrollo de la personalidad antes de alcanzar la madurez.

fixative *n.* fijador, sustancia usada para endurecer muestras de exámenes patológicos.

fixed *a.* fijo-a; decidido-a [*resolved*] resuelto; arreglado-a, determinado-a; compuesto-a; ___ **fee** / honorario ___ o definido; ___ **term** / plazo ___.

flabby *a.* blando-a, flojo-a; *pop.* fofo-a.

flaccid *a.* flácido-a; débil, flojo-a; ___ **paralysis** / parálisis ___.

flagellated *a.* flagelado-a, provisto de flagelo o flagelos.

flagelliform *n.* flageliforme, en forma de látigo.

flagellum n. (pl. **flagella**) flagelo, prolongación o cola en la célula de algunos protozoos.

flail chest n. tórax inestable, condición de la pared del tórax causada por la fractura múltiple de costillas.

flake n. escama; copo; **snow** ___ **-s** / copos de nieve.

flaky a. escamoso-a.

flank n. flanco, parte del cuerpo entre las costillas y el borde superior del íleo.

flap n. [sound of wings] aleteo; sonido de alas; cubierta; colgajo.

flare n. brote, irritación rosácea o área difundida; destello, fulgor; ___ **-up** / ___ con irritación; v. brotar, irritar.

flash n. fulguración, destello; **hot** ___ / fogaje, rubor.

flashback n. retrogresión; retroversión; retrospección y actualización de imágenes pasadas.

flashlight n. linterna eléctrica.

flask n. frasco, pomo.

flat a. plano-a, llano-a; extendido-a.

flatfoot n. pie plano.

flatulence n. flatulencia, distensión y molestias abdominales por exceso de gas en el tracto gastrointestinal.

flatus n. flato, pop. aventación, gas o aire en los intestinos.

flatworm n. gusano plano que se aloja en los intestinos.

flavor n. sabor, gusto.

flaw n. falta, defecto, falla.

flea n. pulga, insecto chupador de sangre; ___ **bite** / picadura de ___.

fleeting a. pasajero, que pasa rápidamente.

flesh n. carne, tejido muscular suave del cuerpo; ___ **wound** / herida superficial.

fleshless a. descarnado-a.

flex v. flexionar, doblar.

flexibility n. flexibilidad, propiedad de flexionar.

flexion n. flexión, acto de flexionar o de ser flexionado.

flexor n. flexor, músculo que hace flexionar una articulación.

flexure n. flexura, pliegue o doblez de una estructura u órgano; **hepatic** ___ / ___ hepática, ángulo derecho del colon; **sigmoid** ___ / sigmoidea, curvatura del colon que antecede al recto; **splenic** ___ / ___ esplénica, ángulo izquierdo del colon.

flicker v. fluctuar, vacilar; [to quiver] oscilar; causar una sensación visual de contraste con interrupción de la luz.

flight n. escape, fuga; vuelo; trayectoria; viaje aéreo.

flight of ideas n. fuga de ideas, interrupciones en el pensamiento y la expresión de palabras.

float n. flotador; v. flotar.

floaters n., pl. flotadores, manchas visuales, máculas.

floating a. flotante, libre, sin adhesión; ___ **ribs** / costillas ___ **-s**.

flocculation n. floculación, precipitación o aglomeración en forma de copos de partículas usu. invisibles.

floor n. piso, suelo.

flora n. flora, grupo de bacterias que se alojan en un órgano; **intestinal** ___ / ___ intestinal.

florid a. florido-a; encarnado-a; de color rojo vivo.

floss n. seda floja; **dental** ___ / hilo dental.

flour n. harina.

flow n. flujo, salida; riego; [menstrual] pop. pérdida; v. fluir; correr; derramar; **blood** ___ / riego sanguíneo; **laminar** ___ / ___ laminar; **turbulent** ___ / ___ turbulento.

flower n. flor, órgano reproductor de la planta.

flowmeter n. medidor de flujo.

fluctuate v. fluctuar, cambiar.

fluctuation n. fluctuación. 1. acto de fluctuar, variación de un curso a otro; 2. sensación de movimiento ondulante producido por líquidos en el cuerpo que se percibe en un examen de palpación.

fluid n. líquido, fluido; secreción. See chart on this page.

fluid balance n. balance hídrico.

fluid retention n. retención de líquido.

fluke n. duela, gusano de la orden Trematoda; **blood** ___ / ___ sanguínea; **intestinal** ___ / ___ intestinal; **liver** ___ / ___ hepática; **lung** ___ / ___ pulmonar.

Fluids	Fluido
amniotic	amniótico
cerebrospinal	cefalorraquídeo
extracellular	extracelular
extravascular	extravascular
interstitial	intersticial
intracellular	intracelular
seminal	seminal
serous	seroso
synovial	sinovial

fluorescence *n.* fluorescencia, propiedad de emisión de luminosidad de ciertas sustancias cuando son expuestas a cierto tipo de radiación, tal como los rayos-x.

fluorescent *a.* fluorescente, rel. a la fluorescencia; ___ **antibody** / anticuerpo ___; ___ **troponemal antibody absorption test** / técnica del anticuerpo ___.

fluoridation *n.* fluoridización, adición de fluoruro al agua.

fluoride *n.* fluoruro, combinación de flúor con un metal o metaloide.

fluorine *n.* flúor, elemento químico gaseoso.

fluoroscope *n.* fluoroscopio, instrumento que hace visibles los rayos-x en una pantalla fluorescente.

fluoroscopy *n.* fluoroscopía, uso del fluoroscopio para examinar los tejidos y otras estructuras internas del cuerpo.

fluorosis *n.* fluorosis, exceso de absorción de flúor.

flush *n.* rubor; [*cleansing*] irrigación; [*to empty out*] vaciar; irrigar; ruborizarse, sonrojarse.

flutter *n.* aleteo, acción similar al movimiento de las alas de los pájaros;**atrial** ___ / ___ auricular; ___ **and fibrillation** / fibrilación y ___; **ventricular** ___ / ___ ventricular; *v.* aletear, sacudir; agitarse.

flux *n.* flujo excesivo proveniente de una cavidad u órgano del cuerpo.

fly *n.* mosca; *vi.* volar.

foam *n.* espuma.

focal *a.* focal, rel. a un foco.

focus *n., L.* (*pl.* **foci**) foco; *v.* enfocar.

fold *n.* pliegue de un margen; **aryepiglottic** ___ / ___ ariepiglótico; **gastric** ___ / ___ gástrico; **gluteal** ___ / ___ glúteo.

folic acid *n.* ácido fólico, miembro del complejo de vitaminas B.

follicle *n.* folículo, saco, bolsa, depresión o cavidad excretora; **atretic** ___ / ___ atrésico; **gastric** ___ / ___ gástrico; **hair** ___ / ___ piloso; **ovarian** ___ / ___ ovárico; **thyroid** ___ / ___ tiroideo.

follicular *a.* folicular, rel. a un folículo; ___ **phase** / fase ___.

folliculitis *n.* foliculitis, infl. de un folículo, gen. un folículo piloso.

follow *v.* seguir, continuar; ___ **-up** / acción continuada, seguimiento, (estudio, procedimiento del caso); ___ **-up evaluation** / evaluación del proceso evolutivo; **to ___ through** / continuar el procedimiento; llevar hasta el final; continuar la observación de un caso.

fomes *n., L.* (*pl.* **fomites**) fomes, cualquier sustancia que puede absorber y luego transmitir agentes infecciosos.

fontanel, fontanella *n.* fontanela, *pop.* mollera, parte suave en el cráneo del recién nacido que normalmente se cierra al desarrollarse los huesos craneales.

food *n.* alimento; comida; **dietetic** ___ / ___ dietética; ___ **additives** / aditivos alimenticios; ___ **contamination** / contaminación de ___ -s; ___ **handling** / manipulación de ___ -s; ___ **poisoning** / intoxicación alimenticia; ___ **requirements** / requisitos alimenticios; ___ **supplements** / alimentos enriquecidos; **organic** ___ / ___ orgánico.

Food and Drug Administration *n.* Administración de Alimentos y Drogas, institución oficial en los Estados Unidos con regulaciones concernientes a alimentos, drogas, cosméticos y disposiciones médicas.

foolishness *n.* tontería, bobería.

foot *n.* (*pl.* **feet**) pie; **athlete's** ___ / ___ de atleta; **flat** ___ / ___ plano.

foot and mouth disease *n.* fiebre aftosa, enfermedad viral propia de animales vacunos y equinos, y que es raramente trasmitida al ser humano, se caracteriza por la erupción de pequeñas vesículas en la lengua, la boca y los dedos de las manos y pies.

foot-drop *n.* pie caído.

footprint *n.* impresión o huella del pie, pisada.

footsore *a.* que presenta molestia o dolor en el pie.

footstep *n.* paso, pisada; [*print*] huella del pie.

for *prep.* [*intended for the use of*] para, **an antibiotic ___ the infection** / un antibiótico ___ la infección; [*in exchange for*] por; **a thermometer ___ taking the temperature** / un termómetro ___ tomar la temperatura; [*for the benefit of*] para; **do it ___ her** / hágalo, hazlo ___ ella; ___ **the time being** / ___ ahora, ___ el momento; **the medicine is ___ the patient** / la medicina es ___ el paciente; [*for the purpose of*] para; **you pay a dollar ___ each pill** / paga un dólar ___ cada pastilla; [*for the sake of*] por.

foramen *n.* foramen, orificio, pasaje, abertura; **intervertebral** ___ / ___ intervertebral; **jugular** ___ / ___ yugular; **optic** ___ / ___ óptico; **ovale** ___ / ___ oval; **sciatic,**

greater ___ / ___ sacrociático mayor; **sciatic, lesser** ___ / ___ sacrociático menor;

forbid *vi.* prohibir, impedir; **God** ___ ! / !no lo permita Dios!.

force *n.* fuerza, vigor, energía; *v.* forzar, violentar, obligar; *v.* **to ___ out** / echar a la fuerza; **to ___ through** / hacer penetrar a la fuerza.

forceps *n.* fórceps, pinza en forma de tenaza que se emplea para sujetar y manipular tejidos o partes del cuerpo.

forearm *n.* antebrazo.

forebrain *n.* prosencéfalo, porción anterior de la vesícula primaria cerebral de donde se desarrollan el diencéfalo y el telencéfalo.

forecast *n.* pronóstico, predicción; *v.* predecir, pronosticar.

forefinger *n.* dedo índice.

forefoot *n.* antepié, parte anterior del pie.

foregut *n.* intestino anterior, porción cefálica del tubo digestivo primitivo en el embrión.

forehead *n.* frente.

foreign *a.* extranjero-a; extraño-a.

foreign bodies *n., pl.* cuerpos extraños, máculas, materia o pequeños objetos ajenos al lugar en que se alojan.

forensic *a.* forense, rel. a asuntos legales; ___ **laboratory** / laboratorio ___; ___ **medicine** / medicina legal; ___ **physician** / médico ___;

foreplay *n.* estímulo erótico que precede al acto sexual.

foresee *vi.* prever; prevenir

foreseen *a., pp.* of **to foresee**, previsto-a.

foresight *n.* precaución, previsión.

foreskin *n.* prepucio. **prepuce.**

forever *adv.* siempre, para siempre, por siempre.

forge *v.* falsificar, falsear

forger *n.* falsificador, -a, falsario-a.

forget *vi.* olvidar; olvidarse de; ___ **it** / olvídese, olvídate de eso; no se preocupe, no te preocupes.

forgetful *a.* olvidadizo-a; negligente.

forgive *vi.* perdonar.

fork *n.* tenedor; bifurcación.

forked *a.* bifurcado-a.

form *n.* forma; [*document*] formulario; *v.* formar, dar forma; establecer.

formaldehyde *n.* formaldehído, antiséptico.

formalin *n.* formalina, solución compuesta de formaldehído.

formation *n.* formación; composición; conjunto.

forme fruste *n. Fr.* forma frustrada, enfermedad abortada o manifestada de manera atípica.

formication *n.* formicación, sensación de hormigueo en la piel.

formula *n.* fórmula, forma prescrita o modelo a seguir.

fornix *n., L.* (*pl.* **fornices**) fórnix. 1. estructura en forma de arco; 2. concavidad en forma de bóveda semejante a la vagina.

forth *adv.* [*forward*] hacia adelante; [*out, away*] afuera, hacia afuera.

forthcoming *a.* venidero-a; disponible.

fortify *v.* fortalecer, fortificar.

fossa *n., L.* (*pl.* **fossae**) fosa, cavidad, hueco, depresión; ___ **glenoid** / ___ glenoidea; ___ **interpeduncular** / ___ interpeduncular; ___ **jugular** / ___ yugular; ___ **mandibular** / ___ mandibular; ___ **nasal** / ___ nasal; ___ **navicular** / ___ navicular.

fourchette *n. Fr.* horquilla, comisura posterior de la vulva.

fovea *n.* fóvea, fosa o depresión pequeña, esp. en referencia a la fosa central de la retina.

foxglove *n.* dedalera, nombre común de Digitalis purpurea.

fraction *n.* fracción, parte separable de una unidad.

fracture *n.* fractura, rotura; *pop.* quebradura. See chart on page 388.

fragility *n.* fragilidad, con disposición a romperse o quebrarse con facilidad.

fragment *n.* fragmento, parte; *v.* fragmentar, romper, dividir en pedazos.

frambesia, yaws *n.* frambesia, enfermedad cutánea tropical infecciosa que se manifiesta con lesiones aframbuesadas ulcerosas.

frame *n.* armazón. estructura de soporte; [*eyeglasses*] armazón. **claw type traction** ___ / armazón de tracción en garra; [*orthopedics*] **traction** ___ / armazón de tracción.

frank *a.* obvio-a, rel. a una condición física presente.

frantic *a.* frenético-a.

fraternal twins *n., pl.* mellizos fraternales, desarrollados de dos óvulos fecundados separadamente.

freckle *n.* peca, mácula pigmentada que se manifiesta en el exterior de la piel esp. en la cara.

freckled *a.* pecoso-a.

free *a.* libre, suelto-a; [*of charge*] gratis; ___ **association** / ___ asociación; **-ly** *adv.* libremente.

freedom *n.* libertad, independencia; *v.* **to have ___ to** / tener ___ para.

freeze *n.* helada; congelación; ___ **dried** / liofilizado; ___ **drying** / liofilización; *vi.*

Fractures	Fracturas
avulsion	por avulsión
blow-out	por estallamiento
butterfly	en mariposa
closed	cerrada
comminuted	conminuta
complete	completa
compressed	por compresión
depressed	con hundimiento
greenstick	de tallo verde
hairline	de raya fina
impacted	impactada
incomplete	incompleta
mallet	en martillo
open	expuesta
pathologic	patológica
perforating	perforante
spiral	espiral
stress	de sobrecarga
T	en T
wedge	en cuña

congelar, helar; congelarse, helarse; **to ___ to death** / morirse de frio.

freezing *n.* congelación; **___ point** / punto de ___.

fremitus *n.* fremitus, frémito, vibración detectable por palpación o auscultación tal como las vibraciones del pecho al toser.

French *n.* [*language*] francés; [*native*] francés, francesa; *a.* francés, francesa.

frenectomy *n.* frenectomía, excisión de un frenillo.

frenulum, frenum *n., L.* (*pl.* **frenulla**) frenulum, pliegue membranoso que impide los movimientos de un órgano o parte; **___ of the tongue** / frenillo de la lengua.

frenzy *n.* locura, frenesí, extravío, arrebato.

frequency *n.* frecuencia

frequent *a.* frecuente, habitual, regular; **-ly** *adv.* frecuentemente, con frecuencia.

fresh *a.* fresco-a, reciente.

freshen *v.* refrescar; renovar; refrescarse; renovarse.

Freudian *a.* freudiano, rel. a las doctrinas de Sigmund Freud, neurólogo vienés (1856-1939).

friable *a.* friable, que se pulveriza o rompe fácilmente.

friction *n.* fricción, rozamiento; **___ rub** / roce de ___.

fried *a. pp.* of **to fry**, frito-a.

fright *n.* espanto, temor excesivo.

frightened *a.* asustado-a, atemorizado-a.

frigid *a.* frígido-a.

frigidity *n.* frígidez, frialdad, esp. de la mujer incapaz de responder a estímulos sexuales.

frigolabile *a.* frigolábil, que se puede alterar fácilmente por el frío.

frigorific *a.* frigorífico-a, que genera frío.

frigotherapy *n.* frigoterapia, terapia de frío.

frivolous *a.* frívolo-a; tonto-a; vano-a.

Frohlich's syndrome *n.* síndrome de Frolich, distrofia adipogenital manifestada en infantilismo sexual con cambios en las características sexuales secundarias.

front *n.* frente; **in ___ of** / en ___ de, delante de.

frontal *a.* frontal, rel. a la frente; **___ bone** / hueso ___; **___ muscle** / músculo ___; **___ sinuses** / senos ___ -es.

frost *n.* escarcha, helada.

frostbite *n.* quemadura por frío.

froth *n.* espuma; *v.* echar espuma, espumar; **to ___ at the mouth** / echar ___ por la boca.

frozen *a. pp.* of **to freeze**, congelado-a; *v.* **to become ___** / congelarse, helarse.

frozen section *n.* corte por congelación, espécimen de tejido fino que se toma y congela inmediatamente para ser usado en el diagnóstico de tumores.

fructose *n.* fructosa, azúcar de frutas; lebulosa; **___ intolerance** / intolerancia a la ___.

fructosuria *n.* fructosuria, fructosa en la orina.

fruit *n.* fruta; *v.* **to eat ___ -s** / comer ___ -s.

fruitful *a.* productivo-a; provechoso-a.

frustrated *a.* frustrado-a.

frustration *n.* frustración.

fry *v.* freír.

fulfill *v.* cumplir; llevar a cabo; realizar.

fulguration *n.* fulguración, uso de corriente eléctrica para destruir tejido vivo.

full *a.* completo-a; lleno-a, pleno-a; **___ answer** / respuesta ___; **___ payment** / pago total; **in ___** / completamente, por completo.

full-grown *a.* completamente desarrollado-a; crecido-a.

full term *n.* a término, [*in obstetrics*] embarazo a término, de 38 a 41 semanas de duración incluyendo el nacimiento.

fulminant *a.* fulminante, que aparece súbitamente con extrema intensidad tal como un dolor o enfermedad.

fume *v.* humear, emitir vapores o gases.

fumes *n., pl.* vapores.

fumigant *n.* fumigante, agente usado en la fumigación.

fumigation *n.* fumigación, exterminación por medio de vapores.

fuming *a.* fumante, que desprende vapores visibles.

fun *n.* diversión, entretenimiento; *v.* **to have ___ /** divertirse, entretenerse.

function *n.* función; facultad; *v.* funcionar, desempeñar un trabajo.

functional *a.* funcional, de utilidad o valor práctico.

functional disease *n.* enfermedad funcional, desorden o trastorno que no tiene una causa orgánica conocida.

functioning *n.* funcionamiento.

fundectomy *n.* fundectomía, excisión del fondo del útero o de cualquier otro órgano.

fundus *n.* fondo, la parte más distante al orificio de entrada de un órgano; ___ **of stomach /** del estómago; ___ **uteri /** ___ del útero.

funeral *n.* funeral, entierro; ___ **parlor /** funeraria.

fungal, fungous *a.* fungoso-a, rel. a hongos o causado por éstos.

fungate *v.* reproducirse rápidamente como los hongos.

fungemia *n.* fungemia, presencia de hongos en la sangre.

fungicide *n.* fungicida, exterminador de hongos.

fungiform *a.* fungiforme, en forma de hongo.

fungistasis *n.* fungistasis, acto de impedir o arrestar el desarrollo de hongos.

fungitoxic *a.* fungitóxico, de efecto tóxico en los hongos.

fungus *n., L.* (*pl.* **fungi**) hongo.

funicular *a.* funicular, rel. al cordón umbilical o espermático.

funiculitis *n.* funiculitis, infl. del cordón espermático.

funnel *n.* embudo.

furfuraceous *a.* furfuráceo-a, escamoso-a, o que se asemeja a escamas.

furious *a.* furioso-a; enfurecido-a.

furor *n.* furor, ira extrema.

furosemide *n.* furosemida, diurético.

furrow *n.* surco; **atrioventricular ___ / ___** atrioventricular; **digital ___ / ___** digital; **gluteal ___ / ___** gluteal.

furuncle *n.* furúnculo; *pop.* grano enterrado.

furunculosis *n.* furunculosis, condición que resulta por la presencia de furúnculos.

furunculous *a.* foruncular, rel. a un forúnculo.

fuse *v.* fundir, fusionar, derretir un metal por medio de calor.

fusiform *a.* fusiforme, en forma de huso.

fusion *n.* fusión. 1. reacción termonuclear en la cual núcleos atómicos de luz se unen para formar átomos más potentes; 2. acto de fusionar o fundir; **nuclear ___ / ___** nuclear.

future *n.* futuro, porvenir.

fuzzy *a.* 1. nublado-a, que no es claramente visible; 2. velloso-a, cubierto de pelusa.

f

g

G *abbr.* **constant of gravitation** / constante de gravitación.

g *abbr.* **gender** / género; **glucose** / glucosa; **grain** / grano.

gadfly *n.* tábano, moscardón; moscón.

Gaenslen test, sign *n.* examen de Gaenslen, procedimiento que se usa para determinar malfuncionamiento sacroilíaco.

gag *n.* abrebocas, instrumento para mantener la boca abierta durante ciertas intervenciones quirúrgicas; ___ **reflex** / reflejo de arqueada.

gage *v.* medir, calibrar.

gain *n.* ganancia, ventaja; provecho; *v.* ganar; **to** ___ **weight** / aumentar de peso.

gainful *a.* ventajoso-a, provechoso-a.

gait *n.* marcha, andar; **cerebellar** ___ / ___ cerebelosa; **compensated gluteal** ___ / ___ compensada glútea; **crutch** ___ / ___ con muletas; **dorsiflexor** ___ / ___ de dorsiflexión; **drag-to** ___ / ___ de arrastre; **duck** ___ / ___ de pato; **equine** ___ / ___ equina; **festinating** ___ / ___ festinante; **gastrocnemius** ___ / ___ gemelar; **hemiplegic** ___ / ___ hemipléjica; **petit pas** ___ / ___ en pequeños pasos; **scissors** ___ / ___ en tijeras; **spastic** ___ / ___ espástica; **steppage** ___ / ___ en estepaje; **tabetic** ___ / ___ tabética; **three point** ___ / ___ en tres apoyos; **Treadelenburg or gluteal** ___ / ___ de Treadelenburg o glútea; **two point** ___ / ___ en dos apoyos; **uncompensated gluteal** ___ / ___ glútea descompensada; **waddling** ___ / ___ de ánade.

galactagogue *n.* galactagogo, galactógeno, agente que promueve la secreción de leche.

galactase *n.* galactasa, enzima presente en la leche.

galactocele *n.* galactocele, quiste de la mama que contiene leche.

galactophoritis *n.* galactoforitis, infl. de los conductos lácteos.

galactophorous *a.* galactóforo-a, que conduce la leche o la lleva.

galactopoiesis *n.* galactopoyesis, producción de leche.

galactorrhea *n.* galactorrea. 1. secreción excesiva de leche; 2. continuación de secreción de leche a intervalos después que el período de lactancia ha terminado.

galactose *n.* galactosa, monosacárido derivado de la lactosa por acción de una enzima o un ácido mineral; ___ **cataract** / catarata de ___ .

galactosemia *n.* galactosemia, ausencia congénita de la enzima necesaria para la conversión de galactosa a glucosa o sus derivados.

galactosuria *n.* galactosuria, orina con apariencia lechosa.

galactotherapy *n.* galactoterapia. 1. tratamiento dirigido a un lactante mediante administración de medicamentos a la madre; 2. uso terapéutico de la leche en una dieta especial.

galacturia *n.* galacturia, aspecto lechoso en la orina.

gall *n.* bilis, hiel; ___ **ducts** / conductos biliares.

gallbladder *n.* vesícula biliar; ___ **attack** / ataque de la vesícula.

gallium *n.* galio, metal.

gallop *n.* galope, ritmo cardíaco que simula el galope de un caballo y que se oye cuando hay fallo del corazón.

gallop rhythm *n.* ritmo de galope, sonido anormal del corazón percibido en casos de taquicardia.

gallstone *n.* cálculo biliar; **calcium oxalate** ___ / ___ de oxalato de calcio; **cholesterol** ___ / ___ de colesterol; **cystine** ___ / ___ de cistina; **fibrin** ___ / ___ de fibrina; **pigment** ___ / ___ de pigmento.

galvanic *a.* galvánico-a, rel. al galvanismo; ___ **battery** / batería; ___ **cell** / célula ___; ___ **current** / corriente ___ .

galvanism *n.* galvanismo, uso terapéutico de corriente eléctrica directa.

galvanocautery *n.* galvanocauterización, electrocauterization.

galvanometer *n.* galvanómetro, instrumento que mide la corriente por acción electromagnética.

gamete *n.* gameto, célula sexual masculina o femenina; ___ **intrafallopian transfer** / transferencia de ___ a los tubos de Falopio.

gametocide *n.* gametocida, agente que destruye gametos.

gametocyte *n.* gametocito, célula que al dividirse produce gametos tal como el parásito de la malaria cuando se divide y pasa al mosquito portador.

gametogenesis *n.* gametogénesis, desarrollo de gametos.

gamma benzene hexachloride *n.* hexacloruro de gamma-benceno, insecticida poderoso utilizado contra la sarna.

gamma globulin *n.* gamma globulina, tipo de anticuerpo producido en el tejido linfático o sintéticamente.

gamma rays *n., pl.* rayos gamma, rayos emitidos por sustancias radioactivas.

gammagraphy *n.* gammagrafía, registro de rayos gamma después de la administración de isótopos radioactivos.

gammopathy *n.* gammopatía, trastorno manifestado por un exceso de inmunoglobulinas como resultado de una proliferación anormal de células linfoides.

gangliectomy *n.* gangliectomía, ganglionectomía, excisión de un ganglio.

gangliocyte *n.* gangliocito, célula ganglionar.

ganglioglioma *n.* ganglioglioma, ganglioneuroma, tumor caracterizado por un gran número de células ganglionares.

ganglioma *n.* ganglioma, tumor de un ganglio, esp. linfático.

ganglion *n.* (*pl.* **ganglia**) ganglio. 1. masa de tejido nervioso en forma de nudo; 2. quiste en un tendón o en una aponeurosis, que se observa a veces en la muñeca, en el talón o en la rodilla; ___ **-a, basal** / ___ -s basales; ___ , **carotid** / ___ carotídeo; ___ , **celiac** / ___ celíaco.

ganglioneuroma *n.* ganglioneuroma, neuroma compuesto de células ganglionares.

ganglionic blockade *n.* bloqueo ganglionar.

gangrene *n.* gangrena, destrucción de un tejido debido a riego sanguíneo interrumpido gen. por infección bacteriana y putrefacción.

gangrenous *a.* gangrenoso, rel. a la gangrena.

gap *n.* laguna, vacío; intervalo, abertura.

Gardner's syndrome *n.* síndrome de Gardner. 1. múltiple poliposis del colon asociado con riesgo de carcinoma del colon; 2. tumor de tejido blando de la piel.

gargle *n.* gargarización; *v.* hacer gárgaras.

gargoylism *n.* gargolismo, condición hereditaria caracterizada por anormalidades físicas, en algunos casos con retraso mental.

garlic *n.* ajo.

gas *n.* gas, sustancia con propiedades de expansión indefinida; **mustard** ___ / ___ de mostaza; **nerve** ___ / ___ neurotóxico; **tear** ___ / ___ lacrimógeno.

gaseous *a.* gaseoso-a, rel. a o de la naturaleza del gas.

gasoline *n.* gasolina; ___ **poisoning** / envenenamiento por ___ .

gastradenitis *n.* gastradenitis, infl. de las glándulas del estómago.

gastralgia *n.* gastralgia, dolor de estómago.

gastrectasis, gastrectasia *n.* gastrectasia, dilatación del estómago.

gastrectomy *n.* gastrectomía, extirpación de una parte o de todo el estómago.

gastric *a.* gástrico-a, rel. o concerniente al estómago; **acid** / ácido ; **analysis** / gastroanálisis; ___ **arteries** / arterias ___; ___ **by-pass** / derivación ___; **digestion** ___ / digestión ___; **emptying** / vaciamiento ___; ___ **feeding** / alimentación ___; ___ **fistula** / fístula ___; ___ **glands** / glándulas ___; ___ **juice** / jugo ___; ___ **lavage** / lavado ___; ___ **stapling** / cirugía de reducción ___ para adelgazar; **ulcer** ___ / úlcera ___; ___ **vertigo** / vértigo ___ .

gastrin *n.* gastrina, hormona segregada por el estómago.

gastritis *n.* gastritis, infl. del estómago; **acute** ___ / ___ aguda; **chronic** ___ / ___ crónica.

gastroanalysis *n.* gastroanálisis, análisis del contenido del estómago.

gastroanastomosis *n.* gastroanastomosis, anastomosis entre las dos porciones de un estómago en reloj de arena.

gastrocele *n.* gastrocele, hernia del estómago.

gastrocolitis *n.* gastrocolitis, infl. del estómago y del colon.

gastrocolostomy *n.* gastrocolostomía, anastomosis del estómago y el colon.

gastroduodenal *a.* gastroduodenal, rel. al estómago y el duodeno.

gastroduodenitis *n.* gastroduodenitis, infl. del estómago y el duodeno.

gastroduodenoscopy *n.* gastroduodenoscopía, uso del endoscopio para examinar visualmente el estómago y el duodeno.

gastroenteritis *n.* gastroenteritis, infl. del estómago y el intestino.

gastroenteroanastomosis *n.* gastroenteroanastomosis, unión quirúrgica del estómago al intestino delgado.

gastroenterocolitis *n.* gastroenterocolitis, infl. del estómago y el intestino delgado.

gastroepiploic *a.* gastroepiploico-a, rel. al estómago y el epiplón.

gastroesophageal *a.* gastroesofágico-a, rel. al estómago y al esófago; ___ **hernia** /

hernia ___; ___ **reflux disease** / enfermedad de reflujo ___ .

gastroesophagitis *n.* gastroesofagitis. V. esophagogastritis.

gastrogavage *n.* gastrogavaje, alimentación artificial al estómago por tubo o a través de una abertura.

gastroileostomy *n.* gastroileostomía, anastomosis entre el estómago y el íleo.

gastrointestinal *a.* gastrointestinal; rel. al estómago y el intestino; ___ **barrier** / barrera ___; ___ **bleeding** / sangramiento___; ___ **decompression** / descompresión ___; ___ **tract** / tracto___ .

gastrojejunostomy *n.* gastroyeyunostomía, anastomosis del estómago y el yeyuno.

gastrolith *n.* gastrolito, concreción en el estómago.

gastrolithiasis *n.* gastrolitiasis, cálculos en el estómago.

gastromalacia *n.* gastromalacia, ablandamiento de las paredes del estómago.

gastromegaly *n.* gastromegalia, agrandamiento del estómago.

gastroplication *n.* gastroplicación, sutura de un pliegue de la pared del estómago para reducir el tamaño del mismo.

gastrorrhagia *n.* gastrorragia, hemorragia estomacal.

gastrorrhaphy *n.* gastrorrafia, sutura o perforación del estómago.

gastroschisis *n.* gastrosquisis, hendidura en la pared abdominal debida a ruptura de la membrana amniótica.

gastrospasm *n.* gastroespasmo, contracciones espasmódicas de las paredes del estómago.

gastrostaxis *n.* gastrostaxis, sangramiento de la membrana mucosa del estómago.

gastrostomy *n.* gastrostomía, creación de una fístula gástrica.

gastrotopic *a.* gastrotópico-a, que afecta al estómago.

gastrula *n.* gástrula, etapa primitiva del desarrollo embriónico.

gauge *n.* medida; *v.* medir.

Gauss sign *n.* Gauss, signo de, movimiento marcado en el útero durante las primeras semanas del embarazo.

gauze *n.* gasa: **absorbable** ___ / ___ absorbible; **absorbent** ___ / ___ absorbente; **antiseptic** ___ / ___ antiséptica; ___ **compress** / compresa de ___ .

gay *n.* homosexual; ___ **bowel syndrome** / síndrome intestinal del ___ .

gel *n.* jalea.

gelatin *n.* gelatina.

gelatinous *a.* gelatinoso-a, de consistencia semejante a la gelatina o que la contiene.

gemmation *n.* gemación, método de fisión en el cual la célula progenitora produce un botón que contiene cromatina, el cual se desprende para crear un gémulo.

gemulo *n.* gémula, pequeño botón, producto de la gemación.

gender *n.* género, denominación del sexo masculino o femenino; ___ **identity** / identidad de ___; ___ **role** / representación de ___ .

gene *n.* gen, gene, unidad básica de rasgos hereditarios; **dominant** ___ / ___ dominante; ___ **frequency** / frecuencia del ___; **lethal** ___ / ___ letal; **recessive** ___ / ___ recesivo; **sex-linked** ___ / ___ ligado al sexo.

genealogic tree *n.* árbol genealógico, gráfico que muestra la descendencia ancestral.

general *a.* general; ___ **appearance** / aspecto___; ___ **condition** / estado ___; ___ **practitioners** / médicos de familia; ___ **treatment** / tratamiento___ .

generalization *n.* generalización.

generalize *v.* generalizar.

generation *n.* generación. 1. acción de crear un nuevo organismo; 2. producción por proceso natural o artificial; 3. conjunto de personas nacidas dentro de un período de unos treinta años aproximadamente.

generator *n.* generador, máquina que convierte energía mecánica en eléctrica.

generic *n.* nombre común de un producto o medicamento no patentado; *a.* genérico-a, rel. al género; ___ **name** / nombre genérico.

genesis *n.* génesis, acto de creación, reproducción y desarrollo.

genetic *a.* genético-a, rel. a la génesis y a la genética; ___ **amplification** / amplificación ___; ___ **association** / asociación ___; ___ **code** / patrón ___; ___ **counseling** / asesoramiento ___; ___ **determinant** / determinante ___; ___ **engineering** / construcción ___; ___ **epidemiology** / epidemiología ___; ___ **fitness** / acondicionamiento ___; ___ **load** / carga ___; ___ **marker** / marcador ___; ___ **substrate** / substrato___ .

genetics *n.* genética, rama de la biología que estudia la herencia y las leyes que la gobiernan; **medical** ___ / ___ médica.

genicular *a.* genicular, rel. a la rodilla.

geniculate *a.* geniculado-a. 1. doblado-a, como una rodilla; 2. rel. al ganglio del nervio facial; ___ **body** / cuerpo ___; ___ **ganglion** / ganglio ___; ___ **neuralgia** / neuralgia ___ .

genioplasty *n.* genioplastia, reconstrucción plástica de la mandíbula.

genital *a.* genital, rel. a los genitales;___ **ambiguity** / ambigedad ___; ___ **cord** / cordón ___; ___ **corpuscles** / corpúsculos ___; ___ **furrow** / surco ___; ___ **herpes** / herpes ___; ___ **phase** / fase ___; ___ **tract** / tracto___; ___ **wart** / verruga ___ .

genitals, genitalia *n., pl.* genitales, órganos de la reproducción.

genitourinary *a.* genitourinario, rel. a los órganos reproductivos y urinarios.

genocide *n.* genocidio, exterminación sistemática de un grupo étnico.

genodermatosis *n.* genodermatosis, una condición de la piel de origen genético.

genom, genome *n.* genoma, el conjunto básico completo de cromosomas haploides en un organismo.

genomic *a.* genómico-a, rel. a un genoma; ___ **clone** / clon ___ .

genotoxic *a.* genotóxico-a, rel. a una sustancia tóxica nociva al material genético de las células.

genotype *n.* genotipo, constitución genética de un organismo.

gentamicin *n.* gentamicina, antibiótico efectivo en varios tipos de bacterias gram-negativas.

gentian violet *n.* violeta de genciana, colorante para teñir tejidos y microorganismos que permiten el estudio microscópico.

gentle *a.* suave, sutil, tierno-a; moderado-a; **-ly** *adv.* suavemente, sutilmente, tiernamente; moderadamente.

genucubital *a.* genucubital, rel. a los codos, las rodillas y su posición; ___ **position** / posición ___ .

genuine *a.* auténtico-a, genuino-a; legítimo-a.

genupectoral *a.* genupectoral, rel. a las rodillas y el tórax y su posición; ___ **position** / posición ___ .

genus *n.* (*pl.* **genera**) género, categoría perteneciente a una clasificación biológica.

genu valgum, knock knee *n.* genu valgum, curvatura anormal de las rodillas hacia adentro y separación de los tobillos al caminar que comienza en la infancia a causa de una deficiencia ósea.

genu varum, bow-leg *n.* piernas arqueadas, *pop.* zambo-a, curvatura anormal de las rodillas hacia afuera.

geographic *a.* that shows physically, natural or superficial markings; ___ **keratitis** / queratitis ___; ___ **retinal atrophy** / atrofia retinal ___; ___ **skull** / cráneo ___ .

geographic tongue *n.* lengua geográfica, lengua caracterizada por áreas desnudas rodeadas de epitelio grueso que simulan áreas terrestres.

geophagia, geophagism, geophagy *n.* geofagia, geofagismo, propensión a comer sustancias terrosas tales como tierra o barro.

geriatrics *n.* geriatría, rama de la medicina que trata de las enfermedades y de los problemas que se manifiestan en la vejez.

germ *n.* germen, microorganismo o bacteria esp. causante de enfermedades.

German measles *n.* rubela, rubéola; *pop.* sarampión de tres días, infección viral benigna muy contagiosa en los niños de 3 a 10 años. Puede causar trastornos serios en el desarrollo del feto al contraerla la madre; ___ **vaccination** / vacunación antirubeólica.

germ-free *n.* axénico.

germinal *a.* germinal, rel. a o de la naturaleza de un germen o gérmenes; ___ **cell** / célula ___; ___ **disk** / disco ___; ___ **epithelium** / epitelio ___; ___ **localization** / localización ___; ___ **vesicle** / vesícula o núcleo ___ .

germination *n.* germinación, brote de una planta o desarrollo de una persona o animal.

germinoma *n.* germinoma, neoplasma de tejido o células germinales usu. localizado en los testículos u ovarios.

geromorphism *n.* geromorfismo, senilidad prematura.

gerontology *n.* gerontología. V. **geriatrics.**

gestalt *n.* gestalt, teoría que mantiene que la conducta responde a la percepción íntegra de una situación y no es posible analizarla atendiendo sólo a las partes componentes de la misma.

gestation *n.* embarazo, gestación, estado de gravidez; **abdominal** ___ / ___ abdominal; **ectopic** ___ / ___ ectópica; **interstitial** ___ / ___ intersticial; **multiple** ___ / ___ múltiple; **prolonged** ___ / ___ prolongada; **secondary** ___ / ___ secundaria; **secondary abdominal** ___ / ___ abdominal secundaria; **tubal** ___ / ___ tubárica; **tubo-ovarian** ___ / ___ tubo-ovárica; **uterotubaric** ___ / ___ útero-tubárica.

gesticulate *v.* gesticular, expresar por medio de gestos o señas.

gesticulation *n.* gesticulación, seña, gesto, ademán.

gesture *n.* gesto, ademán.

get *vi.* obtener, adquirir, conseguir; [*communication*]; **to ___ across** / lograr comunicarse, hacer comprender; **to ___ ahead** / prosperar; **to ___ back something** / recobrar; **to ___ back** / volver; [*to swallow*] **to ___ down** / tragar; [**steps**] **to ___ down** / bajar; **to ___ into** / meterse; **to ___ it over** / acabar de una vez; **to ___** [*someone, something*] **out of the way** / sacar de, quitar de, apartar de; **to ___ sick** / enfermarse; **to ___ underway** / empezar, comenzar; **to ___ up** / levantarse; **to ___ well** / curarse, sanarse.

giant *a.* gigante, de un tamaño grande anormal; **___ cell** / célula ___; **___ cell tumor** / tumor de células ___ -s.

giardiasis *n.* giardiasis, infección intestinal común causada por la *Giardia lamblia* que se trasmite por contaminación de alimentos, de agua o por contacto directo.

gibbosity *n.* gibosidad, corcova, condición de joroba.

Giemsa stain *n.* coloración de Giemsa, usada en frotis de sangre en análisis microscópicos.

Gifford reflex *n.* reflejo de Gifford, contracción pupilar como reacción al cierre de los párpados cuando están abiertos forzadamente.

gigantism *n.* gigantismo, desarrollo en exceso del cuerpo o de una parte de éste; **___ , acromegalic** / ___ acromegálico; **___ , eunuchoid** / eunucoide, gigantismo acompañado de características e insuficiencia sexual propias del eunuco; **___ , normal** / ___ normal, desarrollo normal de los órganos sexuales y proporción normal de los órganos y partes del cuerpo, gen. causado por secreción excesiva de la glándula pituitaria.

Gilles de la Tourette syndrome *n.* síndrome de Gilles de la Tourette, enfermedad de la infancia que afecta más a los varones que a las hembras y que se cree ser de naturaleza neurológica; se manifiesta por anomalías musculares y a veces en la pubertad por expresar obscenidades involuntariamente.

Gillies operation *n.* operación de Gillies, técnica quirúrgica para reducir la fractura del hueso y el arco cigomático.

Gimbernat's ligament *n.* ligamento de Gimbernat, membrana que se adhiere por un extremo al ligamento inguinal y por otro al pubis.

ginger *n.* jengibre.

gingiva *n.* (*pl.* **gingivae**)gingiva, encía, porción de tejido que rodea el cuello de los dientes.

gingival *a.* gingival, rel. a la gingiva.

gingivectomy *n.* gingivectomía, resección de la encía.

gingivitis *n.* gingivitis, infl. de las encías.

girdle *n.* faja, cinturón; **pelvic ___** / cinturón pélvico; **scapular or shoulder ___** / cinturón torácico.

gitalin *n.* gitalina, glucósido extraído de la digitalis.

give *vi.* dar; **___ birth** / dar a luz; **to ___ and take** / hacer concesiones mutuas; **to ___ out** / repartir; **to ___ up** / renunciar a, perder la esperanza; darse por vencido.

given *a., pp.* of **to give**, dado-a; **___ name** / nombre de pila.

glacial *a.* glacial, rel. al. hielo o semejante al mismo.

glad *a.* alegre, contento-a; *v.* **to be ___ of** / alegrarse de; **to be ___ to** / tener mucho gusto en; **-ly** *adv.* con mucho gusto; con satisfacción; alegremente.

glance *n.* mirada, ojeada, vistazo; *v.* dar un vistazo, dar una ojeada; **at first ___** / a primera vista.

gland *n.* glándula, órgano que segrega o secreta sustancias que realizan funciones fisiológicas específicas o que eliminan productos del organismo; **eccrine ___** / ___ ecrina; **endocrine ___** / ___ endocrina; **swollen ___** / ___ inflamada.

glans *n.* glande, masa redonda de estructura similar a una glándula situada en la extremidad del pene (glans penis) y del clítoris (glans clitorides).

glare *n.* resplandor, deslumbramiento, relumbrón; *v.* mirar con intensidad.

glaring *a.* deslumbrante, intenso-a; brillante.

Glasgow coma scale *n.* escala de coma de Glasgow, método para evaluar el grado de un estado de coma.

glass *n.* vidrio, cristal; **magnifying ___** / lente de aumento.

glasses *n., pl.* lentes, espejuelos, gafas; **bifocal ___** / ___ bifocales; **trifocal ___** / ___ trifocales.

glaucoma *n.* glaucoma, enfermedad de los ojos producida por hipertensión del globo ocular, atrofia de la retina y ceguera; **absolutum ___** / ___ absoluto, etapa final del glaucoma agudo que resulta en ceguera;

chronic ___ / ___ crónico; **congential** ___ / ___ congénito; **juvenile** ___ / ___ juvenil, se manifiesta en niños mayores y jóvenes sin agrandamiento del globo ocular; **infantile** ___ / ___ infantil, se manifiesta a partir del nacimiento o desde los tres años.

glenohumeral *a.* glenohumeral, rel. al húmero y la cavidad glenoide; ___ **joint** / articulación ___; ___ **ligaments** / ligamentos ___ .

glenoid *a.* glenoideo-a, con apariencia de fosa o cuenca; ___ **cavity** / cavidad ___; ___ **fossa** / fosa ___ .

glia *n.* glía. V. **neuroglia**.

gliacyte *n.* gliacito, célula de una neuroglía.

glide *v.* resbalar; deslizarse.

glimpse *n.* mirada fugaz.

glioblastoma *n.* glioblastoma, tipo de tumor cerebral.

gliocytoma *n.* gliocitoma, tumor de células de neuroglia.

glioma *n.* glioma, neoplasma del cerebro compuesto de células de neuroglia.

gliomyoma *n.* gliomioma, combinación de glioma y mioma.

glioneuroma *n.* glioneuroma, glioma combinado con neuroma.

gliosarcoma *n.* gliosarcoma, glioma con abundancia de células fusiformes.

global warming *n.* calentamiento global, aumento de los niveles de gases tales como el dióxido de carbono que provoca el alce de la temperatura de la tierra y que puede afectar muchos sistemas biológicos, incluyendo la salud del ser humano.

globin *n.* globina, proteína que constituye la hemoglobina.

globule *n.* glóbulo, pequeña masa esférica.

globulin *n.* globulina, una de las cuatro proteínas más importantes que componen el plasma; **antilymphocyte** ___ / ___ antilinfocítica; **gamma** ___ / gamma ___ .

globulinuria *n.* globulinuria, presencia de globulina en la orina.

globus *n.* globo, esfera; ___ **hystericus** / ___ histérico, sensación subjetiva de tener una bola en la garganta.

glomerular *a.* glomerular, rel. a un glomérulo; en forma de racimo; ___ **cyst** / quiste ___; ___ **filtration rate** / índice de filtración ___; ___ **nephritis** / nefritis ___ .

glomerulonephritis *n.* glomerulonefritis, enfermedad de Bright, infl. del glomérulo renal.

glomerulosclerosis *n.* glomeruloesclerosis, proceso degenerativo del glomérulo renal que se asocia con arterioesclerosis y diabetes.

glomerulus *n., L. (pl.* **glomeruli**) glomérulo, colección de capilares en forma de bola pequeña localizados en el riñón.

glomus *n., L. (pl.* **glomera**) glomo, bola, grupo de arteriolas conectadas directamente a las venas, ricas en inervación.

gloom *n.* tristeza, desaliento.

gloomy *a.* triste, abatido-a.

glossa *n.* glosa, lengua.

glossalgia *n.* glosalgia, dolor en la lengua.

glossectomy *n.* glosectomía, excisión parcial o completa de la lengua.

glossitis *n.* glositis, infl. de la lengua; **acute** ___ / ___ aguda, asociada con estomatitis.

glossodynia *n.* glosodinia, glossalgia.

glossopathy *n.* glosopatía, enfermedad de la lengua.

glossoplasty *n.* glosoplastia, cirugía plástica de la lengua.

glossoplegia *n.* glosoplejía, parálisis total o parcial de la lengua.

glossorrhaphy *n.* glosorrafía, sutura de la lengua.

glossotomy *n.* glosotomía, incisión de la lengua.

glossy skin *n.* liodermia, apariencia brillante de la piel, síntoma de atrofia o traumatismo de los nervios.

glottal *a.* glótico-a; ___ **stop** / oclusión ___ .

glottis *n.* glotis, hendidura en la parte superior de la laringe entre las cuerdas vocales verdaderas; aparato vocal de la laringe.

glottitis *n.* glotitis. V. **glossitis**.

glove *n.* guante; **to handle with kid** ___ **-s** / tratar con mucho cuidado, tratar delicadamente; *v.* **to fit like a** ___ / ajustar.

glucagon *n.* glucagón, una de dos hormonas producidas por los islotes de Langerhans cuya función consiste en aumentar la concentración de glucosa en la sangre y que tiene un efecto antiinflamatorio.

glucagonoma *n.* glucagonoma, tumor que secreta glucagón.

glucocorticoid *n.* glucocorticoide, grupo de hormonas segregadas por la corteza suprarrenal que intervienen en el proceso metabólico del organismo y tienen un efecto antiinflamatorio.

glucogenesis *n.* glucogénesis, proceso de desdoblamiento del glucógeno.

gluconeogenesis *n.* gluconeogénesis. 1. formación hepática de glucógeno a partir de fuentes distintas de los carbohidratos; 2. formación de azúcar por desdoblamiento de glucógeno.

g

glucose *n.* glucosa, dextrosa, azúcar de fruta, fuente principal de energía en organismos vivos; **blood level of** ___ / nivel de ___ en la sangre; ___ , **tolerance test** / prueba de tolerancia a la ___ .

glucose-6-phosphate dehydrogenase *n.* glucofosfato de deshidrogenasa, enzima presente en el hígado y los riñones necesaria en la conversión de glicerol a glucosa.

glucoside, glycoside *n.* glucósido, compuesto natural o sintético que al hidrolizarse libera azúcar.

glucosuria, glycosuria *n.* glucosuria, presencia excesiva de glucosa en la orina; **diabetic** ___ / ___ diabética; **pituitary** ___ / ___ pituitaria; **renal** ___ / ___ renal.

glucuronic acid, glycuronic acid *n.* ácido glucurónico, ácido de efecto desintoxicante en el metabolismo humano.

glue *n.* cola, goma de pegar; ___ **ear** / oído tupido o tapado con cerumen; ___ **-sniffing** / inhalación de ___ .

gluey *a.* gomoso-a, viscoso-a, glutinoso-a.

glutamate *n.* glutamato, sal de ácido glutámico.

glutamic-oxaloacetic transaminase *n.* transaminasa glutámica oxaloacética, enzima presente en varios tejidos y líquidos del organismo cuya concentración elevada en el suero indica daño cardíaco o hepático.

glutamic-pyruvic transaminase *n.* transaminasa glutámica pirúvica, enzima cuyo aumento en la sangre es indicio de daño cardíaco o hepático.

gluteal *a.* glúteo-a, rel. a las nalgas; ___ **fold** / pliegue ___ ; ___ **reflex** / reflejo ___ .

gluten *n.* gluten, materia vegetal albuminoidea; ___ **-free diet** / dieta libre de ___ .

glycemia *n.* glicemia, glucemia, concentración de glucosa en la sangre.

glycerin *n.* glicerina, glicerol, alcohol que se encuentra en las grasas.

glychoprotein *n.* glucoproteína, compuesto de carbohidrato y proteína.

glycine *n.* glicina, ácido aminoacético, aminoácido no esencial.

glycocholic acid *n.* ácido glicocólico, combinación de glicina y ácido cólico.

glycogen *n.* glucógeno, polisacárido usu. almacenado en el hígado que se convierte en glucosa según lo necesite el organismo; ___ **storage disease** / hepatina, almacenamiento de glucógeno en el hígado.

glycogenolysis *n.* glucogenolisis, proceso químico que tiene lugar en el hígado y los músculos y que convierte el glucógeno en glucosa.

glycolic *a.* glucolítico-a, que descompone o digiere los azúcares.

glycolysis *n.* glicólisis, subdivisión de azúcar en compuestos más simples.

glycopenia *n.* glucopenia. V. **hypoglycemia**.

glycopexic *n.* glucopéxico, que fija o acumula azúcar.

glycophilia *n.* glucofilia, estado en el cual una cantidad muy pequeña de dextrosa produce hiperglucemia.

glycorrhachia *n.* glucorraquia, presencia de glucosa en el líquido cefalorraquídeo.

gnashing *n.* rechinamiento de los dientes.

gnat *n.* [*insect*] jején.

gnatho *n.* gnato, el punto más bajo de la línea media de la mandíbula.

gnathoplasty *n.* gnatoplastia, cirugía plástica de la mandíbula.

gnosia *n.* gnosia, facultad de reconocer y distinguir objetos y personas.

go *vi.* ir; irse; **to** ___ **after** / seguir; **to** ___ **about** / andar, caminar; [*to accompany*] **to** ___ **along with** / acompañar; **to** ___ **against** / ir en contra de; **to** ___ **ahead** / adelantar; emprender; **to** ___ **along with a decision** / aceptar, aprobar una decisión; **to** ___ **bad** / echarse a perder; **to** ___ **back** / volver, retroceder; **to** ___ **crazy** / enloquecer; **to** ___ **in or into** / entrar; **to** ___ **deep into** / ahondar; **to** ___ **down with** / enfermarse, caer enfermo-a; [*distance*] **to** ___ **far** / ir lejos; [*to succeed*] tener éxito, progresar; **to** ___ **on** / continuar; **to** ___ **over** / examinar, estudiar; **to** ___ **through** / examinar o estudiar con cuidado; **to let** ___ / soltar, dejar; **to let oneself** ___ / soltarse; dejarse; relajarse.

goat *n.* cabra; ___ **milk** / leche de ___ .

goblet cell *n.* célula caliciforme secretora que se localiza en el epitelio del tubo digestivo y del tubo respiratorio.

godchild *n.* ahijado-a.

godfather *n.* padrino.

godless *n.* ateo-a; incrédulo-a.

godmother *n.* madrina.

goggle-eyed *a.* de ojos saltones.

goiter *n.* bocio, engrosamiento de la glándula tiroides; **congenital** ___ / ___ congénito; **endemic, colloid** ___ / ___ endémico, coloide; **exophtalmic** ___ / ___ exoftálmico; **toxic** ___ / ___ tóxico (de síntomas similares a la tirotoxicosis); **wandering** ___ / ___ móvil.

gold *n.* oro.

gonad *n.* gónada, glándula productora de gametos: los ovarios en la mujer y los testículos en el hombre.

gonadal *a.* gonadal, rel. a una glándula gónada; ___ **dysgenesis** / distenesia, malformación ___ .

gonadectomy *n.* gonadectomía, excisión de una glándula sexual.

gonadopathy *n.* gonadopía, enfermedad de las gónadas.

gonadotropin *n.* gonadotropina, hormona estimulante de las gónadas; **chorionic** ___ / ___ coriónica, presente en la sangre y orina de la mujer durante el embarazo, base de la prueba del embarazo; ___ **of the anterior pituitary** / ___ hipofisaria.

gonadotropin-releasing hormone *n.* hormona que estimula la secreción de gonadotropina.

gonalgia *n.* gonalgia, dolor en la rodilla.

gonarthritis *n.* gonartritis, infl. de la articulación de la rodilla.

gonion *n.* gonión, punto extremo inferior, posterior y lateral del ángulo de la mandíbula.

goniopuncture *n.* goniopuntura, tratamiento de glaucoma por punción en la cámara anterior del ojo.

goniotomy *n.* goniotomía, procedimiento para tratar el glaucoma congénito.

gonococcal *a.* gonocócico; rel. a los gonococos; ___ **arthritis** / artritis ___; ___ **conjunctivitis** / conjuntivitis ___ .

gonococcus *n.* (*pl.* **gonococci**) gonococo, microorganismo de la especie *Neisseria gonorrhoeae*, causante de la gonorrea.

gonorrhea *n.* gonorrea, enfermedad infecciosa catarral contagiosa de la mucosa genital.

gonorrheal *a.* gonorreico-a, rel. a la gonorrea; ___ **arthritis** / artritis ___; ___ **ophthalmia** / oftalmia ___ .

good *a.* bueno-a; **all in** ___ **time** / todo a su debido tiempo; **in** ___ **time** / a buen tiempo, puntual; *v.* **good!** / muy bien!; ___ **afternoon** / buenas tardes; ___ **behavior** / buena conducta, buen comportamiento; ___ **-bye** / adiós; ___ **cause** / causa justificada; ___ **luck** / buena suerte; ___ **morning** / buenos días, buen día; ___ **night** / buenas noches; **in** ___ **faith** / de___fe; **to be** ___ **at** / tener talento para; **to do someone** ___ / hacer bien a alguien; **to put in a** ___ **word** / recomendar.

Good Samaritan Law *n.* Ley del buen samaritano, protección legal al facultativo o a otras personas que prestan ayuda médica en casos de emergencia.

Goodell sign, *n.* Goodell, signo de, ablandamiento del cuello uterino, posible indicación de embarazo.

gooseflesh *n. pop.* carne de gallina.

gout *n.* gota, enfermedad hereditaria causada por defecto del metabolismo de ácido úrico.

gracilis *n.* gracilis, músculo largo interno del muslo.

grade *n.* grado. 1. medida o evaluación estándar; 2. en la patología del cáncer, indicación de la fase de la enfermedad.

gradient *a.* gradiente, línea que indica aumento o disminución en una variable.

Graefe operation *n.* Graefe, operación de. 1. operación de la catarata por incisión de la esclerótica, distinción de la cápsula e iridectomía; 2. iridectomía para glaucoma.

Graefe's sign *n.* Graefe, signo de, fallo del párpado superior en seguir el movimiento del globo del ojo hacia abajo.

graft *n.* injerto, tejido u órgano usado en un trasplante o implante; *v.* injertar. See chart on page 398.

graftable *a.* injertable.

graftage *n.* práctica de hacer injertos.

grain *n.* grano, cereal.

gram *n.* gramo, unidad de medida métrica.

gramicidin *n.* gramicidina, antibiótico producido por *Bacillus brevis*, localmente activo contra bacterias gram-positivas.

grammar *n.* gramática.

gram-molecule *n.* molécula gramo, el peso en gramos de una sustancia igual a su peso molecular.

gram-negative *n.* gram-negativo, resultado de la aplicacion del método de Gram de decoloración de una bacteria o tejido por medio de alcohol.

gram-positive *n.* gram-positivo, retención del color o resistencia a la decoloración en la aplicación del método de Gram.

Gram's method *n.* método de Gram, proceso de coloración de bacterias para identificarlas en un análisis.

granular *a.* granuloso-a, granulado-a, hecho o formado de gránulos; ___ **cell tumor** / tumor celular ___; ___ **conjunctivitis** / conjuntivitis ___; ___ **corneal dystrophy** / distrofia ___ de la córnea; ___ **cortex** / corteza ___; ___ **endoplasmic reticulum** / retículo endoplásmico ___; ___ **leukocyte** / leucocito___; ___ **ophthalmia** / oftalmia ___ .

Grafts	Injertos
accordion g.	i. en acordeón
allogeneic g.	i. alogénico
autologous g.	i. autólogo
autoplastic g.	i. autoplástico
bone g	i. óseo
choriollantoic g.	i. coriolantoideo
corneal g.	i. de la córnea
dermal g.	i. dérmico
fat g.	i. adipose
free g.	i. libre
heterologous g.	i. heterólogo
heteroplastic g.	i. heteroplástico
heterotopic g.	i. heterotópico
homologous g.	i. homólogo
homoplastic g.	i. homoplástico
isoplastic g.	i. isoplástico
mucosal g.	i. mucoso
nerve g.	i. de nervio
orthotopic g.	i. ortotópico
pedicle g.	i. pediculado
sieve g.	i. en criba
skin g.	i. de piel
tendon g.	i. tendinoso
zooplastic g.	i. zooplástico

granular cast *n.* cilindro granuloso, cilindro urinario visto en nefropatías degenerativas o de tipo inflamatorio.

granulation *n.* granulación, masa redonda y carnosa que se forma en la superficie de un tejido, membrana u órgano; ___ **tissue** / tejido de ___ .

granule *n.* gránulo, partícula pequeña formada de gránulos; **acidophil** ___ / ___ acidófilo, que acepta colorantes ácidos; **basophil** ___ / ___ basófilo, que acepta colorantes básicos.

granulocyte *n.* granulocito, leucocito que contiene gránulos.

granulocytopenia *n.* granulocitopenia, deficiencia de granulocitos en la sangre.

granulocytosis *n.* granulocitosis, aumento excesivo de granulocitos en la sangre.

granuloma *n.* granuloma, tumor o neoplasma de tejido granular; **foreign body** ___ / ___ de

cuerpo extraño; **infectious** ___ / ___ infeccioso; **inguinal** ___ / ___ inguinal; **venereum** ___ / ___ ulcerativo de los genitales.

granulomatosis *n.* granulomatosis, granuloma múltiple.

granulomatous *a.* granulomatoso-a, que tiene las características de un granuloma; ___ **colitis** / colitis ___; ___ **encephalomyelitis** / encefalomielitis ___; ___ **enteritis** / enteritis ___; ___ **inflammation** / inflamación ___ .

granulopenia *n.* granulopenia. V. **granulocytopenia**.

granulosa *n.* granulosa, membrana ovárica de células epiteliales que rodea el folículo ovárico.

granulosa cell tumor *n.* tumor de la granulosa.

granulosa-teca cell tumor *n.* tumor de células de la granulosa-teca, tumor ovárico de células que provienen del folículo de Graaf.

grape *n.* uva.

grape sugar *n.* dextrosa, azúcar de uva y de otras frutas.

graphology *n.* grafología, estudio de la escritura como indicación de la personalidad del paciente y como ayuda en el diagnóstico de enfermedades nerviosas.

grass *n.* hierba, yerba.

grateful *a.* agradecido-a.

gratefulness *n.* gratitud.

gravamen *n.* agravio, motivo de queja.

grave *a.* severo-a, serio-a, peligroso-a.

Graves' disease *n.* enfermedad de Graves, hipertiroidismo. *Syn.* **exophthalmic goiter**.

graveyard *n.* cementerio, camposanto.

gravida *n.* mujer embarazada, preñada, encinta, en estado.

gravidity *n.* gravidez, embarazo.

gravity *n.* fuerza de gravedad.

gravy *n.* salsa, jugo de carne.

gray *n.* color gris; *a.* gris; ___ **cataract** / catarata ___; ___ **columns** / columnas ___ -es; ___ **degeneration** / degeneración ___; ___ **fibers** / fibras ___ -es; ___ **hepatization** / hepatización ___; ___ **induration** / induración ___; ___ **matter** / sustancia ___ .

gray matter *n.* materia o sustancia gris, tejido nervioso muy vascularizado de color gris pardo compuesto de células nerviosas y fibras nerviosas amielínicas.

great *a.* grande, grandioso-a; **in** ___ **detail** / muy minucioso; **it is going** ___ / todo va muy bien.

green *n.* verde.

green blindness *n.* ceguera al color verde.
green pepper *n.* pimiento verde.
greet *v.* saludar; recibir.
greeting *n.* saludo.
grid *n.* rejilla.
grief *n.* pesar, aflicción.
grief reaction *n.* reacción de aflicción.
grief-stricken *a.* desconsolado-a; afligido-a; acongojado-a; lleno-a de pesar.
grievance *n.* queja; agravio.
grieve *v.* afligirse, apenarse.
grievous *a.* penoso-a, doloroso-a.
grilled *a.* asado-a a la parrilla.
grime *n.* mugre, tizne.
grind *vi.* moler; triturar; picar.
grinder *n.* [*dental*] molar, *pop.* muela; pulverizador.
grinder's disease *n.* enfermedad de los pulmones producida por inhalación de polvo.
grinding wheel *n.* [*dental*] disco de esmeril.
grip *n.* apretón de la mano; *v.* agarrar, apretar.
grip, grippe *n.* gripe,*Mex.* gripa; influenza.
griseofulvin *n.* griseofulvina, antibiótico usado en el tratamiento de algunas enfermedades de la piel.
gristle *n.* cartílago.
groan *v.* gemir; quejarse.
groggy *a.* atontado-a, vacilante, tambaleante.
groin *n.* ingle.
groove *n.* surco, ranura; **bicipital** ___ / ___ bicipital; **costal** ___ / ___ costal.
gross *a.* grave; grueso-a, denso-a; grotesco-a; ___ **negligence** / imprudencia o negligencia ___ .
gross anatomy *n.* anatomía macroscópica, estudio de los órganos y partes del cuerpo que se ven a simple vista.
ground *n.* base; suelo; terreno; *a. pp.* of **to grind,** molido-a.
ground substance *n.* sustancia fundamental que llena los espacios intercelulares de los huesos, cartílagos y tejido fibroso.
group *n.* grupo, conglomerado; **support** ___ / ___ de soporte.
group therapy *n.* terapia de grupo.
grow *vi.* crecer, desarrollar; **to** ___ **old** / envejecer.
growth *n.* desarrollo, crecimiento, multiplicación; proliferación.
growth hormone *n.* hormona del crecimiento, secreción de la glándula pituitaria que estimula el crecimiento.
grumous *a.* grumoso-a, coagulado-a.
gryposis *n.* griposis, curvatura anormal esp. rel. a una uña.

guaiacol *n.* guayacol, antiséptico y anestésico.
guanethidine *n.* guanetidina, agente usado en el tratamiento de la hipertensión.
guarantee *n.* garantía; *v.* garantizar; acreditar.
guard *v.* [*protect*] guardar, proteger, cuidar; guardarse, cuidarse; **to** ___ **against** / tomar precauciones, cuidarse de, guardarse de.
guarded *a.* de cuidado; guardado-a; vigilado-a; protegido-a; **in** ___ **condition** / de pronóstico reservado.
guardian *n.* guardián-a, custodio-a; tutor-a.
gubernaculum *n., L.* gubernaculum, dirección o guía.
guess *n.* suposición. *v.* adivinar, suponer; acertar.
guest *n.* invitado-a, huésped, comensal; parásito.
guidance *n.* guía, consejo, dirección.
guide *n.* guía, cualquier instrumento o mecanismo que dirige a otro para conducirlo a su objetivo; *v.* guiar.
guideline *n.* pauta, guía, directriz.
Guillain-Barré syndrome *n.* Guillan-Barré, síndrome de, enfermedad neurológica rara que se evidencia por parálisis ascendente que comienza por las extremidades y puede llegar rápidamente a los músculos respiratorios en dos o tres semanas causando fallo respiratorio.
guillotine *n.* guillotina, instrumento quirúrgico.
guinea pig *n.* conejillo de Indias.
gullet *n.* esófago; *pop.* garguero, gaznate.
gulp down *v.* engullir, tragar apresuradamente.
gum *n.* encía. V. **gingiva;** goma; **chewing** ___ / goma de mascar, *pop.* chicle.
gumboil *n.* absceso en la encía, flemón.
gumma *n.* (*pl.* **gummata**) goma, tumor sifilítico.
gummy *a.* pegajoso-a, gomoso-a, viscoso-a.
gun *n.* escopeta; revólver; pistola.
gunshot wound *n.* herida de bala.
gurney *n.* camilla.
gush *v.* salir a borbotones, derramar, verter.
gustation *n.* gustación, sentido del gusto.
gustatory *a.* gustativo-a, rel. al gusto; ___ **agnosia** / agnosia ___; ___ **aura** / aura ___; ___ **hyperhidrosis** / hiperhidrosis ___; ___ **rhinorrhea** / rinorrea ___ .
gut *n.* intestino, *pop.* tripas.
gutta *n.* (*pl.* **guttae**) gutta, gota.
gutta-percha *n.* gutapercha, látex vegetal seco y purificado que se usa en tratamientos dentales y médicos.
guttural *a.* gutural.
gymnastics *n.* gimnasia, calistenia.
gynandroid *n.* ginandroide, persona de características hermafroditas que muestra la apariencia del sexo opuesto.

g

gynecologic, gynecological *a.*
ginecológico-a, rel. al estudio de enfermedades
del tracto reproductivo femenino.

gynecologic operative procedures *n.*
procedimientos quirúrgicos ginecológicos.

gynecologist *n.* ginecólogo-a, especialista en
ginecología.

gynecology *n.* ginecología, estudio de los
trastornos que afectan los órganos reproductivos
femeninos.

gynecomastia *n.* ginecomastia, desarrollo
excesivo de las glándulas mamarias en el
hombre.

gyrus *n., L.* (*pl.* **giri**) circunvolución, porción
elevada de la corteza cerebral; **Broca's** ___ / ___
de Broca, tercera, frontal inferior; **frontal,
superior** ___ / ___ frontal superior; **inferior,
lateral occipital** ___ / ___ occipital inferior
lateral; **superior occipital** ___ / ___ occipital
superior.

h

H *abbr.* **heroin** / heroína; **hydrogen** / hidrógeno; **hypermetropia** / hipermetropía; **hypodermic** / hipodérmico.

h *abbr.* **height** / altura; **hour** / hora; **horizontal** / horizontal.

habilitate *v.* habilitar, equipar.

habit *n.* hábito, uso, costumbre; adicción al uso de una droga o bebida; *v.* **to be in the ___ of** / tener la costumbre de; acostumbrarse a; habituarse; *pop.* [*drugs*] to kick the ___ / dejar la adicción; curarse.

habit-forming *a.* adictivo-a, rel. a una sustancia que envicia, que crea una adicción.

habit training *n.* entrenamiento de hábitos, enseñanza impartida a los niños para realizar actividades básicas tales como comer, dormir, vestirse, asearse y usar el servicio sanitario.

habitual *a.* habitual, usual, acostumbrado-a; **-ly** *adv.* habitualmente.

hacking cough *n.* tos seca recurrente.

had *pp.* of **to have**.

haggard *a.* ojeroso-a; desfigurado-a; desaliñado-a.

hair *n.* pelo, cabello, vello; **axillary ___** / ___ axilar; **curly ___** / ___ rizado; **gray ___** / ___ cana; **pubic ___** / vello púbico; **straight ___** / ___ lacio, liso; **wavy ___** / ___ ondeado.

hairball *n.* bola de pelo, tipo de bezoar.

hairbrush *n.* cepillo para el cabello.

hair bulb *n.* bulbo piloso.

hair follicle *n.* folículo piloso.

hairless *a.* pelón -ona, pelado-a, calvo-a.

hairline *n.* raya del pelo; línea fina; trazo fino; **___ fracture** / fractura de línea fina.

hair remover *n.* depilatorio.

hair root *n.* raíz del pelo.

hair transplantation *n.* trasplante de pelo, trasplante de epidermis que contiene folículos pilosos de otra parte del cuerpo.

hairy *a.* peludo-a, velludo-a; **___ tongue** / lengua velluda, lengua infectada de hongos parásitos.

half *n.* mitad, medio; **___ and ___** / a mitades, en igual proporción; **___ as much** / la mitad; **___ brother** / medio hermano; **___ -hour** / media hora; **___ sister** / media hermana; **___ -starved** / medio muerto de hambre; **in ___** / en dos mitades.

half-life *n.* 1. vida media, tiempo requerido para que la mitad de una sustancia ingerida o inyectada en el organismo se elimine por medios naturales; 2. semidesintegración, tiempo requerido por una sustancia radioactiva para perder la mitad de su radioactividad por desintegración.

halide *n.* haloide, haluro, sales producidas por la combinación de un elemento halógeno y un metal.

halitosis *n.* halitosis, mal aliento.

halitus *n.* hálito, aire aspirado.

hall *n.* vestíbulo; recepción; pasillo.

hallucinate *v.* alucinar, desvariar.

hallucination *n.* alucinación, alucinamiento, sensación subjetiva que no tiene precedencia o estímulo real; **auditory ___** , **imaginary perception of sounds** / ___ auditiva, percepción imaginaria de sonidos; **gustatory ___** , **imaginary sensation of taste** / ___ gustativa, sensación imaginaria del gusto; **haptic ___** , **imaginary perception of pain, temperature, or skin sensations** / ___ táctil, percepción imaginaria de dolor, de temperatura o de sensaciones en la piel; **motor ___** , **imaginary movement of the body** / ___ de movimiento, percepción imaginaria de movimiento del cuerpo; **olfactory ___** , **imaginary smells** / ___ olfativa, de olores imaginarios.

hallucinatory *a.* alucinante, alucinador-a.

hallucinogen *n.* alucinógeno, droga que produce alucinaciones o desvaríos tal como LSD, peyote, mescalina y otras.

hallucinosis *n.* alucinosis, delirio alucinatorio crónico; **acute alcoholic ___** / ___ alcohólica, manifestación de temor patológico acompañado de alucinaciones auditivas.

hallux *n., L.* (*pl.* **halluces**) dedo gordo del pie; **___valgus** / ___ valgus, desviación del dedo gordo hacia los otros dedos; **___varus** / ___ varus, separación del dedo gordo de los demás dedos.

halo *n.* aureola. 1. área del seno de tono más oscuro que rodea el pezón; 2. círculo de luz.

halothane *n.* halótano, anestésico administrado por inhalación, nombre comercial Fluotane.

ham *n.* 1. corva de la pierna, región poplítea detrás de la rodilla; 2. jamón.

hamartoma *n.* hamartoma, nódulo de tejido superfluo semejante a un tumor usualmente benigno.

hamate bone *n.* hueso medio del carpo de la muñeca.

hammer *n.* martillo.1. huesecillo del oído medio; 2. instrumento empleado en exámenes físicos; **___ finger or toe** / dedo en garra;

percussion ___ / ___ de percusión; **reflex** ___ / ___ de reflejo.

hamstring *n.* 1. tendones de la corva; 2. músculos flexores y aductores de la parte posterior del muslo.

hand *n.* mano; **close at** ___ / muy de cerca; **give me a** ___ / ayúdeme, ayúdame; ___ **deformities, acquired** / deformidades adquiridas de la ___; ___ **rest** / apoyo de la ___; **in good** ___ **-s** / en buenas manos; **on the other** ___ / por otra parte; **to have a free** ___ / tener libertad para, tener carta blanca; **to have one's** ___ **-s tied** / tener atadas las manos, sin poder hacer nada; **to keep one's** ___ **-s off** / no meterse; **to shake** ___ **-s** / dar la ___; *v.* **to** ___ **in a report** / presentar un informe; **to** ___ **out information** / facilitar información; **to** ___ **out news** / facilitar noticias.

handful *n.* puñado, manojo.

handicap *n.* impedimento; obstáculo, desventaja; **handicapped person** / persona desvalida, inválida, baldada, impedida.

handle *n.* asa, mango; *v.* tratar, manejar, manipular; ___ **with care** / trátese con cuidado.

handling *n.* manejo, manipulación.

handmade *a.* hecho a mano.

handpiece *n.* [*dental*] pieza de mano.

handsome *a.* guapo-a, hermoso-a, distinguido-a.

handwriting *n.* escritura a mano.

handy *a.* a la mano; conveniente; cercano-a.

hang *vi.* colgar, suspender, ahorcar; ahorcarse.

hanging *n.* suspensión, colgajo; ejecución en la horca.

hangnail *n.* uñero, uña encarnada.

hangover *n.* malestar después de una borrachera.

hang-up *n.* obsesión o problema que irrita.

Hanot's disease *n.* enfermedad de Hanot, cirrosis biliar, cirrosis hipertrófica del hígado acompañada de ictericia.

Hansen's disease *n.* enfermedad de Hansen. *Syn.* **leprosy**.

haploid *n.* haploide, célula sexual que contiene en el cromosoma la mitad de las características somáticas de la especie.

happen *v.* suceder, acontecer, ocurrir.

happening *n.* suceso, hecho, acontecimiento; **What is ?** ___ / ¿Qué sucede?, ¿qué pasa?

happiness *n.* alegría, felicidad.

happy *a.* contento-a, alegre, feliz.

haptoglobin *n.* haptoglobina, mucoproteína que se une a la hemoglobina libre en el plasma.

haptometer *n.* haptómetro, instrumento para medir la agudeza del sentido del tacto.

harass *v.* acosar, perturbar, hostigar, hostilizar.

harassment *n.* acosamiento, perturbación, vejamen.

hard *a.* duro-a, endurecido-a, sólido; trabajoso-a, difícil; [*bone*] osificado; ___ **of hearing** / medio sordo; *v.* **to grow** ___ / endurecerse; [*parturition*]; ___ **labor** / parto laborioso; **-ly** *adv.* a duras penas, dificilmente, escasamente.

hard bone *n.* hueso compacto.

hardbound *a.* estreñido-a.

harden *v.* endurecer, solidificar.

hardening *n.* endurecimiento, solidez.

hard feelings *n., pl.* resentimiento.

hard contact lens *n.* lentes de contacto duros.

hardheaded *a.* obstinado-a, terco-a, testarudo-a.

hard palate *n.* paladar óseo.

hard pressed *a.* acosado-a, apremiado-a.

hardship *n.* sufrimiento, privación, penalidad.

harelip *n.* labio leporino, deformidad congénita a nivel del labio superior causada por falta de fusión del proceso nasal interno y el lateral maxilar; ___ **suture** / sutura del ___.

harelipped *a.* labihendido-a, que tiene labio leporino.

harm *n.* daño, mal, perjuicio; *v.* dañar, perjudicar.

harmful *a.* perjudicial, dañino-a.

harmless *a.* inofensivo-a, inocuo-a.

harmonize *v.* armonizar; [*relations*] llevarse bien.

harmony *n.* armonía, reunión o comunicación agradable.

harness *n.* cinturón corrector.

harvest *n.* recolección, obtención o separación de bacterias u otros microorganismos de un cultivo; cosecha.

hashish *n.* hachís, *pop.* yerba, narcótico de efecto eufórico extraído de la marihuana.

hate, hatred *n.* odio, aversión; *v.* odiar, repudiar.

haustrum *n., L.* haustrum, cavidad o saco, esp. el del colon.

have *vi.* *aux.* haber; tener; **to** ___ **to** / tener que.

haversian system *n.* sistema de Havers, serie de cánículos o pequeños conductos y láminas en formación concéntrica que forman la base estructural del hueso compacto.

hay fever *n.* fiebre del heno, asma del heno, catarro del heno, catarro primaveral, alergia causada por un agente irritante externo, gen. polen.

hazard *n.* riesgo, peligro; **a** ___ **to your health** / un ___ para su salud.

hazardous *a.* arriesgado-a, peligroso-a.

head *n.* 1. cabeza; 2. parte principal de una estructura; **from** ___ **to toe** / de la ___ a los pies; ___ **birth** / presentación cefálica; ___ **drop** / caída de la ___; ___ **injury** / traumatismo del cráneo, golpe en la ___; ___ **of the family** / ___ de familia; *v.* **to nod one's** ___ / asentir con la ___.

headache *n.* cefalalgia, dolor de cabeza, jaqueca.

headrest *n.* apoyo para la cabeza, cabezal.

headshrinker *n.* psiquiatra.

headstrong *a.* voluntarioso-a, testarudo-a.

heal *v.* curar, sanar, recobrar la salud; [*a wound*] cicatrizar; curarse, sanarse; recobrarse.

healer *n.* curador-a; curandero-a.

healing *n.* 1. curación, recuperación de la salud; ___ **process** / proceso de ___; 2. curanderismo.

health *n.* salud; [*government*] **behavioral** ___ / conducta saludable; **dental** ___ / higiene dental; **Department of** ___ / Ministerio de Salud o Salubridad; ___ **and medical assistance** / asistencia médico-sanitaria; ___ **assessment** / evaluación del estado de ___; ___ **authorities** / autoridades de Sanidad; ___ **care** / atención o cuidado de la ___; ___ **care provider** / profesional de atención de la ___; ___ **care reform** / reforma al sistema de ___; ___ **care system** / sistema sanitario; ___ **center** / centro de ___, centro de higiene sanitaria; ___ **certificate** / certificado de ___; ___ **education** / educación médica; ___ **facilities** / instituciones de ___; ___ **food** / alimento sano; ___ **habits** / hábitos sanitarios; ___ **laws** / estatutos sanitarios; ___ **personnel** / profesionales médicos y de asistencia pública; ___ **physicist** / biofísico; ___ **planning** / planeamiento de métodos de ___; ___ **risk assessment** / evaluación de riesgo sanitario; ___ **services** / servicios o atención de la ___; ___ **services for the aged** / servicios de ___ a los ancianos; ___ **statistics** / estadísticas de ___ salud mental; ___ **status** / estado de ___; **home** ___ **care** / cuidado de ___ en el hogar; **mental** ___ / ___ mental; **occupational** ___ / atención médica laboral; **rural** ___ / ___ rural; **uncertain** ___ / ___ precaria; **urban** ___ / ___ urbana.

healthy *a.* sano-a, saludable, fornido-a.

hear *vi.* oír, escuchar.

hearing *n.* audición, oído; ___ **acuity** / agudeza auditiva; ___ **aid** / instrumento auditivo; ___ **level** / umbral auditivo; ___ **loss** / pérdida de la audición.

heart *n.* corazón, órgano muscular cóncavo cuya función es mantener la circulación de la sangre; ruidos cardíacos; **congenital** ___ **disease** / anomalías congénitas del ___; **distant** ___ **sounds** / ruidos cardíacos apagados; **enlarged** ___ / cardiomegalia; **fetal** ___ **sounds** / ruidos cardíacos fetales; ___ **atrium** / aurícula cardíaca; ___ **attack** / ataque al ___; ___ **block** / bloqueo del ___; ___ **block, atrioventricular** / bloqueo auriculoventricular, interrupción en el nódulo A-V; ___ **block, bundle-branch** / bloqueo de rama; ___ **block, interventricular** / bloqueo interventricular; ___ **block, partial** / bloqueo parcial; ___ **block, sinoatrial** / bloqueo senoauricular, interferencia completa o parcial del paso de impulsos del nódulo senoauricular; ___ **catherization** / cateterización o cateterismo cardíaco; ___ **disease** / cardiopatías; ___ **failure, congestive** / insuficiencia cardíaca congestiva, colapso o fallo cardíaco; ___ **failure, low output** / deficiencia en mantener un flujo sanguíneo adecuado; ___ **failure, left** / insuficiencia ventricular izquierda, deficiencia en mantener un gasto normal del ventrículo izquierdo; ___ **failure, right-sided** / insuficiencia del ventrículo derecho; ___ **-healthy** / cardiosaludable; ___ **hypertrophy** / hipertrofia del ___; ___ **murmur** / soplo cardíaco; ___ **output** / gasto cardíaco; ___ **pacemaker** / estimulador cardíaco, marcapasos; ___ **palpitation** / palpitación cardíaca; ___**pump, nuclear powered** / bomba del ___ de fuerza nuclear; ___ **rate** / frecuencia cardíaca; ___ **reflex** / reflejo cardíaco; ___ **scan** / escán cardíaco; ___ **shadow** [*as in x-ray*] / silueta cardíaca; ___ **sound** / ruido del ___; ___ **specialist** / cardiólogo; ___ **transplant** / trasplante del ___; ___ **valve** / válvula del ___; **hypertensive** ___ **disease** / cardiopatía por hipertensión; **low** ___ **output** / gasto bajo; **reduplication of** ___ **sounds** / desdoblamiento de ruidos cardíacos.

heartbeat *n.* latido del corazón, [*rapid*] palpitación; **ectopic** ___ / ___ ectópico.

heartburn *n.* acedía, acidez, *pop.* ardor en el estómago; agruras.

heart-lung machine *n.* máquina corazón-pulmón, máquina cardiopulmonar que se usa para mantener artificialmente las funciones del corazón y de los pulmones.

heat *n.* calor; **conductive** ___ / ___ de conducción; **dry** ___ / ___ seco; ___**cramps** / espasmo muscular (debido a trabajos realizados

en altas temperaturas); ___ **exhaustion** / colapso
por calor; ___ **loss** / pérdida de ___; ___
prostration / insolación con colapso; ___
sensitive / sensible al calor; ___ **stable** /
termoestable; ___ **stroke** / insolación; ___ **unit** /
caloría; ___ **therapy** / termoterapia; **to be
in** ___ / estar en celo; *v.* calentar; dar calor.

heater *n.* calentador; aparato de calefacción;
electric ___ / ___ eléctrico.

heating pad, electric *n.* almohadilla
eléctrica.

heavier *a.* muy pesado; *comp.* más pesado que.

heaviness *n.* pesadez, pesantez, peso; [*sleep*]
sueño pesado, modorra; [*feelings*] abatimiento,
decaimiento.

heavy *a.* pesado-a, grueso-a, fornido-a; ___ **chain
disease** / enfermedad de red o cadena; ___
drinker / bebedor, que bebe demasiado; ___
food / alimento indigesto; ___ **liquid** / líquido
espeso; ___ **meal** / comida fuerte; ___ **period** /
hipermenorrea; ___ **sleep** / sueño profundo; ___
traffic / tráfico denso;

hectic *a.* hético-a, febril; agitado-a; consumido-a,
tísico-a.

heel *n.* talón, calcañal, parte posterior redondeada
del pie.

hefty *a.* fuerte, macizo-a.

height *n.* altura, alto; estatura.

Heimlich maneuver *n.* maniobra de Heimlich,
técnica que se usa para sacar o forzar la
expulsión de un cuerpo extraño que impide el
paso del aire de la tráquea o la faringe.

helical *a.* helicoideo-a, en forma de hélice o
espiral.

heliophobia *n.* heliofobia, temor exagerado al
sol de personas que han sufrido de insolación.

heliotherapy *n.* helioterapia, exposición o baños
de sol con propósito terapéutico.

helium *n.* helio, elemento gaseoso inerte
empleado en tratamientos respiratorios y en
cámaras de descompresión para facilitar el
aumento o disminución de la presión del aire.

helminth *n.* helminto, gusano que se localiza en
el intestino humano.

helminthiasis *n.* helmintiasis, condición
parasítica intestinal.

helminthicide *n.* helminticida, vermicida,
medicamento que extermina parásitos.

help *n.* ayuda, asistencia, socorro, auxilio; *v.*
ayudar, asistir, auxiliar; remediar.

helper *n.* ayudante, asistente, auxiliar.

helpful *a.* útil, provechoso-a.

helpless *a.* desamparado-a, indefenso-a;
desvalido-a, abandonado-a.

hemacytometer *n.* hemacitómetro, instrumento
contador de las células sanguíneas.

hemafecia *n.* hemafecia, presencia de sangre en
las heces fecales.

hemagglutination *n.* hemoaglutinación,
aglutinación de células rojas sanguíneas.

hemagglutinin *n.* hemoaglutinina, anticuerpo
de células rojas o hematíes que causa
aglutinación.

hemangioblastoma *n.* hemangioblastoma,
hemangioma localizado generalmente en el
cerebelo.

hemangioma *n.* hemangioma, tumor benigno
formado por vasos capilares en racimo que
producen una marca de nacimiento de color rojo
púrpura en la piel.

hemangiosarcoma *n.* hemangiosarcoma,
tumor maligno del tejido vascular.

hemarthrosis *n.* hemartrosis, derrame de sangre
en la cavidad de una articulación.

hematemesis *n.* hematemesis, vómito de
sangre.

hematherapy, hemotherapy *n.*
hematerapia, hemoterapia, uso terapéutico de la
sangre.

hematic *n.* hemático, droga usada en el
tratamiento de anemia; *a.* hemático-a,
relacionado con la sangre.

hematochezia *n.* hematoquezia, presencia de
sangre en el excremento.

hematocolpos *n.* hematocolpos, retención del
flujo menstrual en la vagina debido a
imperforación del himen.

hematocrit *n.* hematócrito. 1. aparato
centrifugador que se usa en la separación de
células y partículas del plasma; 2. promedio de
eritrocitos en la sangre.

hematocyst *n.* hematoquiste. 1. quiste
sanguinolento; 2. hemorragia dentro de un
quiste.

hematogenesis *n.* hematogénesis. *v.*
hematopoiesis.

hematologic, hematological *a.*
hematológico-a, rel. a la sangre; ___ **studies** /
estudios ___ -s. See chart on page 405.

hematologist *n.* 1. especialista en hematología;
2. especialista en diagnóstico de pruebas
sanguinea y tratamiento de enfermedades de las
sangre.

hematology *n.* hematología, ciencia que estudia
la sangre y los órganos que intervienen en la
formación de ésta.

hematoma *n.* hematoma, hinchazón por sangre
coleccionada fuera de un vaso; *pop.* chichón;

Hematologic Values	Valores Hematológicos
bleeding time	tiempo de sangramiento
coagulation time	tiempo de coagulación
erythrocyte sedimentation	sedimentación de eritrocitos
hematocrit	promedio de eritrocitos
hemoglobin	hemoglobina
partial thromboplastin time	tiempo parcial de tromboplastin
arterial blood pH	pH de la sangre arterial
prothrombin time	tiempo de protrombina

pelvic ___ / ___ pélvico; **subdural** ___ / derrame subdural.

hematomyelia *n.* hematomielia, derrame de sangre dentro de la médula espinal.

hematopoiesis, hemopoiesis *n.* hematopoyesis, hemopoyesis, formación de sangre.

hemianalgesia *n.* hemianalgesia, insensibilidad al dolor en un lado del cuerpo.

hemianopia, hemianopsia *n.* hemianopia, hemianopsia, pérdida de la visión en la mitad del campo visual de uno o ambos ojos.

hemiataxia *n.* hemiataxia, falta de coordinación muscular que afecta un lado del cuerpo.

hemiatrophy *n.* hemiatrofia, atrofia de la mitad de un órgano o de la mitad del cuerpo.

hemiballism *n.* hemibalismo, lesión en el cerebro que afecta a la mitad del cuerpo con movimientos involuntarios rápidos sin coordinación, esp. en las extremidades superiores.

hemicolectomy *n.* hemicolectomía, extirpación de una mitad del colon.

hemihypertrophy *n.* hemihipertrofia unilateral con desarrollo excesivo de la mitad del cuerpo.

hemilaminectomy *n.* hemilaminectomía, extirpación de un lado de la lámina vertebral.

hemiparalysis *n.* hemiparálisis, parálisis de un lado del cuerpo.

hemiparesis *n.* hemiparesis, debilidad muscular que afecta un lado del cuerpo.

hemiparetic *a.* hemiparético-a, rel. a la hemiparesis o de la naturaleza de la misma.

hemiplegia *n.* hemiplejía, parálisis gen. ocasionada por una lesión cerebral que afecta la parte del cuerpo opuesta al hemisferio cerebral afectado.**alternating** ___ / ___ alternante;

cerebral ___ / ___ cerebral; **crossed** ___ / ___ cruzada; **double** ___ / ___ doble; **facial** ___ / ___ facial; **spastic** ___ / ___ espástica.

hemiplegic *a.* hemipléjico-a, que sufre de hemiplejía.

hemisphere *n.* hemisferio, mitad de una estructura u órgano de forma esférica.

hemithorax *n.* hemitórax, cada mitad del tórax.

hemobilia *n.* hemobilia, sangramiento en los conductos biliares.

hemoblastosis *n.* hemoblastosis, desórdenes proliferativos de los tejidos que forman la sangre.

hemochromatosis, iron storage disease *n.* hemocromatosis, trastorno del metabolismo férrico acompañado por exceso de depósitos de hierro en los tejidos que causa anomalías de pigmentación de la piel, cirrosis hepática y diabetes.

hemoclasis, hemoclasia *n.* rotura, desgarro, [*hemolysis*] disolución u otro tipo de destrucción de eritrocitos.

hemoconcentrate *v.* hemoconcentrar, concentrar hematíes.

hemoconcentration *n.* hemoconcentración, concentración de hematíes a causa de una disminución del volumen líquido sanguíneo.

hemocytoblast *n.* hemocitoblasto, célula sanguínea primitiva de la cual se derivan las demás.

hemocytometer *n.* hemocitómetro, instrumento usado para el conteo de glóbulos rojos en un definido volumen de sangre.

hemodialysis *n.* hemodiálisis, proceso de diálisis usado para eliminar sustancias tóxicas de la sangre.

hemodialyzer *n.* hemodializador, riñón artificial, aparato que se usa en el proceso de diálisis.

hemodilution *n.* hemodilución, aumento del plasma sanguíneo en relación al de los glóbulos rojos.

hemodynamics *n.* hemodinamia, el estudio de la dinámica de la circulación de la sangre.

hemoglobin *n.* hemoglobina, la proteína de mayor importancia en la sangre a la que da color y por la que se transporta el oxígeno.

hemoglobinemia *n.* hemoglobinemia, presencia de hemoglobina libre en el plasma sanguíneo.

hemoglobinuria *n.* hemoglobinuria, presencia de hemoglobina en la orina; **epidemic** ___ / ___

epidémica; **intermittent** ___ / ___ intermitente;
malarial ___ / ___ en malaria; **paroxysmal
cold** ___ / ___ paroxística fría; **paroxysmal
nocturnal** ___ / ___ paroxística nocturna;
postparturient ___ / ___ de la posparturienta;
toxic ___ / ___ tóxica.

hemogram *n.* hemograma, representación
gráfica de un conteo sanguíneo diferencial.

hemolith *n.* hemolito, concreción en un vaso
sanguíneo.

hemolysis *n.* hemólisis, ruptura de eritrocitos
con liberación de hemoglobina en el plasma;
immune ___ / ___ inmune; **venom** ___ / ___
venenosa.

hemolytic *a.* hemolítico-a, rel. a hemólisis o que
la produce; ___ **disorder** / trastorno ___.

hemolytic anemia *n.* anemia hemolítica,
anemia congénita causada por agentes tóxicos de
eritrocitos frágiles de forma esferoidal.

hemolytic disease of the newborn *n.*
hemólisis en el recién nacido, trastorno gen.
causado por la incompatibilidad del factor Rh.Rh
factor.

hemolytic uremic syndrome *n.* síndrome
hemolítico urémico, con anemia hemolítica y
trombocitopenia, presentando un cuadro con
fallo renal agudo; en la infancia se presenta con
síntomas de sangrado gastrointestinal, hematuria,
oliguria, y de anemia hemolítica.

hemolyze *v.* hemolizar, producción de hemólisis
o liberación de la hemoglobina de los glóbulos
rojos.

hemophilia *n.* hemofilia, condición hereditaria
caracterizada por deficiencia de coagulación y
tendencia a sangrar.

hemophiliac *a.* hemofílico-a, persona afectada
por hemofilia.

hemophilus, haemophilus *n.* hemófilo,
bacteria anaeróbica gram-negativa del género
Haemophilus.

hemophobia *n.* hemofobia, temor patológico a
la sangre.

hemopneumothorax *n.* hemoneumotórax,
acumulación de sangre y de aire en la cavidad
pleural.

hemoptysis *n.* hemoptisis, expectoración
sanguinolenta de color rojo vivo.

hemorrhage *n.* hemorragia, derrame profuso de
sangre;**cerebral** ___ / ___ cerebral, accidente
cerebrovascular; **concealed** ___ / ___ oculta;
internal ___ / ___ interna;
intracranial ___ / ___ intracraneana;
intraventricular ___ / ___ intraventricular;

nasal ___ / ___ nasal; **petechial** ___ / ___
petequial; **postpartum** ___ / ___ puerperal.

hemorrhagic *a.* hemorrágico-a.

hemorrhoid *n.* hemorroide, *pop.* almorrana,
masa de venas dilatadas en la pared rectal;
external ___ / ___ -s externas, fuera del esfínter
anal; **internal** ___ / ___ interna;
prolapsed ___ / ___ de prolapso, protrusión de
almorranas internas por el ano.

hemorrhoidectomy *n.* hemorroidectomía,
extirpación de hemorroides.

hemosalpinx *n.* hemosálpinx, acumulación de
sangre en las trompas de Falopio.

hemosiderin *n.* hemosiderina, compuesto
insoluble de hierro derivado de la hemoglobina
que se almacena para ser usado en la formación
de hemoglobina en el momento necesario.

hemosiderosis *n.* hemosiderosis, depósitos de
hemosiderina en el hígado y el vaso.

hemospermia *n.* hemospermia, presencia de
sangre en el semen.

hemostasis *n.* hemostasis, hemostasia,
detención o contención (artificial o natural) de
sangramiento.

hemostat *n.* hemóstato, instrumento o
medicamento que se emplea para contener un
sangramiento.

hen *n.* gallina; [*broth*] caldo de.

heparin *n.* heparina, sustancia que actúa como
anticoagulante.

heparinization *n.* heparinización, proceso de
administrar heparina.

heparinize *n.* heparinizar, evitar la coagulación
por medio del uso de heparina.

hepatectomy *n.* hepatectomía, extirpación de
una parte o de todo el hígado.

hepatic *a.* hepático-a, rel. al hígado; ___ **coma** /
coma ___; ___ **duct** / ducto ___; ___ **lobes** /
lóbulos o subdivisiones ___ -s; ___ **veins** /
venas ___.

hepatitis *n.* hepatitis, infl. del hígado;
amebic ___ / ___ amébica; **active
chronic** ___ / ___ crónica activa;
cholestatic ___ / ___ colestática; **drug-
induced** ___ / ___ inducida por drogas;
epidemic ___ / ___ epidémica;
fulminating ___ / ___ fulminante; **fulminating
chronic** ___ / ___ fulminante crónica;
fulminant ___ / ___ aguda fulminante; ___
A / ___ A, viral, afecta primordialmente a los
niños; ___ **B** / ___ B, causada por un virus y
trasmitida en líquidos del organismo; saliva,
lágrimas, semen; **infectious** ___ / ___ infecciosa

o viral; **non-A, non-B** ___ / ___ no A, no B, asociada con transfusiones de sangre; **serum** ___ / ___ sérica; **persistent chronic** ___ / ___ persistente crónica.

hepatocholangiogastrostomy *n.* hepatocolangiogastrostomía, establecimiento de drenaje de las vías biliares hacia el estómago.

hepatocyte *n.* hepatocito, célula del hígado.

hepatojugular reflex *n.* reflejo hepatoyugular, ingurgitación de las venas yugulares producida por el hígado en casos de insuficiencia cardíaca derecha.

hepatolenticular degeneration *n.* degeneración hepatolenticular.

hepatologist *n.* hepatólogo-a, especialista en trastornos hepáticos.

hepatology *n.* hepatología, estudio del hígado.

hepatomegaly *n.* hepatomegalia, agrandamiento del hígado.

hepatorenal *a.* hepatorrenal, rel. a los riñones y el hígado.

hepatosplenomegaly *n.* hepatosplenomegalia, agrandamiento del hígado y del bazo.

hepatotoxicity *n.* hepatotoxicidad, la tendencia de un fármaco o producto tóxico a dañar el hígado.

hepatotoxin *n.* hepatotoxina, toxina destructora de células hepáticas.

herb *n.* yerba, hierba, planta clasificada como medicinal o usada como condimento; ___ **tea** / infusión.

here *adv.* aquí; ___ **and now** / ahora mismo; ___ **and there** / aquí y allá.

hereditary *a.* hereditario-a; que se trasmite por herencia.

heredity *n.* herencia, trasmisión de características o rasgos genéticos de padres a hijos.

heredofamilial *a.* herencia familiar, rel. a cualquier enfermedad o condición cuya manifestación indica un proceso heredado.

hermaphrodite *n.* hermafrodita, persona cuyo cuerpo presenta los tejidos ovárico y testicular combinados en un mismo órgano o separadamente.

hermaphroditism *n.* hermafroditismo, condición de hermafrodita.

hermetic *a.* hermético-a, que no deja pasar el aire.

hernia *n.* hernia, protrusión anormal de un órgano o víscera a través de la cavidad que la contiene; **cystic** ___ / ___ cística; **femoral** ___ / femoral, que se protrude dentro del canal femoral;

hiatus ___ / ___ hiatal, a través del hiato esofágico del diafragma; **incarcerated** ___ / ___ incarcerada, gen. causada por adherencias; **inguinal** ___ / ___ inguinal, de una víscera con protrusión en la ingle o el escroto; **lumbar** ___ / ___ lumbar, protrusión en la región lumbar; **reducible** ___ / ___ reducible, que puede tratarse por manipulación; **scrotal** ___ / ___ escrotal; **sliding** ___ / ___ por deslizamiento, de una víscera intestinal; **strangulated** ___ / ___ estrangulada, que obstruye los intestinos; **umbilical** ___ / ___ umbilical; **ventral** ___ / ___ ventral, protrusión a través de la pared abdominal. See chart on page 140.

hernial, herniated *a.* herniado-a, rel. a una hernia o que padece de ella; ___ **sac** / saco de la hernia, bolsa peritoneal en la cual desciende la hernia.

herniation *n.* herniación, desarrollo de una hernia; ___ **of nucleus pulposus** / ___ del núcleo pulposo, prolapso o ruptura del disco intervertebral.

herniography *n.* herniografía, radiografía de una hernia usando un medio de contraste.

herniorrhaphy *n.* herniorrafía, reconstrucción o reparación quirúrgica de una hernia.

heroic *a.* heroico-a, rel. a medicamentos de acción muy intensa.

heroin, diacetylomorphine *n.* heroína, diacetilomorfina, narcótico adictivo derivado de la morfina; ___ **addict** / heroinómano-a.

heroinism *n.* heroinismo, heroinomanía, adicción a la heroína.

herpangina *n.* herpangina, enfermedad infecciosa, epidémica en el verano, que afecta las membranas mucosas de la garganta.

herpes *n.* herpes, enfermedad inflamatoria viral dolorosa de la piel que se manifiesta con erupción y ampollas; ___ **genitales** / ___ de los genitales; ___ **ocular** / ___ ocular; ___ **simplex** / ___ simple, de simples vesículas que recurren una y otra vez en la misma área de la piel; ___ **zoster,** *pop.* **shingles** / ___ zóster, erupción dolorosa a lo largo de un nervio, *pop.* culebrilla.

herpetic *a.* herpético-a, rel. al herpes o de naturaleza similar; ___ **gingivostomatitis** / gingivostomatitis ___, infl. de la boca y las encías causada por herpes simple.

hesitant *a.* indeciso-a, vacilante.

hesitate *v.* vacilar, mostrarse indeciso-a; **Don't** ___ **to call us** / No deje, no dejes de llamarnos; no vacile, no vaciles en llamarnos.

(h)

heterogeneous *a.* heterogéneo-a, de naturaleza diferente.

heterograft *n.* heteroinjerto, injerto de un donante de especie o tipo diferente al del receptor.

heterologous *a.* heterólogo-a; derivado de un organismo o especie diferente.

heteroplasia *n.* heteroplasia, presencia anormal de tejido en un área diferente a la que le corresponde según su origen.

heteroplastia *n.* heteroplastia, trasplante de tejido obtenido de un donante que pertenece a una especie diferente.

heterosexual *n.* heterosexual, inclinación sexual hacia el sexo opuesto.

heterosexuality *n.* heterosexualidad.

heterotaxia *n.* heterotaxia, posición anormal o irregular de vísceras o partes del cuerpo.

heterotopia *n.* heterotopía, desplazamiento de un órgano o parte de la posición normal.

heterotopic *a.* heterotópico-a, rel. a la heterotopía.

heuristic *a.* heurístico-a, que descubre una investigación o la estimula.

hiatus *n.* hiatus, abertura, orificio, fisura.

hibernoma *n.* hibernoma, tumor benigno localizado en la cadera o en la espalda.

hiccough, hiccups *n.* hipo, contracción involuntaria del diafragma y la glotis.

hidden *a. pp.* of **to hide,** oculto-a, escondido-a, latente.

hide *vi.* esconder; ocultar; esconderse.

hideous *a.* horrible; abominable.

hidradenitis *n.* hidradenitis, infl. de las glándulas sudoríparas.

hidrosis *n.* hidrosis, sudor excesivo.

high *a.* alto-a, elevado-a; **___ blood pressure /** presión alta; **___ -calorie diet /** dieta rica en calorías; **___ cholesterol /** **___** nivel de colesterol; **___ color /** de color subido; **___ nuclear waste /** desechos nucleares de alta radioactividad; **___ -residue diet /** dieta **___** en residuos (fibras, celulosas); **___ -risk /** **___** peligro o riesgo; **___ -risk behavior /** conducta o actividades de **___** riesgo; **-ly** *adv.* altamente, sumamente, excesivamente.

high altitude sickness *n.* enfermedad de la altura, trastorno por altura excesiva manifestado en dificultades respiratorias por imposibilidad de adaptarse a la disminución de la presión del oxígeno.

highlight *v.* destacar, realzar, subrayar.

high-risk groups *n.* *pl.* pacientes o personas con alto riesgo de contraer una determinada enfermedad debido a factores genéticos o conductales; **___ in HIV /** personas de actividades sexuales múltiples sin adecuada protección; drogadictos que intercambian agujas y jeringuillas; feto *in utero* o infante lactante de madre drogadicta o infectada por el virus.

hike *n.* caminata; *v.* **to go on a ___ /** ir a caminar, ir andando.

hilum, hilus *n., L. (pl.* **hila**) hilio, depresión o apertura en un órgano que sirve de entrada o salida a nervios, vasos y conductos.

hindwater *n.* aguas posteriores, líquido amniótico.

hinge *n.* bisagra; **___ joint /** coyuntura; **___ movement /** movimiento de bisagra; **___ position /** posición de gozne.

hint *n.* insinuación; indicación.

hip *n.* cadera, región lateral de la pelvis; **___ dislocation /** dislocación de la **___**; **___ dislocation, congenital /** dislocación congénita de la **___**; **___ joint /** articulación de la **___**; **___ snapping ___ /** **___** de resorte; **total ___ replacement /** restitución total de la **___**.

hip-joint disease *n.* trastorno de la articulación de la cadera, coxartropatía.

hippocampus *n. (pl.* **hippocampi**) hipocampo, circunvolución de materia gris que forma la mayor parte de la corteza cerebral olfatoria.

hippocratic facies *n.* facies hipocrática, máscara facial que precede a la muerte.

hippocratic oath *n.* juramento hipocrático, juramento ético de la medicina.

hirsute *a.* hirsuto-a, peludo-a.

hirsutism *n.* hirsutismo, desarrollo excesivo de pelo en áreas no comunes, esp. en la mujer.

histamine *n.* histamina, sustancia que produce efecto dilatador en los vasos capilares y estimula la secreción gástrica.

histidine *n.* histidina, aminoácido esencial en el crecimiento y en la restauración de los tejidos.

histocompatibility *n.* histocompatibilidad, estado en el cual los tejidos de un donante son aceptados por el receptor; **major ___ complex /** complejo de **___** mayor.

histologist *n.* histólogo-a, especialista en histología.

histology *n.* histología, estudio de los tejidos orgánicos.

histoplasmin *n.* histoplasmina, sustancia que se usa en la prueba cutánea de histoplasmosis.

histoplasmosis *n.* histoplasmosis, enfermedad de las vías respiratorias causada por el hongo *Histoplasma capsulatum.*

histrionic *a.* histriónico-a, dramático-a.

HIV *n.* **human immunodeficiency virus**,VIH, virus de inmunodeficiencia humano, retrovirus del SIDA. Se transmite a travésde relaciones sexuales o por intercambio de agujas y jeringuillas con una persona infectada. Puede transmitirse también a través de una transfusión de sangre obtenida de donantes infectados. El virus puede ser transmitido igualmente al feto *in utero*, durante el parto o al recién nacido en la lactancia a través de la leche materna de una madre afectada.

hives *n., pl.* ronchas, erupción alérgica.

hoarse *a.* ronco-a; áspero-a.

hoarseness *n.* ronquera, manifestación en la voz de una afección de la laringe.

Hodgkin's disease *n.* enfermedad de Hodgkin, presencia de tumores malignos en los nódulos linfáticos y el bazo.

hold *vi.* aguantar, sujetar; detener, mantener; sostener; contener; **to get ___ of** / agarrar; **to ___ an interview** / tener una entrevista; **to ___ off** / mantener a distancia; **to ___ responsible** / hacer responsable.

hole *n.* hueco, agujero.

holistic *a.* holístico-a, rel. a un todo o unidad.

holistic medicine *n.* medicina holística, sistema médico que considera al ser humano integrado como una unidad funcional.

hollow *a.* hueco-a, cóncavo-a.

hollow back *n.* lordosis.

holocrine *a.* holocrino-a, rel. a las glándulas secretorias.

holodiastolic *a.* holodiastólico-a, rel. a una diástole completa.

hologram *n.* holograma, producción de una holografía.

holography *n.* holografía, figura tridimensional de un objeto por medio de una imagen fotográfica.

holosystolic *a.* holosistólico-a, rel. a una sístole completa.

Holter monitoring *n.* monitoreo de Holter (de funda al hombro), electrocardiografía ambulatoria.

home *n.* casa, hogar;**broken ___** / hogar deshecho.

homeopathic *a.* homeopático-a, rel. a la homeopatía.

homeopathy *n.* homeopatía, curación por medio de medicamentos diluidos en cantidades ínfimas que producen efectos semejantes a los síntomas producidos por la enfermedad.

homogeneous *a.* homogéneo-a, semejante, de la misma naturaleza.

homograft *n.* homoinjerto, transplante tomado de la misma especie o tipo.

homologous *a.* homólogo-a, similar en estructura y origen pero no en funcionamiento.

homophobia *n.* homofobia, temor o repulsión a los homosexuales.

homophobic *a.* homofóbico-a, que tiene repulsión o temor a homosexuales.

homosexual *n.* homosexual, invertido-a, atracción sexual por las personas del mismo sexo.

homotonic *a.* homotónico-a, de la misma tensión.

homotopic *a.* homotópico-a, que ocurre en o corresponde al mismo lugar o parte.

homozygote *n.* homocigoto-a, que presenta alelos idénticos en una característica o en varias.

homozygous *a.* homocigótico-a, rel. a un homocigoto.

homunculus *n.* homúnculo-a, enano-a sin deformidades y proporcionado-a en todas las partes del cuerpo.

honest *a.* honesto-a, honrado-a.

honey *n.* miel de abeja.

hook *n.* gancho.

hookworm *n.* uncinaria, lombriz de gancho, nematodo del intestino; **___ disease** / enfermedad de la **___**.

hope *n.* esperanza; *v.* esperar, tener esperanzas.

hopelessness *n.* estado de desesperanza; desesperación.

hordeolum *n.* hordeolo, orzuelo.

horizontal *n.* *a.* horizontal; **___ position** / posición acostada.

hormonal *a.* hormonal, rel. a una hormona o que actúa como tal.

hormone *n.* hormona, sustancia química natural del cuerpo que produce o estimula la actividad de un órgano; **growth ___** / **___** del crecimiento; **___ therapy** / terapia hormonal; **___ receptor** / receptor hormonal.

hornet *n.* avispa, avispón.

hospice *n.* hospicio.

hospital *n.* hospital.

hospitalization *n.* hospitalización.

hospitalize *v.* hospitalizar, ingresar en un hospital; dar ingreso en un hospital.

host *n.* [*parasite*] huésped, organismo que sostiene o alberga a otro llamado parásito; **___ defenses** / defensas del **___**.

hostage *n.* rehén.

hostile *a.* hostil; enemigo-a.

hostility *n.* hostilidad, agravio, animosidad.

hot *a.* caliente, de temperatura alta; contaminado-a por material radioactivo; ___ **flashes** / fogaje, sofoco; rubores, bochorno.

hot line *n.* línea telefónica de emergencia.

hour *n.* hora; **by the** ___ / por hora; **-ly** *adv.* a cada hora

house *n.* casa, vivienda, domicilio; ___ **call** / visita médica;

household *n.* familia.

housewife *n.* ama de casa, madre de familia.

housework *n.* tareas domésticas, trabajo de la casa.

how *adv.* cómo, cuánto; ___ **are you?** / ¿Cómo está?, ¿Cómo estás?; ___ **late?** / ¿Hasta qué hora?; ___ **many?** / ¿Cuántos-as?; ___ **often?** / ¿Cuántas veces?, ¿Con qué frecuencia?

however *adv.* sin embargo, no obstante.

huge *a.* inmenso-a; enorme.

hum *n.* susurro; tarareo; zumbido; *v.* [*music*] tararear; zumbar; murmurar, susurrar.

human *a.* humano-a, rel. a la humanidad.

human immunodeficiency virus *n.* virus de inmunodeficiencia humana, retrovirus del SIDA.

humanity *n.* humanidad.

humeral *a.* humeral, rel. al húmero.

humerus *n.*, *L.* (*pl.* **humeri**) húmero, hueso largo del brazo.

humid *a.* húmedo-a, que contiene humedad.

humidifier *n.* humectante, humedecedor, aparato que controla y mantiene la humedad en el aire de una habitación.

humidity *n.* humedad.

humor *n.* humor. 1. cualquier forma líquida en el cuerpo; **aqueous** ___ / ___ acuoso, líquido claro en las cámaras del ojo; **crystalline** ___ / ___ cristalino, sustancia que forma el cristalino; **vitreus** ___ / ___ vítreo, sustancia transparente semilíquida localizada entre el cristalino y la retina; 2. secreción; 3. disposición de carácter; *v.* **to be in bad** ___ / estar de mal ___; **to be in good** ___ / estar de buen ___.

humoral *a.* humoral, rel. a los fluidos del cuerpo.

hump *n.* joroba, corcova, jiba.

hunchback *n.* corcova, joroba, deformación con curvatura de la espina dorsal.

hunger *n.* hambre.

hungry *a.* hambriento-a; **to be** ___ / tener hambre; **to go** ___ / pasar hambre.

Huntington's chorea *n.* corea de Huntington, *Syn.* **chorea**.

Hunt's neuralgia, syndrome *n.* neuralgia de Hunt. neuralgia.

hurdle *n.* obstáculo.

hurry *n.* prisa, apuro; **Are you in a** ___? / ¿Tiene prisa?, ¿tienes prisa?; *v.* apresurar; **to** ___ **him, her in** / traerlo, traerla inmediatamente.

hurt *vi.* lastimar, herir, hacer daño, dañar.

husband *n.* esposo, marido.

hyalin *n.* hialina, sustancia proteínica producto de la degeneración de amiloides, hialoides y coloides.

hyaline *a.* hialino-a, vítreo-a o casi transparente; ___ **cast** / cilindro ___, que se observa en la orina; ___ **membrane disease** / enfermedad de la membrana ___, trastorno repiratorio que se manifiesta en recién nacidos.

hyalinization *n.* hialinización, conversión a una sustancia semejante al vidrio.

hyalinosis *n.* hialinosis, degeneración hialina.

hyalitis *n.* hialitis, infl. del humor vítreo.

hyaloid *a.* hialoide, hialoideo-a, semejante al vidrio.

hyaluronic acid *n.* ácido hialurónico, presente en la sustancia del tejido conjuntivo, actúa como lubricante y agente conector.

hybrid *a.* híbrido-a, rel. al producto de un cruzamiento de diferentes especies en animales y plantas.

hybridization *n.* hibridación, cruzamiento de especies.

hybridoma *n.* hibridoma, célula somática híbrida capaz de producir anticuerpos.

hydatid *n.* hidátide, quiste que se manifiesta en los tejidos esp. en el hígado; *a.* hidatídico, rel. a un tumor enquistado; ___ **disease** / equinococcosis; ___ **mole** / quiste ___ en el útero que produce hemorragia.

hydramnion *n.* hidramnios, exceso de líquido amniótico.

hydrate *v.* hidratar, combinar un cuerpo con el agua.

hydrated *a.* hidratado-a, que contiene agua o está húmedo.

hydrocele *n.* hidrocele, acumulación de líquido esp. en la túnica vaginal del testículo.

hydrocelectomy *n.* hidrocelectomía, extirpación de un hidrocele.

hydrocephalus *n.* hidrocéfalo, acumulación de líquido cefalorraquídeo en los ventrículos del cerebro.

hydrochloric acid *n.* ácido clorhídrico o hidroclórico, constituyente del jugo gástrico.

hydrocortisone *n.* hidrocortisona, hormona corticosteroide producida por la corteza suprarrenal.

hydroelectric *a.* hidroeléctrico-a, rel. a la electricidad y el agua.

hydrogen *n.* hidrógeno; ___ **concentration** / concentración de ___.

hydrogen peroxide *n.* peróxido de hidrógeno, agua oxigenada, limpiador y desinfectante.

hydrolysis *n.* hidrólisis, disolución química de un compuesto por acción del agua.

hydrolyze *v.* hidrolizar.

hydromyelia *n.* hidromielia, aumento de líquido cefalorraquídeo en el canal central de la médula espinal.

hydronephrosis *n.* hidronefrosis, distensión en la pelvis renal y cálices a causa de una obstrucción.

hydrophilic *a.* hidrofílico-a, que tiene tendencia a retener agua.

hydrophobia *n.* hidrofobia, 1. temor excesivo al agua; 2. *pop.* rabia.

hydropic *a.* hidrópico-a, rel. a la hidropesía.

hydropneumothorax *n.* hidroneumotórax, acumulación de líquido y de gas en la cavidad pleural.

hydrops, hydropsy *n.* hidropesía, hidropsia o edema.

hydrosalpinx *n.* hidrosálpinx, acumulación de fluído seroso en la trompa de Falopio.

hydrostatic *a.* hidrostático-a, rel al equilibrio de líquidos, o a la presión ejercida por un líquido estacionario.

hydrotherapy *n.* hidroterapia, uso terapéutico del agua con aplicaciones externas en el tratamiento de enfermedades.

hydrothorax *n.* hidrotórax, colección de fluído en la cavidad pleural sin producir inflamación.

hydroureter *n.* hidrouréter, distensión por obstrucción del uréter.

hydroxyapatite *n.* hidroxiapatita, forma de fosfato de calcio, compuesto inorgánico presente en los dientes y los huesos.

hygiene *n.* higiene, estudio de la salud y la conservación de un cuerpo sano; **mental** ___ / ___ mental; **oral** ___ / ___ oral; **public** ___ / ___ pública.

hygienic *a.* higiénico-a, sanitario-a, rel. a la higiene.

hygienist *n.* higienista, especialista en higiene; **dental** ___ / ___ dental, técnico en profiláctica dental.

hygroma *n.* hidroma, saco o bursa que contiene líquido.

hymen *n.* himen, repliegue membranoso que cubre parcialmente la entrada de la vagina.

hymenectomy *n.* himenectomía, excisión del himen.

hymenotomía *n.* himenotomía, incisión del himen.

hyoglossal *a.* hioglosal, rel. al hioides y la lengua.

hyoglossus *n.* hiogloso, músculo de la lengua de acción retractora y lateral.

hyoid *a.* hioideo-a, rel. al hueso hioides.

hyoid bone *n.* hioides, hueso en forma de herradura situado en la base de la lengua.

hypalgesia, hypalgia *n.* hipalgesia, hipalgia, disminución en la sensibilidad del dolor.

hyperacidity *n.* hiperacidez, acidez excesiva.

hyperactive *a.* hiperactivo-a, excesivamente activo-a.

hyperactivity *n., pl.* actividad excesiva; desorden caracterizado por actividad excesiva que se manifiesta en niños y adolescentes acompañado de irritabilidad e incapacidad de mantener la atención.

hyperacuity *n.* desarrollo anormal de uno de los sentidos esp. la vista o el olfato.

hyperacute *a.* sobreagudo-a, extremadamente agudo-a.

hyperalbuminosis *n.* hiperalbuminosis, exceso de albúmina en la sangre.

hyperalimentation *n.* hiperalimentación, sobrealimentación por vía intravenosa.

hyperbilirubinemia *n.* hiperbilirrubinemia, exceso de bilirrubina en la sangre.

hypercalcemia *n.* hipercalcemia, cantidad excesiva de calcio en la sangre.

hypercapnia *n.* hipercapnia, cantidad excesiva de dióxido de carbono en la sangre.

hyperchloremia *n.* hipercloremia, exceso de cloruros en la sangre.

hyperchlorhydria *n.* hipercloridria, secreción excesiva de ácido clorhídrico por células que recubren el estómago.

hypercholesterolemia *n.* hipercolesterolemia, cholesteremia, cholesterolemia.

hyperchromatic *a.* hipercromático-a, con exceso de colorante o pigmentación.

hypercoagulability *n.* hipercoagulabilidad, aumento anormal de la coagulabilidad.

hyperemesis *n.* hiperemesis, vómitos excesivos.

hyperemia *n.* hiperemia, exceso de sangre en un órgano, tejido o parte.

hyperesthesia *n.* hiperestesia, aumento exagerado de la sensibilidad sensorial.

hyperflexion *n.* hiperflexión, flexión excesiva de una articulación, gen. causada por un traumatismo.

hyperfunction *n.* hiperfunción, funcionamiento excesivo.

hypergammaglobulinemia *n.* hipergammaglobulinemia, exceso de gamma globulina en la sangre.

hyperglycemia *n.* hiperglucemia, aumento excesivo de azúcar en la sangre.

hyperglycemic *a.* hiperglucémico-a, que sufre de hiperglucemia, o rel. a la misma.

hyperglycosuria *n.* hiperglucosuria, exceso de azúcar en la orina.

hyperhidrosis *n.* hiperhidrosis, sudor excesivo.

hyperhydration *n.* hiperhidratación, aumento excesivo del contenido de agua en el cuerpo.

hyperinsulinism *n.* hiperinsulinismo, exceso de secreción de insulina en la sangre causando hipoglicemia.

hyperkalemia *n.* hipercalemia, hiperpotasemia, aumento excesivo de potasio en la sangre.

hyperkinesia *n.* hipercinesia, aumento en exceso de actividad muscular.

hyperlipemia *n.* hiperlipemia, cantidad excesiva.

hyperlipidemia *n.* hiperlipidemia, exceso de lipidos en la sangre.

hypermenorrhea *n.* hipermenorrea, período excesivo en cantidad y duración.

hypermobility *n.* hipermobilidad, movilidad excesiva.

hypernatremia *n.* hipernatremia, cantidad excesiva de sodio en la sangre.

hypernephroma *n.* hipernefroma, tumor de Grawitz, neoplasma del parénquima renal.

hyperopia *n.* hiperopia, hipermetropía. V. **farsightedness.**

hyperorexia *n.* hiperorexia, apetito excesivo.

hyperosmia *n.* hiperosmia, sensibilidad olfativa exagerada.

hyperostosis *n.* hiperostosis, desarrollo excesivo del tejido óseo.

hyperpituitism *n.* hiperpituitarismo, actividad excesiva de la glándula pituitaria.

hyperplasia *n.* hiperplasia, proliferación excesiva de células normales en un tejido.

hyperapnea *n.* hiperapnea, aumento de la respiracíon en rapidez y profundidad.

hyperpyrexia *n.* hiperpirexia, temperatura del cuerpo excesivamente alta.

hyperreflexia *n.* hiperreflexia, reflejos exagerados.

hypersalivation *n.* hipersalivación, excesiva secreción de las glándulas salivales.

hypersalpingo-oophorectomy *n.* histerosalpingo-ooforectomía, excison del útero, de los tubos uterinos y de los ovarios.

hypersecretion *n.* hipersecreción, secreción excesiva.

hypersensibility *n.* hipersensibilidad, sensibilidad excesiva al efecto de un antígeno o a un estímulo.

hypersensitive *a.* hipersensible, hiperestísico-a.

hypersplenism *n.* hiperesplenismo, funcionamiento exagerado del bazo.

hypertelorism *n.* hipertelorismo, distancia exagerada en la localización de órganos o partes.

hypertension *n.* hipertensión, presión arterial alta; **benign** ___ / ___ benigna; **essential** ___ / ___ esencial; **malignant** ___ / ___ maligna; **portal** ___ / ___ portal; **primary** ___ / ___ primaria; **renal** ___ / ___ renal.

hypertensive *a.* hipertensivo-a, hipertenso-a. 1. que causa elevación en la presión; 2. rel. a la hipertensión o que padece de ella.

hyperthermia *n.* hipertermia. V. **hyperpyrexia.**

hyperthyroidism *n.* hipertiroidismo, actividad excesiva de la tiroides.

hypertonic *a.* hipertónica-a, rel. a, o caracterizado por aumento de tonicidad o tensión.

hypertrophy *n.* hipertrofia, desarrollo excesivo o agrandamiento anormal de un órgano o parte; **cardiac** ___ / ___ cardíaca, corazón agrandado; **compensatory** ___ / ___ compensatoria, como resultado de un defecto físico.

hypertropia *n.* hipertropia, tipo de estrabismo.

hyperuricemia *n.* hiperuricemia, exceso de ácido úrico en la sangre.

hyperventilation *n.* hiperventilación, respiración excesivamente rápida y profunda con expiración del aire igualmente rápida.

hyperviscosity *n.* hiperviscosidad, viscosidad excesiva.

hyphema *n.* hifema. 1. ojo inyectado; 2. sangramiento en la cámara anterior del ojo.

hypnagogic *a.* hipnagógico-a. 1. adormecedor-a, que induce el sueño; 2. que experimenta alucinaciones o sueños antes de perder el conocimiento o de pasar a un sueño profundo.

hypnosis *n.* hipnosis, estado sugestivo durante el cual la persona sometida responde a mandatos siempre que éstos no contradigan convicciones arraigadas.

hypnotherapy *n.* hipnoterapia, tratamiento terapéutico con práctica de hipnosis.

hypnotism *n.* hipnotismo, práctica de la hipnosis.

hypnotize *v.* hipnotizar, producir hipnosis.

hypoadrenalism *n.* hipoadrenalismo, desorden causado por deficiencia de la glándula suprarrenal.

hypoalbuminemia *n.* hipoalbuminemia, deficiencia de albúmina en la sangre.

hypocalcemia *n.* hipocalcemia, nivel de calcio en la sangre anormalmente bajo.

hypocapnia *n.* hipocapnia, disminución del dióxido de carbono en la sangre.

hypochlorhydria *n.* hipocloridria, deficiencia en la secreción de ácido clorhídrico en el estómago, condición que puede indicar una fase primaria de cáncer.

hypocholesteremia *n.* hipocolesteremia, disminución de colesterol en la sangre.

hypochondria *n.* hipocondría, excesiva preocupación por la salud propia, con síntomas imaginarios de enfermedades.

hypochondriac *n. a.* hipocondríaco-a, hipocóndrico-a, que cree haber contraído alguna enfermedad cuando goza de salud y se preocupa por ello.

hypochondrium *n.* hipocondrio, parte del abdomen a cada lado del epigastrio.

hypochromatism *n.* hipocromatismo, falta o disminución de color o pigmentación, esp. en el núcleo de la célula.

hypochromia *n.* hipocromía, deficiencia de hemoglobina en la sangre.

hyphochromic *a.* hipocrómicó-a rel. a la hipocromía.

hypocyclosis *n.* hipociclosis, deficiencia en la acomodación visual; **lenticular** ___ / ___ por deficiencia muscular o rigidez del cristalino.

hypodermic *a.* hipodérmico-a, que se aplica por debajo de la piel.

hypofibrinogenemia *n.* hipofibrinogenemia, contenido bajo de fibrinógeno en la sangre.

hypofunction *n.* hipofunción, deficiencia en el funcionamiento de un órgano.

hypogammaglobulinemia *n.* hipogammaglobulinemia, nivel anormalmente bajo de gamma globulina en la sangre; **acquired** ___ / ___ adquirida, que se manifiesta después de la infancia.

hypogastrium *n.* hipogastrio, área inferior media y anterior del abdomen.

hypoglossal *a.* hipoglosal, rel. a una posición debajo de la lengua.

hypoglossal nerve *n.* nervio hipogloso.

hypoglycemia *n.* hipoglicemia, hipoglucemia, disminución anormal del contenido de glucosa en la sangre.

hypoglycemic *a.* hipoglicémico-a, hipoglucémico-a, que produce o tiene relación con la hipoglicemia; ___ **agents** / agentes ___ -s; ___ **shock** / choque ___ .

hypoinsulism *n.* hipoinsulinismo, deficiencia en la secreción de insulina.

hypokalemia *n.* hipocalemia, deficiencia en el contenido de potasio en la sangre.

hypokinesia *n.* hipocinesia, disminución de la actividad motora.

hypolipoproteinemia *n.* hipolipoproteinemia, demasiado aumento de lipoproteínas en la sangre.

hyponamia *n.* hipomanía, manía moderada.

hyponatremia *n.* hiponatremia, deficiencia en el contenido de sodio en la sangre.

hypopharynx *n.* hipofaringe, parte de la faringe situada bajo el borde superior de la epiglotis.

hypophysectomy *n.* hipofisectomía, extirpación de la glándula pituitaria.

hypophysis *n.* hipófisis, glándula pituitaria,cuerpo epitelial localizado en la base de la silla turca.

hypopituitarism *n.* hipopituitarismo, condición patológica debida a disminución de la secreción de la glándula pituitaria.

hypoplasia *n.* hipoplasia, desarrollo incompleto de un órgano o parte.

hypoplastic *a.* hipoplástico-a, rel. a la hipoplasia.

hypoprothrombinemia *n.* hipoprotrombinemia, deficiencia en la cantidad de protrombina en la sangre.

hyporeflexia *n.* hiporreflexia, reflejos débiles.

hypospadias *n.* hipospadias, anomalía congénita de la uretra masculina que consiste en el cierre incompleto de la cara ventral de la uretra en distintos grados de longitud. (En la mujer la uretra tiene salida a la vagina.)

hypotelorism *n.* hipotelorismo, dismunición anormal de la distancia entre dos órganos o partes.

hypotension *n.* hipotensión, presión arterial baja.

hypotensive *a.* hipotensivo-a, hipotenso-a, rel. a la presión baja o que sufre de ella.

hypothalamus *n.* hipotálamo, parte del diencéfalo.

hypothermia *n.* hipotermia, temperatura baja.

hypothesis *n.* (*pl.* **hypotheses**) hipótesis, suposición asumida en el desarrollo de una teoría.

hypothrombinemia *n.* hipotrombinemia, deficiciencia de trombina en la sangre que causa una tendencia a sangrar.

hypothyroid *a.* hipotiroideo-a, rel. al hipotiroidismo.

hypothyroidism *n.* hipotiroidismo, deficiencia en el funcionamiento de la tiroides.

hypotonic *a.* hipotónico-a. 1. rel. a la deficiencia en tonicidad muscular; 2. de presión osmótica más baja en comparación con otros elementos.

hypoventilation *n* hipoventilación, reducción en la entrada de aire a los pulmones.

hypovolemia *n.* hipovolemia, disminución del volumen de la sangre en el organismo.

hypoxemia *n.* hipoxemia, insuficiencia de oxígeno en la sangre.

hysterectomy *n.* histerectomía, extirpación del útero; **abdominal** ___ / ___ abdominal, a través del abdomen; **total** ___ / ___ total, del útero y del cuello uterino; **vaginal** ___ / ___ vaginal, a través de la vagina.

hysteria *n.* histeria, neurosis extrema.

hysteric, hysterical *a.* histérico-a, rel. a la histeria o que padece de ella; *v.* **to get** ___ / ponerse ___; ___ **laughter** / risa ___; **-ly** *a.* histéricamente.

hysterics *n.* histerismo, histeria.

hysteroid *n.* histeroide, semejante a la histeria.

hysteromania *n.* histeromanía, ninfomanía.

hysterosalpingography *n.* histerosalpingografía, radiografía del útero y de los oviductos por medio de material de contraste.

hysteroscopy *n.* histeroscopía, examen endoscópico de la cavidad uterina.

hysterotomy *n.* histerectomía, incisión del útero.

i

I *abbr.* símbolo químico del iodo. *pron.* yo, primera persona del singular.

i *abbr.* **iatric** / iátrico; **immune** / inmune; **implant** / implante; **impotence** / impotencia; **incomplete** / incompleto.

iatric *a.* iátrico-a, rel. a la medicina, a la profesión médica, o a los que la ejercen.

iatrogenic *a.* yatrógeno-a, iatrogénico-a, rel. a un trastorno o lesión producido por un tratamiento o por una instrucción errónea del facultativo; ___ **pneumothorax** / neumotórax ___; ___ **transmission** / transmisión ___.

ibuprofen *n.* ibuprofén, agente antiinflamatorio, antipirético y analgésico usado en el tratamiento de artritis reumatoidea.

ice *n.* hielo; ___ **cap,** ___ **bag** / bolsa de ___; ___ **cream** / helado; ___ **water** / agua helada, agua con ___; ___ **treatment** / aplicación de ___; **My hands are like** ___ / Tengo las manos heladas.

ichthyosis *n.* ictiosis, dermatosis congénita caracterizada por sequedad y peladura escamosa esp. de las extremidades.

icing *n.* aplicación de hielo.

icteric *a.* ictérico-a, rel. a la ictericia.

icterogenic *a.* icterogénico-a, causante de ictericia.

icterohepatitis *n.* icterohepatitis, hepatitis asociada con ictericia.

icterus *n.* icterus, ictericia. V. **jaundice.**

icterus gravis *n.* atrofia amarilla aguda del hígado.

icterus neonatorum *n.* ictericia del recién nacido.

ictus *n.* ictus, ataque súbito.

id *n.* id. 1. término en psicoanálisis que con el *ego* y el *superego* forma parte del inconsciente freudiano y actúa como reservorio de la energía psíquica y el libido; 2. sufijo que indica ciertas erupciones secundarias de la piel que aparecen distantes de la sede de la infección primaria.

idea *n.* idea, concepto; **fixed** ___ / ___ fija.

ideal *n. a.* ideal; perfecto-a.

ideation *n.* ideación, proceso de formación de ideas. **paranoid** ___ / ___ paranoide.

idée fixe *n., Fr.* idea fija.

identical *a.* idéntico-a, igual, mismo-a.

identical twins *n., pl.* gemelos idénticos formados por la fertilización de un solo óvulo.

identification *n.* identificación; proceso en el cual una persona adopta inconscientemente características semejantes a otra persona o grupo; ___ **papers** / documento oficial de identidad.

identify *v.* identificar; reconocer.

identity *n.* identidad, reconocimiento propio; ___ **crisis** / crisis de ___.

ideology *n.* ideología, formación de conceptos e ideas.

ideomotion *n.* ideomoción, actividad muscular dirigida por una idea predominante.

idiocracy *n.* idiocracia, tendencia a someterse a ciertos hábitos o drogas.

idiocy *n.* idiotez, deficiencia mental.

idiogram *n.* idiograma, gráfico representativo de los cromosomas de una célula en particular.

idiopathic *a.* idiopático-a. 1. rel. a la idiopatía; 2. que tiene origen espontáneo; ___ **aldosteronism** / aldosteronismo ___; ___ **infants hypercalcemia** / hipercalcemia ___ en los niños; ___ **neuralgia** / neuralgia ___; ___ **pulmonary fibrosis** / fibrosis pulmonar ___; ___ **subglottic stenosis** / estenosis subglótica ___.

idiopathy *n.* idiopatía, enfermedad espontánea o de origen desconocido.

idiosyncrasy *n.* idiosincrasia. 1. características individuales; 2. reacción peculiar de cada persona a una acción, idea, medicamento, tratamiento o alimento.

idiot *a.* idiota, imbécil.

idiotropic *a.* idiotrópico-a. *Syn.* **egocentric.**

idioventricular *a.* idioventricular, rel. a los ventrículos o que afecta exclusivamente a éstos.

ignorance *n.* ignorancia.

ignorant *a.* ignorante.

ignore *v.* desatender, ignorar, desconocer, no hacer caso.

ileal *a.* ileal, rel. al íleon; ___ **arteries** / arterias ___ -es; ___ **orifice** / orificio ___; ___ **ureter** / uréter ___; ___ **veins** / venas ___ -es.

ileal bypass *n.* desviación quirúrgica del íleon.

ileectomy *n.* ilectomía, excisión parcial o total del íleon.

ileitis *n.* ileítis, infl. del íleon; **regional** ___ / ___ regional;

ileocecal *a.* ileocecal, rel. al íleon y al ciego; ___ **valve** / válvula ___.

ileocecostomy *n.* ileocecostomía, anastomosis quirúrgica del íleon al ciego.

ileocolitis *n.* ileocolitis, infl. de la mucosa del íleon y el colon.

ileocolostomy *n.* ileocolostomía, anastomosis del íleon y el colon.

ileocystoplasty *n.* ileocistoplastia, sutura de un segmento del íleon a la vejiga para aumentar la capacidad de ésta.

ileoproctostomy *n.* ileoproctostomía, anastomosis entre el íleon y el recto.

ileosigmoidostomy *n.* ileosigmoidostomía, anastomosis del íleon al colon sigmoide.

ileostomy *n.* ileostomía, anastomosis del íleon y la pared abdominal anterior.

ileotransversostomy *n.* ileotransversostomía, anastomosis del íleon y el colon transverso.

ileum *n.* (*pl.* **ilea**) íleon, porción distal del intestino delgado que se extiende desde el yeyuno al ciego.

iliac *a.* ilíaco-a, rel. al ilion; ___ **bone** / hueso ___; ___ **colon** / colon ___; ___ **crest** / cresta ___; ___ **muscle** / músculo ___.

iliofemoral *a.* iliofemoral, rel. al ilion y el fémur.

iliohypogastric *a.* iliohipogástrico, rel. al ilion y el hipogastrio.

ilioinguinal *n.* ilioinguinal, rel. a las regiones inguinal e ilíaca.

iliolumbar *a.* iliolumbar, rel. a las regiones ilíaca y lumbar; ___ **artery** / arteria ___; ___ **vein** / vena ___.

ilium *n.* (*pl.* **ilia**) ilion, porción del ilíaco.

Ilizarov technique *n.* Ilizarov, técnica de, controlación de osteogenesis con alargamiento del hueso y corrección de deformidades angulares, y de rotación cortando la capa exterior del hueso sin penetrar la cavidad medular.

ill *a.* enfermo-a, insano-a; *v.* **to be** ___ / estar enfermo-a; **to become** ___ / enfermarse; **to feel** ___ / sentirse indispuesto-a; sentirse mal.

ill-advised *a.* mal aconsejado; mal informado-a; desacertado; imprudente.

ill-behaved *a.* de mala conducta.

ill health *n.* mala salud; *v.* **to be in** ___ / no estar bien de salud;

ill-mannered *a.* descortés.

ill-tempered *a.* de mal carácter, de mal genio.

illegal *a.* ilegal.

illegible *a.* ilegible.

illegitimate *a.* ilegítimo-a.

illicit *a.* ilícito, ilegal.

illiterate *a.* analfabeto-a.

illness *n.* enfermedad, dolencia.

illumination *n.* iluminación; **dark field** ___ / iluminación lateral u oblicua del campo oscuro.

illusion *n.* ilusión, interpretación imaginaria de impresiones sensoriales.

illusory *a.* ilusorio-a, rel. a la ilusión.

illustration *n.* ilustración, gráfico.

image *n.* imagen, figura; representación; **body** ___ / ___ del cuerpo propio; **direct** ___ / ___ directa; **double** ___ / ___ doble; **electric** ___ / ___ eléctrica; **inverted** ___ / ___ invertida; **latent** ___ / ___ latente; **mirror** ___ / ___ de espejo; **optic** ___ / ___ óptica; **radiographic** ___ / ___ radiográfica; **real** ___ / ___ real.

imaginary *a.* imaginario-a, ilusorio-a.

imagination *n.* imaginación.

imaging *n.* creación de imágenes.

imbalance *n.* desequilibrio.

imbalanced *a.* desequilibrado.

imbecile *a.* imbécil.

imbed *v.* embed.

imbibition *n.* imbibición, absorción de un líquido.

imbricated *a.* imbricado-a, en forma de capas.

imitable *a.* imitable.

imitate *v.* imitar, copiar.

imitation *n.* imitación, copia.

immature *a.* inmaturo-a, inmaduro-a; prematuro-a; sin madurez.

immediate *a.* inmediato-a, cercano-a; **-ly** *adv.* inmediatamente, en seguida.

immerse *v.* sumergir, hundir.

immersion *n.* inmersión, sumersión de un cuerpo o materia en un líquido.

immigrant *n.* inmigrante.

imminent *a.* inminente; irremediable.

immobile *a.* inmóvil, estable, fijo-a; que no se puede mover.

immobility *n.* inmovilidad, sin movimiento.

immobilization *n.* inmovilización.

immobilize *v.* inmovilizar.

immoderate *a.* inmoderado-a, sin moderación.

immoral *a.* inmoral, corrompido-a, vicioso-a.

immorality *n.* inmoralidad.

immortal *a.* inmortal, imperecedero-a.

immune *a.* inmune, resistente a contraer una enfermedad; ___ **adherence** / adherencia ___; ___ **adsorption** / adsorción ___; ___ **complex** / complejo ___; ___ **paralysis** / parálisis ___; ___ **reaction** / reacción ___; ___ **response** / respuesta ___.

immune system *n.* sistema inmunológico.

immunity *n.* inmunidad. 1. condición del organismo de resistir a un determinado antígeno por activación de anticuerpos específicos; 2. resistencia creada por el organismo en contra de una enfermedad específica; **acquired** ___ / ___ adquirida; **active** ___ / ___ activa; **adoptive** ___ / ___ adoptiva; **antiviral** ___ / ___ antivírica; **artificial** ___ / ___ artificial; **bacteriophage** ___ / ___ bateriófaga; **concomitant** ___ / ___ concomitante; **general** ___ / general ___; **group** ___ / ___ de grupo; **inborn** ___ / ___ nata; **innate** ___ / ___ innata; **maternal** ___ / ___ materna; **natural** ___ / ___ natural; **passive** ___ / ___ pasiva.

immunization *n.* inmunización, proceso para activar la producción de inmunidad en el organismo en contra de una determinada enfermedad. See chart on this page.

immunize *v.* inmunizar, hacer inmune.

immunoassay *n.* inmunoanálisis, proceso para determinar la capacidad de una sustancia para actuar como antígeno y anticuerpo en un tejido; **enzyme** ___ / ___ enzimático.

immunochemotherapy *n.* inmunoquimioterapia, proceso combinado de inmunoterapia y quimioterapia aplicado en el tratamiento de ciertos tumores malignos.

immunocompetency *n.* inmunocompetencia, proceso de alcanzar inmunidad después de la exposición a un antígeno.

immunocompromised *a.* inmunocomprometido-a, rel. a una persona con un sistema inmunológico deficiente.

immunocyte *n.* inmunocito. *v.* lymphocyte.

immunodeficiency *n.* inmunodeficiencia, reacción inmune celular inadecuada que limita la habilidad de responder a estímulos antigénicos; **severe combined** ___ **disease** / enfermedad grave de ___ combinada.

immunoelectrophoresis *n.* inmunoelectroforesis, uso de electroforesis como técnica para investigar el número y tipo de proteínas y anticuerpos presentes en los líquidos del organismo.

immunofluorescence *n.* inmunofluorescencia, método que usa anticuerpos marcados con fluorescina para localizar antígenos en los tejidos.

immunogen *n.* inmunógeno, sustancia que produce inmunidad; **targeted** ___ / ___ específico.

immunoglobuline *n.* inmunoglobulina. 1. proteína de origen animal que pertenece al grupo del sistema de respuesta inmune; 2. uno de los

Immunizations			Immunizaciones		
Age	Vaccine	Method	Edad	Vacuna	Método
2 months	DTP diphteria tetanus pertussis OPV oral poliovirus	vaccination	2 meses	DTP difteria tetanus pertusis o tos ferina OPV oral de la polio	vacuna por vía oral
4 months	DTP	vaccination	4 meses	DTP	vacuna
6 months	OPV	by mouth	6 meses	VOP	por vía oral
15 months	MMR measles mumps rubella	vaccination	15 meses	SPR sarampión paperas rubéola	vacuna por vía oral
18 months	DTP OPV	vaccination by mouth	18 meses	DTP VOP	vacuna por vía oral
2 years	Hib haemophilus	vaccination	2 años	Hib hemófilo influenza b	vacuna
4-6 years	DTP OPV	vaccination by mouth	4-6 años	DTP VOP	vacuna por vía oral

cinco tipos de gamma globulina capaz de actuar como anticuerpo.

immunologic *a.* inmunológico-a, rel. a la inmunología; ___ **competence** / competencia ___; ___ **deficiency** / deficiencia ___; ___ **disease** / enfermedad ___; ___ **enhancement** / realce ___; ___ **mechanism** / mecanismo ___; ___ **paralysis** / parálisis ___; ___ **pregnancy test** / prueba ___ del embarazo; ___ **tolerance** / tolerancia ___.

immunologist *n.* inmunólogo-a, especialista en inmunología.

immunology *n.* inmunología, rama de la medicina que estudia las reacciones del cuerpo a cualquier invasión extraña, tal como la de bacterias, virus o transplantes.

immunoprotein *n.* inmunoproteína, proteína que actúa como anticuerpo.

immunoreaction *n.* inmunoreacción, reacción de inmunidad entre antígenos y anticuerpos.

immunostimulant *n.* inmunoestimulante, agente capaz de inducir o estimular una respuesta inmune.

immunosuppressant *n.* inmunosupresor, agente capaz de suprimir una respuesta inmune.

immunotherapy *n.* inmunoterapia, inmunización pasiva del paciente por medio de anticuerpos preformados (suero o gamma globulina).

immunotyping *n.* tipificación inmunológica.

impact *n.* colisión, impacto; efecto; golpe; *v.* impactar, fijar, rellenar, asegurar; incrustar.

impacted tooth *n.* diente impactado.

impaction *n.* impacción. 1. condición de estar alojado o metido con firmeza en un espacio limitado; 2. impedimento de un órgano o parte.

impair *v.* dañar; debilitar, desmejorar.

impaired *a.* impedido-a, baldado-a; desmejorado-a, debilitado-a.

impalpable *n.* impalpable.

impartial *a.* imparcial.

impatient *a.* impaciente; *v.* **to get, to become** ___ / impacientarse, perder la paciencia.

impede *v.* impedir, obstruir.

impediment *n.* impedimento, obstáculo, obstrucción.

impenetrable *a.* impenetrable, que no puede ser penetrado.

imperative *n.* inperativo; *a.* imperativo-a; requerido-a.

imperfect *n.* tiempo imperfecto; *a.* imperfecto-a; defectuoso-a.

imperfection *n.* imperfección, deformidad, defecto.

imperforate *a.* imperforado-a; ___ **hymen** / himen ___.

imperil *v.* poner en peligro, arriesgar, hacer daño.

impermeable *a.* impermeable, impenetrable, que no deja pasar líquidos.

impersonal *a.* impersonal.

impetigo *n.* impétigo, infección bacteriana de la piel que se caracteriza por pústulas dolorosas de tamaño diferente que al desecarse forman costras amarillentas; ___ **contagiosa** / ___ contagioso; ___ **neonatorum** / ___ del neonato; ___ **vulgaris** / ___ vulgar.

impetuous *a.* impetuoso-a.

implant *n.* implante, cualquier material insertado o injertado en el cuerpo; *v.* implantar, injertar, insertar.

implantation *n.* implantación, inserción o fijación de una parte o tejido en un área del cuerpo.

implanted *a. pp.* of **to implant**, implantado-a.

implementation *n.* implementación

implication *n.* implicación.

implosion *n.* implosión. 1. colapso violento hacia adentro como sucede en la evacuación de un vaso; 2. método de tratamiento para el miedo debido a una fobia.

imply *v.* implicar, insinuar.

importance *n.* importancia.

important *a.* importante.

impose *v.* imponer.

impossible *a.* imposible.

impotence *n.* impotencia, incapacidad de tener o mantener una erección.

impotent *a.* impotente.

impractical *a.* poco práctico-a.

impregnate *n.* impregnar; saturar.

impression *n.* impresión. 1. huella en una superficie; 2. el efecto producido en la mente a través de estímulos externos; 3. copia de la configuración de una parte o del total del arco dental, de dientes individuales, o para uso en una restauración de caries dentales.

impressive *a.* impresionante.

improbable *a.* improbable.

improper action *n.* acción incorrecta.

improve *v.* mejorar; adelantar; mejorarse, recuperarse; restablecerse.

improved *a. pp.* of **to improve**, mejorado-a, recuperado-a.

improvement *n.* mejoría, restablecimiento, recuperación.

improvise *v.* improvisar.
improvised *a.* improvisado-a.
impulse *n.* impulso; fuerza súbita impulsiva;
  cardiac ___ / ___ cardíaco;
  excitatory ___ / ___ excitante;
  inhibitory ___ / ___ inhibitorio;
  nervous ___ / ___ nervioso; *v.* **to act on** ___ /
  dejarse llevar por un ___.
impulsive *a.* impulsivo-a; irreflexivo-a.
impure *a.* impuro-a; contaminado-a, adulterado-a.
in *prep.* [*inside of*] dentro de; [*in time*] con; [*in the*
  night, day, etc.] durante, por; [*in place*] en; *adv.*
  dentro; adentro; ___ **the care of** / al cuidado
  de; ___ **the meantime** / mientras tanto.
in articulo mortis *adv. L.* in articulo mortis, a
  la hora de la muerte, al instante de morir.
in-dwelling catheter *n.* catéter permanente.
in-grown hair *n.* pelo que crece en ángulo
  anormal, revirtiendo el crecimiento hacia
  adentro.
in situ *a. L.* in situ. 1. en el lugar normal; 2. que
  no se extiende más allá del sitio en que se
  origina.
in utero *a. L.* in utero, dentro del útero.
in vitro *a. L.* in vitro, dentro de una vasija de
  vidrio, término aplicado a pruebas de laboratorio.
in vivo *a. L.* in vivo, en el cuerpo vivo.
inability *n.* inhabilidad, incapacidad.
inaccurate *a.* inexacto-a, incorrecto-a.
inaction *n.* inacción, fallo en responder a un
  estímulo.
inactive *a.* inactivo-a, pasivo-a.
inactivity *n.* inactividad; **physical** ___ / ___
  física.
inadequate *a.* inadecuado-a, impropio-a.
inanimate *a.* inanimado-a, sin vida, falto de
  animación.
inanition *n.* inanición; debilidad; desnutrición.
inarticulate *a.* inarticulado-a, incapaz de
  articular palabras o sílabas.
inborn *a.* innato-a, cualidad congénita.
incandescent *a.* incandescente, con brillo de
  luz.
incapable *a.* incapaz.
incapacitate *v.* incapacitar, imposibilitar,
  inhabilitar.
incapacitated *a.* incapacitado-a.
incarcerated *a.* constricto-a; encarcelado-a;
  limitado-a.
incase *v.* encajar, encajonar.
incasement *n.* encajonamiento, encerramiento.
incentive *n.* incentivo, estímulo; incitante,
  estimulante.

incessant *a.* incesante, constante.
incest *n.* incesto.
incestuous *a.* incestuoso-a.
inch *n.* pulgada.
incidence *n.* incidencia; frecuencia.
incidental *a.* incidental, casual.
incinerate *v.* incinerar.
incipient *a.* incipiente, principiante, que
  comienza a existir.
incise *v.* cortar, hacer un corte.
incised *a.* cortado-a, inciso-a.
incision *n.* incisión, corte, cortadura.
incisor *n.* diente incisivo.
incisura *n. L.* incisura, corte, raja.
inclination *n.* inclinación.
inclusion *n.* inclusión, acto de contener una cosa
  dentro de otra; ___ **bodies** / cuerpos de ___,
  presentes en el citoplasma de ciertas células en
  casos de infección.
incoherence *n.* incoherencia, falta de
  coordinación de las ideas.
incoherent *a.* incoherente, que no coordina las
  ideas.
income *n.* ingreso, entrada; ___ **tax** / impuestos.
incompatibility *n.* incompatibilidad.
incompatible *a.* incompatible.
incompetent *a.* incompetente, incapacitado-a.
incomplete *a.* incompleto-a.
inconsiderate *a.* desconsiderado-a.
inconsistency *n.* inconsistencia.
inconsistent *a.* inconsistente.
incontinence *n.* incontinencia, emisión
  involuntaria, inhabilidad de controlar la orina o
  las heces fecales; **bowel** ___ / ___ intestinal;
  fecal ___ / ___ fecal; **overflow** ___ / ___ por
  rebozamiento; **reflex** ___ / ___ de reflejo;
  urinary ___ / ___ urinaria; **urinary**
  stress ___ / ___ urinaria de esfuerzo.
incontinent *a.* incontinente, rel. a la
  incontinencia.
inconvenience *n.* inconveniencia.
inconvenient *a.* inconveniente.
incoordinate *a.* incoordinado, sin coordinación.
incoordination *n.* falta de coordinación.
incorporate *v.* incorporar, añadir.
incorrect *a.* incorrecto-a.
increase *v.* aumentar, agrandar.
increment *n.* incremento.
incretion *n.* incresión, secreción interna o
  endocrina.
incrustation *n.* incrustación, formación de una
  postilla o costra.
incubation *n.* incubación. 1. período de latencia
  de una enfermedad antes de manifestarse; 2.

mantenimiento de un ambiente especial ajustado a las necesidades de recién nacidos, esp. prematuros; ___ **period** / período de ___.

incubator *n.* incubadora, receptáculo usado para asegurar las condiciones óptimas en el cuidado de prematuros.

incudectomy *n.* incudectomía, excisión del incus.

incurable *a.* incurable, que no tiene cura.

incus *n. L.* incus, huesecillo del oído medio.

indecision *n.* indecisión; irresolución.

indecisive *a.* indeciso-a; irresoluto-a.

indefinite *a.* indefinido-a; indeterminado-a.

indemnity *n.* indemnización, resarcimiento; ___ **benefits** / beneficios de ___; ___ **insurance** / seguro de ___.

independent *a.* independiente.

indeterminate *a.* indeterminado-a, desconocido-a.

index *n.* índice; sumario.

indicate *v.* indicar, señalar.

indicated *a.* indicado-a; apropiado-a.

indication *n.* indicación; señal.

indicator *n.* indicador, señalador.

indifferent *a.* indiferente.

indigenous *a.* autóctono-a, indígena.

indigestion *n.* indigestión.

indirect *a.* indirecto-a; ___ **fracture** / fractura ___; ___ **hemagglutination test** / prueba de hemaglutinación ___; ___ **immunofluorescence** / inmunofluorescencia ___; ___ **laryngoscopy** / laringoscopía ___; ___ **nuclear division** / división nuclear ___; ___ **reacting bilirubine** / bilirubina reactiva ___; ___ **transfusion** / transfusión ___; ___ **vision** / visión ___.

indispensable *a.* indispensable, necesario-a.

indispose *vr.* indisponerse, enfermarse.

indisposed *a.* maldispuesto-a; indispuesto-a; *v.* **to become** ___ / enfermarse.

indisposition *n.* indisposición, desorden o enfermedad pasajera.

indissoluble *a.* indisoluble.

individual *n.* individuo; *a.* individual.

individuality *n.* individualidad.

indivisible *a.* indivisible.

indolent *a.* indolente, perezoso-a; inactivo-a, lento-a en desarrollarse, tal como sucede en ciertas úlceras.

induce *v.* inducir, provocar, suscitar, ocasionar.

induced *a. pp.* of **to induce,** inducido-a, provocado-a.

induction *a.* inducción, acción o efecto de inducir.

induration *n.* induración, endurecimiento que puede suceder en tejidos blandos como en el tejido de las membranas mucosas.

inebriation *n.* embriaguez, intoxicación.

ineffective *a.* inefectivo-a; inútil.

inefficient *a.* deficiente; ineficaz.

inert *a.* inerte, rel. a la inercia.

inertia *n.* incercia, falta de actividad.

inexperience *n.* inexperiencia, sin experiencia.

infancy *n.* infancia, menor de edad, primera edad, período desde el nacimiento hasta los primeros dos años.

infant *n.* infante, lactante.

infanticide *n.* infanticidio.

infantile *a.* infantil, pueril; ___ **acropustulosis** / acropustulosis ___; ___ **autism** / autismo ___; ___ **eczema** / eczema ___; ___ **hypothyroidism** / hipotiroidismo ___; ___ **osteomalacia** / osteomalacia ___; ___ **paralysis** / parálisis ___; ___ **purulent conjunctivitis** / conjuntivitis purulenta ___; ___ **scurvy** / escorbuto ___; ___ **spinal muscular atrophy** / atrofia muscular ___ de la espina dorsal.

infantilism *n.* infantilismo, manifestación de características infantiles en la edad adulta.

infarct, infarction *n.* infarto, necrosis de un área de tejido por falta de irrigación sanguínea (isquemia); **bland** ___ / ___ blando; **cardiac** ___ / ___ cardíaco; **cerebral** ___ / ___ cerebral; **hermorrhagic** ___ / ___ hemorrágico; **myocardial** ___ / ___ del miocardio; **pulmonary** ___ / ___ pulmonar.

infect *v.* infectar; infectarse.

infected *a.* infectado-a.

infection *n.* infección, invasión del cuerpo por microorganismos patógenos y la reacción y efecto que éstos provocan en los tejidos; **acute** ___ / ___ aguda; **airborne** ___ / ___ aerógena; **chronic** ___ / ___crónica; **contagious** ___ / ___ contagiosa; **cross** ___ / ___ hospitalaria; **fungus** ___ / ___ de hongos parásitos; **hospital acquired** ___ / ___ intrahospitalaria; **initial or primary** ___ / ___ inicial o primaria; **massive** ___ / ___ masiva; **opportunistic** ___ / enfermedad oportunista infecciosa; **pyogenic** ___ / ___ piogénica; **secondary** ___ / ___ secundaria; **subclinical** ___ / ___ subclínica; **systemic** ___ / ___ sistémica; **water-borne** ___ / ___ hídrica.

infectious *a.* infeccioso-a, rel. a una infección; ___ **agent** / agente ___; ___ **disease** / enfermedad ___.

infecundity *n.* infecundidad, esterilidad.
infer *v.* inferir, deducir.
inferior *a.* inferior.
inferiority complex *n.* complejo de inferioridad.
infertility *n.* infertilidad, inhabilidad de concebir o procrear.
infestation *n.* infestación, invasión del organismo por parásitos.
infibulation *n.* infibulación; circuncisión en la mujer.
infiltrate *v.* infiltrar, penetrar.
infiltration *n.* infiltración, acumulación de sustancias extrañas en un tejido o célula.
infirmary *n.* enfermería, establecimiento de salud local donde se atiende a personas enfermas o lesionadas.
infirmity *n.* enfermedad.
inflame *v.* inflamar; inflamarse.
inflammation *n.* inflamación, reacción de un tejido lesionado.
inflammatory *a.* inflamatorio-a, rel. a la inflamación; **___ bowel disease /** enfermedad ___ de los intestinos.
inflation *n.* inflación, distensión.
inflection *n.* inflexión, torcimiento.
inflict *v.* infligir, causar sufrimiento.
inflow *n.* flujo, afluencia, entrada.
influenza *n.* influenza, infección viral aguda del tracto respiratorio.
inform *v.* informar, comunicar, avisar.
information *n.* información; informe.
informed consent *n.* consentimiento informado.
infraclavicular *a.* infraclavicular, localizado debajo de la clavícula.
infraction *a.* infracción, fractura ósea incompleta sin desplazamiento.
infradiaphragmatic *a.* infradiafragmático-a, localizado debajo del diafragma.
infraorbital *a.* infraorbital, infraorbitario-a, localizado debajo de la órbita.
infrared rays *n., pl.* rayos infrarrojos.
infrascapular *n.* infraescapular, localizado debajo de la escápula.
infrequent *a.* infrecuente, raro-a.
infundibulum *n.* (*pl.* **infundibula**) infundíbulo. 1. estructura en forma de embudo; 2. cada una de las divisiones de la pelvis renal; 3. prolongación corta del ventrículo derecho de donde procede la arteria pulmonar.
infusion *n.* infusión. 1. introducción lenta, por gravedad, de líquidos en una vena; 2. sumersión de un elemento en agua para obtener los principios activos solubles.
ingest *v.* ingerir.
ingestant, ingesta *n.* alimentación oral.
ingestion *n.* ingestión, proceso de ingerir alimentos.
ingredient *n.* ingrediente, componente.
ingrowing *a.* rel. a una parte que crece hacia adentro y no hacia afuera, en forma opuesta a lo normal.
ingrown hair *n.* pelo que crece en ángulo anormal, revirtiendo el crecimiento hacia adentro.
ingrown nail *n.* e uña que crece en ángulo anormal, revirtiendo el crecimiento hacia adentro.
inguinal *a.* inguinal, rel. a la ingle; **___ canal /** conducto, canal ___; **___ hernia /** hernia ___; **___ ligament /** ligamento ___; **___ ring /** anillo ___.
inhalant *n.* inhalante, medicamento administrado por inhalación.
inhalation *n.* inhalación, aspiración de aire o vapor a los pulmones; **smoke ___ / ___ de** humo.
inhale *v.* inhalar, aspirar.
inherent *a.* inherente, rel. a una cualidad natural o innata.
inherit *v.* heredar.
inheritance *n.* herencia. V. **heredity.**
inherited *a.* heredado-a, rel. a la herencia.
inhibit *v.* inhibir; inhibirse, cohibirse.
inhibition *n.* inhibición, interrupción o restricción de una acción o hábito.
inhibitor *n.* inhibidor, agente que causa una inhibición; **fusion ___ / ___ de** fusión.
initial *a.* inicial, primero-a.
initiate *v.* iniciar, comenzar, empezar.
inject *v.* inyectar, acto de introducir líquidos en un tejido, vaso o cavidad por medio de un inyector.
injection *n.* inyección, acción de inyectar una droga o líquido en el cuerpo. See chart on page 422.
injector *n.* inyector, jeringa, dispositivo que se usa para inyectar.
injure *v.* dañar; lastimar, herir.
injured *a. pp.* of **to injure,** lastimado-a, dañado-a; herido-a.
injury *n.* lesión, lastimadura; herida; **degloving ___ /** herida de avulsión; **___ -free /** ileso-a.
ink *n.* tinta.
inlaid *a.* incrustado-a; embutido-a.
inlay *n.* incrustación.

Injection	Inyección
booster shot	de refuerzo
depot	de depósito, con medicamento de liberación lenta
hypodermic	hipodérmica o subcutánea
insulin	de insulina
intraarticular	intraarticular o de punción lumbar
intradermic	intradérmica
intramuscular	intramuscular
intrafecal	intrafecal
intravenous	intravenosa
selective	selectiva
sensitizing	de sensibilización
test	de prueba

inlet *n.* entrada, acceso.

innate *a.* innato-a, inherente.

inner *a.* interior.

innervate *v.* inervar, estimular un área o parte con energía nerviosa.

innervation *n.* inervación.1. acto de inervar;2. distribución de nervios o de energía nerviosa en un órgano o área.

innocent *a.* inocente.

innocuous *a.* inocuo-a, que no daña.

inoculable *a.* inoculable, que puede ser transmitido por inoculación.

inoculate *v.* inocular, inmunizar, vacunar.

inoculation *n.* inoculación, vacunación, inmunización, acción de administrar sueros, vacunas u otras sustancias para producir o incrementar inmunidad a una enfermedad determinada.

inoculum *n.* (*pl.* **inocula**) inóculo, la sustancia introducida por inoculación.

inoperable *a.* inoperable, que no puede tratarse quirúrgicamente.

inorganic *a.* inorgánico-a; que no pertenece a organismos vivos.

inosculating *n.* comunicación directa, anastomosis.

inotropic *a.* inotrópico-a, que afecta la intensidad o energía de las contracciones musculares.

input-output chart *n.* hoja de balance.

inquest *n.* encuesta, investigación oficial.

insalubrious *a.* insalubre; antihigiénico-a.

insane *a.* loco-a, demente.

insanitary *a.* antihigiénico-a.

insanity *n.* locura, demencia.

insanity defense *n.* defensa por demencia.

insatiable *a.* insaciable, insatisfecho-a.

insect *n.* insecto.

insecticide *n.* insecticida.

insecurity *n.* inseguridad.

insemination *n.* inseminación, fertilización de un óvulo.

insensible *n.* insensible, que carece de sensibilidad.

inseparable *a.* inseparable.

insertion *n.* inserción. 1. acto de insertar; 2. punto de unión de un músculo y un hueso.

inside *prep.* por dentro, hacia adentro; adentro.

insider *n.* persona bien informada.

insidious *a.* insidioso-a, rel. a una enfermedad que se desarrolla gradualmente sin producir síntomas obvios.

insight *n.* conocimiento; penetración; *v.* **to get an ___ into** / formarse una idea de; hacer un estudio detenido.

insignificant *a.* insignificante, sin importancia.

insipid *a.* insípido-a, sin sabor; *pop.* soso-a.

insist *v.* insistir; **to ___ on** / ___ en; **to ___ that** / ___ en que.

insolation *n.* insolación. V. **sunstroke**.

insoluble *a.* insoluble, que no se disuelve.

insomnia *n.* insomnio, desvelo.

inspection *n.* inspección.

inspiration *n.* inspiración.

inspiratory *a.* inspiratorio-a, rel a la inspiración;___**capacity** / capacidad ___; ___ **reserve volume** / reserva de volumen ___; ___ **stridor** / estridor ___

instability *n.* inestabilidad.

install *v.* instalar, colocar.

installation *n.* instalación; montaje.

instant *n.* instante; *a.* instantáneo-a, inmediato-a; urgente.

instep *n.* empeine, parte anterior del pie.

instillation *n.* instilación, goteo de un líquido en una cavidad o superficie.

instinct *n.* instinto.

instinctive *a.* instintivo-a.

institution *n.* institución; fundación; establecimiento; [*mental*] asilo, manicomio; [*home for the aged*] asilo de ancianos.

instruct *v.* instruir, enseñar, dar instrucciones.

instrument *n.* instrumento.

insufficiency *n.* insuficiencia, falta de; **adrenal ___** / ___ suprarrenal;

cardiac ___ / ___ cardíaca; **coronary** ___ / ___ coronaria; **hepatic** ___ / ___ hepática; **mitral** ___ / ___ mitral; **pulmonary valvular** ___ / ___ pulmonar-valvular; **renal** ___ / ___ renal; **respiratory** ___ / ___ respiratoria; **valvular** ___ / ___ valvular; **venous** ___ / ___ venosa.

insufficient *a.* insuficiente.

insufflate *v.* insuflar, soplar hacia el interior de una cavidad, parte u órgano.

insula *n.* ínsula, lóbulo central del hemisferio cerebral.

insulin *n.* insulina. hormona secretada en el páncreas; ___ **dependent** / insulinodependiente.

insuline shock *n.* choque insulínico, hipoglicemia severa que se manifiesta en forma de sudor, temblores, ansiedad, vértigo y diplopia, que puede ser seguida por delirio, convulsiones y colapso.

insulinemia *n.* insulinemia, exceso de insulina en la sangre.

insulinogenesis *n.* insulinogénesis, producción de insulina.

insurance *n.* seguro; compañía de seguros;*Mex.* aseguranza; **disability** ___ / ___ por incapacidad; ___**policy** / póliza de ___; **life** ___ / ___ de vida; **medical** ___ / ___ médico.

insure *v.* asegurar; asegurarse.

intake *n.* **ingestion.**

integration *n.* integración. 1. actividad anabólica; 2. el proceso de combinarse en un ser o entidad total.

integrity *n.* integridad.

intelligence *n.* inteligencia.

intelligent *a.* inteligente, listo-a.

intense *a.* intenso-a.

intensify *v.* intensificar.

intensity *n.* intensidad.

intensive *a.* intensivo-a.

intention *n.* intención. 1. meta o propósito; 2. proceso natural en la curación de heridas.

intentional *a.* intencional, a propósito.

interaction *n.* interacción; **drug** ___ / ___ de medicamentos.

intercalated *a.* intercalado-a, colocado-a entre dos partes o elementos.

intercostal *a.* intercostal, entre dos costillas;___ **membranes** / membranas ___ -es ; ___ **nerves** / nervios ___ -es; ___ **space** / espacio ___.

intercourse *n.* [*sexual*] coito, relaciones sexuales; intercambio, comunicación.

intercurrent *a.* intercurrente, que aparece en el curso de una enfermedad y que la modifica.

interdigitation *n.* interdigitación, entrecruzamiento de partes esp. los dedos.

interest *n.* interés; *v.* **to take an** ___ **in** / interesarse por.

interfere *v.* interferir.

interference *n.* interferencia, anulación o colisión entre dos partes.

interferon *n.* interferón, proteína natural liberada por células expuestas a la acción del virus que se usa en el tratamiento de infecciones y neoplasmas.

interfibrillar *a.* interfibrilar, localizado entre fibrillas.

interim *n., L.* interim, entretanto.

interior *a.* interior.

interlobitis *n.* interlobitis, infl. de la pleura que separa dos lóbulos pulmonares.

interlobular *a.* interlobular, que occurre entre dos lóbulos de un órgano.

intermediary *a.* intermediario-a, situado entre dos cuerpos.

intermediate *a.* intermedio-a, situado entre dos extremos; después del principio y antes del final.

intermittent *a.* intermitente, que no es continuo; ___ **positive-pressure breathing** / ventilación ___ bajo presión positiva; ___ **pulse** / pulso ___.

intern *n.* interno-a; médico-a interno-a.

internal *a.* interno-a, dentro del cuerpo; ___ **bleeding** / hemorragia ___

internalization *n.* internalización, proceso inconsciente por el cual una persona adapta las creencias y valores de otra persona o de la sociedad en que vive.

International Red Cross *n.* Cruz Roja Internacional, organización mundial de asistencia médica.

International unit *n.* unidad internacional, medida de una sustancia definida aceptada por la Conferencia Internacional de Unificación de Fórmulas

interosseous *a.* interóseo-a, entre huesos o que conecta los huesos.

interpret *v.* interpretar, traducir oralmente.

interpretation *n.* interpretación.

interpreter *n.* intérprete.

interruption *n.* interrupción.

intersection *n.* intersección, punto común de dos líneas que se atraviesan.

interstices *n., pl.* intersticios, intervalos o pequeños espacios.

interstitial *a.* intersticial, rel. a los espacios dentro de un tejido, órgano o célula; ___ **cell**

stimulating hormone / hormona ___ que estimula células; ___ **cystitis** / cistitis ___; ___ **disease** / enfermedad ___; ___ **emphysema** / enfisema ___; ___ **fluid** / fluido ___; ___ **gastritis** / gastritis ___; ___ **growth** / crecimiento ___; ___ **hernia** / hernia ___; ___ **nephritis** / nefritis ___; ___ **pregnancy** / embarazo ___.

intertrigo *n.* intértrigo, dermatitis irritante que ocurre entre o debajo de los pliegues de la piel.

interval *n.* intérvalo; espacio; período de tiempo.

intervene *v.* intervenir; asistir; supervisar.

interventricular *a.* interventricular, localizado entre los ventrículos; ___ **optum** / tabique ___ del corazón.

intervertebral disk *n.* disco intervertebral.

interview *n.* entrevista.

intestinal *a.* intestinal, rel. a los intestinos; ___ **bypass surgery** / desviación quirúrgica ___; ___

flora / flora ___; ___ **juice** / jugo ___; ___ **obstruction** / obstrucción ___; ___ **perforation** / perforación ___.

intestine *n.* intestino, tubo digestivo que se extiende del píloro al ano; **large** ___ / ___ grueso; **small** ___ / ___ delgado.

intima *n., L.* (*pl.* **intimae**) íntima, la membrana o túnica más interna de las capas de un órgano tal como en un vaso capilar.

intimal *a.* íntimal, rel. a la íntima.

intolerance *n.* intolerancia, incapacidad de soportar dolor o los efectos de una droga.

intorsion *n.* intorsión, rotación del ojo hacia adentro.

intoxicate *v.* intoxicar.

intoxication *n.* intoxicación, envenenamiento o estado tóxico producido por una droga o sustancia tóxica. See Appendix A. See chart on this page.

Intoxication-Poisoning	Intoxicación-Envenenamiento
alcali poisoning-ingestion of an alcali or ammoniac	ingestión de una sustancia alcalí-amoníaco, legía
caffeinism-excessive ingestion of products containing caffeine	cafeinismo-envenenamiento por ingestion excesiva de productos conteniendo cafeína
carbon monoxide-absorbtion of carbon monoxide causing a toxic condition that can be lethal	monóxido de carbono-envenenamiento por absorción e inhalación de monóxido de carbono que puede ser letal.
cyanide poisoning-inhalation of smoke or ingestion of cyanide industrial chemicals	envenenamiento de cianuro-inhalación de humo o ingestión de sustancias químicas industriales
ergotism-ingestion of ergot-infected grain products that cause diarrhea, vomiting and even alteration of the heart rhythm	ergotismo-consumo de productos de grano infestado por ergot que pueden causar diarrea y hasta alteración del ritmo cardíaco
alcohol intoxication- excessive ingestion of alcohol, can be habit forming and cause serious physical and psychological problems	intoxicación alcohólica-ingestión excesiva de alcohol puede ser adictiva y causar serios problemas físicos y psicológicos
lead poisoning-by ingestion or inhalation of paints that contain lead, or containers of water such as water pipes and water tanks	envenenamiento por plomo-por ingestión o absorción, causado por pinturas que contienen plomo, o por contenedores de agua tal como tuberías y tanques
mercury poisoning-poisoning by ingesting mercury, causing acute kidney damage, vomiting and diarrhea that could be lethal	envenenamiento por mercurio-puede causar daño severo al riñón, vómito y diarrea que pueden ser letales
nicotine poisoning-inhalation and ingestion of great amounts of nicotine	envenenamiento por nicotina-inhalación e ingestión de una gran cantidad de nicotina
overdose of drugs-salicylates, neuroleptics, antidepressants, and opiates prescribed or obtained illegally	sobredosis de drogas-salicilatos, neurolépticos, antidepresivos, opiados, prescritos u obtenidos ilegalmente
contaminated shellfish	mariscos contaminados
ophidism-poisoning by snakes, bees, ants, spiders, producing an injected venom	ofidismo-envenenamiento causado por la ponzoña de una abeja, hormiga, avispa, o araña negra o el veneno de una serpiente
strong cleaning substances mixed with strong acids	sustancias limpiadoras fuertes mezcladas con ácidos

intra-abodominal *a.* intrabdominal, localizado dentro del abdomen.

intra-aortic *a.* intraórtico-a, rel. a o situado dentro de la aorta.

intra-arterial *a.* intra-arterial, dentro de una arteria.

intra-articular *a.* intra-articular, dentro de una articulación.

intracapsular *a.* intracapsular, dentro de una cápsula.

intracellular *a.* intracelular, dentro de una célula o células.

intracranial *a.* intracraneal, dentro del cráneo.

intrahepatic *a.* intrahepático-a, dentro del hígado; ___ **cholestasis of pregnancy** / colestasis ___ del embarazo.

intralobular *a.* intralobular, dentro de un lóbulo.

intraluminal *a.* intraluminal.1. dentro de la luz o estructura lumínica; 2. semejante al lumen de un vaso arterial o venoso.

intramuscular *a.* intramuscular, dentro del músculo.

intraocular *a.* intraocular, dentro del ojo; ___ **pressure** / presión ___.

intraoperative *a.* intraoperatorio-a, que tiene lugar durante un proceso quirúrgico.

intraosseous *a.* intraóseo-a, dentro de la sustancia ósea.

intrarenal *a.* intrarrenal, que ocurre dentro del riñón; ___ **failure** / insuficiencia ___.

intrauterine *a.* intrauterino-a, dentro del útero; ___ **device** / dispositivo ___.

intravenous *a.* intravenoso-a, dentro de una vena; ___ **infusion** / infusión ___; ___ **injection** / inyección ___.

intravenous pyelogram *n.* pielograma intravenoso, procedimiento de diagnósticos que usa un agente de contraste por medio intravenoso y rayos-x para obtener claras imágenes del tracto urinario.

intraventricular *a.* intraventricular, dentro de un ventrículo.

intrinsic *a.* intrínseco-a, esencial, exclusivo-a. inherente.

intrinsic factor *n.* factor intrínseco, proteína normalmente presente en el jugo gástrico humano.

introducer *n.* intubador, divisa utilizada para intubar.

introitus *n., L.* introito, abertura o entrada a un canal o cavidad.

introspection *n.* introspección, análisis propio o de sí mismo-a.

introversion *n.* inversion, introversión, acto de concentración de una persona en sí misma, con disminución del interés por el mundo externo.

intubation *n.* intubación, inserción de un tubo en un conducto o cavidad del cuerpo.

intumesce *v.* intumecer, engrosar, agrandar.

intumescence *n.* intumescencia, engrosamiento.

intumescent *a.* engrosado-a, que se va hinchando.

intussusception *n.* intususcepción, invaginación tal como la de una porción del intestino que causa una obstrucción intestinal.

invade *v.* invadir, penetrar; atacar.

invaginate *v.* invaginar, replegar una porción de una estructura en otra parte de la misma.

invagination *n.* invaginación, proceso de inclusión de una parte dentro de otra.

invalid *a.* inválido-a; debilitado-a; incapacitado-a.

invariable *a.* invariable, que no cambia.

invasion *n.* invasión, acto de invadir.

invasive *a.* invasor-a, invasivo-a; que invade tejidos adyacentes; **non-** ___ / no ___.

inverse, inverted *a.* inverso-a, invertido-a.

inversion *n.* inversión, proceso de volverse hacia adentro; ___ **of chromosomes** / ___ de cromosomas; ___ **of the uterus** / ___ del útero; **paracentric** ___ / ___ paracéntrica; **pericentric** ___ / ___ pericéntrica; **visceral** ___ / ___ visceral.

invert *v.* invertir.

investigation *n.* investigación, indagación.

investment *n.* revestimiento, cubierta.

invisible *a.* invisible, que no puede verse a simple vista.

involuntary *a.* involuntario-a.

involution *n.* involución, cambio retrógrado.

involutional melancholia *n.* melancolía involucional, trastorno emocional depresivo que se observa en mujeres de 40 a 55 años y en hombres de 50 a 65 años.

involved *a.* complicado, enredado; *v.* **to be** ___ / ___ estar involucrado; **to get** ___ / involucrarse o meterse en.

iodine *n.* iodo, yodo. 1. elemento no metálico que pertenece al grupo halógeno usado como componente en medicamentos para contribuir al desarrollo y funcionamiento de la tiroides;

2. tintura de yodo usada como germicida y desinfectante.

iodism *n.* yodismo, envenenamiento por yodo.

iodize *v.* yodurar, tratar con yodo.

iododerma *n.* yododerma, afección cutánea.

iodophilia *n.* yodofilia, afinidad por el yodo, como se manifiesta en algunos leucocitos.

ion *n.* ion, átomo o grupo de átomos provistos de carga eléctrica.

ionization *n.* ionización, disociación de compuestos en los iones que los componen.

ionizing radiation *n.* radiación por ionización.

ipecac, syrup of *n.* jarabe de ipecacuana, emético y expectorante.

ipsilateral *a.* ipsilateral, ipsolateral, que afecta el mismo lado del cuerpo.

irascible *a.* irascible, que se irrita fácilmente.

iridectomy *n.* iridectomía, extirpación de una parte del iris.

iridology *n.* iridología, estudio del iris y de los cambios que éste sufre en el curso de una enfermedad.

iris *n.* iris, membrana contráctil del humor acuoso del ojo situada entre el cristalino y la córnea, que regula la entrada de la luz.

iritis *n.* iritis, infl. del iris.

iron *n.* hierro; *v.* **to have an ___ constitution** / tener una constitución de hierro.

iron-deficiency anemia *n.* anemia por deficiencia de hierro.

iron lung *n.* pulmón de hierro, máquina que se usa para producir respiración artificial.

irradiate *v.* irradiar; exponer a o tratar por uso de radiación.

irradiation *n.* irradiación, uso terapéutico de radiaciones.

irrational *n.* irracional.

irreducible *a.* irreducible, que no puede reducirse.

irregular *a.* irregular.

irrelevant *a.* ajeno-a, no pertinente, que no tiene relación con lo que se discute; que no viene al caso.

irrigate *v.* irrigar, lavar con un chorro de agua.

irrigation *n.* irrigación, acto o proceso de irrigar.

irritability *n.* irritabilidad, propiedad de un organismo o tejido de reaccionar al ambiente.

irritable *n.* irritable, que reacciona con irritación a un estímulo; **___ bowel syndrome** / síndrome de irritación intestinal.

irritate *v.* irritar.

irritation *n.* irritación, reacción extrema a un dolor o a una condición patológica.

ischemia *n.* isquemia, insuficiencia de riego sanguíneo a un tejido o parte; **silent ___** / **___** silenciosa.

ischemic *a.* isquémico-a, que padece de isquemia o rel. a la misma.

ischium *n., L. (pl.* **ischia)** isquion, parte posterior de la pelvis.

ischuria *n.* iscuria, retención o suspensión de orina.

island *n.* isla, nombre dado a un grupo celular o a un tejido aislado.

isolate *v.* aislar, separar.

isolated *a.* aislado-a, separado-a.

isolation *n.* aislamiento. 1. proceso de aislar o separar; 2. la separación física de organismos infectados de otros con el fin de evitar la contaminación; **behavioral ___** / **___** conductual; **exclusion ___** / **___** de exclusión; **infectious ___** / **___** de infección; **___ ward** / sala de **___**.

isometric *a.* isométrico-a, de dimensiones iguales.

isometropia *n.* isometropía, la misma refracción en los dos ojos.

isoniazid *n.* isoniazida, medicamento antibacteriano usado en el tratamiento de tuberculosis.

isosthenuria *n.* isostenuria, condición de insuficiencia renal.

isotonic *a.* isotónico-a, que tiene la misma tensión que otra dada; **___ exercise** / ejercicio **___**.

isotope *n.* isótopo, elemento químico que pertenece a un grupo de elementos que presentan propiedades casi idénticas, pero que difiere de éstos en el peso atómico.

issue *n.* emisión; cuestión; **___ of blood** / pérdida de sangre; **to avoid the ___** / esquivar la cuestión; *v.* brotar, fluir; emitir.

issued *a.* expedido-a, emitido-a.

issuing *n.* salida.

isthmectomy *n.* istmectomía, extirpación de la parte media de la tiroides.

isthmus *n.* istmo. 1. conducto estrecho que conecta dos cavidades o dos partes mayores; 2. constricción entre dos partes de un órgano o estructura; **aortic ___** / **___** de la aorta; **___ of auditory tube** / **___** del tubo auditivo; **___ of the encephalon** / **___** del encéfalo; **___ of the eustachian tube** / **___** de la trompa de Eustaquio; **___ of the fauces** / **___** de las fauces; ___ **of the ureter** / ___ de la uretra; **pharyngeal** ___ / ___ de la faringe; **tubaric** ___ / ___ tubárico.

it *pron. neut.* they; **it is** / eso es; es; **it's** *contr.* of **it** and **is**; **the best of** ___ / lo mejor; **the worst of** ___ / lo peor.

itch *n.* picazón.

itching *n.* sensación de picazón.

itself *pron., m.* (él) mismo, si mismo; *f.* (ella) misma; si misma.

ivy *n.* hiedra.

ixodes *n.* ixodes, género que incluye garrapatas y otros ácaros.

ixodiasis *n.* ixodiasis, lesiones cutáneas debidas a la picadura de cierta clase especial de garrapata.

j

j *abbr.* **joint** / articulación;

jab *n.* pinchazo, punzada; golpe corto; *v.* pinchar; dar golpes cortos.

jacket *n.* forro; corsé, soporte del tronco y de la espina dorsal usado para corregir deformidades.

Jacksonian epilepsy *n.* epilepsia jacksoniana, epilepsia parcial sin pérdida del conocimiento.

Jackson membrane *n.* membrana de Jackson, una membrana vascular delgada que cubre la superficie anterior del colon ascendente.

Jaeger test types *n., pl.* Jaeger, tipos de prueba, líneas de tipos de letras de distintos tamaños para determinar la precisión visual.

jam *n.* conserva, compota; *v.* **to be in a** ___ / estar en apuros.

jamais vu *n. Fr.* jamais vu, nunca visto, percepción de una experiencia familiar o conocida como si fuera una experiencia nueva.

jar *n.* jarro, frasco, pomo, recipiente de cristal.

jargon *n.* jerga, jerigonza; parafasia. V. **paraphasia.**

jasmine *n.* jazmín; ___ **tea** / té de ___.

jaundice *n.* ictericia, derrame biliar por exceso de bilirrubina en la sangre que causa pigmentación amarillo-anaranjada de la piel y otros tejidos y fluidos del cuerpo; **obstructive** ___ / ___ obstructiva, obstrucción de la bilis; icterus.

jaundiced *a.* ictérico-a, rel. a la ictericia o que padece de ella.

jaw *n.* mandíbula, quijada, maxilar inferior;___ **reflex** / reflejo mandibular; ___ **winking** / pestañeo mandibular.

jawbone *n.* hueso maxilar de la mandíbula.

jaw-lever *n.* abrebocas. V. **gag.**

jealous *a.* celosa-a.

jealousy *n.* celos.

jejunal *a.* yeyunal, rel. al yeyuno.

jejunectomy *n.* yeyunectomía, excisión de todo el yeyuno o parte del mismo.

jejunocolostomy *n.* yeyunocolostomía, anastomosis quirúrgica entre el yeyuno y el colon.

jejunostomy *n.* yeyunostomía, creación de una abertura permanente en el yeyuno a través de la pared abdominal.

jejunum *n.* yeyuno, porción del intestino delgado que se extiende del duodeno al íleon.

jelly *n.* jalea, sustancia gelatinosa; **contraceptive** ___ / ___ anticonceptiva; **petroleum** ___ / vaselina.

jerk *n.* sacudida, reflejo súbito, contracción muscular brusca; *a.* [*slang*] tonto-a, imbécil; *v.* sacudir, tirar de, mover bruscamente.

jest *n.* broma, chiste; *v.* bromear.

jet *n.* chorro; avión de propulsión.

jet lag *n.* estado de cansancio que sufren los viajeros aéreos después de jornadas largas a través de diferentes zonas de tiempo.

jitters *n.* [*slang*] nerviosidad.

job *n.* trabajo, empleo; [*task*] tarea.

jog *v.* correr acompasadamente como medio de ejercicio físico.

jogger *n.* corredor-a.

jogging *n.* acción de correr como medio de ejercicio.

join *v.* unir, juntar; [*as a member*] hacerse miembro, hacerse socio-a; [*meet*] encontrarse.

joint *n.* articulación, coyuntura, punto de unión entre dos huesos; **arthrodial** ___ / -artrodia, que permite un movimiento de deslizamiento; **ball-and-socket** ___ / ___ esferoidea, que permite movimientos en varias direcciones; **hip** ___ / ___ de la cadera; ___ **efussion** / derrame articular; ___ **inflammation** / arthritis; ___ **freely movable** / ___ con facilidad de movimiento, diartrosis; ___ **fluid** / líquido sinfial; ___ **pain** / artralgia; ___ **replacement** / artroplastia; **knee** ___ / ___ de la rodilla; **sacroiliac** ___ / ___ sacroilíaca; **shoulder** ___ / ___ del hombro.

joint capsule *n.* cápsula articular, cubierta en forma de bolsa que envuelve una articulación.

joint mice *n.* partículas sueltas de cartílago o hueso que se alojan generalmente en algunas articulaciones.

jolly *a.* alegre, jovial.

jolt *n.* sacudida, tirón.

journal *n.* diario.

jovial *n.* jovial, alegre.

jowl *n.* cachete, carrillo.

joy *n.* alegría.

judge *n.* juez, magistrado-a; *v.* juzgar, hacer juicio.

judgment *n.* juicio; decisión, opinión.

jug *n.* jarro.

jugular *a.* yugular, rel. a las venas yugulares; ___ **foramen** / foramen ___; ___ **fossa** / fosa ___; ___ **gland** / glándula ___; ___

glomus / glomo ___; ___ **nerve** / nervio ___; ___ **pulse** / pulso ___; ___ **venous arch** / arco venoso ___.

jugular veins *n.* venas yugulares, venas que llevan la sangre de la cabeza y del cuello al corazón.

juice *n.* jugo, zumo, líquido extraído o segregado; **apple** ___ / ___ de manzana; **carrot** ___ / ___ de zanahoria; **gastric** ___ / ___ gástrico; **grape** ___ / ___ de uva; **grapefruit** ___ / ___ de toronja; **intestinal** ___ / ___ intestinal; **pancreatic** ___ / ___ pancreático; **pineapple** ___ / ___ de piña; **plum** ___ / ___ de ciruela.

juiciness *n.* jugosidad.

juicy *a.* jugoso-a.

jump *n.* salto, brinco; *v.* saltar, brincar.

jumpy *a.* inquieto-a, intranquilo-a.

junction *n.* unión, entronque, punto de contacto de dos partes.

juncture *n.* juntura; coyuntura.

junkie *a. slang*, [*rel. to drug addiction*], vicioso; a, narcómano-a, *Mex.* tecato-a.

jurisprudence, medical *n.* jurisprudencia médica, ciencia del derecho judicial que se aplica a la medicina.

Jurkat cells *n., pl.* células de Jurkat, línea de células T que se usan en la investigación inmunológica.

just *a.* justo-a; preciso-a, exacto-a; **-ly** adv. justamente.

justice *n.* justicia.

justify *v.* justificar.

juvenile *a.* juvenil, joven; ___ **arthritis** / artritis ___; ___ **cataract** / catarata ___; ___ **delinquency** / delincuencia ___; ___ **myoclonic epilepsy** / epilepsia mioclónica ___; ___ **on-set diabetes** / principio de diabetes ___; ___ **pelvis** / pelvis ___; ___ **periodontitis** / periodontitis ___; ___ **plantar dermatitis** / dermatitis plantar ___.

juvenile absence epilepsy *n.* epilepsia juvenil de ausencia, síndrome de epilepsia generalizado que se presenta durante la adolescencia caracterizida por episodios de convulsiones con pérdida del conocimiento y convulsiones clónicas.

juvenile rheumatoid arthritis *n.* artritis reumatoidea juvenil. rheumatism.

juxtaglomerular *a.* yuxtaglomerular, junto a un glomérulo.

juxtaglomerular apparatus *n.* aparato yuxtaglomerular, grupo de células localizadas alrededor de arteriolas aferentes del riñón, que intervienen en la producción de renina y en el metabolismo del sodio.

juxtaglomerular cells *n.* células yuxtaglomerulares, localizadas cerca de o junto a glomérulos del riñón.

juxtaposition *n.* yuxtaposición, aposición; posición adyacente.

K

k

K *abbr.* **kalium** / potasio.

k *abbr.* **kilogram** / kilogramo.

kala-azar *n.* kala-azar, infestación visceral por un protozoo.

kalemia *n.* potasemia, presencia de potasio en la sangre.

kaliuresis *n.* caliuresis, aumento en la excreción de potasio en la orina.

kallikrein *n.* calicreína, enzima potente de acción vasodilatadora.

Kanner syndrome *n.* Kanner, síndrome de, autismo infantil.

kaolin *n.* caolín, silicato de aluminio hidratado, agente de cualidades absorbentes de uso interno y externo.

Kaposi's disease *n.* enfermedad de Kaposi, neoplasma maligno localizado en las extremidades inferiores de hombres adultos que se desarrolla rápidamente en casos de SIDA.

Karvonen method *n.* Karvonen, método de, método de calcular el espectro máximo del índice cardíaco durante pruebas de ejercicios de tolerancia.

karyocyte *n.* cariocito, célula nucleada.

karyogamy *n.* cariogamía, conjugación celular con unión de dos núcleos.

karyogenesis *n.* cariogénesis, desarrollo del núcleo de la célula.

karyolysis *n.* cariolisis, disolución del núcleo de una célula.

karyolytic *a.* cariolítico-a, rel. a cariolisis o que la causa.

karyon *n.* carión, núcleo celular.

karyotype *n.* cariotipo, cromosoma característico de un individuo o de una especie.

Katz formula *n.* Katz, fórmula de, fórmula para obtener la velocidad media de sedimentación de los eritrocitos.

Kawasaki disease *n.* Kawasaki, enfermedad de, enfermedad infantil febril aguda. Los síntomas más destacados son conjuntivitis, lesiones bucales, enrojecimiento, infl. y exfoliación de la epidermis en los dedos de las manos y los pies. Estos síntomas distinguen esta enfermedad entre otras como la escarlatina y el síndrome de choque tóxico.

Kegel exercises *n.* Kegel, ejercicios de, ejercicios que consisten en alternar contracciones y relajamiento de los músculos perineales con el fin de controlar mejor la incontinencia.

keep *vi.* [*a record*] mantener; [*guard*] guardar; **to ___ down** / limitar; **to ___ from** / abstenerse de, guardarse de, evitar; **to ___ off** / alejarse, apartarse; **to ___ on** / continuar; **to ___ quiet** / estarse quieto-a, quedarse callado-a; **to ___ up** / mantener, continuar.

keeping *n.* cuidado, custodia.

Kelly operation *n.* Kelly, operación de. 1. histerectomía abdominal subtotal; 2. operación para corregir la incontinencia urinaria poniendo suturas en la vagina debajo del cuello de la vejiga.

keloid *n.* queloide, cicatriz de tejido grueso rojizo que se forma en la piel después de una incisión quirúrgica o de una herida.

keloidosis *n.* queloidosis, formación de queloides.

kelp *n.* cenizas de un tipo de alga marina rica en yodo.

keratectomy *n.* queratectomía, incisión de una parte de la córnea.

keratin *n.* queratina, proteína orgánica insoluble que es un elemento componente de las uñas, la piel y el cabello.

keratinization *n.* queratinización, proceso por el cual las células se vuelven callosas por dépositos de queratina.

keratinous *a.* queratinosa-a, rel. a o de la naturaleza de la queratina.

keratitis *n.* queratitis, infl. de la córnea; **interstitial ___ / ___** intersticial; **mycotic ___ / ___** micótica, queratomicosis, infección fungal de la córnea; **trophic ___ / ___** trófica, causada por el virus del herpes.

keratocele *n.* queratocele, hernia de la membrana anterior de la córnea.

keratoconjunctivitis *n.* queratoconjuntivitis, infl. de la córnea y la conjuntiva.

keratoconus *n.* queratocono, deformidad de forma cónica de la córnea.

keratoderma *n.* queratoderma, queratodermia, hipertrofia del estrato córneo de la piel, esp. en las regiones de las palmas de las manos y las plantas de los pies.

keratohemia *n.* queratohemia, presencia de sangre en la córnea.

keratolysis *n.* queratolisis. 1. exfoliación de la epidermis; 2. anomalía congénita por la cual se muda la piel periódicamente; **___ neonatorum / ___** neonatal.

keratolytic *n.* queratolítico, agente que provoca exfoliación.

keratoma *n.* queratoma, callosidad, tumor córneo.

keratomalacia *n.* queratomalacia, degeneración de la córnea causada por deficiencia de vitamina A.

keratoplasty *n.* queratoplastia, cualquier modificación de la córnea por medio de cirugía plástica.

keratorrhexis *n.* queratorrexis, rotura de la córnea debido a un trauma o a una úlcera perforante.

keratoscope *n.* queratoscopio, instrumento para examinar la córnea.

keratoses *n.* queratoses, enfermedad no contagiosa de la piel con escamación y posible inflamación.

keratosis *n.* queratosis, condición callosa de la piel tal como callos y verrugas; **actinic** ___ / ___ actínica, lesión solar precancerosa; **blenorrhagic** ___ / ___ blenorrágica, manifestada en la palma de las manos y los pies con erupción escamosa.

keratotomy *n.* queratotomía, incisión a través de la córnea.

keratous *a.* queratoso-a, semejante a la córnea.

kernicterus *n.* kernícterus, forma de ictericia del recién nacido.

ketoacidosis *n.* cetoacidosis, acidosis causada por el aumento de cuerpos cetónicos en la sangre.

ketoaciduria *n.* cetoaciduria, acidosis causada por el aumento de cuerpos cetónicos en la orina.

ketogenesis *n.* cetogénesis, producción de acetona.

ketone bodies *n.* cuerpos cetónicos o acetónicos, comúnmente llamados acetonas, productos desintegrados de las grasas en el catabolismo celular.

ketonemia *n.* cetonemia, concentración de cuerpos cetónicos en el plasma.

ketosis *n.* cetosis, producción excesiva de cuerpos acetónicos como resultado del metabolismo incompleto de ácidos lípidos; acidosis.

key *n.* llave; [*clue, reference*] clave.

kick *n.* patada, puntapié *v.* patear, dar puntapiés; [*addiction*] **to ___ the habit [to abstain or stay away]** / dejar la droga.

kid *n.* [*child*] niño, niña, chiquillo, chiquilla.

kidney *n.* riñón, órgano par situado a cada lado de la región lumbar y que sirve de filtro al organismo; **artificial** ___ / ___ artificial; ___**cancer** / cáncer del ___; ___ **dialysis** / dialysis del ___; **disease** / enfermedad del ___; ___**failure** / fallo renal; ___ **stones** / piedras o cálculos renales, *pop.* piedras en los riñones; **polycystic** ___ / ___ poliquístico. See illustration on page 432.

kill *v.* matar; [*germs*] exterminar; **to ___ time** / pasar el tiempo.

killer cell *n.* linfocito citolítico o linfocito citocida.

kilo *n.* kilogramo, kilo.

kilometer *n.* kilómetro.

kind *n.* clase, tipo; *a* bondadoso-a; **to be so ___ as to** / tener la bondad de; **-ly** *adv.* ___ / bondadosamente.

kindness *n.* bondad.

kindred *n.* parentesco.

kinesiology *n.* cinesiología, estudio de los músculos y los movimientos musculares.

kinesitherapy *n.* cinesiterapia, tratamiento por medio de movimiento o ejercicios.

kinesthesia *n.* cinestesia, experiencia sensorial, sentido y percepción de un movimiento.

kinetic *n.* cinético-a, rel. al movimiento.

kingdom *n.* reino, categoría en la clasificación de animales, plantas y minerales.

kinship *n.* [*family relationship*] parentesco.

kit *n.* equipo.

kitchen *n.* cocina.

klebsiella *n.* klebsiela, bacilo gram-negativo asociado con infecciones respiratorias y del tracto urinario.

Klebs-Löffler bacillus *n.* bacilo de Klebs-Löffler, bacilo de la difteria.

kleptomania *n.* cleptomanía, deseo incontrolable de robar.

kleptomaniac *n.* *a.* cleptómano-a, persona afectada por cleptomanía; rel. a la cleptomanía.

knead *v.* amasar, sobar.

kneading *n.* amasijo, proceso de masaje y frotación.

knee *n.* rodilla, articulación del fémur, la tibia y la patela; ___ **ankle foot orthosis** / ortosis de la ___ y tobillo; ___ **dislocation** / dislocación de la ___; ___ **joint** / articulación de la ___; ___ **protector** / rodillera; ___ **reflex** / reflejo de la ___; **locked** ___ / ___ bloqueada.

kneecap *n.* rótula.

knee jerk *n.* reflejo de la rodilla que se produce con el toque de un martillo de goma en el ligamento de la patela.

knife *n.* cuchillo.

knob *n.* protuberancia, bulto.

knock-knee *n.* V. genu valgum.

knot *n.* nudo; **surgical** ___ / ___ quirúrgico.

know *vi.* saber, [*to be acquainted*] conocer; **to ___ how to** / *saber + inf*; **to ___ of** / tener noticias de, estar enterado-a de.

knowledge *n.* conocimiento; **to the best of my ___** / a mi entender, por lo que sé; *v.* **to have ___ of** / saber.

knuckle *n.* nudillo.

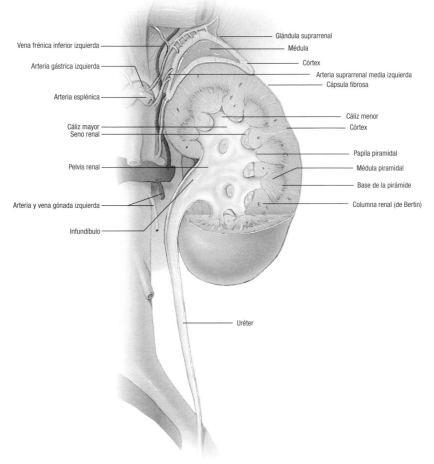

Vena frénica inferior izquierda

Arteria gástrica izquierda

Arteria esplénica

Cáliz mayor
Seno renal

Pelvis renal

Arteria y vena gónada izquierda

Infundíbulo

Glándula suprarrenal
Médula
Córtex
Arteria suprarrenal media izquierda
Cápsula fibrosa

Cáliz menor
Córtex

Papila piramidal
Médula piramidal
Base de la pirámide
Columna renal (de Bertin)

Uréter

Riñón izquierdo y glándula suprarrenal

Koch's bacillus *n.* bacilo de Koch, *Mycobacterium tuberculosis,* causa de la tuberculosis en los mamíferos.

kolpitis *n.* colpitis, infl. de la mucosa vaginal.

Koplic spots *n.* Koplic, manchas de, pequeños puntos blancuzcos rodeados por un anillo rojo que aparece en la parte interna de las mejillas en la fase temprana del sarampión.

Krukenberg tumor *n.* tumor de Krukenberg, tumor maligno del ovario, gen. bilateral y frecuentemente secundario a un cáncer del tracto gastrointestinal.

Kussmaul breathing *n.* respiración de Kussmaul, respiración jadeante y profunda vista en casos de acidosis diabética.

kwashiorkor *n.* Kwashiorkor, deficiencia proteínica o desnutrición durante la infancia que se manifiesta después del destete esp. en áreas tropicales y subtropicales.

kyphosis, hunchback *n.* cifosis, exageración en la curvatura posterior de la espina dorsal que da lugar a una corcova.

kyphotic *a.* cifótico-a; *pop.* corcovado-a, que sufre de una corcova; ___ **pelvic** / pelvis ___.

l

L *abbr.* **liter** / litro.

l *abbr.* **left** / izquierdo-a; **lethal** / letal; **light** / ligero-a; **lower** / más bajo.

label *n.* etiqueta; *v.* poner etiquetas.

labial *a.* labial, rel. a los labios; ___ **branches of mental nerve** / ramas labiales del nervio mentoniano; ___ **glands** / glándulas labiales; ___ **hernia** / hernia ___; ___ **occlusion** / oclusión ___; ___ **splint** / férula ___; ___**veins** / venas labiales.

labial glands *n.* glándulas labiales, situadas entre la mucosa labial y el músculo orbicular de la boca.

labile *a.* lábil, inestable, frágil, que cambia o se altera fácilmente.

lability *n.* labilidad, condición de inestabilidad.

labiochorea *n.* labiocorea, espasmo crónico de los labios y trastornos del lenguaje que se derivan de esa condición.

labioversion *n.* labioversión, posición incorrecta de un diente que se sale de la línea normal de oclusión hacia los labios.

labium *n., L.* (*pl.* **labia**) labio. 1. borde carnoso; 2. estructura semejante a un labio; **labia majora and labia minora** / ___ mayor y ___ menor.

labor *n.* parto; **active** ___ / ___ activo; **after** ___ / después del ___; **before** ___ / antes del ___; **complicated** ___ / ___ complicado; **contractions during** ___ / contracciones durante el ___; **dry** ___ / ___ seco; **during** ___ / durante el ___; **hard** ___ / ___ laborioso; **induction of** ___ / ___ inducido; ___ **pains** / dolores de ___; ___ **room** / sala de ___; **painless** ___ / ___ sin dolor; **stages of** ___ / etapas del ___; *v.* **to be in** ___ / estar de parto; **childbirth**.

laboratory *n.* laboratorio; ___ **findings** / resultados del análisis; ___ **technician** / técnico de ___.

labored *a.* laborioso-a, trabajoso-a; ___ **breathing** / respiración jadeante.

laborious *a.* laborioso-a, trabajoso-a.

labyrinth *n.* laberinto. 1. red de conductos del oído interno cuya función relaciona la audición con el equilibrio del cuerpo; 2. conductos y cavidades que forman un sistema comunicándose entre sí.

labyrinthectomy *n.* laberintectomía, excisión del laberinto.

labyrinthine *a.* laberíntico-a, rel. a un laberinto; ___ **artery** / arteria ___; ___ **fistula** / fístula ___; ___ **nystagmus** / nistagmo ___; ___ **veins** / venas ___; ___ **vertigo** / vértigo ___.

labyrinthitis *n.* laberintitis. 1. infl. aguda o crónica del laberinto; 2. otitis interna.

lacerate *v.* lacerar, desgarrar.

laceration *n.* laceración, desgarro.

lachrymogenous *a.* lacrimógeno-a, que produce lágrimas.

lachrymose *a.* lacrimoso-a, lagrimoso-a.

lack *n.* falta, carencia; necesidad; falta de; ___ **of food** / ___ de alimentos; ___ **of medication** / falta de o carencia de medicina; ___ **of orientation** / ___ de orientación; *v.* carecer de; faltar; **they** ___ **everything** / carecen de todo.

lacrimal *a.* lagrimal, rel. a las lágrimas y a los órganos y partes relacionados con éstas; ___ **apparatus** / aparato ___; ___ **artery** / arteria ___; ___ **bone** / hueso ___; ___ **canaliculus** / canículo ___; ___ **duct** / conducto ___; ___ **fossa** / fosa ___; ___ **gland** / glándula ___; ___ **nerve** / nervio ___; ___ **papilla** / papila; ___ **punctum** / punto ___; ___ **sac** / saco ___; ___ **vein** / vena ___.

lacrimation *n.* lagrimeo, producción de lágrimas.

lacrimotomy *n.* lacrimotomía, incisión del conducto o saco lacrimal.

lactacidemia *n.* lactacidemia, exceso acumulado de ácido láctico en la sangre.

lactase *n.* lactasa, enzima intestinal que hidroliza la lactosa y produce dextrosa y galactosa.

lactation *n.* lactancia, crianza; secreción de leche.

lactial *a.* lácteo-a, rel. a la leche.

lactic acid *n.* ácido láctico.

lactiferous *a.* lactífero-a, que segrega y conduce leche; ___ **ducts** / conductos ___; ___ **sinus** / senos ___.

lacto-ovovegetarian *a.* lacto-ovovegetariano-a; que sigue una dieta de vegetales, huevos y productos lácteos.

lacto-vegetarian *a.* lactovegetariano, que sigue una dieta de vegetales y productos lácteos.

lactocele *n.* lactocele. V. **galactocele**.

lactogen *n.* lactógeno, agente que estimula la producción o secreción de leche.

lactose, lactine *n.* lactosa, lactina, azúcar de leche; ___ **deficiency** / intolerancia a la ___.

lacuna *n.* L. (*pl.* **lacunae**) lacuna, laguna, depresión pequeña tal como las cavidades del cerebro.

lady *n.* dama, señora

lag *n.* atraso, retraso; [*slow growth*] latencia; ___ time / período de latencia.

laid up *a.* inactivo-a; *pop.* en cama; enfermo-a.

laity *n.* [*nonprofessional*] lego.

La Leche League *n.* La Liga de la Leche, organización que promueve la lactancia materna.

lallation, lambdacism *n.* lalación, lambdacismo. 1. defecto y cambio fonético de la *l* por la *r*; 2. balbuceo, tartamudeo infantil.

Lamaze technique, Lamaze method *n.* método de Lamaze, procedimiento de parto natural con adiestramiento de la madre en técnicas respiratorias que facilitan el proceso del parto.

lamb *n.* cordero-a, oveja, borrego-a.

lamb chop *n.* chuleta de cordero.

lamb's wool *n.* lana de cordero.

lame *a.* cojo-a, lisiado-a; *v.* **to go** ___ / cojear, andar cojeando.

lamella *n.* laminilla. 1. capa fina; 2. disco que se inserta en el ojo para aplicar un medicamento.

lament *n.* lamento, queja; lamentarse, quejarse.

lamina *n.*, *L.* (*pl.* **laminae**) lámina, placa o capa fina; ___ **arcus vertebrae** / ___ del arco vertebral; ___ **basalis choroidae** / ___ basal de la coroide; ___ **limitans anterior corneae** / ___ elástica anterior de la córnea; ___ **limitans posterior corneae** / ___ elástica posterior de la córnea; ___ **multiform of cerebral cortex** / ___ multiforme de la corteza cerebral.

laminar *a.* laminar, laminado-a, rel. a láminas; formado por capas.

laminated *a.* laminado-a, que está formado por una o varias láminas.

laminectomy *n.* aminectomía, extirpación de una o varias láminas vertebrales.

lamp *n.* lámpara; **infrared** ___ / ___ infrarroja; **lamplight** / luz de una ___; **slit** ___ / ___ de hendidura; **sun** ___ / ___ solar.

lancet, lance *n.* lanceta, instrumento quirúrgico; *v.* abrir con una lanceta.

lancinating *a.* lancinante, rel. a un dolor agudo con sensación de pinchazos.

Landry paralysis, Landry syndrome *n.* Landry, parálisis de, síndrome de Landry. Guillain-Barré syndrome.

Landztainer's classification *n.* clasificación de Landztainer, diferenciación de grupos sanguíneos; O-A-B-AB.

language *n.* lenguaje; ___ **skills** / habilidades lingísticas.

languid *a.* lánguido-a, débil, flojo-a; decaído-a.

languidness *n.* languidez, decaimiento.

lanolin *n.* lanolina, sustancia purificada que se obtiene de la lana de la oveja y se usa en pomadas.

lantern *n.* linterna, farol.

lanugo *n.* lanugo, vellosidad, pelusilla suave que cubre el cuerpo del feto.

lap *n.* regazo, falda; **mother's** ___ / el ___, la ___ de la madre.

laparocele *n.* laparocele, hernia abdominal.

laparoendoscopy *n.* laparoendoscopía, introducción de un laparoscopio en el abdomen para llevar a cabo distintos procedimientos.

laparoscope *n.* laparoscopio, instrumento usado para visualizar la cavidad peritoneal.

laparoscopy *n.* laparoscopía, examen de la cavidad peritoneal por medio de un laparoscopio.

laparotomy *n.* aparotomía, incisión y abertura del abdomen.

lapse *n.* [*time*] lapso, intervalo de tiempo.

lard *n.* manteca, grasa de origen animal.

large *a.* grande, grueso-a, abultado-a; ___ **intestine** / intestino grueso.

larger, largest *a.*, *comp.*, *sup.* of large, más grande; mayor; **the tumor is** ___ **now** / el tumor está más grande ahora.

larva *n.*, *L. larvae*larva, primera fase o forma de ciertos organismos tal como los insectos.

larval *a.* larval, larvado-a, rel. a una larva.

larvate *a.* larvado-a. rel. a un síntoma atípico o insidioso.

larvicide *n.* larvicida, agente que destruye las larvas, esp. las de los insectos.

laryngeal *a.* laríngeo-a; ___ **papillomatosis** / papilomatosis ___; ___ **prominence** / prominencia ___; ___ **reflex** / reflejo ___, tos producida por irritación de la laringe; ___ **stenosis** / estenosis ___; ___ **syncope** / síncope ___; ___ **ventricle** / ventrículo ___; ___ **web** / red ___.

laryngectomy *n.* aringectomía, extirpación de la laringe.

laryngitis *n.* laringitis. 1. infl. de la laringe; 2. afonía, ronquera.

laryngopharyngitis *n.* laringofaringitis, infl. de la laringe y la faringe.

laryngopharynx *n.* laringofaringe, porción inferior de la faringe.

laryngoplasty *n.* aringoplastia, reconstrucción plástica de la laringe.

laryngoscope *n.* laringoscopio, instrumento usado para examinar la laringe.

laryngoscopy *n.* laringoscopía, examen de la laringe; **direct** ___ / ___ directa, por medio de un laringoscopio; **indirect** ___ / ___ indirecta, por medio de un espejo.

laryngospasm *n.* laringoespasmo, espasmo de los músculos de la laringe.

laryngotomy *n.* aringotomía, incisión de la laringe.

larynx *n.* laringe. 1. parte del tracto respiratorio situado en la parte superior de la tráquea; 2. órgano de la voz.

laser *n.* laser. 1. sigla del inglés "Light Amplification by Stimulated Emission of Radiation" (amplificación de la luz por estimulación de emisión de radiación); 2. bisturí microquirúrgico usado en la cauterización de tumores.

laser beams *n., pl.* rayos de laser, rayos de luz por efecto radioactivo de calor intenso que se usan para destruir tejidos o separar partes.

laser skin resurfacing *n.* renovación de la superficie de la piel a través de láser.

lassitude *n.* lasitud, languidez, agotamiento.

last *a.* último-a; final, pasado-a; ___ **night** / anoche; **the** ___ **treatment** / el ___ tratamiento; **the** ___ **word** / la ___ palabra.

late *a.* tardío-a, último-a; *adv.* tarde; ___ **auditory evoked response** / respuesta auditiva evocada ___; ___ **dumping syndrome** / síndrome de vaciamiento ___; **luteal phase dysphoria** ___ / fase luteal ___ de la disforia; **to be** ___ / atrasarse, retrasarse; **-ly** *adv.* últimamente, hace poco.

latency *n.* latencia, acto de permanecer latente; ___ **period** / período de ___.

latent *a.* latente, presente pero no activo-a; sin síntomas aparentes; sin manifestación.

later *a., comp.* of *late. adv.* más tarde, luego, después.

lateral *a.* lateral, rel. a un lado o costado.

lateral humeral epicondylitis *n.* epicondilitis humeral lateral, codo de tenista.

lateroflexion *n.* lateroflexión, flexión lateral o de inclinación hacia un costado.

latest *a., sup.* de late, último; **at the** ___ / a más tardar; **the** ___ **drug on the market** / el medicamento más reciente en el mercado.

latex *n.* látex, sustancia derivada de ciertas plantas de semillas que contienen un elemento de goma natural; en muchos casos puede causar alergia.

lather *n.* jabonadura, espuma de jabón.

latter *pron.* éste, ésta; el, la más reciente, el más moderno, la más moderna.

laugh *n.* risa; *v.* reír; **to** ___ **at** / reírse de, mofarse.

laughter *n.* risa, carcajada.

lavage *n.* lavado, irrigación de una cavidad.

lavatory *n.* [*basin*] lavatorio, lavabo, lavamanos; [*restroom*] inodoro, servicio, baño, excusado.

law *n.* ley, regla, norma.

lawsuit *n.* pleito legal, litigio.

lawyer *n.* abogado-a, *Mex.* licenciado-a.

lax *a.* laxo-a, suelto-a, relajado-a.

laxative *n.* laxante, laxativo, purgante suave.

laxity *n.* laxitud, aflojamiento, flojedad; relajación.

lay *n.* laico, secular; *vi.* poner, colocar; **to** ___ **aside** / desechar apartar; **to** ___ **off** / suspender, despedir.

layer *n.* capa, estrato.

laying *n.* colocación, acto de colocar.

laziness *n.* pereza, holgazanería, haraganería.

lazy *a.* perezoso-a, flojo-a, holgazán, holgazana, haragán, haragana.

lazy eye *n.* ambliopía, falta de coordinación en la percepción de la profundidad visual.

lead *n.* 1. plomo; ___ **apron** / delantal de ___, usado como protección a radiaciones; ___ **poisoning** / envenenamiento por ___; 2. conductor, tal como la guía que se usa en una electrocardiografía; *vi.* conducir *v.* llevar de la mano, guiar.

leading *a.* principal, primero-a, más importante.

leaf *n.* hoja.

leak *n.* [*of gas*] escape; [*water*] gotera, filtración; salirse, derramarse, escaparse.

lean *a.* [*meat*] magro-a, sin grasa; [*without flesh*] enjuto, flaco-a; seco-a; *v.* [*aptitude*] **to** ___ **toward** / tener propensión o disposición hacia algo o hacia alguien [*on, against*] apoyarse, recostarse, arrimarse a [*over*] inclinarse.

learn *v.* aprender; [*to have knowledge of*] saber; [*to learn about something new*] tener noticias de, enterarse de.

learning *n.* aprendizaje; **cognitive** ___ / ___ cognitivo; **incidental** ___ / ___ incidental; **latent** ___ / ___ latente; ___ **disability** / impedimento en el ___; **passive** ___ / ___ pasivo; **state dependent** ___ / ___ dependiente del estado.

leather *n.* cuero, piel curtida.

leave *n.* [*of absence*] licencia, permiso de ausencia del trabajo; *vi.* [*to go away from*] salir;

[*to give up*] dejar, renunciar; descontinuar, abandonar; **to ___ alone** / dejar en paz; **to ___ behind** / dejar atrás; **to ___ off** / dejar fuera.

Leber disease *n.* enfermedad de Leber, tipo de atrofia hereditaria que causa degeneración del nervio óptico y que afecta a los hombres.

lecithin *n.* lecitina, elemento esencial en el metabolismo de las grasas presente en los tejidos de los animales, esp. el tejido nervioso.

lecture *n.* conferencia, disertación.

ledge *n.* borde.

leech *n.* sanguijuela, gusano anélido acuático chupador de sangre; **artificial ___** / ventosa.

left *a.* izquierdo-a; **___ -hand** / mano izquierda; **___side** / lado **___**; **to the ___** / a la izquierda.

left-handed *a.* zurdo-a.

leg *n.* pierna, extremidad inferior que se extiende de la rodilla al tobillo; **___ injuries** / traumatismos de la **___**; *v.* **to pull one's ___** / tomar el pelo.

legal *a.* legal, legítimo-a, de acuerdo con la ley; **___ blindness** / ceguera **___**; **___ medicine, forensic medicine** / medicina **___**; **___ suit** / litigio, demanda, pleito.

legionnaire's disease *n.* enfermedad de los legionarios, enfermedad infecciosa grave, a veces letal, que se caracteriza por pulmonía, tos seca, dolor muscular y a veces síntomas gastrointestinales.

legislation, medical *n.* legislación médica.

legitimacy *n.* legitimidad.

legitimate *a.* legítimo-a, auténtico-a.

legume *n.* legumbre

leiomyofibroma *n.* leiomiofibroma, tumor benigno compuesto de tejido conectivo fibroso y muscular liso.

leiomyoma *n.* leiomioma, tumor benigno compuesto esencialmente de tejido muscular liso.

leiomyosarcoma *n.* leiomiosarcoma, tumor formado por leiomioma y sarcoma.

leisure *n.* holganza, ociosidad; **at ___** / a conveniencia, cómodamente; *a.* **___ hours** / tiempo libre, horas desocupadas.

lema *n.* legaña, lagaña, secreción de los ojos.

lemon *n.* [*fruit*] limón; [*tree*] limonero.

lemonade *n.* limonada.

lend *v.* prestar; **to ___ a hand** / prestar ayuda, ayudar, dar ayuda.

Lenegre syndrome *n.* Lenegre, síndrome de, fibrosis del sistema conductivo intracardíaco que se caracteriza gen. como fibrosis idiopática del nódulo atrioventricular.

length *n.* longitud, largo; extensión, distancia; **___ of time** / período de tiempo; **___ of stay** [*in a hospital*] / tiempo de internamiento.

lengthen *v.* alargar, extender, dilatar, prolongar.

lengthy *a.* largo-a; prolongado-a.

lenient *a.* indulgente, lenitivo-a; consentidor-a.

lens *n.* 1. lente; **achromatic ___** / **___** acromático; **adherent ___** / **___** adherido; **biconcave ___** / **___** bicóncavo; **biconvex ___** / **___** biconvexo; **bifocal ___** / **___** bifocal; **contact ___** / **___** de contacto, lentillas; **dislocation of ___** / dislocación del **___**; **___ implantation, intraocular** / **___** -s intraoculares; **trifocal ___** / **___** -s trifocales; 2. cristalino, lente transparente del ojo.

lent *a. pp.* of **to lend** prestado-a.

lenticula *n.* lente pequeño.

lenticular *a.* lenticular, rel. a un lente.

lentiform *a.* lentiforme, en forma de lente.

lentiginosis *n.* lentiginosis, presencia de un gran número de léntigos.

lentigo *n.* léntigo, mácula de la piel; **malignant ___** / **___** maligno; **múltiple ___** / **___** múltiple; **senile ___** / **___** senil.

lentil *n.* lenteja.

leper *a.* leproso-a, lazarino-a; que sufre de lepra.

leprechaunism *n.* leprecaunismo, condición hereditaria con características de enanismo acompañadas por retardo físico y mental, trastornos endocrinos y susceptibilidad a infecciones.

leprosy *n.* lepra, enfermedad infecciosa conocida también como enfermedad de Hansen causada por el bacilo *Mycobacterium leprae* caracterizada por lesiones cutáneas de pústulas y escamas.

leptomeninges *n.* leptomeninges, las membranas más finas del cerebro; la piamadre y la aracnoide.

leptomeningitis *n.* leptomeningitis, infl. de las leptomeninges.

lesbian *n.* lesbiana, mujer homosexual.

lesbianism *n.* lesbianismo, homosexualidad femenina.

lesion *n.* lesión, herida, contusión; **degenerative ___** / **___** degenerativa; **depressive ___** / **___** depresiva; **diffuse ___** / **___** difusa; **functional ___** / **___** funcional; **gross ___** / **___** grosera; **peripheral ___** / **___** periférica; **precancerous ___** / **___** precancerosa;

systemic ___ / ___ sistemática; **toxic** ___ / ___ tóxica; **traumatic** ___ / ___ traumática; **vascular** ___ / ___ vascular; **whiplash** ___ / ___ de latigazo. See chart on page 162.

less *a. comp.* menos, menor; ___ **and** ___ / cada vez menos; ___ **complicated** / ___ complicado; ___ **difficult** / ___ difícil; **more or** ___ / más o menos; *adv.* menos, en grado menor; *sufijo* menos, sin.

lessen *v.* aliviar, aminorar, disminuir, acortar; **a pill to** ___ **the pain** / una pastilla para ___ el dolor.

lesser *a. comp.* of *less* menor; más pequeño.

lesson *n.* lección, enseñanza, instrucción.

let *vi.* permitir, dejar, conceder; ___ **us go** / vámonos; ___ **us + inf.** / vamos a + *inf*; **to** ___ **be** / dejar tranquilo-a; **to** ___ **blood** / hacer sangrar; **to** ___ **down** / dejar bajar; dejar caer; desilusionar, abandonar; **to** ___ **go** / soltar; **to** ___ **in** / dejar entrar, admitir; **to** ___ **out** / dejar salir.

lethal *a.* letal, mortal; ___ **dose** / dosis ___; ___ **factor** / factor ___; ___ **gene** / gene ___; ___ **mutation** / mutación ___.

lethargic, lethargical *a.* letárgico-a, aletargado-a.

lethargy *n.* letargo, estupor.

letter *n.* letra; carta; ___ **opener** / abrecartas.

lettuce *n.* lechuga.

leucine *n.* leucina, aminoácido esencial en el crecimiento y metabolismo.

leucinuria *n.* leucinaria, presencia de leucina en la orina.

leucocoria *n.* leucocoria, pupila de aspecto blanco producto de una catarata.

leukapheresis *n.* leucaferesis, separación de leucocitos de la sangre de un paciente con subsecuente retransfusión al mismo paciente.

leukemia *n.* leucemia, cáncer de la sangre; **acute lymphocytic** ___ / ___ linfoncítica aguda; **aleukemic** ___ / ___ aleucémica; **chronic granulocytic** ___ / ___ granulocítica crónica; **chronic** ___ / ___ crónica; **chronic myeloid** ___ / ___ mieloide crónica; **eosinophilic** ___ / ___ eosinofílica; **lymphocytic** ___ / ___ linfocítica; **monocytic** ___ / ___ monocítica.

leukemic *a.* leucémico-a, rel. a la leucemia o que padece de ella.

leukemoid *n.* leucemoide, semejante a la leucemia.

leukoblast *n.* leucoblasto, leucocito inmaduro.

leukocitosis *n.* leucocitosis, aumento temporal de leucocitos en la sangre que ocurre gen.

durante el acto de digerir y durante el embarazo; **absolute** ___ / ___ absoluta; **mononuclear** ___ / ___ mononuclear; **polynuclear** ___ / ___ polinuclear; **relative** ___ / ___ relativa.

leukocyte *n.* leucocito, glóbulo blanco, célula importante en la defensa y reparación del organismo; **acidophil** ___ / ___ acidófilo, que cambia de color con ácidos colorantes; **basophil** ___ / ___ basófilo, que cambia de color con colorantes básicos; **lymphoid** ___ / ___ linfoide, sin gránulos; **neutrophil** ___ / ___ neutrófilo, de afinidad con colorantes neutros; **polymorphonuclear** ___ / ___ polimorfonucleado, con núcleos de más de un lóbulo.

leukoencephalitis *n.* leucoencefalitis, infl. de la sustancia blanca.

leukoencephalopathy *n.* leucoencefalopatía, cambios progresivos en la materia blanca del cerebro encontrados en niños que padecen de leucemia y que se asocian a lesiones producidas por radiación y quimioterapia.

leukopathia *n.* leucopatía, albinismo, falta de pigmentación.

leukopenia *n.* leucopenia, número anormalmente bajo de glóbulos blancos.

leukoplakia *n.* leucoplasia, áreas de color opaco en la membrana mucosa de la lengua gen. de carácter precanceroso.

leukorrhea *n.* leucorrea, flujo vaginal blancuzco.

leukosis *n.* leucosis, formación anormal de leucocitos.

leukotrichia *n.* leucotriquia, blancura del cabello.

levator *n.* 1. elevador, músculo que eleva o levanta una parte; 2. instrumento quirúrgico para levantar una depresión en una fractura del cráneo.

level *n.* nivel, plano; ___ **of consciousness** / ___ de conciencia; *v.* nivelar, ajustar; ___ **of health** / estado de salud.

leveling *n.* nivelación.

levocardia *n.* levocardia, transposición de las vísceras abdominales y conservación de la posición normal del corazón en el lado izquierdo del tórax.

levodopa *n.* levodopa, sustancia química usada en el tratamiento de la enfermedad de Parkinson.

levulose *n.* levulosa. V. **fructose**.

lewd *a.* lujurioso-a, deshonesto-a, libidinoso-a, obsceno-a.

lewdness *n.* lujuria, impudicia, sensualidad, lascivia.

lexical *a.* léxico-a, rel. al vocabulario.

liability *n.* riesgo, responsabilidad de pago.

liable *a.* responsable, sujeto-a a cargos.

liar *n. a.* embustero-a, mentiroso-a.

liberation *n.* liberación.

liberty *n.* libertad; **to be at** ___ **to** / tener ___ para.

libidinous *a.* libidinoso-a, rel. al libido.

libido *n.* libido. 1. impulso sexual, consciente o inconsciente; 2. en psicoanálisis, la fuerza o energía que determina la conducta del ser humano.

Libman-Sacks endocarditis, Libman Sacks syndrome *n.* Libman-Sacks, síndrome de, endocartitis verrugosa no bacteriana que se asocia con lupus eritematoso diseminado.

librarian *n.* bibliotecario-a.

library *n.* biblioteca.

lice *n., pl.* piojos.

license, licence *n.* licencia, permiso; **medical** ___ / ___ para ejercer la medicina.

licensure *n.* autorización, permiso legal para ejercer la medicina o ejecutar actos sólo permitidos a médicos o personal médico.

lichen *n.* liquen, lesiones o erupciones de la piel no contagiosas de forma papular; **atrophic sclerotic** ___ / ___ esclerotico atrófico; ___ **scrofulosorum** / ___ escrofularia; ___ **planus** / ___ plano; ___ **urticatus** / ___ de urticaria; **ulcerative** ___ / ___ ulcerativo.

licit *a.* lícito-a, permitido-a.

lick *v.* lamer; golpear, *pop.* dar una tunda.

lid *n.* 1. párpado del ojo; 2. tapa, tapadera.

lidocaine *n.* lidocaína, anestésico.

lie *n.* mentira, embuste; ___ **detector** / polígrafo, detector de ___ -s; *v.* mentir; *v.* tenderse; **to** ___ **down** / echarse, acostarse, descansar.

lienal artery *n.* arteria esplénica.

lientery *n.* lientería, diarrea que muestra partículas de alimento no digerido.

life *n.* vida, modo de vivir, existencia; ___ **expectancy** / expectativa de ___, promedio de ___; ___ **insurance** / seguro de ___; ___ **preservers,** ___ **support devices** / aparatos para prolongar la ___; ___ **-saving measure** / medida para prolongar o salvar la ___; ___ **span** / longevidad; ___ **-threatening** / que puede causar la muerte.

life insurance *n.* seguro, póliza de seguro; *Mex. A.* aseguranza.

lifeless *a.* muerto-a, sin vida.

lifetime *n.* toda la vida, curso de la vida; *a.* vitalicio-a.

lift *v.* levantar, alzar, elevar; ___ **your hand** / levante, levanta la mano; **to give one a** ___ / ayudar, animar, alentar.

lifting *n.* acto de levantar, levantamiento.

ligament *n.* ligamento. 1. banda de fibras de tejido conjuntivo que protege las articulaciones y evita que sufran torceduras o luxaciones; 2. banda protectora de fascias y músculos que conectan o sostienen vísceras; **acromioclavicular** ___ / ___ acromioclavicular; **alveolo-dental** ___ / ___ alveolodentario; **anococcygeal** ___ / ___ anococcígeo; **brachiocubital** ___ / ___ braquiocubital; **capsular** ___ / ___ capsular; **gastrocholic** ___ / ___ gastrocólico; **glossoepiglottic** ___ / ___ glosoepiglótico; **hepatoduodenal** ___ / ___ hepatoduodenal; **iliofemoral** ___ / ___ iliofemoral; ___ **tear** / desgarre del ___; **long plantar** ___ / ___ largo del plantar; **palmar** ___ / ___ palmar; **radiocubital** ___ / ___ radiocubital; **sternoclavicular** ___ / ___ esternoclavicular; **trapezoid** ___ / ___ trapezoide.

ligate *v.* ligar, aplicar una ligadura.

ligature, ligation *n.* ligadura; acción o proceso de ligar.

light *n.* luz; lumbre; ___ **absorption** / absorción de la ___; ___ **adaptation** / adaptación de la ___; ___ **perception** / percepción de la ___; ___ **reflex** / reflejo de la ___; ___ **therapy** / fototerapia; *a.* ligero-a, liviano-a claro-a, pálido-a; ___ **-headed** / [*dizzy*] mareado-a; **-ly** *adv.* ligeramente, levemente.

lighten *v.* iluminar, prender la luz; [*color*] aclarar.

lightening *n.* [*childbirth*] aligeramiento, descenso del útero en la cavidad pélvica, gen. en la etapa final del embarazo.

lighter *a. comp.* más ligero-a, más claro-a, más pálido-a.

likable *a.* agradable, amable, simpático-a.

like *a.* parecido-a, igual, semejante; [*to look alike*] **The boy looks** ___ **the father** / El niño se parece al padre; **to look** ___ / parecerse a; *v.* **I** ___ **this medicine** / Me gusta esta medicina; **to** ___ **someone, something** / gustar, agradar; *prep.* como; *adv.* como si, del mismo modo.

lima beans *n., pl.* habas de lima.

limb *n.* 1. extremidad, miembro del cuerpo; 2. porción terminal o distal de una estructura; ___

amputation / amputación de una ____; ____
   rigidity / rigidez de la ____ o del miembro.
limber *a.* flojo-a, flexible.
limbic *a.* marginal.
limbic system *n.* sistema límbico, grupo de
   estructuras cerebrales.
limbus *n.* limbo, filo o borde de una parte; ____
   corneae / ____ de la córnea.
lime *n.* 1. lima. ____ **juice** / jugo, zumo de ____; 2.
   cal, óxido de calcio.
liminal *a.* liminal, casi imperceptible.
limit *n.* límite, frontera; **assimilation** ____ / ____ de
   asimilación; ____ **of perception** / umbral
   perceptivo; **saturation** ____ / ____ de saturación.
limitation *n.* limitación, restricción; ____ **of**
   motion / ____ de movimiento.
limited *a.* limitado-a, restricto-a; ____ **activity** /
   actividad ____; ____ **autopsy** / autopsia parcial.
limp *n.* cojera, flojera; *v.* cojear, renquear,
   renguear.
linden tea *n.* té de flores de tilo.
line *n.* línea; rasgo; arruga; límite o guía.
linear *a.* lineal, semejante a una línea.
linen *n.* lienzo, lino; **bed** ____ / ropa de cama.
linger *v.* [*to suffer*] consumirse, padecer
   lentamente; [*to delay*] demorarse.
lingering *v.* prolongación, tardanza, morosidad;
   a. prolongado-a, retardado-a, moroso-a.
lingua *n., L.* (*pl.* **linguae**) lengua o estructura
   semejante a la lengua.
lingual *a.* lingual, rel. a la lengua.
lingula *n.* língula, proyección o estructura en
   forma de lengeta.
liniment *n.* linimento, untura de uso externo.
lining *n.* túnica, capa, forro, cubierta,
   revestimiento.
linitis *n.* linitis, V. **gastritis**.
link *n.* eslabón, vínculo.
linkage *n.* vínculo, unión, asociación de genes.
lint *n.* 1. fibra de algodón; 2. partículas
   desprendidas de la ropa.
lip *n.* labio, parte externa de la boca.
lipectomy *n.* ipectomía, excisión de tejido graso;
   submental ____ / ____ submental, del cuello.
lipedema *n.* lipedema, infl. crónica, gen. en las
   extremidades inferiores en las mujeres, debido a
   acumulación de exceso de grasa y líquido en los
   tejidos subcutáneos.
lipemia *n.* lipemia, presencia anormal de grasa en
   la sangre.
lipid, lipide *n.* lípido, sustancia orgánica que no
   se disuelve en el agua pero que es soluble en
   alcohol, éter o cloroformo.

lipoarthritis *n.* lipoartritis, infl. de tejidos
   adiposos de la rodilla.
lipodystrophy *n.* lipodistrofia, trastorno del
   metabolismo de las grasas;
   cephalothoracic ____ / ____ cefalotorácica;
   insulin ____ / ____ insulínica; **intestinal** ____ / ____
   intestinal.
lipofuscinosis *n.* lipofuscinosis,
   almacenamiento anormal de cualquiera de los
   pigmentos adiposos.
lipogenesis *n.* lipogénesis, producción de grasa.
lipoid *n.* lipoide, sustancia que se asemeja a la
   grasa.
lipoinfiltration *n.* lipoinfiltración,
   procedimiento quirúrgico que consiste en
   infiltración de grasa en áreas de hendidura o
   deficiencia.
lipolysis *n.* lipólisis, descomposición de las
   grasas.
lipoma *n.* lipoma, tumor de tejido adiposo.
lipomatosis *n.* lipomatosis. 1. condición
   causada por depósito excesivo de grasa; 2.
   lipomas múltiples.
lipomatous *a.* lipomatoso-a, obeso-a.
lipopenia *n.* lipopenia, disminución de grasas en
   la sangre y en el organismo.
lipoproteins *n., pl.* lipoproteínas, proteínas
   combinadas con compuestos lípidos que
   contienen una concentración alta de colesterol.
liposarcoma *n.* liposarcoma, tumor maligno que
   contiene elementos grasos.
liposis *n.* obesidad, acumulación excesiva de
   grasa en el cuerpo.
liposoluble *a.* liposoluble, que se disuelve en
   sustancias grasas.
liposuction *n.* liposucción, proceso de extraer
   grasa por medio de alta presión al vacío.
lipotrophy *n.* lipotrofía, aumento de la grasa del
   cuerpo.
lip reading *n.* lectura labial, interpretación del
   movimiento de los labios.
lipuria *n.* lipuria, presencia de lípidos en la orina.
liquefy *v.* licuar, disolver; descoagular.
liquid *n.* líquido, fluido; **heavy** ____ / ____
   espeso; ____ **balance** / balance de ____; ____
   retention / retención de ____.
liquor *n.* 1. licor, líquido acuoso que contiene
   sustancias medicinales; 2. término general
   aplicado a algunos líquidos del cuerpo.
lisping *n.* ceceo, sustitución de sonidos debido a
   un defecto en la articulación de las palabras, tal
   como el sonido de la *z* por la *c*, o el sonido de la
   c por la *s*.

list *n.* lista; **casualty** ___ / lista de accidentados.

listen *v.* escuchar, atender, prestar atención.

listless *a.* apático-a, lánguido-a, sin ánimo; indiferente.

liter *n.* litro.

lithiasis *n.* litiasis, formación de cálculos, esp. biliares o del tracto urinario.

lithium *n.* litio, elemento metálico usado como tranquilizante para tratar casos severos de psicosis.

lithotomy *n.* itotomía, incisión en un órgano o conducto para extraer cálculos.

lithotripsy *n.* litotripsia, trituración de cálculos en el riñón, el uréter, la vejiga y la vesícula biliar.

lithotriptor *n.* litotriturador, aparato o mecanismo para triturar cálculos; **extracorporal shock wave** ___ / ___ extracorporal con ondas de choque.

lithuresis *n.* lituresis, arenilla en la orina.

litter *n.* [*stretcher*] camilla; *v.* tirar basura.

little *a.* [*size*] pequeño-a; [*quantity*] poco, muy poco, un poquito; ___ **by** ___ / poco a poco.

live *v.* vivir, existir; ___ **birth** / nacimiento con vida.

livedo *n.* livedo, mancha en la piel, frecuentemente azulada o morada, similar a un morado.

livelihood *n.* vida; existencia; subsistencia.

lively *a.* vivo-a; vivaracho-a, animado-a.

liver *n.* hígado, glándula mayor del cuerpo que segrega bilis y sirve de estabilizador y productor de azúcar, enzimas, proteínas y colesterol además de eliminar las sustancias tóxicas del organismo; **enlarged** ___ / ___ agrandado; **infantile biliary** ___ **cirrhosis** / cirrosis biliar infantil; ___ **circulation** / circulación hepática; ___ **cirrhosis** / cirrosis hepática; ___ **damage** / lesión hepática; ___ **failure** / insuficiencia hepática; ___ **function tests** / pruebas funcionales hepáticas; ___ **spots** / manchas hepáticas.

livid *a.* lívido-a; *pop.* amoratado-a.

lividity *n.* lividez, descoloración que resulta de la gravitación de sangre; **post mortem** ___ / ___ cadavérica.

living *n.* vida; con vida; modo de vivir; **cost of** ___ / costo de ___ ; ___ **expenses** / gastos de mantenimiento; ___ **under stress** / ___ agitada, ___ con estrés.

living will *n.* testamento hecho por una persona en completo estado de salud en el que dispone que en caso de peligro de muerte no se use ningún medio artificial para prolongarle la vida.

load *n.* carga, peso; ___ **dose** / dosis de ___; *v.* cargar, recargar.

loading *n.* carga por administración de una sustancia en una prueba metabólica; ___ **test** / prueba de carga.

loan *n.* préstamo; *v.* prestar.

lobar *a.* lobar, lobular, rel. a un lóbulo; ___ **pneumonia** / pulmonía ___.

lobby *n.* salón de entrada, sala de espera, vestíbulo.

lobe *n.* lóbulo, porción redondeada y más o menos delimitada de un órgano; **middle** ___ **syndrome** / síndrome del ___ medio del pulmón.

lobectomy *n.* obectomía, excisión de un lóbulo; **complete** ___ / ___ completa; **left lower** ___ / ___ izquierda anterior; **partial** ___ / ___ parcial.

lobotomy *n.* obotomía, incisión de un lóbulo cerebral con el fin de aliviar ciertos trastornos mentales.

lobster *n.* langosta.

lobular *a.* lobular, rel. a un lóbulo.

lobule *n.* lobulillo, lóbulo pequeño.

local *a.* local, rel. a una parte aislada; ___ **anesthesia** / anestesia ___; ___ **application** / aplicación ___; ___ **recurrence** / reaparición ___.

localization *n.* localización. 1. rel. al punto de origen de una sensación; 2. determinación de la procedencia de una infección o lesión.

localize, locate *v.* localizar.

lochia *n.* loquios, flujo serosanguíneo del útero en las primeras semanas después del parto.

lock *n.* cerradura; *v.* cerrar, trancar; encerrar, cerrar con llave; encerrarse, trancarse; cerrarse.

lockjaw *n.* tétano; pasmo. V. **tetanus**.

locomotion *n.* locomoción.

loculated, locular *a.* locular, rel. a un lóculo.

loculus *n.* (*pl.* **loculi**) lóculo, cavidad pequeña.

locus *n.* 1. lugar, sitio; 2. localización de un gene en el cromosoma.

logagraphia *n.* logagrafía, incapacidad de reconocer palabras escritas o habladas.

logamnesia *n.* logamnesia, afasia sensorial.

logaphasia *n.* logafasia, afasia motora, gen. causada por una lesión cerebral.

logic *a.* lógico-a, acertado-a.

logical *a.* lógico-a, preciso-a, exacto-a.

logopedics *n.* logopedia, estudio y tratamiento de la voz.

logoplegia *n.* logoplejía, parálisis de los órganos del lenguaje.

loin *n.* flanco, ijar, ijada, parte inferior de la espalda y de los costados entre las costillas y la pelvis.

long *a.* largo-a, extenso-a, prolongado-a; **How __ ago?** / ¿Cuánto tiempo hace?; **__ after** / mucho después; **__ ago** / hace tiempo; **__ -distance** / larga distancia; **__ -standing** / de larga duración; **not __ before** / poco tiempo antes.

longevity *n.* longevidad, ancianidad, duración larga de la vida.

longing *n.* deseo, anhelo, ansia.

longitudinal *a.* longitudinal, a lo largo del eje del cuerpo.

longus *a.* largo-a, extenso-a.

look *n.* [*appearance*] aspecto, apariencia, cara; mirada, ojeada. *v.* mirar; revisar; **to __ bad** / tener mal aspecto; **to __ for** / buscar; **to __ through** / examinar con cuidado; **to take a __ at** / mirar, echar una mirada.

loop *n.* asa; estructura en forma de lazo semejante a la curvatura de una cuerda.

loose *a.* suelto-a, desatado-a, libre; **__ bowels** / deposiciones blandas o aguadas; *v.* desatar, desprender, aflojar.

loose associations *n.* disociación de ideas.

lordosis *n.* lordosis, curva exagerada; aumento exagerado hacia adelante de la concavidad de la columna lumbar.

lose *vi.* perder.

loss *n.* pérdida; **at a __** / confundido-a; **__ of balance** / __ del equilibrio; **__ of blood** / __ de sangre; **__ of consciousness** / __ del conocimiento; **__ of contact with reality** / __ del contacto con la realidad; **__ of grip** / __ de la retención; **__ of hearing** / __ de la audición; **__ of memory** / __ de la memoria; **__ of motion** / __ del movimiento; **__ of muscle tone** / __ de la tonicidad muscular; **__ of vision** / __ de la visión.

lost *a. pp.* of **to lose,** perdido-a, desorientado-a, extraviado-a.

lotion *n.* loción, ablución.

Lou Gehrig disease *n.* Lou Gehrig, enfermedad de, atrofia muscular progresiva.

loud *a.* ruidoso-a, escandaloso-a.

loupe *n.* lupa binocular, lente convexa de aumento usada esp. por cirujanos y oculistas.

louse *n.(pl.* **lice)** piojo, insecto parásito que se aloja en el pelo, trasmisor de enfermedades infecciosas tales como la fiebre tifoidea.

love *n.* amor, cariño, afecto; *v.* amar, querer; **to fall in __** / enamorarse; **to fall in __ with** / enamorarse de.

low *a.* bajo-a; [*in spirits*] abatido-a; **__ opinion** / mala opinión.

lower *a. comp.* of low, inferior; bajo-a; *v.* bajar, poner más bajo; [*in quantity, price*] reducir, disminuir; **__ esophageal sphincter** / esfínter esofágico __; **__ extremity** / extremidad __; **to __ the arm** / __ el brazo.

loyal *a.* leal, fiel, constante.

lozenge *n.* pastilla que se disuelve en la boca.

lubricant *n.* lubricante, agente oleaginoso que al lubricar disminuye la fricción entre dos superficies; **oil-based __** / __ oleaginoso; **waterbased __** / __ acuífero.

lubricate *v.* lubricar, untar, saturar una superficie con un líquido, especialmente aceite.

lubrication *n.* lubrificación, lubricación.

lucid *a.* lúcido-a, claro-a, inteligible; cuerdo-a.

lucidity *n.* claridad, esp. mental.

lucidness *n.* lucidez, claridad mental.

luck *n.* suerte, dicha; casualidad; **good __** / buena __; **out of __** / de mala suerte; **worse __** / pear o la peor __.

lucky *a.* afortunado-a, dichoso-a; *v.* **to be __** / tener suerte.

lues *n.* lúes, sífilis.

luetic *a.* luético-a, sifilítico-a, rel. a o que padece de sífilis.

lukewarm *a.* tibio-a, templado-a; [*feelings*] indiferente.

lumbago *n.* lumbago, dolor en la parte inferior de la espalda.

lumbar *a.* lumbar, región de la espalda entre el tórax y la pelvis; **__ puncture** / punción __; **__ vertebrae** / vértebras __ -es.

lumbrisosis *n.* lumbricosis, infestación por lombrices.

lumen *n.* lumen. 1. unidad de flujo luminoso; 2. espacio en una cavidad, canal, conducto u órgano.

luminal *a.* luminal, rel. a la luz de un conducto.

luminescence *n.* luminosidad, emisión de luz sin producción de calor.

luminous *a.* luminoso-a, rel. a la luminosidad

lump *n.* bulto, protuberancia, chichón; [*in the throat*] nudo en la garganta; [*of sugar*] terrón de azúcar.

lumpectomy *n.* tumorectomía, extirpación de un tumor gen. de la mama.

lunacy *n.* locura, demencia.

lunar *a.* lunar, rel. a la luna.

lunatic *a.* lunático-a, demente, loco-a.

lunch *n.* almuerzo, comida del mediodía.

lung *n.* pulmón, órgano par de la respiración contenido dentro de la cavidad pleural del tórax que se conecta con la faringe a través de la tráquea y la laringe;**air containing** ___ / ___ aireado; ___ **abscess** / absceso pulmonar; ___ **cancer** / cáncer del ___; ___ **capacities** / volumen pulmonar; ___ **collapse** / colapso del ___; ___ **diseases** / neumopatías; ___ **elasticity** / elasticidad pulmonar; ___ **hemorrhage** / hemorragia pulmonar; **quiet** ___ / ___ silencioso.

lungworm *n.* gusano nematodo que infesta los pulmones.

lupus *n.* lupus, enfermedad crónica de la piel de origen desconocido que causa lesiones degenerativas locales; **anticoagulant** ___ / ___ anticoagulante; ___ **vulgaris** / ___ vulgar; **marginal** ___ / ___ marginado.

lupus erythematosus, discoid *n.* lupus eritematoso discoide, condición caracterizada por placas escamosas de bordes enrojecidos que causa irritación de la piel.

lupus erythematosus, systemic *n.* lupus eritematoso sistémico, condición caracterizada por episodios febriles que afecta las vísceras y el sistema nervioso.

lust *n.* lujuria, codicia, deseo incontenible.

luteal *a.* lúteo, rel. al cuerpo lúteo.

lutein *n.* luteína, pigmento amarillo que se deriva del cuerpo lúteo, de la yema del huevo y de las células adiposas.

luteinizing hormone *n.* hormona luteinizante producida por la pituitaria anterior que estimula la secreción de hormonas sexuales por los testículos (testosterona) y el ovario (progesterona) e interviene en la formación de esperma y óvulos.

luteoma *n.* luteoma, tumor del cuerpo lúteo.

luxation *n.* luxación, dislocación.

lycopene *n.* licopina, pigmento vegetal muy abundante en tomates y zanahorias.

lycopenemia *n.* licopenemia, aumento de licopinas en la sangre, que resulta en un color amarillo-anaranjado de la piel.

lye *n.* lejía; ___ **poisoning** / envenenamiento por ___.

lying *a.* acostado-a; recostado-a; extendido-a.

Lyme disease *n.* Lyme, enfermedad de, trastorno inflamatorio que afecta a múltiples sistemas del cuerpo, y que es causado por una garrapata. Ocurre mayormente en el este de los Estados Unidos durante la primavera y el verano. La erradicación inmediata de las garrapatas del cuerpo evita el contagio.

lymph *n.* linfa, líquido claro que se encuentra en los vasos linfáticos; ___ **nodes** / ganglios linfáticos.

lymphadenectomy *n.* infadenectomía, extirpación de vasos linfáticos y ganglios.

lymphadenitis *n.* linfadenitis, infl. de los ganglios linfáticos.

lymphadenopathy *n.* linfadenopatía, enfermedad que afecta los nódulos linfáticos; **axillary** ___ / ___ axilar; **cervical** ___ / ___ cervical; **generalized** ___ / ___ generalizada; **mediastinal** ___ / ___ mediastínica; **supraclavicular** ___ / ___ supraclavicular.

lymphangiectasis *n.* linfagiectasis, dilatación de los vasos linfáticos.

lymphangiogram *n.* linfangiograma, representación filmada de ganglios y vasos linfáticos usando un medio de contraste inyectado.

lymphangitis *n.* linfangitis, infl. de vasos linfáticos.

lymphatic *a.* linfático-a, rel. a la linfa; ___ **spaces** / espacios ___-s; ___ **system** / sistema ___.

lymphedema *n.* linfedema, edema causado por una obstrucción en los vasos linfáticos.

lymphemia *n.* linfemia, presencia en la sangre circulante de un número elevado de linfocitos extremadamente grandes, de sus precursores, o de ambos.

lymphoblast *n.* linfoblasto, forma primitiva del linfocito.

lymphoblastoma *n.* linfoblastoma, linfoma maligno formado por linfoblastos.

lymphocyte *n.* linfocito, célula linfática; ___ **B cell** / ___ B, importante en la producción de anticuerpos.

lymphocyte T *n.* linfocitos de células T, linfocitos diferenciados en el timo que dirigen la respuesta inmunológica y alertan a las células B a responder a los antígenos; **cytotoxic** ___ / ___ citotóxicos, ayudan a exterminar células extrañas como en el rechazo de órganos transplantados; ___ **T helper** / ayudante de ___, inductores, aumentan la producción de anticuerpos de las células B; **supressor** ___ / represores de ___, detienen la producción de anticuerpos de las células B.

lymphocytosis *n.* linfocitosis, cantidad excesiva de linfocitos en la sangre periférica.

lymphogranulomatosis, Hodgkin's disease *n.* linfogranulomatosis, enfermedad de Hodgkin, granuloma infeccioso del sistema linfático.

lymphogranuloma venereum *n.* linfogranuloma venéreo, enfermedad viral trasmitida sexualmente que puede producir elefantiasis de los genitales y estrechez rectal.

lymphohistyocytosis *n.* linfohistiocitosis, proliferación o infiltración de histiocitos y linfocitos.

lymphoid *a.* linfoide, que se asemeja al tejido linfático.

lymphoma *n.* linfoma, neoplasma del tejido linfático.

lymphomatoid *n.* linfomatoide, rel. a un linfoma o semejante a éste.

lymphopenia, lymphocytopenia *n.* linfopenia, linfocitopenia, disminución en el número de linfocitos en la sangre.

lymphoreticular *a.* linforreticular, rel. a células reticuloendoteliales de los nódulos linfáticos.

lymphosarcoma *n.* linfosarcoma, neoplasma maligno del tejido linfoide.

lysergic acid diethylamide *n.* dietilamida del ácido lisérgico.

lysin *n.* lisina, anticuerpo que disuelve o destruye células y bacterias.

lysinogen *n.* lisinógeno, agente que tiene la propiedad de producir lisinas.

lysis *n.* lisis.1. proceso de destrucción o disolución de glóbulos rojos, bacterias o cualquier antígeno por medio de lisina;2. desaparición gradual de los síntomas de una enfermedad.

m

m *abbr.* **male** / hombre; **malignant** / maligno; **married** / casado-a; **mature** / maduro; **melts at** / se derrite a; **minute** / minuto; **molecular weight** / peso molecular; **morphine** / morfina.

macerate *v.* macerar; suavizar una materia por medio de inmersión en un líquido.

maceration *n.* maceración, descomposición y ablandamiento de tejidos y órganos en el agua u otros líquidos.

machine *n.* aparato, máquina.

macroblepharia *n.* macroblefaria, tamaño excesivamente grande del párpado.

macrocephalia *n.* macrocefalia, cabeza anormalmente grande.

macrocephalic *a.* macrocefálico-a, megalocefálico-a, de cabeza anormalmente grande.

macrocosm *n.* macrocosmo. 1. el universo como representación del ser humano; 2. el universo considerado como un todo.

macrocythemia *n.* macrocitemia, macrocitosis, glóbulos rojos anormalmente grandes.

macroglossia *n.* macroglosia, agrandamiento excesivo de la lengua.

macrognathia *n.* macrognatia, mandíbula demasiado grande.

macromolecule *n.* macromolécula, molécula de tamaño grande tal como la de una proteína.

macrophage, macrophagus *n.* macrófago, célula mononuclear fagocítica; ___ **migration** / migración de ___ -s.

macroscopic *a.* macroscópico-a, que se ve a simple vista, antónimo de microscópico.

macrospore *n.* macroespora, espora grande.

macula, macule *n.* mácula, pequeña mancha descolorida de la piel.

macula lutea, yellow spot *n.* mácula lútea, pequeña zona amarillenta situada en el centro de la retina.

macular *a.* macular, rel. a una mácula.

maculopapular *a.* maculopapular, rel. a máculas y pápulas.

mad *a.* [*insane*] loco-a, demente, perturbado-a; [*moody*] enojado-a, furioso-a; *v.* **to become** ___ / enloquecer; enloquecerse, enfurecerse; volverse loco-a; enojarse.

made *v. pret. pp.* of **to make**, hecho-a, producido-a.

madhouse *n.* manicomio, asilo de locos.

maggot *n.* larva de un insecto.

magistral *a.* magistral, rel. a medicamentos que se preparan de acuerdo a indicaciones médicas.

magma *n.* magma. 1. suspensión de partículas en una cantidad pequeña de agua; 2. sustancia viscosa compuesta de material orgánico.

magnesia *n.* magnesia, óxido de magnesio; **milk of** ___ / leche de ___.

magnesium *n.* magnesio; ___ **sulfate** / sulfato de ___.

magnet *n.* imán.

magnetic *a.* magnético-a; ___ **field** / campo ___.

magnetic resonance imaging *n.* imágenes por resonancia magnética, procedimiento por imágenes basado en el análisis cualitativo de la estructura química y biológica de un tejido.

magnetism *n.* magnetismo, propiedad de atracción y repulsión magnéticas.

magnetize *v.* magnetizar, imantar.

magnetoelectricity *n.* magnetoelectricidad, electricidad inducida por medios magnéticos.

magnification *n.* magnificación, ampliación de un objeto.

magnifier *n.* amplificador; vidrio de aumento.

magnify *v.* amplificar, agrandar, ampliar, aumentar.

magnifying glass *n.* lente de aumento; lupa.

magnitude *n.* magnitud.

mail *n.* correo, correspondencia; *v.* **to** ___ **a letter** / echar una carta al ___

maim *v.* mutilar; estropear; lisiar.

main *a.* principal; esencial; **-ly** *adv.* principalmente, esencialmente.

maintenance *n.* mantenimiento; [*feeding*] alimentación; sostén, apoyo; [*of a building*] conservación, mantenimiento.

make *vi.* hacer; [*money*] ganar; [*earn*] **How much do you** ___? / ¿Cuánto gana usted?, ¿cuánto ganas tú?; **to** ___ **a prescription** / llenar, preparar una receta; **to** ___ **believe** / fingir; **to** ___ **fun of** / burlarse de; **to** ___ **known** / declarar; **to** ___ **mistakes** / hacer errores; equivocarse; **to** ___ **no difference** / no tener importancia; **to** ___ **sense** / tener sentido; **to** ___ **sure** / asegurarse; **to** ___ **up** [*time*] / recobrar el tiempo perdido; **to** ___ **up one's mind** / decidirse.

mal *n.* enfermedad, trastorno, desorden.

malabsorption syndrome *n.* síndrome de malabsorción, condición gastrointestinal con trastornos múltiples causada por absorción inadecuada de alimentos.

malacia *n.* malacia, reblandecimiento o pérdida de consistencia en órganos o tejidos.

malacoplakia *n.* malcoplaquia, formación de áreas blandas en la membrana mucosa de un órgano hueco.

maladjusted *a.* inadaptado-a, incapaz de adaptarse al medio social y de soportar tensiones.

malady *n.* enfermedad, trastorno, desorden.

malaise *n.* malestar, indisposición, molestia.

malar *a.* malar, rel. a la mejilla o a los pómulos.

malar bone *n.* pómulo, hueso en ambos lados de la cara.

malaria *n.* malaria, infección febril aguda a veces crónica causada por protozoos del género *Plasmodium* y trasmitida por el mosquito *Anófeles*.

malariacidal *a.* malaricida, que destruye parásitos de malaria.

malassimilation *n.* malasimilación, asimilación deficiente.

maldigestion *n.* indigestión.

male *n.* varón; hombre; macho; ___ **nurse** / enfermero.

malformation *n.* deformación, anomalía o enfermedad esp. congénita.

malfunction *n.* disfunción, funcionamiento defectuoso; *v.* funcionar mal.

malice *n.* malicia, malos deseos.

malicious *a.* malicioso-a.

malignancy *n.* 1. cualidad de malignidad; 2. tumor canceroso.

malignant *a.* maligno-a, pernicioso-a, de efecto destructivo.

malignant hyperthermia *n.* hipertermia maligna, brote de fiebre extremadamente alta llegando a alcanzar 106°F ó 41+ C. *Syn.* **fulminating hyperpirexia.**

malignant melanoma *n.* melanoma maligno, neoplasma maligno pigmentoso que puede originarse en cualquier parte de la piel aunque muy raramente en la mucosa. El melanoma maligno tiene la capacidad de hacer metástasis a otras partes de la piel y la linfa, los pulmones, el hígado y el cerebro. El melanoma benigno tiene la apariencia de un lunar o verruga pigmentada.

malinger *v.* fingirse enfermo-a; fingir una enfermedad.

malingerer *n.* simulador-a, persona que finge o exagera los síntomas de una enfermedad.

malleable *a.* maleable.

malleolus *n.* (*pl.* **malleoli**) maléolo, protuberancia en forma de martillo tal como la que se ve a ambos lados de los tobillos.

mallet finger *n.* dedo de la mano en martillo.

mallet toe *n.* dedo del pie en martillo.

malleus *n.* (*pl.* **mallei**) malleus, uno de los huesecillos del oído medio.

malnourished *a.* desnutrido-a, malnutrido-a.

malnutrition *n.* malnutrición; mala alimentación; deficiencia nutricional.

malocclusion *n.* maloclusión, mordida defectuosa.

malposition *n.* posición inadecuada.

malpractice *n.* negligencia profesional.

malpresentation *n.* presentación anormal del feto durante el parto.

malrotation *n.* malarotación, rotación anormal o defectuosa de un órgano o parte.

malt *n.* malta; **malted milk** / leche malteada.

maltose *n.* maltosa, tipo de azúcar.

malunion *n.* malaunión, fijación imperfecta de una fractura.

mamma *n.* mama, glándula secretora de leche en la mujer localizada en la parte anterior del tórax.

mammal *n.* animal mamífero.

mammalgia *n.* mamalgia, dolor en la mama.

mammaplasty, mammoplasty *n.* mamaplastia, mamoplastia, cirugía plástica de los senos; **augmentation** ___ / ___ de aumento; **reconstructive** ___ / ___ de reconstrucción; **reduction** ___ / ___ de reducción.

mammary *a.* mamario-a, rel. a los pechos o senos; ___ **glands** / glándulas ___ -s.

mammectomy, mastectomy *n.* mamectomía, mastectomía, excisión de la mama o de una porción de la glándula mamaria.

mammillary *a.* mamilar, que se asemeja a un pezón.

mammillated *a.* mamilado-a, que presenta protuberancias similares a un pezón.

mammilliplasty *n.* mamiliplastia, operación plástica del pezón.

mammillitis *n.* mamilitis, infl. del pezón.

mammitis, mastitis *n.* mastitis, infl. de la mama.

mammogram *n.* mamograma, rayos-x de la mama.

mammography *n.* mamografía, rayos-x de la glándula mamaria.

mammoplasty *n.* mamoplastia, operación plástica de la mama.

man *n.* (*pl.* **men**) hombre.

manageable *a.* manejable; dócil.

manager *n.* administrador-a, gerente-a.

mandatory *a.* necesario-a, requerido-a.

mandible *n.* mandíbula, hueso de la quijada en forma de herradura.

mandibular *a.* mandibular, rel. a la mandíbula.

maneuver *n.* maniobra, movimiento preciso hecho con la mano.

mange *n.* sarna, roña.

mangy *a.* sarnoso-a, roñoso-a.

manhandle *v.* maltratar.

manhood *n.* virilidad; edad viril.

mania *n.* manía, trastorno emocional caracterizado por excitación excesiva, ansiedad y altas y bajas de espíritu.

maniac *a.* maníaco-a, persona afectada de manía.

manic-depressive psychosis *n.* psicosis maníaco-depresiva cíclica, condición caracterizada por estados de depresión y manía.

manifest *v.* manifestar; expresar; revelar; manifestarse, revelarse.

manifestation *n.* manifestación; revelación.

manikin *n.* maniquí, figura representativa del cuerpo humano.

manipulate *v.* manipular, manejar.

manipulation *n.* manipulación, tratamiento por medio del uso diestro de las manos.

manliness *n.* masculinidad, virilidad.

manly *a.* varonil.

manner *n.* manera, modo; hábito, costumbre; [*behavior*] **bad** ___ **-s** / malos modales.

mannerism *n.* manerismo, expresión peculiar en la manera de hablar, de vestir o de actuar.

manometer *n.* manómetro, instrumento para medir la presión de líquidos o gases.

manslaughter *n.* homicidio sin premeditación.

mantle *n.* manto, capa.

manual *a.* manual, manuable.

manubrium *n.* (*pl.* **manubria**) manubrium, estructura en forma de mano.

many *a., pron.* muchos-as; tantos, tantas; **a great** ___ / muchos, muchas; **as** ___ **as** / tantos-as como, igual número de.

marasmus *n.* marasmo, emaciación debida a malnutrición, esp. en la infancia.

march *n.* marcha, progreso; *v.* marchar, poner en marcha.

margarine *n.* margarina.

margin *n.* margen, borde.

marginal *a.* marginal; **a** ___ **case** / un caso ___.

margination *n.* marginación, acumulación y adherencia de leucocitos a las paredes de los vasos capilares en un proceso inflamatorio.

marijuana, marihuana *n.* mariguana. *Cannabis sativa*.

marital *a.* matrimonial, marital; ___ **relations** / relaciones ___ **-es**.

marjoram *n.* mejorana.

mark *n.* marca, seña, señal, signo; *v.* marcar; señalar.

marker *n.* marcador, indicador.

marmalade *n.* mermelada, conserva de frutas.

marriage *n.* matrimonio; [*ceremony*] boda, casamiento.

married *a.* casado-a; ___ **couple** / matrimonio; ___ **life** / vida conyugal, vida matrimonial.

marrow *n.* médula, tejido esponjoso que ocupa las cavidades medulares de los huesos; *pop.* tuétano; ___ **aspiration** / aspiración de la ___; ___ **cellularity** / celularidad medular; ___ **failure** / insuficiencia medular; ___ **infiltration** / infiltración medular; ___ **injury** / lesión medular; ___ **puncture** / punción de la ___ ósea; ___ **transplant** / transplante de la ___.

marsupialization *n.* marsupialización, conversión de una cavidad cerrada a una forma de bolsa abierta.

masculation *n.* masculación, desarrollo de características masculinas.

masculine *a.* masculino-a, viril.

masculinization *n.* masculinización. virilización.

mash *v.* mezclar ingredientes; amasar.

mashed *a. pp.* of **to mash**, [*vegetables*] ___ **potatoes** / puré de patatas.

mask *n.* máscara. 1. cubierta de la cara; 2. aspecto de la cara, esp. como manifestación patológica; **death** ___ / mascarilla; **pregnancy** ___ / manchas en la cara durante el embarazo; **surgical** ___ / cubreboca.

masked *a.* enmascarado-a; oculto-a.

masochism *n.* masoquismo, condición anormal de placer sexual por abuso infligido a otros o a sí mismo-a.

mass *n.* masa, cuerpo formado de partículas coherentes.

massage *n.* masaje, proceso de manipulación del cuerpo por medio de fricciones; **cardiac** ___ / ___ cardíaco de resucitación; *v.* dar masaje, sobar.

masseter *n.* músculo masetero, músculo principal de la masticación.

masseur, masseuse *n. Fr.* masajista, persona que da masajes.

massive *a.* maciso-a, abultado-a.

mastadenitis *n.* mastadenitis, infl. de una glándula mamaria. *Syn.* **mastitis**.

mastadenoma *n.* mastadenoma, tumor de la mama, tumor del seno.

mastalgia *n.* mastalgia, V. **mammalgia**.

mast cell tumor *n.* mastocitoma, tumor compuesto de mastocitos.

mastectomy *n.* mastectomía. V. **mammectomy**.

masticate *v.* masticar, mascar.

mastication, chewing *n.* masticación.

masticatory *a.* masticatorio-a, rel. a la masticación.

mastitis *n.* mastitis**chronic cystic** ___ / ___ cística crónica; **glandular** ___ / ___ glandular; **granulomatous** ___ / ___ granulomatosa; **lacteal** ___ / ___ lacteal; **neonatorum** ___ / ___ del neonato; **puerperal** ___ / ___ puerperal; **suppurative** ___ / ___ supurativa.

mastitis, cystic *n.* mastitis cística, enfermedad fibroquística de la mama.

mastocytoma *n.* mastocitoma, acumulación de mastocitos con apariencia de un neoplasma.

mastocytosis *n.* mastocitosis, mastocitos neoplásicos que aparecen en varios tejidos como urticaria pigmentosa.

mastoid *n.* mastoides, apófisis del hueso temporal; *a.* 1. mastoideo-a, rel. a la mastoides o que ocurre en la región del proceso mastoideo; 2. semejante a una mama.

mastoid antrum *n.* antro mastoideo, cavidad que sirve de comunicación entre el hueso temporal, el oído medio y las células mastoideas.

mastoid cells *n., pl.* células mastoideas, bolsas de aire en la prominencia mastoidea del hueso temporal.

mastoiditis *n.* mastoiditis, infl. de las células mastoideas.

mastopathy *n.* mastopatía, afección de las glándulas mamarias.

mastopexy *n.* mastopexia, corrección plástica del seno pendular.

masturbate *v.* masturbarse.

masturbation *n.* masturbación, autoestimulación y manipulación de los genitales para obtener placer sexual.

match *n.* semejante; [*by pairs*] pareja; [*game*] juego, partido; copia; *v.* igualar, asemejar, [*colors*] armonizar, hacer juego.

matching *n., a.* semejante, igual; ___ **pair** / compañero-a, pareja.

material *n.* materia; asunto; *a.* material; esencial.

maternal *a.* maternal, materno-a, rel. a la madre; ___ **fetal exchange** / intercambio maternofetal; ___ **welfare** / bienestar materno.

maternity *n.* maternidad; ___ **hospital** / hospital de ___.

mating *n.* emparejamiento de sexos opuestos esp. para la reproducción.

matricide *n.* matricidio.

matrilineal *a.* de línea materna, descendiente de la madre.

matrix *n.* matriz; molde.

matter *n.* materia, sustancia; asunto; **as a** ___ **of fact** / en realidad; **gray** ___ / ___ gris; **Let's take care of this** ___ / Vamos a hacernos cargo de este asunto; **What is the** ___ **?** / ¿Qué pasa?, ¿qué ocurre?

mattress *n.* colchón.

maturate *v.* madurar; sazonar; supurar.

mature *a.* [*fruit*] maduro-a; sazonado-a.

maturity *n.* madurez; etapa de desarrollo completo.

maxilla *n.* maxila, hueso del maxilar superior.

maximum *a., sup.* máximo.

may *v. aux.* poder, [*possibility*]; **it** ___ **be** / puede ser; [*permission*] ___ **I see you?** / ¿Puedo verlo-a?, ¿puedo verte?; ___ **I come in?** / ¿Puedo entrar?

maybe *adv.* quizás, tal vez.

maze *n.* laberinto.

me *pron.* me, mí; **Come with** ___ / Venga, ven conmigo; **The doctor is going to see** ___ / El doctor me va a ver; **The medicine is for** ___ / La medicina es para mí.

meager *a.* escaso-a, insuficiente, pobre.

meal *n.* comida; **at** ___ **time** / a la hora de la ___.

mean *n.* media, índice, término medio; ___ **corpuscular hemoglobin** / índice corpuscular de hemoglobina; *a.* malo-a, desconsiderado-a, de mal humor.

meaning *n.* significado.

measles *n.* sarampión; *pop. Mex.* tapetillo de los niños, enfermedad sumamente contagiosa esp. en niños de edad escolar causada por el virus de la rubéola.

measles immune serum globulin *n.* suero de globulina preventivo contra el sarampión, se inyecta en uno de los cinco días siguientes a la exposición al contagio.

measles virus vaccine, live *n.* vacuna antisarampión de virus vivo, de uso en la inmunización contra el sarampión.

measure *n.* medida, dimensión, capacidad de algo; *v.* medir.

meat *n.* carne; **roast** ___ / ___ asada.

meatal *a.* meatal, concerniente al meato.

447

meatus *n.* meato, pasaje, abertura, apertura.

mechanic *n.* mecánico-a.

mechanical *a.* mecánico-a.

mechanism *n.* mecanismo. 1. respuesta involuntaria a un estímulo; **defense** ___ / ___ de defensa; **implementation** ___ / ___ de ejecución; **pain** ___ / ___ del dolor; 2. estructura semejante a una máquina.

meconium *n.* meconio,primera fecalización del recién nacido.

medial *a.* medial, localizado-a hacia la línea media.

median *n.* mediana; ___ **plane** / plano medio.

mediastinal *a.* mediastínico-a, rel. al mediastino.

mediastinitis *n.* mediastinitis, infl. del tejido del mediastino.

mediastinoscopy *n.* mediastinoscopía, examen del mediastino por medio de un endoscopio.

mediastinum *n.* mediastino. 1. cavidad entre dos órganos; 2. masa de tejidos y órganos que separa los pulmones.

mediate *v.* mediar, interceder.

mediator *a.* mediador-a; intercesor-a.

medic *n.* técnico-a entrenado para dar primeros auxilios.

Medicaid *n.* Asistencia Médica, programa del gobierno de los Estados Unidos que provee asistencia médica a los pobres.

medical *a.* médico-a; medicinal, curativo-a; ___ **assistance** / asistencia ___; ___ **examiner** / médico forense; ___ **history** / historia clínica; ___ **records** / registros ___ -s; [*patient's record*] expediente del paciente; ___ **staff** / cuerpo médico; ___ **student** / estudiante de medicina.

medical record *n.* expediente médico.

medical record linkage *n.* conexión del expediente médico. 1. cualquier información que conecte al paciente con su expediente médico; 2. colección de datos de la historia clínica de un paciente proporcionada por varias fuentes; 3. cualquier dato referente a un paciente participante en un estudio clínico que pueda revelar su identidad como sujeto participante.

medical waste *n.* deshechos de efectos médicos.

Medicare *n.* Programa de asistencia médica del gobierno de los Estados Unidos a personas desde los 65 años de edad o a adultos incapacitados para trabajar.

medicate *v.* recetar, medicinar.

medication *n.* medicina, medicamento; *pop.* remedio.

medicinal *a.* medicinal, rel. a la medicina, o con propiedades curativas.

medicine *n.* medicina. 1. ciencia que se dedica al mantenimiento de la salud por medio de tratamienos de curación y prevención de enfermedades; **aerospace** ___ / ___ del espacio; **clinical** ___ / ___ clínica; **community** ___ / ___ comunal, al servicio de la comunidad; **environmental** ___ / ___ ecológica; **forensic** ___ / ___ forense; **legal** ___ / ___ legal; ___ **chest** / botiquín; **nuclear** ___ / ___ nuclear; **preventive** ___ / ___ preventiva; **socialized** ___ / ___ socializada; **sports** ___ / ___ deportiva; **tropical** ___ / ___ tropical; **veterinary** ___ / ___ veterinaria; 2. una droga o medicamento.

medicine man *n.* curandero.

medicine woman *n.* curandera.

medicolegal *a.* médicolegal, rel. a la medicina en relación con las leyes.

mediolateral *a.* mediolateral, rel. a la parte media y a un lado del cuerpo.

medium *n.* (*pl.* **media**) medio. 1. intermediario-a, elemento mediante el cual se obtiene un resultado; 2. sustancia que transmite impulsos; 3. sustancia que se usa en un cultivo de bacterias.

medulla *n.* médula, *pop.* tuétano, parte interna o central de un órgano; ___ **oblongata** / ___ oblongata, bulbo raquídeo, porción de la médula localizada en la base del cráneo; ___ **ossium, bone marrow** / ___ ósea.

medullar, medullary *a.* medular, rel. a la médula.

medulloblastoma *n.* meduloblastoma, neoplasma maligno localizado en el cuarto ventrículo y en el cerebelo, que puede invadir las meninges.

meet *n.* reunión; concurso; *vi.* encontrar; reunirse con; **I am glad to** ___ **you** / Mucho gusto en conocerlo-a.

meeting *n.* reunión, junta. 1. partes que se unen, tales como las partes de un hueso a las márgenes de una herida; 2. reunión de un grupo de personas.

megabladder, megalocystis *n.* megalocisto, vejiga distendida.

megacaryocyte *n.* megacariocito; célula ósea grande esencial en la producción de plaquetas.

megacephalic *a.* megacefálico-a. **macrocephalia**.

megacolon *n.* megacolon, colon anormalmente agrandado.

megadose *n.* megadosis, una dosis de una sustancia nutritiva que supera exageradamente la cantidad diaria recomendada.

megaesophagus *n.* megaesófago, dilatación anormal de la parte inferior del esófago.

megalomania *n.* megalomanía, delirio de grandeza.

megalophobia *n.* megalofobia, miedo a los objetos grandes.

megavitamin *n.* megavitamina, dosis de vitamina en exceso de la cantidad normal requerida diariamente.

meibomian cyst *n.* quiste meibomiano, quiste del párpado.

meiosis *n.* meiosis, proceso de subdivisión celular que resulta en la formación de gametos.

melancholia *n.* melancolía, depresión acentuada.

melancholic *a.* melancólico-a, rel. a la melancolía.

melanin *n.* melanina, pigmento oscuro de la piel, el pelo y partes del ojo.

melanocyte *n.* melanocito, célula que produce melanina.

melanoma *n.* melanoma, tumor maligno compuesto de melanocitos.

melanosis *a.* melanosis, condición que se caracteriza por la pigmentación oscura presente en varios tejidos y órganos.

melanuria *n.* melanuria, presencia de pigmentación oscura en la orina.

melasma gravidarum *n.* melasma gravídico. chloasma.

melena *n.* melena, masa de heces fecales negruscas y pastosas que contiene sangre digerida.

mellow *a.* dulce, suave, tierno-a.

melon *n.* melón.

melt *v.* derretir, disolver.

member *n.* miembro. 1. órgano o parte del cuerpo; 2. socio-a de una organización.

membrane *n.* membrana, capa fina que sirve de cubierta o protección a una cavidad, estructura u órgano; **elastic** ___ / ___ elástica; **mucous** ___ / ___ mucosa; **nuclear** ___ / ___ nuclear; **permeable** ___ / ___ permeable; **placental** ___ / ___ de la placenta; **semipermeable** ___ / ___ semipermeable; **synovial** ___ / ___ sinovial; **tympanic** ___ / ___ timpánica.

membranous *a.* membranoso-a, rel. a una membrana o de la naturaleza de ésta.

memorandum *n.* memorando, nota.

memorial *n.* memoria, recuerdo.

memorize *v.* memorizar, aprender de memoria.

memory *n.* memoria, retentiva, facultad de la mente para registrar y recordar experiencias; **bad** ___ / mala ___; **good** ___ / buena ___; **short-term** ___ / ___ inmediata; *v.* **Do you have a good** ___ **?** / ¿Tiene, tienes buena ___ ?; **to have memories from** / tener recuerdos de; **to lose the** ___ / perder la ___.

menace *n.* amenaza; *v.* amenazar, atemorizar.

menarche *n.* menarca, inicio de la menstruación.

mend *v.* reparar, componer, mejorar.

mendable *a.* reparable, componible.

mendelism *n.* mendelismo, principios que explican la trasmisión genética de ciertos rasgos.

meningeal *a.* meníngeo-a, rel. a las meninges.

meninges *n., pl.* meninges, las tres capas de tejido conjuntivo que rodean al cerebro y a la médula espinal.

meningioma *n.* meningioma, neoplasma vascular gen. benigno de desarrollo lento que se origina en las meninges.

meningism *n.* meningismo, irritación congestiva de las meninges gen. de naturaleza tóxica con síntomas similares a los de la meningitis pero sin inflamación.

meningismus *n. L.* meningismus. V. **meningism**.

meningitic *a.* meningítico-a, rel. a las meninges.

meningitis *n.* meningitis, infl. de las meninges cerebrales o espinales; **cryptococcal** ___ / ___ criptocócica; **viral** ___ / ___ viral.

meningocele *n.* meningocele, protrusión de las meninges a través del cráneo o de la espina dorsal.

meningococcus *n.* meningococo, uno de los microorganismos causantes de la meningitis cerebral epidémica.

meningoencephalitis *n.* meningoencefalitis, cerebromeningitis, infl. del encéfalo y de las meninges.

meningoencephalocele *n.* meningoencefalocele, protrusión del encéfalo y de las meninges a través de un defecto en el cráneo.

meningomyelitis *n.* meningomielitis, infl. de la médula espinal y las membranas que la cubren.

meningomyelocele *n.* meningomielocele, protrusión de la médula espinal y las meninges a través de un defecto en la columna vertebral.

meniscectomy *n.* meniscectomía, extirpación de un menisco.

meniscus *n.* (*pl.* **menisci**) menisco, estructura cartilaginosa de forma lunar.

menometrorrhagia *n.* menometrorragia, sangrado anormal entre menstruaciones.

menopause *n.* menopausia, cambio de vida en la mujer adulta, terminación de la etapa de reproducción y disminución de la producción hormonal.

menorrhagia *n.* menorragia, períodos o reglas muy abundantes.

menorrhalgia *n.* menorralgia, menstruación dolorosa.

menorrhea *n.* menorrea, flujo menstrual normal.

menses *n.* menses, menstruo, menstruación, período, regla.

menstrual *a.* menstrual, rel. a la menstruación; ___ **cycle** / ciclo ___; ___ **disorder** / trastorno ___.

menstruate *v.* menstruar.

menstruation *n.* menstruación, flujo sanguíneo periódico de la mujer.

mental *a.* mental, rel. a la mente; ___ **age** / edad ___; ___ **disorder** / trastorno ___; ___ **deficiency** / retraso ___; ___**handicap** / minusvalía ___; ___ **health** / salud ___; ___ **hygiene** / higiene ___; ___ **illness** / enfermedad ___; ___ **retardation** / retraso ___; ___ **test** / examen de capacidad ___.

mentality *n.* mentalidad, capacidad mental.

mentation *n.* actividad mental.

menthol *n.* mentol, sustancia que se obtiene del alcanfor de menta y que tiene efecto sedante.

mentum *n.* mentón, barbilla, prominencia de la barba.

mephenytoin *n.* mefenitoina, anticonvulsivo sumamente tóxico que se usa en combinación con otras drogas.

meralgia *n.* meralgia, dolor en el pie que puede extenderse hasta el muslo; ___ **paresthetic** / ___ parestética.

merbromin *n.* merbromina, polvo rojo inodoro, soluble en agua, usado como germicida.

merciful *a.* misericordioso-a, compasivo-a.

merciless *a.* inhumano-a, despiadado-a.

mercurial *a.* mercurial, perteneciente o rel. al mercurio.

mercurochrome *n.* mercurocromo, nombre registrado de la merbromina.

mercury *n.* mercurio, metal líquido volátil; ___ **poisoning** / envenenamiento por ___.

mercy *n.* misericordia, compasión; ___ **killing** / eutanasia.

merergacia *n.* merergacia, tipo de trastorno psíquico caracterizado por cierto grado de inestabilidad emocional y ansiedad.

merge *v.* unir, unificar.

meridian *n.* meridiano, línea imaginaria que conecta los extremos opuestos del axis en la superficie de un cuerpo esférico.

mescaline *n.* mescalina, alcaloide alucinogénico, *pop.* peyote.

mesectoderm *n.* mesectodermo, masa de células que componen las meninges.

mesencephalon *n.* mesencéfalo, el cerebro medio en la etapa embrionaria.

mesenchyme *n.* mesénquima, red de células embrionarias que forman el tejido conjuntivo y los vasos sanguíneos y linfáticos en el adulto.

mesenteric *a.* mesentérico-a, concerniente al mesenterio.

mesentery *n.* mesenterio, repliegue del peritoneo que fija el intestino a la pared abdominal posterior.

mesial *a.* mesial. V. **medial**.

mesion *n.* mesión, plano imaginario medio que divide el cuerpo en dos partes simétricas.

mesmerism *n.* mesmerismo, uso del hipnotismo como método terapéutico.

mesocardia *n.* mesocardia, desplazamiento anormal del corazón hacia el centro del tórax.

mesocolon *n.* mesocolon, mesenterio que fija el colon a la pared abdominal posterior.

mesoderm *n.* mesodermo, capa media germinativa del embrión situada entre el ectodermo y endodermo de la cual provienen el tejido óseo, el muscular, los vasos sanguíneos y linfáticos, y las membranas del corazón y abdomen.

mesothelium *n.* mesotelio, capa celular del mesodermo embrionario que forma el epitelio que cubre las membranas serosas en el adulto.

mess *n.* lío, confusión; *v.* **to make a** ___ / hacer un ___; desordenar, revolver, ensuciar.

message *n.* mensaje, recado.

messy *a.* revuelto-a, desordenado-a, sucio-a.

metabolic *a.* metabólico-a, rel. al metabolismo; ___ **rate** / índice ___.

metabolism *n.* metabolismo, suma de los cambios fisicoquímicos que tienen efecto a continuación del proceso digestivo; **constructive** ___ / anabolismo, asimilación; **destructive** ___ / ___ destructivo, catabolismo; **basal** ___ / ___ basal, el nivel más bajo del gasto de energía; **protein** ___ / ___ de proteínas, digestión de proteínas y conversión de éstas en aminoácidos.

metabolite *n.* metabolito, sustancia producida durante el proceso metabólico.

metacarpal *a.* metacarpiano-a, rel. al metacarpio.

metacarpus *n.* metacarpo, la parte formada por los cinco huesecillos metacarpianos de la mano.

metal *n.* metal; ___ **fume fever** / fiebre por aspiración de vapores metálicos;

metallic *a.* metálico-a, rel. a un metal o de la naturaleza de éste.

metamorphosis *n.* metamorfosis. 1. cambio de forma o estructura; 2. cambio degenerativo patológico.

metanephrine *n.* metanefrina, catabolito de epinefrina que se encuentra en la orina.

metaphase *n.* metafase, una de las etapas de la división celular.

metaphysis *n.* metáfisis, zona de crecimiento del hueso.

metastasis *n.* metástasis, extensión de un proceso patológico de un foco primario a otra parte del cuerpo a través de los vasos sanguíneos o linfáticos como se observa en algunos tipos de cáncer.

metastasize *v.* metastatizar, esparcirse por metástasis.

metastatic *a.* metastásico-a, rel. a la metástasis.

metatarsial *a.* metatarsiano-a, rel. al metatarso.

metatarsus *n.* metatarso, la parte formada por los cinco huesecillos del pie situados entre el tarso y los dedos.

meteorism *n.* meteorismo, abdomen distendido causado por acumulación de gas en el estómago o los intestinos.

methadone *n.* metadona, droga sintética potente de acción narcótica menos intensa que la morfina.

methanol, wood alcohol *n.* metanol, alcohol de madera.

method *n.* método, procedimiento; proceso; tratamiento.

meticulous *a.* meticuloso-a.

metopic *a.* metópico-a, frontal, rel. a la frente.

metria *a.* metria, infl. del útero durante el puerperio.

metric *a.* métrico-a; ___ **system** / sistema ___.

metritis *n.* metritis, infl. de la pared uterina.

metroflebitis *n.* metroflebitis, infl. de las venas uterinas.

micrencephaly *n.* micrencefalia, cerebro anormalmente pequeño.

microabscess *n.* microabsceso, absceso diminuto.

microanatomy *n.* microanatomía, histología.

microbe *n.* microbio, microorganismo, organismo diminuto.

microbial, microbian *a.* microbiano-a, rel. a los microbios.

microbicide *n.* microbicida, agente exterminador de microbios.

microbiology *n.* microbiología, ciencia que estudia los microorganismos.

microcephaly *n.* microcefalia, cabeza anormalmente pequeña de origen congénito.

microcheiria *n.* microquiria, trastorno en el cual las manos son de un tamaño más pequeño que lo normal.

micrococcus *n.* micrococo, microorganismo.

microcolon *n.* microcolon, colon anormalmente pequeño.

microcosmus *n.* microcosmo. 1. universo en miniatura; 2. cualquier entidad o estructura considerada en sí misma un pequeño universo.

microcurie *n.* microcurie, unidad de radiación.

microdrip *n.* microgotero, un instrumento para administrar una cantidad precisa pequeña de una sustancia por medio intravenoso.

microfiche *n.* microficha, ficha en la que se acumulan datos para ser vistos bajo un lente amplificador.

microfilm *n.* microfilm, microfilme, película que contiene información reducida a un tamaño mínimo.

microgenitalia *n.* microgenitalia, escaso desarrollo de los genitales externos.

microglia cells *n.* células de microglia, pequeñas células intersticiales migratorias que pertenecen al sistema nervioso.

micrognathia *n.* micrognatia, mandíbula inferior anormalmente pequeña.

micrography *n.* micrografía, estudio microscópico.

microgyria *n.* microgiria, pequeñez o escaso desarrollo de las circunvoluciones cerebrales.

microinvasion *n.* microinvasión, invasión de tejido celular adyacente a un carcinoma localizado que no puede verse a simple vista.

microlithiasis *n.* microlitiasis, pequeñas concreciones excretadas en ciertos órganos.

micromelia *n.* micromelia, extremidades anormalmente pequeñas.

ⓜ

micromelic *a.* micromélico-a, rel. a la micromelia.

micrometer *n.* micrómetro, instrumento para medir distancias cortas.

micronucleus *n.* micronúcleo, el núcleo más pequeño de una célula que posee más de un núcleo.

microorganism *n.* microorganismo, organismo que no puede verse a simple vista.

microphage *n.* micrófago. *v.* phagocyte.

microphallus *n.* microfalo, pene anormalmente pequeño.

microscope *n.* microscopio, instrumento óptico con lentes que amplifican objetos que no pueden verse a simple vista; **electron** ___ / ___ electrónico; **light** ___ / ___ con luz o lumínico.

microscopic *a.* microscópico-a, rel. al microscopio.

microscopy *n.* microscopía, examen que se realiza con un microscopio.

microsome *n.* microsoma, elemento fino granular del protoplasma.

microsomia *n.* microsomía, cuerpo anormalmente pequeño de proporciones normales.

microsurgery *n.* microcirugía, operación efectuada con el uso de microscopios quirúrgicos e instrumentos minúsculos de precisión.

microtome *n.* micrótomo, instrumento de precisión que se usa en la preparación de secciones finas de tejido para ser examinadas bajo el microscopio.

microtomy *n.* microtomía, corte de secciones finas de tejido.

microwave *n.* microonda, onda corta electromagnética de frecuencia muy alta.

miction *n.* emisión de orina.

micturate *v.* orinar.

middle *n.* medio, centro; **in the** ___ **of** / en el ___ de.

middle age *n.* mediana edad, madurez.

middle ear *n.* oído medio, parte del oído situada más allá del tímpano.

middle finger *n.* el dedo cordial.

middle lobe syndrome *n.* síndrome del lóbulo medio del pulmón.

midget *n.* enano-a.

midgut *n.* intestino medio del embrión.

midline *n.* línea media del cuerpo.

midnight *n.* medianoche.

midplane *n.* plano medio.

midriff *n.* diafragma.

midsection *n.* sección media.

midstream specimen *n.* especimen de orina que se toma después de comenzar la emisión y poco antes de terminarse.

midwife *n.* comadrona, partera, mujer que se especializa en el cuidado y atención de la salud de mujeres durante el embarazo, el parto y el postpartum.

midwifery *n.* partería.

midyear *n.* mediados de año.

migraine *n.* migraña, jaqueca, ataques severos de dolor de cabeza que gen. se manifiestan en un solo lado acompañados de visión alterada y en algunos casos de náuseas y vómitos.

migrans thrombophlebitis *n.* tromboflebitis migratoria, tromboflebitis de progreso lento de una vena a otra.

migration *n.* migración, movimiento de las células de un lugar a otro.

migratory cell *n.* célula migratoria, célula que tiene locomoción.

migratory pneumonia *n.* neumonía migratoria, tipo de neumonía que aparece en diferentes partes del pulmón.

mild *a.* [*pain*] leve, tolerable; moderado-a, indulgente.

mildew *n.* moho, añublo.

milia neonatorum *n.* milia neonatorum, pequeños quistes no patógenos vistos a veces en los recién nacidos.

miliary *a.* miliar, caracterizado-a por pequeños tumores o nódulos.

miliary tuberculosis *n.* tuberculosis miliar, enfermedad que invade el organismo a través de la sangre y se caracteriza por la formación de tubérculos diminutos en los órganos afectados.

milieu *n.* medio ambiente.

milk *n.* leche; **boiled** ___ / ___ hervida; **clotted** ___ / ___ cuajada; **condensed** ___ / ___ condensada; **dry** ___ / ___ en polvo; **evaporated** ___ / ___ evaporada; **albumina** / lactoalbúmina; ___ **ascites** / ascites seudoquilosa; ___ **of magnesia** / ___ de magnesia; **mother's** ___ / leche materna; **skim** ___ / ___ desnatada; **sterilized** ___ / ___ esterilizada.

milking *n.* ordeño, maniobra para forzar sustancias fuera de un tubo.

milk leg *n.* flegmasia cerúlea dolorosa, trombosis de una de las venas de la pierna (gen. femoral) que manifiesta dolor agudo, infl., sianosis y edema, que puede producir un problema circulatorio severo.

milky *a.* lechoso-a, lácteo-a.

mimetic, mimic *a.* mimético-a, que imita.

mind *n.* mente, entendimiento; ___ **-body medicine** / medicina psicosomática; *v.* atender, tener en cuenta; **to bear in** ___ / tener presente; **to be out of one's** ___ / volverse loco-a; **to make up one's** ___ / decidirse; **to speak one's** ___ / dar una opinión; dar su parecer.

miner *n.* minero.

mineral *n.* mineral, elemento inorgánico; *a.* mineral; ___ **water (carbonated)** / agua ___ efervescente.

mineralization *n.* mineralización, depósitos de minerales en los tejidos.

mineralocorticoid *n.* mineralocorticoide, tipo de hormona liberada por la glándula suprarrenal que participa en la regulación del volumen de la sangre.

minilaparotomy *n.* minilaparotomía, un tipo de intervención pélvica para uso de diagnóstico o con el propósito de esterilización por medio de ligación de las trompas.

minimal *a. comp.* mínimo-a, más pequeño-a.

minimal dose *n.* dosis mínima, la menor dosis necesaria para producir un efecto determinado.

minimal lethal dose *n.* dosis letal mínima, la menor dosis de una sustancia que puede ocasionar la muerte.

minimize *v.* aliviar, atenuar, mitigar; reducir al mínimo; **This pill is to** ___ **the pain** / Esta pastilla es para ___ el dolor.

minister *n.* ministro; pastor.

minor *n.* [*in age*] menor de edad; *a.* [*smaller, youngest*] menor, más pequeño; **a** ___ **problem** / un problema sin importancia; ___ **burn** / quemadura leve; ___ **surgery** / cirugía menor.

minority *n.* minoría, minoridad.

mint *n.* [*herb*] menta.

minute *n.* [*time*] minuto, momento; *a.* menudo-a, mínimo-a, diminuto-a.

miosis *n.* miosis, contracción excesiva de la pupila.

miracle *n.* milagro, prodigio.

miraculous *a.* milagroso-a, prodigioso-a.

mirror *n.* espejo.

misadventure *n.* infortunio, desgracia; accidente.

misanthropy *n.* misantropía, aversión a la humanidad.

misbehave *v.* portarse mal, conducirse mal.

misbehaved *a.* malcriado-a, majadero-a; mal educado-a.

misbehavior *n.* mala conducta, mal comportamiento.

miscalculate *v.* hacer un error o falta; equivocarse.

miscalculation *n.* error, falta, equivocación.

miscarriage *n.* aborto, malparto, expulsión del feto por vía natural.

miscegenation *n.* mestizaje, cruzamiento de razas o de culturas.

miscible *a.* capaz de mezclarse o disolverse.

misdiagnosis *n.* diagnóstico equivocado o erróneo.

misery *n.* sufrimiento, pena; desesperación; miseria.

misfit *n.* mal adaptado-a; *v.* no sentar bien, desajustar.

misfortunate *a.* desdichado-a, desgraciado-a.

misfortune *n.* desdicha, desgracia.

misguide *v.* dirigir mal, aconsejar mal.

misguided *a.* mal aconsejado-a, mal dirigido-a.

misinform *v.* dar una información errónea.

misinformed *a.* mal informado-a.

misjudge *v.* juzgar mal, tener una opinión errónea.

misleading *a.* engañoso-a, descaminado-a, erróneo-a.

misogamy *n.* misogamia, aversión al matrimonio.

misogyny *n.* misoginia, aversión a las mujeres.

misplace *v.* extraviar, poner algo fuera de lugar.

miss *n.* señorita, jovencita; *v.* [*to fail, to overlook*] perder; **to** ___ **an appointment** / perder el turno; [*sentiment*] to ___ **one's family** / echar de menos a la familia; [*to skip*] to ___ **a period** / faltar la regla, faltar el período.

misshape *v.* deformar, desfigurar.

misshaped, misshapen *a.* deforme, desfigurado-a.

missing *a.* desaparecido-a; extraviado-a.

mission *n.* misión; destino.

mistake *n.* error, equivocación, desacierto, falta; *vi.* equivocar, entender mal, confundir; *vr.* equivocarse, confundirse.

mistaken *a. pp.* of **to mistake**; equivocado-a, desacertado-a, incorrecto-a

mister *n.* señor.

mistimed *a.* inoportuno, fuera de tiempo.

mistranslation *n.* traducción incorrecta.

mistrustful *a.* desconfiado-a, receloso-a.

mistyping of blood *n.* error the emparejamiento de sangre; **blood transfusion** ___ / error de emparejamiento en una transfusión sanguínea; *pop.* error de "tipaje".

misunderstand *vi.* no comprender, entender mal.

mitigate *v.* mitigar, aliviar, calmar.

mitigated *a.* mitigado-a, aliviado-a, calmado-a; disminuido-a.

mitochondria *n.* mitocondria, filamentos microscópicos del citoplasma que constituyen la fuente principal de energía de la célula.

mitogen *n.* mitógeno, sustancia que induce mitosis celular.

mitogenesis, mitogenia *n.* mitogénesis, causa de la mitosis celular.

mitosis *n.* mitosis, división celular que da lugar a nuevas células y reemplaza tejidos lesionados.

mitral *a.* mitral, rel. a la válvula mitral o bicúspide ___ **disease** / enfermedad de la válvula ___ del corazón; ___ **incompetence** / insuficiencia ___; ___ **murmur** / soplo; ___ **orifice** / orificio ___; ___ **valve insuficiency** / insuficiencia de la válvula ___; ___ **valve prolapse** / prolapso de la válvula ___ , cierre defectuoso de la válvula ___.

mitral regurgitation *n.* regurgitación mitral, flujo sanguíneo retrógrado del ventrículo izquierdo a la aurícula izquierda causado por lesión de la válvula mitral.

mitral stenosis *n.* estenosis mitral, estrechez del orificio izquierdo aurículo-ventricular.

mitral valve *n.* válvula mitral, válvula aurículoventricular izquierda del corazón.

mittelschmerz *n.* dolor en el vientre relacionado con la ovulación que ocurre gen. a mitad del ciclo menstrual.

mix *v.* mezclar, juntar, asociar.

mixed *a.* mezclado-a, asociado-a.

mixture *n.* mezcla, mixtura; poción.

mnemonics *n.* mnemónica, adiestramiento de la memoria por medio de asociación de ideas y otros recursos.

moan *n.* quejido, gemido, queja, lamento; *vr.* quejarse, lamentarse.

mobility *n.* movilidad.

mobilization *n.* movilización.

mobilize *v.* movilizar; movilizarse, moverse.

modality *n.* modalidad, cualquier método de aplicación terapeútica.

mode *n.* 1. moda, manera, valor repetido con mayor frecuencia en una serie; 2. modo.

model *n.* modelo, patrón, molde.

moderated *a.* moderado-a, mesurado-a; [*price*] módico, [*weather*] templado; ___ **temperature** / temperatura ___.

moderation *n.* moderación, sobriedad.

modern *a.* moderno-a, reciente.

modest *a.* modesto-a, recatado-a.

modification *n.* modificación, cambio.

modify *v.* modificar, cambiar.

modulation *n.* modulación, acto de ajustar o adaptar tal como ocurre en la inflexión de la voz.

moiety *n.* mitad, una de las porciones de un todo.

molar *n.* diente molar, muela.

mold *n.* moho, cualquier moho.

molding *n.* amoldamiento de la cabeza del feto para adaptarla a la forma y tamaño del canal del parto.

mole *n.* mancha, lunar.

molecular *a.* molecular, rel. a una molécula; ___ **biology** / biología ___.

molecule *n.* molécula, unidad mínima de una sustancia.

molest *v.* dañar físicamente, vejar; humillar; asaltar.

mollusc, mollusk *n.* (*pl.* **mollusca**) molusco.

moment *n.* momento, instante.

momentary *a.* momentáneo-a.

momentum *n.* L. momentum; ímpetu; fuerza de movimiento.

monarticular *a.* monarticular, que concierne o afecta a una sola articulación.

money *n.* dinero; moneda; divisas.

mongoloid *a.* mongoloide, rel. al mongolismo o que sufre del mismo.

moniliasis *n.* moniliasis. V. **candidiasis**.

monitor *n.* monitor. 1. instrumento electrónico usado para monitorear una función; 2. persona que supervisa una función o actividad; *v.* monitorear, chequear sistemáticamente con un instrumento electrónico una función orgánica, tal como los latidos del corazón.

monitoring *n.* monitoreo, acción de monitorear; **blood pressure** ___ / ___ de la presión arterial; **cardiac** ___ / ___ cardíaco; **fetal** ___ / ___ del corazón fetal.

monochromatic *a.* monocromático-a, de un solo color.

monoclonal *a.* monoclonal, rel. a un solo grupo de células; ___ **antibodies** / anticuerpos ___ -es.

monocular *a.* monocular, rel. a un solo ojo.

monocyte *n.* monocito, glóbulo blanco mononuclear granuloso.

monogamy *n.* monogamia, unión matrimonial legal con una sola persona.

mononuclear *a.* mononuclear, que tiene un solo núcleo; ___ **cell** / célula ___.

mononucleosis *n.* mononucleosis, presencia de un número anormalmente elevado de leucocitos mononucleares en la sangre;

infectious ___ / ___ infecciosa, infección viral aguda.

monosaccharide *n.* monosacárido, azúcar simple.

monotone *n.* monotonía.

monotonous *a.* monótono-a.

monozygotic twins *n., pl.* gemelos monocigóticos con características genéticas idénticas.

monster *n.* monstruo.

month *n.* mes.

monthly *a.* mensual; *adv.* mensualmente.

mood *n.* humor, disposición, estado de ánimo; **changeable** ___ **-s** / cambios de humor, cambios de disposición; ___ **disorders** / cambios de estado de ánimo; **to be in a sad** ___ / sentirse triste; **to be in the** ___ **to** / tener ganas de.

moody *a.* malhumorado-a; propenso-a a cambios de ánimo.

moon *n.* luna; **moonlight** / luz de la ___ .

moonface *n.* cara de luna, cara llena redonda característica de pacientes sometidos a un tratamiento prolongado de un esteroide.

moonlighter *n.* persona que tiene más de un empleo.

moral *a.* moral, honesto-a, honrado-a.

morality *n.* ética, rectitud, moral.

morbid *a.* mórbido, insano-a, morbosa-a, rel. a una enfermedad.

morbidity *n.* morbidez, morbosidad, enfermedad.

mordacious *a.* mordaz, satírico-a.

more *a.* más; *adv.* más; **more and more** / cada vez ___ ; **once** ___ / una vez ___ ; [*before numeral*] ___ **than a hundred** / ___ de cien ; [*before a verb*] ___ **than** / más de lo que ___ ; ___ **than he needs** / más de lo que necesita.

moreover *adv.* además, además de eso; también.

morgue *n. Fr.* morgue, necrocomio, depósito temporal de cadáveres.

moribund *a.* moribundo-a, cercano-a a la muerte, agonizante.

morning *n.* mañana, madrugada; **early in the** ___ / muy de ___ ; **Good** ___ / buenos días, buen día; **in the** ___ / por la ___ , en la ___ ; ___ **stiffness** / rigidez matutina muscular y de las articulaciones; **tomorrow** ___ / ___ por la ___ .

morning sickness *n.* trastorno matutino de náuseas y vómitos que sufren algunas mujeres en la primera etapa del embarazo.

moron *n.* morón-a, persona con retraso mental de un cociente intelectual de 50 a 70.

morphine *n.* morfina, alcaloide que se obtiene del opio y se usa como analgésico y sedante.

morphinism *n.* morfinismo, condición morbosa ocasionada por la adicción a la morfina.

mortal *a.* mortal, mortífero-a, fatal, letal.

mortality *n.* mortalidad, mortandad. 1. estado de ser mortal; 2. índice de mortalidad.

mortify *v.* mortificar; mortificarse, sentirse mortificado-a.

mortuary *n.* mortuorio, funeraria.

mórula *n.* mórula, masa esférica y sólida de células que resulta de la división celular del óvulo fecundado.

mosaic *n.* mosaico, la presencia en una persona de distintos tejidos adyacentes derivados de la misma célula como resultado de mutaciones.

mosaicism *n.* mosaicismo, así como en un mosaico, los cromosomas son genéticamente mutadores diferentes que pueden establecer características distintas en humanos, tal como se muestra en la fisonomía por diferencias de sexo.

mosquito *n.* mosquito.

most *a. sup.* de **more**, el, la más; lo más; el, la mayor; el mayor número de, la mayor parte de; *adv.* más, muy, a lo sumo; **-ly** sumamente, principalmente.

mother *n.* madre, mamá.

motherhood *n.* maternidad.

mother-in-law *n.* suegra.

motility *n.* movilidad.

motion *n.* movimiento; [*sign*] seña, indicación; moción; ___ **sickness** / mareo producide por movimiento.

motionless *a.* sin movimiento, inmóvil.

motivate *v.* motivar, animar.

motivation *n.* motivación, estimulación externa.

motive *n.* motivo; ánimo, fuerza mayor.

motor *n.* motor, agente que produce o induce movimiento; *a.* motor-a, que causa movimiento.

motor development *n.* desarrollo motor.

motor neuron *n.* neurona motora, células nerviosas que conducen impulsos que inician las contracciones musculares.

mottled *a.* moteado-a, descolorido-a.

mountain *n.* montaña.

mourn *v.* estar de duelo; guardar luto.

mouse *n.* (*pl.* **mice**) ratón, [*small*] ratoncito.

moustache *n.* bigote.

mouth *n.* boca. 1. cavidad bucal; 2. abertura de cualquier cavidad; **by** ___ / por vía bucal; **Open your** ___ / Abra, abre la boca.

mouthwash *n.* antiséptico bucal; enjuague.

move *n.* movimiento; paso; *v.* mover; mudar; ___ **your fingers** / Mueva, mueve los dedos; ___ **your hand** / Mueva, mueve la mano; **to** ___

about, to ___ **around** / caminar, andar, ir; **to** ___ **away** / irse, trasladarse, mudarse; **to** ___ **down** / bajar.

movement *n.* movimiento, moción, acción, maniobra; [*of the intestines*] evacuación, defecación.

much *a.* mucho-a; abundante; *adv.* excesivamente, demasiado, en gran cantidad; **as** ___ **as** / tanto como; **How** ___**?** / ¿Cuánto?; **not as** ___ **as before** / no tanto como antes; **How** ___ **does it hurt?** / ¿Cuánto le duele?; **too** ___ / en exceso, demasiado.

mucin *n.* mucina, glucoproteína, ingrediente esencial del mucus.

mucocele *n.* mucocele, dilatación de una cavidad ósea debida a una acumulación de secreción mucosa.

mucocutaneous *a.* mucocutáneo-a, rel. a la membrana mucosa y la piel.

mucoid *n.* mucoide, glucoproteína similar a la mucina; *a.* de consistencia mucosa.

mucomembranous *a.* mucomembranoso-a, rel. a la membrana mucosa.

mucosa *n.* mucosa, membrana mucosa. **alveolar** ___ / ___ alveolar; **bronchial** ___ / ___ bronquial; **esophageal** ___ / ___ esofágica; **gastric** ___ / ___ gástrica; **laryngeal** ___ / ___ laríngea; **lingual** ___ / ___ lingual; ___ **of colon** / ___ del colon; ___ **of mouth** / ___ de la boca or bucal; ___ **of nose** / ___ nasal o de la nariz; ___ **of pharynx** / ___ de la nariz; ___ **of renal pelvis** / ___ de la pelvis renal; ___ **of small intestine** / ___ del intestino delgado; ___ **of stomach** / ___ del estómago or estomacal; ___ **of (urinary) bladder** / ___ de la vejiga urinaria; **nasal** ___ / ___ nasal; **olfactory** ___ / ___ olfatoria; **pharyngeal** ___ / ___ faríngea; **vaginal** ___ / ___ de la vagina.

mucosal *a.* mucosal, rel. a cualquier membrana mucosa.

mucosity *n.* mucosidad.

mucous *a.* mucoso-a, flemoso-a; ___ **colitis** / colitis ___.

mucous membrane *n.* membrana mucosa, láminas finas de tejido celular que cubren aberturas o canales que comunican con el exterior.

mucus *n.* moco, mucosidad, sustancia viscosa segregada por las membranas y glándulas mucosas.

multicellular *a.* multicelular, que consiste de muchas células.

multifactorial *a.* multifactorial, rel. a varios factores.

multifocal *a.* multifocal, rel. a más de un foco.

multilocular *a.* multilocular, V. **multicelular**.

multiparity *n.* multiparidad. 1. condición de una mujer que ha tenido más de un parto logrado; 2. parto múltiple.

multiparous *n.* multípara, mujer que ha parido más de una vez.

multiple *a.* múltiple, más de uno; ___ **family therapy** / terapia familiar ___; ___ **organ failure** / fallo ___ de órganos; ___ **personality** / personalidad ___.

multiple sclerosis *n.* esclerosis múltiple, enfermedad progresiva lenta del sistema nervioso central causada por pérdida de la capa de mielina que cubre las fibras nerviosas del cerebro y de la médula espinal.

mummification *n.* momificación, conversión a un estado similar al de una momia tal como en la gangrena seca o en el estado de un feto que muere y permanece en la matriz.

mumps *n.* paperas, parotiditis, enfermedad febril aguda de alta contagiosidad que se caracteriza por la infl. de las glándulas parótidas y otras glándulas salivales.

mural *a.* mural, rel. a las paredes de un órgano o parte.

muriatic *n.* muriático, derivado de sal común; ácido muriático.

murmur *n.* soplo, ruido; sonido breve raspante, esp. un sonido anormal del corazón. See chart on this page.

muscle *n.* músculo, tipo de tejido fibroso capaz de contraerse y que permite el movimiento de las

Murmur	Soplo
aortic, regurgitant	aórtico, regurgitante
bronchial	bronquial
cardiac	cardíaco
continuous	continuo
crescendo	creciente
diastolic	diastólico
endocardial	endocardial
exocardial	exocardial
functional	funcional
mitral	mitral
pansystolic	pansistólico
presystolic	presistólico
systolic	sistólico

partes y los órganos del cuerpo;
cardiac ___ / ___ cardíaco; **flexor** ___ / ___
flexor; **involuntary, visceral** ___ / ___
involuntario, visceral; **loss of** ___ **tone** / pérdida
de la tonicidad muscular; ___ **building** /
desarrollo muscular; ___ **relaxants** / relajadores
musculares, medicamentos para aliviar espasmos
musculares; ___ **strain** / distensión
muscular; ___ **toning** / tonicidad muscular;
striated, voluntary ___ / ___ estriado,
voluntario.

muscular *a.* muscular, musculoso-a, rel. al
músculo; ___ **atrophy** / atrofia ___; ___
contractions / contracciones ___ -es; ___
dystrophy / distrofia ___; ___ **rigidity** /
rigidez ___.

muscularis *n.* muscularis, capa muscular de un
órgano.

musculature *n.* musculatura; aparato muscular
del cuerpo.

musculoskeletal *a.* musculoesquelético-a, rel.
a los músculos y el esqueleto.

musculotendinous *a.* musculotendinoso-a,
que está formado por músculo y tendón.

mushroom *n.* hongo, seta, champiñón; ___
poisoning / envenenamiento por ___ -s.

musophobia *n.* musofobia, miedo a los ratones.

mussel *n.* almeja.

must *v. aux.* deber, ser necesario, tener que; **You
must take the medication** / Usted debe, tú
debes tomar la medicina.

mustard *n.* mostaza.

mutagen *n.* mutágeno, sustancia o agente que
causa mutación.

mutant *a.* mutante, rel. a un organismo que ha
pasado por mutaciones.

mutation *n.* mutación, alteración, cambios
espontáneos o inducidos en la estructura
genética.

mute *n.* mudo-a.

mutilate *v.* mutilar, cortar, cercenar.

mutilation *n.* mutilación.

mutism *n.* mutismo, mudez.

mutter *v.* murmurar, musitar; decir entre dientes;
pop. cuchichear.

my *a.* mi, mis; mío-a, míos-as.

myalgia *n.* mialgia, dolor muscular.

myasis *n.* miiasis, cualquier infección causada
por la larva de insectos dípteros que infecta una
cavidad cualquiera del organismo.

myasthenia *n.* miastenia, debilidad
muscular; ___ **gravis** / ___ grave.

myatonia *n.* miatonía, deficiencia o pérdida del
tono muscular.

mycetoma *n.* micetoma, infección causada por
hongos parásitos que afectan a la piel, al tejido
conjuntivo y a los huesos.

mycobacterium *n.* L. *Mycobacterium*, especie
de bacterias gram-positivas en forma de
bastoncillo que incluyen las causantes de la lepra
y la tuberculosis.

mycology *n.* micología, estudio de hongos y de
las enfermedades que ellos producen.

mycoplasmas *n., pl.* microplasmas, la más
diminuta forma de organismos vivos libres a la
cual pertenecen los virus que causan
enfermedades como la pulmonía y la faringitis.

mycosis *n.* micosis, cualquier enfermedad
causada por hongos; ___ **fungoide** / ___
fungosa.

mycotic *a.* micótico-a, rel. a la micosis.

mycotoxicosis *n.* micotoxicosis, condición
sistémica tóxica causada por toxinas creadas por
hongos.

mycotoxins *n., pl.* micotoxinas, toxinas
producidas por hongos parásitos.

mydriasis *n.* midriasis, dilatación prolongada de
la pupila del ojo.

mydriatic *a.* midriático-a, que causa dilatación
de la pupila del ojo.

myectomy *n.* miectomía, extirpación de una
porción de un músculo.

myelatelia *n.* mielatelia, defecto en el desarrollo
de la espina dorsal.

myelauxe *n.* mielauxa, hipertrofia de la espina
dorsal.

myelin *n.* mielina, sustancia de tipo grasoso que
cubre las fibras nerviosas.

myelination, myelinization *n.*
mielinización, crecimiento de mielina alrededor
de una fibra nerviosa.

myelinolysis *n.* mielinólisis, enfermedad que
destruye la mielina alrededor de ciertas fibras
nerviosas; **acute** ___ / ___ aguda; ___
transverse / ___ transversa.

myelitis *n.* mielitis, infl. de la espina dorsal.

myeloblast *n.* mieloblasto, una célula no
madura en la serie granulocítica, generalmente
presente en la médula ósea.

myeloblastemia *n.* mieloblastemia, la
presencia de mieloblastos en la sangre.

myelocele *n.* mielocele, hernia de la médula
espinal a través de la columna vertebral.

myeloclast *n.* mieloclasto, una célula que
destruye las vainas de mielina de las células
nerviosas del sistema nervioso central.

myelocyst *n.* mieloquiste, un quiste compuesto
de células nerviosas que se desarrolla en un
canal del sistema nervioso central.

myelocyte *n.* mielocito, leucocito granular de la médula ósea presente en la sangre en ciertas enfermedades.

myelocytic *a.* mielocítico-a, rel. a mielocitos; ___ **leukemia** / leucemia ___.

myelocytoma *n.* mielocitoma, una acumulación de mielocitos en ciertos tejidos, presente en ciertas enfermedades.

myelodysplasia *n.* mielodisplasia, desarrollo anormal de la columna vertebral.

myelofibrosis *n.* mielofibrosis, fibrosis de la médula ósea.

myelogenic, myelogenous *a.* mielógeno-a, que se produce en la médula.

myelogenic sarcoma *n.* sarcoma que se origina en la médula ósea.

myelogram *v.* mielograma, radiografía de la médula usando un medio de contraste.

myelography *n.* mielografía, radiografía de la columna vertebral con inyección de medio de contraste en la región subaracnoidea.

myeloid *n.* mieloide; *a.* rel. a la médula espinal o similar a la médula espinal o a la médula ósea; ___ **tissue** / médula roja.

myeloleukemia *n.* mieloleucemia, una forma de leucemia en la cual las células anormales provienen de tejido mielopoyético.

myeloma *n.* mieloma. 1. cualquier tumor de la médula espinal u ósea; 2. tumor formado por el tipo de células que se encuentran en la médula ósea; **multiple** ___ / ___ múltiple.

myelomeningocele *n.* mielomeningocele, hernia de la médula espinal y de las meninges con protrusión a través de un defecto en el canal vertebral.

myelopathy *n.* mielopatía, cualquier condición patológica de la médula espinal o de la médula ósea;

myeloproliferative *a.* mieloproliferativo-a, que se caracteriza por una proliferación de la médula ósea dentro o fuera de la médula.

myeloschisis *n.* mielosquisis, secuela de espina bífida.

myelosuppression *n.* mielosupresión, producción reducida de eritrocitos y de plaquetas en la médula ósea.

myesthesia *n.* miestesia, sensaciones en un músculo de cualquier tipo.

myocardial, myocardiac *a.* miocárdico-a, rel. al miocardio; ___ **contraction** / contracción del miocardio; ___ **diseases** / miocardiopatías.

myocardial infarction *n.* infarto cardíaco, necrosis de células del músculo cardíaco debido a un bloqueo del abastecimiento de sangre que lo irriga, condición usu. conocida como "ataque al corazón".

myocardiography *n.* miocardiografía, trazado de los movimientos del músculo cardíaco.

myocardiopathy *n.* miocardiopatía. V. **cardiomyopathy**.

myocarditis *n.* miocarditis, infl. del miocardio.

myocardium *n.* miocardio, capa media de la pared cardíaca.

myoclonus *n.* mioclonus, contracción o espasmo muscular tal como se manifiesta en la epilepsia.

myocyte *n.* miocito, célula del tejido muscular.

myodystrophy *n.* miodistrofia, distrofia muscular.

myofibril *n.* miofibrilla, fibrilla diminuta delgada del tejido muscular.

myofibroma *n.* miofibroma, tumor compuesto de elementos musculares.

myofilament *n.* miofilamento, filamentos microscópicos que constituyen las fibrillas musculares.

myogenic *a.* miogénico-a, que se origina en un músculo.

myoglobin *n.* mioglobina, pigmento del tejido muscular que participa en la distribución de oxígeno.

myography *n.* miografía, gráfico que registra la actividad muscular.

myolysis *n.* miolisis, destrucción de tejido muscular.

myoma *n.* mioma, tumor benigno compuesto de tejido muscular. ___ **previum** / ___ previo.

myomectomy *n.* miomectomía. 1. excisión de una porción de un músculo o de tejido muscular; 2. extirpación de un tumor miomatoso localizado gen. en el útero.

myometrium *n.* miometrio, pared muscular del útero.

myonecrosis *n.* mionecrosis, necrosis del tejido muscular.

myoneural *a.* mioneural, rel. a una terminación nerviosa en un músculo; ___ **junction** / unión ___.

myopathy *n.* miopatía, cualquier enfermedad muscular; **ocular** ___ / ___ ocular.

myope *n.* miope, persona que tiene miopía.

myopia *n.* miopía, defecto del globo ocular por el cual los rayos de luz hacen foco enfrente de la retina, lo que causa dificultad para ver objetos a distancia.

myopic *a.* miope. 1. que padece de miopía; 2. rel. a la miopía.

myorrhexia *n.* miorexia, desgarro en cualquier músculo.

myosin *n.* miosina, la proteína más abundante del tejido muscular.

myositis *n.* miositis, infl. de uno o de más músculos.

myotomy *n.* miotomía, sección o disección de un músculo.

myotonia *n.* miotonía, condición muscular con aumento en rigidez y contractibilidad muscular y disminución de relajamiento.

myringectomy, myringodectomy *n.* miringectomía, extirpación de la membrana timpánica o de una parte de ésta.

myringitis *n.* miringitis, infl. del tímpano.

myringoplasty *n.* miringoplastia, cirugía plástica de la membrana del tímpano.

myxedema *n.* mixedema, condición causada por deficiencia funcional de la tiroides.

myxoma *n.* mixoma, tumor compuesto de tejido conjuntivo.

n

abbr. **nasal** / nasal; **nerve** / nervio; **nitrogen** / nitrógeno; **normal** / normal; **number** / número.

Nabothian cysts *n., pl.* quistes de Naboth, quistes pequeños gen. benignos formados por obstrucción de las glándulas secretoras de mucus del cuello uterino.

nail *n.* 1. uña de los dedos del pie o de la mano; **ingrown** ___ / uñero, ___ encarnada; ___ **scratch** / arañazo; ___ **biting** / comerse la uñas; 2. clavo. **pin.**

nailbed *n.* matriz de la uña, porción de epidermis que cubre la uña.

naive *a.* ingenuo-a; cándido-a; inocente.

naked *a.* desnudo-a, descubierto-a; *pop.* en cuero, en pelota; **with the** ___ **eye** / a simple vista; *v.* **to strip** ___ / desnudarse.

name *n.* nombre; [*first name and surname*] nombre completo, nombre y apellido; **What is your** ___? / ¿Cómo se llama usted?, ¿cómo te llamas tú?, ¿cuál es su, tu nombre?

nanism *n.* nanismo. V. **dwarfism.**

nanocephaly *n.* nanocefalia, desarrollo anormal de la cabeza caracterizada por su pequeñez.

nanocormia *n.* nanocormia. V. **microsomia.**

nanomelia *n.* nanomelia. V. **micromelia.**

nap *n.* siesta; *v.* **to take a** ___ / echar una ___, dormir una ___.

nape *n.* nuca, cerviz, parte posterior del cuello; *pop.* pescuezo, cogote.

napkin *n.* servilleta.

narcissism *n.* narcisismo. 1. amor excesivo a si mismo; 2. placer sexual derivado de la contemplación del propio cuerpo.

narcoanalysis *n.* narcoanálisis, tratamiento de psicoterapia usado originalmente en casos de psicosis de guerra, y también en el tratamiento de trauma infantil. *Syn.* **narcosynthesis.**

narcohypnosis *n.* narcohipnosis, hipnosis inducida por el uso de narcóticos.

narcolepsy *n.* narcolepsia, padecimiento crónico de accesos de sueño.

narcoleptic *a.* narcoléptico-a, rel. a la narcolepsia o que padece de ella.

narcosis *n.* narcosis. 1. letargo y alivio de dolor por el efecto de narcóticos; 2. drogadicción.

narcotherapy *n.* narcoterapia, psicoterapia que se lleva a cabo bajo el efecto de un sedativo o narcótico.

narcotic *a.* narcótico-a, estupefaciente de efecto analgésico que puede producir adicción; ___ **blockade** / bloqueo ___; ___**reversal** / reversión ___.

narcotism *n.* narcotismo. *v.* narcosis.

naris *n.* (*pl.* **nares**) naris, orificios o ventanas de la nariz.

narrow *a.* angosto-a, estrecho-a.

nasal *a.* nasal, rel. a la nariz; ___ **cavity** / cavidad ___; ___**congestion** / congestión ___; ___ **discharge** / secreción ___; ___ **drip** / goteo ___; ___ **hemorrhage** / epistaxis, hemorragia ___; ___ **instillation** / instilación ___, moquera; ___ **meatus** / meato ___; ___**polyp** / pólipo ___; ___ **septum** / tabique ___.

nascent *a.* 1. naciente, incipiente; 2. liberado de un compuesto químico.

nasion *n.* nasión, punto medio de la sutura nasofrontal.

nasogastric *a.* nasogástrico-a, rel. a la nariz y el estómago; ___ **tube** / tubo ___.

nasolabial *a.* nasolabial, rel. a la nariz y al labio.

nasopharynx *n.* nasofaringe, parte de la faringe localizada sobre el velo del paladar. See illustration on page 461.

nasty *a.* agresivo-a, de mal carácter; ___ **illness** / enfermedad grave, seria; ___ **weather** / mal tiempo.

natal *a.* natal, rel. a la natalidad.

natality *a.* natalidad, índice de nacimientos en una comunidad.

natimortality *n.* natimortalidad, índice de mortalidad de muertes perinatales y natales en proporción la mortalidad.

nationality *n.* nacionalidad.

native *n.* nativo-a, [*indigenous*] indígena; *a.* nativo-a, autóctono-a; ___ **born** / nacido-a en; oriundo-a de; ___ **tongue** / lengua materna.

nativity *n.* natividad, nacimiento.

natremia *n.* natremia, presencia de sales de sodio en la sangre.

natriuretic *n.* natriurético-a, diuretic.

natural *a.* natural; sencillo-a; ___ **childbirth** / parto ___; **-ly** *adv.* naturalmente.

natural parents *n., pl.* madre y padre biológicos.

nature *n.* naturaleza.

naturopath *n.* naturópata, persona que practica la naturopatía.

naturopathy *n.* naturopatía, tratamiento terapéutico por medio de recursos naturales.

naughtiness *n.* malacrianza, travesura, majadería.

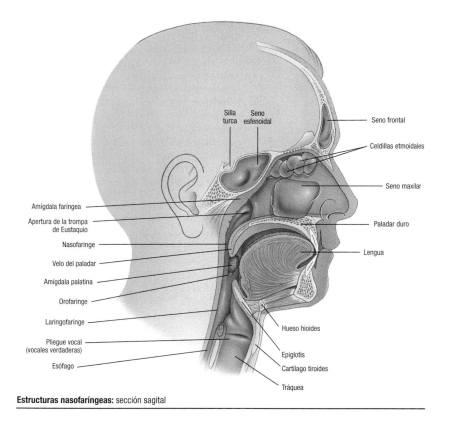

Silla turca | Seno esfenoidal | Seno frontal | Celdillas etmoidales | Seno maxilar | Amígdala faríngea | Apertura de la trompa de Eustaquio | Paladar duro | Nasofaringe | Lengua | Velo del paladar | Amígdala palatina | Orofaringe | Laringofaringe | Hueso hioides | Pliegue vocal (vocales verdaderas) | Epiglotis | Esófago | Cartílago tiroides | Tráquea

Estructuras nasofaríngeas: sección sagital

naughty *a.* travieso-a, majadero-a.

nausea *n.* náusea, asco, ganas de vomitar.

nauseate *v.* dar o causar náuseas, dar asco; **to be nauseated** / tener náuseas.

nauseating *a.* nauseabundo-a.

nauseous *a.* nauseoso-a. 1. propenso a tener náuseas; 2. que produce náusea o asco.

navel *n.* ombligo.

navicular *n.* navicular, hueso escafoide; *a.* en forma de nave; ___ **abdomen** / abdomen ___; ___ **bone** / hueso ___; ___ **fossa of urethra** / fosa ___ de la uretra.

near *a.* cercano-a, próximo-a, a corta distancia; **a ___ relative** / un pariente ___; [*almost*] casi; *prep.* cerca de, junto a; [*at hand*] a la mano; [*toward*] ___ **the right** / hacia la derecha, cerca de la derecha; **-ly** *adv.* casi, por poco; **He, she ___ died** / él, ella por poco se muere.

nearsighted *a.* miope, corto-a de vista.

nearsightedness *n.* miopía. myopia.

neat *a.* pulcro-a, cuidadoso-a, aseado-a; [*very pleasing*] bueno-a.

nebula *n.* nébula, opacidad ligera de la córnea.

nebulization *n.* nebulización, atomización, conversión de un líquido a una nube de vapor.

nebulizer *n.* nebulizador, atomizador de líquido.

nebulous *a.* nebuloso-a.

necessary *n.* necesidad; *a.* necesario-a, indispensable; **It is ___** / Es necesario; **what is ___** / lo necesario; **whatever is ___** / lo que sea necesario.

necessity *n.* necesidad.

neck *n.* cuello, pescuezo. 1. parte del cuerpo que une la cabeza al tronco; 2. región de un diente entre la corona y la raíz.

necklace *n.* collar, gargantilla.

neck of uterus *n.* cuello uterino.

necrobiosis *n.* necrobiosis, degeneración gradual de células y tejidos como resultado de cambios debidos al desarrollo, el envejecimiento y el uso.

necrogenic *a.* necrógeno-a, rel. a la muerte; que se forma o compone de materia muerta.

necrology *n.* necrología, estudio de estadísticas referentes a la mortalidad.

necrophilia *n.* necrofilia. 1. atracción mórbida por los cadáveres; 2. relación sexual con un cadáver.

necrophobia *n.* necrofobia, temor anormal a la muerte y a los cadáveres.

necropsy *n.* necropsia. autopsy.

necrose *v.* necrosar, causar o experimentar necrosis.

necrosis *n.* necrosis, muerte parcial o total de las células que forman un tejido tal como ocurre en la gangrena; **acute massive liver** ___ / ___ hepática masiva aguda; **acute retinal** ___ / ___ aguda de la retina; **aseptic** ___ / ___ aséptica; **caceous** ___ / ___ caseosa; **central** ___ / ___ central; **coagulation** ___ / ___ de coagulación; **cystic medial** ___ / ___ cística media; **fat** ___ / ___ grasa; **focal** ___ / ___ focal; **ischenic** ___ / ___ isquémica; **laminar cortical** ___ / ___ laminar cortical; ___**of epiphysis** / ___ epifisaria; **progressive emphysematous** ___ / ___ progresiva enfisematosa; **progressive outer retinal** ___ / ___ externa progresiva de la retina; **renal papillary** ___ / ___ renal papilar; **simple** ___ / ___ simple; **subcutaneous fat** ___ **of newborn** / ___ de tejidos grasos subcutáneos del neonato; **suppurative** ___ / ___ supurativa; **total** ___ / ___ total.

necrotic *a.* necrótico-a, rel. a la necrosis o a un tejido afectado por ésta.

necrotize *v.* necrosar, causar la muerte, producir necrosis.

need *n.* necesidad; **a person in** ___ / un-a necesitado-a; *v.* necesitar.

needle *n.* aguja; **hypodermic** ___ / ___ hipodérmica;

needless *a.* inútil, innecesario.

needy *n.*, *pl.* necesitados; **the** ___ / los ___; *a.* necesitado-a; pobre;

negation *n.* negación.

negative *a.* negativo-a; ___ **culture** / cultivo ___ ; **-ly** *adv.* negativamente.

negative predictive value *n.* valor pronóstico de un diagnóstico con resultado negativo.

negative transference *n.* transferencia negativa, en el análisis psicológico, el resultado de casos de transferencia que se caracterizan por hostilidad de parte del paciente hacia el analista.

negativism *n.* negativismo, conducta caracterizada por una actuación opuesta a la sugerida.

neglect *n.* negligencia, descuido, desamparo.

neglectful *a.* negligente, descuidado-a.

negligence *n.* negligencia, descuido.

negligent *a.* negligente, descuidado-a.

neighbor *n.* vecino-a.

nemathelminth *n.* nematelminto, gusano intestinal de forma redondeada que pertenece al orden de los *Nemathelmintes.*

nematocide *n.* nematocida, agente que destruye nematodos.

Nematoda *n., L. Nematoda*, clase de gusanos del orden de los *Nemathelmintes.*

nematode *n.* nematodo, gusano de la clase *Nematoda.*

nematodiasis *n.* nematodiasis, infección por parásitos nematodos.

nematology *n.* nematología, estudio de los gusanos de la clase *Nematoda.*

neoarthrosis, nearthrosis *n.* neoartrosis, neartrosis, articulación artificial o falsa.

neologism *n.* neologismo. 1. vocablos a los cuales el paciente mental atribuye nuevos significados no relacionados con el verdadero; 2. vocablo al cual se le atribuye un giro nuevo.

neomycin *n.* neomicina, antibiótico de espectro amplio.

neonatal *a.* neonatal, rel. a las primeras seis semanas después del nacimiento.

neonate *n.* neonato-a, recién nacido-a, de seis semanas o menos de nacido-a.

neonatologist *n.* neonatólogo-a, especialista en neonatología.

neonatology *n.* neonatología, estudio y cuidado de los recién nacidos.

neoplasia *n.* neoplasia, formación de neoplasmas.

neoplasm *n.* neoplasma, crecimiento anormal de tejido nuevo tal como un tumor.

neoplastic *a.* neoplástico-a, rel. a un neoplasma.

neoplastic growth *n.* neoplasia o tumor.

neovascularization *n.* neovascularización, proliferación anormal de nuevos vasos sanguíneos como reacción a la isquemia.

nephew *n.* sobrino.

nephralgia *n.* nefralgia, dolor en el riñón.

nephrectomy *n.* nefrectomía, extirpación de un riñón.

nephric *a.* néfrico-a, renal.
nephritic *n.* nefrítico-a, rel. a la nefritis o afectado por ella.
nephritis *n.* nefritis, infl. del riñón; **acute** ___ / ___ aguda; **analgesic** ___ / ___ analgésica; **chronic** ___ / ___ crónica; **focal** ___ / ___ focal; **glomerular** ___ / ___ glomerular; **hemorrhagic** ___ / ___ hemorrágica; **hereditary** ___ / ___ hereditaria; **immune complex** ___ / ___ de complejo inmune; **interstitial** ___ / ___ intersticial; **lupus** ___ / ___ lipomatosa; **suppurative** ___ / ___ supurativa; **syphilitic** ___ / ___ sifilítica.
nephrocalcinosis *n.* nefrocalcinosis, depósitos de calcio en los túbulos renales que pueden causar insuficiencia renal.
nephrocele *n.* nefrocele, hernia del riñón.
nephrogram *n.* nefrograma, radiografía del riñón.
nephrolithiasis *n.* nefrolitiasis, presencia de cálculos renales.
nephrolithotomy *n.* nefrolitotomía, incisión en el riñón para extraer cálculos renales.
nephrology *n.* nefrología, estudio del riñón y de las enfermedades que lo afectan.
nephroma *n.* nefroma, tumor del riñón.
nephromegaly *n.* nefromegalia, extrema hipertrofia de los riñones.
nephron *n.* nefrona, unidad funcional y anatómica del riñón.
nephropathy *n.* nefropatía, cualquier enfermedad del riñón.
nephropexy *n.* nefropexia, fijación de un riñón flotante.
nephrosclerosis *n.* nefroesclerosis, endurecimiento del sistema arterial y del tejido intersticial del riñón.
nephrosis *n.* nefrosis, afección renal degenerativa asociada con gran cantidad de proteína en la orina, niveles bajos de albúmina en la sangre y edema pronunciado.
nephrostomy *n.* nefrostomía, formación de una fístula en el riñón o en la pelvis renal.
nephrotic syndrome *n.* síndrome nefrótico, afección del riñón caracterizada por un exceso de pérdida de proteína.
nephrotomography *n.* nefrotomografía, tomografía del riñón.
nephrotomy *n.* nefrotomía, incisión en el riñón.
nephrotoxic *a.* nefrotóxico, que destruye células renales.
nephrotoxin *n.* nefrotoxina, toxina que destruye células renales.

nerve *n.* nervio, cada una de las fibras libres o fibras en haz que conectan al cerebro y la médula espinal con otras partes y órganos del cuerpo; ___ **block** / bloqueo del ___; ___ **cells** / neuronas; ___ **degeneration** / degeneración nerviosa; ___ **ending** / terminación del ___; ___ **fiber** / fibra nerviosa; ___ **tissue** / tejido nervioso; **pinched** ___ / ___ pellizcado.
nervous *a.* nervioso-a, ansioso-a, excitable; ___ **breakdown** / colapso ___, crisis ___; ___ **debility** / fatiga ___; ___ **disorder** / trastorno ___; ___ **impulse** / impulso ___; ___ **system** / sistema ___.
nervousness *n.* nerviosismo, nerviosidad.
nervus *n., L. (pl.* **nervi**) nervio.
nest *n.* nido de células, masa de células en forma de nido de pájaro.
nestiatria *n.* nestiatría, terapia con ayuno.
network *n.* red, encadenación; arreglo de fibras en forma de malla.
neural *a.* neural, rel. al sistema nervioso; ___ **arch** / arco ___; ___ **crest** / cresta ___; ___ **cyst** / quiste ___; ___**folds** / pliegues neurales; ___ **plate** / placa ___.
neural hearing loss *n.* pérdida neural de la audición debida a una lesión del octavo nervio craneal.
neuralgia *n.* neuralgia, dolor intenso a lo largo de un nervio; **atypical facial** ___ / ___ facial atípica; **atypical trigeminal** ___ / ___ trigeminal atípica; **facial** ___ / ___ facial; **glossopharyngeal** ___ / ___ glosofaríngea; **hallucinatory** ___ / ___ halucinatoria.
neuralgic *a.* neurálgico-a, rel. a la neuralgia.
neurapraxia *n.* neurapraxia, parálisis temporal de un nervio sin causar degeneración.
neurasthenia *n.* neurastenia, término asociado con un estado general de irritabilidad y agotamiento nervioso; **angiopathic** ___ / ___ angiopática; **gravis** ___ / ___ grave; **praecox** ___ / ___ precoz; **primary** ___ / ___ primaria; **pulsating** ___ / ___ pulsativa.
neurasthenic *a.* neurasténico-a, rel. a o con síntomas de neurastenia.
neurectomy *n.* neurectomía, corte de un segmento del nervio.
neurilemma *n.* neurilema, membrana fina que cubre una fibra nerviosa.
neurinoma *n.* neurinoma, neoplasma benigno de las capas que rodean un nervio.
neuritis *n.* neuritis, infl. de un nervio.
neuro-ophthalmology *n.* neurooftalmología, rama de la oftalmología que se especializa en la

parte del sistema nervioso relacionada con la visión.

neuroanatomy *n.* neuroanatomía, estudio anatómico del sistema nervioso.

neuroblast *n.* neuroblasto, célula nerviosa primitiva.

neuroblastoma *n.* neuroblastoma, tumor maligno del sistema nervioso formado en gran parte por neuroblastos.

neurocyte *n.* neurocito. *v.* neuron.

neurocytoma *n.* neurocitoma, neoplasma, gen. intraventricular.

neurodermatitis *n.* neurodermatitis, trastorno de lesiones cutáneas blanquecinas que gen. se observan en personas nerviosas, y que suelen ser crónicas, diseminadas o localizadas.

neurodermatosis *n.* neurodermatosis, erupción crónica cutánea de origen desconocido que se caracteriza por una picazón intensa en áreas localizadas.

neuroectoderm *n.* neuroectodermo, tejido embrionario del cual se deriva el tejido nervioso.

neuroendocrinology *n.* neuroendocrinología, estudio del sistema nervioso y su relación con las hormonas.

neurofibroma *n.* neurofibroma, tumor del tejido fibroso que cubre un nervio periférico.

neurofibromatosis *n.* neurofibromatosis, condición que se caracteriza por la manifestación de múltiples neurofibromas a lo largo de los nervios periféricos.

neurogenic, neurogenetic *a.* neurogenético. 1. que se origina en el sistema nervioso; 2. rel. a neurogenesis; ___ **atrophy** / atrofia ___.

neuroglia *n.* neuroglia, células que sirven de sostén y constituyen el tejido intersticial del sistema nervioso.

neurohypophysis *n.* neurohipófisis, porción nerviosa posterior de la glándula pituitaria.

neurolepsis *n.* neurolepsia, estado alterado de la conciencia producido por drogas antipsicóticas; el paciente muestra síntomas de ansiedad e indiferencia.

neuroleptic *n.* neuroléptico, agente tranquilizante, pertenece a la clase psicotrópica de fármacos usada en el tratamiento de psicosis, esp. esquizofrenia; **anesthesia** ___ / anestesia con el uso de un ___.

neuroleptic malignant syndrome *n.* síndrome maligno de neurolepsis causado por el uso de agentes neurolépticos y que se manifiesta en síntomas de hipertermia, pérdida del conocimiento y otras reacciones graves

relacionadas con el sistema nervioso central que pueden ocasionar la muerte.

neurologist *n.* neurólogo-a, especialista del sistema nervioso.

neurology *n.* neurología, rama de la medicina que estudia el sistema nervioso.

neurolysin *n.* neurolisina, anticuerpo inyectable que se obtiene de una sustancia cerebral. *Syn.* **neurotoxin.**

neurolysis *n.* neurólisis. 1. proceso de librar un nervio de anejos inflamatorios; 2. destrucción de tejido nervioso.

neuroma *n.* neuroma, tumor constituido principalmente por fibras y células nerviosas; **acoustic** ___ / ___ acústico.

neuromagnetic field *n.* campo neuromagnético.

neuromalacia *n.* neuromalacia, reblandecimiento patológico de un tejido nervioso.

neuromatosis *n.* neuromatosis, la presencia de neuromas múltiples.

neuromeningeal *a.* neuromeníngeo, rel. al tejido nervioso y las meninges.

neuromuscular *a.* neuromuscular, rel. a nervios y músculos; ___ **blocking agents** / agentes bloqueadores neuromusculares; ___ **relaxant** / relajador ___; ___ **system** / sistema ___

neuron *n.* neurona, célula que constituye la unidad básica funcional del sistema nervioso.

neuropacemaker *n.* neuromarcapasos, instrumento para estimular eléctricamente la médula espinal.

neuropathology *n.* neuropatología, ciencia que estudia las enfermedades nerviosas.

neuropathy *n.* neuropatía, trastorno o cambio patológico en los nervios periféricos; **autonomic** ___ / ___ autónoma; **motor** ___ / ___ motora.

neuropharmacology *n.* neurofarmacología, estudio farmacológico del efecto de drogas en el sistema nervioso.

neurophysiology *n.* neurofisiología, fisiología del sistema nervioso.

neuropil *n.* neurópilo, red de fibras nerviosas (dendritas y neuritas) y de las células de la glia interrumpidas por sinapsis en partes del tejido nervioso.

neuropore *n.* neuroporo, apertura embriónica al exterior del canal neural.

neuropsychopharmacology *n.* neurosicofarmacología, estudio de medicamentos y del efecto que causan en el tratamiento de trastornos mentales.

neuroradiology *n.* neurorradiología, radiología del sistema nervioso.

neurosarcocleisis *n.* neurosarcocleisis, intervención quirúrgica para aliviar la neuralgia que consiste en la resección de una pared del canal óseo, llevando el nervio y transplantándolo en tejidos blandos.

neurosis *n.* neurosis, condición que se manifiesta principalmente por ansiedad y por el uso de mecanismos de defensa. See chart on this page.

neurosurgeon *n.* neurocirujano-a, especialista en neurocirugía.

neurosurgery *n.* neurocirugía, del sistema nervioso.

neurosyphilis *n.* neurosífilis, sífilis que afecta el sistema nervioso central; **tabetic** ___ / ___ tabética.

neurotic *a.* neurótico-a, que sufre de neurosis.

neurotomy *n.* neurotomía, disección o división de un nervio.

neurotoxic *a.* neurotóxico-a, que ejerce un efecto tóxico sobre el sistema nervioso. ___ **agent** / ___ agente.

neurotoxicity *n.* neurotoxicidad. 1. la capacidad de una sustancia o agente de destruir o lesionar el tejido nervioso; 2. acción tóxica destructiva, sistema nervioso.

neurotoxin *n.* neurotoxina, cualquier toxina que se asienta específicamente sobre tejido nervioso.

neurotransmitter *n.* neurotransmisor, neurorregulador, sustancia química que modifica la transmisión de impulsos a través de una sinapsis entre nervios o entre un nervio y un músculo; **adrenergic** ___ / ___ adregénico; **cholinergic** ___ / ___ colinérgico.

neurotropic atrophy *n.* atrofia neurotrópica, sinónimo de atrofia neurogénica, anomalía de la piel, tejidos subcutáneos y huesos debida a lesiones de nervios periféricos.

neurotropy, neurotropism *n.* neurotropía, neurotropismo, atracción de organismos patógenos y elementos nocivos, venenos y sustancias nutritivas hacia los centros nervíosos.

neurovascular *a.* neurovascular, rel. a los sistemas nervioso y vascular.

neutral *a.* neutral.

neutralization *n.* neutralización, proceso de anular o contrarrestar la acción de un agente.

neutralize *v.* neutralizar; contrarrestar.

neutropenia *n.* neutropenia. V. **agranulocytosis**.

neutrophil *n.* neutrófilo, leucocito-fagocito que se tiñe con colorantes neutrales.

neutrophilia *n.* neutrofilia, aumento de neutrófilos en la sangre.

neutrotaxis *n.* neutrotaxis, estimulación de neutrófilos con una sustancia que los atrae o repele.

never *adv.* nunca, jamás; ___ **fear** / pierda cuidado; ___ **mind** / no importa.

nevertheless *adv.* sin embargo, no obstante.

nevus *n.* (*pl.* **nevi**) nevo, lunar, marca de nacimiento. **comedonicus** ___ / ___ comedónico; **compound** ___ / ___ compuesto; **dysplastic** ___ / ___ de displasia, con algunas células malignas; **faun tail** ___ / ___ de cola de fauno; **flammeus** ___ / ___ flamante; **junction, junctional** ___ / ___ de unión; **melanocytic** ___ / ___ melanocítico; **sebaceous** ___ / ___ sebáceo.

new *a.* nuevo-a; **What is new?** / ¿Qué hay de ___ ?.

newborn *n.* neonato-a, infante nacido a las 37 semanas de una gestación normal.

news *n., pl.* noticias; **bad** ___ / malas ___; **good** ___ / buenas ___; *v.* **to break the** ___ / dar la noticia.

newspaper *n.* diario, periódico.

next *a.* próximo-a, siguiente; ___ **door** / al lado; ___ **of kin** / el pariente más cercano; ___ **to nothing** / casi nada; **The table is** ___ **to the bed** / La mesa está al lado de la cama; **Who is** ___? / ¿Quién es el, la ___?.

nexus *n.* (*pl.* **nexus**) nexo, conexión, unión.

niacin *n.* ácido nicotínico.

nice *a.* delicado-a, fino-a, bueno-a; **-ly** *adv.* finamente, delicadamente; **nicely done** / bien hecho.

neurosis	neurosis
accidental	accidental
anxiety	de ansiedad
cardiac	cardíaca
character	del carácter
combat	de guerra
compensation	de compensación
compulsive	compulsiva
depressive	depresiva
hypochondriacal	hipocondríaca
hysterical	histérica
obsessional	obsesiva
obsessive-compulsive	obsesiva-compulsiva
occupational	ocupacional
post-traumatic	post-traumática

niche *n.* nicho, depresión o defecto pequeño esp. en la pared de un órgano hueco.

nicotine *n.* nicotina, alcaloide tóxico, ingrediente principal del tabaco.

nictitation *n.* nictitación, acto de guiñar.

nidation *n.* nidación, fijación del huevo fecundado en la mucosa uterina.

nidus *n.* (*pl.* **nidi**) nido.

niece *n.* sobrina.

night *n.* noche; **by** ___ / de noche, por la noche; **Good** ___ / Buenas noches; **last** ___ / anoche; ___ **before last** / anteanoche.

night-blindness *n.* ceguera nocturna. *v.* nyctalopia.

nightfall *n.* atardecer, anochecer.

nightgown *n.* bata de dormir, camisa o camisón.

nightmare *n.* pesadilla.

night vision *n.* visión nocturna. V. **scotopia.**

night watch *n.* guardia nocturna.

nihilism *n.* nihilismo, en psiquiatría una idea ilusoria en la cual nada es real o inexistente.

nipple *n.* pezón; [*of male*] tetilla; [*nursing bottle*] mamadera, tetera; **cracked** ___ / ___ agrietado; **engorged** ___ / ___ enlechado; **retracted** ___ / ___ retractado.

nitric acid *n.* ácido nítrico.

nitrogen *n.* nitrógeno; **authentic, legitimate** ___ / ___ auténtico, legítimo; **blood urea** ___ / concentración plasmática de urea; **illegitimate** ___ / ___ ilegítimo; ___ **monoxid** / ___ monóxido de ___; **residual** ___ / ___ residual.

nitroglycerine *n.* nitroglicerina, nitrato de glicerina usado como vasodilatador esp. en la angina de pecho.

no *adv.* no, de ningún modo, de ninguna manera; **no good** / no vale; ___ **one** / nadie; **Say yes or** ___ / Diga, di que sí o que no.

Nocardia *n. Nocardia*, microorganismo grampositivo que causa nocardiosis.

nocardiosis *n.* nocardiosis, infección generalmente pulmonar causada por *Nocardia* que puede expandirse a varias partes del cuerpo.

nocturia, nycturia *n.* nocturia, nicturia, frecuencia aumentada de emisión de orina esp. durante la noche.

nocturnal *a.* nocturno-a, nocturnal, de noche; ___ **emission, emiction** / micciones ___ s orinarse en la cama; emisión ___ involuntaria de semen.

nod *v.* inclinar la cabeza; aprobar.

node *n.* nudo, nódulo, ganglio; **lymphatic** ___ / ___ linfático;

milker's ___ / ___ de los ordeñadores; **singer's** ___ / ___ vocal o de los cantantes; **syphilis** ___ / ___ sifilítico; **vermis** ___ / ___ del vermis.

nodose *a.* nudoso-a, formado por nódulos o protuberancias.

nodular *a.* nodular, semejante a un nudo.

nodule *n.* nódulo o nudo pequeño; **solitary** ___ / ___ solitario; **subcutaneous** ___ / ___ subcutáneo.

noise *n.* ruido; *v.* **to make** ___ / hacer ___.

noiseless *a.* callado-a, tranquilo-a.

noise pollution *n.* polución de ruido.

noisy *a.* ruidoso-a, turbulento-a, bullicioso-a.

noma *n.* noma, úlcera, estomatitis gangrenosa en la cara interna de la mejilla.

nomadic *a.* nómada, errante.

nomenclature *n.* nomenclatura, terminología.

nominal *a.* nominal; ___ **aphasia** / afasia ___.

non compos mentis *a. L.* non compos mentis, mentalmente incompetente.

none *pron.* nadie, ninguno-a.

noninvasive *a.* no invasor, que no se propaga o invade.

nonparous *a.* nulípara. V. **nulliparous.**

nonsense *n.* tontería, bobería, disparate.

nonspecific *a.* sin especificación.

nonviable *n.* que no puede sobrevivir.

noodle *n.* fideo, tallarín; pasta.

noon *n.* mediodía.

norm *n.* norma, regla.

normal *a.* normal, natural, regular.

normalization *n.* normalización, regreso al estado normal.

normoblast *n.* normoblasto, célula roja precursora de los eritrocitos en los humanos.

normocalcemia *n.* normocalcemia, nivel normal de calcio en la sangre.

normoglycemia *n.* normoglucemia, concentración normal de azúcar en la sangre.

normokalemia *n.* normopotasemia, nivel normal de potasio en la sangre.

normotensive *a.* normotenso-a, de presión arterial normal.

normothermia *n.* normotermia, temperatura normal.

normotonic *a.* normotónico-a, de tono muscular normal.

normovolemia *n.* normovolemia, volumen normal de la sangre.

nose *n.* nariz; **bridge of the** ___ / tabique nasal, puente de la nariz; **running** ___ / nariz destilante; coriza.

nosebleed *n.* sangramiento por la nariz.

nosocomial *a.* nosocomial, rel. a un hospital o clínica; ___ **infection** / infección ___, enfermedad adquirida en un hospital.

nostalgia *n.* nostalgia, tristeza, añoranza.

nostril *n.* naris, fosa nasal, ventana o ala de la nariz.

not *adv.* no, de ningún modo; ___ **at all** / de ninguna manera; **Why not?** / ¿Por qué no?

notalgia *n.* notalgia, dolor en la espalda.

notch *n.* incisión, incisura, ranura, escotadura; **suprasternal** ___ / ___ supraesternal.

note *n.* nota, apunte, aviso; **progress** ___ **-s** / informe del progreso clínico; *v.* notar, apreciar; **to take** ___ **of** / tomar ___ de, darse cuenta de, observar.

nothing *n.* nada, niguna cosa; *adv.* en nada, de ningún modo, de ninguna manera.

notice *n.* aviso, informe, nota; observación; *v.* notar, hacer caso, observar.

noticeable *a.* notorio-a, que se distingue.

notification *n.* notificación, aviso, información.

notify *v.* avisar, informar, notificar; ___ **your doctor at once** / Avise a su médico en seguida.

notion *n.* noción, concepto, opinión.

notochord *n.* notocordio, sostén fibrocelular del embrión que se convierte más tarde en la columna vertebral.

noun *n.* nombre, sustantivo.

nourish *v.* alimentar, nutrir, sustentar.

nourishable *a.* nutritivo-a, alimenticio-a.

nourishing *a.* alimenticio-a, nutritivo-a.

nourishment *n.* alimento, nutrición, sustento.

novice *a.* principiante, novicio-a.

novocaine *n.* novocaína, anestésico.

now *adv.* ahora, ahorita, en este momento, actualmente; **from** ___ **on** / de ___ en adelante; **just** ___ / ___ mismo, hace un momento; ___ **and then** / de vez en cuando; ___ **then** / ahora bien.

nowadays *adv.* hoy en día, al presente.

no way *adv.* de ningún modo, de ninguna manera.

nowhere *adv.* en ninguna parte; ___ **else** / en ninguna otra parte.

nubile *a.* núbil. rel. a la madurez sexual femenina.

nucha *n.* nuca, parte posterior del cuello.

nuchal brace *n.* braguero de cuello.

nuclear *a.* nuclear. 1. rel. al núcleo de la célula; 2. rel. a la fuerza atómica.

nuclear envelope *n.* envoltura nuclear, forma que toman las dos membranas nucleares que envuelven al núcleo de la célula al examinarse bajo el microscopio electrónico.

nuclear magnetic resonance *n.* resonancia magnética nuclear.

nuclear medicine *n.* medicina nuclear, rama de la medicina que concierne el empleo de radionúclidos para usos de diagnóstico y servicios terapéuticos.

nucleated *a.* nucleado-a, que posee un núcleo.

nucleic acid *n.* ácido nucleico.

nucleolus *n.* nucléolo, pequeña estructura esférica en el núcleo celular.

nucleopetal *a.* nucleópeto-a, que se mueve en dirección al núcleo.

nucleotide *n.* nucleótido, unidad estructural de ácido nucleico.

nucleus *n.* (*pl.* **nuclei, nucleuses**) núcleo, parte esencial de una célula; ___ **pulpous** / ___ pulposo, masa gelatinosa contenida dentro de un disco intervertebral.

nude *a.* desnudo-a, *pop.* en cuero, en cuero vivo.

nudity *n.* desnudez.

nuisance *n.* molestia, incomodidad, estorbo; **What a** ___ **!** / ¡Qué lata!.

null *a.* nulo-a, sin valor, inútil; ___ **hypothesis** / hipótesis ___.

nulligravida *n.* nuligrávida, mujer que nunca ha concebido.

nulliparous *n.* nulípara, mujer que nunca ha dado a luz un feto con vida.

numb *a.* [*extremity*] entumecido-a, adormecido-a; aturdido-a; **my fingers are** ___ / mis dedos están ___ **-s**; **I feel** ___ / Me siento entumecido-a; me siento aturdido-a.

numb chin syndrome *n.* síndrome del mentón entumecido, pérdida de sensación y parestesia con calambre en un lado del mentón y el labio inferior como resultado de una condición de infiltración neoplásica del nervio mental ipsilateral obstruido por un mioloma o un carcinoma de la mama o de la próstata.

number *n.* número, cifra.

numbness *n.* [*in a part*] entumecimiento, adormecimiento; [*confusion*] aturdimiento, entorpecimiento.

numerous *a.* numeroso-a.

numskull *a.* mentecato-a, tonto-a.

nun *n.* monja, hermana religiosa.

nurse *n.* enfermero-a; **chief** ___, **head** ___ / jefe-a de ___ **-s**; **community health** ___ / ___ de salud pública; ___ **aid** / asistente de ___; ___ **anesthetist** / ___ anestesista; ___ **practitioner** / practicante de ___; **surgical** ___ / ___ de cirugía; *v.* [*care*] cuidar a una persona enferma; [*breast-feeding*] amamantar, dar el pecho, dar de mamar.

nursery *n.* guardería; [*in a hospital*] sala de niños recién nacidos.

nursing *n.* 1. cuidado de los enfermos; 2. lactancia.

nut *n.* [*fruit*] nuez; [*mad*] loco-a, maniático-a; [*screw*] tuerca.

nutrient *n.* alimento, nutriente, sustancia nutritiva.

nutriment *n.* nutrimento, alimento, sustancia nutritiva.

nutrition *n.* nutrición, mantenimiento, alimentación.

nutritious *a.* nutritivo-a, alimenticio-a, que proporciona nutrición.

nutritive *a.* nutritivo-a, sustancioso-a, alimenticio-a.

nutty *a.* abundante en nueces, con sabor a nueces; *pop.* [*crazy*] loco-a, chiflado-a.

nyctalopia *n.* nictalopía, visión imperfecta bajo iluminación baja.

nympha *n.* ninfa, labio interior de la vulva.

nymphectomy *n.* ninfectomía, excisión parcial o total de la labia menor.

nymphomania *n.* ninfomanía, fuego uterino, deseo sexual mórbido en la mujer.

nymphomaniac *a.* ninfómana, mujer afectada por ninfomanía.

nystagmography *n.* nistagmografía, técnica para registrar nistagmo.

nystagmus *n.* nistagmo, espasmo involuntario del globo ocular; **palatal** ___ / ___ palatal.

O

O *abbr.* **oculus** / ojo; **oral** / oral; **orally** / oralmente, por la boca; **oxygen** / oxígeno.

oath *n.* juramento, promesa; **Hippocratic** ___ / ___ hipocrático; **under** ___ / bajo ___; *v.* **to take an** ___ / jurar, prestar ___.

oatmeal *n.* harina de avena.

obedience *n.* obediencia.

obedient *a.* obediente.

obese *a.* obeso-a, excesivamente grueso-a.

obesity *n.* obesidad, grasa excesiva en el cuerpo; **alimentary** ___ / ___ alimentaria; **endogenous** ___ / ___ endógena; **exogenous** ___ / ___ exógena.

obey *v.* obedecer; **You must** ___ / usted debe ___, tú debes ___.

obfuscation *n.* ofuscación, confusión mental.

object *n.* objeto, cosa; *v.* objetar, oponerse, tener inconveniente.

objective *n.* objetivo, propósito; *a.* objetivo-a, rel. a la percepción de fenómenos y sucesos tal como se manifiestan en la vida real; ___ **sign** / señal ___; ___ **symptoms** / síntomas ___ -s; **-ly** *adv.* objetivamente.

obligate *v.* obligar, exigir.

obligation *n.* obligación, deber, compromiso.

obligatory *a.* obligatorio-a.

oblique *a.* oblicuo-a, diagonal.

obliquity *n.* oblicuidad, estado de estar inclinado-a.

obliterate *v.* obliterar, anular, destruir.

obliteration *n.* obliteración, destrucción; oclusión por degeneración o por cirugía.

obscure *a.* oscuro-a; oculto-a, escondido-a.

observation *n.* observación, examen, estudio.

observe *v.* observar, estudiar, examinar.

obsession *n.* obsesión, preocupación excesiva con una idea o emoción fija.

obsessional *a.* obsesivo-a, rel. a una obsesión o causante de ésta.

obsessive-compulsive *n.* estado neurótico obsesivo-compulsivo con repetición morbosa de acciones como desahogo de tensiones y ansiedades.

obsolete *a.* obsoleto-a, anticuado-a, en desuso, inactivo-a.

obstacle *n.* obstáculo, *pop.* traba.

obstetric *a.* obstétrico-a, rel. a la obstetricia.

obstetrician *n.* obstetra, partero-a, tocólogo-a, especialista en obstetricia.

obstetrics *n.* obstetricia, rama de la medicina que se refiere al cuidado de la mujer durante el embarazo y el parto.

obstinate *a.* obstinado-a, *pop.* cabeza dura, cabeciduro-a.

obstipation *n.* obstipación, estreñimiento rebelde.

obstruct *v.* obstruir, impedir.

obstructed *a.* obstruido-a, tupido-a.

obstruction *n.* obstrucción, bloqueo, obstáculo, impedimento; **intestinal** ___ / ___ intestinal.

obstructive lung disease, chronic *n.* obstrucción crónica del pulmón que impide la entrada libre del aire a causa de un estrechamiento físico o funcional del árbol bronquial.

obtain *v.* obtener, adquirir, conseguir.

obturation *n.* obturación, obstrucción o bloqueo de un pasaje.

obturator *a.* obturador-a, bloqueador-a, que obstruye una abertura.

obtuse *a.* obtuso-a. 1. que le falta agudeza mental; 2. romo-a, mellado-a.

obvious *a.* obvio-a, evidente.

occasion *n.* ocasión, circunstancia, casualidad; *v.* causar, ocasionar.

occasional *a.* infrecuente, casual, accidental; **-ly** *adv.* a veces; de vez en cuando, ocasionalmente.

occipital *a.* occipital, rel. a la parte posterior de la cabeza; ___ **bone** / hueso ___; ___ **condyle** / cóndilo ___; ___ **lobe** / lóbulo ___.

occipitofrontal *a.* occipitofrontal. rel. al occipucio y la frente.

occipitoparietal *a.* occipitoparietal, rel. a los huesos y lóbulos occipital y parietal.

occipitotemporal *a.* occipitotemporal, rel. a los huesos occipital y temporal.

occiput *n.* occipucio, porción postero-inferior del cráneo.

occlusion *n.* oclusión, cierre, obstrucción; **coronary** ___ / ___ coronaria; **pupillar** ___ / ___ de la pupila.

occult *a.* oculto-a, desconocido-a; escondido-a.

occult blood *n.* sangre oculta, presencia de sangre en cantidad tan ínfima que no puede verse a simple vista.

occupation *n.* ocupación, trabajo, profesión, oficio, ___ **neurosis** / neurosis del trabajo, de la profesión.

occupational *a.* ocupacional, rel. a una ocupación; ___ **health** / salud ___; ___ **injuries** / lesiones laborales; ___ **therapist** / terapista ___; ___ **therapy** / terapia ___.

occupy *v.* ocupar, llenar.

occurrence *n.* ocurrencia, suceso, acontecimiento; **of frequent ___** / que sucede con frecuencia.

octogenarian *n.* octogenario-a, persona de ochenta años de edad o más; *a.* octogenario-a.

ocular *a.* ocular, visual, rel. a los ojos o a la vista. **___ foreign body ___** / cuerpo extraño; **___ movements** / movimientos **___**; **ataxia** / ataxia **___**; **___cone** / cono **___**; **vertigo ___** / vértigo **___**.

oculist *n.* oculista. V. **ophthalmologist.**

oculography *n.* oculografía, método que registra la posición y movimiento de los ojos.

oculogyric *a.* oculógiro-a, rel. a la rotación del globo ocular.

oculomotor *a.* oculomotor, rel. al movimiento del globo ocular.

oculus *L.* oculus, ojo, órgano de la visión.

odd *a.* extraño-a, irregular, raro-a, inexacto-a; **an ___ case** / un caso **___**; **___or even** / nones o pares; **thirty ___ pills** / treinta píldoras más o menos, treinta y tantas píldoras; **at ___ times** / en momentos imprevistos, a horas imprevistas.

Oddi's sphincter *n.* Oddi, esfínter de, músculo circular contráctil localizado al nivel de la incisura angular del estómago y de los conductos pancreáticos.

odontalgia *n.* odontalgia, dolor de dientes; dolor de muelas.

odontectomy *n.* odontectomía, extracción de una pieza dental.

odontogenesis *n.* odontogénesis, proceso de desarrollo dentario.

odontoid *a.* odontoideo-a, semejante a un diente.

odontologist *n.* odontólogo-a, dentista o cirujano-a dental.

odontology *n.* odontología, estudio de los dientes y del tratamiento de las enfermedades dentales.

odontoplasty *n.* procedimiento quirúrgico que se usa para mejorar el control de placas y cuidado de las encías.

odor *n.* olor.

odorless *a.* sin olor, inodoro-a.

odorous *a.* oloroso-a, fragante.

odynophobia *n.* odinofobia, temor excesivo al dolor.

Oedipus complex *n.* complejo de Edipo, amor patológico del hijo a la madre acompañado de celos y antipatía al padre.

of *prep.* de; [*possession*] **___ the** / del, de la; [*telling time*] / menos; **call at a quarter ___ six** / Llame, llama a las seis **___** cuarto.

off *adv.* fuera de aquí, lejos; **___ and on** / a veces, a intervalos; **___ the record** / confidencial; *v.* [*work*] **to be ___** / ausente, [*without work*] sin trabajo; **the operation is ___** / se ha suspendido la operación; **to put ___** / aplazar, posponer, diferir; **to turn ___** / cerrar, apagar; *int.* ¡fuera!, ¡salga!, ¡sal!

offence, offense *n.* ofensa, agravio, afrenta.

offend *v.* ofender, insultar, agraviar.

offensive *a.* ofensivo-a.

offer *n.* oferta, ofrecimiento.

office *n.* oficina; **doctor's ___** / consulta, consultorio; [*business*] **___**; **hours** / horas de **___**; horas de consulta.

official *a.* oficial, autorizado-a.

offspring *n.* descendencia, sucesión, hijos.

often *adv.* con frecuencia, frecuentemente, a menudo; **how ___?** / ¿Cuántas veces?; **as ___ as needed** / tantas veces como sea necesario; **not ___** / pocas veces; **too ___** / demasiadas veces.

oil *n.* aceite; **castor ___** / **___** de ricino; **cod liver ___** / **___** de hígado de bacalao; **mineral ___** / **___** mineral; **olive ___** / **___** de oliva; **salad ___** / **___** para ensalada; *v.* aceitar, lubricar, engrasar, untar con aceite.

oily *a.* grasoso-a, grasiento-a, oleaginoso-a, lubricante.

ointment *n.* ungento, pomada, unto, untura; medicamento oleaginoso semisólido de uso externo.

old *a.* viejo-a, anciano-a; antiguo-a; **an ___ man** / un anciano, un hombre **___**; **an ___ method** / un método antiguo; **How ___ are you?** / ¿Cuántos años tiene, tienes?; **I am fifty years ___** / Tengo cincuenta años; **___ wives' tale** / cuento de **___** -s.

oleaginous *a* oleaginoso-a, aceitoso-a, derivado del aceite o rel. al mismo.

oleomargarine *n.* oleomargarina, margarina.

olfaction *n.* olfacción. 1. el acto de oler; 2. el sentido del olor.

olfactory *a.* olfatorio-a, rel. al sentido del olfato.

oligodactylia *n.* oligodactilia, carencia del número normal de dedos en las manos o los pies.

oligodendrocyte *n.* oligodendrocito, célula de la neuroglia que participa en pocos aunque delicados procesos.

oligodendroglia *n.* oligodendroglia, células de la neuroglia que forman o mantienen el tejido del sistema nervioso central.

oligodontia *n.* oligodoncia, condición hereditaria que resulta en un numéro menor de dientes que el normal.

oligohemia, oligemia *n.* oligohemia. **hypovolemia.**

oligohydramnios *n.* oligohidramnios, bajo nivel de líquido amniótico al término de la gestación.

oligomenorrhea *n.* oligomenorrea, deficiencia en la menstruación.

oligospermia *n.* oligospermia, disminución del número de espermatozoos en el semen.

oliguria *n.* oliguria, disminución en la formación de orina.

olive *n.* oliva. 1. materia gris localizada detrás de la médula oblongata; 2. color aceitunado, verde oliva; 3. árbol del olivo; 4. aceituna.

omalgia *n.* omalgia, dolor en el hombro.

omen *n.* agero.

omental *a.* omental, rel. a un omento o formado por él.

omentectomy *n.* onentectomía, extirpación total o parcial de un omento.

omentitis *n.* omentitis, infl. del omento.

omentum *n.* omento, repliegue del peritoneo que conecta el estómago con ciertas vísceras abdominales.

ominous *a.* ominoso-a, nefasto-a.

omission *n.* omisión; exclusión.

omit *v.* omitir, suprimir, excluir.

omnivorous *a.* omnívoro-a, que come alimentos de origen vegetal y animal.

omphalectomy *n.* onfalectomía, extirpación del ombligo.

omphalic *n.* onfálico-a, rel. al ombligo.

omphalitis *n.* onfalitis, infl. del ombligo.

omphalocele *n.* onfalocele, hernia congénita del ombligo.

on *prep.* sobre, encima, en, hacia; [*before inf.*] después de; al; ___ **an average** / por término medio; ___ **the contrary** / al contrario; ___ **the left foot** / en el pie izquierdo; ___ **the right eye** / en el ojo derecho; ___ **the table** / sobre la mesa, encima de la mesa; *adv.* ___ **account of** / a causa de; ___ **all sides** / por todos lados; *v.* **to be** ___ **call** / estar de guardia; **caught** ___ / atrapado-a en; ___ **condition that you come back** / con tal de que vuelva; **later** ___ / más tarde; **off and** ___ / a intervalos, de vez en cuando; ___ **and** ___ / continuamente, sin cesar, sin parar; ___ **purpose** / a propósito; [*function*] funcionando; **The machine is on** / El aparato está funcionando; *a.* [*clothing*] puesto-a; **She has the robe on** / Ella tiene la bata ___; [*after a verb*]; **Go** ___! / ¡Siga, sigue!; ¡Continúe, continúa!.

onanism *n.* onanismo, coito interrumpido.

once *n.* una vez; *adv.* **all at** ___ / al mismo tiempo, de pronto; **at** ___ / en seguida, ahora mismo; ___ **in a while** / algunas veces, de vez en cuando.

oncogenesis *n.* oncogénesis, formación y desarrollo de un tumor.

oncogenic *a.* oncogénico-a, rel. a la oncogénesis.

oncologist *n.* oncólogo-a. especialista en oncología.

oncology *n.* oncología, rama de la medicina que estudia los neoplasmas.

oncolysis *n.* oncólisis, destrucción de las células de un tumor.

oncotic *a.* oncótico-a, rel. a una tumefacción o la causa de ésta.

oncotomy *n.* oncotomía, incisión en un tumor, absceso o quiste.

one *n.* [*number*] uno; *a.* un, uno-a, solo, único-a; **just** ___ / solamente uno; **only** ___ **form** / una sola forma; **from** ___ **day to another** / de un día a otro; **he is** ___ **good patient** / él es un buen paciente; *pron.* **the only** ___ / el único, la única; **the** ___ **I have** / el que tengo; **this** ___ / éste; ___**and all** / todos; ___**of them** / ___ de ellos.

one-eyed *n.* tuerto-a.

oneiric *a.* onírico-a, rel. a los sueños.

oneirism *n.* onirismo, estado de ensoñación; soñar despierto.

onerous *a.* oneroso-a, gravoso-a.

onicopathy *n.* onicopatía, cualquier enfermedad de la uña.

oniomania *n.* oniomanía, psicosis de urgencia de gastar dinero.

onion *n.* cebolla.

onlay *n.* injerto, esp. en la reparación de defectos óseos.

only *a.* único-a, solo-a; *adv.* sólo, solamente.

onomatomania *n.* onomatomanía, repetición obsesiva de palabras.

onychectomy *n.* oniquectomía, extirpación de una uña.

onychia *n.* oniquia, infl. de la matriz de una uña.

onychosis *n.* onicosis, enfermedad o deformidad de las uñas.

oocyte *n.* oocito, ovocito, el óvulo antes de la madurez.

oogenesis *n.* oogénesis, formación y desarrollo del óvulo.

ookinesis *n.* oocinesis, mitosis del óvulo en el ovario embriónico durante la maduración y fecundación.

oophorectomy *n.* ooforectomía, excisión parcial o total de un ovario.

oophoritis *n.* ooforitis, infl. de un ovario.

oophorocystosis *n.* ooforocistosis, formación de un ovario cístico.

oophoropexy *n.* ooforopexia, fijación o suspensión de un ovario desplazado.

oosperm *n.* oospermo, óvulo fecundado.

ooze *v.* exudar, supurar.

oozing *n.* exudado; supuración.

opacification *n.* opacificación, proceso de opacar.

opacity *n.* opacidad, falta de transparencia.

opaque *a.* opaco-a, sin brillo, que no deja pasar la luz.

open *a.* abierto-a, descubierto-a, destapado-a, libre de paso; ___ **heart surgery** / operación a corazón ___; *v.* abrir, descubrir, destapar, abrir paso; cortar, rajar.

open reduction *n.* reducción abierta, [*in fractures*] técnica de reducir fracturas con exposición de la dislocación o del hueso.

opening *n.* abertura, orificio de entrada o salida.

operable *a.* operable, que puede tratarse con cirugía.

operate *v.* operar, intervenir, proceder.

operating room *n.* sala de operaciones, quirófano.

operation *n.* operación, intervención quirúrgica, procedimiento quirúrgico.

operculum *n.* opérculo. 1. cubierta o tapadera; 2. una de las partes del cerebro que cubre la ínsula.

operon *n.* operon, sistema de genes combinados en el cual el gene operador regula los demás genes estructurales.

ophthalmia *n.* oftalmía. 1. conjuntivitis severa; 2. infl. interna del ojo.

ophthalmic *a.* oftálmico-a, visual, rel. al ojo; ___ **nerve** / nervio ___; ___ **solutions** / soluciones ___ -s.

ophthalmitis *n.* oftalmitis, condición inflamatoria del ojo.

ophthalmologist *n.* oftalmólogo-a, médico oculista especializado en trastornos y enfermedades de la vista.

ophthalmology *n.* oftalmología, rama de la medicina que trata del estudio del ojo y trastornos de la vista.

ophthalmoneuritis *n.* oftalmoneuritis, infl. del nervio óptico.

ophthalmopathy *n.* oftalmopatía, enfermedad de los ojos.

ophthalmoplasty *n.* oftalmoplastia, cirugía plástica del ojo.

ophthalmoplegia *n.* oftalmoplegia, parálisis de un músculo ocular.

ophthalmoscope *n.* oftalmoscopio, instrumento usado para visualizar el interior del ojo.

ophthalmoscopy *n.* oftalmoscopía, examen del ojo con un oftalmoscopio.

opiate *n.* opiáceo, opiato, cualquier droga derivada del opio; ___ **abstinence syndrome** / síndrome provocado por la abstinencia de opio o sus derivados.

opinion *n.* opinión, juicio, parecer; *v.* **to have an** ___ / opinar, hacer juicio, dar el parecer; **to be of the same** ___ / estar de acuerdo, acordar.

opinionated *a.* obstinado-a, inflexible.

opioids *n. pl.* drogas que no son derivadas del opio pero pueden producir efectos similares a éste.

opisthotonos *n.* opistótonos, espasmo tetánico de los músculos de la espalda por el cual los talones se viran hacia atrás y el tronco se proyecta hacia adelante.

opium *n.* opio, *Papaver somniferum*, narcótico, analgésico, estimulante venenoso y alucinógeno cuya adicción produce deteriorización física y mental.

opiumism, opiomania *n.* opiomanía. 1. adicción al uso de opio o sus derivados; 2. condición física deteriorada por el uso de opio.

opponent *n.* oponente, antagonista, contrario-a; *a.* opuesto-a, contrario-a.

opportune *a.* oportuno-a, conveniente.

opportunist *n.* oportunista.

opportunistic *a.* oportunista.

opportunistic infectious disease *n.* enfermedad oportunista infecciosa, infección parasítica oportunista, producida por un microorganismo gen. no dañino, que no causa una enfermedad severa o prolongada pero se convierte en patógeno cuando la inmunidad del organismo ha sido ya quebrantada.

opportunity *n.* oportunidad, ocasión.

oppose *v.* oponer, resistir; oponerse, resistirse.

opposite *a.* opuesto-a, adverso-a, contrario-a.

opposition *n.* oposición, objeción.

oppress *v.* oprimir, afligir, agobiar; apretar.

oppression *n.* opresión, pesadez; **an** ___ **in the chest** / una ___, una sofocación en el pecho.

oppressive *a.* opresivo-a, sofocante, molesto-a, gravoso-a.

opsoclonus *n.* opsoclono, movimiento irregular del ojo, esp. relacionado con algunos casos de trastorno cerebral.

opsonin *n.* opsonina, anticuerpo que al combinarse con un antígeno hace que éste sea más suceptible a los fagocitos.

optic, optical *a.* óptico-a, rel. a la visión; ___ **disk** / disco ___, punto ciego de la retina; ___ **illusion** / ilusión ___; ___**nerve** / nervio ___.

optics *n.* óptica, ciencia que estudia la luz y la relación de ésta con la visión.

optimist *a.* optimista.

optimum *a.* óptimo-a, el mejor, la mejor; ___ **temperature** / temperatura ___.

option *n.* opción, alternativa.

optometer *n.* optómetro, instrumento usado para medir el poder de refracción del ojo.

optometrist *n.* optometrista, optómetra, profesional que practica la optometría.

optometry *n.* optometría, práctica de examinar los ojos para determinar la agudeza visual y para la prescripción de lentes correctivos y otros auxilios visuales.

or *conj.* o, u (*used instead of o before words beginning in o or ho*).

oral *a.* oral, bucal, rel. a la boca; verbal, hablado; ___ **contraceptive** / píldora contraceptiva; ___ **diagnosis** / diagnóstico bucal; ___ **hygiene** / higiene bucal.

orange *n.* naranja; ___ **grove** / naranjal; **orangeade** / naranjada.

orbicular *a.* orbicular, circular; ___ **ciliaris** / ___ de los párpados; ___ **muscle** / músculo ___, rodea una pequeña abertura tal como la de la boca; ___ **oris** / ___ de los labios.

orbit *n.* órbita, cavidad ósea de la cara que contiene los ojos.

orbital *a.* orbital. rel. a la órbita; ___ **fractures** / fracturas ___ -es.

orchidectomy *n.* orquidectomía, orquectomía, extirpación de un testículo.

orchiditis, orchitis *n.* orquiditis, orquitis, infl. de los testículos.

orchidopexy, orchiopexy *n.* orquidopexia, orquipexia, procedimiento por el cual se baja y se fija al escroto un testículo que no ha descendido.

orchiotomy *n.* orquiotomía, incisión en un testículo.

order *n.* orden, reglamento, disposición; **in** ___ **that** / para que, a fin de que; **in** ___ **to** / para; *v.* ordenar, disponer, mandar; [*arrange*] arreglar; **to be in good** ___ / estar en buen estado; **to get out of** ___ / descomponerse.

orderly *n.* asistente de enfermero-a.

ordinary *a.* ordinario-a, corriente, común.

orexigenic *a.* orexígeno-a, que estimula el apetito.

organ *n.* órgano, parte del cuerpo que realiza una función específica; **end** ___ / ___ terminal; ___ **displacement** / desplazamiento de un ___; ___ **transplant** / transplante de un ___.

organelle *n.* organelo, organito, órgano diminuto de los organismos unicelulares.

organic *a.* orgánico-a. 1. rel. a un órgano u órganos; 2. rel. a organismos de origen vegetal o animal; ___ **disease** / enfermedad ___.

organism *n.* organismo, ser vivo.

organization *n.* organización; asociación.

organize *v.* organizar, disponer, arreglar.

organogenesis *n.* organogénesis, desarrollo y crecimiento de un órgano.

organomegaly *n.* organomegalia, agrandamiento de los órganos viscerales.

orgasm *n.* orgasmo, clímax sexual.

orient *n.* oriente, este.

oriental *a.* oriental.

orientation *n.* orientación, dirección.

orifice *n.* orificio, salida, boquete, abertura.

origin *n.* origen, principio.

original *n.* original, prototipo; *a.* original; primitivo-a.

originality *n.* originalidad.

originate *v.* originar, engendrar; provenir de.

originator *n.* originador, productor.

ornithine *n.* ornitina, aminoácido que aunque no está presente en las proteínas desempeña un papel importante en el ciclo de la urea.

orofacial *a.* orofacial, rel. a la boca y a la cara.

oropharynx *n.* orofaringe, parte central de la faringe.

Oroya fever *n.* Oroya, fiebre de, fiebre (calentura) muy elevada que se observa en el Perú y se manifiesta con anemia perniciosa y extrema sensibilidad del tejido hemopoyético.

orphan *n.* huérfano-a.

orphanage *n.* orfanato, hospicio, asilo de huérfanos.

orthocephalic *a.* ortocefálico-a, que posee un cráneo normal proporcionado al cuerpo, con un índice cefálico vertical entre 70 y 75.

orthochromatic *a.* ortocromático-a, de color normal o que acepta coloración sin dificultad.

orthodiagraph *n.* ortodiágrafo, aparato radiográfico que determina con precisión la forma, posición y tamaño de órganos internos u objetos extraños en el cuerpo.

orthodontia *n.* ortodoncia, rama de la odontología que trata las irregularidades dentales por medio de procedimientos correctivos.

orthomyxovirus *n.* ortomixovirus, familia de virus a la cual pertenecen los tres grupos de virus de la influenza.

orthopedia, orthopedics *n.* ortopedia, rama de la medicina que trata de la prevención y corrección de trastornos en los huesos, articulaciones, músculos, ligamentos y cartílagos.

orthopedic *a.* ortopédico-a, rel. a la ortopedia; ___ **shoes** / calzado ___ ; ___ **surgery** / cirugía ___.

orthopedist *n.* ortopédico-a, ortopedista, especialista en ortopedia.

orthopnea *n.* ortópnea, dificultad para respirar excepto en posición erecta.

orthopsychiatry *n.* ortopsiquiatría, rama de la psiquiatría que comprende psiquiatría infantil, pediatría e higiene mental y se dedica a la prevención y tratamiento de trastornos psicológicos en niños y adolescentes.

orthoptics *n.* ortóptica, el estudio y corrección de trastornos de la visión binocular y los movimientos oculares.

orthoscopic *a.* ortoscópico, rel. a los instrumentos que se usan para corregir distorsiones ópticas.

orthosis *n.* ortosis, corrección de una deformidad o impedimento.

orthotonos, orthotonus *n.* ortótonos, espasmo como el del tétano que se caracteriza por una rigidez en línea recta de la nuca, las extremidades y el cuerpo.

orthotopic *a.* ortotópico-a, que ocurre en una posición normal o correcta.

os *n., L.* (*pl.* **ossa**) os, hueso.

oscillate *v.* oscilar; fluctuar.

oscillation *n.* oscilación, movimiento de vaivén, tal como el de un péndulo.

oscillatory *a.* oscilatorio-a, que oscila.

oscillopsia *n.* oscilopsia, visión oscilante durante el progreso de la esclerosis múltiple.

Osgood-Schlatter disease *n.* Osgood-schlatter, enfermedad de, infl. de la apófisis.

osmolar *a.* osmolar, de naturaleza o propiedad osmótica.

osmology *n.* osmología. estudio de los olores.

osmoreceptor *n.* osmorreceptor. 1. grupo de células cerebrales que reciben estímulos olfatorios; 2. grupo de células en el hipotálamo que responden a cambios en la presión osmótica de la sangre.

osmosis *n.* osmosis, difusión de un solvente a través de una membrana semipermeable interpuesta entre soluciones de concentración diferente.

osmotic *a.* osmótico-a, rel. a la osmosis.

osseous *a.* óseo-a, rel. a los huesos; ___ **tissue** / tejido ___.

ossicle *n.* huesillo, osículo.

ossific *a.* osífico-a, rel. a la formación del tejido óseo.

ossification *n.* osificación, proceso de desarrollo óseo.

ossification, ostosis *n.* osificación. 1. conversión de una sustancia en hueso; 2. desarrollo del hueso.

ossify *v.* osificar, transformarse en hueso.

osteal *a.* óseo-a, rel. a los huesos.

osteitis *n.* osteítis, ostitis, infl. de un hueso; ___ **fibrosa cystica** / ___ fibrosa cística, con degeneración fibrosa y manifestación de quistes y nódulos en el hueso.

ostensive *a.* ostensivo-a, evidente, aparente.

osteoaneurysm *n.* osteoaneurisma, aneurisma que ocurre en un hueso.

osteoarthritis *n.* osteoartritis, hipertrofia degenerativa del hueso y de las articulaciones esp. en la vejez.

osteoarthropathy *n.* osteoartropatía, enfermedad gen. dolorosa que afecta las articulaciones y los huesos.

osteoblast *n.* osteoblasto, célula desarrollada aisladamente en una lacuna de la sustancia ósea.

osteoblastoma *n.* osteoblastoma. V. **osteoma**.

osteocarcinoma *n.* osteocarcinoma, cáncer del hueso.

osteocartillaginous *a.* osteocartilaginoso-a, rel. a la formación de huesos y cartílagos.

osteochondral *n.* osteocondral, rel. a o compuesto de hueso y cartílago.

osteochondritis *n.* osteocondritis, infl. del hueso y del cartílago.

osteochondroma *n.* osteocondroma, tumor compuesto de elementos óseos y cartilaginosos.

osteoclast *n.* osteoclasto, célula gigante multinucleada que participa en la formación de tejido óseo y reemplaza al cartílago durante la osificación.

osteocyte *n.* osteocito, célula ósea desarrollada.

osteodystrophy *n.* osteocito, célula ósea desarrollada.

osteodystrophy *n.* osteeodistrofia, hipertrofia múltiple degenerativa con formación defectiva del hueso.

osteogenesis *n.* osteogénesis. V. **ossification**.

osteoid *a.* osteoide, rel. o semejante a un hueso.

osteology *n.* osteología, rama de la medicina que estudia la estructura y funcionamiento de los huesos.

osteoma *n.* osteoma, tumor formado de tejido óseo.

osteomalacia *n.* osteomalacia, reblandecimiento de los huesos debido a la pérdida de calcio en la matriz del hueso.

osteomyelitis *n.* osteomielitis, infección del hueso y de la médula ósea.

osteomyelodysplasia *n.* osteomielodisplasia, desplazamiento óseo caracterizado por estrechez de la capa ósea, un aumento de la cavidad medular, leucopenia y fiebre.

osteonecrosis *n.* osteonecrosis, destrucción y muerte del tejido óseo.

osteopath *n.* osteópata, especialista en osteopatía.

osteopathy *n.* osteopatía. 1. sistema terapéutico médico con énfasis en la relación entre los órganos y el sistema muscular esquelético que hace uso de la manipulación como medio de corrección; 2. cualquier enfermedad de los huesos.

osteopenia *n.* osteopenia, disminución de la calcificación ósea.

osteophyte *n.* osteófito, prominencia ósea.

osteoplastic *a.* osteoplástico-a. 1. rel. a la formación de un hueso; 2. cirugía plástica de un hueso.

osteoporosis *n.* osteoporosis, pérdida en la densidad del hueso.

osteosarcoma *n.* osteosarcoma, sarcoma óseo o que contiene tejido óseo.

osteosynthesis *n.* osteosíntesis, fijación quirúrgica de un hueso mediante el uso de un medio mecánico tal como una placa o un clavo.

osteotomy *n.* osteotomía, cortar o serruchar un hueso.

ostial *a.* ostial, rel. o concerniente a un orificio o abertura.

ostium *n., L.* (*pl.* **ostia**) ostium, pequeña abertura.

ostium primum *L.* ostium primum, apertura que comunica las dos aurículas del corazón fetal y que se empequeñece gradualmente.

ostomy *n.* ostomía, creación de una abertura entre un órgano y la piel como medio de salida exterior, tal como se efectúa en colostomías e ileostomías.

otalgia, otodynia, otoneuralgia *n.* otalgia, otodinia, otoneuralgia, dolor de oídos.

Ota's nevus *n.* Ota, nevus de, nevus que puede desarrollarse en melanoma.

otectomy *n.* otectomía, extirpación del contenido estructural del oído medio.

other *a.* otro-a, diferente, nuevo-a; **every ___ day** / un día sí y otro no; *pron.* **the ___ one** / el otro, la otra; **the ___ ones** / los otros, las otras.

otherwise *adv.* de otra manera, de otro modo, por otra parte.

otic *a.* ótico-a, rel. al oído.

oticodinia *n.* oticodinia, vértigo causado por una enfermedad del oído.

otitis *n.* otitis, infl. del oído externo, medio o interno.

otolaryngologist *n.* otolaringólogo-a, especialista en otolaringología.

otolaryngology *n.* otolaringología, estudio de la garganta, nariz y oídos.

otologist *n.* otólogo-a, especialista en enfermedades del oído.

otology *n.* otología, rama de la medicina que estudia el oído, su función y las enfermedades que lo afectan.

otoneurology *n.* otoneurología, estudio del oído interno en su relación con el sistema nervioso.

otoplasty *n.* otoplastia, cirugía plástica del oído.

otorrhagia *n.* otorragia, sangramiento por el oído.

otosclerosis *n.* otosclerosis, sordera progresiva debida a la formación de tejido esponjoso en el laberinto del oído.

otoscope *n.* otoscopio, instrumento para examinar el oído.

otoscopy *n.* otoscopia, uso del otoscopio en un examen del oído.

ototomy *n.* ototomía, incisión en el oído.

ototoxic *a.* ototóxico-a, que tiene efecto tóxico en el octavo par craneal o en los órganos de la audición.

ouch *int.* ay!

ought *v.* deber, deber de + *inf.*; ser necesario, tener la obligación de + *inf*; **you ___ to take the med** / debe, debes tomar la medicina.

ounce *n.* onza.

oust *v.* expulsar, sacar, echar fuera.

out *adv.* afuera, fuera; [*light, appliance*] apagado-a [*unconscious*] inconsciente, sin conocimiento;___ **of** / ___ de; **three ___ of ten cases** / tres de diez casos; **___ of work** / sin trabajo, sin empleo, desempleado-a; *v.* **to be ___** / estar ausente; **to go ___** / salir; **get ___!** / ,salga!, ,sal!.

outbreak *n.* erupción; [*of an epidemic*] brote epidémico.

outbreathe *v.* dejar sin aliento; *pop.* dejar sin resuello.

outburst *n.* erupción; estallido; arranque; manifestación abrupta, brote.

outcome *n.* resultado, consecuencia; [*good*] éxito.

outdated *a.* anticuado-a.

outdo *vi.* superar, exceder.

outdoors *a.* al aire libre; externo-a; *adv.* afuera de la casa.

outer *a.* externo-a; exterior.

outfit *n.* traje, equipo, habilitación.

outflow *n.* derrame, salida, flujo.

outgoing *n.* salida, ida, partida; a. saliente, cesante; expansivo-a.

outgrow *vi.* sobrepasar, crecer más.

outgrowth *n.* excrecencia, bulto.

outlet *n.* orificio de salida; [*electric*] tomacorriente.

outlive *v.* sobrevivir, vivir más que; durar más.

outlook *n.* punto de vista, expectativa, opinión.

outnumber *v.* exceder en número.

outpass *v.* pasar más allá de; avanzar.

outpatient *n.* paciente externo, paciente de consulta externa, paciente no hospitalizado.

outpour *n.* derramamiento, chorro; *v.* chorrear, derramar, verter.

output *n.* rendimiento; producción; salida; ___ **failure** / fallo en el ___.

outrageous *a.* [*shocking*] atroz; increíble.

outright *a.* sincero-a, franco-a, cabal; *adv.* francamente, sinceramente.

outroot *v.* sacar de raíz, desarraigar, extirpar.

outside *n.* exterior, apariencia; *prep.* fuera de, más allá de.

outspoken *a.* franco-a, que habla sin rodeos.

outstretch *v.* extender, alargar, expandir.

outweigh *v.* pesar más que; exceder.

oval *a.* oval; rel. al óvulo.

oval window *n.* ventana oval; abertura del oído medio.

ovarian *a.* ovárico-a, rel. a los ovarios.

ovariectomy *n.* ovariectomía. V. **oophorectomy**.

ovary *n.* ovario, órgano reproductor femenino que produce el óvulo.

over *a.* acabado-a, terminado-a; *prep.* sobre, encima, por; a través de; *adv.* por encima, de un lado; a otro; al otro lado; al revés ___ **again** / otra vez; ___ **and** ___ **again** / muchas veces; *v.* [*years*] **to be** ___ / tener más de; **It is** ___ / ya se pasó, ya se acabó; **turn** ___ / vuélvase, vuélvete.

overact *v.* exagerar.

overanxious *a.* demasiado inquieto-a, excitado-a, muy ansioso-a.

overbearing *a.* insoportable.

overbite *n.* sobremordida.

overboil *v.* hervir demasiado, hervir más de lo necesario.

overburden *v.* agobiar, sobrecargar.

overcareful *a.* demasiado cuidadoso-a, *pop.* puntilloso-a.

overcharge *n.* precio excesivo, recargo de precio; *v.* sobrecargar, cobrar demasiado.

overclosure *n.* sobrecierre, cierre de la mandíbula antes de que los dientes superiores e inferiores se junten.

overcoat *n.* abrigo, sobretodo.

overcome *vi.* vencer, rendir; sobreponerse;**you must ___ this** / debe sobreponerse, debes sobreponerte a esto; **you must ___ this sickness** / debe, debes ___ a esta enfermedad.

overcompensation *n.* sobrecompensación, intento exagerado de ocultar sentimientos de inferioridad o de culpa.

overcorrection *n.* sobrecorrección, acción de corregir en exceso un defecto visual por medio de lentes.

overdose *n.* dosis excesiva; dosis tóxica; sobredosis.

overdue *a.* retrasado-a, tardío-a.

overeat *vi.* comer con exceso; hartarse.

overexposure *n.* superexposición; exposición excesiva.

overextension *n.* sobreextensión.

overfeed *vi.* sobrealimentar, alimentar en exceso.

overflow *n.* rebosamiento; derramamiento; *pop.* desparramo.

overgrown *a.* demasiado crecido-a, muy grande o agrandado-a.

overgrowth *n.* proliferación excesiva.

overhear *vi.* oir por casualidad; alcanzar a oir.

overjoyed *a.* rebosante de alegría.

overnight *n.* velada, la noche completa; *adv.* durante la noche; la noche pasada.

overpowering *a.* abrumador-a; irresistible.

overproduction *n.* superproducción.

overreact *v.* reaccionar en exceso.

overresponse *n.* sobrerespuesta, reacción excesiva a un estímulo.

oversight *n.* descuido, equivocación, inadvertencia.

overtime *n.* tiempo suplementario; horas extras de trabajo.

overweigh *v.* pesar más que; sobrecargar.

overweight *n.* peso excesivo, sobrepeso.

overwhelm *v.* abrumar; colmar.

overwork *n.* trabajo excesivo, trabajo en exceso.

ovicular, ovoid *a.* ovicular, en forma de huevo.

oviduct *n.* oviducto, conducto uterino; trompas de Falopio.

ovotestis *n.* ovotestis, glándula hermafrodita que contiene tejido ovárico y testicular.

ovulation *n.* ovulación, liberación periódica del óvulo o gamete por el ovario.

ovulatory *a.* ovulatorio-a, rel. al proceso de ovulación.

ovum *n.* (*pl.* **ova**) óvulo, gamete fecundado.

oxalic acid *n.* ácido oxálico.

oxidant *a.* oxidante, que causa oxidación o rel. a ésta.

oxidation *n.* oxidación, combinación de una sustancia con oxígeno.

oxidize *v.* oxidar, combinar con oxígeno.

oximeter *n.* oxímetro, instrumento para medir la cantidad de oxígeno en la sangre.

oxygen *n.* oxígeno, elemento o gas incoloro e inodoro no metálico que circula libremente en la atmósfera; ___ **deficiency** / falta de ___; ___ **distribution** / distribución de ___; ___ **treatment** / tratamiento de ___.

oxygen tent *n.* cámara de oxígeno, tienda de oxígeno.

oxygen therapy *n.* terapia de oxígeno, tratamiento de oxígeno por el cual se distribuye una concentración de oxígeno para aliviar la respiración del paciente por medio de un catéter nasal, tienda, cámara o máscara.

oxygenation *n.* oxigenación, saturación de oxígeno.

oxygenator *n.* oxigenador, instrumento para oxigenar la sangre gen. usado durante cirugía.

oxygenotherapy *n.* oxigenoterapia, uso terapéutico del oxígeno.

oxyhemoglobin *n.* oxihemoglobina, sustancia de color rojo brillante que se forma cuando los glóbulos rojos se combinan permanentemente con el oxígeno.

oxytocin *n.* oxitocina, ocitocina, hormona pituitaria que estimula las contracciones del útero.

oyster *n.* ostra, ostión.

p

P *abbr.* part / parte; **phosphorous** / fósforo;
plasma / plasma; **population** / población;
positive / positivo; **posterior** / posterior;
postpartum / postpartum; **pressure** / presión;
psychiatry / psiquiatría; **pulse** / pulso.
pabulum *n., L.* pabulum, alimento o sustancia
alimenticia.
pace *n.* marcha, paso, el andar; *v.* andar, marchar.
pacemaker, pacer *n.* marcapasos,
estabilizador del ritmo cardíaco;
internal ___ / ___ interno;
temporary ___ / ___ temporal.
pachyderma *n.* paquidermia. V. **elephantiasis.**
pachygyria *n.* paquigiria, circunvoluciones
gruesas en la corteza cerebral.
pacifier *n.* chupete, tetera, teto.
pacify *v.* apaciguar, tranquilizar.
pack *n.* envoltura. 1. cubierta fría o caliente en la
cual se envuelve el cuerpo; 2. compresa; *v.* [*to
wrap*] envolver.
packing *n.* tapón, taponamiento. 1. acto de llenar
una cavidad con gasa o algodón; 2. envoltura.
pad *n.* cojín, almohadilla; *v.* [*to fill*] rellenar.
padding *n.* relleno.
paid *v. pp.* **to pay,** pagado.
pain *n.* [*ache*] dolor; [*suffering*] sufrimiento, pena;
[*colicky*] cólico. See chart on page 100.
painful *a.* doloroso-a, penoso-a, aflictivo-a. ___
menstrual period / menstruación ___; ___
intercourse / dispareunia, relaciones
sexuales ___ -as; ___ **urination** / dolor al orinar.
painkiller *n.* calmante, sedante, remedio, pastilla
para el dolor.
painless *a.* sin dolor; [*easy*] fácil.
paint *n.* pincelación, aplicación a la piel de una
solución medicinal; *v.* pintar, aplicar una
solución.
pair *n.* par, pareja.
pajama *n.* piyama, pijama.
palatable *a.* sabroso-a, apetitoso-a; gustoso-a.
palatal myoclonus *n.* mioclono palatino,
contracciones rítmicas del paladar, los músculos
faciales y el diafragma debido a lesiones
cerebrales.
palatal reflex *n.* reflejo palatino, deglución
estimulada por el paladar.
palate *n.* paladar; velo del paladar; *pop.* cielo de
la boca;**bony** ___ / ___ óseo; **hard** ___ / ___
duro; **soft** ___ / ___ blando.

palatine *a.* palatino, rel. al paladar.
pale *a.* pálido-a, descolorido-a.
paleface *n.* rostro pálido, carapálida.
palindromic *a.* palindrómico-a, recurrente.
palliative *a.* paliativo-a, lenitivo-a, que alivia.
pallid *a.* pálido-a, descolorido-a.
pallor *n.* palidez.
palm *n.* palma, parte inferior de la mano; ___ **oil** /
aceite de ___ .
palmar *a.* palmar, rel. a la palma de la mano.
palpable *a.* palpable.
palpate *v.* palpar, acto de palpación.
palpation *n.* palpación, acto de tocar y examinar
con las manos un área del cuerpo.
palpitate *v.* palpitar, latir.
palpitation *n.* palpitación, latido; pulsación;
aleteo rápido.
palsy *n.* perlesía, parálisis, pédida temporal o
permanente de la sensación, de la función o
control de movimiento de una parte del cuerpo;
cerebral ___ / ___ cerebral,parálisis parcial y
falta de coordinación muscular debida a una
lesión cerebral congénita.
paludism *n.* paludismo, enfermedad infecciosa
febril gen. crónica, transmitida por la picadura
de un mosquito *Anófeles* infectado por un
protozooario *Plasmodium.*
pamper *v.* mimar; malcriar.
pampered *a. pp.* of **to pamper,** mimado-a,
consentido-a.
pamphlet *n.* folleto.
pampiniform *a.* pampiniforme, semejante a la
estructura de un zarcillo de la vid.
panacea *n.* panacea, remedio para todas las
enfermedades.
panarteritis *n.* panarteritis, infl. de las capas de
una arteria.
panarthritis *n.* panartritis. 1. infl. de varias
articulaciones del cuerpo; 2. infl. de los tejidos
de una articulación.
pancreas *n.* pancreas, glándula del sistema
digestivo que secreta externamente el jugo
pancreático e interiormente la insulina y el
glucagón; ___ **transplant** / transplante del ___ .
pancreatalgia *n.* pancreatalgia, dolor en el
páncreas.
pancreatectomy *n.* pancreatectomía, excisión
parcial o total del páncreas.
pancreatic *a.* pancreático-a, rel. al
páncreas; ___ **cyst** / quiste ___; ___ **duct** /
conducto ___; ___ **juice** / jugo ___; ___
neoplasms / neoplasmas ___ -s.
pancreatic function test *n.* prueba del
funcionamiento del páncreas.

pancreaticoenterostomy *n.* pancreaticoenterostomía, anastomosis entre el conducto pancreático y el intestino.

pancreatin *n.* pancreatina, enzima digestiva del páncreas.

pancreatitis *n.* pancreatitis, infl. del páncreas; **acute** ___ / ___ aguda; **hemorrhagic, acute** ___ / ___ hemorrágica aguda.

pancytopenia *n.* pancitopenia, disminución anormal del número de células sanguíneas.

pandemic *a.* pandémico-a, de contagiosidad epidémica en un área geográfica extensa.

panendoscope *n.* panendoscopio, instrumento óptico usado para examinar la vejiga.

pang *n.* dolor agudo penetrante.

panglossia *n.* panglosia, verborrea.

panhidrosis *n.* panhidrosis, transpiración generalizada.

panhypopituitarism *n.* panhipopituitarismo, deficiencia de la pituitaria anterior.

panhysterectomy *n.* panhisterectomía, excisión total del útero.

panic *n.* pánico, temor excesivo; ___ **attacks** / ataques de ___; *v.* tener un miedo excesivo; sobrecogerse de pánico.

panicked *a. pp.* of **to panic,** sobrecogido-a de pánico; *pop.* muerto-a de miedo.

panniculitis *n.* paniculitis, infl. del panículo grasoso.

panniculus *n.* panículo, capa de tejido adiposo; ___ **adiposus** / ___ adiposo; ___ **carnosus** / ___ carnoso.

pannus *n.* L. pannus, paño, membrana de tejido granulado que cubre una superficie normal.

pansinusitis *n.* pansinusitis, infl. de los senos paranasales de un lado o de ambos.

pant *v.* jadear, resollar.

panting *n.* jadeo, respiración rápida.

pants *n., pl.* pantalones, calzones.

Papanicolaou test, Pap smear *n.* prueba de Papanicolaou (frotis, unto), recolección de mucosa de la vagina y del cuello uterino para detectar un cáncer incipiente.

papaya *n.* papaya, *Cuba* frutabomba.

paper *n.* papel; **toilet** ___ / ___ higiénico.

papilla *n. (pl.* **papillae)** papila, protuberancia esp. en la lengua; **acoustic** ___ / ___ acústica; **dermal** ___ / ___ dérmica; **duodenal** ___ / ___ duodenal; **filiform** ___ / ___ filiforme; **lacrimal** ___ / ___ lagrimal; **lingual** ___ / ___ lingual.

papillary *a.* papilar, rel. a una papila.

papillary carcinoma *n.* carcinoma papilar, tumor de la tiroides caracterizado por tener varias tumoraciones en forma de dedos.

papilledema *n.* papiledema, edema del disco óptico.

papilliforme *a.* papiliforme, similar a una papila.

papillitis *n.* papilitis, infl. del disco óptico.

papilloma *n.* papiloma, tumor epitelial benigno.

papillomatosis *n.* 1. desarrollo de numerosos papilomas; 2. proyecciones de papilares.

papovavirus *n.* papovavirus, miembro de un grupo de virus de gran importancia en el estudio del cáncer.

papular *a.* papular, rel. a una pápula.

papule *n.* pápula, protuberancia en la piel compuesta de materia sólida.

papulosquamous *a.* papuloescamoso-a, rel. a pápulas y escamas; ___ **skin diseases** / enfermedades cutáneas ___ -s.

para-amino benzoic acid *n.* para-amino ácido benzóico, un factor en el complejo de vitamina B usado como facto.

paracentesis *n.* paracéntesis, punción para obtener o eliminar líquido de una cavidad.

paraffin *n.* parafina.

parainfluenza viruses *n., pl.* virus de parainfluenza, virus asociados con infecciones respiratorias, esp. en los niños.

parallax *n.* paralaje, posición de desplazamiento aparente de un objeto de acuerdo con la posición del observador.

paralysis *n.* parálisis, pérdida parcial o total de movimiento o de función de una parte del cuerpo; **accomodation** ___ / ___ de acomodación; **alcoholic** ___ / ___ alcohólica; **amyotrofic** ___ / ___ amiotrófica; **ascending** ___ / ___ ascendente; **central** ___ / ___ central; **cold induced** ___ / ___ por enfriamiento; **diver's** ___, *pop.* **bends** / ___ de los buzos; **hysterical** ___ / ___ histérica; **motor** ___ / ___ motor; **peripheral fascial** ___ / ___ periférica facial; **rapidly progressive** ___ / ___ galopante.

paralytic *a.* paralítico-a, inválido-a; impedido-a, rel. a o que sufre de parálisis; ___ **ileus** / parálisis del intestino.

paralyze *v.* paralizar, inmovilizar.

paralyzer *a.* paralizador, que causa parálisis.

paramagnetic *a.* paramagnético-a, rel. a una sustancia susceptible al magnetismo.

paramedic *n.* paramédico-a, profesional con entrenamiento para ofrecer asistencia médica esp. de emergencia.

parametrium *n.* parametrio, tejido celular suelto alrededor del útero.

paramyotonia *n.* paramiotonía, miotonía atópica caracterizada por espasmos musculares y tonicidad anormal de los músculos. **ataxic** ___ / ___ atáxica; **congenital** ___ / ___ congénita; ___ **disorder** / trastorno de ___; **symptomatic** ___ / ___ sintomática.

paranasal *a.* paranasal, adyacente a la cavidad nasal.

paranasal sinuses *n., pl.* senos paranasales, cualquiera de las cavidades aéreas en los huesos adyacentes a la cavidad nasal.

paranasal sinus radiography *n.* radiografía de los senos paranasales que comprende los senos frontales: esfenoide, maxilar y etmoide.

paranoia *n.* paranoia, trastorno mental caracterizado por delirio de persecución o de grandeza.

paranoid *a.* paranoico-a, persona afectada por paranoia.

parapancreatic *a.* parapancreático-a, adyacente al páncreas.

paraparesis *n.* paraparesis, parálisis parcial esp. de las extermidades inferiores.

paraphasia *n.* parafasia, tipo de afasia que se caracteriza por el uso incoherente de palabras.

paraphimosis *n.* parafimosis. 1. constricción del prepucio detrás del glande del pene; 2. retracción del párpado por detrás del globo ocular.

paraplegia *n.* paraplejía, parálisis de la parte inferior del tronco y de las piernas. **cerebral infantile** ___ / ___ cerebral infantil; **familiar, spasmodic** ___ / ___ espasmódica, familiar; **spasmodic, spastic** ___ / ___ espasmódica, espástica.

paraplegic *a.* parapléjico-a, rel. a, o afectado por paraplejía.

parapsychology *n.* parapsicología, estudio de fenómenos psíquicos tales como la telepatía y la percepción extrasensorial.

pararectal *a.* pararrectal, adyacente al recto.

parasite *n.* parásito, organismo que vive a expensas de otro.

parasite and stool ova exam *n.* análisis de huevos y parásitos en las heces fecales

parasitic *a.* parasítico-a, parasitario-a.

parasitism *n.* parasitismo, infección de parásitos.

parasitology *n.* parasitología, estudio de los parásitos.

parasomnia *n.* parasomnia, término que se refiere a cualquier trastorno sufrido durante el sueño, enuresis, pesadillas, sonambulismo, etc.

parasternal *a.* parasterno-a, adyacente al esternón.

parasympathetic *a.* parasimpático, rel. a una de las dos ramas del sistema nervioso autónomo; ___ **nervous system** / sistema nervioso autónomo.

parasympatholytic *a.* parasimpatolítico, que destruye o bloquea las fibras nerviosas del sistema nervioso parasimpático.

parasystole *n.* parasístole, irregularidad en el ritmo cardíaco.

parathormone *n.* hormona paratiroidea, hormona reguladora del calcio.

parathyroid *n.* paratiroides, grupo de glándulas endocrinas pequeñas situadas junto a la tiroides; ___ **hormone** / hormona ___ , reguladora de calcio; *a.* paratiroideo-a, localizado-a cerca de la tiroides.

parathyroidectomy *n.* paratiroidectomía, extirpación de una o más de las glándulas paratiroideas.

paratyphoid *n.* paratífica, fiebre similar a la tifoidea.

paravertebral *a.* paravertebral, situado-a al lado de la columna vertebral.

parched *a.* reseco-a.

paregoric *n.* paregórico, narcótico, calmante derivado del opio.

parenchyma *n.* parénquima, partes funcionales de un órgano.

parent *n.* padre o madre; *pl.* ___ -s / padres.

parenteral *a.* parenteral, rel. a la introducción de medicamentos o sustancias en el organismo por otra vía que no sea la del canal alimenticio; ___ **hyperalimentation** / sobrealimentación intravenosa.

parenthood *n.* paternidad o maternidad.

paresis *n.* paresia, parálisis parcial o leve.

paresthesia *n.* parestesia, sensación de hormigueo o de calambre que se asocia a una lesión de un nervio periférico.

paretic *a.* parético-a, rel. o afectado por paresis.

parietal *a.* parietal, rel. al hueso parietal; rel. a la pared de una cavidad.

parietal bone *n.* hueso parietal, uno de los dos huesos situados en la parte superior y lateral del cráneo.

Parkinson's disease *n.* enfermedad de Parkinson, atrofia o degeneración de los nervios cerebrales que se manifiesta con temblores, debilidad muscular progresiva, cambios en el habla, la manera de andar y la postura.

parodynia *n.* parodinia, parto difícil.

paronychia *n.* paroniquia, infl. del área adyacente a la uña.

parotid *n.* parótida, glándula secretora de saliva localizada cerca del oído.

parotiditis *n.* parotiditis, parotitis. V. **mumps.**

paroxysm *n.* paroxismo, ataque. 1. espasmo o convulsión; 2. síntomas que se repiten y se intensifican.

paroxysmal nocturnal dyspnea *n.* disnea paroxística nocturna, que gen. despierta al paciente inesperadamente y es causada por congestíon pulmonar.

paroxysmal tachycardia *n.* taquicardia paroxística, episodios de palpitaciones que comienzan y terminan abruptamente, pero también pueden durar horas y a veces varios días y pueden ser recurrentes.

pars *n. L.* pars, parte, porción.

parsley *n.* perejil.

part *n.* parte, porción; [*component of an instrument*] pieza; **-ly** *adv.* parcialmente, en parte.

parthenogenesis *n.* partenogénesis, reproducción en la cual el óvulo se desarrolla sin ser fecundado por un espermatozoo; **artificial** ___ / ___ **artificial.**

partial *a.* parcial; **-ly** *adv.* parcialmente.

partial lung colapse *n.* colapso parcial del pulmón.

participate *v.* participar, tomar parte.

particle *n.* partícula, porción ínfima de una materia.

particular *a.* particular; **-ly** *adv.* particularmente.

parturient *a.* parturienta, mujer que acaba de dar a luz o está en el acto de dar a luz.

parturifacient *n.* parturifaciente, droga que induce el parto.

parturition *n.* parto, alumbramiento.

parumbilical *a.* paraumbilical, adyacente al ombligo.

parvovirus *n.* parvovirus, grupo de virus patógenos que originan enfermedades en animales aunque no en personas.

pass *v.* pasar, aprobar; **to** ___ **away** / morir, fallecer; **to** ___ **on** / contagiar, pegar; **to** ___ **out** / desmayarse; **to** ___ **over** / pasar por, atravesar.

pass away *v.* fallecer, morir.

passage *n.* pasaje. 1. conducto o meato; 2. evacuación del intestino.

passing *a.* [*fleeting*] pasajero; **a** ___ **pain** / un dolor ___ .

passion *n.* pasión, emoción intensa.

passionate *a.* apasionado-a.

passive *a.* pasivo-a; sumiso-a; inactivo-a, que no es espontáneo o activo; ___ **exercise** / ejercicio ___ .

passive movement *n.* movimiento pasivo, movimiento creado por una persona asistente que ayuda al paciente a realizar movimientos sin que el paciente tenga que hacer esfuerzo muscular alguno.

passive smoker *n.* fumador-a pasivo-a, persona que inhala el humo producido por un fumador-a próximo-a; **he smokes and his wife is a** ___ / él fuma y su esposa es una ___ .

passivity *n.* pasividad, estado anormal de dependencia de otros.

past *n.* pasado. *a.* pasado-a.

pasta *n.* pasta, preparación de sustancias medicinales gen. para aplicar a la epidermis.

pasteurization *n.* pasteurización, proceso de destrucción de microorganismos nocivos por medio de la aplicación de calor regulado.

patch *n.* placa, mancha. 1. pequeña porción de tejido que se caracteriza por pigmentación diferente a la del área que lo rodea; 2. parche, adhesivo aplicado para proteger heridas; ___ **test** / prueba alérgica.

patella *n. L.* patella, rótula.

patellectomy *n.* patelectomía, excisión de la patela.

patellofemoral *a.* patelofemoral, rel. a la rótula y el fémur.

patency *n.* permeabilidad. V. **permeability**.

patent *n.* patente, producto de marca autorizada o derecho exclusivo; ___ **medicine** / medicina de ___ ; *a.* patente; accesible; abierto-a.

paternal *a.* paterno, rel. al padre.

paternity *n.* paternidad.

paternity test *n.* prueba de la paternidad, comparación del tipo sanguíneo de un niño o niña con el de un hombre para comprobar si éste puede ser el padre.

path *n.* vía, curso.

pathetic *a.* patético-a.

pathogen *n.* patógeno, agente capaz de producir una enfermedad.

pathogenesis *n.* patogénesis, origen y desarrollo de una enfermedad.

pathogenic *a.* patógeno-a, que causa una enfermedad.

pathognomonic *a.* patognomónico-a, rel. a un signo o síntoma característico de una enfermedad.

pathologic, pathological *a.* patológico-a, rel. a o producido por enfermedades.

pathology *n.* patología, ciencia que estudia la naturaleza y causa de las enfermedades.

pathophysiology *n.* patofisiología, estudio de los efectos de una enfermedad en los procesos fisiológicos.

pathway *n.* curso, comunicación; senda.

patience *n.* paciencia.

patient *n.* paciente, enfermo-a, ___discharge / alta, egreso del___; ___'s care / cuidado del ___; private ___ / ___ privado-a; self-paying ___ / ___ solvente; -ly *adv.* con paciencia, pacientemente.

patrilineal *a.* de descendencia paterna; rel. a rasgos heredados del padre.

patronize *v.* tratar con condescendencia.

pattern *n.* patrón, modelo, tipo.

patulous *a.* abierto-a, distendido-a.

pause *n.* pausa, interrupción; paro; compensatory ___ / ___ compensatoria; *v.* to give ___ / dar que pensar.

pay *vi.* pagar; to ___ attention / prestar atención; to ___ in cash / ___ al contado.

payment *n.* pago.

pea *n.* chícharo, guisante.

peace *n.* paz; ___ of mind / tranquilidad de espíritu; *v.* to be at ___ / estar en paz, tranquilizarse; to keep, to hold one's ___ / quedarse tranquilo-a.

peaceful *a.* pacífico-a; tranquilo-a, calmado-a.

peach *n.* melocotón, *H.A.* durazno.

peak *n.* [*sickness*] crisis, [*diagram*] cresta; cima, punta.

peanut *n.* maní, *Mex.* cacahuete; ___ butter / mantequilla de ___ .

pear *n.* pera.

peau d'orange *n. Fr.* piel de naranja, condición cutánea que asemeja la cáscara de naranja y que es señal importante en el cáncer de la mama.

pectin *n.* pectina, carbohidrato que se obtiene de la cáscara de frutas cítricas y de manzana.

pectoral *a.* pectoral, rel. al pecho.

pectus *n. L.* pecho, tórax.

peculiar *a.* peculiar.

pedal *a.* pedal; rel. al pie.

pederasty *n.* pederastia, relación homosexual anal esp. entre un hombre adulto y un muchacho.

pediatric *a.* pediátrico-a, rel. a la pediatría.

pediatrician *n.* pediatra, médico-a especialista en enfermedades de la infancia.

pediatrics *n.* pediatría, rama de la medicina relacionada con el cuidado y desarrollo de los niños y el tratamiento de las enfermedades que los afectan.

pedicle *n.* pedículo, porción estrecha que conecta un tumor o colgajo con su base.

pediculosis *n.* pediculosis, infestación de piojos.

pedodontist *n.* dentista infantil.

pedophilia *n.* pedofilia, atracción mórbida sexual de un adulto hacia los niños.

peduncle *n.* pedúnculo, conexión en forma de tallo.

pedunculated *a.* pediculado-a, pedunculado-a, rel. a o provisto de pedúnculo.

pedunculus *n. L.* pedúnculo.

peel *n.* [*fruits*] cáscara, hollejo, corteza; *v.* pelar; [*to shed skin*] despellejarse, pelarse.

peeling *n.* peladura; chemical ___ / ___ química; exfoliation.

pellagra *n.* pelagra, enfermedad causada por deficiencia de niacina y caracterizada por dermatitis, trastornos gastrointestinales y finalmente mentales.

pelvic *a.* pélvico-a, pelviano-a, rel. a la pelvis.

pelvic inflammatory disease *n.* enfermedad inflamatoria de la pelvis.

pelvis *n.* pelvis. 1. cavidad en la parte inferior del tórax formada por los huesos de la cadera, el sacro y el cóccix; 2. cavidad en forma de vasija o copa.

pemphigoid *a.* penfigoideo, semejante al pénfigo con diferencias clínicas.

pemphigus *n. L.* pénfigo, término usado para definir una variedad de dermatosis, cuya característica común consiste en la manifestación de ampollas que se infectan y revientan.

pendent, pending *a.* [*hanging*] pendiente, colgante, suspenso-a, dependiente; [*waiting*] pendiente.

pendulous *a.* pendular, que oscila o cuelga.

peneal, penial *a.* peneano-a, rel. al pene.

penetrate *v.* penetrar, pasar, atravesar.

penetrating *a.* [*as a pain*] penetrante, agudo-a.

penetration *n.* penetración. 1. acción de penetrar; 2. paso de radiación a través de una sustancia.

penicillin *n.* penicilina, antibiótico que se obtiene directa o indirectamente de un grupo de cultivos del hongo de la especie *Penicillium.*

penile *a.* peneal.

penis *n.* pene, parte exterior del aparato reproductor masculino que contiene la uretra y a través de la cual pasan el semen y la orina.

people *n.* [*of a nation*] pueblo; [*population*] población, personas, habitantes; gente.

pepper *n.* [*spice*] pimienta; pimiento.

peppermint *n.* hierbabuena, yerbabuena.

pepsin *n.* pepsina, enzima principal del jugo gástrico.

peptic ulcer *n.* úlcera péptica, ulceración de las membranas mucosas del esófago, estómago o duodeno causada por acidez excesiva en el jugo gástrico y producida por tensión aguda o crónica; ___ **perforation** / perforación de la ___ .

per *prep.* por; ___ **rectum** / ___ el recto, ___ vía rectal.

perceive *v.* darse cuenta de, percibir, advertir.

percentage *n.* porcentaje, tanto por ciento.

perception *n.* percepción, acción de reconocer conscientemente un estímulo sensorial; **extrasensory** ___ / ___ extrasensorial.

perceptivity *n.* perceptibilidad, capacidad de percibir.

perceptual *a.* perceptivo-a, que recibe o transmite sensaciones.

percuss *v.* percutir, producir una percusión.

percussion *n.* percusión, procedimiento de palpación de toque firme en la superficie del cuerpo para producir sensaciones vibratorias que indiquen el estado de una parte interior determinada; **auscultatory** ___ / ___ auscultatoria.

percutaneous *a.* percutáneo-a, aplicado-a a través de la piel.

percutaneous transluminal angioplasty *n.* angioplastia transluminal percutánea, proceso de dilatación de una arteria por medio de un balón inflado a presión.

perfect *a.* perfecto-a, completo-a, acabado-a; **-ly** *adv.* perfectamente, completamente.

perfectionism *n.* perfeccionismo, tendencia al fervor exagerado en la ejecución de actividades sin distinción de importancia entre las mismas.

perfectionist *a.* perfeccionista.

perforate *v.* perforar, abrir un agujero.

perforation *n.* perforación, agujero.

perform *v.* llevar a cabo, realizar, hacer; **to ___ an operation** / operar, intervenir quirúrgicamente.

perfusion *n.* perfusión, pasaje de un líquido o sustancia a través de un conducto.

perianal *a.* perianal, situado alrededor del ano.

pericardial, pericardiac *a.* pericárdico-a, pericardial, rel. al pericardio; ___ **effusion** / derrame ___; ___ **window** / resección ___, creación de una apertura en el pericardio.

pericardiectomy *n.* pericardiectomía, excisión parcial o total del pericardio.

pericarditis *n.* pericarditis, infl. del pericardio; **constrictive** ___ / ___ constrictiva; **fibrinous** ___ / ___ fibrinosa.

pericardium *n.* pericardio, membrana delicada de capa doble en forma de saco que envuelve el corazón y el inicio de los grandes vasos.

peril *n.* peligro, riesgo.

perimetrium *n.* perimetrio, membrana exterior del útero.

perinatal *n.* perinatal, rel. a o que ocurre antes, durante o inmediatamente después del nacimiento.

perinatologist *n.* perinatólogo-a, especialista en perinatología.

perinatology *n.* perinatología, estudio del feto y del recién nacido durante el período perinatal.

perineal *a.* perineal, rel. al perineo.

perinephric *a.* perinefrítico-a, rel. a o cercano al riñón.

perineum *n.* perineo, suelo pelviano delimitado anteriormente por la raíz del escroto en el hombre y la vulva en la mujer y posteriormente por el ano.

period *n.* período. 1. intervalo de tiempo; época; **incubation** ___ / ___ de incubación; **latency** ___ / ___ de latencia; 2. período, menstruación, menses, regla; 3. *gr.* punto.

periodic *a.* periódico-a.

periodical *n.* publicación, periódico.

periodontal *a.* periodontal, localizado alrededor de un diente.

periodontics *n.* periodoncia, rama de la odontología que estudia las enfermedades que atacan las áreas que envuelven los dientes.

periosteum *n.* periosteo, membrana fibrosa gruesa que cubre la superficie de los huesos excepto la superficie articular.

peripheral *a.* periférico-a, rel. a la periferia.

peripheral nervous system *n.* sistema nervioso periférico, nervios situados fuera del sistema nervioso central.

periphery *n.* periferia, parte de un cuerpo fuera del centro.

perishable *a.* perecedero-a, de fácil descomposición debido al contenido orgánico.

peristalsis *n.* peristalsis, contracciones ondulantes de estructuras tubulares tal como el canal alimenticio, cuyo movimiento fuerza el contenido almacenado hacia afuera en dirección descendiente.

peristaltic *a.* peristáltico-a, rel. a la peristalsis.

peritoneal *a.* peritoneal, rel. al peritoneo; ___ **cavity** / cavidad ___ .

peritoneal fluid *n.* fluido peritoneal, fluido excretado por las células del peritoneo.

peritoneoscopy *n.* peritoneoscopía, examen del peritoneo por medio de un peritoneoscopio. V. **laparoscopy.**

483

peritoneoscope *n.* peritoneoscopio *Syn.* **laparoscope**

peritoneum *n.* peritoneo, membrana que cubre la pared abdominal y las vísceras.

peritonitis *n.* peritonitis, infl. del peritoneo.

peritonsillar *a.* periamigdalino-a, que rodea o está cerca de una amígdala.

periungual *a.* periungueal, localizado cerca de una uña.

periurethral *a.* periuretral, alrededor de la uretra.

perlèche *n. Fr.* perlèche, *pop.* boquera, infección en la comisura de los labios y manifestaciones de infl. y fisuras, gen. causada por desnutrición.

permanent *a.* permanente; **-ly** *adv.* permanentemente.

permeability *n.* permeabilidad, cualidad de ser permeable; **capillary** ___ / ___ capilar.

permeable *a.* permeable, que permite el paso de sustancias a través de una membrana u otras estructuras.

permissible *a.* permisible; permitido-a.

permit *n.* permiso, consentimiento; *v.* permitir, autorizar.

pernicious *a.* pernicioso-a, nocivo-a, destructivo-a.

peroxide, hydrogen *n.* peróxido de hidrógeno, agua oxigenada.

perpendicular *a.* perpendicular.

persecution *n.* persecución, acosamiento.

perseveration *n.* perseveración, tipo de trastorno mental que se manifiesta con repetición anormal de palabras y acciones.

persist *v.* persistir, perseverar, insistir.

persistence *n.* persistencia, insistencia, constancia.

person *n.* persona.

persona *n.* persona, personalidad adoptada que encubre la verdadera.

personal *a.* personal, privado-a.

personality *n.* personalidad, rasgos, características y conducta individual que distinguen a una persona de otras; **anal** ___ / ___ anal; **antisocial** ___ / ___ antisocial; **compulsive** ___ / ___ compulsiva; **extroverted** ___ / ___ extrovertida; **introverted** ___ / ___ introvertida; **neurotic** ___ / ___ neurótica; **paranoid** ___ / ___ paranoica; **psychopathic** ___ / ___ psicopática; **split** ___ / ___ desdoblada; **schizoid** ___ / ___ esquizoide.

personality disorder *n.* trastorno de la personalidad, término general para un grupo de trastornos de conducta caraacterizados por alteración de los patrones de percepción y cognición; **attention deficit disorder** / ___ de falta de atención; **depression disorder** / ___ de depresión; **addictive disorder** / ___ de adicción; **adjustment disorder** / ___ de ajuste; **cyclothymic disorder** / ___ ciclotímico; **eating disorder** / ___ de deglución; **mood disorder** / ___ de cambios emocionales; **panic disorder** / ___ de pánico; **phobic disorder** / ___ de fobias.

personnel *n.* personal; **medical** ___ / equipo médico, cuerpo facultativo.

perspective *n.* perspectiva.

perspiration *n.* sudor, transpiración.

perspire *v.* sudar, transpirar.

persuade *v.* persuadir.

persuasion *n.* persuasión, técnica terapéutica que consiste en un acercamiento racional al paciente para orientarle en sus actuaciones.

pertaining *a.* perteneciente; referente a.

pertubation *n.* pertubación, acto de insuflar oviductos para hacerlos permeables.

perturbation *n.* perturbación. 1. sentimiento de inquietud; 2. variación anormal de un estado regular a otro.

pertussis, whooping cough *n.* pertusis, tosferina, enfermedad infantil infecciosa que se inicia con un estado catarral seguido de una tos seca persistente.

perversion *n.* perversión, desviación depravada, gen. de índole sexual.

pervert *n.* pervertido-a, persona que manifiesta alguna forma de perversión.

pervious *a.* pervio-a, permeable.

pes *n., L.* (*pl.* **pedes**) pie o estructura similar a éste.

pessary *n.* pesario, dispositivo de goma en forma de copa que se inserta en la vagina y se usa como soporte del útero.

pessimism *n.* pesimismo, propensión a juzgar situaciones negativamente.

pessimist *n.* pesimista, persona que muestra pesimismo.

pessimistic *a.* pesimista.

pest *n.* 1. insecto nocivo; 2. peste. V. **plague.**

pesticide *n.* pesticida, exterminador de insectos y roedores.

pet *n.* 1. animal doméstico favorito; 2. niño-a mimado-a.

petechia *n.* (*pl.* **petechiae**) petequia, mancha hemorrágica pequeña que se manifiesta en la piel y las mucosas en casos de estado febril esp. en la tifoidea.

petit mal *n. Fr.* petit mal, ataque epiléptico benigno con pérdida del conocimiento pero sin convulsiones.

petrified *a.* petrificado-a, convertido-a en piedra.

peyote *n.* peyote, planta de la que se extrae la mescalina, droga alucinatoria.

phage *n.* bacteriófago.

phagocyte *n.* fagocito, célula que ingiere y destruye otras células, sustancias y partículas extrañas.

phagocytic *a.* fagocítico-a, fagocitario-a, rel. a fagocitos.

phagocytosis *n.* fagocitosis, proceso de ingestión y digestión realizado por fagocitos.

phalanx *n.* (*pl.* phalanxes, phalanges) falange, uno de los huesos largos de los dedos de los pies o las manos.

phallic *a.* fálico, rel. al pene.

phantasm *n.* fantasma, ilusión óptica, aparición.

phantom *n.* fantasma, fantoma. 1. imagen mental; 2. patrón transparente del cuerpo y sus partes.

pharmaceutical *a.* farmacéutico-a, rel. a la farmacia.

pharmaceutics *n.* preparaciones farmacéuticas.

pharmacist *n.* farmacéutico-a, boticario-a.

pharmacokinetics *n.* farmacocinética, estudio *in vivo* del metabolismo y acción de las drogas.

pharmacology *n.* farmacología, estudio de drogas, medicamentos, su naturaleza, origen, efectos y usos.

pharmacopeia *n.* farmacopea, compendio de drogas, agentes químicos y medicamentos regidos por una autoridad oficial que sirve de estándar en la preparación y dispensación de productos farmacéuticos.

pharmacy *n.* farmacia, botica.

pharyngitis *n.* faringitis, infl. de la faringe.

pharynx *n.* faringe, pasaje del aire de las fosas nasales a la laringe y de la boca al esófago en el tracto alimenticio.

phase *n.* fase, estado de desarrollo, estado transitorio.

phasic *a.* fásico-a, rel. a una fase.

phenobarbital *n.* fenobarbital, hipnótico, sedante, nombre comercial Luminal.

phenomenon *n.* (*pl.* **phenomena**) fenómeno. 1. evento o manifestación de cualquier índole; 2. síntoma objetivo de una enfermedad.

phenotype *n.* fenotipo, características visibles de un organismo como resultado de interacción entre el ambiente y los factores hereditarios.

phimosis *n.* fimosis, estrechamiento del orificio del prepucio que impide que éste pueda extenderse hacia atrás sobre el glande.

phlebitis *n.* flebitis, infl. de una vena, trastorno común esp. en las extremidades.

phlebogram *n.* flebograma, trazado del pulso venoso.

phlebolith *n.* flebolito, depósito calcáreo en una vena.

phlebotomy *n.* flebotomía, venotomía, incisión en una vena para sacar sangre.

phlegm *n.* flema. 1. mucus; 2. uno de los cuatro humores del cuerpo.

phlegmon *n.* flemón, infl. del tejido celular.

phobia *n.* fobia, temor exagerado e irracional.

phobic *a.* fóbico-a, rel. a la fobia.

phonation *n.* fonación, emisión de la voz.

phone *n.* teléfono; ___ **call** / llamada telefónica.

phonetic *a.* fonético-a, rel. a la voz y a los sonidos articulados.

phonetics *n.* fonética, ciencia que estudia la articulación de los sonidos y su pronunciación.

phoniatrics *n.* foniatría, estudio de la fonación.

phonocardiogram *n.* fonocardiograma, representación gráfica que describe los sonidos del corazón.

phonogram *n.* fonograma, representación gráfica de la intensidad de un sonido.

phonoscope *n.* fonoscopio, instrumento para registrar los sonidos del corazón.

phosphate *n.* fosfato, sal del ácido fosfórico.

phosphorus *n.* fósforo, elemento no metálico que se encuentra en alcaloides.

photocoagulation *n.* fotocoagulación, proceso usado en cirugía óptica por el cual un rayo intenso de luz controlada (laser) produce una coagulación localizada.

photophobia *n.* fotofobia, intolerancia a la luz.

phototherapy *n.* fototerapia, exposición a los rayos del sol o a una luz artificial con propósito terapéutico.

phrase *n. gr.* frase.

phrenetic *a.* frenético-a, maníaco-a.

phthiriasis *n.* ftiriasis. V. **pediculosis.**

phylaxis *n.* filaxis, autodefensa del organismo.

physic *n.* medicamento, esp. un catártico o purgante.

physical *a.* físico-a, rel. al cuerpo y su condición; ___ **examination** / examen ___; ___ **fitness** / acondicionamiento ___; ___ **therapist** / terapeuta ___; ___ **therapy** / terapia ___ .

physician *n.* médico-a; **attending** ___ / ___ de cabecera; **consulting** ___ / ___ consultante, consultor; **family** ___ / ___ de familia; ___ **on call** / ___ de guardia; **primary** ___ / ___ de asistencia primaria; **referring** ___ / ___ recomendante.

physiognomy n. fisionomía, semblante, rasgos faciales.

physiologist n. fisiólogo-a, especialista en fisiología.

physiology n. fisiología, ciencia que estudia las funciones de los organismos vivos y los procesos químicos o físicos que los caracterizan.

physiotherapy n. fisioterapia, tratamiento por medio de agentes físicos como agua, calor o luz.

physique n. físico, presencia, figura.

phytobezoar n. fitobezoar, concreción formada por fibra vegetal que se deposita en el estómago o el intestino y no se digiere.

pia mater n. L. piamáter, piamadre, membrana vascular fina, la más interna de las meninges.

pian n. frambesia.

pica n. pica, deseo insaciable de ingerir sustancias que no son comestibles.

pick n. [axe] pico; [choice] selección; v. seleccionar, escoger; **to ___ out** / sacar, entresacar; **to ___ up** / recoger; captar.

picture n. fotografia; lámina; retrato.

piece n. pedazo, parte.

pierce v. agujerear, perforar.

piercing a. penetrante, agudo-a.

pigeon-toed a. patizambo-a.

pigment n. pigmento, colorante.

pigmentation n. pigmentación, coloración.

piles n., pl. almorranas, hemorroides.

piliation n. piliación, formación y desarrollo de pelo.

pill n. pastilla, píldora; **birth control ___** / la píldora, píldora de control del embarazo; **pain ___** / calmante, sedativo, ___ para el dolor; **sleeping ___** / sedativo, ___ para dormir.

pillar n. columna, pilar.

pillow n. almohada; [inflatable] almohadilla, cojín.

pilus n., L. (pl. **pili**) pilus, pelo.

pimple n. barrillo, [blackhead] espinilla, grano de la cara.

pin n. clavo ortopédico, pieza de metal o hueso que se usa para unir partes de un hueso fracturado.

pinch n. pellizco; v. pellizcar; comprimir, apretar.

pinched nerve n. nervio pellizcado.

pineal a. pineal, en forma de piña o cono.

pineal gland n. glándula o cuerpo pineal.

pink a. rosado-a, sonrosado-a.

pinkeye n. conjuntivitis catarral, oftalmia purulenta.

pinna n. L. pinna, pabellón de la oreja.

pipet, pipette n. pipeta, probeta, tubo de ensayo.

pit n. hueco, hoyo; [seed] semilla de frutas.

pitch n. tono, diapasón, cualidad de un sonido de acuerdo con la frecuencia de las ondas que lo producen.

pith n. médula, parte principal.

pitiful a. lastimoso-a, pobre.

pituitary gland n. glándula pituitaria. hypophysis.

pity n. lástima, compasión; **what a ___** ! / ¡qué ___ !

pivot n. pivote, eje, parte que sostiene la corona de un diente.

place n. lugar, sitio; **in ___ of** / en ___ de; v. colocar; **to put in ___** / colocar en su ___ .

placebo n. placebo, sustancia anodina sin valor medicinal gen. usada en experimentos por comparación; **___ controlled trial** / prueba controlada por ___ .

placenta n. placenta, órgano vascular que se desarrolla en la pared del útero a través del cual el feto se nutre de la madre por medio del cordón umbilical; **early, previa ___** / **___** previa, anterior al feto en relación con la apertura externa del cuello uterino, lo que puede causar una hemorragia grave.

placental a. placentario-a, de la placenta, rel. a la placenta; **___ insufficiency** / insuficiencia ___ .

plague n. peste. 1. peste bubónica, infección epidémica transmitida por la picadura de pulgas de ratas; 2. enfermedad epidémica que causa alta mortalidad.

plain a. común, ordinario-a.

plan n. plan, planificación; intento; v. planear.

plane n. plano. 1. superficie lisa y plana; 2. superficie relativamente lisa formada por un corte imaginario o un corte real a través de una parte del cuerpo; **axial ___** / **___** axial; **coronal ___** / **___** coronal, frontal; **sagittal ___** / **___** sagital.

planned parenthood n. planificación familiar.

planning n. planeamiento, planificación; organización; **family ___** / **___** familiar.

plant a. planta; **medicinal ___** / **___**, yerba medicinal.

plantar a. plantar, rel. a la planta del pie; **___ reflex** / reflejo plantare; Babinski's sign.

plaque, placque n. placa; plaqueta. 1. cualquier superficie de la piel o membrana mucosa; 2. plaqueta sanguínea.

plasma n. plasma, componente líquido de la sangre y linfa que se compone en su mayor parte (91%) de agua; **___ proteins** / proteínas sanguíneas.

plaster *n.* yeso, emplaste, molde; ___ **cast** / vendaje enyesado, tablilla de ___ .

plastic *n.* plástico; *a.* plástico-a

plasticity *n.* plasticidad, capacidad para moldearse.

plastic surgery *n.* cirugía plástica, proceso quirúrgico para reparar o reconstruir estructuras del cuerpo.

plate *n.* placa. 1. estructura lisa tal como una lámina ósea; 2. pieza de metal que se usa como soporte de una estructura.

platelet *n.* plaqueta, elemento celular esencial en la coagulación de la sangre.

platinum *n.* platino.

play *v.* jugar; [*an instrument*] tocar.

play therapy *n.* terapia infantil aplicada en un ambiente de juguetes y juegos infantiles por medio de los cuales se estimula a los niños a revelar conflictos interiores.

please *int.* por favor; **come in!** ___! / ¡entre, entra por favor!; *v.* gustar, agradar, satisfacer; tener placer, tener gusto en.

pleasing *a.* agradable, placentero-a, gustoso-a.

pleasure principle *n.* principio del placer, conducta dirigida a satisfacer deseos propios y evadir el dolor.

pledget *n.* tapón de algodón absorbente o de gasa.

pleomorphism *n.* pleomorfismo, cualidad de asumir o tener formas diferentes.

plethora *n.* plétora, exceso de cualquiera de los líquidos del organismo.

plethysmography *n.* pletismografía, registro de las variaciones de volumen que ocurren en una parte u órgano en relación con la cantidad de sangre que pasa sobre los mismos.

pleura *n.* pleura, membrana doble que cubre los pulmones y la cavidad torácica; **parietal** ___ / ___ parietal; **visceral** ___ / ___ visceral.

pleural *a.* pleural, rel. a la pleura; ___ **cavity** / cavidad ___; ___ **effusion** / derrame ___ .

pleuralgia *n.* pleuralgia, dolor en la pleura o en un costado.

pleurisy *n.* pleuresía, infl. de la pleura.

pleuritic *a.* pleurítico-a, rel. a o de la naturaleza de la pleuresía.

pleuritis *n.* pleuritis. pleurisy.

pleuroscopy *n.* pleuroscopía, examen de la cavidad pleural a través de una incisión en el tórax.

plexiform *a.* plexiforme, en forma de plexo o red.

plexus *n.* plexo, red de nervios o de vasos sanguíneos o linfáticos.

pliability *n.* flexibilidad; docilidad.

plica *n.* (*pl.* **plicae**) plica, doblez o pliegue.

plicate *v.* doblar, plegar.

plug *n.* tapón.

plumbism *n.* plumbismo, envenenamiento crónico con plomo.

plural *a. gr.* plural, más de uno en número.

pluripotent, pluripotential *a.* pluripotencial, que puede tomar más de un curso de acción.

pneumatic *a.* neumático-a, rel. al aire o a la respiración.

pneumatization *n.* neumatización, formación de cavidades llenas de aire en un hueso esp. en el hueso temporal.

pneumatocele *n.* neumatocele. 1. hernia de tejido pulmonar; 2. saco o tumor que contiene gas.

pneumococcal *a.* neumocócico-a, rel. a la neumonía o que la causa.

pneumococcus *n, L.* (*pl.* **pneumococci**) neumococo, microorganismo o tipo de bacteria gram-positiva que causa neumonía aguda y otras infecciones del tracto respiratorio superior.

pneumocystis carinii pneumonia *n.* neumonía neumocística carinii, tipo de pulmonía aguda intersticial causada por el bacilo *Pneumocysti carinii*, considerada una de las infecciones oportunistas comunes del SIDA.

pneumoencephalography *n.* neumoencefalografia, rayos-x del cerebro por medio de aire o gas inyectado para permitir distinguir visualmente la corteza y los ventrículos cerebrales.

pneumomediastinum *n. L.* neumomediastinum, presencia de gas o de aire en los tejidos del mediastino.

pneumonia *n.* pulmonía, neumonía, enfermedad infecciosa causada por bacterias o virus presentes en el tracto respiratorio superior; **double** ___ / ___ doble; ___ **lobar** / ___ lobar; **staphylococcal** ___ / ___ estafilocócica.

pneumonic *a.* neumónico-a, rel. a los pulmones o a la neumonía.

pneumonic plague *n.* peste neumónica, forma de peste con síntomas de esputos sanguíneos, escalofríos y fiebre (calentura) alta que puede ser letal.

pneumonitis *n.* neumonitis. V. **pneumonia.**

pneumothorax *n.* neumotórax, acumulación de aire o gas en la cavidad pleural que resulta en colapso del pulmón afectado;

spontaneous ___ / ___ espontáneo;
tension ___ / ___ por tensión.
pocket n. saco, bolsa; [*clothing*] bolsillo.
pockmark n. marca, señal o cicatriz. 1. marca de una pústula; 2. señal que deja la viruela.
podiatrist n. podiatra, especialista en podiatría.
podiatry n. podiatría, diagnóstico y tratamiento de afecciones de los pies.
point n. punto, punta.
poison n. veneno; [*insect, reptile bite*] ponzoña; substancia tóxica; ___ ivy / hiedra venenosa.
poisoning n. envenenamiento.
poisonous a. venenoso-a; tóxico-a.
polar a. polar, rel. a un polo.
polarity n. polaridad. 1. cualidad de poseer polos; 2. presentación de efectos opuestos en dos extremos o polos.
polarization n. polarización.
pole n. polo. 1. cada uno de los extremos opuestos de un cuerpo u órgano o de una parte esférica u oval.
policy n. póliza; reglamento; insurance ___ / ___ de seguros.
polio, poliomyelitis n. polio, poliomielitis, parálisis infantil, enfermedad contagiosa que ataca el sistema nervioso central y causa parálisis en los músculos esp. de las piernas.
poliovirus n. poliovirus, agente causante de la poliomielitis.
polite a. cortés.
pollen n. polen.
pollute v. contaminar, corromper.
pollution n. polución, contaminación; air ___ / ___ del aire; water ___ / ___ del agua.
poly n. poli, leucocito polimorfonuclear.
polyarthritis n. poliartritis, infl. de varias articulaciones.
polyarticular a. poliarticular, que afecta varias articulaciones.
polyclinic n. policlínica, hospital general.
polycystic a. poliquístico-a, que está formado-a por varios quistes; ___ kidney disease / enfermedad ___ del riñón; ___ ovarian syndrome / síndrome ___ ovárico.
polycythemia n. policitemia, aumento excesivo de glóbulos rojos; ___ rubra / ___ vera secundaria, ___ vera; primary ___ / ___ primaria.
polydactyly n. polidactilia, condición anormal de poseer más de cinco dedos en la mano o el pie.
polydipsia n. polidipsia, sed insaciable.
polygamy n. poligamia, práctica de poseer más de un cónyuge a la vez.

polygraph n. polígrafo, instrumento para obtener diversas pulsaciones arteriales y venosas simultáneamente.
polyhydramnios n. polihidramnios, exceso de líquido amniótico.
polymorphonuclear a. polimorfonucleado-a, que tiene un núcleo lobular complejo.
polymorphonuclear leukocyte n. leucocito polimorfonucleado, granulocito con núcleo de lóbulos múltiples.
polymyalgia n. polimialgia, condición caracterizada por dolor en distintos músculos; ___ rheumatica / ___ reumática.
polymyopathy n. polimiopatía, cualquier enfermedad que afecta varios músculos simultáneamente.
polymyositis n. polimiositis. V. dermatomyositis.
polyneuropathy n. polineuropatía, enfermedad que afecta varios nervios a la vez.
polyp n. pólipo, cualquier protuberancia o bulto que se desarrolla de una membrana mucosa.
polypectomy n. polipectomía, excisión de un pólipo.
polyposis n. poliposis, formación numerosa de pólipos.
polysaccharide n. polisacárido, carbohidrato que puede disolverse en agua.
polyunsaturated a. poli-nosaturado, que denota un ácido graso.
polyvalent a. polivalente, que tiene efecto en contra de más de un agente.
pomade n. pomada, sustancia medicinal semisólida para uso externo.
pons n. L. pons, formación de tejido que sirve de puente entre dos partes.
pontiac fever n. legionnaire's disease.
poor a. pobre, necesitado-a; deficiente; in ___ condition / en mala condición, en mal estado.
popliteal a. poplíteo-a, área posterior de la rodilla.
popper n. pop. nombre atribuído a algunas drogas adictivas.
population n. población, habitantes de un área.
porcine a. porcino-a, rel. al cerdo.
pore, porus n. poro, abertura diminuta tal como la de una glándula sudorípara.
pork n. cerdo, puerco; ___ chop / chuleta o costilla de ___ .
porosis n. porosis, formacion de una cavidad.
porous a. poroso-a, permeable.
porphyria n. porfiria, defecto metabólico congénito que se caracteriza por exceso de porfirina en la sangre, en la orina y en las heces

fecales, causando numerosos trastornos físicos y psiquiátricos.

porphyrin *n.* porfirina, compuesto que ocurre en el protoplasma y que es la base de los pigmentos respiratorios en los animales y las plantas.

porta *n. L.* porta, entrada, esp. la parte de un órgano por donde penetran vasos sanguíneos y nervios.

portacaval *a.* portacava, rel. a la vena porta y la vena cava inferior.

portal *a.* portal, rel. al sistema portal.

portal circulation *n.* circulación portal, curso por el cual la sangre entra al hígado por la vena porta y sale por la vena hepática.

portal hypertension *n.* hipertensión portal, aumento de la presión en la vena porta debido a una obstrucción.

portal vein *n.* vena porta, vena formada por varias ramas de venas que provienen de órganos abdominales.

portion *v.* porción.

position *n.* posición. 1. actitud o postura del cuerpo; **anatomic** ___ / ___ anatómica; **central** ___ / ___ central; **decubitus** ___ / ___ decúbito; **deep** ___ / ___ dentro de, profunda; **distal** ___ / ___ distal; **genupectoral** ___ / ___ genupectoral; **inferior** ___ / ___ inferior; **lateral** ___ / ___ lateral, de un lado; **lithotomy** ___ / ___ de litotomía; **lying down** ___ / ___ yacente, acostada; **medial** ___ / ___ media; **posterior** ___ / ___ posterior, detrás de; **prone** ___ / ___ prona, boca abajo; **superficial** ___ / ___ superficial; **superior** ___ / ___ superior, encima de; **supine** ___ / ___ supina, boca arriba; **upright** ___ / ___ erecta; 2. posición y presentación del feto.

positive *a.* positivo-a, afirmativo-a.

positivity *n.* positividad, manifestación de una reacción positiva.

possess *v.* poseer, tener.

possessed *a.* poseído-a, dominado-a por una idea o pasión.

possession *n.* posesión.

possessive *n. gr.* adjetivo o pronombre posesivo; *a.* posesivo-a.

posterior *a.* posterior. 1. rel. a la parte dorsal o trasera de una estructura; 2. que continúa.

posthumous *a.* póstumo, que ocurre después de la muerte.

posthypnotic *a.* posthipnótico-a, que sigue al estado hipnótico.

post ictal *a.* post ictal, después de un ataque.

post mature *a.* postmaduro-a, rel. a un recién nacido después de un embarazo prolongado.

postmortem *n. L.* post mortem, después de la muerte; autopsia.

postnasal *a.* postnasal, detrás de la nariz.

postnasal drip *n.* goteo postnasal.

postoperative *a.* postoperatorio-a, que ocurre después de la operación; ___ **care** / cuidado ___; ___ **complication** / complicación ___ .

postpartum *n. L.* postpartum, después del parto; ___ **blues** / estado de depresión que sigue al parto; ___ **pituitary insufficiency** / insuficiencia pituitaria del ___ .

postpartum period, puerperium *n.* puerperio, período de aproximadamente seis semanas después del parto durante el cual los órganos de la madre vuelven a su estado normal.

postpartum psychosis *n.* psicosis del postpartum.

postpone *v.* posponer, demorar, aplazar.

postprandial *a.* postprandial, después de una comida.

postsurgical pain treatment *n.* tratamiento de dolor posoperatorio.

postural *a.* postural, rel. a la postura del cuerpo; ___ **hypotension** / hipotensión ___, descenso de la presión arterial en posición erecta.

posture *n.* postura, posición del cuerpo.

potable *a.* potable, salubre, que puede beberse.

potassium *n.* potasio, mineral que se encuentra en el cuerpo combinado con otros, esencial en la conducción de impulsos nerviosos y actividad muscular.

potato *n.* patata, *H.A.* papa.

potbelly *n.* panza, barriga.

potency *n.* fuerza, potencia.

potent *a.* potente, fuerte; eficaz.

potential *a.* potencial, que existe en forma de cierta capacidad o disposición.

potion *n.* poción, dosis de líquido medicinal.

pouch *n.* bolsa, saco, cavidad.

poultice *n.* cataplasma, emplasto.

pound *n.* libra, medida de peso; *v.* machacar, golpear.

pour *v.* verter, vaciar, derramar.

poverty *n.* pobreza, carencia.

powder *n.* polvo; **powdered** *a.* en polvo.

power *n.* poder, fuerza.

pox *n.* enfermedad eruptiva de la piel caracterizada por manifestación de vesículas que se convierten en pústulas.

P

practical *a.* práctico-a.

practice *n.* práctica; costumbre;
 private ___ / ___ privada; *v.* practicar.

prandial *a.* prandial, rel. a las comidas.

preagonal *a.* preagónico-a; moribundo-a, al borde de la muerte.

preanesthetic *n.* preanestésico, agente preliminar que se administra con anticipación a la anestesia general.

precancerous *a.* precanceroso-a, susceptible a o que puede convertirse en un cáncer.

precarious *a.* precario-a.

precaution *n.* precaución.

precede *v.* preceder, anteceder.

precipitate *n.* precipitado, depósito de partes sólidas que se asientan en una solución; *a.* precipitado-a, que sucede con rapidez.

precise *a.* preciso-a, correcto-a.

precision *n.* precisión, exactitud.

precocious *a.* precoz, de un desarrollo más avanzado que el normal para la edad; ___ **child** / niño-a ___ .

precocity *n.* precocidad, desarrollo de rasgos físicos o facultades mentales más avanzados que lo normal en comparación con la edad cronólogica.

precursor *n.* precursor-a, predecesor-a, manifestación tal como la aparición de un síntoma o señal antes de desarrollarse una enfermedad; *a.* precursor-a, predecesor-a; preliminar.

predict *v.* predecir.

predictable *a.* predecible.

predispose *v.* predisponer.

predisposed *a.* predispuesto-a, que tiene susceptibilidad o tendencia a contraer una enfermedad.

predisposition *n.* predisposición, inclinación a desarrollar una condición o enfermedad debido a factores genéticos, ambientales o psicológicos.

predominant *a.* predominante.

preeclampsia *n.* preeclampsia, condición tóxica que se ve en la última etapa del embarazo y que se manifiesta con hipertensión, albuminuria y edema.

prefer *v.* preferir, seleccionar.

preferable *a.* preferible, favorito-a.

preference *n.* preferencia.

prefix *n. gr.* prefijo.

pregnancy *n.* embarazo, gravidez, estado de gestación; **ectopic** ___ / ___ ectópico; **extrauterine** ___ / ___ extrauterino; **incomplete** ___ / ___ incompleto;

interstitial ___ / ___ intersticial; **false** ___ / ___ falso; **multiple** ___ / ___ múltiple; **prolonged** ___ / ___ prolongado; **surrogate** ___ / ___ subrogado; **tubal** ___ / ___ tubárico.

pregnant *a.* embarazada, encinta, en estado de gestación; grávida.

prehensile *a.* prensil, adaptado para agarrar o asir.

prejudice *n.* prejuicio.

preliminary *a.* preliminar.

premature *a.* [*newborn*] prematuro-a, nacido antes de llegar a término.

prematurity *n.* prematurez, condición del feto antes de alcanzar el término de treinta y siete semanas de la gestación.

premedication *n.* premedicación.

premenstrual *n.* premenstrual, antes de la menstruación; ___ **tension** / tensión ___ .

premenstrual syndrome *n.* síndrome premenstrual, síndrome que se manifiesta días anteriores a la menstruación y que se caracteriza por irritabilidad, retención de líquidos y tensión emocional.

premonition *n.* premonición, presentimiento.

premunition *n.* premunición, inmunidad a una infección específica debida a la presencia previa del agente que la causa en el organismo.

prenatal *a.* prenatal, anterior al nacimiento; ___ **care** / cuidado ___ .

preoccupation *n.* preocupación.

preoccupied *a.* preocupado-a.

preoccupy *v.* preocupar; preocuparse.

preoperative care *n.* cuidado preoperatorio, cuidado preliminar a la operación.

prep *abbr.* término que se usa esp. para referirse a todo lo relacionado con el proceso preoperatorio.

preparation *n.* preparación. 1. acción de preparar algo; 2. un medicamento que se prepara para ser administrado.

prepare *v.* preparar.

prepared childbirth *n.* parto natural. V. natural childbirth.

preposition *n. gr.* preposición.

prepubescent *a.* prepubescente, anterior a la pubertad.

prepuce *n.* prepucio, pliegue de piel sobre el glande del pene.

prerenal *a.* prerrenal. 1. situado frente al riñón; 2. que tiene lugar en la circulación antes de llegar al riñón.

presacral *a.* presacro, frente al sacro.

presbiopia *n.* presbiopía, presbicia, condición de la visión que ocurre en la vejez a causa de una deficiencia en la elasticidad del cristalino.

prescribe *v.* prescribir, recetar.
prescribed *a. pp.* of **to prescribe**, recetado, ordenado-a.
prescription *n.* receta; ___ **tablet, pad** / formulario.
presence *n.* [*looks*] presencia, aspecto; [*attendance*] asistencia.
present *n.* 1. [*gift*] regalo, obsequio; 2. *gr.* tiempo presente; **at** ___ / actualmente; *v.* **to be** ___ / asistir, estar presente; **-ly** *adv.* ahora, actualmente.
presentation *n.* presentación. 1. reporte oral; 2. posición del feto en el útero según se detecta en un examen, o posición de salida en relación al canal del parto en el momento del nacimiento; **breech** ___ / ___ de nalgas; **brow** ___ / ___ de cejas o frente; **cephalic** ___ / ___ de cabeza; **face** ___ / ___ de cara; **footling** ___ / ___ de pies; **shoulder** ___ / ___ de hombro; **transverse** ___ / ___ transversa.
preservation *n.* preservación, conservación.
preservative *n.* preservativo, conservador. 1. agente que se añade a un alimento o medicamento para impedir el desarrollo de bacterias; 2. profiláctico.
preserve *v.* preservar, conservar.
press *v.* hacer presión, comprimir, oprimir.
pressor *a.* presor, que tiende a aumentar la presión sanguínea.
pressure *n.* presión, tensión, compresión; **arterial** ___ / ___ arterial, presión o tensión de la sangre sobre las paredes de los vasos capilares; **atmospheric** ___ / ___ atmosférica, la que ejerce la masa de aire alrededor de la tierra; **central venous** ___ / ___ central venosa, presión de la sangre en la aurícula derecha del corazón; **diastolic** ___ / ___ diastólica, presión arterial durante la diástole; **intracranial** ___ / ___ intracraneana o intracraneal, presión ejercida dentro de la cavidad craneana; **intrathoracic** ___ / ___ intratorácica, presión dentro del tórax; **osmotic** ___ / ___ osmótica; osmosis; **partial** ___ / ___ parcial, la que ejerce uno de los gases de una composición mixta; **pulse** ___ / ___ de pulso; **systolic** ___ / ___ sistólica, presión arterial durante la contracción de los ventrículos; **venous** ___ / ___ venosa, la de la sangre en las venas; *v.* hacer presión, presionar.
pressure point *n.* punto de presión, área donde puede sentirse el pulso o hacer presión para contener un sangramiento.
pressure sore *n.* úlcera de decúbito.

pretend *v.* pretender, fingir, aparentar.
preterit *n. gr.* pretérito, tiempo pasado.
preterm *n.* pretérmino, lo que concierne a sucesos anteriores a completar el término de treinta y siete semanas en un embarazo.
prevalence *n.* prevalencia, número de casos en una población afectados por la misma enfermedad en un tiempo determinado.
prevent *v.* prevenir, precaver, evitar.
preventive *a.* preventivo-a; ___ **health services** / servicios de salud ___ -s.
prevertebral *a.* prevertebral, situado enfrente de una vértebra.
previous *a.* previo-a, anterior.
priapism *n.* priapismo, erección prolongada y dolorosa del pene a consecuencia de una enfermedad.
price *n.* precio, valor, costo.
prick *n.* pinchazo; punzada; picadura, aguijón; *v.* picar, punzar, aguijonear, pinchar.
prickly heat *n.* salpullido, sarpullido.
priest *n.* sacerdote, padre, cura.
primarily *adv.* primeramente; principalmente, primordialmente.
primary *a.* inicial, primario-a, rel. al contacto o atención de un caso en su principio; ___ **physician** / médico de cabecera, facultativo que atiende al paciente inicialmente, esp. un pediatra o médico de familia.
primary care *n.* atención inicial del paciente.
prime *a.* primero-a, principal; *v.* **to be in one's** ___ / estar en la flor de la vida.
primitive *a.* primitivo-a; embriónico-a.
primordial *a.* primordial, esencial.
principal *a.* principal, más importante.
principle *n.* principio. 1. ingrediente esencial de un compuesto químico; 2. regla; orden.
print *n.* impresión, marca.
prior *n.* antecesor, predecesor; *a.* previo-a; ___ **to** / anterior a, antes de.
priority *n.* prioridad, preferencia, precedencia.
prism *n.* prisma.
privacy *n.* vida privada; aislamiento.
private *a.* privado-a, particular, exclusivo-a; ___ **hospital** / clínica; ___ **practice** / consulta particular; ___ **room** / cuarto ___; **-ly** *adv.* privadamente.
privation *n.* privación, necesidad.
privilege *n.* privilegio, derecho.
privileged *a.* confidencial, privilegiado-a; reservado-a; ___ **information** / información ___ o reservada.
probability *n.* probabilidad.

probable *a.* probable, casi posible; **-ly** *adv.* probablemente.

probe *n.* sonda, instrumento flexible que se usa para explorar cavidades o conductos y para medir la penetración de una herida; **hollow** ___ / ___ acanalada.

problem *n.* problema; cuestión; trastorno; ___ **solving** / solución de ___ -s.

problematic *a.* problemático-a; dificultoso-a.

procedure *n.* procedimiento; **clinical** ___ / ___ clínico; **invasive** ___ / ___ invasivo; **noninvasive** ___ / ___ no invasivo; **surgical** ___ / ___ quirúrgico; **therapeutic** ___ / ___ terapéutico.

proceed *v.* proceder, continuar, seguir adelante, avanzar.

process *n.* proceso, método, sistema.

procreate *v.* engendrar, procrear, reproducir.

procreation *n.* procreación, reproducción.

proctalgia *n.* proctalgia, dolor en el recto y el ano.

proctitis *n.* proctitis, infl. de la mucosa del recto y del ano.

proctologist *n.* proctólogo-a, especialista en proctología.

proctology *n.* proctología, estudio del colon, recto y ano, de las enfermedades que los afectan y su tratamiento.

proctoscope *n.* proctoscopio, espéculo rectal, tipo de endoscopio usado para examinar el recto.

procure *v.* procurar, tratar de obtener.

prodromal *a.* prodrómico-a, rel. a la fase inicial de una enfermedad.

prodrome *n.* pródromo, señal o síntoma preliminar.

produce *n.* producto, esp. vegetales, frutas y legumbres; producción; *v.* producir, crear; causar.

product *n.* producto; resultado, efecto.

production *n.* producción, rendimiento.

productive *a.* productivo-a, fecundo-a.

profession *n.* profesión, carrera, oficio.

professional *n.* profesional, facultivo-a; ___ **care** / cuidado ___; ___ **help** / asistencia ___; *a.* profesional; facultivo-a.

profile *n.* perfil, bosquejo, esbozo; **biochemical** ___ / ___ bioquímico; **physical** ___ / ___ físico.

profit *n.* beneficio, ganancia; ventaja.

profunda *a., L* (*pl.* **profunda**) muy interior, en referencia esp. a algunas arterias.

profundus *n., L.* profundo, interior.

profuse *a.* profuso-a; abundante; **-ly** *adv.* profusamente; abundantemente.

progeny *n.* descendencia, prole.

progesterone *n.* progesterona, hormona esteroide segregada por los ovarios.

prognathous *a.* prognato-a, que tiene la mandíbula prominente.

prognose *v.* pronosticar o predecir el desarrollo de una enfermedad.

prognosis *n.* pronóstico, evaluación del curso probable de una enfermedad.

prognosticate *v.* pronosticar.

progress *n.* progreso; *v.* **to make** ___ / progresar, mejorar.

progressive *a.* progresivo-a, que avanza.

projection *n.* proyección. 1. protuberancia; 2. mecanismo por el cual el (la) paciente atribuye inconscientemente a otras personas u objetos las cualidades y sentimientos propios que rechaza.

prolapse *n.* prolapso, caída de un órgano o parte.

proliferation *n.* proliferación, multiplicación en número por reproducción esp. de células similares.

proliferous, prolific *a.* prolífero-a, que se reproduce fácilmente.

prolong *v.* prolongar, extender; retardar.

prolongation *n.* prolongación, extensión.

prominence *n.* prominencia, proyección; *pop.* bulto.

promise *n.* promesa; *v.* prometer, dar la palabra.

promontory *n.* promontorio, elevación.

prompt *a.* puntual, a tiempo.

pronate *v.* pronar, poner el cuerpo o parte del mismo en posición prona.

prone *a.* acostado-a, postrado-a. 1. en posición acostada boca abajo; 2. con la mano virada, apoyada en el dorso; 3. propenso, susceptible a contraer una enfermedad.

pronoun *n. gr.* pronombre.

pronounce *v.* pronunciar, articular sonidos de letras.

pronunciation *n.* pronunciación.

proof *n.* prueba, comprobación; *v.* probar, demostrar.

propagate *v.* propagar, diseminar.

propagation *n.* propagación, reproducción.

proper *a.* propio-a, particular, apropiado-a.

property *n.* propiedad, cualidad, característica, atributo. See chart on page 211.

prophase *n.* profase, primera fase en la mitosis celular.

prophylactic *n.* profiláctico. 1. agente o método para evitar infecciones; 2. contraceptivo.

prophylaxis *n.* profilaxis, medidas para prevenir enfermedades o su propagación.

proportion *n.* proporción, tamaño determinado, medida.

proprietary medicine *n.* medicamento de patente.

proprioceptive *a.* propioceptivo-a, que recibe estímulos.

proprioceptor *n.* propioceptor, terminación nerviosa receptora que responde a estímulos y transmite información de los movimientos y posiciones del cuerpo.

proptosis *n.* proptosis, desplazamiento de un órgano hacia adelante tal como el globo ocular.

proscribe *v.* prohibir, cancelar.

prosencephalon *n.* prosencéfalo, porción anterior de la vesícula cerebral de la que se desarrollan el diencéfalo y el telencéfalo.

prostate *n.* próstata, glándula masculina que rodea el cuello de la vejiga y la uretra.

prostatectomy *n.* prostatectomía, excisión parcial o total de la próstata.

prostatic *a.* prostático-a, rel. a la próstata; ___ **hypertrophy** / hipertrofia ___, agrandamiento benigno de la próstata debido a la vejez.

prostatic specific antigen *n.* antígeno prostático específico, examen sanguíneo para evaluar los antígenos prostáticos específicos en la circulación.

prostatism *n.* prostatismo, trastorno debido a una obstrucción del cuello de la vejiga por agrandamiento de la próstata.

prostatitis *n.* prostatitis, infl. de la próstata.

prosthesis *n.* prótesis, reemplazo de una parte del cuerpo con un sustituto artificial.

prosthetics *n.* prostética, rama de la cirugía que se dedica al reemplazo de partes del cuerpo.

prostitution *n.* prostitución.

prostrate *a.* postrado-a. 1. en posición prona o supina; 2. débil, abatido-a; *v.* postrar; abatir; *vr.* postrarse; abatirse, debilitarse.

prostration *n.* postración, debilidad, abatimiento.

protean *n.* protéico, que se manifiesta en distintas formas.

protect *v.* proteger, cuidar.

protection *n.* protección, cuidado.

protective *a.* protector-a.

protective isolation *n.* aislamiento protector, estado que se recomienda en casos de pacientes de baja resistencia o inmunidad.

protein *n.* proteína, complejo compuesto nitrogenado esencial en el desarrollo y preservación de los tejidos del cuerpo; ___ **balance** / balance de las ___ -s; ___ **concentration** / ___ concentración de ___ .

proteinaceous *a.* proteináceo-a, de la naturaleza de o semejante a una proteína.

proteinemia *n.* proteinemia, proteínas en la sangre.

proteinosis *n.* proteinosis, acumulación en exceso de proteínas en los tejidos.

proteinuria *n.* proteinuria, presencia de proteínas en la orina.

prothrombin *n.* protrombina, una de las cuatro proteínas principales del plasma junto a la albúmina, la globulina y el fibrinógeno.

protocol *n.* protocolo, notas oficiales de un procedimiento.

protoplasm *n.* protoplasma, parte esencial de la célula que incluye el citoplasma y el núcleo.

prototype *n.* prototipo, modelo, ejemplo.

protozoon *n.* (*pl.* **protozoa**) protozoo, organismo unicelular.

protraction *n.* protracción, tracción hacia afuera, como en la mandíbula.

protrude *v.* sobresalir; salirse de su lugar.

protruding *a.* saliente.

protuberance *n.* protuberancia, prominencia.

proud *a.* orgulloso-a, arrogante.

prove *v.* demostrar, comprobar, probar.

provide *v.* proveer, dar, abastecer.

providence *n.* providencia.

provision *n.* provisión, abastecimiento.

provisional *a.* provisional, interino; **-ly** *adv.* provisionalmente, por lo pronto.

proximal *a.* cerca del punto de referencia.

prune *n.* ciruela pasa.

pruriginous *a.* pruriginoso-a, rel. a prurigo.

prurigo *n.* prurigo, condición cutánea crónica inflamatoria que se caracteriza por pápulas pequeñas y picazón intensa.

pruritus *n.* prurito, comezón, picazón.

pseudoaneurysm *n.* pseudoaneurisma, condición semejante a la dilatación de un aneurisma.

pseudocyesis *n.* pseudociesis. V. **pseudopregnancy**.

pseudocyst *n.* pseudoquiste, formación semejante a la de un quiste.

pseudogout *n.* seudogota, condición artrítica recurrente con síntomas similares a los de la gota.

pseudopregnancy *n.* embarazo falso o imaginario.

psoriasis *n.* psoriasis, dermatitis crónica que se manifiesta con manchas rojas cubiertas de escamas blancas.

psyche *n.* psique, proceso mental consciente o inconsciente.

psychedelic *a.* psicodélico-a, rel. a substancias o drogas que pueden inducir alteraciones perceptuales tales como alucinaciones y delirios.

psychiatric *a.* psiquiátrico-a, siquiátrico-a.

psychiatrist *n.* psiquiatra, siquiatra, especialista en psiquiatría.

psychiatry *n.* psiquiatría, rama de la medicina que estudia los trastornos mentales.

psychic *a.* psíquico-a, rel. a la mente o psique.

psychoactive *a.* psicoactivo-a, que afecta la condición mental.

psychoanalysis *n.* psicoanálisis, método de análisis psicológico creado por Sigmund Freud que se vale de la interpretación de los sueños y de la libre asociación de ideas para hacer al paciente consciente de conflictos reprimidos y tratar de ajustar su conducta emocional.

psychoanalyst *n.* psicoanalista, analista.

psychoanalyze *v.* psicoanalizar, sicoanalizar.

psychobiology *n.* psicobiología, estudio de la psique en relación con otros procesos biológicos.

psychodrama *n.* psicodrama, método de terapia psíquica en el cual se dramatizan situaciones conflictivas de la vida del paciente con la participación de éste.

psychological *a.* psicológico-a, rel. a la psicología.

psychologist *n.* psicólogo-a, profesional que practica la psicología.

psychology *n.* psicología, sicología, ciencia que estudia los procesos mentales y la conducta de un individuo.

psychomotor *a.* psicomotor-a, rel. a acciones motoras como resultado de actividades mentales.

psychopath *n.* psicópata, persona que padece de trastornos mentales.

psychopathology *n.* psicopatología, rama de la medicina que trata de las causas y naturaleza de las enfermedades mentales.

psychopharmacology *n.* psicofarmacología, estudio del efecto de drogas y medicamentos en la mente y la conducta.

psychophysiological *a.* psicofisiológico-a, rel. a la influencia mental sobre procesos físicos tal como se manifiesta en algunos desórdenes y enfermedades.

psychosis *n.* psicosis, trastorno mental severo de origen orgánico o emocional en el cual el paciente pierde contacto con la realidad y sufre de alucinaciones o aberraciones mentales; **alcoholic** ___ / ___ alcohólica; **depressive** ___ / ___ depresiva; **drug** ___ / ___ por drogas; **manic-depressive** ___ / ___

maníaco depresiva; **organic** ___ / ___ orgánica; **senile** ___ / ___ senil; **situational** ___ / ___ situacional; **toxic** ___ / ___ tóxica; **traumatic** ___ / ___ traumática.

psychosocial *a.* psicosocial, rel. a factores psicológicos y sociales.

psychosomatic *a.* psicosomático-a, rel. al cuerpo y a la mente; ___ **symptom** / síntoma ___ .

psychotherapy *n.* psicoterapia, tratamiento de trastornos mentales o emocionales por medios psicológicos tales como el psicoanálisis.

psychotic *a.* psicótico-a, rel. a o que sufre de una psicosis.

psychotropic drugs *n.* drogas psicotrópicas, compuestos químicos que afectan la estabilidad mental.

ptosis *n. Gr.* ptosis, prolapso de un órgano o parte, esp. visto en el párpado superior.

puberty *n.* pubertad, adolescencia, desarrollo de las características sexuales secundarias y comienzo de la capacidad reproductiva.

pubescense *n.* pubescencia. 1. principio de la pubertad; 2. aparición de la vellosidad.

pubic *a.* púbico-a, rel. al pubis; ___ **hair** / vello ___ .

pubis *n.* (*pl.* **pubes**) pubis, región púbica, estructura ósea frontal de la pelvis.

public *a.* público-a.

public health *n.* salubridad pública, rama de la medicina que se dedica a la atención social, física y mental de los miembros de una comunidad.

pudendum *n.* (*pl.* **pudenda**) pudendum, órganos genitales externos, esp. los femeninos.

puerile *a.* pueril, infantil.

puerperal *a.* puerperal, concerniente al puerperio.

puerperium *n.* puerperio. V. **post partum**.

pull *n.* tirón; *v.* tirar, halar, arrancar, sacar; **to** ___ **in** / tirar hacia adentro; **to** ___ **oneself together** / calmarse; **to** ___ **through** [*as in a sickness*] / recuperarse; **to** ___ **up one's knees** / levantar las rodillas.

pulley *n.* polea.

pulmonary, pulmonic *a.* pulmonar, pulmónico-a, rel. al pulmón o a la arteria pulmonar; ___ **alveolar proteinosis** / proteinosis alveolar ___ ; ___ **artery wedge pressure** / presión diferencial de la arteria ___ ; ___ **edema** / edema ___ ; ___ **embolism** / embolia ___ ; ___ **emphysema** / enfisema ___ ; ___ **insufficiency** /

insuficiencia ___; ___ **stenosis** /
estenosis ___; ___ **valve** / válvula ___; ___
vein / vena ___ .

pulp *n.* pulpa. 1. parte blanda de un órgano; 2.
quimo; 3. pulpa dental, parte central blanda de
un diente.

pulsatile *a.* pulsátil, de pulsación rítmica.

pulsation *n.* pulsación, latido rítmico tal como el
del corazón.

pulse *n.* pulso, dilatación arterial rítmica que gen.
coincide con los latidos cardíacos;
alternating ___ / ___ alternante;
bigeminal ___ / ___ bigeminado;
bounding ___ / ___ saltón; **dorsalis**
pedis ___ / ___ de la arteria dorsal del pie;
femoral ___ / ___ femoral; **filiform** ___ / ___
filiforme; **full** ___ / ___ lleno;
irregular ___ / ___ irregular;
peripheral ___ / ___ periférico; ___ **pressure** /
presión del pulso, diferencia entre la presión
sistólica y la diastólica; **radial** ___ / ___ radial;
rapid ___ / ___ rápido; **regular** ___ / ___
regular; **water hammer** ___ / ___ en martillo de
agua. See chart on page 213.

pulverize *v.* pulverizar, reducir a polvo, hacer
polvo.

pump *n.* bomba; **intravenous** ___ / ___
intravenosa; **oxigenator** ___ / ___ oxigenadora;
stomach ___ / ___ gástrica; *v.* bombear; **to** ___
out / ___ hacia afuera, sacar por bomba.

pumping *n.* bombeo; **heart** ___ / ___ del
corazón; **stomach** ___ / ___ estomacal.

punch *n.* sacabocados, instrumento quirúrgico que
se usa para perforar o cortar un disco o un
segmento de tejido.

punctuate *n.* puntuar, acto de perforar un tejido
con un instrumento afilado.

puncture *n.* punción, perforación; *v.* punzar,
pinchar; agujerear.

puncture wound *n.* herida por perforación con
un instrumento afilado.

pungent *a.* pungentivo-a, acre; penetrante.

pupil *n.* pupila, abertura contráctil del iris que da
entrada a la luz.

pupillary *a.* pupilar, rel. a la pupila.

pure *a.* puro-a, sin contaminación.

purgation *n.* purgación, evacuación mediante el
uso de un medicamento purgativo.

purgative *n.* purgante, catártico, agente que
causa evacuación intestinal; ___ **enema** / enema,
lavativa, lavabo; ___ **saline** / ___ salino.

purge *n.* purga, medicamento o catártico; *v.* 1.
purgar o limpiar; 2. forzar la evacuación de los
intestinos por medio de un purgante.

purification *n.* purificación, destilación.

purified *a.* depurado-a, purificado-a; ___ **water** /
agua ___ .

purify *v.* purificar, destilar.

purple *n.* color púrpura; morado.

purpose *n.* propósito, intención.

purposeful *a.* intencional, con intención;
determinado-a.

purpura *n.* púrpura, condición caracterizada por
manchas rojizas o de color púrpura en la piel,
debidas al escape de sangre a los tejidos;
thrombocytopenic ___ / ___ trombocitopénica.

purulence *n.* purulencia, pus.

purulent *a.* purulento-a, que está supurando.

pus *n.* pus, excreción, fluido amarillento espeso
que se forma por supuración;___**discharge** /
supuración; ___ **-like** / purulento-a.

push *n.* empujón; pujo; ___ **button** / botón de
llamada; *v.* [*as to bear down*] pujar.

pustule *n.* pústula, costra, elevación pequeña de
la piel que contiene pus;*pop.* postilla.

put *vi.* poner; **to** ___ **in** / poner dentro de, echar
en, meter; **to** ___ **off** / aplazar, cancelar; **to** ___
on [*clothes*] / ponerse la ropa, vestirse; **to** ___
out [*light, fire*] / apagar; **to** ___ **together** / unir,
juntar; **to** ___ **up with** / aguantar, soportar,
tolerar.

putrefaction *n.* putrefacción, condición de ser
pútrido-a, corrompido-a.

putrid *a.* pútrido-a, corrompido-a.

pyelogram *n.* pielograma, radiografía de la
pelvis renal y uréter usando un medio de
contraste.

pyelolithotomy *n.* pielolitotomía, incisión para
extraer un cálculo de la pelvis renal.

pyelonephritis *n.* pielonefritis, infl. del riñón y
de la pelvis renal.

pyeloplastia *n.* pieloplastia, operación de
reparación plástica de la pelvis renal.

pyelostomy *n.* pielostomía, formación o
establecimiento de una abertura en la pelvis
renal para desviar la orina hacia el exterior.

pyelotomy *n.* pielotomía, incisión de la pelvis
renal.

pyloric *a.* pilórico, rel. al píloro.

pyloroplasty *n.* piloroplastia, reparación del
píloro.

pylorus *n.* píloro, abertura u orificio circular
entre el estómago y el duodeno.

pyocyte *n.* piocito, corpúsculo de pus.

pyoderma *n.* pioderma, cualquier enfermedad de
la piel que presenta supuración.

pyogenic *a.* piógeno-a, purulento-a.

pyorrhea *n.* piorrea, periodontitis.

pyramid *n.* pirámide, estructura semejante a un cono, tal como la médula oblongata.

pyrectic, pyretic *a.* pirético-a, rel. a la fiebre.

pyretolysis *n.* piretolisis. 1. reducción de fiebre; 2. proceso de curación que se acelera con la fiebre.

pyrexia *n.* pirexia, condición febril.

pyrogen *n.* pirógeno, sustancia que produce fiebre.

pyromania *n.* piromanía, obsesión con el fuego; manía incendiaria.

pyuria *n.* piuria, presencia de piocitos en la orina.

q

q. *abbr.* **quantity** / cantidad; **quaque** / cada.

quack *n.* charlatán, persona que pretende tener cualidades o conocimientos para curar enfermedades.

quackery *n.* curanderismo, charlatanería.

quadrangle *n.* cuadrángulo, figura geométrica formada por cuatro ángulos.

quadrant *n.* cuadrante, cuarta parte de un círculo.

quadrate *a.* cuadrado, que tiene cuatro lados iguales; ___ **lobe** / lóbulo cuadrado; ___ **lobule** / lobulillo cuadrado.

quadratus *n. L.* quadratus. 1. músculo de cuatro lados; 2. figura de cuatro lados.

quadriceps *n.* cuadríceps, músculo de cuatro cabezas, extensor de la pierna.

quadriplegia *n.* cuadriplegia, parálisis de las cuatro extremidades.

quadriplegic *a.* cuadriplégico, que sufre de parálisis en las cuatro extremidades.

quadruplet *a.* cuádruple, cada uno de los cuatro hijos nacidos en un parto múltiple.

quake *n.* [*earthquake*] temblor de tierra, terremoto, sismo, estremecimiento; *v.* temblar.

qualification *n.* calificación; [*competence*] capacidad.

qualified *a.* competente, capaz.

qualify *v.* calificar; capacitar.

qualitative *a.* cualitativo-a, rel. a cualidad o clase.

qualitative test *n.* prueba cualitativa.

quality *n.* cualidad, propiedad.

quantitative test *n.* prueba cuantitativa.

quantity *n.* cantidad.

Quant sign *n.* signo de Quant, hendidura en forma de T que aparece en el hueso occipital y que se ve en casos de raquitismo.

quantum *n. L.* quantum, unidad de energía.

quarantine *n.* cuarentena, período de cuarenta días durante los cuales se restringen las actividades de personas o animales para prevenir la propagación de una enfermedad contagiosa.

quarrel *n.* pelea, riña, disputa, querella; *v.* reñir, disputar, pelear.

quartan *a.* cuartana, que recurre cada cuatro días tal como la fiebre palúdica.

quarter *n.* cuarto, cuarta parte de un todo.

quash *v.* suprimir, sofocar.

quaver *n.* vibración, temblor; *v.* vibrar, temblar.

queasy *a.* nauseabundo-a; ___ **stomach** / naúseas, asco.

Queckensted sign *n.* signo de Queckensted, falta de aumento en la presión del líquido cerebroespinal cuando hay compresión de las venas del cuello; en personas saludables, la presión aumenta rápidamente cuando ocurre la compresión.

queer *a.* raro-a, excéntrico-a; [*slang*] homosexual, invertido, maricón.

quench *v.* extinguir, apagar; [*thirst*] saciar.

quenching *n.* [*thirst*] el acto de saciar; [*extinguishing*] el acto de extinguir, o disminuir.

query *n.* pregunta; duda.

quest *n.* indagación, búsqueda, pesquisa.

question *n.* pregunta; cuestión, problema; *v.* interrogar, preguntar.

questionnaire *n.* cuestionario.

quick *a.* rápido-a, ligero-a, [*alert*] listo-a; ___ **-frozen** / congelado-a al instante; **-ly** *adv.* pronto, rápidamente, al instante.

quicken *v.* acelerar; animar, avivar, estimular.

quickening *n.* 1. animación; 2. percepción por la madre del primer movimiento del feto en el útero.

quiescent *a.* quiescente, en estado de reposo; inactivo-a.

quiet *a.* quieto-a, sosegado-a, tranquilo-a; *v.* calmar, tranquilizar.

quinidine *n.* quinidina, alcaloide derivado de una *Cinchona* que se usa en irregularidades cardíacas.

quinine *n.* quinina, alcaloide que se obtiene de la corteza de una *Cinchona* usado como antiséptico y antipirético esp. en el tratamiento de paludismo, tifoidea y malaria.

quininism *n.* quininismo, chinchonismo, intoxicación de sales de quinina.

quintan *n.* quintana, fiebre recurrente cada cinco días.

quintuplet *a.* quíntuple, cada uno de los cinco hijos nacidos en un parto múltiple.

quit *v.* desistir, dejar, parar.

quota *n.* cuota.

quotidian *a.* cotidiano-a, de todos los días; ___ **malaria.** / malaria ___

quotient *n.* cuociente, cociente, cifra que resulta de una división; **achievement** ___ / ___ de realización; **blood** ___ / ___ sanguíneo; **growth** ___ / ___ de crecimiento; **intelligence** ___ / ___ de inteligencia.

q

r

R *abbr.* **radioactive** / radioactivo; **resistance** / resistencia; **respiration** / respiración; **response** / respuesta, reacción.

rabbi *n.* rabí, rabino.

rabbit *n.* conejo-a; ___ **test** / prueba del embarazo.

rabbit fever *n.* fiebre de conejo. *Syn.* **tularemia.**

rabid *a.* rabioso-a, rel. a la rabia o afectado por ella.

rabies *n.* rabia. V. **hydrophobia.**

race *n.* raza, grupo étnico diferenciado por características comunes heredadas.

racemose *a.* racimoso-a, racimado-a, similar a un racimo de uvas.

rachicentesis *n.* raquicentesis, punción lumbar.

rachiotomy *n.* raquiotomía. V. **laminectomy.**

rachis *n.* raquis, la columna vertebral.

rachitic *a.* raquítico-a. rel. al raquitismo; débil, endeble.

rachitism, rhachitis, rachitis *n.* raquitismo, enfermedad por deficiencia que afecta el desarrollo óseo en los adolescentes, causada por falta de calcio, fósforo y vitamina D.

racial *a.* racial, étnico-a, de la raza; ___ **prejudice** / prejuicio ___; ___ **immunity** / inmunidad ___, tipo de inmunidad natural de los miembros de una raza.

racial immunity *n.* inmunidad racial.

rad *n.* rad. 1. dosis de radiación absorbida; 2. rad, *abbr.* of radix, raíz.

radial *a.* radial. 1. rel. al hueso del radio; 2. que se expande en todas direcciones a partir de un centro.

radiant *a.* radiante, que emite rayos.

radiate *v.* irradiar, expandirse.

radiation *n.* radiación. 1. emisión de materiales o partículas radioactivas; 2. propagación de energía; 3. emisión de rayos desde un centro común; ___ **dosage** / dosis de ___; ___ **hazards** / riesgos y peligros causados por una ___; ___ **therapy** / radioterapia; **electromagnetic** ___ / ___ electromagnética; **infrared** ___ / ___ por rayos infrarrojos; **ionizing** ___ / ___ ionizante; **ultraviolet** ___ / ___ de rayos ultravioleta.

radiation oncology *n.* uso de radiación en el tratamiento de neoplasmas.

radiation sickness *n.* enfermedad por radiación causada por exposición a rayos-x o a materiales radioactivos.

radiation therapy *n.* terapia de radiación, tratamiento de un tumor o enfermedad por medio de radiaciones de radium o radon. *Syn.* **Radiotherapy.**

radical *n. gr.* raíz de una palabra; *a.* radical, dirigido a erradicar la raíz de una enfermedad o de todo tejido enfermo; ___ **treatment** / tratamiento ___ .

radicle *n.* radícula, estructura semejante a una raíz.

radicular *a.* radical, rel. a la raíz u origen.

radiculectomy *n.* radiculectomía, excisión de la raíz de un nervio, esp. de la raíz de un nervio espinal.

radiculitis *n.* radiculitis, infl. de la raíz de un nervio.

radiculomyelopathy *n.* radiculomielopatía, enfermedad que afecta la médula espinal y la raíz de los nervios espinales.

radiculoneuritis, Guillain-Barré syndrome *n.* radiculoneuritis, síndrome de Guillain-Barré, infl. de las raíces de los nervios espinales.

radiculoneuropathy *n.* radiculoneuropatía, condición patológica de los nervios y sus raíces.

radiculopathy *n.* radiculopatía, cualquier enfermedad de las raíces de los nervios espinales.

radioactive *a.* radiactivo-a, rel. a la radiactividad o que la posee.

radioactive iodine excretion test *n.* prueba radiactiva del yodo, evaluación de la función de la tiroides por medio del uso de yodo radiactivo.

radioactivity *n.* radiactividad, propiedad de ciertos elementos de producir radiaciones.

radiobiology *n.* radiobiología, estudio del efecto de la radioactividad en tejidos vivos.

radiocarbon *n.* carbono radiactivo.

radiocardiography *n.* radiocardiografía, registro gráfico de una sustancia radioactiva durante su paso a través del corazón.

radiocontrast media *m.* medio de contraste de sustancia radioactiva usado en el proceso de efectuar varios tipos de pruebas para diagnóstico.

radiocurable *a.* radiocurable, que se puede curar por medio de radioterapia.

radiodermatitis *n.* radiodermatitis, dermatitis causada por la exposición a radiaciones.

radiodiagnosis *n.* radiodiagnosis, diagnosis por medio de rayos-x.

radioelement *n.* radioelemento, cualquier elemento que tiene propiedades radiactivas.

radiography *n.* radiografía, uso de rayos-x para producir imágenes en placas o en una pantalla fluorescente.

radioimmunity *n.* radioinmunidad, disminución de la sensibilidad a las radiaciones.

radioimmunoassay *n.* radioinmunoensayo.

radioisotope *n.* radioisótopo, isótopo radioactivo.

radiologic *a.* radiológico-a, rel. a la radiología.

radiologist *n.* radiólogo-a, especialista en radiología.

radiology *n.* radiología, ciencia que trata de los rayos-x o rayos que provienen de sustancias radiactivas, esp. para uso médico.

radiolucent *a.* radiolúcido-a, que permite el paso de la mayor parte de rayos-x.

radionecrosis *n.* radionecrosis, desintegración de tejidos por radiación.

radionuclear venography *n.* venografía radionuclear, estudio de las venas por medio de rayos gamma.

radionuclide imaging *n.* V. **scintigraphy.**

radiopaque *a.* radioopaco-a, que no deja pasar rayos-x u otra forma de radiación; ___ **dye** / colorante ___ .

radiopharmaceutical agents *n.* radiofármacos, drogas radioactivas usadas en el tratamiento y diagnóstico de enfermedades.

radioreceptor *n.* radiorreceptor, receptor que recibe energía radiante como la de los rayos-x, de la luz o del calor.

radioresistance *n.* radiorresistencia, resistencia a los efectos de una radiación.

radioresistant *a.* radiorresistente, que tiene la propiedad de resistir efectos radioactivos.

radioscopy *n. v.* radioscopia, examen de las estructuras internas del cuerpo por medio de rayos-x y de rayos emitidos por electrones y positrones conocidos como rayos roentgen.V. **fluoroscopy.**

radiosensitive *a.* radiosensitivo-a, que es afectado por o que responde a un tratamiento de radiación.

radiotherapy *n.* radioterapia, tratamiento de una enfermedad por medio de rayos-x o por otras sustancias radioactivas.

radish *n.* rábano.

radium *L.* radium, radio, elemento metálico radioactivo y fluorescente usado en algunas de sus variaciones en el tratamiento de tumores malignos; ___ **needle** / aguja de radio, divisa en forma de aguja que contiene radio usado en radioterapia.

radium therapy *n.* radioterapia, terapia con el uso de radio.

radius *n.* radio. 1. hueso largo del antebrazo; 2. línea recta que une el centro y cualquier punto de la circunferencia.

radon *n.* radón, elemento radiactivo gaseoso.

rage *n.* rabia, ira, cólera.

rain *n.* lluvia; *v.* llover.

raise *v.* levantar; [*increase*] aumentar, subir.

raisin *n.* pasa, uva seca.

rale *n.* estertor, sonido anormal originado en el pulmón que se percibe durante la auscultación; **coarse** ___ / ___ áspero; **crackling** ___ / ___ crujiente; **crepitant** ___ / ___ crepitante; **dry** ___ / ___ seco; **moist** ___ / ___ húmedo.

rambling *a.* sin orden ni concierto.

ramification *n.* ramificación, distribución en ramas.

ramify *v.* ramificar; ramificarse.

ramus *n., L* (*pl.* **rami**) rama, bifurcación, división.

rancid *a.* rancio-a, de olor desagradable; que denota descomposición.

rancor *n.* rencor, resentimiento.

random control test *n.* prueba de control sin método.

random test *n.* prueba al azar.

range *n.* escala de diferenciación, amplitud, margen; ___ **of motion** / amplitud de movimiento; ___**of colors** / gama de colores; ___ **of vision** / campo visual.

ranine *n.* ranino-a, rel. a la ránula o parte inferior de la lengua.

ranula *n.* ránula, quiste situado debajo de la lengua causado por la obstrucción de un canal glandular.

rape *n.* violación; *v.* violar, abusar sexualmente.

raphe *n.* rafe, línea de unión de dos mitades simétricas de una estructura tal como la lengua.

rapid *a.* rápido-a, veloz; ___ **eye movement** / movimientos oculares ___; **-ly** *adv.* rápidamente

rapid respiration *n.* taquipnea, respiración excesivamente rápida.

rapidity *n.* rapidez, velocidad.

rapidly progressive sickness *n.* enfermedad rápidamente progresiva.

rapport *n.* relación armoniosae entendimiento, congenio amistoso entre dos personas.

raptus *L.* raptus, arrebato, ataque súbito violento.

rare *a.* raro-a; único-a; **-ly** *adv.* raramente, casi nunca.

rash, rasche *Fr. n.* rasche, erupción; **diaper** ___ / eritema de los pañales; **heat** ___ /

r

salpullido; **hemorrhagic** ___ / ___ hemorrágica; **maculopapular** ___ / ___ maculopapular; **papular** ___ / ___ papular; **squamous** ___ / ___ escamosa.

raspberry *n.* frambuesa; ___ **mark** / marca de nacimiento de color rosado.

rasura *n.* rasura, raspadura, limadura.

rat *n.* rata.

rate *n.* tasa, índice; **at any** ___ / de todos modos; no obstante; **at the** ___ **of** / a razón de; **birth** ___ / ___ de natalidad; **birth death** ___ / í. de mortinatalidad; **case fatality** ___ / índice de letalidad de casos; **death** ___ / ___ de mortalidad; **intrinsic** ___ / frecuencia intrínseca; *v.* estimar, evaluar, tasar.

rather *adv.* algo, un tanto; bastante; más bien.

ratify *v.* ratificar, confirmar.

rating *n.* evaluación; clasificación, determinación.

ratio *L.* relación, proporción, razón, expresión de la cantidad de una sustancia en relación con otra.

ration *n.* ración, porción alimenticia.

rational *a.* racional, cuerdo-a, basado-a en la razón.

rationale *n.* razón fundamental.

rationalization *n.* racionalización, mecanismo de defensa por el cual se justifica la conducta o actividades propias con explicaciones que aunque razonables no se ajustan a la realidad.

rattlesnake *n.* serpiente de cascabel; ___ **poison** / veneno de la ___ .

Rauwolfia serpentina *n. Rauwolfia serpentina*, planta tropical de la cual se obtiene la reserpina, extracto que se usa en el tratamiento de hipertensión y en algunos casos de trastornos mentales.

rave *v.* delirar, hablar irracionalmente.

raw *a.* crudo-a; [*skin*] en carne viva; [*fruit*] sin madurar; [*material*] materia prima.

ray *n.* rayo.

Raynaud's disease *n.* síndrome de Raynaud. V. **acrocyanosis.**

Raynaud's phenomenon *n.* fenómeno de Raynaud, síntomas asociados con el síndrome de Raynaud.

razor *n.* navaja, cuchilla.

reabsorb *v.* reabsorber.

reach *n.* alcance; **within** ___ / al ___ de; *v.* alcanzar, obtener.

react *v.* reaccionar, responder a un estímulo.

reaction *n.* reacción, respuesta; **allergic** ___ / ___ alérgica; **anaphylactic** ___ / ___ anafiláctica; **anxiety** ___ / ___ de ansiedad; **chain** ___ / ___ en cadena; **conversion** ___ / ___ de conversión; **immune** ___ / ___ inmune; **runaway** ___ / ___ de escape.

reactivate *v.* reactivar, volver a activar.

reactivation *n.* reactivación, el acto de volver a activar.

reactive *a.* reactivo-a, que tiene la propiedad de reaccionar o de causar una reacción.

reactive depression *n.* reacción depresiva psicótica a consecuencia de una experiencia traumática.

reactivity *n.* reactividad, manifestación de una reacción.

read *vi.* leer; ___ **the letters** / Lea, lee las letras.

reader *n.* lector, lectora.

reading *n.* lectura; ___ **glasses** / anteojos, espejuelos, gafas para leer; ___ **disorders** / trastornos o impedimentos en la ___ .

ready *a.* listo-a, preparado-a; *v.* **to get** ___ / prepararse, arreglarse.

reaffirm *v.* reafirmar, asegurar.

reagent *n.* reactivo, agente que produce una reacción.

reagin *n.* reagina, anticuerpo usado en el tratamiento de alergias que estimula la producción de histamina.

real *a.* real, verdadero-a, cierto-a; **-ly** *adv.* realmente, verdaderamente, ciertamente.

realistic *a.* verdadero-a, realista.

reality *n.* realidad.

reality principle *n.* principio de realidad, método de orientación del paciente hacia el mundo externo para provocar el reconocimiento de objetos y actividades olvidadas, esp. dirigido a personas severamente desorientadas.

reality therapy *n.* terapéutica por realidad, método por el que se enfrenta al paciente con la realidad ayudándolo a aceptarla.

realize *v.* realizar; llevar a cabo; darse cuenta de.

reanimate *v.* reanimar, revivir.

rear *a.* posterior, trasero-a.

reason *n.* razón; justificación; *v.* razonar; justificar; ___ **for admission** / razón de ingreso.

reasonable *a.* razonable; justificado-a; sensato-a; ___ **care** / cuidado justificado; ___ **charge** / honorarios ___ -s; ___ **cost** / costo ___ .

reassessment *n.* estimado; reevaluación; ___ **of the case** / reevaluación del caso.

reassure *v.* asegurar, alentar, restablecer la confianza.

reattach *v.* volver a juntar, volver a unir.

reattachment *n.* acción de volver a unir, re-unión; acción de repegar; ___ **of amputated fingers** / re-unión de dedos amputados.

reawaken *v.* volver a despertar.

rebel *n.* rebelde.

rebellion *n.* rebelión.

rebound *n.* rebote, regreso a una condición previa después que el estímulo inicial se suprime; *v.* rebotar, repercutir.

rebound phenomenon *n.* fenómeno de rebote, movimiento intensificado de una parte hacia adelante cuando se elimina la fuerza inicial contra la cual ésta hacía resistencia.

recalcification *n.* recalcificación, restauración de compuestos de calcio en los tejidos.

recall *v.* recordar; reclamar; hacer volver; acordarse de.

recede *v.* disminuir, [*water*] bajar, retroceder.

receipt *n.* recibo, carta de pago.

receive *v.* recibir, admitir; acoger; aceptar.

recent *a.* reciente; moderno; nuevo-a; **-ly** *adv.* recientemente, hace poco tiempo.

receptaculum *L.* (*pl.* **receptacula**) receptaculum, receptáculo, recipiente.

receptionist *n.* recepcionista.

receptive *a.* receptivo-a, acogedor-a.

receptor *n.* receptor, terminación nerviosa que recibe un estímulo y lo transmite a otros nervios; **auditory** ___ / ___ auditivo; **contact** ___ / ___ de contacto; **mechanoreceptor** / mecanoreceptor; **chemoreceptor** / quimorreceptor; **proprioceptive** ___ / ___ propioceptivo; **sensory** ___ / ___ sensorial; **taste** ___ / ___ gustativo; **temperature** ___ / ___ de temperatura.

recess *n.* suspensión; cavidad, espacio vacío.

recession *n.* recesión, retirada, retroceso patológico de tejidos tal como la retracción de la encía.

recessive *a.* recesivo-a. 1. que tiende a retraerse; 2. en genética, rel. al gene que permanece latente.

reciding *a.* disminuido, que va disminuyendo; [*memory*] desvanecida, [*hair*] disminuido.

recidivism *n.* recidiva, reincidencia, tendencia a recaer en una condición, enfermedad o síntoma previo.

recipe *n.* receta, prescripción.

recipient *n.* 1. receptor; vasija; recipiente; 2. persona que recibe una transfusión, un implante de tejido o un órgano de un donante. 3. [*as in organ receiver*] receptor, [*mail*] destinatario-a.

reciprocal *a.* recíproco-a, mutuo-a.

reciprocity *n.* reciprocidad.

reckless *a.* descuidado-a, imprudente.

recklessness *n.* descuido; indiferencia; imprudencia; temeridad.

reclaim *v.* reclamar.

reclamation *n.* reclamación.

recline *n.* reclinación; *v.* reclinar, inclinar; recostarse.

reclined position *n.* posición en decúbito.

reclining *a.* recostado-a, inclinado-a.

recognition *n.* reconocimiento, estado de ser reconocido.

recognize *v.* reconocer; admitir.

recollection *n.* recuerdo, memoria.

recombination *n.* recombinación.

recommend *v.* recomendar; aconsejar.

recommendation *n.* recomendación.

recompense *n.* recompensa, compensación, reparación.

recompression *n.* recompresión, vuelta a la presión ambiental normal.

reconcile *v.* reconciliar; reconciliarse; resignarse, conformarse.

reconciliation *n.* reconciliación, conformidad.

reconsider *v.* recapacitar; volver a considerar.

reconstitution *n.* reconstitución, restitución de un tejido a la forma inicial.

reconstruct *v.* reconstruir, reparar, restablecer.

reconstruction *v.* reconstrucción.

record *n.* registro; [*medical history*] historia clínica, expediente; informe; **off the** ___ / confidencialmente; **patient** ___ / ___ del paciente; **to go on** ___ / expresar públicamente; *v.* registrar, inscribir.

recorder *n.* registrador-a, anotador-a; archivero-a; **tape** ___ / grabador-a.

recording *n.* registro, [*tape*] grabación.

recoup *v.* recuperar; recobrar; recuperarse, recobrarse; restablecerse.

recourse *n.* recurso, auxilio.

recover *v.* recobrar, recuperar, restablecer; restablecerse, recobrarse, reponerse.

recovery *n.* recuperación, restablecimiento, recobro, mejoría; **past** ___ / sin remedio, sin cura; ___ **room** / sala de ___ .

recovery room *n.* sala de recuperación.

recreation *n.* recreo, pasatiempo, entretenimiento.

recrudescence *n.* recrudescencia, relapso, reaparición de síntomas.

rectal *a.* rectal, del recto, rel. al recto; ___ **abscess** / absceso ___; ___ **biopsy** / biopsia ___; ___ **inflammation** / inflamación ___; ___ **lump** / protuberancia, bulto ___; ___ **prolapse** / prolapso ___ .

rectification *n.* rectificación, corrección; enmienda.

rectify *v.* rectificar, corregir, enmendar.

rectocele *n.* rectocele, hernia del recto con protrusión en la vagina.

rectosigmoid *a.* rectosigmoide, rel. al sigmoide y al recto.

rectovaginal *a.* rectovaginal, rel. a la vagina y el recto.

rectovesical *a.* rectovesical, rel. al recto y la vejiga.

rectum *n.* recto, la porción distal del intestino grueso que se extiende de la flexura sigmoidea al ano.

rectus *L.* (*pl.* **recti**) músculo recto; ___ **muscles** / músculos ___, grupo de músculos rectos tales como los situados alrededor del ojo y en la pared abdominal.

recumbent *a.* yacente, acostado-a, recostado-a, reclinado-a, recumbente; acostado-a de espalda ___ **position** / posición ___ .

recuperate *v.* recuperar, recobrar las fuerzas; recuperarse, reponerse.

recuperation *n.* recuperación, restablecimiento.

recur *v.* repetir, volver a ocurrir; recaer, repetirse.

recurrence *n.* recidiva. 1. reaparición de síntomas después de una remisión; 2. relapso, recaída.

recurrent *a.* recurrente, que reaparece temporalmente; repetido-a, constante; ___ **cystitis** / cistitis ___; ___ **pain** / dolor constante.

red *n., a.* rojo; ___ **cell** / glóbulo rojo, hematíe, eritrocito; **Congo** ___ / ___ Congo; **scarlet** ___ / ___ escarlata.

red-eyed *a.* de ojos enrojecidos; con los ojos inyectados.

red-faced *a.* ruborizado-a, con la cara encendida.

red-hot *a.* muy caliente, candente.

redden *v.* enrojecer, teñir de rojo.

reddish *a.* rojizo-a, enrojecido-a.

redhead *a.* pelirrojo-a.

redness *n.* enrojecimiento.

redress *v.* volver a vendar; poner un nuevo vendaje; remediar.

reduce *v.* reducir, rebajar; disminuir. 1. restaurar a la situación normal, tal como un hueso fracturado o dislocado; 2. disminuir la potencia al dar hidrógeno o quitarle oxígeno a un compuesto; 3. bajar de peso.

reducible *a.* reducible, susceptible a la reducción.

reducing diet *n.* régimen para bajar de peso

reducing exercises *n., pl.* ejercicios para adelgazar, ejercicios para bajar de peso.

reducing factor *n.* factor que afecta el proceso de peso.

reductase *n.* reductasa, enzima que actúa como catalítico en el proceso de reducción.

reduction *n.* reducción, baja, disminución; rebaja.

reduction mammaplasty *n.* cirugía plástica de reducción del seno, con mejoramiento a la posición y apariencia.

reductor *n.* reductor, agente que causa reducción en otras sustancias.

reeducation *n.* reeducación, enseñanza con entrenamiento para recobrar funciones motoras o mentales.

reedy nail *n.* uña estriada, a nail having longitudinal ridges and furrows.

refer *v.* referir, atribuir, asignar, referirse a.

reference *n.* referencia; ___ **values** / valores de ___ .

referral *n.* recomendación; remisión; ___ **and consultation** / ___ y consulta.

refill *n.* repuesto; repetición; relleno; repetición de una receta; *v.* reponer; repetir; rellenar.

refine *v.* refinar, purificar.

reflect *v.* reflejar; **to** ___ **upon** / reflexionar.

reflection *n.* reflexión. 1. acomodamiento o vuelta hacia atrás tal como una membrana que después de llegar a la superficie de un órgano se repliega sobre sí misma; 2. rechazo de la luz u otra forma de energía radiante de una superficie; 3. introspección.

reflex *n.* reflejo, respuesta motora involuntaria a un estímulo; **Achilles tendon** ___ / ___ del tendón de Aquiles; ___ **action** / acto, acción ___; ___**arch** / arco ___; **behavior** ___ / ___ adquirido; **chain** ___ / ___ en cadena; **conditioned** ___ / ___ condicionado; **instinctive** ___ / ___ instintivo; **patellar** ___ / ___ patelar o rotuliano; **radial** ___ / ___ radial; **rectal** ___ / ___ rectal; **stretch** ___ / ___ de estiramiento; **unconditioned** ___ / ___ no condicionado; **vagal** ___ / ___ vagal.

reflexogenic *n.* reflexógeno, agente que causa un reflejo.

reflux *n.* reflujo, flujo retrógrado; **abdominojugular** ___ / ___ abdominoyugular; **esophageal** ___ / ___ esofágico; **hepatojugular** ___ / ___ hepatoyugular; **intrarenal** ___ / ___ intrarenal; **ureterorenal** ___ / ___ ureterorenal.

reform *n.* reforma, cambio; *v.* reformar, cambiar; reformarse.

refract *v.* refractar, desviar. 1. cambiar una dirección tal como la de un rayo de luz al pasar de un medio a otro de diferente densidad; 2. rectificar anormalidades de refracción en el ojo y corregirlas.

refraction *n.* refracción, acto de refractar; **ocular.** ___ / ___ ocular

refractive surgery *n.* cirugía refractiva, corrección del cristalino del ojo.

refractivity *n.* refractividad, habilidad de refractar.

refractory *a.* refractario-a. 1. resistente a un tratamiento; 2. que no responde a un estímulo.

refresh *v.* refrescar; renovar, revivir; refrescarse; renovarse.

refreshing *a.* refrescante.

refreshment *n.* refresco; refrigerio.

refrigerant *a.* refrigerante; antipirético-a.

refrigerate *v.* refrigerar, mantener en el frío.

refrigeration *n.* refrigeración, reducción del calor a una temperatura fría por medios externos.

refringent *a.* refringente, rel. a la refracción o que la causa.

refuge *n.* refugio; asilo; *v.* **to take** ___ / refugiarse.

refugee *n.* refugiado-a.

refusal *n.* rechazo, negación.

refuse *n.* desecho, basura; desperdicios; *v.* rehusar, rechazar, denegar; ___ **the hospital food** / ___ la comida del hospital; ___ **to take the medication** / rehusar tomar la medicina.

regain *v.* recuperar, recobrar; **to** ___ **consciousness** / recobrar el conocimiento.

regard *n.* respeto, consideración; **in** ___ **to** / respecto a; **regards** / recuerdos.

regarding *prep.* respecto a.

regenerate *v.* regenerar.

regeneration *n.* regeneración, restauración, renovación.

regime *n.* régimen, regla, plan, esp. en referencia a una dieta o ejercicio físico.

region *n.* región, parte del cuerpo más o menos delimitada.

regional *a.* regional; ___ **medical programs** / programas médicos ___ -es.

registration *n.* registro, inscripción; [*courses*] matrícula.

regression *n.* regresión, retrogresión. 1. vuelta a una condición anterior; 2. apaciguamiento de síntomas o de un proceso patológico.

regret *n.* sentimiento de pesar; remordimiento; sentir, lamentar, deplorar; **I** ___ **to tell you** / siento decirle, decirte.

regrettable *a.* lamentable; infortunado-a.

regular *a.* regular, común, **-ly** *adv.* regularmente, con regularidad.

regularity *n.* regularidad, normalidad.

regulate *v.* regular, ordenar.

regulation *n.* regulación, norma o regla.

regulator *n.* regulador-a.

regurgitant *a.* regurgitante, rel. a la regurgitación.

regurgitate *v.* regurgitar.

regurgitation *n.* regurgitación. 1. acto de devolver o expulsar la comida de la boca; 2. flujo retrógrado de la sangre a través de una válvula defectuosa del corazón; **aortic** ___ / ___ aórtica; **mitral** ___ / ___ de la válvula mitral; **valvular** ___ / ___ valvular.

rehabilitate *v.* rehabilitar, ayudar a recobrar funciones normales por medio de métodos terapéuticos.

rehabilitation *n.* rehabilitación, acto de rehabilitar.

rehabilitee *n.* *a.* rehabilitado-a.

rehydration *n.* rehidratación, restablecimiento del balance hídrico del cuerpo.

reimplantation *n.* reimplantación. 1. restauración de un tejido o parte; 2. restitución de un óvulo al útero después de extraerlo y fecundarlo *in vitro*.

reinfection *n.* reinfección, infección subsecuente por el mismo microorganismo.

reinforce *v.* reforzar; fortalecer.

reinfusion *n.* reinfusión, reinyección de suero sanguíneo o líquido cefalorraquídeo.

reinnervation *n.* reinervación, injerto de un nervio para restaurar la función de un músculo.

reinoculation *n.* reinoculación, inoculación subsecuente con el mismo microorganismo.

reject *n.* rechazar, rehusar.

rejection *n.* rechazo, reacción inmunológica de incompatibilidad a células de tejidos transplantados; **acute** ___ / ___ agudo; **chronic** ___ / ___ crónico; **hyperacute** ___ / ___ hiperagudo.

rejuvenate *v.* rejuvenecer; rejuvenecerse.

rejuvenescense *n.* rejuvenecimiento.

relapse *n.* recidiva, recaída, reincidencia; *v.* recaer, volver a sufrir una enfermedad o los síntomas de ésta después de cierta mejoría.

relapsing fever *n.* fiebre recurrente.

relate *v.* relacionar; establecer una relación; relacionarse.

related *a.* relacionado-a; emparentado-a.

relation *n.* relación; comparación.

relationship *n.* relación; parentesco, lazo familiar.

relative *n.* pariente, familiar; *a.* relativo-a; *gr.* pronombre relativo.

r

relax *v.* relajar el cuerpo, reducir tensión; relajarse; aflojar; descansar.

relaxant *n.* relajante, tranquilizante; droga que reduce la tensión.

relaxation *n.* relajación, acto de relajar o de relajarse; reposo, descanso.

relaxed *a.* relajado-a.

release *n.* información; liberación; *v.* soltar, librar, desprender; [*to inform*] informar, dar a conocer.

releasing hormone *n.* hormona estimulante.

reliability *n.* confiabilidad; calidad de confianza.

reliable *a.* [*person*] formal, responsable; seguro-a.

relief *n.* alivio, mejoría; ayuda, auxilio; what a ___! / ¡ay, qué ___ !; *v.* to be on ___ / recibir asistencia social.

relieve *v.* [*pain*] aliviar, mejorar.

religion *n.* religión.

religious *a.* religioso-a.

reluctance *n.* renuencia, aversión, disgusto.

reluctant *a.* renuente; resistente; contrario-a.

rely *v.* depender, contar con, confiar en.

remain *v.* permanecer; to ___ in bed / guardar cama.

remainder *n.* resto, residuo.

remains *n., pl.* restos, despojos.

remake *v.* rehacer.

remark *n.* observación, nota, advertencia; *v.* observar, indicar, advertir.

remarkable *a.* extraordinario-a, notable.

remedial *a.* remediador-a, reparador-a, curativo-a.

remedy *n.* remedio, cura, medicamento; *v.* remediar, curar.

remember *v.* recordar, acordarse; ___ correctly! / ¡Acuérdese, acuérdate bien!; Don't you ___? / ¿No se acuerda?, ¿no te acuerdas?

remind *v.* recordar, advertir.

remineralization *n.* remineralización, reemplazo de minerales perdidos en el cuerpo.

reminisce *v.* recordar; divagar.

reminiscense *n.* memoria, recordatorio, reminiscencia.

remission *n.* remisión. 1. disminución o cesación de los síntomas de una enfermedad; 2. período de tiempo durante el cual los síntomas de una enfermedad disminuyen.

remittent *a.* remitente, que se repite a intervalos.

remodeling *n.* restauración.

remorse *n.* remordimiento.

remote *a.* remoto-a, distante.

removable *a.* separable, mudable.

removal *n.* extirpación, remoción.

remove *v.* sacar; quitar, extraer; extirpar.

renal *a.* renal, rel. a o semejante al riñón; ___ cell carcinoma, / carcinoma de células renales; ___ clearance / aclaración ___ aclaramiento ___; ___ clearance test / prueba de aclaramiento o depuración ___; ___ colic / cólico nefrítico, cólico renal; ___ failure / insuficiencia renal; ___ failure, acute / insuficiencia ___ aguda; ___ function test / prueba funcional ___; ___ gammagraphy / gamagrafía, barrido ___; ___ hypertensión ___ / hipertensión de origen renal; ___ insufficiency / insuficiencia ___; ___ involvement / [*participation*] intervención ___; ___ papillary necrosis / necrosis papilar ___; ___ pelvis / pelvis ___; ___ replacement therapy ___ / diálisis, terapia de reemplazo; ___ scanning / gammagrafía renal, barrido renal; ___ transplantation / transplante ___ .

renal ballottement *n.* peloteo renal, maniobra para mover por presión el riñón y determinar la forma, tamaño y mobilidad del riñón.

renew *v.* renovar.

renin *n.* renina, enzima segregada por el riñón que interviene en la regulación de la presión arterial.

renogram *n.* renograma, proceso de monitoreo del índice de eliminación sanguínea a través del riñón usando una sustancia radioactiva inyectada previamente.

renovate *v.* reformar, renovar.

reopen *v.* volver a abrir, abrir de nuevo.

repair *n.* reparación, restauración; *v.* reparar, restaurar.

repeat *n.* repetir, reiterar.

repellent *a.* repelente.

repercussion *n.* repercusión. 1. penetración o dispersión de una inflamación, tumor o erupción; 2. peloteo.

replace *v.* reemplazar, reponer, substituir.

replacement *n.* reemplazo, substitución, repuesto.

replete *a.* repleto-a, lleno-a en exceso.

replication *n.* reproducción, duplicación.

reply *n.* contestación, respuesta; *v.* contestar, responder.

repolarization *n.* repolarización, restablecimiento de la polarización de una célula o de una fibra nerviosa o muscular después de su depolarización.

report *n.* informe, reporte; *v.* informar, reportar.

reprehensible *a.* reprensible, reprobable, censurable.

repress *v.* reprimir.

repression *n.* represión. 1. inhibición de una acción; 2. mecanismo de defensa por el que se eliminan del campo de la conciencia deseos e impulsos en conflicto.

reproduce *v.* reproducir; reproducirse.

reproducer *n.* reproductor.

reproduction *n.* reproducción; **sexual** ___ / ___ sexual.

reproductive *a.* reproductivo-a, rel. a la reproducción.

repudiate *v.* repudiar, repeler.

repugnant *a.* repugnante, repulsivo-a.

repulsion *n.* repulsión, aversión, repugnancia.

repulsive *a.* repulsivo-a, chocante.

reputation *n.* reputación, fama, nombre.

reputed *a.* reputado-a, distinguido-a, de buena fama.

request *n.* petición, encargo; solicitud; *v.* pedir, hacer una petición, [*of supplies*] encargar.

require *v.* requerir, solicitar.

required *a.* requerido-a, necesario-a; mandatorio-a.

requirement *n.* requerimiento.

requisite *n.* requisito.

res ipsa loquitur *L.* res ipsa loquitor, evidente, que habla por sí mismo.

rescind *v.* rescindir, anular; terminar.

rescue *v.* salvar, rescatar, librar; ___ **method** / método de ___, de salvamento.

research *n.* investigación, indagación, pesquisa; *v.* investigar, indagar, hacer investigaciones.

resect *n.* resecar. 1. cortar una porción de un órgano o tejido; 2. hacer una resección.

resection *n.* resección, extirpación de una porción de órgano o tejido; **bloc** ___ / ___ en bloque; **gastric** ___ / ___ gástrica; **transurethral** ___ / ___ transuretral; **wedge** ___ / ___ en cuña.

resectoscope *n.* resectoscopio, instrumento quirúrgico provisto de un electrodo cortante como el que se usa para la resección de la próstata a través de la uretra.

resectoscopy *n.* resectoscopía, resección de la próstata con un resectoscopio.

resemblance *n.* semejanza, parecido.

resemble *v.* tener semejanza; parecerse a.

resentment *n.* resentimiento, rencor.

reserpine *n.* reserpina, derivado de la *Rauwolfia serpentina* que se usa principalmente en el tratamiento de la hipertensión y de desórdenes emocionales.

reservation *n.* reservación, reserva.

reserve *n.* reserva, sustancia, objeto o idea que se guarda para uso futuro; *v.* reservar; conservar, guardar.

reserved *a.* reservado-a, [*personality*] reservado-a, callado-a.

reside *v.* residir, vivir.

residency *n.* residencia, período de entrenamiento médico especializado que se hace gen. en un hospital.

resident *n.* médico-a residente, que cursa una residencia.

residual *a.* residual, restante, remanente; ___ **function** / función ___; ___ **urine** / orina ___ .

residue *n.* residuo; ___ **diet, high** / dieta de ___ alto; ___ **diet, low** / dieta de ___ bajo.

resign *v.* renunciar, resignar, desistir; resignarse.

resilience *n.* elasticidad. V. **elasticity**.

resilient *a.* elástico-a.

resin *a.* resina, sustancia vegetal insoluble en el agua aunque soluble en alcohol y éter que tiene una variedad de usos medicinales y dentales.

resist *v.* resistir; rechazar.

resistance *n.* resistencia, oposición; capacidad de un organismo para resistir efectos dañinos; **initial** ___ / ___ inicial; **acquired** ___ / ___ adquirida; **peripheral** ___ / ___ periférica; *v.* **to offer** ___ / oponerse; hacer resistencia.

resistant *a.* resistente; **fast** ___ / resistencia a un colorante.

resolute *a.* resuelto-a, determinado-a.

resolution *n.* resolución. 1. terminación de un proceso inflamatorio; 2. habilidad de distinguir detalles pequeños y sutiles tal como se hace a través de un microscopio; 3. descomposición sin supuración.

resolve *v.* resolver. 1. encontrar una solución; 2. descomponer, analizar, separar en componentes.

resonance *n.* resonancia, capacidad de aumentar la intensidad de un sonido; **normal** ___ / ___ normal; **vesicular** ___ / ___ vesicular; **vocal** ___ / ___ vocal.

resonant *a.* resonante, que da un sonido vibrante a la percusión.

resorcinol *n.* resorcinol, agente usado en el tratamiento de acné y otras dermatosis.

resorption *n.* resorción, pérdida total o parcial de un proceso, tejido o exudado por resultado de reacciones bioquímicas tales como lisis y absorción.

resort *n.* recurso; **health** ___ / lugar de recuperación física; **the last** ___ / el último ___; *v.* acudir, pedir ayuda, recurrir.

resource *n.* recurso, medio.

r

respect *n.* respeto, consideración; *v.* respetar, considerar.

respectable *a.* respetable, acreditado-a.

respiration *n.* respiración, proceso respiratorio; **abdominal** ___ / ___ abdominal; **aerobic** ___ / ___ aeróbica; **accelerated** ___ / ___ acelerada; **anaerobic** ___ / ___ anaeróbica; **diaphragmatic** ___ / ___ diafragmática; **air hunger, gasping** ___ / ___ jadeante; **labored** ___ / ___ laboriosa.

respirator *n.* respirador, aparato para purificar el aire que se inhala o para producir respiración artificial; **chest** ___ / ___ torácico.

respiratory *a.* respiratorio-a, rel. a la respiración; ___ **airway** / conducto, pasaje ___; ___ **alkalosis** / alkalosis ___; ___ **arrhythmia** / arritmia ___; ___ **ataxia** / ataxia ___; ___ **bronchioles** / bronquíolos ___; ___ **capacity** ___ / capacidad; ___ **care unit** / unidad de cuidado ___; ___ **distress syndrome** / síndrome de dificultad ___; ___ **enzyme** / enzima ___; ___ **failure, acute** / insuficiencia ___ aguda; ___ **failure, chronic** / insuficiencia ___ crónica; ___ **function tests** / pruebas de función ___; ___ **inhibitor** / inhibidor ___; ___ **lobule** / lóbulo ___; ___ **metabolism** / metabolismo ___; ___ **mucosa** / mucosa ___; ___ **quotient** / cociente ___; ___ **rate** / índice ___; ___ **sounds** / ruidos ___; ___ **system** / sistema ___; ___ **tract infections and diseases** / infecciones y enfermedades de las vías ___ -s.

respiratory acidosis *n.* acidosis respiratoria, causada por retención de dioxido de carbono debido a hipoventilación.

respiratory center *n.* centro respiratorio, área en la médula oblongata que regula los movimientos respiratorios.

response *n.* respuesta. 1. reacción o cambio de un órgano o parte a un estímulo; **immune** ___ / ___ inmune; 2. reacción de un paciente a un tratamiento.

responsibility *n.* responsabilidad.

responsible *a.* responsable.

rest *n.* descanso, reposo; residuo, resto; ___ **cure** / cura de reposo; *v.* decansar, reposar.

restenosis *n.* reestenosis, recurrencia de estenosis después de cirugía correctiva.

restful *a.* tranquilo-a, quieto-a.

resting *a.* inactivo-a, en reposo, en estado de descanso.

restitutio ad integrum *L.* restitutio ad integrum, recuperación total de la salud.

restoration *n.* restauración, restitución, restablecimiento, acción de restituir algo a su estado original.

restorative *n.* restaurativo, agente que estimula la restauración.

restore *v.* restituir, restablecer.

restraint *n.* restricción; confinamiento; ___ **in bed** / ___ en cama; **mechanical** ___ / ___ mecánica; **medicinal** ___ / ___ con uso de medicamentos.

restrict *v.* restringir, confinar.

restricted *a.* limitado-a, confinado; ___ **area** / área ___ .

restroom *n.* servicio, aseos, *Lat. Am.* inodoro, cuarto de baño.

result *n.* resultado, conclusión.

resuscitate *v.* resucitar; reanimar.

resuscitation *n.* resucitación. 1. devolver la vida; reanimar el corazón; 2. respiración artificial.

resuscitator *n.* resucitador, aparato automático de asistencia respiratoria.

retain *v.* retener, guardar; quedarse con.

retainer *n.* [*dentistry*] aro, freno de retención.

retardate *a.* retardado-a, retrasado-a, atrasado-a.

retardation *n.* retraso, atraso, retardo anormal de una función motora o mental; **psychomotora** ___ / ___ psicomotor. V. **mental retardation**.

retch *n.* arcada, basca, contracciones abdominales espasmódicas que preceden al vómito.

rete *L.* (*pl.* **retia**) rete; red; **network**.

retention *n.* retención, conservación; **fluid** ___ / ___ de líquido; **gastric** ___ / ___ gástrica; ___ **enema** / enema de ___; **urinary** ___ / ___ urinaria.

reticular *a.* reticular, retiforme, en forma de red.

reticulation *n.* reticulación, disposición reticular.

reticulocyte *n.* reticulocito, célula roja inmadura, eritrocito en red o gránulos que aparece durante la regeneración de la sangre; ___**count** / recuento de ___ .

reticulocytopenia, reticulosis *n.* reticulocitopenia, reticulosis, disminución anormal del número de reticulocitos en la sangre.

reticulocytosis *n.* reticulocitosis, sobreaumento de nuevos reticulocitos circulantes en la corriente sanguínea como regeneración activa de la sangre, estimulantes de la médula ósea después del tratamiento de anemia hemolítica genética o por adaptación ambiental.

reticuloendothelial system *n.* sistema reticuloendotelial, red de células fagocíticas (excepto leucocitos circulantes) esparcidas por todo el cuerpo que intervienen en procesos tales como la formación de células sanguíneas, destrucción de grasas, eliminación de células gastadas y restauración de tejidos que son participantes esenciales en el proceso inmunológico del organismo.

reticuloendothelioma *n.* reticuloendotelioma, tumor del sistema reticuloendotelial.

reticuloendothelium *n.* reticuloendotelio, tejido del sistema reticuloendotelial.

reticulohistiocytoma *n.* reticulohistiocitoma, agregación de células granulares y gigantes.

reticulopenia *n.* reticulopenia. V. **reticulocytopenia.**

reticulum *n.* retículo. 1. red de nervios y vasos sanguíneos; 2. tejido reticular.

Retin-A *n.* Retin-A, nombre comercial del ácido retinoico, medicamento usado en el tratamiento de acné.

retina *n.* retina, la capa más interna del ojo que recibe imágenes y transmite impulsos visuales al cerebro; **detachment of the ___ /** desprendimiento de la ___ .

retinaculum *n.* retináculo, estructura que retiene un órgano o un tejido en su lugar.

retinal *a.* de la retina, retiniano-a; rel. a la retina; **___ degeneration /** deterioro retiniano, deterioración retiniana; **___ perforation /** perforación ___ .

retinitis *n.* retinitis, infl. de la retina.

retinoblastoma *n.* retinoblastoma, tumor maligno de la retina gen. hereditario.

retinol *n.* retinol, vitamina A1.

retinopathy *n.* retinopatía, cualquier condición anormal de la retina.

retinoscopy *n.* retinoscopía, determinación y evaluación de errores visuales de refracción.

retinosis *n.* retinosis, proceso degenerativo de la retina.

retire *v.* retirar; [*from work*] retirarse, jubilarse; [*to bed*] irse a acostar.

retired *a. pp.* of **to retire**, retirado-a; [*from work*] jubilado-a, retirado-a; [*withdrawn*] reservado-a; [*secluded*] alejado-a, apartado-a.

retiree *n.* jubilado-a; retirado-a.

retract *v.* retraer, retractar; retraerse, volverse hacia atrás.

retractile *a.* retráctil, retractable.

retraction *n.* retracción, encogimiento, contracción; acto de echarse hacia atrás;

clot ___ / ___ del coágulo; uterine ___ / ___ uterina;

retractor *n.* retractor. 1. instrumento para separar los bordes de una herida; 2. tipo de músculo que retrae una parte u órgano.

retrieval *n.* recuperación de algo.

retroaction *n.* retroacción, acción retroactiva.

retroactive *a.* retroactivo-a, de acción retroactiva.

retroauricular *a.* retroauricular, rel. a o situado detrás de la oreja o aurícula.

retrocecal *a.* retrocecal, rel. a o situado detrás del ciego.

retrocession *n.* retroceso.

retroflexion *n.* retroflexión, flexión de un órgano hacia atrás.

retrograde *a.* retrógrado-a, que se mueve hacia atrás o retorna al pasado; **___ amnesia /** amnesia ___; **___ aortography /** aortografía ___; **___ pyelography /** pielografía ___ .

retrogression *n.* retrogresión, regreso a un estado más primitivo de desarrollo.

retrolental *a.* retrolental, situado detrás del cristalino; **___ fibroplasia /** fibroplasia ___ .

retroperitoneal *a.* retroperitoneano-a, rel. a o situado detrás del peritoneo.

retroplasia *n.* retroplasia. V. **anaplasia.**

retrospective *a.* retrospectivo-a; **___ study /** estudio ___ .

retroversion *n.* retroversión, inclinación o vuelta hacia atrás; **___ of the uterus /** desplazamiento del útero hacia atrás.

retrovirus *n.* retrovirus, virus que pertenece al grupo ácido ARN, algunos de los cuales son oncogénicos; **human endogenous ___ / ___** endógeno humano.

retry *v.* ensayar de nuevo.

return *n.* regreso, retorno; *v.* regresar.

Retzius, space of *n.* espacio de Retzius, área entre la vejiga y los huesos del pubis.

reunion *n.* reunión, unión de partes o tejidos esp. en un hueso fracturado o en partes de una herida al cicatrizar.

revascularization *n.* revascularización, proceso de restauración de la sangre a una parte del cuerpo después de una lesión o una derivación quirúrgica.

reversal *n.* reversión, restitución a un estado anterior.

review *n.* revisión, análisis, repaso; **admission ___ /** revisión de ingresos; **case ___ / ___ del caso; ___ of systems / ___**

r

de sistemas; [*literary*] reseña; *v.* repasar, volver a ver.

revise *v.* revisar, repasar, mirar con detenimiento.

revision *n.* revisión.

revitalize *n.* revitalizar, vivificar, volver a dar fuerzas.

revive *v.* revivir.

revivification *n.* revivificación, renovación de vida y fuerzas después de un padecimiento.

revulsion *n.* revulsión.

revulsive *a.* revulsivo-a, rel. a la revulsión o que la causa.

Reye's syndrome *n.* síndrome de Reye, enfermedad aguda que se manifiesta en niños y adolescentes con edema agudo en órganos importantes esp. en el cerebro y el hígado.

Rh blood group *n.* grupo sanguíneo Rh.

Rh genes *n., pl.* genes Rh, determinantes de los distintos tipos sanguíneos Rh.

rhabdomyosarcoma *n.* rabdomiosarcoma, tumor maligno de fibras musculares estriadas que afecta gen. los músculos esqueléticos.

rhachitis *n.* raquitismo. V. **rickets.**

rheum, rheuma *n.* 1. reuma, secreción catarral o acuosa por la nariz; 2. reumatismo.

rheumatic *a.* reumático-a, rel. a o afectado por reumatismo.

rheumatic fever *n.* fiebre reumática, fiebre o condición acompañada de dolores en las articulaciones que puede dejar como secuela trastornos cardíacos y renales.

rheumatism *n.* reumatismo, enfermedad aguda crónica caracterizada por infl. y dolor en las articulaciones.

rheumatoid *a.* reumatoide, de naturaleza semejante al reumatismo.

rhinal *a.* rinal, rel. a la nariz.

rhinitis *n.* rinitis, infl. de la mucosa nasal.

rhinolaryngitis *n.* rinolaringitis, infl. simultánea de las mucosas nasales y laríngeas.

rhinopharyngitis *n.* rinofaringitis, infl. de la nasofaringe.

rhinophyma. *n.* rinofima, acné rosácea aguda en el área de la nariz.

rhinoplasty *n.* rinoplastia, cirugía plástica de la nariz.

rhinorrhea *n.* rinorrea, secreción mucoso-líquida por la nariz.

rhinoscopy *n.* rinoscopía, examen de los pasajes nasales a través de la nasofaringe o de los orificios nasales.

rhizotomy *n.* rizotomía, división o transección de la raíz de un nervio.

rhodopsin *n.* rodopsina, pigmento de color rojo púrpura que se encuentra en los bastoncillos de la retina y que facilita la visión en luz tenue.

rhythm *n.* ritmo, regularidad en la acción o función de un órgano u órganos del cuerpo tal como el corazón.

rhythmical *a.* rítmico-a.

rhytidectomy *n.* ritidectomía, estiramiento de la piel de la cara por medio de cirugía plástica.

rib *n.* costilla, uno de los huesos de una serie de doce pares que forman la pared torácica.

riboflavin *n.* riboflavina, vitamina B2, componente del complejo vitamínico B esencial en la nutrición.

ribonucleoprotein *n.* ribonucleoproteína, sustancia que contiene proteína y ácido ribonucleico.

rich *a.* [*wealth*] rico-a, opulento-a; [*food*] sabroso-a; muy sazonado-a, muy condimentado-a.

rickets *n.* raquitismo. V. **rachitism**.

rickettsia *n.* ricketsia, rickettsia, uno de los organismos gram-negativos que se reproducen solamente en células huéspedes de pulgas, piojos, garrapatas y ratones, y que se transmiten a humanos a través de las mordidas de éstos.

ridge *n.* borde, reborde, elevación prolongada.

rifampicin *n.* rifampicina, sustancia semisintética, antibacteriana que se usa en el tratamiento de la tuberculosis pulmonar.

right *n.* justicia; derecho; *a.* derecho-a, rel. a la parte derecha del cuerpo; recto-a, correcto-a; ___ -handed / diestro-a, que usa con preferencia la mano derecha; on the ___ side / al costado o lado derecho; [*health*] sano-a; the ___ medication / la medicina necesaria; the ___ treatment / el tratamiento adecuado; [*in a problem*]; taking the ___ direction / la solución indicada; everything is all ___ / todo está bien; ___ or wrong / con o sin razón; *adv.* bien, correctamente; mismo; It is going all ___ / Todo sigue bien; ___ here / aquí mismo.

right to refuse treatment *n.* derecho a rehusar tratamiento, el derecho que tiene el (la) paciente de negarse a recibir tratamiento en contra de su voluntad.

right to treatment *n.* derecho a recibir tratamiento, el derecho que tiene el (la) paciente de recibir atención médica de una institución de salud que ha asumido la responsabilidad de tratar al paciente.

rights of the patient *n., pl.* derechos del paciente.

rigid *a.* rígido-a, tieso, inmóvil.

rigidity *n.* rigidez, tesura, inmovilidad, inflexibilidad; **cadaveric** ___ / ___ cadavérica, rigor mortis.

rigor *n.* rigor. 1. escalofrío repentino con fiebre alta; 2. tesura, inflexibilidad muscular.

ring *n.* anillo, círculo; *vi.* sonar; zumbar.

ringing *a.* resonante, retumbante; ___ **ears** / tintineo, zumbido, ruido en los oídos.

ringworm *n.* tiña.

rip *v.* rasgar, desgarrar.

ripe *a.* [*fruit*] maduro-a; [*boil, cataract*] madurado-a.

ripen *v.* madurar; madurarse.

ripening *n.* reblandecimiento, dilatación tal como la del cuello uterino durante el parto.

ripping *n.* laceración, rasgadura; descosedura.

rise *n.* ascensión, subida, salida, crecimiento; *vi.* ascender, subir; [*from bed*] levantarse o salir de la cama.

risk *n.* riesgo, peligro; ___ **of contamination** / riesgo o peligro de contaminación; ___ **factors** / factores de ___; **high-** ___ **groups** / grupos de alto ___; **potential** ___ / ___ posible; ___ **of infection** / ___ de infección; ___ **of injury** / ___ de una lesión; ___ **of violence** / ___ de violencia; *v.* poner en peligro; arriesgarse.

risky *a.* arriesgado-a, peligroso-a.

risorious *n.* risorio, músculo que se inserta en la comisura de la boca.

ristocetin *n.* ristocetina, antibiótico que se usa en el tratamiento de infecciones producidas por un estreptococo gram-positivo.

Ritalin hydrochloride *n.* clorhidrato de Ritalin, estimulante y antidepresivo benigno.

ritual *n.* ritual, rito.

rivalry *n.* rivalidad; competencia.

roach *n.* cucaracha.

road *n.* camino, carretera; curso.

roast *a.* asado-a ___ **meat** / carne ___; *v.* asar, hornear.

robe *n.* [*dressing gown*] bata.

robust *a.* robusto-a, vigoroso-a.

rod *n.* bastoncillo; varilla.

rodent *n.* roedor; *a.* roedor-a; ___ **ulcer** / úlcera ___, que destruye poco a poco.

rodenticide *n.* rodenticida, agente que destruye roedores.

roentgenography *n.* radiografía.

role *n.* [*theatre*] papel; *v.* **to play the** ___ **of** / hacer el ___ de.

role model *n.* prototipo, modelo.

roll *n.* panecillo; *v.* rodar.

Romberg's sign *n.* signo de Romberg, oscilación del cuerpo que indica inhabilidad de mantener el equilibrio en posición erecta, con los pies juntos y los ojos cerrados.

rongeur *Fr.* rongeur, fórceps o pinzas para extraer astillas de hueso y tejidos endurecidos.

room *n.* cuarto, sala; **bath** ___ / ___ de baño; **delivery** ___ / sala de partos; **operating** ___ / sala de operaciones, quirófano; **the patient's** ___ / ___ del paciente; **recovery** ___ / sala de recuperación; ___ **temperature** / temperatura ambiente; **waiting** ___ / sala de espera.

root *n.* raíz; radical.

Rorschach test *n.* prueba de Rorschach, prueba psicológica por la cual se revelan rasgos de la personalidad a través de la interpretación de una serie de borrones de tinta.

rosary *n.* rosario, estructura que se asemeja a cuentas enlazadas.

rose water *n.* agua de rosa.

rosemary *n.* romero.

roseola *n.* roséola, condición de la piel caracterizada por manchas rosáceas de varios tamaños.

rosette *F.* rosette, células en formación semejante a una rosa.

rostral *a.* rostral, rel. o semejante a un rostro.

rostrum *L.* rostro. 1. cara; 2. pico, proyección.

rosy *a.* rosado-a, de color de rosa.

rot *v.* podrirse, pudrirse, echarse a perder.

rotary *a.* rotatorio-a; giratorio-a.

rotate *v.* rotar, girar, voltear.

rotation *n.* rotación; **fetal** ___ / ___ de la cabeza del feto.

rotator *n.* rotador; *a.* rotador-a.

rotten *a.* podrido-a, putrefacto-a, corrompido-a; [*tooth*] cariado-a.

rough *a.* [*surface, skin*] áspero-a, escabroso-a; [*character*] rudo-a. grosero-a; *v.* **to have a** ___ **time** / pasarla mal.

round *a.* redondo-a, circular; ___ **-shouldered** / cargado de espaldas; **all year** ___ / todo el año.

route *n.* ruta.

routine *n.* rutina, hábito, costumbre; *a.* rutinario-a.

rub *n.* 1. fricción, frote, frotación, masaje; 2. sonido producido por el roce de dos superficies secas que se detecta en auscultación; *v.* frotar, hacer penetrar un ungüento o pomada en la piel; friccionar; **to** ___ **off** / limpiar frotando; borrar; **to** ___ **down** / dar un masaje.

rubber *n.* goma; ___ **bulb** / perilla de ___; ___ **gloves** / guantes de ___ .

rubbing *n.* masaje.

r

rubbing alcohol *n.* alcohol para fricciones.

rubefacient *n.* enrojecedor, agente que enrojece la piel.

rubella *n.* rubéola, sarampión alemán; *pop. Mex.* pelusa, enfermedad infecciosa viral que se manifiesta con dolor de garganta, fiebre y una erupción rosácea y que puede ocasionar serios trastornos fetales si la madre la contrae durante los primeros tres meses del embarazo.

rubella virus vaccine, live *n.* vacuna de virus vivo contra la rubéola.

rubescent *a.* ruborizado-a, que se enrojece.

rubor *n.* rubor, enrojecimiento de la piel.

rudiment *n.* rudimento. 1. órgano parcialmente desarrollado; 2. órgano o parte que ha perdido total o parcialmente su función anterior.

ruga *n. L.* (*pl.* **rugae**) arruga, pliegue.

rugose *a.* arrugado-a, lleno-a de arrugas.

rugosity *n.* rugosidad, arruga.

rule *n.* régimen, regla, precepto; ___ **s and regulations** / según el reglamento; **as a** ___ / por lo general; *v.* gobernar, administrar; **to** ___ **out** / prohibir, desechar; **to be ruled by one's emotions** / dejarse llevar por las emociones.

rumble *n.* ruido sordo; estruendo.

run *n.* carrera; *vi.* correr, hacer correr; **to** ___ **a fever** / tener calentura.

rupture *n.* [*hernia*] ruptura; [*bone*] rotura, fractura; [*boil*] reventazón; *v.* reventar, romper, fracturar; abrirse, reventarse, romperse, fracturarse.

rush *n.* precipitación, agolpamiento, torrente; oleada; **with a** ___ / de golpe, de repente; *v.* darse prisa; **to** ___ **in** / entrar de golpe, entrar con precipitación.

rusty *a.* oxidado-a.

rye *n.* centeno.

S

S *abbr.* **sacral** / sacral; **section** / sección; **stimulus** / estímulo; **subject** / sujeto; **sulphur** / sulfuro, azufre.

s *abbr.* **second** / segundo; **singular** / singular.

Sabin vaccine *n.* vacuna de Sabin, vacuna oral contra la poliomielitis.

sac *n.* saco, bolsa; estructura u órgano en forma de saco o bolsa.

saccades *n.* sacades. V. **nystagmus.**

saccharide *n.* sacárido, compuesto químico que pertenece a una serie de carbohidratos que incluye los azúcares.

saccharine *n.* sacarina, sustancia sumamente dulce, agente dulcificante artificial, *a.* sacarino-a, azucarado-a.

saccule *n.* sáculo, saco o bolsa pequeña.

saclike *a.* en forma de saco.

sacral *a.* sacral, rel. al sacro o situado cerca de éste; **plexus** ___ / plexo ___; ___ **nerves** / nervios ___ -es.

sacralization *n.* sacralización, fusión de la quinta vértebra lumbar con el sacro.

sacrifice *n.* sacrificio; *v.* sacrificar.

sacroilitis *n.* sacroilitis, infl. de la articulación sacroilíaca.

sacrolumbar *a.* sacrolumbar, rel. a las regiones sacral y lumbar.

sacrum *n.* sacro, hueso triangular formado por cinco vértebras fusionadas en la base de la espina dorsal y entre los dos huesos de la cadera.

sad *a.* triste, desconsolado-a.

saddle back *n.* espalda caída. lordosis.

sadism *n.* sadismo, perversión por la cual se obtiene placer sexual infligiendo dolor físico o psicológico a otros.

sadist *n.* sadista, persona que practica sadismo.

sadistic *a.* sádico-a, rel. al sadismo.

sadness *n.* tristeza, melancolía.

sadomasochism *n.* sadomasoquismo, derivación de placer sexual infligiendo dolor físico a si mismo o a otros.

sadomasochist *n.* sadomasoquista, persona que practica sadomasoquismo.

safe *a.* seguro-a, sin peligro; sin riesgo; **-ly** *adv.* seguramente; sin peligro.

safety *n.* seguridad, protección; ___ **pin** / imperdible.

sag *v.* perder elasticidad, perder la forma; combarse; pandearse; [*to weaken*] debilitarse.

sage *n.* salvia.

sagittal *a.* sagital, semejante a una saeta; ___ **plane** / plano ___, paralelo al eje longitudinal del cuerpo.

said *a. pp.* of **to say**, dicho; dicho-a, citado-a, antes mencionado.

salacious *a.* lascivo-a, libidinoso-a.

salad *n.* ensalada.

salary *n.* sueldo, salario.

salicylate *n.* salicilato, cualquier sal de ácido salicílico; ___ **poisoning** / envenenamiento por aspirina.

salicylic acid *n.* ácido salicílico, ácido cristalino blanco derivado del fenol.

salicylism *n.* salicilismo, condición tóxica causada por ingestión excesiva de ácido salicílico.

salient *a.* saliente, pronunciado-a.

saline *a.* salino-a; ___ **cathartic** / purgante ___; ___ **solution** / solución ___, agua destilada con sal.

saliva *n.* saliva, secreción de las glándulas salivales que envuelve y humedece el bolo alimenticio en la boca y facilita la deglución.

salivant *a.* salivoso-a, rel. a la saliva.

salivary glands *n., pl.* glándulas salivales o salivares.

salivation *n.* salivación. 1. acto de secreción de saliva; 2. secreción excesiva de saliva.

Salk vaccine *n.* vacuna de Salk, vacuna contra la poliomielitis.

sallow *a.* pálido-a, lívido-a.

salmon *n.* salmón.

salmonella *n.* Salmonela, género de bacterias gram-negativas de la familia *Enterobacteriaceae* que causan fiebres entéricas, otras infecciones gastrointestinales y septicemia.

salmonellosis *n.* salmonelosis, infección causada por ingestión de comida contaminada por bacterias del género Salmonela.

salpingectomy *n.* salpingectomía, extirpación de una o de ambas trompas de Falopio.

salpingitis *n.* salpingitis, infl. de las trompas de Falopio.

salpingo-oophorectomy *n.* salpingo-ooforectomía, extirpación de un ovario y un tubo uterino.

salpingoplasty *n.* reparación plástica de las trompas de Falopio.

salpinx *n., Gr.* (*pl.* **salpinges**) trompa, estructura similar a la trompa de Eustaquio o a la trompa de Falopio.

salt *n.* sal, cloruro de sodio; **iodized** ___ / ___ yodada; **low- ___ diet** / dieta hiposódica; **noniodized** ___ / ___ corriente; ___ **-free diet** / dieta libre de ___ o sin ___; ___ **shaker** / salero; **smelling** ___ **-s** / ___ -es aromáticas; *v.* salar, echar sal; [*to season with*] condimentar con sal, sazonar.

salty *a.* salado-a, salobre, salino-a.

salubrious *a.* salubre, saludable.

salutary *a.* saludable.

salve *n.* ungento, pomada.

same *a.* mismo-a, idéntico-a, igual.

sample *n.* espécimen, muestra; *v.* probar; sacar o tomar una muestra.

sampling *n.* muestreo; hacer muestras; selección partitiva; **random** ___ / ___ al azar.

sanatorium *n.* sanatorio, institución de rehabilitación física o mental.

sanction *n.* sanción, pena.

sand *n.* arena.

sandy *a.* arenoso-a.

sane *a.* sano-a; [*mentally*] cuerdo-a.

sanguine *a.* sanguíneo-a. 1. rel. a la sangre; 2. de complexión rosácea, con disposición alegre.

sanguineous *a.* sanguíneo-a, rel. a la sangre o de abundante sangre.

sanguinolent *a.* sanguinolento-a, que contiene sangre.

sanitarian *n.* sanitario-a, persona entrenada en problemas de salubridad.

sanitarium *n.* sanatorio, institución de salud de rehabilitación física o mental.

sanitary *a.* higiénico-a; ___ **napkin** / servilleta ___ absorbente, toalla ___ .

sanitation *n.* saneamiento, sanidad.

sanity *n.* cordura, sensatez, bienestar mental.

sap *n.* savia, jugo natural de algunas plantas.

saphenous *a.* safeno-a, rel. a las venas safenas.

saphenous veins *n., pl.* venas safenas, dos venas superficiales de la pierna.

sapphism *n.* safismo, lesbianismo.

saprophyte *n.* saprófito, organismo vegetal que vive en materia orgánica pútrida.

sarcoidosis *n.* sarcoidosis. V. **Schaumann's disease.**

sarcoma *n.* sarcoma, neoplasma maligno formado por tejido conectivo; **chondroblastic** ___ / ___ condroblástico; **fibropastic** ___ / ___ fibroblástico; **gastric** ___ / ___ gástrico; **lymphatic** ___ / ___ linfático; **medullary** ___ / ___ medular; **myelogenic** ___ / ___ mielógeno; **osteogenic** ___ / ___ óseo; **prostatic** ___ / ___ prostático; **pulmonary** ___ / ___ pulmonar; **renal** ___ / ___ renal; **soft tissue** ___ / ___ de tejido blando.

sardonic laugh *n.* risa sardónica, contracción espasmódica de los músculos risorios en forma de una sonrisa.

sat *a. pp.* of **to sit**, sentado-a.

satellite *n.* satélite, estructura asociada con otra o situada cerca de ella.

satiate *v.* saciar.

satiated *a.* saciado-a.

satiety *n.* saciedad, hartura, hartazgo.

satisfactory *a.* satisfactorio-a.

satisfied *a.* satisfecho-a, contento-a.

satisfy *v.* satisfacer.

saturate *v.* saturar; empapar.

saturated *a.* saturado-a, empapado-a, incapaz de absorber o recibir una sustancia más allá de un límite; ___ **solution** / solución ___ .

saturation *n.* saturación, acto de saturar; ___ **index** / índice de ___; ___ **time** / tiempo de ___ .

sauce *n.* salsa; [*dressing*] aderezo.

sausage *n.* salchicha; chorizo.

save *v.* salvar, [*energy, money*] ahorrar; [*time*] aprovechar el tiempo.

say *vi.* decir; **You don't say!** / ¡No me diga!, ¡no me digas!

scab *n.* costra, escara.

scabies *n.* sarna, infección cutánea parasitaria muy contagiosa que causa picazón.

scald *n.* escaldadura, quemadura de la piel causada por vapor o por un líquido caliente; *v.* lavar en agua hirviendo, quemar con un líquido caliente.

scale *n.* 1. escala, balanza; 2. escama, costra, lámina que se desprende de la piel seca.

scaling *n.* peladura.

scalp *n.* cuero cabelludo; ___ **dermatoses** / dermatosis del ___ .

scalpel *n.* escalpelo; bisturí, instrumento quirúrgico.

scaly *a.* escamoso-a.

scan, scintiscan *n.* tomografía, escán; rastreo, proceso que reproduce la imagen de un tejido u órgano específico usando un detector de la sustancia radiactiva tecnecio 99 m. inyectada como medio de contraste; **bone** ___ / ___ de los huesos; **brain** ___ / ___ del cerebro; **heart** ___ / ___ cardíaco; **lung** ___ / ___ pulmonar; **thyroid** ___ / ___ de la tiroide.

scanner *n.* escáner.

scanning *n.* exploración, barrido, escrutinio y registro por medio de un instrumento de detección de la emisión de ondas radiactivas de una sustancia específica que ha sido inyectada y que se concentra en partes o tejidos en observación.

scant *a.* escaso-a, parco-a, insuficiente.

scanty *a.* escaso-a, limitado-a, no abundante.

scaphoid *a.* escafoide, en forma de bote esp. en referencia al hueso del carpo y al del tarso.

scapula *n.* escápula, hueso del hombro.

scar *n.* cicatriz, marca en la piel; *v.* cicatrizar.

scare *v.* asustar, atemorizar.

scarification *n.* escarificación, acto de hacer punturas o raspaduras en la piel.

scarlet fever, scarlatina *n.* escarlatina, enfermedad contagiosa aguda caracterizada por fiebre y erupción con enrojecimiento de la piel y la lengua.

scatology *n.* escatología. 1. estudio de las heces fecales; 2. obsesión con el excremento y las inmundicias.

scatter *v.* esparcir, diseminar; dispersar, desparramar.

scattered *a.* esparcido-a, diseminado-a; desparramado-a, regado-a.

scene *n.* escena, escenario.

scent *n.* olor; aroma, perfume.

Schaumann's disease *n.* enfermedad de Schaumann, enfermedad crónica manifestada con pequeños tubérculos esp. en los pulmones, los nódulos linfáticos, los huesos y la piel.

schedule *n.* horario; *v.* hacer un horario; programar.

schema *n.* esquema, plan, planeamiento.

schematic *a.* esquemático-a, rel. a un esquema.

Schilling test *n.* prueba de Schilling, uso de vitamina B$_{12}$ radioactiva en el diagnóstico de anemia perniciosa primaria.

Schistosoma *n. Schistosoma*, esquistosoma, duela, especie de trematodo cuyas larvas entran en la sangre del huésped por contacto con agua contaminada a través del tubo digestivo o la piel.

schistosomiasis *n.* esquistosomiasis, infestación producida por la duela.

schizoid *a.* esquizoide, semejante a la esquizofrenia.

schizophrenia *n.* esquizofrenia, desintegración mental que transforma la personalidad con varias manifestaciones psicóticas tales como alucinaciones, retraimiento y distorsión de la realidad.

schizophrenic *a.* esquizofrénico-a, rel. a la esquizofrenia o que padece de ella.

sciatica *n.* ciática, neuralgia que se irradia a lo largo del nervio ciático.

sciatic nerve *n.* nervio ciático, nervio que se extiende desde la base de la columna vertebral a lo largo del muslo y se ramifica en la pierna y el pie.

scintigraphy *n.* escintigrafía, técnica de diagnóstico que emplea radioisótopos para obtener una imagen bidimensional de la distribución de un radiofármaco en un área designada del cuerpo.

scintillate *v.* escintilar, centellear, brillar.

scintiscan *n.* escintiescán, gammagrama, registro de la imagen bidimensional de la distribución interior de un radiofármaco en un área seleccionada previamente para fines de diagnóstico.

scirrhous *a.* escirroso-a, duro-a, rel. a un escirro.

scirrhus *n.* escirro, tumor canceroso duro.

scissors *n., pl.* tijeras.

sclera, sclerotica *n.* esclerótica, parte blanca del ojo compuesta de tejido fibroso.

scleritis *n.* escleritis, infl. de la esclerótica.

scleroderma *n.* escleroderma, esclerodermia, induración y casi total atrofia de la epidermis.

scleroma *n.* escleroma, área endurecida y circunscrita de tejido granuloso en la piel o en la membrana mucosa.

sclerosing solutions *n. pl.* soluciones esclerosantes.

sclerosis *n.* esclerosis, endurecimiento progresivo de los tejidos y órganos; **Alzheimer's** ___ / ___ de Alzheimer; **amyotrophic lateral** ___ / ___ lateral amiotrófica; **arterial** ___ / ___ arterial; **multiple** ___ / ___ múltiple.

sclerotherapy *n.* escleroterapia, tratamiento con una solución química que se inyecta en las várices para producir esclerosis.

sclerotic *a.* esclerótico-a, rel. a la esclerosis o afectado por ella.

scoliosis *n.* escoliosis, desviación lateral pronunciada de la columna vertebral.

scoop *n.* paletada, cucharada.

scorch *v.* chamuscar, quemar, abrasar.

score *n.* valoración, evaluación; *v.* llevar la cuenta; [*in a game*] anotar.

scorpion *n., Gr.* escorpión, alacrán; ___ **sting** / picadura de ___ .

scotoma *n., Gr. (pl.* **scotomata***)* escotoma, área del campo visual en la cual existe pérdida parcial o total de la visión.

scotopia *n.* escotopia, visión nocturna, adaptación visual a la oscuridad.

scotopic *a.* escotópico-a, rel. a la escotopia; ___ **vision** / visión ___ .

scrape *n.* raspadura, rasponazo, raspado; *v.* raspar, rasguñar.

scraper *n.* descarnador, raspador.

scratch *n.* rasguño, arañazo; *v.* raspar, rascar, rascarse; ___ **test** / prueba del rasguño, gen. para uso en pruebas alérgicas.

scream *n.* grito, chillido; *v.* gritar, chillar.

screech *v.* chillar.

screen *n.* pantalla; *v.* examinar sistemáticamente un grupo de casos; escrutar; **toxicology** ___ / protocolo toxicológico.

screening *n.* escrutinio, averiguación, selección; **biochemical** ___ / serie selectiva bioquímica; **multiphasic** ___ / ___ múltiple; **prescriptive** ___ / ___ prescrito.

screw *n.* tornillo, rosca.

scribble *n.* garabato.

scrofula *n.* escrófula, tuberculosis de la glándula linfática.

scrofuloderma *n.* escrofuloderma, *pop.* lamparón, tipo de escrófula cutánea.

scrotal *a.* escrotal, rel. al escroto.

scrotum *n.* escroto, saco o bolsa que envuelve o contiene los testículos.

scrub *v.* limpiar, fregar, restregar; ___ **nurse** / enfermera de cirugía.

scrubbing *n.* limpieza rigurosa de las manos y brazos antes de la cirugía.

scruple *n.* escrúpulo.

scrupulous *a.* escrupuloso-a.

scrupulousness *n.* escrupulosidad.

scrutiny *n.* escrutinio.

scum *n.* espuma; escoria.

scurvy *n.* escorbuto, enfermedad causada por deficiencia de vitamina C que se manifiesta con anemia, encías sangrantes y un estado general de laxitud.

seal *n.* sello; *v.* cerrar herméticamente.

seam *n.* costura, línea de costura.

search *n.* búsqueda, investigación; registro; *v.* buscar, registrar; investigar.

seasickness *n.* mareo; mareo por movimiento.

season *n.* estación; temporada; *v.* [*cooking*] sazonar.

seasonal affective disorders *n., pl.* trastornos afectivos estacionales.

seasoned *a.* sazonado-a; ___ **foods** / alimentos ___ -s.

seat *n.* asiento; localidad.

sebaceous *a.* sebáceo-a, seboso-a, rel. al sebo o de la naturaleza de éste; ___ **cyst** / quiste ___; ___ **gland** / glándula ___ .

seborrhea *n.* seborrea, trastorno de las glándulas sebáceas, caracterizado por una secreción excesiva de sebo.

seborrheic *a.* seborréico-a, rel. to seborrhea; ___ **blepharitis** / blefaritis ___; ___ **dermatitis** / dermatitis ___; ___ **keratosis** / queratosis ___ .

sebum *n.* sebo, secreción espesa que segregan las glándulas sebáceas.

second *n.* segundo; *a.* segundo-a.

secondary *a.* secundario-a.

secretagogue, secretogogue *n.* secretogogo, agente que estimula la secreción glandular.

secrete *v.* secretar, segregar.

secretion *n.* secreción. 1. producción de un tejido o sustancia como resultado de una actividad glandular; **purulent** ___ / ___ purulenta; 2. sustancia producida por secreción.

secretory *a.* secretor-a, que tiene la propiedad de secretar; ___ **capillaries** / capilares secretores; ___ **carcinoma** / carcinoma ___; ___ **fiber** / fibra ___; ___ **nerve** / nervio ___ .

section *n.* sección, porción, parte; *v.* cortar; seccionar.

sectioning *n.* el acto de seccionar, dividir, cortar.

secure *a.* seguro-a; *v.* asegurar.

security *n.* seguridad; ___ **measures** / medidas de ___ .

sedation *n.* sedación, acción o efecto de calmar o sedar; *v.* **to put under** ___ / dar un sedante, calmante o soporífero.

sedative *n.* calmante, sedante, agente con efectos tranquilizantes.

sedentary *a.* sedentario-a. 1. de poca actividad física; 2. rel. a la posición sentada.

sediment *n.* sedimento, materia que se deposita en el fondo de un líquido.

sedimentation *n.* sedimentación, acción o proceso de depositar sedimentos; ___ **rate** / índice de ___ .

see *vi.* ver; **I see!** / ¡Ya veo!; **Let's** ___ / Vamos a ver; **to** ___ **to it** / atender, ver que, hacer que.

seed *n.* semilla, simiente.

seeing *n.* vista, visión.

seen *a. pp.* of **to see**, visto-a.

segment *n.* segmento, porción, sección.

segmentation *n.* segmentación, acto de dividir en partes.

Seguin's signal symptom *n.* Seguin, síntoma de, contracción involuntaria de los músculos antes de un ataque epiléptico.

seizure *n.* ataque repentino, acceso; ___ **activity** / actividad convulsiva.

seldom *adv.* rara vez, con rareza, raramente.

select *v.* seleccionar, escoger.

selection *n.* selección, elección.

self *n.* el yo; *pron.* uno-a mismo-a; *a.* sí mismo-a; mismo-a; propio-a; ___ **-assurance** / confianza en ___; ___ **-centered** / egoísta, egocéntrico-a; ___ **-conscious** / concentrado-a en ___, cohibido-a; ___ **-contained** / autónomo; [*personality*] reservado-a; ___ **-contamination** / autocontaminación; ___ **-control** / dominio de ___; ___ **-defense** / defensa propia; ___ **-delusion, deception** / engaño a ___; ___ **-denial** / abnegación; ___ **-determination** / autodeterminación; ___ **-distrust** / falta de confianza en ___; ___ **-esteem** / amor propio, reconocimiento de valores propios; ___ **-identity** / conciencia de la identidad del yo; ___ **-induced** / auto-inducido-a; ___ **-medication** / automedicación; ___ **-pity** / compasión por ___; *v.* **to be** ___ **-sufficient** / valerse por ___ .

selfish *a.* egoísta.

sella turcica *n.* silla turca, depresión en la superficie superior del esfenoide que contiene la hipófisis.

semantics *n.* semántica, estudio del significado de las palabras.

semen *n.* semen, esperma, secreción espesa blanca segregada por los órganos reproductivos masculinos.

semester *n.* semestre.

semicoma *n.* semicoma, estado comatoso leve.

semidisintegration *n.* semidesintegración, tiempo requerido por una sustancia radiactiva para perder la mitad de la radioactividad por desintegración.

seminal *a.* seminal, rel. a una semilla o que consiste de una semilla.

seminiferous *a.* seminífero-a, que produce semen.

seminuria *n.* seminuria, presencia de semen en la orina.

semiotic *n.* semiótico-a, rel. a los síntomas o señales de una enfermedad.

semiotics *n.* semiótica, rama de la medicina que trata de las señales y síntomas de una enfermedad.

send *vi.* enviar, mandar.

senescence *n.* senescencia, senectud, proceso de envejecimiento.

senile *a.* senil, rel. a la vejez esp. en lo que afecta a las funciones mentales y físicas.

senility *n.* senilidad, cualidad de ser senil.

senior citizen *n.* persona mayor; jubilado-a.

sensation *n.* sensación, percepción de una estimulación por un órgano sensorial.

sense *n.* sentido, facultad de percibir por medio de los órganos sensoriales; **common** ___ / ___ común; ___ **of hearing** / ___ del oído; ___ **of humor** / ___ del humor; ___ **of sight** / ___ de la vista; ___ **of smell** / ___ del olfato; ___ **of taste** / ___ del gusto; ___ **of touch** / ___ del tacto; *v.* sentir.

sensibility *n* sensibilidad, capacidad de recibir sensaciones.

sensiferous *a.* sensífero-a, que causa, transmite o conduce sensaciones.

sensitive *a.* sensitivo-a, sensible.

sensitivity *n.* sensibilidad, susceptibilidad.

sensitivity training *n.* entrenamiento de la sensibilidad o capacidad sensorial.

sensitization *n.* sensibilización, acto de hacer sensible o sensorial.

sensorial *a.* sensorial, sensitivo-a; que se percibe por los sentidos.

sensorimotor *a.* sensitivomotor, rel. a las actividades motoras y sensitivas del cuerpo.

sensory *a.* sensorial, sensorio-a, rel. a las sensaciones o los sentidos; ___ **acuity level** / nivel de agudeza ___; ___ **aphasia** / afasia ___; ___ **epilepsy** / epilepsia ___; ___ **ganglion** / ganglio ___; ___ **image** / imagen ___; ___ **integration** / integración ___; ___ **overload** / sobrecarga ___; ___ **processing** / procesamiento ___ .

sensory nervous system *n.* sistema nervioso sensorial.

sensory threshold *n.* umbral sensorial.

sensual *a.* sensual, carnal.

sensuous *a.* sensual.

sentiment *n.* sentimiento.

separate *v.* separar, dividir.

separation *n.* separación, división; selección.

sepsis *n., L.* sepsis, condición tóxica producida por una contaminación bacteriana.

septal *a.* septal, rel. a un septum; ___ **deviation** / desviación ___ .

septate *a.* septado-a, rel. a una estructura dividida por un septum.

septectomy *n.* septectomía, escisión parcial o total del tabique nasal.

septic *n.* séptico-a, rel. a la sepsis; ___ **shock** / choque ___ .

septicemia, blood poisoning *n.* septicemia, envenenamiento de la sangre, invasión de la sangre por microorganismos virulentos.

septimetritis *n.* septimetritis, infl. del útero debido a sepsis.

septostomy *n.* septostomía, apertura quirúrgica de un septum.

septum *n., L. (pl.* **septa**) septum, tabique o membrana que divide dos cavidades o espacios; **ventricular** ___ / ___ventricular;

sequela *n. (pl.* **sequelae**) secuela, condición que resulta de una enfermedad, lesión o tratamiento.

sequence *n.* secuencia, sucesión.

sequester *v.* secuestrar, aislar.

sequestration *n.* secuestro, aislamiento. 1. acto de aislar; 2. formación de un sequestrum.

sequestrum *n.* sequestrum, secuestro, fragmento de un hueso necrosado que se separa de un hueso sano adyacente.

serene *a.* sereno-a, tranquilo-a.

serial *a.* en serie.

series *n.* serie, grupo de espécimenes en una secuencia.

serious *a.* serio-a; complicado-a; **-ly** *adv.* seriamente.

seroconversion *n.* seroconversión, desarrollo de anticuerpos como respuesta a una infección o a la administración de una vacuna.

serologic, serological *a.* serológico-a, rel. a un suero; ___ **test** / prueba ___ .

serology *n.* serología, ciencia que estudia las propiedades de los sueros.

seroma *n.* seroma, acumulación gen. subcutánea de suero sanguíneo que produce una hinchazón que se asemeja a un tumor.

seronegative *a.* seronegativo-a, que presenta una reacción negativa a pruebas serológicas.

seropositive *a.* seropositivo-a, que presenta una reacción positiva a pruebas serológicas.

seropositivity *n.* seropositividad, resultado positivo en un examen serológico.

serosa *n.* membrana serosa.

serosanguineous *a.* serosanguíneo-a, de naturaleza serosa y sanguínea.

serositis *n.* serositis, infl. de una membrana serosa, signo importante en enfermedades del tejido conjuntivo tal como el lupus sistémico eritematoso.

serotype *n.* serotipo, tipo de microorganismo que se determina por las clases y combinaciones de antígenos presentes en la célula.

serotyping *n.* determinación del serotipo.

serous *a.* seroso-a, que produce o contiene suero.

serpiginous *n.* serpiginoso-a, sinuoso-a, de movimiento semejante a una serpiente.

serrated *a.* serrado-a, endentado-a, con proyección similar a los dientes de un serrucho.

serum *n.* suero, líquido seroso. 1. elemento del plasma que permanece líquido y claro después de la coagulación; 2. cualquier líquido seroso; 3. suero inmune de animales o personas que se inocula para producir inmunizaciones pasivas o temporales.

services *n.* servicios; **emergency** ___ / ___ de emergencia; **extended care facility** ___ / ___ de cuidado o atención extendida; **preventive health** ___ / ___ de salud preventiva.

sesamoid *a.* sesamoideo, semejante a una pequeña masa o semilla incrustada en una articulación o cartílago.

sessile *a.* sésil, insertado o fijo en una base ancha que carece de pedúnculo.

session *n.* sesión.

set *n.* conjunto, equipo; grupo; instrumentos y accesorios; [*surgical*] instrumental quirúrgico; **it is all** ___ / todo está arreglado; *vi.* poner, colocar; [*a broken bone*] encasar, fijar, ajustar; ___ **a fracture** / componer una fractura.

setback *n.* recaída; retraso, contrariedad.

setting *n.* [*environment*] ambiente; montaje.

settle *v.* asentar, fijar; asegurar.

settlement *n.* [*account*] arreglo, ajuste.

sever *v.* cortar, romper; separar.

several *a.* varios-as, muchos-as, algunos-as.

severe *a.* grave, severo-a; ___ **acute respiratory syndrome** / síndrome respiratorio agudo ___ .

severe combined immunodeficiency disease *n.* enfermedad grave de inmunodeficiencia combinada, una de las enfermedades genéticas raras que se caracteriza por el desarrollo defectivo de las células que generan anticuerpos.

sew *vi.* coser.

sewage *n.* aguas de alcantarilla, cloacas.

sewing *n.* costura, puntada.

sex *n.* sexo; ___ **determination** / determinación del ___; ___ **disorders** / trastornos o anomalías sexuales; ___ **distribution** / distribución según el ___ .

sex-linked *a.* 1. relacionado con el sexo; 2. que se refiere a cromosomas sexuales o es transmitido por ellos.

sexual *a.* sexual, rel. al sexo; ___ **assault** / agresión ___; ___ **behavior** / conducta ___; ___ **characteristics** / características ___ -es; ___ **development** / desarrollo ___; ___ **health** / salud ___; ___ **intercourse** / relaciones ___ -es, coito; ___ **life** / vida ___; ___ **maturity** / madurez ___; **-ly** *adv.* sexualmente; ___ **transmitted disease.** / enfermedad transmitida ___ . See chart on page 517.

sexuality *n.* sexualidad, características de cada sexo.

S

Sexual Disorders	Trastornos Sexuales
erotomania	erotomania
exhibitionism	exhibicionismo
fetishism	fetichismo
frotteurism	froterismo
masochism	masoquismo
nymphomania	ninfomanía
paraphilia	parafilia
pedophilia	pedofilia
sadism	sadismo
satyromania	satiromanía
transvestic fetishism	fetichismo trasvestido
voyeurism	voyeurismo, mironismo

shade *n.* sombra.

shadow *n.* sombra; opacidad.

shaft *n.* caña. V. **diaphysis.**

shake *vi.* agitar; [*hands*] dar la mano; [*from cold*] temblar, tiritar de frío;___ **well before using /** agítese bien antes de usarse;

shaken *a.* sacudido-a; afectado-a; debilitado-a.

shakes *n. pl.* temblores, *pop.* tembladera; escalofríos; fiebre intermitente.

shaking palsy *n.* parálisis agitante.Parkinson's disease.

shaky *a.* vacilante, temeroso-a; [*untrustworthy*] que no merece confianza.

shall *v. aux.* deber.

shaman *n.* curandero.

shamanism *n.* curanderismo.

shame *n.* vergenza; **What a** ___ ! / ¡Qué pena!, ¡Qué lástima!; *v.* avergonzar.

shameful *a.* vergonzoso-a, penoso-a.

shank *n.* canilla de la pierna.

shape *n.* forma, aspecto; condición [*health*] **in bad** ___ / enfermo-a; destruido-a; **out of** ___ / deformado-a, imperfecto [*physically*] desajuste físico; *v.* formar, moldear.

sharp *a.* [*pain*] agudo-a; [*instrument*] afilado-a.

shave *v.* afeitar; afeitarse.

shears *n., pl.* tijeras.

sheath *n.* cubierta, capa o membrana protectora.

shed *vi.* [*blood, tears*] derramar; [*light*] dar, esparcir; difundir; [*skin, hair*] mudar; pelar; soltar; descamar.

shedding *n.* [*hair*] exfoliación; [*skin*] peladura.

sheep *n.* oveja, carnero.

sheet *n.* lámina, hoja de metal; [*bedclothes*] sábana.

shelf *n.* anaquel, estructura en forma horizontal alargada.

shell *n.* cáscara; concha marina.

shellfish *n.* molusco; marisco.

shield *n.* escudo, cubierta.

shift *n.* cambio de posición, desviación; [*work period*] turno; *v.* cambiar, desviar.

shigellosis *n.* shigelosis, disentería bacilar.

shinbone *n.* espinilla, borde anterior de la tibia.

shingles *n. pop.* culebrilla, herpes zóster, erupción inflamatoria de la piel con vesículas o ampollas gen. localizadas en el tronco.

shirt *n.* camisa; **under** ___ / camiseta.

shiver *n.* estremecimiento, escalofrío, temblor; *v.* tener escalofríos; tiritar de frío; estremecerse.

shock, choc *n., Fr.* shock, choque, estado anormal generado por una insuficiencia circulatoria sanguínea que puede causar descenso en la presión arterial, pulso rápido, palidez, temperatura anormalmente baja y debilidad; **anaphylactic** ___ / ___ anafiláctico; **endotoxic** ___ / ___ endotóxico; **septic** ___ / ___ séptico; ___ **therapy, electric /** terapia electroconvulsiva.

shoe *n.* zapato, calzado; **cast** ___ / ___ en escayola; **orthopedic** ___ **-s /** calzado ortopédico.

short *a.* corto-a; [*time*] breve; [*height*] bajo-a; **in a** ___ **time /** en breve, dentro de poco; **on** ___ **notice /** en corto plazo; ___ **of breath /** falto-a de respiración.

shortage *n.* carencia, falta, déficit.

shorten *v.* acortar.

shortsightedness, nearsightedness *n.* miopía.

shot *n.* tiro, disparo, [*wound*] balazo; [*injection*] inyección.

should *v. aux. cond. pret.* of *shall,* deber.

shoulder *n.* hombro, unión de la clavícula, la escápula y el húmero.

shout *n.* grito, alarido; *v.* gritar.

show *vi.* mostrar, enseñar, manifestar; revelar.

shower *n.* ducha; *v.* ducharse, darse una ducha.

shrimp *n.* camarón.

shrink *n. pop.* psiquiatra o alienista, psicólogo; *vi.* encoger; encogerse.

shudder *v.* estremecerse.

shunt *n.* desviación, derivación, *shunt*; **low-flow** ___ / derivación de flujo lento; *v.* desviar, derivar.

shut *vi.* cerrar.

shy *a.* tímido-a, temeroso-a; cauteloso-a.

Shy-Drager syndrome *n.* Shy-Drager, síndrome de, enfermedad neurodegenerativa vista en personas de edad media y mayores de edad, que afecta el sistema nervioso autónomo y se caracteriza por hipotensión crónica ortostática, con pérdida del conocimiento, impotencia, incontinencia y arrítmia cardíaca.

sialadenitis, sialoadenitis *n.* sialoadenitis, infl. de una glándula salival.

sialogogue *n.* sialagogo, agente que estimula la secreción salival.

sialogram *n.* sialograma, rayos-x del conducto de la glándula salival.

sick *n.* *a.* enfermo-a; ___ **leave** / licencia por enfermedad.

sickly *a.* enfermizo-a, achacoso-a, endeble.

sickness *n.* enfermedad, dolencia, mal; **acute African sleeping** ___ / ___ africana del sueño; **altitude** ___ / mal de altura; **beriberi** ___ / de Ceylon; **bleeding** ___ / hemofilia; **car** ___ / cinetosis, mareo; **decompression** ___ / ___ de los buzos; **falling** ___ / epilepsia; **gall** ___ / anaplasmosis; **green** ___ / clorosis, cloroanemia; **milk** ___ / brucelosis; **morning** ___ / trastorno de las embarazadas; **motion** ___ / ___ de los viajeros; **radiation** ___ / ___ por radiación.

side *n.* lado, costado; **by the** ___ **of** / al ___ de; **right** ___ / ___ derecho; **left** ___ / ___ izquierdo; ___ **effect** / efecto secundario, reacción gen. adversa a un medicamento, tratamiento o droga.

sideways *a.* de lado.

sieve *n.* colador; *v.* colar, pasar por un tamiz.

sight *n.* vista; **at first** ___ / a primera ___ .

sigmoid *a.* sigmoide, sigmoideo. 1. que tiene forma de sigmoid; 2. rel. al colon sigmoide.

sigmoidoscope *n.* sigmoidoscopio, instrumento tubular largo que se usa para examinar la flexura sigmoide.

sigmoidoscopy *n.* sigmoidoscopía, uso de un sigmoidoscopio para examinar la flexura sigmoide.

sign *n.* señal, signo, indicación, manifestación objetiva de una enfermedad; **vital** ___ **-s** / signos vitales.

signature *n.* 1. firma; 2. parte de una receta médica que contiene las instrucciones.

significance *a.* significado; **of no** ___ / sin importancia.

significant *a.* importante, significativo-a.

signify *v.* significar.

sign language *n.* lenguaje mímico por señales. V. **dactylology.**

silence *n.* silencio.

silent *a.* silencioso-a.

silicon *n.* silicio, elemento no metálico encontrado en la tierra.

silicone *n.* silicón, silicona, compuesto orgánico que se usa en lubricantes, productos sintéticos, cirugía plástica y en prótesis.

silicosis *n.* silicosis, inhalación de partículas de polvo.

silk *n.* seda.

silly *a.* tonto-a.

silver *n.* plata; ___ **nitrate** / nitrato de ___ .

similar *a.* similar, semejante, parecido-a.

simmer *v.* cocer a fuego lento.

simple *a.* simple, sencillo-a; **-ly** *adv.* simplemente, meramente.

simplify *v.* simplificar.

simulate *v.* fingir, simular, pretender.

simulation *n.* simulación, fingir un síntoma o enfermedad.

since *adv.* desde; ___ **then, ever** ___ / ___ entonces; ___ **when?** / ¿___ cuándo?

sinew *n.* tendon.

single *a.* sencillo-a, simple, solo-a; [*unmarried*] soltero-a.

singular *a.* singular, único.

singultus *n., L.* hipo.

sinoatrial *a.* sinoatrial, rel. a la región del seno auricular.

sinoatrial, sinoauricular node *n.* nódulo sinusal o senoauricular, localizado en la unión de la vena cava y la aurícula derecha, y que se considera el punto de origen de los impulsos que estimulan los latidos del corazón.

sinogram *n.* sinograma, radiografía de un seno paranasal usando un medio de contraste.

sinuous *a.* sinuoso-a, ondulado-a.

sinus *n., L.* sinus, seno, cavidad de abertura estrecha; ___ **rhythm** / ritmo sinusal.

sinusal *a.* sinusal, rel. a un sinus.

sinusitis *n.* sinusitis, infl. de la mucosa de un seno o cavidad, esp. los senos paranasales.

sinusoid *n.* sinusoide, conducto diminuto que lleva sangre a los tejidos de un órgano; *a.* rel. a un sinus.

sip *n.* sorbo, trago; *v.* sorber.

siphon *n.* sifón.

sister *n.* hermana; ___ **-in-law** / cuñada.

sit *vi.* sentar, asentar; **to** ___ **down** / sentarse.

situated *a.* situado-a, localizado-a.

situation *n.* situación, localización.

situs *n., L.* situs, posición, sitio.

size *n.* tamaño; [*garments*] talla.

Sjogrens' Syndrome *n.* Sjogren, síndrome de, trastorno autoinmune que resulta en escasa

S

secreción salivar y lacrimal causando sequedad en la boca y los ojos.

skeletal *n.* esquelético-a.

skeleton *n.* esqueleto, armazón ósea del cuerpo.

skew *n.* movimiento oblicuo-a, movimiento sesgado-a, de lado.

skill *n.* destreza, habilidad.

skin *n.* piel, epidermis, cutis; *pop.* pellejo; **sagging facial** ___ / cutis colgante; ___ **cancer** / cáncer de la ___; ___ **chafing** / fricción de la ___; ___ **diseases** / enfermedades de la ___, dermatosis ; ___ **graft** / injerto de la ___; ___ **rash** / erupción cutánea, urticaria ; ___ **rejuvenation** / rejuvenecimiento de la ___; ___ **tests** / pruebas cutáneas; ___ **ulcer** / úlcera cutánea. See illustration on this page.

skinny *a.* flaco-a, delgado-a, descarnado-a.

skip *v.* omitir, pasar por alto; [*jump*] saltar.

skirt *n.* falda.

skull *n.* cráneo; calavera, estructura ósea de la cabeza; **base of the** ___ / base del ___; ___ **fractures** / fracturas del ___ .

slant *n.* inclinación, plano inclinado; *v.* inclinar; [*words*] distorsionar; inclinarse.

slanted *a.* oblicuo-a, inclinado-a; sesgado-a.

slap *n.* bofetada, manotazo; *v.* pegar, dar una bofetada, dar un manotazo.

sleep *n.* sueño; **balmy** ___ / ___ reparador; ___ **apnea** / apnea intermitente que ocurre durante el sueño; ___ **cycles** / ciclos del ___; ___ **disorders** / trastornos del ___; ___ **stages** / fases del ___; **twilight** ___ / ___ crepuscular; *vi.* dormir; dormirse; **to** ___ **soundly** / ___ profundamente.

sleepiness *n.* somnolencia, adormecimiento.

sleeping pill *n.* soporífero, somnífero, pastilla para dormir.

sleeping sickness *n.* enfermedad del sueño, dolencia aguda endémica de África que se manifiesta con fiebre, letargo, escalofríos, pérdida de peso y debilidad general, causada por un protozoo transmitido por la picadura de la mosca tsetse.

sleepwalking *n.* sonambulismo.

sleeve *n.* manga; **Put up your** ___ / Súbase, súbete la manga.

slender *a.* esbelto-a; delgado-a.

slice *n.* pedazo, tajada, rebanada.

slide *n.* diapositiva, laminilla, [*specimen holder*] portaobjeto; *v.* deslizarse.

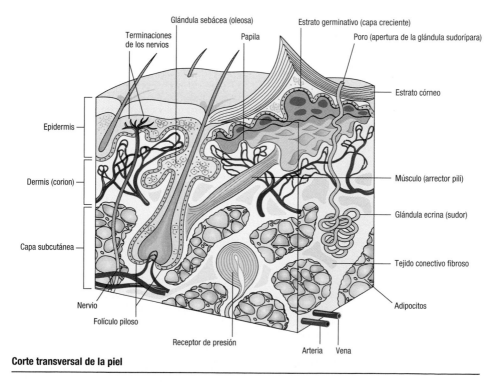

Corte transversal de la piel

sliding *n.* deslizamiento.

slight *a.* ligero-a, leve; —— **fever** / fiebrecita, fiebre —— .

slim *a.* delgado-a; esbelto-a; insuficiente; **a** —— **chance** / poco probable.

slimy *a.* viscoso-a; enlodado-a.

sling *n.* cabestrillo, soporte de vendaje.

slip *v.* resbalarse.

slippery *a.* resbaladizo-a, resbaloso-a.

slipping *n.* el acto de resbalar.

slit *n.* incisión, hendidura, rajadura; *v.* **to make a** —— / hacer una incisión, hacer una hendidura; rajar, cortar en tiras.

slope *n.* inclinación; declive; *v.* estar inclinado-a; estar en declive.

slough *n.* esfacelo, masa de tejido muerto que se ha desprendido de un tejido vivo.

slow *a.* lento-a, pausado-a, despacioso-a; [*clock*] atrasado, retrasado; *v.* **to** —— **down** / ir más despacio; tener más calma; **-ly** *adv.* lentamente, pausadamente, más despacio.

sluggish *a.* flojo-a, inactivo-a, de movimiento lento.

small *a.* pequeño-a; **smaller** / *comp.* más pequeño; **smallest** / *sup.* el menor, el más pequeño.

smallpox *n.* viruela, enfermedad infecciosa viral que se manifiesta con un cuadro febril agudo y erupción de ampollas y pústulas diseminadas por todo el cuerpo.

smart *a.* inteligente, listo-a.

smear *n.* frotis, unto; *v.* untar, embarrar.

smegma *n.* esmegma, secreción producida por las glándulas sebáceas vista esp. en los órganos genitales exteriores.

smell *n.* 1. olor, aroma; **penetrating** —— / —— penetrante; 2. sentido del olfato; *v.* oler, percibir un olor.

smile *n.* sonrisa; *v.* sonreír.

smiling *a.* risueño-a.

smog *n.* mezcla de niebla y humo.

smoke *n.* humo; —— **inhalation** / inhalación de ——; —— **screen** / cortina de ——; *v.* fumar; **Do not** —— **here** / No fume, no fumes aquí.

smooth *a.* liso-a; [*cutis*] suave, terso-a, delicado-a.

snake *n.* serpiente, culebra; —— **-bite** / mordedura de ——; —— **venom** / ponzoña de ——; **poisonous** —— / —— venenosa.

snap *n.* chasquido, ruido cardíaco relacionado con la apertura de una válvula del corazón, gen. la válvula mitral; **opening** —— / —— de apertura.

sneeze *n.* estornudo; *v.* estornudar.

sniff *v.* olfatear, oler; absorber por la nariz; resoplar.

sniffle *n.* catarro nasal; *v.* sorber repetidamente por la nariz.

snooze *v.* adormecerse.

snore *n.* ronquido; *v.* roncar.

snort *v.* aspirar a través de la mucosa nasal.

snow *n.* nieve; *v.* nevar.

snuff *v.* inhalar; resoplar hacia adentro; **to** —— **up** / tomar por la nariz.

so *adv.* así, de este modo, de esta manera; **it is not** —— / no es ——; **not** —— **much** / no tanto; **so-so** / más o menos, regular; —— **that** / de manera que.

soak *v.* remojar, empapar; **to** —— **in, to** —— **up** / absorber, chupar.

soap *n.* jabón; *v.* enjabonar; **to** —— **oneself** / enjabonarse.

sob *n.* sollozo; *v.* sollozar.

sober *a.* sobrio-a, serio; *v.* **to get** —— / dejar de beber, dejar de tomar bebidas alcohólicas;

sociable *a.* sociable, amigable.

social *a.* social, sociable; —— **behavior** / conducta o comportamiento ——; —— **security** / seguro ——; —— **work** / asistencia ——; —— **worker** / trabajador-a —— .

socialization *n.* socialización, adaptación social.

socialized *a.* socializado-a; —— **medicine** / medicina —— .

society *n.* sociedad; organización social.

sociobiology *n.* sociobiología, ciencia que estudia los factores genéticos como determinantes de la conducta.

sociologist *n.* sociólogo-a, especialista en sociología.

sociology *n.* sociología, ciencia que trata de las relaciones sociales y de los fenómenos de tipo social.

sociopath *n.* sociópata, persona caracterizada por una conducta antisocial.

sock *n.* media, calcetín.

socket *n.* hueco, [*of a bone*] fosa; [*electric*] enchufe.

soda *n.* soda, carbonato de sodio; **baking** —— / bicarbonato de sodio.

sodium *n.* sodio, elemento metálico alcalino que se encuentra en los líquidos del cuerpo.

sodomite *n.* sodomita, persona que comete sodomía.

sodomy *n.* sodomía, término que denota relación sexual entre personas del mismo sexo; bestialidad o felación.

soft *a.* blando-a, suave, delicado-a; [*metals*] flexible, maleable; —— **diet** / dieta ——; —— **drinks** / refrescos, bebidas no alcohólicas; **-ly** *adv.* suavemente, blandamente.

soften v. ablandar, suavizar.

softening n. reblandecimiento, ablandamiento; suavidad.

soggy a. saturado-a, empapado-a.

soil n. tierra, terreno; [*dirt*] suciedad.

solace n. consuelo; solaz; esparcimiento; v. consolar; alegrar.

solar a. solar, rel. al sol.

sole n. suela, planta del pie.

solid a. sólido-a, macizo-a; [*person*] serio-a, formal.

soluble a. soluble.

solution n. solución.

solvent n. solvente, líquido que disuelve o es capaz de producir una solución.

somatic a. somático-a, rel. al cuerpo.

somatization n. somatización. proceso de conversión de experiencias mentales en manifestaciones corporales.

some a. alguno-a; algún, algo de, un poco de; unos, unos cuantos, unas, unas cuantas, algunos-as.

somebody n. alguien; ___ **else** / otra persona.

somehow adv. de algún modo, de alguna manera.

something n. alguna cosa, algo; ___ **else** / otra cosa.

somnambulance, somnambulism n. sonambulismo.

somnambule n. sonámbulo-a, persona que anda mientras está dormida.

somniferous n. soporífero.

somniloquism n. somniloquia, el acto de hablar dormido-a.

somnolence n. somnolencia.

son n. hijo; ___ **-in-law** / yerno; **sonny** / hijito.

sonogram n. sonograma, registro de una imagen producida por ultrasonido.

sonography n. sonografía. ultrasonography.

sonolucent a. sonoluciente, [*ultrasonography*] que puede dar paso a las ondas sonoras sin reflejarlas de nuevo en la fuente de origen.

sonorous a. sonoro-a, resonante, con un sonido vibrante.

soon adv. pronto, dentro de poco, en poco tiempo.

soothe v. calmar, aliviar, mitigar; suavizar.

sophistication n. sofisticación, adulteración de una sustancia.

soporific n. soporífico, agente que produce el sueño.

soporose, soporous a. soporosa, soporoso, en estado de sopor.

sore n. llaga, úlcera, herida; a. [*feeling*] adolorido-a, doloroso-a, con dolor; ___ **all over** / malestar general, dolor en todo el cuerpo; ___ **eyes** / malestar en los ojos, ojos adoloridos; ___ **throat** / dolor de garganta; v. **to be** ___ / estar adolorido-a.

sorrow n. pena, aflicción, pesar, dolor.

sorrowful a. apenado-a, afligido-a, apesadumbrado-a, adolorido-a.

sorry a. apesadumbrado-a; arrepentido-a; **I am** ___ / Lo siento; v. **to be** ___ / arrepentirse de; **to be** ___ **for** [*someone*] / tener lástima de (alguien).

sort n. clase, especie, género; **all** ___ **-s of** / una variedad de; **out of** ___ **-s** / malhumorado-a, indispuesto-a; v. separar, clasificar, distribuir.

soul n. alma, espíritu.

sound n. sonido, ruido; ruido de soplo percibido por auscultación; v. sonar.

soup n. sopa.

sour a. agrio-a, ácido, avinagrado-a.

source n. origen; foco; fuente.

sourness n. agrura, acidez.

south n. sur.

soy n. soja, soya.

space n. área, espacio, segmento, lugar.

spacial a. espacial, rel. al espacio.

span n. lapso, instante, momento; tiempo limitado; intervalo; distancia.

Spanish n. [*language*] español; [*native*] español-a a. español-a; **Spanish-American** / hispanoamericano-a.

spasm n. espasmo, convulsión, contracción muscular involuntaria.

spasmodic a. espasmódico-a.

spastic a. espástico-a, convulsivo-a, espasmódico-a. 1. de naturaleza espasmódica; ___ **colon** / colon espasmódico o espástico; 2. que sufre espasmos.

spasticity n. espasticidad, aumento en la tensión normal de un músculo que causa movimientos rígidos y dificultosos.

spatula n. espátula.

speak vi. hablar; ___ **louder** / hable, habla más alto; ___ **slowly** / hable, habla despacio.

special a. especial, único-a; extraordinario-a; **-ly** adv. especialmente.

specialist n. especialista.

specialize v. especializarse.

specialty n. especialidad.

species n. especie, clasificación de organismos vivos pertenecientes a una categoría biológica.

specific a. específico-a; determinado-a; preciso-a.

specify v. especificar.

specimen *n.* espécimen, muestra.
speck *n.* mácula, mancha.
spectacles *n., pl.* lentes, espejuelos, gafas.
spectrum *n.* (*pl.* **spectra**) espectro. 1. amplitud en la actividad de un antibiótico contra variedades de microorganismos; 2. serie de imágenes que resultan de la refracción de radiación electromagnética;3. banda matizada de rayos solares discernibles a simple vista o con un instrumento sensitivo.
speculate *v.* argumentar, especular.
speculum *n.* espéculo, instrumento para dilatar un conducto o cavidad.
speech *n.* habla, lenguaje; **garbled ___ /** enredada; **___ defect** / defecto del ___; **___ disorder** / trastorno del ___; **___ therapy /** terapéutica del ___ .
spell *n.* ataque súbito; *v.* **to have a ___ /** tener un ataque o acceso de; deletrear; **to ___ a word /** deletrear una palabra.
spend *vi.* [*money*] gastar, [*energy*] gastar, consumir; [*time*] pasar.
sperm *n.* esperma, semen; **decreased ___ count /** conteo disminuido de ___; **___ count /** espermiograma; semen.
spermatic *a.* espermático, rel. al esperma.
spermaticidal, spermaticide *n.* espermaticida, que destruye o causa la muerte de espermatozoos.
spermatocele *n.* espermatocele, quiste del epidídimo que contiene espermatozoos.
spermatogenesis *n.* espermatogénesis, proceso de formación y desarrollo de espermatozoos.
spermatoid *a.* espermatoide, con apariencia de semen.
spermatorrhea *n.* espermatorrea, pérdida involuntaria de esperma.
spermatozoid, spermatozoon *n., Gr.* (*pl.* **spermatozoa**) espermatozoo, célula sexual masculina que fertiliza el óvulo.
spermicidal *n.* espermicida.
spermiogram *n.* espermiograma, evaluación de los espermatozoides en el proceso de determinación de la esterilidad.
sphenoid *n.* esfenoide, hueso situado en la base del cráneo.
sphere *n.* esfera. 1. estructura en forma de globo; 2. ambiente sociológico.
spherical *a.* esférico-a, rel. a una esfera.
spherocyte *n.* esferocito, eritrocito de forma esférica.
spherocytosis *n.* esferocitosis, presencia de esferocitos en la sangre.

spheroid *n.* esferoide, de forma esférica.
spherule *n.* esfera diminuta.
sphincter *n.* esfínter, músculo circular que abre y cierra un orificio.
sphincter of Oddi *n.* Oddi, esfínter de, músculo circular contráctil situado en la apertura intestinal de la bilis y los conductos pancreáticos.
sphincteroplasty *n.* esfinteroplastia, operación plástica de un esfínter.
sphincterotomy *n.* esfinterotomía, corte de un esfínter.
sphygmomanometer *n.* esfigmomanómetro, instrumento para determinar la presión arterial.
spica *n.* espica, tipo de vendaje.
spice *n.* especia, condimento.
spicular *a.* espicular, en forma de aguja.
spicule *n.* espícula, cuerpo en forma de aguja.
spider *n.* araña; **black ___ /** araña negra.
spike *n.* espiga; [*in a graphic*] cresta o elevación brusca.
spill *n.* derrame; *v.* derramar, verter.
spina *n.* spina, espina. 1. protuberancia en forma de espina; 2. la espina o columna vertebral.
spina bifida *n.* espina bífida, malformación congénita en el cierre de un conducto de la estructura ósea de la espina vertebral, con o sin protrusión de las meninges medulares, gen. a nivel lumbar; **occult ___ /** ___ oculta, sin protrusión.
spinach *n.* espinaca.
spinal *a.* espinal, raquídeo-a, rel. a la médula espinal o a la espina o columna vertebral; **___ anesthesia** / anestesia raquídea; **___ canal /** canal raquídeo; **___ cord** / médula ___; **___ fluid** / líquido cefalorraquídeo; **___ fusion /** fusión ___; **___muscular atrophy** / atrofia muscular ___; **___ puncture** / punción ___; **___ shock** / choque ___; **___ stenosis** / estenosis ___.
spinal column *n.* columna o espina vertebral, estructura ósea formada por treinta y tres vértebras que rodean y contienen la médula espinal.
spinal cord *n.* médula espinal, columna de tejido nervioso que se extiende desde el bulbo raquídeo hasta la segunda vértebra lumbar y de la cual parten todos los nervios que van al tronco y a las extremidades; **___ compression /** compresión de la ___ .
spindle *n.* huso. 1. estructura o célula en forma de rodillo; 2. forma que toman los cromosomas durante la mitosis y la meiosis.

spine *n.* columna o espina vertebral; *pop.* espinazo.

spine-shaped *a.* espinoso-a, acantoso-a.

spinous *a.* espinoso-a, en forma de espina.

spiral *a.* espiral, que se envuelve alrededor de un centro o axis.

spirit *n.* 1. espíritu, alma; 2. solución alcohólica de una sustancia volátil.

spiritual healing *n.* cura mental, cura espiritual.

spirochetal *a.* espiroquetósico-a, rel. a espiroquetas.

spirochete *n.* espiroqueta, microorganismo espiral de la especie *Spirochaetales* que incluye el microorganismo causante de la sífilis.

spirometer *n.* espirómetro, instrumento que se usa para medir la cantidad de aire que se inhala y la que se expele del pulmón.

spirometry *n.* espirometría, medida de la capacidad respiratoria tomada por medio de un espirómetro.

spit *n.* saliva, escupo; *vi.* escupir, expectorar.

spittle *n.* saliva; expectoración; salivazo, escupitazo.

splanchnic *a.* esplácnico-a, rel. a las vísceras o que llega a éstas; ___ **nerves** / nervios ___ -s.

spleen *n.* bazo, órgano vascular linfático, situado en la cavidad abdominal; **accesory** ___ / ___ accesorio.

splenectomy *n.* esplenectomía, excisión del bazo.

splenic *a.* esplénico-a, rel. al bazo.

splenoportography *n.* esplenoportografía, radiografía de las venas esplénica y cava usando un medio de contraste radioopaco inyectado en el bazo.

splenorenal *a.* esplenorrenal, rel. al bazo y al riñón.

splenorenal shunt *n.* derivación esplenorrenal, anastomosis de la vena o arteria esplénica a la vena renal esp. en el tratamiento de la hipertensión portal.

splint *n.* férula, tablilla, soporte de madera, metal, plástico, vidrio de fibra o yeso usado para dar apoyo, inmovilizar un hueso fracturado o proteger una parte del cuerpo.

splinter *n.* espina; esquirla; astilla.

split *n.* división, desunión; abertura; *v.* dividir, desunir, separar; dividirse, separarse.

splitting *n.* fragmentación; desdoblamiento.

spoil *v.* echar a perder.

spoken *v. pp.* of **to speak,** hablado.

spoken language *n.* lenguaje hablado.

spondylitis *n.* espondilitis, infl. de una o más vértebras; **ankylosing** ___ / anquilosante, reumatoide.

spondylolisthesis *n.* espondilolistesis, desplazamiento anterior de una vértebra sobre otra, gen. la cuarta lumbar sobre la quinta o ésta sobre el sacro.

spondylolysis *n.* espondilólisis, disolución o destrucción de una vértebra.

spondylopathy *n.* espondilopatía, cualquier enfermedad que afecta las vértebras.

spondylosis *n.* espondilosis. 1. anquilosis vertebral; 2. toda lesión degenerativa de la columna vertebral.

sponge *n.* esponja; *v.* esponjar, remojar con una esponja.

spongy *a.* esponjoso-a; poroso-a.

spontaneous *a.* espontáneo-a.

spoon *n.* cuchara.

spoonful *n.* cucharada.

sporadic *a.* esporádico-a, infrecuente.

spore *n.* espora, célula reproductiva unicelular.

sporicide *n.* esporicida, agente que destruye esporas.

sport *n.* deporte; ___ **-s medicine** / medicina del deporte.

spot *n.* mancha, marca, pápula; **blind** ___ / punto ciego; **liver** ___ / ___ hepática; *v.* [*stain*] manchar; [*notice*] notar.

spotting *n.* manchas de flujo vaginal sanguinolento.

spouse *n.* esposo-a.

sprain *n.* torcedura, esguince, torsión de una articulación con distensión y laceración parcial de los ligamentos; *v.* torcer; torcerse; **to** ___ **one's ankle** / ___ el tobillo.

spray *n.* atomizador de líquido para rociar; *v.* rociar con un líquido.

spread *n.* extensión, diseminación, esparcimiento; *a.* extendido-a, esparcido-a; diseminado-a; *vi.* diseminar; esparcir, extender; diseminarse, esparcirse, extenderse.

sprue *n.* esprue, enfermedad digestiva crónica caracterizada por la inhabilidad de absorber alimentos que contienen gluten.

spur *n.* espolón, protuberancia esp. de un hueso; **calcaneal** ___ / ___ calcáneo.

spurious *a.* espurio-a, falso-a.

sputum *n.* esputo, flema; **bloody** ___ / ___ sanguinolento.

squamous *a.* escamoso-a; ___ **cell** / célula ___ .

square *n.* cuadrado; *a.* cuadrado-a; correcto-a, justo, -a.

squash *n*. calabaza; *v*. aplastar; estrujar.

squat *v*. agacharse; sentarse en cuclillas; acuclillarse.

squeak *n*. chirrido; *v*. chirriar, rechinar.

squeal *n*. chillido, alarido; *v*. chillar.

squeeze *v*. apretar, comprimir; [*cloth, fruit*] exprimir.

squint *n*. estrabismo; acción de encoger los ojos como protección contra una luz intensa, o para tratar de ver mejor. V. **strabismus.**

stab *n*. puñalada; *v*. apuñalar, acuchillar.

stability *n*. estabilidad, permanencia, seguridad.

stabilization *n*. estabilización, acto de hacer algo estable.

stabilize *v*. estabilizar, evitar cambios o fluctuaciones.

stabilizer *n*. estabilizador, agente que estabiliza.

stable *a*. estable, que no fluctúa.

staff *n*. personal de una institución.

stage *n*. [*sickness*] estadío, etapa o período de transición durante el desarrollo de una enfermedad; fase; **in a recuperating ___** / en una fase de recuperación.

stagger *v*. escalonar, saltear, distribuir con una secuencia; vacilar; tambalear; tambalearse.

staging *n*. estadificación, clasificación de la extensión y gravedad durante el proceso de una enfermedad.

stagnation *n*. estancación, estancamiento, falta de circulación en los líquidos.

stain *n*. 1. colorante, tinte; 2. mancha, mácula.

staining *n*. coloración, tintura.

stalk *n*. tallo, estructura alargada que se asemeja al tallo de una planta.

stammer *n*. tartamudeo, balbuceo; *v*. tartamudear, balbucear.

stand *n*. sitio, puesto, situación; *vi*. ponerse o estar de pie; sostenerse; **___ on your toes** / pararse en la punta de los pies; **to ___ back** / retroceder; **to ___ still** / no moverse, estarse quieto-a.

standalone *n*. estandona, droga esteroide anabólica.

standard *n*. estándar, norma, criterio, pauta a seguir; lo normal, lo usual o común; **___ deviation** / desviación **___**; **___ error** / error **___**; **___ of care** / atención o cuidado **___**; **___ procedure** / procedimiento **___**, procedimiento usual establecido.

standardization *n*. estandarización, uniformidad; normalización.

standing *n*. [*position*] de pie; [*pending*] vigente; **___ orders** / órdenes o reglamento vigente.

standstill *n*. paro, cese de actividad.

stapedectomy *n*. excisión del estribo para mejorar la audición.

stapes *n*. estribo, el más interno de los huesecillos del oído.

staphylococcal *a*. estafilocócico-a, rel. a o causado por estafilococos; **___ food poisoning** / intoxicación alimenticia por estafilococos; **___ infections** / infecciones **___** .

staphylococcemia *n*. estafilococemia, presencia de estafilococos en la sangre.

Staphylococcus *n*. *Gr*. estafilococo. 1. especie de bacteria gram-positiva que puede causar diferentes clases de infecciones; incluye parásitos que se alojan en la piel y las mucosas; 2. término aplicado a cualquier micrococo patológico.

staphylotoxin *n*. estafilotoxina, toxina producida por estafilococos.

staple *n*. presilla, grapa; *v*. presillar, engrapar.

star *n*. estrella.

starch *n*. almidón, fécula, elemento principal de los carbohidratos. *v*. almidonar.

starchy *a*. feculento-a; almidonado-a; **___ foods** / alimentos **___** -s, almidones que contienen carbohidratos.

stare *n*. mirada fija; *v*. mirar fijamente.

start *n*. comienzo, principio, inicio; *v*. empezar, comenzar, iniciar; hacer andar o funcionar un aparato; [*motor*] arrancar, poner en marcha.

starvation *n*. desnutrición, inanición, hambre, privación de alimentos.

starve *v*. pasar hambre, privar de alimentos.

stasis *n*. estasis, estancamiento de la circulación de un líquido tal como la sangre y la orina en una parte del cuerpo.

state *n*. estado, condición; **nutritional ___** / **___** nutricional.

station *n*. estación; **nursing ___** / puesto de enfermeras.

stationary *a*. estacionario-a, estacionado-a, que permanece en una posición fija.

statistics *n*. estadística.

stature *n*. estatura, altura.

status *n*. *L*. status, estado o condición; **___ asthmaticus** / **___** asmaticus, condición de un ataque de asma agudo; **___ epilepticus** / **___** epiléptico, serie de ataques sucesivos con pérdida del conocimiento.

stay *n*. estancia; **short ___** / **___** breve; *v*. permanecer; quedarse; **to ___ awake** / desvelarse; **to ___ in bed** / **___** en cama, guardar cama.

steam *n.* vapor.

stearine *n.* estearina, componente blanco y cristalino de las grasas.

steatorrhea *n.* esteatorrea, exceso de grasa en las heces fecales.

stellate *a.* estrellado-a, semejante a una estrella.

stem *n.* tallo, pedúnculo, estructura semejante al tallo de una planta; **brain** ___ / ___ encefálico; ___ **cell** / célula madre.

stenosed *a.* estenosado-a, rel. a una estenosis.

stenosis *n.* estenosis, estrechamiento o contracción anormal de un pasaje; **aortic** ___ / ___aórtica; **pyloric** ___ / ___ pilórica.

stenotic *a.* estenósico-a, producido por o caracterizado por estenosis.

step *n.* paso; [*stairs*] escalón, peldaño; ___ **by** ___ / paso a paso; *v.* **to___ down** / bajar; reducir; **to___ in** / entrar; intervenir; **to___ up** / subir; apurar, acelerar.

steppage *n.* estepaje, alteración en la marcha que resulta de la caída pendular del pie obligando a levantar la rodilla y flexionar el muslo sobre la pelvis.

stereoradiography *n.* estereorradiografía, radiografía tridimensional.

stereotaxis *n.* estereotaxia, técnica de localización de áreas cerebrales usada en procedimientos neurológicos.

stereotype *n.* estereotipo; cliché.

sterile *a.* estéril. 1. que no es fértil; 2. aséptico-a; que no contiene ni produce microorganismos.

sterility *n.* esterilidad, incapacidad de concebir o procrear.

sterilization *n.* esterilización. 1. procedimiento que impide la reproducción; 2. destrucción completa de microorganismos; **dry heat** ___ / ___por calor seco; **gas** ___ / ___ por gas; **vapor** ___ / ___ por vapor.

sterilize *v.* esterilizar.

sternal *a.* esternal, rel. al esternón; ___ **puncture** / punción ___ .

sternocostal *a.* esternocostal, rel. al esternón y las costillas.

steroid *n.* esteroide, compuesto orgánico complejo del cual se derivan varias hormonas como el estrógeno, la testosterona y la cortisona.

stertor *n.* estertor. rale.

stethoscope *n.* estetoscopio, instrumento médico usado en la auscultación.

stew *n.* guisado, cocido; *v.* guisar, cocer.

sticky *a.* pegajoso-a.

stiff *a.* tieso-a, rígido-a; ___ **neck** / cuello ___ .

stigma *n.* estigma, huella. 1. señal específica de una enfermedad; 2. marca o señal en el cuerpo.

still *a.* inmóvil, quieto-a, tranquilo-a.

stillbirth *n.* nacimiento sin vida.

stillborn *a.* mortinato-a, muerto-a al nacer.

Still's disease *n.* enfermedad de Still, artritis reumatoidea juvenil.

stimulant *n.* estimulante, agente que produce una reacción.

stimulate *v.* estimular; motivar; excitar.

stimulation *a.* estimulación; motivación.

stimulus *n.* (*pl.* **stimuli**) estímulo, cualquier agente o factor que produce una reacción; **conditioned** ___ / ___ condicionado; **subliminal** ___ / ___ sublimado.

sting *n.* picadura; **bee-** ___ / picadura de abeja; **wasp** ___ / ___ de avispa.

stink *n.* olor desagradable, mal olor.

stippling *n.* punteado, condición de apariencia con manchas.

stipulate *v.* negociar, estipular.

stir *n.* movimiento; excitación; *v.* revolver, agitar.

stirrup bone *n.* estribo.stapes.

stitch *n.* punto de sutura; *v.* dar puntos.

stock *n.* caldo.

stocking *n.* medias; **elastic** ___ / calceta, media elástica.

stocky *a.* robusto-a.

stoma *n.* estoma, abertura hecha por cirugía, esp. en la pared del abdomen.

stomach *n.* estómago, órgano en forma de saco que forma parte del tubo digestivo; **on an empty** ___ / en ayunas; ___ **-ache** / dolor de ___; ___ **pump** / bomba estomacal; ___ **pumping** / lavado de ___; ___ **ulcer** / úlcera gástrica; *v. pop.* soportar, tolerar.

stomachal *a.* estomacal, rel. al estómago; ___ **tonic** / tónico ___ .

stomal *n.* estomal, rel. a un estoma.

stomatitis *n.* estomatitis, infl. de la mucosa de la boca; **aphthous** ___ / ___ aftosa.

stone *n.* piedra, cálculo.

stool *n.* heces fecales, excremento; ___ **fat** / grasa fecal; ___ **softener** / copro-emoliente.

stop *n.* parada, alto, interrupción; *v.* detener, parar, interrumpir; **to make a** ___ / hacer alto, hacer una parada; detenerse, pararse.

stoppage *n.* bloqueo; obstrucción; taponamiento.

storm *n.* tormenta; intensificación repentina de síntomas de una enfermedad.

strabismus *n.* estrabismo, alineamiento anormal de los ojos debido a una deficiencia muscular; *pop.* bizquera.

straight *a.* derecho-a, recto-a; estirado-a, erguido-a.

straightjacket *n.* camisa de fuerza.

strain *n.* esfuerzo, torcedura, sprain; [*inherited trait*] rasgo, cepa; *v.* forzar; **to ___ a muscle** / torcer un músculo; [*filter*] colar, pasar; esforzarse demasiado; **to ___ the eyes** / forzar la vista.

strainer *n.* colador, coladera.

strand *n.* filamento, hilo; fibra delicada.

strange *a.* extraño-a, raro-a; extranjero-a; no relacionado-a con un organismo o situado-a fuera del mismo.

strangle *v.* estrangular.

strangulated *n.* estrangulado-a; constreñido-a; **___ hernia** / hernia ___ .

strangulation *n.* estrangulación. 1. asfixia o sofocación gen. causada por obstrucción de las vías aéreas; 2. constricción de un órgano o estructura debida a compresión.

strap *n.* faja, banda, correa, tira; *v.* poner una faja; amarrar, atar.

stratification *n.* estratificación, formación en capas.

stratified *a.* estratificado-a, colocado-a en capas; **___ epithelium** / epitelio ___ .

stratum *n.* estrato; capa.

strawberry *n.* fresa; **___ mark** / marca en forma de ___ .

stream *n.* chorro, flujo, corriente.

strength *n.* fuerza, vigor, resistencia.

strep throat *n.* infección y dolor de garganta causados por un estreptococo.

streptococcal *a.* estreptocócico-a, rel. a estreptococos; **___ infections** / infecciones ___ -s.

streptococcemia *n.* estreptococemia, infección de la sangre debida a la presencia de estreptococos.

streptococcus *n.* estreptococo, género de microorganismo de la tribu *Streptococceae*, bacterias gram-positivas que se agrupan en pares o cadenas y que causan enfermedades serias.

streptomycin *n.* estreptomicina, antibiótico que se usa contra infecciones bacterianas.

stress *n.* estrés, tensión emocional, compulsión. 1. factor químico, físico o emocional que provoca un cambio como respuesta inmediata o demorada en las funciones del cuerpo o en sus partes; **___ test** / prueba de esfuerzo; 2. *gr.* énfasis, acento tónico.

stretch *n.* tirón, estirón, esfuerzo; *v.* extender, alargar, estirar; **to ___ forth, to ___ out** / estirarse, extenderse, alargarse; **___ receptor** / receptor de estiramiento.

stretcher *n.* camilla, andas; dilatador, extendedor.

stretching *n.* dilatación, estiramiento.

stria *n.* lista, fibra.

striated *a.* estriado-a, enlistado-a; **___ muscle** / músculo ___ .

stricken *a.* afectado-a súbitamente; afligido-a.

strict *a.* estricto-a; exacto-a.

stricture *n.* estrechez, estrechamiento, constricción.

stridor *n.* stridor, estridor, ruido sordo respiratorio.

strike *n.* golpe, ataque repentino; *vi.* golpear, atacar súbitamente.

string *n.* cuerda, cordel.

string bean *n.* habichuela verde.

stroke *n.* 1. embolia cerebral, apoplejía; ataque súbito; 2. choque, golpe.

stroking *n.* acto de frotar suavemente.

stroma *n.* estroma, armazón de tejido que sirve de soporte a un órgano.

strong *a.* fuerte, fornido-a, robusto-a; **___ -minded** / determinado-a, decidido-a.

strontium *n.* estroncio, elemento químico con propiedades parecidas a las del calcio que se emplea como tónico gástrico y antiséptico.

structural *a.* estructural, rel. a la estructura de un órgano.

structure *n.* estructura; orden.

struggle *n.* lucha, esfuerzo; *v.* luchar, esforzarse.

struma *n. L.* estruma, engrosamiento de la tiroides; *pop.* bocio.

strychnine *n.* estricnina, alcaloide cristalino muy venenoso.

stubborn *a.* obstinado-a, testarudo-a, caprichoso-a; *v.* **to be ___** / obstinarse, encapricharse.

student *n.* estudiante; **medical ___** / ___ de medicina.

study *n.* estudio; **double-blind ___ -ies** / ___ -s de doble incógnita, de doble desconocimiento; *v.* estudiar.

stuff *n.* material, elemento; *v.* embutir, llenar, empaquetar; **to ___ oneself** / hartarse.

stump *n.* muñón, parte que queda de una extremidad amputada.

stun *v.* aturdir, pasmar.

stupid *n.* estúpido-a, imbécil.

stupidity *n.* estupidez.

stupor *n.* estupor, letargo.

sturdy *a.* fuerte, vigoroso-a.

stutter *v.* tartamudear.

stuttering *n.* tartamudeo.

sty *n.* orzuelo, condición inflamatoria de las glándulas sebáceas del párpado.

styloid *a.* estiloide, de forma larga y puntiaguda.

subacromial *a.* subacromial, rel. al acromión o localizado debajo de éste.

subacute *a.* subagudo-a, rel. a una condición que no es ni aguda ni crónica.

subarachnoid *a.* subaracnoideo-a, que ocurre debajo de la membrana aracnoidea o de posición inferior a ésta; ___ **hemorrhage** / hemorragia ___; ___ **space** / espacio ___ .

subatomic *a.* subatómico-a, menor que un átomo.

subcapsular *n.* subcapsular, situado debajo de una cápsula.

subclavian, subclavicular *a.* subclavicular, localizado debajo de la clavícula; ___ **artery** / arteria ___; ___ **steal syndrome** / síndrome del secuestro ___; ___ **vein** / vena ___ .

subclinical *a.* subclínico-a, sin manifestación clínica.

subconscious *n.* subconsciente, subconsciencia, estado durante el cual los procesos mentales que afectan el pensamiento los sentimientos y la conducta ocurren sin que la persona esté consciente de ello; *a.* rel. a. la zona mental en la que la persona no se encuentra totalmente consciente.

subcostal *a.* subcostal, debajo de las costillas.

subculture *n.* subcultivo, cultivo de bacterias que se deriva de otro.

subcutaneous *a.* subcutáneo-a, debajo de la piel.

subdivide *v.* subdividir.

subdue *a.* sumiso-a, dominado-a, subyugado-a; *v.* dominar, subyugar.

subdural *a.* subdural, situado debajo de la dura madre; ___ **hematoma** / hematoma ___; ___ **hemorrhage** / hemorragia ___; ___ **space** / espacio ___ .

subhepatic *a.* subhepático-a, situado debajo del hígado.

subinvolution *n.* subinvolución, involución incompleta; ___ **of uterus** / ___ del útero.

subject *n.* sujeto. 1. término usado en referencia al paciente; 2. tópico; 3. *gr.* sujeto del verbo.

subjective *a.* subjectivo-a; ___ **symptoms** / síntomas ___ -s.

sublethal dose *a.* dosis subletal, cantidad insuficiente de una sustancia para causar la muerte.

sublimate *n.* sublimado, sustancia adquirida por sublimación; *v.* sublimar, depurar.

sublimation *n.* sublimación. 1. cambio de un estado sólido a vapor; 2. término freudiano que se refiere al proceso de transferir un impulso o deseo instintivo a una conducta aceptada socialmente.

sublingual *a.* sublingual, situado-a debajo de la lengua; ___ **gland** / glándula ___ .

subluxation *a.* subluxación, dislocación incompleta.

submandibular *a.* submandibular, debajo de la mandíbula.

submental *a.* submental, debajo del mentón.

submerge *v.* sumergir, colocar debajo de un líquido.

submission *n.* sumisión, sometimiento.

submit *v.* someter; someterse.

submucosa *n.* submucosa, capa de tejido celular situado debajo de una mucosa.

subnormal *a.* subnormal, menos que el promedio normal.

subphrenic *a.* subfrénico-a, situado-a debajo del diafragma; ___ **abscess** / absceso ___ .;

subscapular *a.* subescapular, debajo de la escápula.

subscription *n.* subscripción, parte de la receta médica que da instrucciones para la preparación de un medicamento.

subside *v.* menguar, apaciguar, bajar, cesar.

subsist *v.* subsistir, sobrevivir.

substance *n.* sustancia, líquido; droga; ___ **ground** ___ / ___ fundamental; ___ **abuse** / abuso de drogas; ___ **dependence** / dependencia de drogas; ___ **withdrawal syndrome** / síndrome de abstinencia de drogas.

substantive *n. gr.* substantivo, sustantivo, nombre.

substernal *a.* subesternal, debajo del esternón.

substitute *n.* sustituto-a; reemplazo; *v.* sustituir, reemplazar.

substitution *n.* substitución; ___ **therapy** / terapia por ___ .

substratum *n.* sustrato, fundación, base en la que vive un organismo.

substructure *n.* subestructura, soporte o material que sirve de base.

subtile, subtle *a.* sutil, delicado-a; inadvertido-a, desapercibido-a.

subungual *a.* subungual, debajo de una uña.

succeed *v.* tener éxito, salir bien; lograr.

success *n.* éxito, acierto, triunfo.

successful *a.* afortunado-a, de excelente resultado.

successive *a.* sucesivo-a, consecutivo-a.

succus *n. L.* succus, jugo.

such *a.* tal, semejante; **in** ___ **manner** / en ___ forma.

suck *v.* chupar, [*mother's milk*] mamar; **to ___ out** / chupar sacando; vaciar, extraer.

sucrose *n.* sucrosa, sacarosa que se obtiene de la caña de azúcar o la remolacha.

suction *n.* succión, aspiración; **___ device** / dispositivo de ___ .

sudamen *n.* sudamina, erupción cutánea no inflamatoria que presenta vesículas blanquecinas llenas de líquido acuoso y que se manifiestan después de una sudación copiosa o una enfermedad febril.

sudden *a.* súbito-a, imprevisto-a, repentino-a; **___ death** / muerte ___ .

sudden infant death syndrome *n.* síndrome de muerte infantil súbita, muerte súbita de un bebé menor de un año de edad cuya causa permanece desconocida.

sudor *n.* sudor, secreción de las glándulas sudoríparas.

sudorific *a.* sudorífico-a, que promueve el sudor.

sudoriparous *a.* sudoríparo-a, que secreta sudor; **___ gland** / glándula ___ .

sue *v.* demandar, poner pleito.

suffer *v.* sufrir, padecer; **to ___ from** / padecer de.

suffering *n.* sufrimiento, padecimiento.

sufficient *a.* suficiente; **-ly** *adv.* suficientemente.

suffix *n. gr.* sufijo.

suffocate *v.* sofocar, asfixiar; faltar la respiración.

suffocation *n.* asfixia, paro de la respiración.

suffusion *n.* sufusión, infiltración de un líquido del cuerpo en los tejidos circundantes.

sugar *n.* azúcar, carbohidrato que consiste esencialmente de sucrosa; **beet ___, cane ___** / sucrosa; **fruit ___** / fructosa; **grape ___** / glucosa; **milk ___** / lactosa.

suggest *v.* sugerir, indicar, aconsejar.

suggestion *n.* sugerencia, consejo, indicación; sugestión.

suggestive *a.* sugestivo-a, rel. a la sugestión o que sugiere.

suicidal *a.* suicida, rel. al suicidio o con tendencia al mismo.

suicide *n.* suicidio; suicidarse; **attempted ___** / tentativa o intento de ___ .

sulciform *a.* sulciforme, en forma de surco.

sulcus *n. L.* (*pl.* **sulci**) sulcus, depresión leve, sisura.

sulfa drugs *n.* sulfa, medicamentos del grupo sulfonamida, antibacterianos.

sulfacetamide *n.* sulfacetamida, sulfonamida antibacteriana.

sulfate *n.* sulfato, sal de ácido sulfúrico.

sulfonamides *n., pl.* sulfonamidas, grupo de compuestos orgánicos sulfuro-bacteriostáticos.

sulfur *n.* azufre, sulfuro.

sulfuric *a.* sulfúrico-a, rel. al sulfuro.

sullen *a.* malhumorado-a; resentido-a.

summary *n.* sumario, historia clínica del paciente; **___ of hospital records** / sumario del expediente.

summation *n.* suma total, acción o efecto acumulativo.

sun *n.* sol; **___ -bathing** / baño de ___; **___ -burn** / quemadura de ___, eritema solar; **___ -burnt** / quemado-a, tostado-a por el sol; **___ exposure** / estar expuesto-a al ___; *v.* **to ___ -bathe** / tomar el ___ .

sunscreen *n.* bloqueador de sol, sustancia que bloquea los rayos solares.

sunspot *n.* mancha de sol.

sunstroke *n.* insolación.

superb *a.* magnífico-a, superior.

super ego *n. L.* el yo, término freudiano que se refiere a la parte de la psique que concierne a los valores sociales, morales y éticos.

superfecundation *n.* superfecundación, fertilización sucesiva de dos óvulos que pertenecen al mismo ciclo menstrual en dos actos sexuales distintos.

superfemale *n.* superhembra, organismo femenino que tiene más del número necesario de cromosomas que determinan el sexo.

superfetation *n.* superfetación, fecundación de dos óvulos en el mismo útero en un intervalo de tiempo corto aunque correspondientes a dos períodos menstruales diferentes.

superficial *a.* superficial, rel. a la superficie; **-ly** *adv.* superficialmente.

superinfection *n.* superinfección, infección subsecuente producida gen. por un microorganismo diferente que ocurre durante el curso de una infección presente.

superior *n.* superior, más alto; [*position*] hacia arriba; al exterior.

superiority complex *n.* complejo de superioridad.

supernatural *a.* sobrenatural.

supernumerary *a.* supernumerario-a, en número mayor que el normal.

superolateral *a.* superolateral, en posición superior y lateral.

supersaturate *v.* supersaturar, saturar excesivamente, añadir una sustancia en una cantidad mayor de la que puede ser disuelta normalmente por un líquido.

supersaturated *a.* supersaturado-a.

supersensitiveness *n.* supersensibilidad, hipersensibilidad.

supersonic *a.* supersónico-a, ultrasónico, rel. a ondas de frecuencia demasiado alta para ser captadas por el oído humano.

superstition *n.* superstición.

superstitious *a.* supersticioso-a.

supervise *v.* supervisar, dirigir.

supervisor *n.* supervisor-a, jefe-a.

supine *a.* supino-a, de posición acostada de espalda, boca arriba y con la palma de la mano hacia arriba.

supper *n.* cena, la comida.

supplant *v.* reemplazar, substituir.

supplement *n.* suplemento; *v.* complementar.

supplemental *a.* suplemental, adicional.

supply *n.* abastecimiento; **supplies** / provisiones; *v.* proveer, surtir, abastecer.

support *n.* soporte, sostén.

suppose *v.* suponer.

suppository *n.* supositorio, medicamento semisólido que se inserta en una cavidad natural del cuerpo (vagina, recto).

suppression *n.* supresión. 1. fallo súbito del cuerpo en la producción de una excreción o secreción normal; 2. en psicoanálisis, la inhibición de una idea o deseo.

suppurate *v.* supurar, excretar.

suppuration *n.* supuración, formación o salida de pus.

suppurative *a.* supurativo-a, rel. a la supuración.

supraclavicular *a.* supraclavicular, situado-a encima de la clavícula.

supraglottic *a.* supraglótico-a, situado encima de la glotis.

suprapubic *a.* suprapúbico-a, localizado-a encima del pubis; ___ **catheter** / catéter ___; ___ **cystostomy** / cistostomía ___ .

supratentorial *a.* supratentorial, que ocurre encima del tentorio.

sural *a.* sural, rel. a la pantorrilla.

sure *a.* seguro-a, decidido-a; positivo-a.

surface *n.* superficie; porción o límite exterior de una estructura; ___ **tension** / tensión superficial.

surfactant *n.* surfactante, agente tensoactivo que modifica la tensión superficial de un líquido.

surgeon *n.* cirujano-a.

surgery *n.* cirugía, rama de la medicina que comprende procesos operatorios de reparación, diagnosis de enfermedades y corrección de estructuras del cuerpo. See chart on this page.

Surgery	Cirugía
ambulatory	ambulatoria
arthroscopic	artroscópica
cardiothoracic	cardiotorácica
cosmetic	cosmética
cytoreductive	citorreductiva
conservative	conservadora
corrective	correctiva
endoscopic	endoscópica
excisional	de excisión
exploratory	exploratoria
major	mayor
minor	menor
orthopedic	ortopédica
oral	oral
plastic	plástica
radical	radical
reconstructive	reconstructiva
sustenance	de sustentación, sustento

surgical *a.* quirúrgico-a; ___ **dressing** / vendaje ___ protector; ___ **equipment** / equipo ___; ___ **flaps** / colgajos ___ -s; ___ **incision** / incisión ___; ___ **instruments** / instrumentos ___ -s; ___ **mesh** / malla ___; ___ **resident** / residente de cirugía.

surname *n.* apellido, nombre de familia.

surpass *v.* sobrepasar, exceder.

surplus *n. a.* sobrante, excedente.

surprise *n.* sorpresa.

surrogate *a.* subrogado-a, que sustituye algo o a alguien; *v.* subrogar, sustituir.

surveillance *n.* vigilancia.

survey *n.* encuesta; cuestionario.

survival *n.* supervivencia.

survive *v.* sobrevivir.

survivor *n.* sobreviviente.

survivorship *n.* supervivencia; anualidad, renta o pensión anual.

susceptibility *n.* susceptibilidad.

susceptible *a.* susceptible.

suspect *a.* sospechoso-a.

suspend *v.* suspender, cancelar.

suspicion *n.* sospecha.

sustain *v.* sostener, mantener; [*a wound*] sufrir una herida.

sustained *a.* sostenido-a; ininterrumpido-a; sufrido-a.

sustenance *n.* sustentación, sustento.

suture *n.* sutura; puntada; línea de unión; **absorbable surgical** ___ / ___ absorbible quirúrgica; **bolster** ___ / ___ compuesta; **catgut** ___ / ___ de catgut; **near and far** ___ / ___ de aposición o aproximación; **purse-string** ___ / ___ en bolsa de tabaco; **uninterrupted continuous** ___ / ___ continua, de peletero; **vertical mattress** ___ / ___ de colchonero.

swab *n.* escobillón; *v.* limpiar, fregar.

swaddling band *n.* fajero.

swallow *n.* trago; deglución; *v.* tragar, deglutir.

swallowing *n.* deglución.

Swan-Ganz catheter *n.* catéter de Swan-Ganz, sonda flexible que contiene un balón cerca de la punta y que se emplea para medir la presión sanguínea en la arteria pulmonar.

swaying *n.* vaivén, movimiento acompasado.

sweat *n.* sudor, secreción de las glándulas sudoríparas; **cold** ___ / ___ -es fríos; **night** ___ -s / ___ -es nocturnos; *v.* sudar; hacer sudar.

sweated *a. pp.* of **to sweat**, sudoriento-a; sudoroso-a.

sweat glands *n., pl.* glándulas sudoríparas.

sweating *n.* sudor, perspiración, transpiración.

sweaty *a.* sudado-a, sudoroso-a.

sweep *vi.* barrer; recoger; limpiar.

sweet *a.* dulce, azucarado-a; [*tempered*] dulce, agradable, gentil.

sweet basil *n.* albahaca.

sweeten *v.* endulzar, azucarar.

sweetener *n.* dulcificante.

sweets *n., pl.* golosinas, dulces.

swell *vi.* hinchar, abultar, entumecer, agrandar; hincharse, entumecerse, agrandarse.

swelling *n.* hinchazón; tumefacción; *pop.* bulto, chichón.

swift *a.* ligero-a; fácil, sin complicación; **a** ___ **operation** / una operación fácil, sin complicaciones.

swim *vi.* nadar.

swimmer *n.* nadador-a; ___ **'s ear** / otitis del ___ .

switch *n.* [*instrumento*] cambio; conector eléctrico; *v.* cambiar; **to** ___ **off** / desconectar; cambiar; **to** ___ **on** / conectar.

swollen *a. pp.* of **to swell**, hinchado-a.

swoon *n.* desmayo, síncope; *v.* desfallecer; desmayarse, desvanecerse.

Sydenham's chorea *n.* Sydenham, corea de; tipo de corea menor o reumática, gen. vista en la infancia causada por una infección estreptococa, y que en su comienzo se manifiesta con contracciones musculares de la cara y brazos.

syllable *n. gr.* sílaba.

Sylvian aqueduct *n.* acueducto de Silvius, conducto estrecho que conecta los ventrículos cerebrales tercero y cuarto.

symbiosis *n.* simbiosis, unión estrecha de dos organismos que pertenecen a especies diferentes.

symbiotic *a.* simbiótico-a, rel. a la simbiosis.

symbol *n.* símbolo, representación o señal que sustituye o representa en la práctica otra cosa o idea.

symbolism *n.* simbolismo. 1. uso de símbolos en la práctica para dar una representación a las cosas; 2. anormalidad mental por la cual el paciente percibe todos los sucesos y cosas como reflejos de sus propios pensamientos.

symmetrical *a.* simétrico-a.

symmetry *n.* simetría, correspondencia perfecta entre partes de un cuerpo colocadas en posición opuesta a un centro o axis.

sympathectomy *n.* simpatectomía, extirpación de una porción del simpático.

sympathetic *a.* simpático-a, rel. al sistema nervioso simpático.

sympathetic nervous system *n.* sistema nervioso simpático, abastecedor de los músculos involuntarios, formado por nervios motores y sensoriales.

sympatholytic *a.* simpatolítico-a, que ofrece resistencia a la actividad producida por la estimulación del sistema nervioso simpático.

sympathomimetic *a.* simpatomimético-a, que puede causar cambios fisiológicos similares a los causados por el sistema nervioso simpático.

sympathy *n.* simpatía, asociación, relación. 1. afinidad; 2. relación entre dos órganos afines por la cual una anomalía en uno afecta al otro; 3. afinidad entre la mente y el cuerpo que causa que se afecten entre sí.

symphysis *n.* sínfisis, articulación en la cual las superficies óseas adyacentes se unen por un fibrocartílago; **pubic** ___ / ___ púbica.

symptom *n.* síntoma, manifestación o indicio de una enfermedad según se percibe por el paciente; **constitutional** ___ / ___ constitucional; **delayed** ___ / ___ demorado; **objective** ___ / ___ objetivo; **pathognomic** ___ / ___ patognómico; **presenting** ___ / ___ presente; **prodromal** ___ / ___ prodrómico; **withdrawal** ___ / ___ de supresión.

S

symptomatic *a.* sintomático-a, de la naturaleza de un síntoma o rel. a éste.

symptomatology *n.* sintomatología, conjunto de síntomas que se refieren a una enfermedad o a un caso determinado.

symptomatolytic *a.* sintomatolítico, que elimina los síntomas.

symptom complex *n.* complejo de síntomas concurrentes que caracterizan una enfermedad.

synapse *n.* sinapsis, punto de contacto entre dos neuronas donde el impulso que pasa por la primera neurona origina un impulso en la segunda.

synapsis *n.* sinapsis, aparejamiento de cromosomas homólogos al comienzo de la meiosis.

synaptic *a.* sináptico-a, rel. a la sinapsis.

synarthrosis *n.* sinartrosis, articulación inmóvil en la cual los elementos óseos están fusionados.

syncanthus *n.* sincanto, adhesión del globo ocular a los tejidos de la órbita.

syncheira *n.* sinqueiria, condición por la cual una excitación aplicada a una parte del cuerpo es referida a otra parte.

synchondrosis *n.* sincondrosis, articulación inmóvil de superficies unidas por tejido cartilaginoso.

synchysis *n.* sinquisis, estado de fluidez del humor vítreo; ___ **scintillans** / ___ centelleante.

synclonus *n.* sinclono, espasmo o temblor de varios músculos a la vez.

syncopal *a.* sincopal, rel. a un síncope.

syncope *n.* síncope, desmayo o pérdida temporal del conocimiento; **anginal** ___ / ___ anginoso; **deglutition** ___ / ___ de deglución; **cardiac** ___ / ___ cardíaco; **convulsive** ___ / ___ convulsivo; **hysterical** ___ / ___ histérico; **laryngeal** ___ / ___ laríngeo.

syncytial *a.* sincitial, rel. a un sincitio o que lo constituye.

syncytium *n.* sincitio, masa protoplasmática nucleada que resulta de la fusión celular.

syndactylism *n.* sindactilia, anomalía congénita que consiste en la fusión de dos o más dedos de la mano o los pies.

syndesmitis *n.* sindesmitis. 1. infl. de uno o más ligamentos; 2. infl. de la conjuntiva.

syndesmoma *n.* sindesmoma, tumor del tejido conjuntivo.

syndrome *n.* síndrome, síntomas y señales que caracterizan una enfermedad; **acquired immune deficiency** ___ / ___ de inmunodeficiencia adquirida; **adipose** ___ / ___ adiposo; **adrenogenital** ___ / ___ suprarrenogenital; **battered children** ___ / ___ de niños maltratados; **congenital rubella** ___ / ___ congénito de rubéola; **dumping** ___ / ___ de vaciamiento gástrico rápido; **hepatorenal** ___ / ___ hepatorrenal; **irritable bowel** ___ / ___ de intestino irritado, irritable; **malabsorption** ___ / ___ de malabsorción gastrointestinal; **middle lobe** ___ / ___ del lóbulo medio del pulmón; **nephrotic** ___ / ___ nefrótico; **respiratory stress** ___ / ___ de dificultad respiratoria; **scalded skin** ___ / ___ de escaldadura, quemadura de la epidermis; **sick sinus** ___ / ___ del seno carotídeo; **subclavian steal** ___ / ___ del secuestro subclavicular; **sudden death** ___ / ___ de muerte súbita; **multiple transfusion** ___ / ___ de transfusión múltiple; **premenstrual** ___ / ___ premenstrual; **toxic shock** ___ / ___ de choque tóxico, envenenamiento de la sangre causado por estafilococos; **withdrawal** ___ / ___ de privación.

synechia *n.* sinequia, unión o adherencia anormal de tejidos u órganos esp. referente al iris, al cristalino y a la córnea.

synergic *n.* sinérgico-a, que posee la propiedad de actuar en cooperación.

synergism *n.* sinergismo, correlación o unión armoniosa entre dos o más estructuras o sustancias.

synostosis *n.* sinostosis, unión ósea entre dos huesos adyacentes; **senile** ___ / ___ senil; **tribacillary** ___ / ___ tribacilar.

synovia *n.* sinovia, líquido que lubrica las articulaciones y los tendones.

synovial *a.* sinovial, rel. a la membrana sinovial; ___ **bursa** / bursa ___; ___ **cyst** / quiste ___ .

synovial fluid *n.* líquido sinovial, líquido viscoso transparente.

synovioma *n.* sinovioma, tumor que se origina en una membrana sinovial.

synovitis *n.* sinovitis, infl. de la membrana sinovial; **dry** ___ / ___ seca; **purulent** ___ / ___ purulenta; **serous** ___ / ___ serosa.

synovium *n.* membrana sinovial.

synthesis *n.* síntesis, composición de un todo por la unión de las partes.

synthesize *v.* sintetizar, producir síntesis.

synthetic *a.* sintético-a, rel. a una síntesis o producido por ésta.

syntonic *a.* sintónico-a, rel. a un tipo de personalidad estable que se adapta normalmente al ambiente.

syphilis *n.* sífilis, enfermedad venérea contagiosa que se manifiesta en lesiones cutáneas, usu. transmitida por contacto directo.

syphilitic *n. a.* sifilítico-a, rel. a la sífilis o causado por ella; ___ **macula** / mácula ___ .

syphilology *n.* sifilología, rama de la medicina que se dedica al tratamiento y diagnosis de la sífilis.

syphiloma *n.* tumor sifilítico.

syringe *n.* jeringa, jeringuilla; **disposable** ___ / ___ desechable; **glass cylinder** ___ / ___ con tubo de cristal; **hypodermic** ___ / ___ hipodérmica.

syringobulbia *n.* siringobulbia, presencia de cavidades en la médula oblongata.

syringocele *n.* siringocele. 1. conducto central de la médula espinal; 2. meningomielocele que contiene una cavidad en la médula espinal ectópica.

syringomyelia *n.* siringomielia, enfermedad crónica progresiva de la columna vertebral caracterizada por cavidades llenas de líquido en la región cervical y que a veces se extiende a la médula oblongata.

syrinx *n. Gr.* (*pl.* **syringes**) syrinx. 1. fístula; 2. tubo o conducto.

syrup *n.* jarabe, almíbar.

systaltic *a.* sistáltico-a, que alterna contracciones y dilataciones.

system *n.* sistema, grupo de partes u órganos combinados que constituyen un conjunto que desempeña una o más funciones vitales en el organismo; **cardiovascular** ___ / ___ cardiovascular; **digestive** ___ / ___ digestivo; **endocrine** ___ / ___ endocrino; **genitourinary** ___ / ___ genitourinario; **hematopoietic** ___ / ___ hematopoyético; **immune** ___ / ___ de inmunidad; **lymphatic** ___ / ___ linfático; **nervous** ___ / ___ nervioso; **osseous** ___ / ___ óseo; **portal** ___ / ___ portal; **reproductive** ___ / ___ reproductiós; **respiratory** ___ / ___ respiratorio; **reticuloendothelial** ___ / ___ reticuloendotelial.

systematic *a.* sistemático-a, que se ajusta a un régimen o sistema.

systematization *n.* sistematización, acción de seguir un sistema.

systematize *n.* sistematizar, hacer una síntesis.

systemic *a.* sistémico-a; que afecta el cuerpo en general; ___ **circulation** / circulación ___ ; ___ **disease** / enfermedad diseminada.

systole *n.* sístole, contracción del corazón esp. de los ventrículos; **atrial** ___ / ___ auricular; **premature** ___ / ___ prematura; **ventricular** ___ / ___ ventricular;

systolic *a.* sistólico-a, rel. a la sístole; ___ **murmur** / soplo___ ; ___ **pressure** / presión ___ .

t

T *abbr.* **absolute temperature** / temperatura absoluta; **T+, increased tension** / tensión aumentada; **T-, diminished tension** / tensión disminuida.

tabacism *n.* tabaquismo, intoxicación aguda o crónica causada por una excesiva inhalación de polvo de tabaco.

tabardillo *n. pop.* nombre dado al tifus y la fiebre tifoidea en México y otros países de América Latina.

tabes *n.* tabes, deterioro progresivo del organismo o de una parte del mismo debido a una enfermedad crónica.

tabetic *a.* tabético-a, rel. a tabes o que padece de éste.

table *n.* tabla. 1. capa o lámina ósea; 2. mesa; **examination** ___ / ___ de reconocimiento; **operating** ___ / ___ de operaciones; 3. tabla, colección de datos o de referencia con una variante determinada.

tablespoon *n.* cuchara; _____ -ful / cucharada; Apéndice C.

tablet *n.* tableta, comprimido, dosis en un compuesto sólido; **enteric coated** ___ / ___ de capa entérica.

taboo, tabu *n.* tabú, prohibición; *a.* prohibido-a.

tabular *a.* tabular, dispuesto en forma de tabla o cuadro.

tabulate *v.* tabular, hacer tablas o listas.

tache *n.* tacha, mancha, peca; imperfección.

tachyarrythmia *n.* taquiarritmia, forma de arritmia acompañada de pulso rápido.

tachycardia *n.* taquicardia, aceleración de la actividad cardíaca, gen. a una frecuencia de más de 100 por minuto en una persona adulta; **atrial** ___ / ___ auricular; **ectopic** ___ / ___ ectópica; **en salves** ___ / ___ en salves; **exophthalmic** ___ / ___ exoftálmica; **fetal** ___ / ___ fetal; **paroxysmal atrial** ___ / ___ auricular paroxística; **reflex** ___ / ___ refleja; **sinus** ___ / ___ sinusal; **supraventricular** ___ / ___ supraventricular; **ventricular** ___ / ___ ventricular.

tachyphagia *n.* taquifagia, hábito de hablar muy rápido.

tachypnea *n.* taquipnea, respiración rápida.

tact *n.* tacto; diplomacia, discreción.

tactful *a.* discreto-a.

tactic *n.* táctica.

tactile *a.* táctil, palpable; rel. al sentido del tacto; ___ **discrimination** / discriminación ___; ___ **system** / sistema ___ .

tactless *a.* indiscreto-a.

taenia, tenia *n.* tenia, parásito de la clase *Cestoda* que en la etapa adulta vive en el intestino de los vertebrados.

tag *n.* [*label*] etiqueta.

tail *n.* [*appendage*] cola, rabo.

taint *n.* [*stain*] mancha, mácula; *v.* manchar, podrirse o causar putrefacción; corromperse.

take *vi.* [*to get*] tomar; [*to seize*] coger, agarrar; [*to carry something, to take someone*] llevar; [*to remove*] quitar; **to be taken ill** / enfermarse; **to** ___ **notes** / anotar; **to** ___ **a trip** / viajar; **to** ___ **a walk** / dar un paseo.

talar *a.* talar, rel. al tobillo.

talc *n.* talco.

talcum *n.* polvo.

tale *n.* [*story*] cuento; [*gossip*] *pop.* chisme.

talent *n.* talento, habilidad.

talk *n.* charla, plática; *v.* charlar, hablar, platicar.

tall *a.* alto-a; elevado-a.

talon *n.* talón, parte posterior de un diente molar.

talotibial *a.* talotibial, rel. al talón y la tibia.

talus *n.* (*pl.* **tali**) talón, astrágalo, tubillo.

tambour *n.* tambor. 1. tímpano del oído medio; 2. instrumento de precisión que se usa para registrar y transmitir movimientos ligeros tales como las contracciones peristálticas.

tampon *n.* tapón, gasa o algodón prensado que se aplica o inserta en la vagina u otra cavidad para absorber secreciones.

tamponade *n. Fr.* taponamiento, aplicación de tapones a una herida o cavidad para detener una hemorragia o absorber secreciones; **balloon** ___ / ___ por balón insuflable; **cardiac** ___ / ___ cardíaco, compresión aguda del corazón causada por un exceso de sangre acumulada en el pericardio.

tangible *a.* tangible.

tangle *n.* enredo, confusión; *v.* enredarse; confundirse.

tangled *a.* enredado-a; confundido-a.

tangy *a.* [*smell*] fuerte, penetrante.

tantrum *n.* rabieta; *pop.* berrinche, pataleta.

tap *n.* punción, perforación; acto de perforar un tejido con un instrumento afilado; **bloody** ___ / ___ lumbar hemática; **spinal** ___ / ___ lumbar; *v.* tocar ligeramente; punzar, perforar, hacer una punción; ___ **water** / agua corriente.

tape *n.* [*audiotape*] cinta magnética; [*adhesive*] esparadrapo; ___ **recorder** / grabadora.

tapeworm *n.* tenia, solitaria. taenia, tenia.

tapping *n.* 1. percusión; 2. extracción de fluido.

tarantula *n.* tarántula, araña negra venenosa.

tardive *Fr.* tardío, retardado-a, que tarda en aparecer.

target *n.* 1. [*area*] blanco; 2. objectivo de una investigación; 3. célula "en diana" u órgano afectado por un agente definido (droga u hormona).

tarsal *a.* tarsal, tarsiano-a. 1. rel. al tarso; 2. rel. al tejido conectivo que soporta el párpado del ojo.

tarsal bones *n., pl.* huesos del tarso.

tarsometatarsal *a.* tarsometatarsiano-a, rel. al tarso y al metatarso.

tarsus *n.* tarso, parte posterior del pie situada entre los huesos de la pierna y los huesos metatarsianos.

tart *a.* agrio-a, ácido-a.

task *n.* tarea, labor, trabajo.

taste *n.* gusto; **in good** ___ / de buen ___; ___ **buds** / papilas gustativas; *v.* probar, saborear.

tasteful *a.* gustoso-a, sabroso-a.

tasteless *a.* insípido-a, sin sabor.

tasty *a.* gustoso-a, apetitoso-a, sabroso-a.

tattooing *n.* tatuaje, diseño con colorantes permanentes en la epidermis.

taught *pret. pp.* of **to teach**, enseñado.

tax *n.* impuesto, contribución; *a.* ___ **-exempt** / exento de impuesto; *v.* imponer; cargar, abrumar.

taxis *L.* taxis. 1. manipulación o reducción de una parte u órgano para llevarlo a la posición normal; 2. reflejo direccional del movimiento de un organismo en respuesta a un estímulo.

T cell regulator *n.* célula T reguladora, dirige otras células del sistema inmune a hacer otras funciones especiales cuyo objetivo es el ataque al SIDA.

T cells *n., pl.* linfocitos T, linfocitos diferenciados en el timo que dirigen la respuesta inmunológica y que asisten a los linfocitos B a responder a antígenos; **helper** ___ / ___ inductores, ayudantes, estimulantes de la producción de anticuerpos formados por células que se derivan del linfocito B; **cytotoxic** ___ / ___ citotóxicos, destructores de células extrañas al cuerpo (como en el caso de órganos transplantados); **suppressor** ___ / ___ supresores de la producción de anticuerpos formados por células que se derivan del linfocito B.

T8 cell cytotoxic *n.* célula T8 citotóxica, lleva a cabo las funciones de destrucción de antígenos, ataque y eliminación de células infectadas por virus, parásitos y hongos.

T8 cell suppressor *n.* célula T8 supresora, grupo de células cuya función es de inhibir la respuesta inmune.

tea *n.* té.

teach *vi.* enseñar.

team *n.* equipo; grupo asociado; *v.* **to** ___ **up** / asociarse en cooperación.

teamwork *n.* esfuerzo coordinado; trabajo en coordinación.

tear *n.* lágrima; desgarramiento, desgarro; ___ **gas** / gas lacrimógeno; *vi.* rasgar, desgarrar, romper; **to shed** ___ **-s** / lagrimear, llorar; **to** ___ **off** / arrancar.

tear duct *n.* conducto lacrimal.

tearful *a.* lagrimoso-a.

tearing *n.* lagrimeo.

tease *v.* rasgar, separar un tejido o espécimen con agujas para examinarlo bajo el microscopio.

teaspoon *n.* cucharita; ___ **-ful** / cucharadita.

teat *n.* tetilla. 1. glándula mamaria; 2. pezón.

technetium 99m *n.* technecio 99m., radioisótopo que emite rayos gamma, de uso frecuente en medicina nuclear.

technician *n.* técnico-a, persona entrenada en la administración de tratamientos o pruebas de laboratorio y que gen. actúa bajo la supervisión de un facultativo; **dental** ___ / ___ dental; **electrocardiographic** ___ / ___ electrocardiógrafo-a; **emergency medical** ___ / ___ de emergencia; **medical laboratory** ___ / laboratorista; **radiologic** ___ / ___ radiólogo-a; **respiratory therapy** ___ / ___ de terapia respiratoria.

technique *n.* técnica, método o procedimiento.

technologist *n.* tecnólogo-a, persona experta en tecnología.

technology *n.* tecnología, ciencia que trata de la aplicación de procedimientos técnicos.

tectorium *L.* tectorium, membrana que cubre el órgano de Corti.

tectum *L.* (pl. tectum) estructura en forma de techo.

tedious *a.* tedioso-a, aburrido-a, engorroso-a.

teenage *n.* adolescencia.

teenager *n.* jovencito-a de trece a diecinueve años de edad.

teeth *n., pl.* dientes; **deciduous** ___ / ___ de leche o primera dentición; **permanent** ___ / ___ permanentes; **secondary** ___ / ___ secundarios; **wisdom** ___ / ___ cordales; *pop.* muelas del juicio.

teething *n.* dentición.

tegument *n.* tegumento, la piel.

telangiectasia *n.* telangiectasia, telangiectasis, condición causada por dilatación de los vasos capilares y arteriolas que puede formar un angioma.

telecardiophone *n.* telecardiófono, instrumento que permite escuchar los latidos del corazón.

telemedicine *n.* telemedicina, uso de la televisión como medio de asistencia en el cuidado de la salud.

telemetry *n.* telemetría, información transmitida electrónicamente a distancia.

telencephalon *n.* telencéfalo, porción anterior del encéfalo.

teleopsy *n.* teleopsia, desorden visual por el cual los objetos parecen estar más lejos de lo que están en realidad.

telepathy *n.* telepatía, comunicación aparente de pensamientos de una persona a otra por medios extrasensoriales.

telephone *n.* teléfono; ___ **call** / llamada telefónica; *v.* telefonear, llamar por teléfono.

teleradiography *n.* telerradiografía, rayos-x tomados a dos o más metros de distancia del objectivo para disminuir distorsiones.

television *n.* televisión; ___ **set** / televisor;

tell *vi.* decir; relatar, contar.

telophase *n.* telofase, fase final de un proceso.

temper *n.* carácter, disposición; temple, humor; genio; *v.* **to have bad** ___ / tener mal ___; **to have good** ___ / tener buen ___ .

temperament *n.* temperamento, combinación de la constitución física, mental y emocional de una persona que la distingue de otras.

temperate *a.* moderado-a; sobrio-a, abstemio-a.

temperature *n.* temperatura. 1. grado de calor o frío según se mide en una escala específica; 2. calor natural de un cuerpo vivo; 3. fiebre o calentura; **absolute** ___ / ___ absoluta; **ambient** ___ / ___ ambiental; **axillary** ___ / ___ axilar; **body** ___ / ___ del cuerpo; **critical** ___ / ___ crítica; **maximum** ___ / ___ máxima; **minimum** ___ / ___ mínima; **normal** ___ / ___ normal; **oral** ___ / ___ oral; **rectal** ___ / ___ rectal; **subnormal** ___ / ___ subnormal.

tempest *n.* tempestad, tormenta.

template *n.* patrón, molde.

temple *n.* sien, superficie lisa a cada lado de la parte lateral de la cabeza.

temporal *a.* temporal. 1. rel. a la sien; ___ **bone** / hueso ___; ___ **lobe** / lóbulo ___; 2. rel. al tiempo.

temporary *a.* temporal; pasajero-a; [*transition period*] interino-a; transitorio-a.

temporomandibular joint *n.* articulación temporomaxilar, rel. a la articulación entre la mandíbula y el hueso temporal.

tempting *a.* tentador-a; atractivo-a.

tenacious *a.* tenaz, persistente; determinado-a.

tend *v.* cuidar, atender; vigilar.

tendency *n.* tendencia.

tender *a.* sensitivo-a al tacto o la palpación; ___ **points** / puntos neurálgicos; [*soft*] blando-a, tierno-a

tenderness *n.* blandura; delicadeza. 1. sensibilidad, condición sensible al tacto o palpación; 2. ternura.

tendinitis, tendonitis *n.* tendinitis, tendonitis, infl. de un tendón.

tendinous *a.* tendinoso-a, rel. a o semejante a un tendón.

tendon *n.* tendón, tejido fibroso que sirve de unión a los músculos y los huesos y a otras partes; **deep** ___ **reflexes** / reflejos profundos de los ___ -es; ___ **jerk** / tirón tendinoso; ___ **reflex** / reflejo tendinoso.

tenesmus *n.* tenesmo, condición dolorosa e ineficaz al orinar o defecar.

tennis elbow *n.* codo de tenista.

tenosynovitis *n.* tenosinovitis, infl. de la vaina que cubre un tendón.

tense *a.* tenso-a, rígido-a, tirante, en estado de tensión.

tenseness *n.* tensión.

tension *n.* tensión. 1. acto o efecto de estirarse o ser extendido; 2. grado de estiramiento; 3. sobreesfuerzo mental, emocional o físico; **premenstrual** ___ / ___ premenstrual; 4. expansión de un gas o vapor; **surface** ___ / ___ superficial.

tension headache *n.* dolor de cabeza causado por una tensión nerviosa mental.

tensor *n.* tensor, músculo que estira o hace tensión.

tent *n.* tienda, cámara esp. para cubrir un espacio en el cual se incluye al paciente; **oxygen** ___ / ___ o cámara de oxígeno.

tentaculum *n.* tentáculo, tipo de gancho quirúrgico para sujetar o prensar una parte.

tentative *a.* tentativo-a, experimental, sujeto-a a cambios.

tentorial *a.* tentorial, rel. a un tentorium.

tentorium *L.* tentorium, estructura que se asemeja a una tienda.

tenuous *a.* tenue, delicado-a.

tepid *a.* tibio-a.

teratogen *n.* teratógeno, agente que causa teratogénesis.

teratogenesis *a.* teratogénesis, producción de anomalías severas en el feto.

teratoid *a.* teratoide. 1. semejante a un monstruo; 2. que proviene de un embrión malformado; ___ **tumor** / tumor ___ .

teratology *n.* teratología, estudio de malformaciones en el feto.

teratoma *n.* teratoma, neoplasma que deriva de más de una capa embrionaria y por lo tanto se compone de tejidos de distintas clases.

teres *L.* teres, término empleado para describir ciertos tipos de músculos o ligamentos alargados y cilíndricos.

term *n.* término. 1. período de tiempo de duración efectiva o limitada tal como en el embarazo; 2. vocablo.

terminal *a.* terminal, final.

terminal illness *n.* enfermedad maligna que causa la muerte.

terminate *v.* terminar, acabar.

termination *n.* terminación.

terminology *n.* terminología, nomenclatura.

ternary *a.* ternario-a, que se compone de tres elementos.

terrible *a.* terrible.

terror *n.* terror, pánico.

tertian *a.* terciano-a, que se repite cada tercer día; ___ **fever** / fiebre ___ .

tertiary syphillis *n.* sífilis terciaria, el estado más avanzado de la sífilis.

test *n.* prueba; examen; análisis; **antinuclear antibody** ___ / ___ antinuclear de anticuerpo; **creatinine clearance** ___ / ___ de aclaramiento de creatinina; **endurance** ___ / ___ de resistencia; **fat stool** ___ / ___ de grasa fecal; **follow-up** ___ / ___ subsecuente; **glucose tolerance** ___ / ___ de tolerancia a la glucosa; **liver function** ___ / ___ de función hepática; **outcome of** ___ / resultado de la ___; **pregnancy** ___ / ___ del embarazo; **random** ___ / ___ de control sin método; **respiratory function** ___ / ___ de función respiratoria; **skin** ___ / ___ cutánea; **scratch** ___ / ___ de rasguño, ___ de alergia; **screening** ___ / ___ eliminatoria; **single-blind** ___ / ___ de ciego simple; **stress** ___ / ___ de esfuerzo; ___ **double-blind** / ___ de doble incógnita; ___ **tube** / tubo de ensayo; ___ **type** / ___ de tipo, prueba visual de letras; **thyroid function** ___ / ___ de función

tiroidea; **timed** ___ / ___ de tiempo limitado o medido; **treadmill** ___ / ___ de esfuerzo; **visual** ___ / ___visual; **visual field** ___ / ___ visual de campimetría.

testament *n.* testamento.

tester *n.* probador, ensayador.

testicle *n.* testículo, una de las dos glándulas reproductivas masculinas que produce espermatozoos y la hormona testosterona; **ectopic** ___ / ___ ectópico; **undescended** ___ / ___ no descendido.

testicular *a.* testicular, rel. al testículo;___ **examination** / examen ___ ; ___**tumors** / tumores ___ -es.

testify *v.* declarar, testificar.

testis *n.* *L.* (*pl.* **testes**) testis, testículo.

testosterone *n.* testosterona, hormona producida en el testis estimulante del desarrollo de algunas características masculinas secundarias tales como el vello facial y la voz grave; ___ **implant** / implante de ___ .

test-tube baby *n.* fertilización *in vitro*, embarazo en probeta o que resulta de un óvulo fecundado fuera de la madre en el laboratorio y reimplantado en el útero.

tetanic *a.* tetánico-a, rel. al tétano; ___ **antitoxin** / antitoxina ___; ___ **convulsion** / convulsión ___; ___ **toxoid** / toxoide ___ .

tetanus, lockjaw *n.* tétano, enfermedad infecciosa aguda causada por el bacilo del tétano gen. introducido a través de una lesión y que se manifiesta con espasmos musculares y rigidez gradual de la mandíbula, el cuello y el abdomen.

tetany *n.* tetania, afección neuromuscular que se manifiesta con espasmos intermitentes de los músculos voluntarios asociada con deficiencia paratiroidea y disminución del balance de calcio.

tetracycline *n.* tetraciclina, antibiótico de espectro amplio usado para combatir microorganismos gram-positivos y gram-negativos, ricketsia y cierta variedad de virus.

tetrad *n.* tétrada, grupo de cuatro elementos similares.

tetralogy *n.* tetralogía, término aplicado a una combinación de cuatro factores o elementos.

tetraplegia *n.* tetraplejía, parálisis de las cuatro extremidades.

tetraploid *n.* tetraploide, que posee cuatro grupos de cromosomas.

tetravalent *n.* tetravalente, que posee una valencia química igual a cuatro.

texture *n.* textura, composición de la estructura de un tejido.

thalamic *a.* talámico-a, rel. al tálamo.

thalamus *n.* tálamo, una de las dos estructuras formadas por masas de materia gris que se encuentran en la base del cerebro y que constituyen el centro principal por donde los impulsos sensoriales pasan a la corteza cerebral.

thalassemia *n.* talasemia, grupo de diferentes tipos de anemia hemolítica hereditaria encontrada en poblaciones de la región mediterránea y sureste de Asia; **major** ___ / ___ mayor; **minor** ___ / ___ menor.

thalassophobia *n.* talasofobia, miedo mórbido al mar.

thalassotherapy *n.* talasoterapia, tratamiento de una enfermedad por medio de baños de mar o exposición al aire marino.

thalidomide *n.* talidomida, sedativo e hipnótico, causante probado de malformaciones en niños de madres que tomaron la droga durante el embarazo.

thallitoxicosis *n.* talitoxicosis, envenenamiento incidental de ingestión de sulfato de talio usado en pesticidas.

than *conj.* que; *comp.* que.

thanatology *n.* tanatología, rama de la medicina que trata de la muerte en todos sus aspectos.

thanatomania *n.* tanatomanía, manía suicida o de asesinato.

thanatometer *n.* tanatómetro, instrumento usado para determinar cuando una muerte ocurrió midiendo la temperatura interna del cuerpo.

thank *v.* dar gracias; agradecer.

thankful *a.* agradecido-a.

thanks *n., pl.* gracias; agradecimiento, gratitud.

thaw *n.* deshielo, descongelación; *v.* descongelar, deshelar, derretir.

theca *n.* teca, envoltura o capa que actúa esp. como protectora de un órgano.

thecoma *n.* tecoma, tumor ovárico gen. benigno.

thenar *a.* tenar, rel. a la palma de la mano; ___ **eminence** / eminencia ___; ___ **muscles** / músculos ___ -es.

theoretical *a.* teórico-a, rel. a una teoría.

theory *n.* teoría. 1. conocimientos relacionados con un tema sin verificación práctica de los mismos; 2. especulación u opinión que no ha sido probada científicamente.

therapeutic *a.* terapéutico-a. 1. que tiene propiedades curativas; 2. rel. a la terapéutica; ___ **indications** / indicaciones ___ -s; ___**plasma exchange** / intercambio ___ de plasma.

therapeutics *n.* terapéutica, rama de la medicina que estudia tratamientos y curaciones.

therapist *n.* terapeuta, persona experta en una o más áreas de aplicación de tratamientos en el campo de la salud; **physical** ___ / ___ físico; **speech** ___ / finiatra, logopeda.

therapy *n.* terapia, terapéutica, tratamiento de una enfermedad; **adjuvant** ___ / ___ adjunta; **anticoagulant** ___ / ___ anticoagulante; **behavioral** ___ / ___ de conducta; **biologic** ___ / ___ biológica; **by substitution** ___ / ___ substitutiva; **diathermic** ___ / ___ diatérmica; **electroshock** ___ / electrochoque; **group** ___ / ___ de grupo; **inhalation** ___ / ___ por inhalación; **immune suppressive** ___ / ___ inmunosupresiva; **non-specific** ___ / ___ inespecífica; **occupational** ___ / ___ ocupacional; **oxygen** ___ / ___ de oxígeno; **radiation** ___ / ___ por radiación; **respiratory** ___ / ___ respiratoria; **supportive** ___ / ___ de apoyo; **systemic** ___ / ___ sistémica.

thermal, thermic *a.* termal, térmico-a, rel. al calor o producido por éste.

thermistor *n.* termistor, tipo de termómetro para medir cambios mínimos en la temperatura.

thermocoagulation *n.* termocoagulación, coagulación de tejidos por medio de corrientes de alta frecuencia.

thermodynamics *n.* termodinámica, ciencia que trata de la relación entre el calor y otras formas de energía.

thermograph *n.* termógrafo, detector infrarrojo que registra variaciones de la temperatura corporal según reacciona a los cambios de la circulación sanguínea.

thermography *n.* termografía, registro obtenido con un termógrafo.

thermometer *n.* termómetro, instrumento usado para medir el grado de calor o frío; **Celsius** ___ / ___ de Celsius o centígrado; **clinical** ___ / ___ clínico; **Fahrenheit** ___ / ___ de Fahrenheit; **rectal** ___ / ___ rectal; **self-recording** ___ / ___ de registro automático.

thermonuclear *a.* termonuclear, rel. a reacciones termonucleares.

thermoregulation *n.* termorregulación, regulación del calor o de la temperatura; termotaxis.

thermos *n.* termo.

thermostat *n.* termostato, instrumento regulador de temperaturas.

thermosterilization *n.* termoesterilización, esterilización por medio del calor.

thermotaxis *n.* termotaxis. 1. mantenimiento de la temperatura del cuerpo; 2. reacción de un organismo al estímulo del calor.

thermotheraphy *n.* termoterapia, uso terapéutico del calor.

thesis *n.* (*pl.* **theses**) tesis; postulado.

thick *a.* grueso-a; macizo-a; [*liquid*] espeso-a.

thicken *v.* engrosar, espesar; condensar.

thickness *n.* espesor, densidad; consistencia.

thigh *n.* muslo, porción de la extremidad inferior entre la cadera y la rodilla; ___ **bone** / fémur.

thin *a.* delgado-a, flaco-a; [*liquid*] aguado-a, aclarado-a; [*light*] ligero-a.

thing *n.* cosa, objeto.

think *vi.* pensar; [*believe*] creer; **to** ___ **it over** / pensarlo bien; **to** ___ **nothing of** / tener en poco; **to** ___ **through** / considerar; **to** ___ **well of** / tener buena opinión de.

thinner *n.* solvente, diluyente.

third degree burn *n.* quemadura de tercer grado.

thirst *n.* sed.

thirsty *a.* sediento-a; *v.* **to be** ___ / tener sed.

thoracentesis *n.* toracentesis, punción y drenaje quirúrgicos de la cavidad torácica.

thoracic *a.* torácico-a, rel. al tórax; ___ **cage** / caja o pared ___; ___ **cavity** / cavidad ___; ___ **duct** / conducto ___; ___ **injuries** / traumatismos ___ -s; ___ **neoplasms** / neoplasmas ___ -s.

thoracicoabdominal *a.* toracicoabdominal, rel. al tórax y al abdomen.

thoracolumbar *a.* toracolumbar, rel. a las vértebras torácicas y lumbares.

thoracoplasty *n.* toracoplastia, cirugía plástica del tórax por medio de excisión de costillas para provocar la caída de un pulmón afectado.

thoracostomy *n.* toracostomía, incisión en la pared del tórax usando la abertura como drenaje.

thoracotomy *n.* toracotomía, incisión de la pared torácica.

thorax *n.* tórax, el pecho.

thorough *a.* completo-a, minucioso-a, acabado-a; **-ly** *adv.* completamente, minuciosamente, a fondo.

thought *n.* pensamiento, concepto, idea; *a. pp.* of **to think,** pensado.

thoughtful *n.* atento, solícito-a, esmerado-a.

thread *n.* hilo; fibra, filamento; línea fina. 1. material de sutura; 2. cualquier filamento fino semejante a un hilo; *v.* enhebrar, ensartar; ___ **-like** / hiliforme, fibroso-a, filamentoso-a.

threat *n.* amenaza.

threaten *v.* amenazar.

threatened abortion *n.* amenaza de aborto.

threshold *n.* umbral. 1. grado mínimo necesario de un estímulo para producir un efecto; 2. dosis mínima que puede producir un efecto; **absolute** ___ / ___ absoluto; **auditory** ___ / ___ auditivo; **renal** ___ / ___ renal; **sensory** ___ / ___ sensorio; ___**dose** / dosis mínima; ___**of consciousness** / ___ de la consciencia.

thrill *n.* "thrill", estremecimiento, vibración o ruido especial que se siente por palpación; **aneurysmal** ___ / ___ aneurismal; **aortic** ___ / ___ aórtico; **arterial** ___ / ___ arterial; **diastolic** ___ / ___ diastólico; **presystolic** ___ / ___ presistólico; **systolic** ___ / ___ sistólico; *v.* emocionar, excitar; *v.* emocionarse, excitarse.

thrive *v.* prosperar, progresar.

throat *n.* garganta, área que incluye la faringe y la laringe; ___ **swab** / muestra faríngea.

throat culture *n.* muestra de cultivo del mucus extraído de la garganta y detección en el laboratorio de la presencia o no de agentes infecciosos en el mismo.

throb *n.* latido, pulsación, palpitación; *v.* latir, palpitar, pulsar.

throbbing *a.* palpitante.

thrombectomy *n.* trombectomía, extracción de un trombo.

thrombin *n.* trombina, enzima presente en la sangre extravasada que cataliza en la conversión de fibrinógeno en fibrina.

thrombinogen *n.* trombinógeno. V. **prothrombin.**

thrombin time *n.* tiempo de trombina, espacio de tiempo necesario para que se forme un coágulo de fibrina después de añadirle trombina al plasma citrado.

thromboangiitis *n.* tromboangiitis, infl. de un vaso sanguíneo con trombosis; trombosis de un vaso sanguíneo.

thrombocyte *n.* trombocito, plaqueta.

thrombocytopenia *n.* trombocitopenia, disminución anormal del número de las plaquetas sanguíneas.

thrombocytopenic *a.* trombocitopénico-a, rel. a la trombocitopenia.

thrombocytosis *n.* trombocitosis, aumento excesivo de plaquetas en la sangre.

thromboembolism *n.* tromboembolia, obstrucción de un vaso sanguíneo por un coágulo desprendido del lugar de origen.

thrombogenesis *n.* trombogénesis, formación de cóagulos o trombos.

thrombolysis *n.* trombólisis, lisis o disolución de un coágulo.

thrombolytic *a.* trombolítico-a, rel. a un trombo o que causa la disolución de éste.

thrombophlebitis *n.* tromboflebitis, dilatación de la pared de una vena asociada con trombosis.

thrombophlebitis migrans *n.* tromboflebitis migratoria, tromboflebitis de progreso lento de una vena a otra.

thrombosed *a.* trombosado-a, rel. a un vaso sanguíneo que contiene un trombo.

thrombosis *n.* trombosis, formación, desarrollo y presencia de un trombo; **biliary** ___ / ___ biliar; **cardiac** ___ / ___ cardíaca; **coronary** ___ / ___ coronaria; **embolic** ___ / ___ embólica; **traumatic** ___ / ___ traumática; **venous** ___ / ___venosa.

thrombotic *a.* trombótico-a, rel. a la trombosis o que padece de ella.

thrombus *n.* (*pl.* **thrombi**) trombo, coágulo que causa una obstrucción vascular parcial o total.

throw *vi.* tirar; arrojar.

thrush *n.* muguet, afta, infección fungosa de la mucosa oral que se manifiesta con placas blancas en la cavidad bucal y la garganta.

thumb *n.* dedo pulgar; ___ **sucking** / chuparse el dedo gordo.

thumbnail *n.* uña del pulgar.

thymectomy *n.* timectomía, extirpación del timo.

thymic *a.* tímico-a, rel. al timo.

thymocyte *n.* timocito, linfocito que se origina en el timo.

thymoma *n.* timoma, tumor que se origina en el timo.

thymus *n.* timo, glándula situada en la parte inferior del cuello y anterosuperior de la cavidad torácica que desempeña un papel de importancia en la función inmunológica.

thyroglobulin *n.* tiroglobulina. 1. iodina que contiene glicoproteína secretada por la tiroides; 2. sustancia que se obtiene de tiroides porcinas y se administra como suplemento en el tratamiento de hipertiroidismo.

thyroglossal *a.* tirogloso-a, rel. a la tiroides y a la lengua.

thyroid *n.* glándula tiroides, una de las glándulas endocrinas situadas delante de la tráquea y constituída por dos lóbulos laterales conectados en el centro; ___ **function tests** / pruebas del funcionamiento de la ___; *a.* tiroideo-a, rel. a la tiroides; ___ **cartilage** / cartílago ___; ___

hormones / hormonas ___ -as; ___ **storm** / tormenta ___, crisis ___ .

thyroidectomy *n.* tiroidectomía, extirpación de la tiroides.

thyroidism *n.* tiroidismo, condición por exceso de secreción tiroidea.

thyroiditis *n.* tiroiditis, infl. de la tiroides.

thyroid-stimulating hormone *n.* hormona estimulante de la secreción tiroidea. V. **thyrotropin.**

thyromegaly *n.* tiromegalia, agrandamiento de la tiroides.

thyroparathyroidectomy *n.* tiroparatiroidectomía, excisión de la tiroides y la paratiroides.

thyrotoxicosis *n.* tirotoxicosis, trastorno causado por hipertiroidismo que se manifiesta con agrandamiento de la tiroides, aumento en el metabolismo, taquicardia, pulso rápido e hipertensión.

thyrotropin *n.* tirotropina, hormona estimulante de la tiroides secretada por el lóbulo anterior de la pituitaria; ___ **releasing factor** / factor liberador de la ___; ___ **releasing hormone** / hormona estimulante de ___ .

thyroxine *n.* tiroxina, hormona producida por la tiroides que contiene yodo; se obtiene sintéticamente de la tiroides de animales y se usa en el tratamiento de hipotiroidismo.

tibia *n.* tibia, hueso triangular anterior de la pierna situado debajo de la rodilla.

tibial *a.* tibial, rel. a la tibia o localizado cerca de ella.

tic *n. Fr.* tic, espasmo súbito o involuntario de un músculo que ocurre esp. en la cara; **convulsive** ___ / ___ convulsivo; **coordinated** ___ / ___ coordinado; **douloureux** ___ / ___ doloroso; **facial** ___ / ___ facial.

tick *n.* garrapata, acárido chupador de sangre transmisor de enfermedades; ___ **bite** / picadura de ___ .

tickle *n.* cosquilleo; *v.* hacer cosquillas, cosquillear; sentir un cosquilleo.

tickling *n.* cosquilla.

tidal *a.* rel. al volumen de inspiración y expiración.

tidiness *n.* aseo, pulcritud; limpieza.

tidy *a.* aseado-a, pulcro-a; limpio-a.

tie *n.* ligadura, lazo; conexión *v.* amarrar, atar, enlazar; **to be tied up** / estar muy ocupado-a.

tight *a.* [*fitted*] apretado-a, ajustado-a; [*airtight*] hermético-a; tirante; **a** ___ **situation** / una situación grave; ___ **squeeze** / *pop.* aprieto; *v.* **to hold on** ___ / agarrarse bien.

tighten *v.* apretar, ajustar.

time *n.* tiempo, medida de duración; **a limited ___** / **___** limitado; **at the same ___** / a la vez; **at ___ s** / a veces; **At what ___?** / ¿A qué hora?; **behind ___** / atrasado-a; **bleeding ___** / **___** de sangramiento; **coagulation ___** / **___** de coagulación; **for some ___** / por algún ___; **for the ___ being** / por el momento, por ahora; **from ___to ___** / de vez en cuando; **in due ___** / a su debido ___; **on ___** / a tiempo; **perception ___** / **___** de percepción; **prothrombin ___** / **___** de protrombina; **___ exposure** / **___** de exposición; **___ frame** / espacio de ___; **___ lag** / **___** de latencia; **What ___ is it?** / ¿Qué hora es?; *v.* marcar, medir el tiempo; **to set the ___** / medir el tiempo.

timed *a. pp.* tiempo medido.

timely *a.* oportuno-a.

timer *n.* regulador de tiempo, minutero.

timid *a.* tímido-a.

tincture *n.* tintura, extracto de origen animal o vegetal que contiene alcohol.

tinea *L.* tinea, tiña, infección cutánea fungosa; **___ capital** / **___** capitis; **___ pedis** / **___** pedis; *pop.* pie de atleta; **___ versicolor** / **___**versicolor.

tingle *n.* hormigueo, comezón, sensación de picazón.

tinnitus *n.* zumbido, chasquido, sonido que se siente en el oído.

tint *n.* tinte, colorante; *v.* teñir, colorar, dar color.

tiny *a.* diminuto-a.

tip *n.* punta, extremo; [*light touch*] toque ligero.

tired *a.* cansado-a, fatigado-a.

tiredness *n.* cansancio, fatiga.

tireless *a.* incansable, infatigable.

tiresome *a.* pesado-a, tedioso-a.

tiring *a.* agotador-a, que cansa o fatiga.

tissue *n.* tejido, grupo de células similares de función determinada unidas por una sustancia intercelular que actúan conjuntamente. See chart on this page.

tissue typing *n.* tipificación, clasificación por tipo; tipificación de tejido.

titer, titre *n.* título, la cantidad de una sustancia que se requiere para producir una reacción con un volumen determinado de otra sustancia.

titrate *v.* titular, determinar por titulación.

titration *n.* titulación, determinación de volumen usando soluciones estandarizadas de valor conocido.

toadstool *n.* seta venenosa; hongo venenoso.

Tissue	Tejido
adipose	adiposo
bone, bony	óseo
cartilaginous	cartilaginoso
connective	conectivo
endothelial	endotelial
epithelial	epitelial
erectile	eréctil
fibrous	fibroso
fluid	intersticial
glandular	glandular
granulation	de granulación
lymphoid	linfoide
mesenchymal	mesenquimatoso
muscular	muscular
nervous	nervioso
scar	cicatrizante
subcutaneous	subcutáneo

toast *n.* tostada.

tobacco *n.* tabacco, planta americana de la *Nicotiana tabacum* cuyas hojas preparadas contienen nicotina, sustancia tóxica perjudicial a la salud; **___ smoke pollution** / contaminación por humo de ___; **___ use disorder** / trastorno por uso de ___ .

tocograph *n.* tocógrafo, instrumento para estimar la fuerza de las contracciones uterinas.

tocometer *n.* tocómetro. tocograph.

today *adv.* hoy.

toddler *n.* niño-a que comienza a caminar.

toe *n.* dedo del pie.

toe drop *n.* caída de los dedos del pie.

toe nail *n.* uña de un dedo del pie.

toilet *n.* 1. servicio, inodoro; 2. limpieza relacionada con un procedimiento médico o quirúrgico; **___ paper** / papel higiénico.

toilet training *n.* entrenamiento de los niños para controlar el acto de orinar y de defecar.

tolerable *a.* tolerable.

tolerance *n.* tolerancia, capacidad de soportar una sustancia o un ejercicio físico sin sufrir efectos dañinos, tal como el uso de una droga o una actividad física prolongada.

tolerant *a.* tolerante.

tolerate *v.* tolerar.

tomato *n.* tomate; **___ soup** / sopa de ___ .

tomogram *n.* tomograma, radiografía seccionada de una parte del cuerpo.

tomograph *n.* tomógrafo, máquina radiográfica que se usa para hacer una tomografía.

tomography *n.* tomografía, técnica de diagnóstico por la cual se hacen radiografías de un órgano por secciones del mismo a profundidades distintas; **computed __ / __** computada; **computerized axial __ / __** axial computarizada; **conventional __ / __** convencional; **dynamic computed __ / __** dinámica computada; **electron beam __ / __** con rayos de electrón; **high-resolution computed __ / __** computada de alta resolución; **nuclear magnetic resonance __ / __** de resonancia magnética nuclear; **positron emission __ / __** de emisión por positrón.

tomorrow *adv.* mañana; **day after __ /** pasado __ .

tone *n.* tono. 1. grado normal de vigor y tensión en el funcionamiento de los órganos y músculos de un cuerpo sano; **muscular __ / __** muscular; 2. cualidad definida de un sonido o voz.

tongue *n.* lengua; **black hairy __ / __** negra velluda, lengua infectada de hongos parásitos; **dry __ / __** seca; **geographic __ / __** geográfica; **red __ / __** roja o enrojecida; **sticky __ / __** pegajosa; **__ depressor /** depresor de __ .

tonic *n.* tónico, reconstituyente que restaura la vitalidad del organismo *a.* tónico-a. 1. que restaura el tono normal; 2. caracterizado-a por una tensión continua.

tonicity *a.* tonicidad, cualidad normal de tono o tensión.

tonight *adv.* esta noche.

tonoclonic *a.* tonoclónico-a, rel. a espasmos musculares que son tónicos y clónicos.

tonometer *n.* tonómetro, instrumento usado para medir la tensión o presión esp. intraocular.

tonometry *n.* tonometría, medida de la presión o tensión.

tonsil *n.* amígdala, tonsila; **cerebellar __ / __** cerebelosa; **lingual __ / __** lingual; **palatine __ / __** palatina; **pharyngeal __ / __** faríngea.

tonsillar *a.* tonsilar, rel. a una tonsila; **__ crypt /** cripta __ o amigdalina; **__ fossa /** fosa amigdalina.

tonsillectomy *n.* amigdalectomía, extirpación de las amígdalas.

tonsillitis *n.* amigdalitis, infl. de las amígdalas.

tonsilloadenoidectomy *n.* tonsiloadenoidectomía, extirpación de las adenoides y las amígdalas.

tonus *L.* tonus. V. **tone.**

too *adv.* además; también; asimismo; demasiado.

tooth *n.* (*pl.* **teeth**) diente; **impacted __ / __** impactado; **__ unerupted / __** no erupcionadom. See illustration on this page.

toothache *n.* dolor de muelas.

toothbrush *n.* cepillo de dientes.

toothpaste *n.* pasta de dientes, dentífrico.

tophaceous *a.* tofacio, rel. a un tofo o de naturaleza arenosa.

tophus *n.* tofo. 1. depósito de sal de ácido úrico en los tejidos, gen. visto en casos de gota; 2. cálculo dental.

topical *a.* tópico-a, rel. a un área localizada.

topographic anatomy *n.* anatomía topográfica.

torment *n.* tormento. *v.* **atormentar.**

torpid *a.* tórpido-a, torpe en los movimientos.

torpor *n.* embotamiento; estancamiento, inactividad física.

torque *n., Fr.* torque, fuerza rotatoria.

torsion *n.* torsión, rotación de una parte sobre su propio eje longitudinal; **ovarian __ / __** ovárica; **testicular __ / __** testicular.

torso *n.* torso, el tronco humano.

torticollis *n.* tortícolis, espasmo tonicoclónico de los músculos del cuello que causa torsión cervical e inmovilidad de la cabeza.

tortuous *a.* tortuoso-a; torcido-a; sinuoso-a.

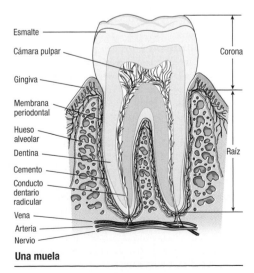

Esmalte

Cámara pulpar

Gingiva

Membrana periodontal

Hueso alveolar

Dentina

Cemento

Conducto dentario radicular

Vena

Arteria

Nervio

Corona

Raíz

Una muela

torture *n.* tortura, gran sufrimiento; castigo.

torus *n. L.* (*pl.* **tori**) torus, eminencia, protuberancia, abultamiento.

total *a.* total; completo-a; *v.* sumar, añadir.

totipotency *n.* totipotencia, habilidad de una célula de regenerarse o desarrollarse en otro tipo de célula.

totipotent *a.* totipotente, que puede generar totipotencia.

touch *n.* 1. sentido del tacto, percepción a través de la piel o de las membranas mucosas; 2. [*act of touching*] toque; *v.* tocar, palpar.

touch-up *n.* retoque.

tourniquet *n.* torniquete, dispositivo usado para aplicar presión sobre una arteria y contener la salida de la sangre.

towel *n.* toalla.

toxemia *n.* toxemia, condición tóxica provocada por la absorción de toxinas que provienen de un foco infeccioso.

toxic *a.* tóxico-a, venenoso-a, rel. a un veneno o de naturaleza venenosa.

toxicity *n.* toxicidad, cualidad de ser venenoso.

toxicological *a.* toxicológico-a, rel. a la toxicología.

toxicologist *n.* toxicólogo-a, especialista en toxicología.

toxicology *n.* toxicología, estudio de los venenos o sustancias tóxicas, los efectos que causan en el organismo y su tratamiento; ___ **screen** / protocolo toxicológico.

toxicosis *n.* toxicosis, estado morboso debido a un veneno.

toxin *n.* toxina, veneno, sustancia nociva de origen animal o vegetal; **bacterial** ___ / ___ bacteriana.

toxin-antitoxin *n.* toxina antitoxina, mezcla casi neutra de toxina diftérica y antitoxina que se usa en inmunizaciones contra la difteria.

toxoid *n.* toxoide, toxina desprovista de toxicidad que al introducirse en el organismo causa la formación de anticuerpos; *a.* toxoide, de naturaleza tóxica o venenosa; **diphtheria** ___ / ___ diftérico; **tetanus** ___ / ___ tetánico.

Toxoplasma *n. Toxoplasma*, género de parásito protozoario.

toxoplasmosis *n.* toxoplasmosis, infección causada por un microorganismo de la familia *Toxoplasma* que invade los tejidos, con síntomas leves de malestar o posible infl. de las glándulas linfáticas; puede ocasionar daños a la vista y al sistema nervioso central.

toy *n.* juguete.

trace *n.* rastro, vestigio. 1. cantidad diminuta de un elemento químico; 2. marca visible; *v.* trazar; rastrear, investigar.

tracer *n.* trazador, radioisótopo que al introducirse en el cuerpo crea un rastro que puede detectarse.

trachea *n.* tráquea, conducto respiratorio entre la parte extrema inferior de la laringe y el comienzo de los bronquios.

tracheal *a.* traqueal, rel. a la tráquea; ___ **stenosis** / estenosis ___ .

tracheitis *n.* traqueítis, infl. de la tráquea.

tracheoesophageal *a.* traqueoesofágico-a, rel. a la tráquea y al esófago.

tracheomalasia *n.* traqueomalasia. reblandecimiento de los cartílagos traqueales.

tracheostenosis *n.* traqueostenosis, estrechez de la tráquea.

tracheostomy *n.* traqueostomía, incisión en la tráquea para permitir el paso de aire en caso de obstrucción.

tracheotomy *n.* traqueotomía, incisión en la tráquea a través de la piel y los músculos del cuello.

trachoma *n.* tracoma, infección viral contagiosa de la conjuntiva y la córnea que se manifiesta con fotofobia, dolor, lagrimeo y, en casos severos, ceguera total.

tracing *n.* trazo, gráfica descriptiva que hace un instrumento al registrar un movimiento.

tract *n.* tracto, tubo, vía, vías, sistema alargado compuesto de tejidos y órganos que actúan coordinadamente para desempeñar una función; **alimentary** ___ / ___ alimenticio; **ascending** ___ / ___ ascendiente; **biliary** ___ / ___ biliar; **digestive** ___ / ___ digestivo; **genitourinary** ___ / ___ genitourinario; **olfactory** ___ / vía olfatoria; **pyramidal** ___ / ___ piramidal; **respiratory** ___ / ___ o vía respiratoria;

traction *n.* tracción. 1. acto de tirar o halar; 2. fuerza que tira con tensión; **cervical** ___ / ___ cervical; **lumbar** ___ / ___ lumbar.

tractor *n.* tractor, instrumento o máquina usada para aplicar tracción.

trademark *n.* marca registrada.

tragus *n.* (*pl.* **tragi**) trago, protuberancia triangular en la parte externa del oído.

train *v.* entrenar; entrenarse.

trained nurse *n.* enfermero-a graduado-a.

training *n.* entrenamiento; adiestramiento.

trait *n.* rasgo o característica; **acquired** ___ / ___ adquirido; **inherited** ___ / ___ heredado.

trance *n.* trance, condición semejante a un estado hipnótico que se caracteriza por la disminución de la actividad motora.

tranquil *a.* tranquilo-a, sereno-a.

tranquility *n.* tranquilidad, descanso.

tranquilizer *n.* tranquilizante, calmante.

transabdominal *a.* transabdominal, a través del abdomen o de la pared abdominal.

transaxial *a.* transaxial, a través del axis de una estructura o parte.

transcapillary *a.* transcapilar, que ocurre a través de las paredes de los capilares.

transcript *n.* expediente; copia.

transcutaneous *a.* transcutáneo-a, a través de la piel; ___ **electrical nerve stimulation** / estimulación eléctrica ___ de un nervio.

transducer *n.* transductor, dispositivo que convierte una forma de energía a otra.

transect *v.* cortar transversalmente.

transection *n.* corte transversal a través del eje largo de un órgano.

transfer *v.* transferir, cambiar.

transfer, transference *n.* transferencia. 1. reorientación que hace el paciente de sentimientos negativos o positivos (esp. reprimidos inconscientemente) hacia otra persona, esp. el psicoanalista; 2. transmisión de síntomas o fluidos de una parte a otra del cuerpo.

transferrin *n.* transferrina, globulina beta en el plasma de la sangre que fija y transporta el hierro.

transfixion *n.* transfixión, acto de atravesar y cortar al mismo tiempo los tejidos blandos de dentro hacia afuera como en la extirpación de tumores o en amputaciones.

transform *v.* transformar, cambiar la apariencia, carácter o estructura.

transformation *n.* transformación, cambio de forma o apariencia.

transfusion *n.* transfusión, acto de transferir un fluido a una vena o arteria; **blood** ___ / ___ de sangre; **direct** ___ / ___ directa; **exchange** ___ / exsanguino-transfusión; **indirect** ___ / ___ indirecta.

transillumination *n.* transiluminación, paso de luz a través de un cuerpo.

transitional *a.* transitorio-a, rel. a transición o cambio.

transitory *a.* transitorio-a, pasajero-a.

translate *v.* traducir.

translator *n.* traductor-a; intérprete.

translocation *n.* translocación, desplazamiento de un cromosoma o parte del mismo hacia otro cromosoma.

translucent *a.* translúcido-a, que deja pasar la luz.

transmigration *n.* transmigración, paso de un lugar a otro tal como las células sanguíneas en diapédesis.

transmissible *a.* transmisible, trasmisible, que puede transmitirse.

transmission *n.* transmisión, acto de transmitir o transferir tal como una enfermedad contagiosa o hereditaria; **droplet** ___ / ___ por instilación; **pathogen** ___ / ___ patógena; **placental** ___ / ___ placentaria; ___**by contact** / ___ por contacto.

transmission electron microscope *n.* microscopio electrónico de transmisión, instrumento usado para visualizar las células con una capacidad superior de un millón más de visualización que el microscopio común.

transmit *v.* transmitir, trasmitir, contagiar; conducir.

transmural *a.* transmural, que ocurre o se administra a través de una pared.

transmutation *n.* transmutación. 1. transformación, cambio evolutivo; 2. cambio de una sustancia en otra.

transocular *a.* transocular, que pasa a través de la órbita ocular.

transonance *n.* transonancia, resonancia transmitida.

transorbital *a.* transorbital, que ocurre o que pasa a través de la cavidad ósea del ojo.

transparency *n.* transparencia; [*slide*] diapositiva.

transparent *a.* transparente.

transpiration *n.* transpiración, perspiración.

transpire *v.* transpirar; [*to perspire*] sudar, transpirar; [*to happen*] suceder, acontecer.

transplacental *a.* transplacental, a través de la placenta.

transplant *n.* trasplante. 1. acto de transferir un órgano o tejido de un donante a un recipiente, o de una parte del cuerpo a otra para sustituir una parte enferma o restituir un órgano a su función normal; 2. parte artificial o natural que se usa como reemplazo; *v.* transplantar.

transplant of the bone marrow *n.* transplante de la medula ósea, injerto de tejido de la médula a pacientes de cáncer después de un agotador tratamiento de quimioterapia o a pacientes que sufren de anemia plástica o en casos severos de leucemia.

transplantation *n.* transplantación, trasplantación, acto de hacer un trasplante;

autoplastic ___ / ___ autoplástica;
heteroplastic ___ / ___ heteroplástica;
heterotopic ___ / ___ heterotópica;
homotopic ___ / ___ homotópica.

transpleural *a.* transpleural, que ocurre o se administra a través de la pleura.

transport *n.* transporte, movimiento de materiales en el cuerpo esp. a través de la membrana celular.

transportation *n.* transporte.

transposition *n.* transposición. 1. desplazamiento de un órgano o parte a una posición opuesta; 2. cambio genético de un cromosoma a otro que resulta a veces en defectos genéticos.

transposition of great vessels *n.* transposición de los grandes vasos, anomalía congénita en la cual la aorta sale del ventrículo derecho mientras que el tronco pulmonar sale del ventrículo izquierdo.

transrectal ultrasound *n.* ultrasonido transrectal, procedimiento que se usa para examinar la próstata por medio de ultrasonido. Se introduce un instrumento por el recto para captar distintas imágenes de la próstata que se proyectan por medio de ondas sonoras emitidas por ecos reproducidos por una computadora (ordenador); ___ **resection prostate /** resección ___ de la próstata.

transsexual *a.* transexual. 1. persona que tiene una urgencia psicológica de pertenecer al sexo opuesto; 2. persona que ha cambiado de sexo sometiéndose a una operación quirúgica.

transudate *n.* transudado, fluido que ha pasado a través de una membrana o ha sido expulsado como resultado de una inflamación.

transurethral *a.* transuretral, que ocurre o se administra a través de la uretra; ___ **resection prostate /** resección ___ de la próstata.

transvaginal *a.* transvaginal, a través de la vagina.

transversal *a.* transversal.

transverse *a.* transversal, atravesado-a; ___ **colon /** colon ___ ; ___ **plain /** plano ___ .

transvestism *n.* trasvestismo, adopción de modales del sexo opuesto, esp. la manera de vestir.

transvestite *n.* transvestido-a, transvestita, persona que practica el transvestismo.

trapezius *n.* trapecio, músculo triangular plano esencial en la rotación de la escápula.

trash *n.* basura, desecho.

trauma *n.* 1. trauma, estado psicológico; 2. traumatismo, si se refiere a una condición física.

traumatic *a.* traumático-a, rel. a un trauma.

traumatism *n.* traumatismo.

traumatize *v.* traumatizar, lesionar, lastimar.

traumatized *a.* traumatizado.

traumatology *n.* traumatología, rama de la cirugía que trata del cuidado de lesiones y heridas.

travel *n.* viaje; *v.* viajar, hacer un viaje.

treadmill *n.* [*physical fitness*] rueda de andar; tapiz rodante.

treatment *n.* tratamiento, método o procedimiento que se usa en la cura de enfermedades, lesiones y deformaciones; **preventive** ___ / ___ preventivo; **symptomatic** ___ / ___ sintomático; ___**plan /** plan o método de ___ .

tree *n.* 1. árbol; 2. estructura anatómica semejante a un árbol.

Trematoda *n. Trematoda,* clase de gusanos parásitos de la especie de los *Platyhelminthes* que incluye la duela y los gusanos planos que infectan el organismo humano.

trematode *n.* trematodo, gusano parásito de la clase *Trematoda.*

tremble *n.* temblor, estremecimiento, movimiento involuntario oscilatorio; *v.* temblar; estremecerse.

tremendous *a.* tremendo-a, formidable.

tremor *n.* temblor, estremecimiento; **alcoholic** ___ / ___ alcohólico; **coarse** ___ / ___ lento y acentuado; **continuous** ___ / ___ continuo; **essential** ___ / ___ esencial; **fine** ___ / ___ de variaciones rápidas; **flapping** ___ / ___ de aleteo; **intention** ___ / ___ intencional; **intermittent** ___ / ___ intermitente; **muscular** ___ / ___ muscular; **physiological** ___ / ___ fisiológico; **rest** ___ / ___ de reposo.

tremulous *a.* trémulo-a, afectado-a por un estremecimiento o que posee las características de un temblor.

trench *n.* trinchera, zanja, foso; ___ **back /** rigidez y dolor de espalda; ___ **fever /** fiebre de ___, fiebre remitente transmitida por piojos; ___ **foot /** pie de ___, infección en los pies por exposición al frío; ___ **-mouth /** infección con ulceración de las mucosas de la boca y la faringe.

trend *n.* tendencia; dirección.

Trendelenburg position *n.* posición de Trendelenburg, posición del paciente en la cual la cabeza descansa en un nivel más bajo que el tronco y las extremidades inferiores.

trepan *n.* trépano, instrumento usado en la trepanación; *v.* trepanar, perforar el cráneo con un trépano.

trepanation *n.* trepanación, perforación del cráneo con un instrumento especial para reducir el aumento de la presión intracraneal causada por fractura, acumulación de sangre o pus.

trephination *n.* trefinación, acto de cortar un tejido o un hueso dando un corte circular o de disco, operación gen. efectuada en el cráneo.

treponema *n.* treponema, parásito de la orden *Spirochaetales* que invade a humanos y animales; ___ **pallidum** / ___ pallidum, parásito causante de la sífilis.

treponemiasis *n.* treponemiasis, infección causada por espiroquetas del género *Treponema*.

triad *n.* triada, grupo de tres elementos que se relacionan entre sí.

triage *Fr.* triage, clasificación y evaluación de víctimas en acontecimientos catastróficos para establecer prioridades según la urgencia del tratamiento y aumentar así el número de sobrevivientes.

trial *n.* prueba, ensayo.

triangle *n.* triángulo.

triangular *a.* triangular.

tribe *n.* tribu, categoría biológica en taxonomía.

triceps *L.* tríceps, músculo de tres porciones o cabezas; ___ **reflex** / reflejo del ___ .

Trichinella *n.* Trichinella, género de gusanos nematodos, parásitos de animales carnívoros.

trichinosis *n.* triquinosis, enfermedad adquirida por la ingestión de carne cruda o mal cocinada, esp. de cerdo, que contiene larvas enquistadas de *Trichinella spiralis*.

trichitis *n.* triquitis, infl. de los bulbos pilosos.

trichobezoar *n.* tricobezoar, concreción o bezoar formado de pelo que se aloja en el intestino o el estómago.

Trichomonas *n.* Trichomonas, parásitos protozoarios que se alojan en el tubo digestivo y en el tracto genitourinario de vertebrados; ___ **vaginalis** / ___ vaginalis, agente causante de la vaginitis.

trichomoniasis *n.* trichomoniasis, infestación por *Trichomonas*.

trichromatic *a.* tricromático-a, compuesto de tres colores.

tricky *a.* engañoso-a; complicado-a.

tricuspid *a.* tricúspide. 1. que posee tres puntas o cúspides; 2. rel. a la válvula tricúspide del corazón; ___ **atresia** / atresia ___; ___ **murmur** / soplo ___ .

trifocal *a.* trifocal; ___ **lenses** / lentes ___ -es.

trigeminal *a.* trigeminal, rel. al nervio trigémino; ___ **cough** / tos ___; ___ **neuralgia** / neuralgia ___; ___ **pulse** / pulso ___ .

trigeminal nerve *n.* nervio trigémino. cranial nerves.

trigeminus *L.* trigeminus, nervio trigémino.

trigger *n.* desencadenamiento; impulso o reacción que inicia otros eventos; ___ **points** / puntos de ___; *v.* desencadenar, iniciar.

trigger zone *n.* área sensitiva que al recibir un estímulo ocasiona una reacción en otra parte del cuerpo.

triglycerides *n., pl.* triglicéridos, combinación que resulta de una molécula de glicerol con tres moléculas de ácidos grasos diferentes; la presencia elevada de triglicéridos se considera un factor importante en el desarrollo de enfermedades cardiovasculares.

trigone *n.* trígono, área de forma triangular.

trigonitis *n.* trigonitis, infl. del trígono de la vejiga urinaria.

trimester *n.* trimestre.

trip *n.* 1. viaje; 2. *slang*, uso de drogas alucinatorias.

triphasic *a.* trifásico-a, que se produce en tres fases o variaciones, esp. en referencia a las corrientes eléctricas.

triple *a.* triple, que consiste de tres componentes.

triplopia *n.* triplopia, trastorno visual por el cual se producen tres imágenes del mismo objeto.

trismus *Gr.* trismus, espasmo de los músculos de la masticación debido a una condición patológica.

trisomic *a.* trisómico-a, caracterizado por trisomía.

trisomy *n.* trisomía, trastorno genético por el cual una persona posee tres cromosomas homólogos por célula en lugar de dos (diploide), lo cual causa deformaciones fetales serias.

triturate *v.* triturar.

triumph *n.* triunfo, éxito; *v.* triunfar, tener éxito.

trochanter *n.* trocánter, una de las dos prominencias exteriores localizadas bajo el cuello del fémur; **greater** ___ / ___ mayor; **lesser** ___ / ___ menor.

trochlea *n.* tróclea, estructura que sirve de polea.

trochlear nerve *n.* nervio troclear. cranial nerves.

trophic *a.* trófico-a, rel. a la nutrición.

tropical *a.* tropical; ___ **diseases** / enfermedades ___ -es; ___ **medicine** / medicina ___ .

tropism *n.* tropismo, tendencia de una célula u organismo a reaccionar de una forma definida (positiva o negativa) en respuesta a estímulos externos.

trouble *n.* aflicción, calamidad, problema; **What is the trouble?** / ¿qué sucede? ¿qué pasa?; *v.* **to be in** ___ / estar en un apuro; **to be worth the** ___ / valer la pena.

troubled *a.* afligido-a, inquieto-a; preocupado-a.

trough *n.* canal o zanja.

trousers *n., pl.* pantalones.

true *a.* verdadero-a, cierto-a, real; verídico-a.

true pelvis *n.* pelvis verdadera o menor, parte inferior contráctil de la pelvis.

truncal *a.* troncal, truncado-a, rel. al tronco.

truncate *a.* truncado-a, que tiene una parte cercenada; amputado-a; *v.* truncar, cortar, amputar.

truncus *L.* truncus, tronco, torso, el cuerpo humano con exclusión de la cabeza y las extremidades.

truss *n.* braguero, faja para mantener una hernia reducida en su lugar; *v.* ligar, amarrar.

trust *n.* confianza, fe; *v.* confiar, creer en.

truth *n.* verdad; realidad; ___ **serum** / suero de la ___ .

truthful *a.* veraz, verdadero-a; **-ly** *adv.* verdaderamente, realmente.

try *n.* prueba, ensayo; *v.* probar, ensayar, hacer una prueba; intentar; **to** ___ **out** / probar, someter a prueba; **to** ___ **on** / probarse.

Trypanosoma *n. Tripanosoma*, género de parásito protozoario que se aloja en la sangre y es transmitido a los vertebrados por insectos vectores.

trypanosomal *a.* tripanosómico-a, rel. a un tripanosoma o que es afectado por éste.

trypanosomiasis *n.* tripanosomiasis, cualquier infección causada por un parásito flagelado del género *Tripanosoma*.

trypsin *n.* tripsina, enzima formada por el tripsinógeno presente en el jugo pancreático.

trypsinogen *n.* tripsinógeno, sustancia inactiva segregada por el páncreas en el duodeno para formar tripsina.

tryptophan *n.* triptófano, aminoácido cristalino presente en las proteínas, esencial a la vida animal.

tsetse fly *n.* mosca tsetsé, insecto del sur de África, transmisor de la enfermedad del sueño.

tub *n.* tina, bañera.

tubal *a.* tubárico-a; ___ **pregnancy** / embarazo ectópico en una trompa de Falopio; ___ **ligation** / ligadura o ligazón de las trompas.

tube *n.* tubo, conducto, trompa; **drainage** ___ / ___ de drenaje; **endotracheal** ___ / ___ endotraqueal; **inhalation** ___ / ___ de inhalación; **intestinal decompression** ___ / sonda intestinal; **nasogastric** ___ / ___ nasogástrico; **tracheotomy** ___ / ___ de traqueotomía; **thoracostomy** ___ / ___ de toracostomía.

tuber *L. tubera*tuber, tuberosidad; nódulo.

tubercle *n.* tubérculo. 1. nódulo pequeño; 2. pequeña prominencia de un hueso; 3. lesión producida por el bacilo de la tuberculosis.

tubercular *a.* tubercular, caracterizado por lesiones tuberosas.

tuberculin *n.* tuberculina, compuesto preparado del bacilo de la tuberculosis usado en las pruebas de diagnóstico de infecciones de la tuberculosis.

tuberculin test *n.* prueba de la tuberculina.

tuberculocidal *a.* tuberculocida, que destruye el bacilo de la tuberculosis.

tuberculosis *n.* tuberculosis, infección bacteriana aguda o crónica causada por el germen *Mycobacterium tuberculosis* que gen. afecta los pulmones pero que también puede afectar otros órganos; **meningeal** ___ / ___ meníngea; **pulmonary** ___ / ___ pulmonar; **spinal** ___ / ___ espinal; ___**in childhood** / ___ infantil; **urogenital** ___ / ___ urogenital.

tuberculous *a.* tuberculoso-a, rel. a o que padece de tuberculosis o que puede causarla.

tuberculum *L.* tuberculum, tubérculo.

tuberosity *n.* tuberosidad, elevación o protuberancia.

tuberous *a.* tuberoso-a, semejante a una tuberosidad.

tuberous sclerosis *n.* esclerosis tuberosa, enfermedad familiar marcada por ataques convulsivos, deficiencia mental progresiva y formación de múltiples tumores cerebrales cutáneos.

tuboabdominal pregnancy *n.* embarazo tuboabdominal.

tubo-ovarian *a.* tuboovárico-a, rel. a la trompa de Falopio y el ovario; ___ **abscess** / absceso ___ .

tubo-ovaritis *n.* tubo-ovaritis, infl. del ovario y la trompa de Falopio.

tuboplasty *n.* tuboplastia, reparación plástica de un conducto esp. de una trompa de Falopio.

tubule *n.* túbulo, conducto o canal pequeño; **collecting** ___ / ___ colector; **renal** ___ / ___ renal; **seminiferous** ___ / conduto seminífero.

tuft *n.* penacho, copete.

tug *n.* tirón; estirón; *v.* halar; estirar.

tugging *n.* tirón, acción de estirar con fuerza o tensión.

tularemia *n.* tularemia, fiebre de conejo, infeción transmitida a las personas por la picadura de un insecto vector o contraída en la manipulación de carne infectada.

tumefaction *n.* tumefacción, tumescencia, proceso de hinchazón.

tumefy *v.* entumecerse, hincharse.

tumid *a.* túmido-a, hinchado-a.

tummy *n.* pancita, barriguita.

tumor *n.* tumor. 1. bulto o hinchazón; 2. crecimiento espontáneo de tejido nuevo en masa que no tiene propósito fisiológico alguno; **diffuse** ___ / ___ difuso; **inflammatory** ___ / ___ inflamatorio; **medullary** ___ / ___ medular; **necrotic** ___ / ___ necrótico; **nonsolid** ___ / ___ no sólido; **radioresistant** ___ / ___ radiorresistente; **radiosensitive** ___ / ___ radiosensitivo; **scirrhous** ___ / ___ escirroso; **undifferentiated** ___ / ___ no diferenciado.

tumor makers, serum *n., pl.* sustancias en el plasma sanguíneo indicativas de la posible presencia de un tumor maligno.

tumor virus *n.* virus tumoroso, capaz de producir cáncer.

tumoricidal *a.* tumoricida, que destruye células tumorales.

tumorigenesis *n.* tumorigénesis, formación de tumores.

tumorous *a.* tumoroso-a, que tiene la apariencia de un tumor.

tuna *n.* [*fish*] atún.

tunic *n.* túnica, membrana protectora; ___ **adventitia** / ___ adventicia; ___ **albuginea** / cápsula albugínea; ___ **externa** / ___ externa; ___ **interna** / ___ interna; ___ **media** / ___ media; ___ **mucosa** / ___ mucosa; ___ **muscularis** / ___ muscular; ___ **serosa** / ___ serosa; ___ **vaginalis** / ___ vaginal.

tunnel *n.* túnel, canal o conducto estrecho; **carpal** ___ / ___ del carpo; **flexor** ___ / ___ flexor; **tarsal** ___ / ___ tarsiano.

tunnel vision *n.* visión en túnel, trastorno frecuente en casos de glaucoma avanzado que produce al paciente una disminución visual considerable tal como si mirara a través de un túnel.

turbid *a.* turbio-a, túrbido-a; nebuloso-a.

turbinated *a.* aconchado-a. 1. en forma de concha o cúpula; 2. rel. a los cornetes nasales.

turgid *a.* túrgido-a; hinchado-a, distendido-a.

turgor *n.* turgor. 1. distensión; 2. tensión celular normal.

turn *n.* vuelta, giro; turno; *v.* voltear, virar, dar vuelta, torcer; **to** ___ **back** / volver, regresar, retroceder; **to** ___ **down** / doblar; desaprobar, rechazar; [*when referring to one's body*] volverse, darse vuelta, virarse; **to** ___ **into** / volverse, convertirse en, transformarse; **to** ___ **out** / resultar; **to** ___ **pale** / palidecer; **to** ___ **red** / enrojecerse.

turned-down *a.* vuelto-a; doblado-a hacia abajo; desaprobado-a; rechazado-a.

turned-up *a.* vuelto-a, doblado-a hacia arriba.

Turner's syndrome *n.* síndrome de Turner, trastorno endocrino congénito que se manifiesta con deficiencia ovárica, amenorrea, estatura baja y la presencia de cromosomas X solamente.

turning *n.* 1. versión, término obstétrico referente a la manipulación del feto en el útero para facilitar el parto; 2. vuelta; *a.* giratorio-a; **the** ___ **point** / la crisis, el momento decisivo.

turnover *n.* cambio; *a.* cambiado-a de posición; *v.* voltear, cambiar de posición; transferir.

tussis *L.* tussis, tos.

tussive *a.* tusivo-a, rel. a la tos o causado por ésta.

T wave *n.* onda T, parte del electrocardiograma que representa la repolarización de los ventrículos.

tweezers *n., pl.* pinzas, tenacillas.

twice *adv.* dos veces; ___ **as much,** ___ **as many** / el doble.

twig *n.* terminación o rama diminuta de un nervio o de una arteria.

twilight *n.* crepúsculo; ___ **sleep** / sueño crepuscular; ___ **state** / estado de somnolencia.

twinge *n.* punzada, dolor agudo.

twinkle *n.* guiñada, pestañeo; *v.* guiñar un ojo; pestañear, parpadear; **in a** ___ / en un momento, en un instante.

twins *n., pl.* gemelos, mellizos, jimaguas, uno de dos hijos nacidos de un mismo embarazo; **dizygotic** ___ / ___ dicigóticos; **identical** ___ / ___ idénticos; **monozygotic** ___ / ___ monocigotos; **Siamese** ___ / ___ siameses; **true** ___ / ___ verdaderos.

twist *n.* torsión, torcedura; sacudida, contorsión; peculiaridad; *v.* [*an ankle*] torcer, virar, doblar.

twitch *n.* tic nervioso espasmódico; sacudida.

tympanectomy *n.* timpanectomía, excisión de la membrana timpánica.

tympanic *a.* timpánico-a, resonante; rel. al
tímpano ⎯ **membrane** / membrana ⎯; ⎯
resonance / resonancia ⎯ .

tympanites *n.* timpanitis, distensión del
abdomen causada por acumulación de gas en los
intestinos.

tympanitic *a.* timpanítico-a, rel. a la timpanitis
o afectado por ésta.

tympanoplasty *n.* timpanoplastia,
reconstrucción del oído medio.

tympanotomy *n.* timpanotomía, incisión de la
membrana timpánica.

tympanum *n.* tímpano, oído medio.

type *n.* tipo, género, clase, modelo o ejemplar
distintivo.

typhlitis *n.* tiflitis, infl. del ciego.

typhoid *a.* tifoideo-a, rel. al tifo o semejante a éste.

typhoid fever *n.* fiebre tifoidea, infección
abdominal aguda que es causada por una
bacteria de la clase *Salmonella* y que se
manifiesta con infl. abdominal, postración, fiebre
alta y dolor de cabeza.

typhus *n.* tifus, tifo, infección aguda causada por
una *Rickettsia* que se manifiesta con fiebre alta,
intensos dolores de cabeza y delirio.

typhus vaccine *n.* vacuna tífica.

typical *a.* típico-a, conforme a un tipo.

typing *n.* tipificación de tejidos, determinación
por tipos; **blood** ⎯ / determinación del grupo
sanguíneo.

u

U *abbr.* **unit** / unidad; **uranium** / uranio; **urology** / urología.

udder *n.* ubre, glándula mamaria de la vaca y otros animales mamíferos.

ugliness *n.* fealdad.

ugly *a.* feo-a.

ulcer *n.* úlcera, llaga o lesión en la piel o en la membrana mucosa con desintegración gradual de los tejidos. See chart on this page.

ulcerate *v.* ulcerar; ulcerarse.

ulcerated *a.* ulcerado-a, de la naturaleza de una úlcera o afectado por ella.

ulceration *n.* ulceración, supuración; proceso de formación de una úlcera.

ulcerative *a.* ulcerativo-a, rel. a una úlcera o caracterizado-a por una condición ulcerosa; ___ **colitis** / colitis ___ .

ulcerogenic *a.* ulcerógeno-a, que produce úlceras.

ulcerous *a.* ulceroso-a, rel. a una úlcera o que la padece.

ulerythema *n.* uleritema, dermatitis eritematosa caracterizada por la formación de cicatrices; ___

Ulcer	Úlcera
chancroidal	chancroide
chronic	crónica
chronic leg varicose	varicosa crónica de la pierna
decubitus	por decúbito
duodenal	duodenal
gastric	gástrica
hemorrhagic	homorrágica
indolent	indolente
marginal	marginal
mycotic	micótica
peptic	péptica
perforating	perforante
phagedenic	fagedénica
rodent	roedora
syphilitic	sifilítica
vesical	vesical

ophryogenes / ___ ofriógeno; ___ **sycosiforme** / ___ sicosiforme.

ulitis *n.* ulitis. gingivitis.

ulna *n.* cúbito. V. **cubitus**.

ulnar *n.* ulnar, rel. al cúbito o a los nervios y arterias relacionados con éste; ___ **nerve dysfunction** / disfunción del nervio ___ .

ulocarcinoma, ulocarcinomata *n.* ulocarcinoma, ulocarcinomata, cáncer de las encías.

ultimate *a.* último-a, final; fundamental.

ultracentrifuge *n.* ultracentrífuga, aparato de fuerza centrífuga que separa y sedimenta las moléculas de una sustancia.

ultrafiltration *n.* ultrafiltración, proceso de filtración que deja pasar pequeñas moléculas pero impide el paso de moléculas mayores.

ultramicroscope *n.* ultramicroscopio, microscopio de campo oscuro capaz de hacer visibles objetos que no se distinguen en un microscopio de luz común.

ultrasonic *a.* ultrasónico-a, supersónico-a; ___ **diagnosis** / diagnóstico por ultrasonido.

ultrasonogram *n.* ultrasonograma, imagen producida por medio de ultrasonografía.

ultrasonography *n.* ultrasonografía, técnica de diagnóstico que emplea ultrasonido para producir imágenes de una estructura o de tejidos del cuerpo.

ultrasound *n.* ultrasonido, ondas de frecuencia superior a las del oído humano que se usan en ultrasonografía en procedimientos terapéuticos y de diagnóstico; **abdominal** ___ / ___ abdominal; **breast** ___ / ___ de la mama; **pregnancy** ___ / ___ del embarazo; **thyroid** ___ / ___ de la tiroides.

ultrasound imaging *n.* imágenes por ultrasonido, captación de imágenes de órganos o tejidos del cuerpo por medio de ultrasonido empleando técnicas de reflejo (ecograma).

ultrastructure *n.* ultraestructura, estructura diminuta que solamente puede distinguirse bajo un microscopio electrónico.

ultraviolet *a.* ultravioleta, que se extiende más allá de la zona violeta del espectro; ___ **rays** / rayos ___ ; ___ **therapy** / terapia de radiación ___ .

ululation *n.* ululación, emisión de gritos o alaridos incoordinados de tipo histérico esp. de pacientes mentales.

umbilical *a.* umbilical, rel. al ombligo; ___ **notch** / ligamento ___ ; ___ **hernia** / hernia ___ .

umbilical cord *n.* cordón umbilical, estructura que sirve de conexión entre el feto y la placenta durante la gestación.

umbilicus, navel *n.* ombligo, depresión en el centro del abdomen que marca el punto de inserción del cordón umbilical.

unable *a.* incapaz, inhábil.

unacceptable *a.* inaceptable, no aprobado-a.

unaccustomed *a.* no usual, no acostumbrado-a, desacostumbrado-a.

unadulterated *a.* natural, puro-a, sin mezcla, no adulterado-a.

unaffected *a.* no afectado-a.

unanimous *a.* unánime.

unanswered *a.* por contestar, no contestado-a.

unassisted *a.* sin ayuda, sin auxilio, desamparado-a.

unattached *a.* suelto-a, sin conexión.

unattended *a.* desatendido-a.

unavoidable *a.* inevitable.

unaware *a.* sin conocimiento de causa; que ignora.

unbearable *a.* insoportable, intolerable, insufrible, imposible de soportar.

unbeliever *a.* incrédulo-a.

unbiased *a.* imparcial, sin prejuicios.

unclog *v.* desbloquear, permeabilizar; destupir, destapar.

uncomfortable *a.* incómodo-a, molesto-a, desagradable.

uncommon *a.* poco común, raro-a, extraño-a.

unconditioned reflex *n.* reflejo no condicionado o natural.

unconditioned response *n.* respuesta no condicionada o reacción no restringida.

unconscious *a.* inconsciente. 1. que ha perdido el conocimiento; 2. que no responde a estímulos sensoriales.

unconsciousness *n.* inconsciencia, pérdida del conocimiento.

uncooperative *a.* poco dócil; que no coopera.

uncover *v.* destapar, descubrir, poner al descubierto.

unction *n.* unción, aplicación de un ungüento o aceite.

unctuous *a.* untuoso-a, oleaginoso-a; grasoso-a.

undecided *a.* indeciso-a, indeterminado-a.

undefined *a.* indefinido-a.

under *a.* inferior; *prep. adv.* debajo, menos, menos que; bajo; ___ **observation** / bajo observación; ___ **treatment** / bajo tratamiento.

underage *a.* menor de edad.

underclothing *n.* ropa interior.

underdeveloped *a.* subdesarrollado-a; en desarrollo.

underdevelopment *n.* subdesarrollo.

underestimate *v.* subestimar; menospreciar.

underfed *a.* desnutrido-a, mal alimentado-a.

undergo *vi.* someterse a; sufrir, padecer, soportar; **to** ___ **surgery** / someterse a una operación.

underline *v.* subrayar.

undermine *v.* dañar, debilitar.

undernourished *a.* desnutrido-a; malnutrido-a.

undernutrition *a.* desnutrición.

undershirt *n.* camiseta.

underside *n.* el lado de abajo.

undersigned *n.* el abajo firmante.

understand *vi.* comprender, entender.

understood *a. pp.* of **to understand** convenido-a, entendido-a, comprendido-a.

undertake *vi.* emprender, iniciar, tomar la iniciativa.

underway *n.* en camino; bajo estudio.

underwear *n.* ropa interior.

underweight *n.* falta de peso, peso deficiente; bajo de peso; de peso insuficiente.

undesirable *a.* indeseable, inaceptable, aborrecido-a.

undetected *a.* no detectado-a, no descubierto-a, inadvertido-a.

undetermined *a.* indeterminado-a.

undeveloped *a.* no desarrollado-a, sin manifestación.

undifferentiation *n.* indiferenciación. V. **anaplasia**.

undigested *a.* no digerido-a, no asimilado-a.

undiluted *a.* no diluido-a, sin diluirse, concentrado-a.

undiminished *a.* sin disminución.

undisclosed *a.* no revelado-a, no dado-a a conocer.

undo *vi.* deshacer, desatar; desabrochar.

undress *v.* desvestirse; quitarse la ropa.

undulant *a.* ondulante; ___ **fever** / fiebre ___, brucellosis.

undulated *a.* ondulado-a, de borde ondulado o irregular.

uneasy *a.* inquieto-a.

unengaged *a.* desencajado-a, fuera de lugar.

unequal *a.* desigual; desproporcionado-a.

unexpected *a.* inesperado-a, imprevisto-a.

unfinished *a.* incompleto-a, sin terminar.

unfit *a.* inepto-a, inhábil, incapaz.

unfitness *n.* ineptitud, incapacidad, incompetencia.

unforeseen *a.* inesperado-a, imprevisto-a.

unfortunate *a.* infeliz, desafortunado-a, desgraciado-a.

unfriendly *a.* poco amistoso-a, poco amigable.

ungrateful *a.* desagradecido-a, ingrato-a.

ungual *a.* ungueal, rel. a una uña.

unguent *n.* ungüento, medicamento preparado para uso externo.

unhappy *a.* infeliz, desgraciado-a.

unharmed, unhurt *a.* ileso-a; *pop.* sano-a y salvo-a.

unhealthy *a.* [*environment*] insalubre, malsano-a; [*person*] enfermizo-a, achacoso-a.

uniarticular *a.* uniarticular, rel. a una sola articulación.

unibasal *a.* unibásico-a, rel. a una sola base.

unicellular *a.* unicelular, de una sola célula.

uniform *n.* [*garment*] uniforme; *a.* uniforme; invariable.

unigravida *a.* unigrávida, mujer embarazada por primera vez.

unilateral *a.* unilateral, rel. a un solo lado.

uninsured *a.* no asegurado-a, sin seguro.

union *n.* unión. 1. acción de unir dos cosas en una; 2. juntura de dos partes cortadas (amputadas) de un hueso o de los bordes de una herida.

uniovular *a.* uniovular, que se desarrolla de un solo óvulo.

uniparous *a.* unípara, mujer que tiene un parto simple.

unipolar *a.* unipolar, de un solo polo, tal como las células nerviosas.

unique *a.* único-a; solo-a; que se distingue de otros.

unit *n.* unidad. 1. estándar de medida; 2. unidad internacional / **international unit**; 3. unidad fisiológica, la más mínima división de un órgano capaz de realizar una función; **motor___** / ___ motora.

unite *v.* unir; reunir.

united *a.* unido-a.

unity *n.* unidad; unión.

universal *a.* universal, general; ___ **antidote** / antídoto ___ .

universal donor *n.* donante universal, persona que pertenece al grupo de sangre tipo O, de factor RH negativo, cuya sangre puede ser dada a personas con sangre tipo ABO con poco riesgo de complicaciones.

universal recipient *n.* recipiente universal, persona que pertenece al grupo de sangre AB.

universe *n.* universo.

university *n.* universidad.

unjust *a.* injusto-a.

unkind *a.* despiadado-a, sin bondad.

unlawful *a.* ilegal, ilícito-a.

unlicensed *a.* no acreditado-a, sin licencia o sin permiso.

unlikely *a.* improbable, dudoso-a.

unlucky *a.* desafortunado-a.

Unna's paste boot *n.* bota de pasta de Unna, compresión que se usa en el tratamiento de úlceras varicosas en la pierna, con vendajes en espiral aplicados y cubiertos con la pasta medicinal de Unna.

unnecessary *a.* innecesario-a.

unobstructed *a.* abierto-a, suelto-a; libre; no obstruido.

unofficial *a.* sin autorización; no oficial, se dice de una droga o medicamento no aprobado por la farmacopea o los formularios vigentes autorizados.

unopened *a.* cerrado-a, tapado-a, sin abrir.

unorganized *a.* desorganizado-a; no estructurado; sin orden.

unreal *a.* ilusorio-a, imaginario-a.

unreasonable *a.* irrazonable, intransigente.

unrest *n.* desasosiego, inquietud; intranquilidad.

unsalted *a.* sin sal, que le falta sal.

unsanitary *a.* insalubre, malsano.

unsaturated *a.* no saturado-a.

unstable *a.* inestable; ___ **angina** / angina ___ ; ___ **bladder** / vejiga ___ .

untiring *a.* incansable.

untreated *a.* no tratado-a.

unwanted *a.* no deseado-a.

up *prep. adv.* arriba, en lo alto.

update *v.* [*to improve*] modernizar; [*documents*] poner al día; arreglar.

upgrade *v.* mejorar.

upgrowth *n.* crecimiento, desarrollo, maduración.

upper *n. pop.* droga estimulante, esp. una anfetamina; *a. comp.* superior, más alto-a.

upper airway obstruction *n.* obstrucción en el conducto aéreo superior.

upper GI *n.* examen radiográfico del estómago y duodeno con ingestión de una sustancia que sirve de medio de contraste.

upper jaw *n.* mandíbula superior.

upper respiratory infection *n.* infección del tracto respiratorio superior.

upper respiratory tract *n.* aparato respiratorio superior compuesto de la nariz, los conductos nasales y la nasofaringe.

upset *a.* indipuesto-a; nervioso-a; disgustado-a; *v.* trastornar; enfadar.

uptake *n.* absorción, fijación o incorporación de alguna sustancia a un organismo vivo; ___ **and storage** / toma y almacenamiento.

551

uranic *a.* uránico-a, rel. a la uremia.
uranium *n.* uranio, elemento metálico pesado.
urate *n.* urato, sal de ácido úrico.
urea *n.* urea, producto del metabolismo de las proteínas, forma en la cual el nitrógeno se excreta por la orina; **hereditary ___ cycle abnormality** / ciclo ureico hereditario anormal.
ureal *a.* ureico-a, rel. o concerniente a la urea.
urelcosis *n.* urelcosis, ulceración de las vías urinarias.
uremia *n.* uremia, condición tóxica causada por insuficiencia renal que produce retención en la sangre de sustancias nitrogenadas, fosfatos y sulfatos.
uremic *a.* urémico-a, rel. a la uremia o causado por ella.
ureter *n.* uréter, uno de los conductos que llevan la orina del riñón a la vejiga.
ureteral *a.* ureteral, uretérico-a, rel. o concerniente al uréter; **___ injury** / lesión ___; **___ reflex** / reflejo ___ .
ureterectasis *n.* ureterectasis, dilatación anormal del uréter.
ureterectomy *n.* ureterectomía, extirpación parcial o total del uréter.
ureteritis *n.* ureteritis, infl. del uréter.
ureterocele *n.* ureterocele, dilatación quística de la porción distal intravesical del uréter debida a una estenosis del orificio ureteral.
ureterocystoneostomy *n.* ureterocistoneostomía. V. **ureteroneocystostomy**.
ureterocystostomy *n.* ureterocistostomía, transplantación de un uréter a otra parte de la vejiga.
ureterography *n.* ureterografía, radiografía del uréter usando un medio radioopaco.
ureteroheminephrectomy *n.* ureteroheminefrectomía, resección de la porción de un riñón y el uréter en ciertos casos de duplicación del tracto urinario superior.
ureterohydronephrosis *n.* ureterohidronefrosis, distensión del uréter y del riñón debida a una obstrucción.
ureteroiliostomy *n.* ureteroiliostomía, anastomosis del uréter a un segmento aislado del íleon.
ureterolithiasis *n.* ureterolitiasis, desarrollo de un cálculo ureteral.
ureterolithotomy *n.* ureterolitotomía, incisión del uréter para extraer un cálculo.
ureteroneocystostomy *n.* ureteroneocistostomía. V. **ureterocystoneostomy**.

ureteronephrectomy *n.* ureteronefrectomía, excisión del riñón y su uréter.
ureteropelvic *a.* ureteropélvico-a, rel. al uréter y a la pelvis; **___ junction obstruction** / obstrucción de la unión ___ .
ureteroplasty *n.* ureteroplastia, cirugía plástica del uréter.
ureteropyeloplasty *n.* ureteropieloplastia, cirugía plástica del uréter y la pelvis renal.
ureterosigmoidostomy *n.* ureterosigmoidostomía, implantación del uréter en el colon sigmoideo.
ureterostomy *n.* ureterostomía, formación de una fístula permanente para drenar un uréter.
ureterotomy *n.* ureterotomía, incisión de un uréter.
ureteroureterostomy *n.* ureteroureterostomía, anastomosis de dos uréteres o de dos extremos del mismo uréter.
urethra *n.* uretra, canal o conducto urinario.
urethral *a.* uretral, rel. a la uretra; **___ catheter** / catéter ___; **___ obstruction** / obstrucción ___; **___ procedure** / procedimiento ___; **___ stricture** / estrechez ___ ; **___ suspension** / suspensión ___; **___ syndrome** / síndrome ___ .
urethralgia *n.* uretralgia, dolor en la uretra.
urethrectomy *n.* uretrectomía, excisión parcial o total de la uretra.
urethritis *n.* uretritis, infl. aguda o crónica de la uretra.
urethrography *n.* uretrografía, rayos-x de la uretra usando una sustancia radioopaca inyectada.
urethroscope *n.* uretroscopio, instrumento para visualizar el interior de la uretra.
urethrotome *n.* uretrótomo, instrumento quirúrgico empleado en una uretrotomía.
urethrotomy *n.* uretrotomía, incisión efectuada para aliviar una estrechez uretral.
urgent *a.* urgente.
uric acid *n.* ácido úrico, producto del metabolismo de las proteínas presente en la sangre y excretado en la orina.
uricemia *n.* uricemia, exceso de ácido úrico en la sangre.
uricosuria *n.* uricosuria, presencia excesiva de ácido úrico en la orina.
urinal *n.* orinal, vasija en que se recoge la orina; *pop.* taza, pato.
urinalysis *n.* urinálisis, examen de orina.
urinary *a.* urinario-a, rel. o concerniente a la orina. **___ calculi** / cálculos ___ -s; **___**

infection / infección renal o ___; ___ **sediments** / sedimentos ___ -s.

urinary bladder *n.* vejiga urinaria, órgano muscular en forma de saco que recoge la orina que secretan los riñones.

urinary system *n.* sistema urinario, órganos y conductos que participan en la producción y excreción de la orina.

urinary tract *n.* vías urinarias. ___ **infections** / infecciones de las ___ .

urinate *n.* orinar, mear.

urination *n.* orina, acto de emisión de la orina; **frequent** ___ / orinar con frecuencia, micción frecuente; *Mex. A. pop.* meadera; **difficult** ___ / orinar con dificultad, micción difícil; **painful** ___ / orinar con dolor, micción dolorosa.

urine *n.* orina, orín, *pop.* aguas menores, líquido ambarino secretado por los riñones que se almacena en la vejiga y se elimina en la uretra. See chart on this page.

uriniferous *a.* urinífero-a, que contiene o conduce orina.

urinogenital *a.* urinogenital. V. **urogenital**.

urinoma *n.* urinoma, tumor o quiste que contiene orina.

urobilinogen *n.* urobilinógeno, pigmento derivado de la reducción de bilirrubina por acción de bacterias intestinales.

urodynamics *n.* urodinámica, estudio del proceso activo patofisiológico de la micción.

urodynia *n.* urodinia, micción dolorosa.

Urine, anomalies	Orina, anomalías
acute retention (inability to urinate)	retención aguda (incapacidad de orinar)
abnormal color	color anormal
abnormal odor	olor anormal
blood in urine	sangre en la orina
midstream changes	cambios a mitad de chorro
frequent urination	micción frecuente
involuntary urine leak	escape o goteo involuntario de orina
little or no urination	escasa o ninguna cantidad de orina
painful urination	micción dolorosa
urge incontinence	micción imperiosa

urogenital *a.* urogenital, rel. a la vía urinaria o al tracto urinario y genital; ___ **diaphragm** / diafragma ___ .

urogram *n.* urograma, rayos-x hechos por urografía.

urography *n.* urografía, rayos-x de una parte de las vías urinarias con el uso de una sustancia radioopaca inyectada; **excretory or descending** ___ / ___ excretora o descendiente; **retrograde** ___ / ___ retrógrada.

urohematonephrosis *n.* urohematonefrosis, condición patológica del riñón en la cual la pelvis se distiende con sangre y orina.

urokinase *n.* urocinasa, enzima presente en la orina que se emplea en la disolución de coágulos.

urolithiasis *n.* urolitiasis, formación de cálculos urinarios y trastornos asociados con su presencia.

urologist *n.* urólogo-a, especialista en urología.

urology *n.* urología, estudio y tratamiento de las enfermedades del aparato genitourinario en el hombre y del tracto urinario en la mujer.

uropathy *n.* uropatía, enfermedades de las vías urinarias.

uropyourether *n.* uropiouréter, acumulación de orina y pus en la pelvis renal.

uroschesis *n.* urosquesis, supresión o retención de orina.

urticaria *n.* urticaria, erupción cutánea gen. alérgica que se manifiesta con ronchas rosáceas, se acompaña de picazón intensa y puede producirse por un factor interno o externo; ___ **pigment** / ___ pigmentosa.

usage *n.* uso, costumbre.

use *n.* uso, utilidad, provecho; *v.* usar, emplear; **off-label** ___ / ___ no aprobado.

useful *a.* útil, provechoso-a, práctico-a.

usual *a.* usual, de costumbre; **-ly** *adv.* usualmente, generalmente.

uterine *a.* uterino-a, rel. al útero o matriz; ___ **bleeding** / sangramiento ___, sangramiento no relacionado con la menstruación; ___ **cancer** / cáncer del útero o de la matriz; ___ **prolapse** / prolapso ___; ___ **rupture** / rotura ___ .

uterosalpingography *n.* uterosalpingografía, examen de rayos-x de la matriz y la trompa de Falopio usando una sustancia radioopaca inyectada.

uterovaginal *a.* uterovaginal, rel. al útero y a la vagina.

uterovesical *a.* uterovesical, rel. al útero y la vejiga urinaria.

uterus *n.* útero, matriz, órgano muscular femenino del aparato reproductivo que contiene

y nutre al embrión y feto durante la gestación;
didelphys ___ / ___ didelfo.

utriculus *L.* (*pl.* **utriculi**) utriculus, pequeña
bolsa; ___ **of vestibular organ** / ___ del oído o del
vestíbulo; ___**prostaticus** / ___ prostático o uretral.

uvea *n.* úvea, túnica vascular del ojo formada por
el iris, el cuerpo ciliar y la coroide.

uveitis *n.* uveítis, infl. de la úvea.

uvula *n.* úvula, *pop.* campanilla, estructura
colgante en el centro posterior del paladar
blando.

uvulitis *n.* uvulitis, infl. de la úvula.

uvulotomy *n.* uvulotomía, sección total o parcial
de la úvula.

U wave *n.* onda U, onda positiva que sigue a la
onda T en el electrocardiograma.

V

V *abbr.* **valve** / válvula; **vein** / vena; **vide (see)** / vea; **vision** / visión; **volume** / volumen.

vacation *n.* vacaciones.

vaccinate *v.* vacunar, inocular.

vaccination *n.* vacunación, inoculación de una vacuna.

vaccine *n.* vacuna, preparación de microorganismos atenuados o muertos que se introduce en el cuerpo para establecer una inmunidad en contra de la enfermedad específica causada por dichos microorganismos; **BCG** ___ / ___ del bacilo Calmette-Guérin, contra la tuberculosis; **chickenpox** ___ / ___ contra la varicela; **DTP (diptheria, tetanus, pertussis)** ___ / ___ triple contra la difteria, tétano y pertusis (tos ferina); **hepatitis A** ___ / ___ contra la hepatitis A; **hepatitis B** ___ / ___ contra la hepatitis B; **influenza** ___ / ___ contra la influenza; **measles virus, inactivated** ___ / ___ antisarampión, inactivada; **measles virus, live attenuated** ___ / ___ antisarampión de virus vivo, atenuada; **pneumococcal polyvalent** ___ / ___ antineumocócica polivalente; **pneumovax** ___ / ___ neumocócica polisacárida; **poliovirus, live oral trivalent** ___ / ___ antipolio trivalente o de Sabin; **rabies** ___ / ___ antirrábica; **Salk's antipoliomyelitis** ___ / ___ antipoliomielítica de Salk; **smallpox** ___ / ___ antivariolosa, antivariólica; **tetanus** ___ / ___ contra el tétano; **typhus** ___ / ___ antitífica; **typhoid** ___ / ___ contra la tifoidea; ___ **reaction** / reacción a la ___ .

vaccinia *n.* vaccina, virus causante de la viruela bovina del cual se obtiene la vacuna contra la viruela.

vacillate *v.* vacilar; fluctuar.

vacillating *a.* vacilante, oscilante, fluctuante.

vacuity *n.* vacuidad, vacío.

vacuole *n.* vacuola, pequeña cavidad o espacio en el protoplasma celular que contiene líquido o aire.

vacuolization *n.* vacuolización, formación de vacuolas.

vacuum *n. L.* vacuum, vacío, espacio desprovisto de materia o aire; *v.* extraer el polvo con una aspiradora; ___ **packed** / envasado-a al vacío.

vagal *a.* vagal, rel. al nervio vago o neumogástrico.

vagina *n.* vagina. 1. conducto en la mujer que se extiende del útero a la vulva; 2. estructura semejante a una vaina.

vaginal *a.* vaginal. 1. que posee forma de vaina; 2. rel. a la vagina; ___ **bleeding** / sangrado ___ , hemorragia ___; ___ **candidiasis** / candidiasis ___; ___ **culture** / cultivo ___; ___ **cysts** / quistes vaginales; ___ **discharge** / flujo ___; ___ **drying treatment** / tratamiento de secamiento ___; ___ **itching** / picazón ___; ___ **wall repair** / reparación de la pared de la ___; ___ **tumor** / tumor ___ .

vaginismus *L.* vaginismus, contracción dolorosa espasmódica de la vagina.

vaginitis *n.* vaginitis, infl. de la vagina; **bacterial** ___ / ___ bacteriana.

vagolytic *a.* vagolítico, rel. al nervo vago.

vagotomy *n.* vagotomía, interrupción del nervio vago.

vagrant *a.* errante; suelto-a; libre.

vague *a.* vago-a, indefinido-a; **-ly** *adv.* vagamente.

vagus *n.* vago, nervio neumogástrico.

vain *a.* vano-a, vanidoso-a; **-ly** *adv.* vanamente, en vano.

valgus *n. L.* valgus, doblado o torcido hacia afuera.

valiant *a.* valiente.

valid *a.* válido-a, valedero-a.

validity *n.* validez.

vallecula *n.* valécula, depresión, surco o fisura esp. en referencia a estructuras anatómicas.

valley fever *n.* fiebre del valle. *Syn.* **coccidioidomycosis.**

valorization *n.* valorización, evaluación.

Valsalva's maneuver *n.* maniobra, experimento de Valsalva, procedimiento para demostrar la permeabilidad de la trompa de Eustaquio o de ajustar la presión del oído medio mediante una espiración forzada con la boca y la nariz tapadas.

valuable *a.* valioso-a, valuable.

value *n.* valor.

valve *n.* (*pl.* **valvae**) válvula, valva, estructura membranosa en un canal u orificio que al cerrarse temporalmente impide el reflujo del contenido que pasa a través de ella; **aortic** ___ / ___ aórtica; **aortic-semilunar** ___ / ___ aórtica semilunar; **atrioventricular left** ___ / ___ auriculoventricular izquierda; **atrioventricular**

right ___ , **tricuspid** / ___ auriculoventricular derecha, tricúspide; **bicuspid or mitral** ___ / ___ bicúspide o mitral; **ileocecal** ___ / ___ ileocecal; **pulmonary** ___ / ___ pulmonar; **pyloric** ___ / ___ pilórica.

valvulae conniventes *n., pl.* válvulas conniventes, pliegues circulares membranosos localizados en el intestino delgado que retardan el paso del contenido alimenticio en el intestino.

valvular *a.* valvular, rel. a una válvula o de su naturaleza; ___ **pulmonary stenosis** / estenosis pulmonar ___ .

valvuloplasty *n.* valvuloplastia, operación plástica de una válvula.

valvulotome *n.* valvulótomo, instrumento quirúrgico que se usa para seccionar una válvula.

vapor *n.* vapor, gas.

vaporization *n.* vaporización. 1. acción o efecto de vaporizar; 2. uso terapéutico de vapores.

vaporize *v.* vaporizar, convertir una sustancia en gas o vapor.

vaporizer *n.* vaporizador, dispositivo para convertir una sustancia en vapor y aplicarla a usos terapéuticos.

variability *n.* variabilidad.

variable *n.* variable, factor que puede variar; *a.* que puede cambiar.

variant *n.* variante, objeto esencialmente igual a otro pero que difiere en la forma; *a.* variable, inconstante, que cambia o varía.

variation *n.* variación, diversidad en las características de objetos que se relacionan entre sí.

varicella *n.* varicela. V. **chickenpox**.

varicocele *n.* varicocele, condición varicosa de las venas del cordón espermático que produce una masa blanda en el escroto.

varicoid *a.* varicoide, que se asemeja a una várice.

varicose *a.* varicoso-a, rel. a las várices o que se les asemeja; ___ **veins** / venas ___ -s.

varicotomy *n.* varicotomía, excisión de una vena varicosa.

variety *n.* variedad.

variola *n.* variola, viruela.

variolic, variolous *a.* variólico-a, rel. a la viruela.

varioliform *a.* varioliforme, semejante a la viruela.

varix *n.* (*pl.* **varices**) várice, vena, arteria o vaso linfático aumentado o dilatado.

varus *n. L.* varus, doblado o torcido hacia adentro.

vary *v.* variar, cambiar; cambiarse; desviarse.

vas *n. L.* (*pl.* **vasa**) vas, vaso.

vascular *a.* vascular, rel. a vasos sanguíneos; ___ **ectasia of the colon** / ectasia ___ del colon; ___ **purpura** / púrpura ___; ___ **skin changes** / cambios cutáneos vasculares; ___ **spasm** / espasmo ___; ___ **system** / sistema ___, todos los vasos del cuerpo esp. los sanguíneos; ___ **tunic** / túnica ___ .

vascularization *n.* vascularización, formación de vasos sanguíneos nuevos.

vasculature *n.* vasculatura, disposición de los vasos sanguíneos en un órgano o parte.

vasculitis *n.* vasculitis, angiitis.

vasculopathy *n.* vasculopatía, cualquier enfermedad de los vasos sanguíneos.

vas deferens *n. L.* vas deferens, conducto excretor de espermatozoides.

vasectomy *n.* vasectomía, excisión parcial y ligadura de los conductos deferentes para impedir la salida de espermatozoides en el semen, procedimiento gen. usado como contraceptivo.

vaseline *n.* vaselina.

vasoactive *a.* vasoactivo, que afecta los vasos sanguíneos.

vasoconstrictive *a.* vasoconstrictivo-a, que causa constricción en los vasos sanguíneos.

vasodilation *n.* vasodilatación, aumento del calibre de los vasos sanguíneos.

vasodilator *n.* vasodilatador, agente que causa vasodilatación; *a.* vasodilatador-a; que causa vasodilatación.

vasomotor *n.* vasomotora, agente que regula las contracciones y la dilatación de los vasos sanguíneos; *a.* vasomotor-a, que causa dilatación o contracción en los vasos sanguíneos; ___ **angina** / angina ___; ___ **rhinitis** / rinitis ___ .

vasopressin *n.* vasopresina, hormona liberada por la pituitaria posterior que aumenta la reabsorción de agua en el riñón elevando la presión arterial.

vasopressor *n.* vasopresor, agente que produce constricción en los vasos sanguíneos; *a.* que tiene efecto vasoconstrictivo.

vasospasm *n.* vasoespasmo; **coronary** ___ / ___ coronario e. V. **angiospasm**.

vasotonic *a.* vasotónico, rel. al tono de un vaso.

vasovagal *a.* vasovagal, rel. a los vasos y al nervio vago.

vasovagal syncope *n.* síncope vasovagal, desmayo súbito breve debido a un trastorno vasomotor y vagal.

vastus *a. L.* vastus, dilatado-a, agrandado-a, extendido-a.

Vater's ampulla *n.* ámpula de Vater, punto de entrada en el duodeno de los conductos excretores biliar y pancreático.

veal *n.* carne de ternera; ___ **chop** / chuleta de ___ .

vector *n.* vector, portador, organismo microbiano transmisor de agentes infecciosos.

vegan *n.* vegetariano en el sentido estricto de la palabra.

vegetable *n.* vegetal.

vegetarian *n.* vegetariano-a, persona cuya dieta consiste principalmente en vegetales; *a.* rel. a los vegetales.

vegetarianism *n.* vegetarianismo, método de alimentación que consiste mayormente en una dieta de vegetales y frutas.

vegetation *n.* vegetación, crecimiento anormal de verrugas o excrecencias en una parte del cuerpo tal como se ve en la endocarditis.

vegetative *a.* vegetativo-a. 1. rel. a funciones de crecimiento y nutrición; 2. rel. a funciones corporales involuntarias o inconscientes.

vehicle *n.* vehículo. 1. sustancia sin acción terapéutica que acompaña a un agente activo en una preparación medicinal; 2. agente de transmisión.

veil *n.* velo. 1. membrana o cubierta fina que cubre una parte del cuerpo; 2. parte de la membrana amniótica que cubre la cara del feto; 3. alteración ligera de la voz.

vein *n.* vena, vaso fibromuscular que lleva la sangre de los capilares al corazón; **spider** ___ **-s** / ___ varicosas.

vena *n. L.* vena.

vena cava *n.* vena cava, una de las dos venas mayores, la vena cava inferior y la vena cava superior, que devuelven la sangre desoxigenada a la aurícula derecha del corazón.

venal *a.* venal, rel. a las venas.

veneer *n.* barniz, enchapado.

venepuncture *n.* venipuntura, punción de una vena.

venereal *a.* venéreo-a, que resulta a consecuencia del acto sexual; ___ **disease** / enfermedad ___; ___**wart** / verruga ___ .

venin-antivenin *n.* veninantivenina, suero antídoto contra el veneno de serpientes.

venin, venine *n.* venina, sustancia tóxica del veneno de serpientes.

venisection *n.* venisección. V. **phlebotomy**.

venoconstriction *n.* venoconstricción, reducción de las paredes venosas.

venogram *n.* venograma, radiografía de las venas usando un medio de contraste; **renal** ___ / ___ renal.

venography *n.* venografía, gráfica e información de un venograma.

venom *n.* veneno, sustancia tóxica.

venomous *a.* venenoso-a, tóxico-a.

veno-occlusive *a.* venoclusivo-a, rel. a una obstrucción venosa.

venotomy *n.* venotomía. V. **phlebotomy**.

venous *a.* venoso-a, rel. a las venas; ___ **blood** / sangre ___; ___ **congestion** / congestión ___; ___ **insufficiency** / insuficiencia ___; ___ **return** / retorno ___; ___ **sinus** / seno ___; ___**thrombo-embolism** / tromboembolismo ___; ___ **thrombosis** / trombosis ___ .

vent *Fr.* vent, abertura.

ventilate *v.* ventilar, airear.

ventilation *n.* ventilación. 1. circulación de aire fresco en una habitación; 2. oxigenación de la sangre; **pulmonary** ___ / ___ pulmonar; 3. expresión franca de conflictos emocionales internos.

ventilator *n.* ventilador; respirador artificial.

ventral *a.* ventral, abdominal, rel. al vientre o a la parte anterior del cuerpo humano.

ventricle *n.* ventrículo, cavidad pequeña esp. una estructura del corazón, el cerebro o la laringe; **fourth** ___ **of the brain** / cuarto ___ cerebral; **larynx** ___ / ___ de la laringe; **lateral** ___ **of the brain** / ___ lateral del cerebro; **left** ___ **of the heart** / ___ izquierdo del corazón; **right** ___ **of the heart** / ___ derecho del corazón; **third** ___ **of the brain** / tercer ___ del cerebro.

ventricular *a.* ventricular, rel. a un ventrículo; ___ **fibrillation** / fibrilación ___; ___ **puncture** / punción ___; ___ **septal defect** / defecto septal ___; ___ **tachycardia** / taquicardia ___ .

ventricular septal defect *n.* defecto del tabique ventricular.

ventriculitis *n.* ventriculitis, infl. de un ventrículo.

ventriculography *n.* ventriculografía. V. **pneumoencephalography**.

ventriculotomy *n.* ventriculotomía, incisión de un ventrículo.

ventrodorsal *a.* ventrodorsal, rel. a las superficies ventral y dorsal.

venule *n.* vénula, vena diminuta que conecta los vasos capilares con venas mayores.

verb *n. gr.* verbo.

verbatim *n. L.* verbatim, al pie de la letra, palabra por palabra.

verdict *n.* veredicto, fallo.

verge *n.* anillo anal; margen; límite; borde; **on the ___ of** / a punto de.

verification *n.* verificación.

verify *v.* comprobar, verificar.

vermicide *n.* vermicida, vermífugo, agente destructor de vermes (gusanos).

vermiform *a.* vermiforme, que tiene la apariencia de un gusano.

vermiform appendix *n.* apéndice vermiforme.

vermilion border *n.* borde bermellón, el margen rosado expuesto del labio.

vermis *n. L.* vermis. 1. gusano parásito; 2. estructura semejante a un gusano tal como el lóbulo medio del cerebelo.

vernal conjunctivitis *n.* conjuntivitis vernal o primaveral, conjuntivitis bilateral acompañada por intensa picazón y fotofobia o evasión de la luz.

vernix *n. L.* barniz; **___ caseosa** / unto sebáceo, secreción que protege la piel del feto.

verruca *n.* (*pl.* **verrucae**) verruga; **plantaris (plantar wart) ___** / **___** plantaris; **seborrheic ___** / **___** seborreica; **filiformis** / **___** filiforme; **___planae juveniles** / **___** planas juveniles; **___ simples** / **___** simple; **vulgaris ___** / **___** vulgaris.

verrucous *a.* verrugoso-a.

versatile *a.* versátil, polivalente; que tiene una variedad de aplicaciones.

version *n.* versión. 1. cambio de dirección de un órgano tal como el útero; 2. cambio de posición del feto en el útero que facilita el parto; **bimanual ___** / **___** bimanual; **bipolar ___** / **___** bipolar; **cephalic ___** / **___** cefálica; **combined ___** / **___** combinada; **external ___** / **___** externa; **spontaneous ___** / **___** espontánea.

vertebra *n.* (*pl.* **vertebrae**) vértebra, cada uno de los treinta y tres huesos que forman la columna vertebral; **cervical ___** / **___** cervical; **coccygeal ___** / **___** coccígea; **lumbar ___** / **___** lumbar; **sacral ___** / **___** sacra; **thoracic ___** / **___** torácica.

vertebral *a.* vertebral, rel. a las vértebras; **___ artery** / arteria **___**; **___ canal** / conducto **___**; **___ ribs** / costillas **___** -es.

vertebrate *n.* vertebrado, que posee columna vertebral o una estructura semejante.

vertebrobasilar *a.* vertebrobasilar, rel. a las arterias vertebral y basilar; **___ circulatory**

disorders / trastornos **___** -es de la circulación; **___ insufficiency** / insuficiencia **___** .

vertex *n.* (*pl.* **vertices**) vértice. 1. cúspide de una estructura, tal como el punto extremo de la cabeza; 2. punto en que concurren los lados de un ángulo.

vertical *a.* 1. vertical, de posición erecta; 2. rel. al vértice; **-ly** *adv.* verticalmente.

vertiginous *a.* vertiginoso-a, rel. al vértigo.

vertigo *n.* vértigo, sensación de rotación en la que se cree que uno gira alrededor del mundo exterior o que éste gira alrededor de uno; **labyrinthine ___** / **___** laberíntico.

verumontanitis *f.* verumontanitis, infl. del verumontanum.

verumontanum *n. L.* verumontanum, elevación en la uretra en el punto de entrada de los conductos seminales.

vesical *a.* vesical, rel. a una vejiga o semejante a ella.

vesication *n.* vesicación 1. formación de ampollas; 2. una ampolla.

vesicle *n.* vesícula. 1. pequeña ampolla; 2. bolsa pequeña de la capa exterior de la piel que contiene líquido seroso.

vesicoureteral *a.* vesicoureteral, rel. a la vejiga urinaria y el uréter.

vesicovaginal *a.* vesicovaginal, rel. a la vejiga urinaria y la vagina.

vesicular *a.* vesicular, rel. a las vesículas.

vessel *n.* vaso, conducto o canal portador de un fluido tal como la sangre y la linfa; **blood ___** / **___** sanguíneo; **collateral ___** / **___** colateral; **great ___ -s** / grandes **___** -s; **lymphatic ___** / **___** linfático.

vestibular *a.* vestibular, rel. a un vestíbulo; **___ bulb** / bulbo **___**; **___ nerve** / nervio **___** .

vestibule *n.* vestíbulo, cavidad que da acceso a un conducto.

vestige *n.* vestigio, resto de una estructura que en una etapa previa de la especie o el embrión, tuvo un desarrollo completo.

vestigial *a.* vestigial, rel. a vestigio; rudimentario-a.

vet *n. pop.* veterinario-a.

veterinarian *n.* veterinario-a, persona especializada en veterinaria; *a.* veterinario-a, rel. a la veterinaria.

veterinary medicine *n.* veterinaria, ciencia que trata de la prevención y cura de enfermedades y lesiones de animales, esp. domésticos.

via *n. L.* vía, tracto, conducto.

viability *n.* cualidad de ser viable.

viable *a.* viable, capaz de sobrevivir, término que se usa gen. en referencia al feto o al recién nacido.

viaduct *n.* viaducto.

vial *n.* frasco, ampolleta.

vibration *n.* vibración, oscilación.

vibrative, vibratory *a.* vibratorio-a, que produce vibración u oscila; ___ **sense** / sentido ___ .

vicarious *a.* vicario-a, que asume el lugar de otro.

vice *n.* vicio; falta, defecto.

vicinity *n.* proximidad, vecindad; barrio.

vicious *a.* [*ridden by vice*] vicioso-a, depravado-a; **-ly** *adv.* viciosamente, malvadamente.

victim *n.* víctima.

vide *n. L.* véase.

video *n.* video; ___ **tape** / videocinta.

view *n.* vista; **in** ___ **of** / en vista de; *v.* mirar, examinar.

viewpoint *n.* punto de vista.

vigil *n.* vigilia. 1. estado de respuesta consciente a un estímulo; 2. insomnio.

vigilance *n.* vigilancia, estado alerta o de atención.

vigor *n.* vigor, fortaleza.

vigorous *a.* vigoroso-a; fuerte; **-ly** *adv.* vigorosamente.

villous *a.* velloso-a, velludo-a.

villus *n.* (*pl.* **villi**) vellosidad, vello, proyección filiforme que crece en una superficie membranosa; **aracnoid** ___ / ___ aracnoidea; **chorionic** ___ / ___ -es coriónicas; **intestinal** ___ / ___ intestinal.

vinegar *n.* vinagre.

violaceous *a.* violáceo-a.

violate *v.* violar, abusar sexualmente.

violence *n.* violencia.

violent *a.* violento-a.

violet *n.* color violeta; *a.* violeta.

viper *n.* víbora.

viral *a.* viral, rel. a un virus; ___ **arthritis** / artritis ___; ___ **croup** / crup ___; ___ **gastroenteritis** / gastroenteritis ___; ___ **hemorrhagic fever** / fiebre hemorrágica ___; ___ **hepatitis** / hepatitis ___; ___ **pneumonia** / neumonía ___; ___ **replication** / replicación ___; ___ **upper respiratory infection** / infección ___ del sistema respiratorio superior.

viremia *n.* viremia, presencia de un virus en la sangre.

virgin *n.* virgen. 1. sustancia sin contaminación; 2. persona que no ha realizado el acto sexual.

virginal *a.* virginal.

virginity *n.* virginidad.

virile *a.* viril, varonil.

virility *n.* virilidad. 1. potencia sexual; 2. estado de poseer características masculinas.

virilization *n.* virilización, masculinización, proceso por el cual se desarrollan en la mujer características masculinas gen. debido a un trastorno hormonal o al suplemento artificial de hormonas masculinas.

virion *n.* virión, partícula viral madura que constituye la forma extracelular infecciosa de un virus.

virology *n.* virología, ciencia que estudia los virus.

virtual *a.* virtual, de existencia aparente, no real.

virulence *n.* virulencia. 1. poder de un organismo de causar determinadas enfermedades en el huésped; 2. cualidad o estado de ser virulento.

virulent *a.* virulento-a, nocivo-a, extremadamente tóxico.

virus *n.* virus, microorganismo ultramicroscópico capaz de causar enfermedades infecciosas; **attenuated** ___ / ___ atenuado; **Cocsackie** ___ / ___ de Cocsackie; **cytomegalic** ___ / ___ citomegálico; **ECHO** ___ / ___ ECHO; **enteric** ___ / ___ entérico; **herpes** ___ / ___ herpético; **pox** ___ / ___ variólico o de Pox; **respiratory syncytial** ___ / ___ sincitial respiratorio; **tumor** ___ / ___ oncogénico.

viscera *n., pl.* vísceras, órganos internos del cuerpo, esp. del abdomen.

visceral *a.* visceral, rel. a las vísceras.

visceromegaly *n.* visceromegalia, agrandamiento anormal de una víscera.

viscosity *n.* viscosidad, cualidad de ser viscoso, esp. la propiedad de los líquidos de no fluir libremente debido a la fricción de las moléculas.

viscous *a.* viscoso-a, gelatinoso-a, pegajoso-a.

viscus *n. L.* (*pl.* **viscera**) víscera.

visible *a.* visible, aparente, evidente; **-ly** *adv.* visiblemente, evidentemente; aparentemente.

vision *n.* visión. 1. sentido de la vista; 2. capacidad de percibir los objetos por la acción de la luz a través de los órganos visuales y los centros cerebrales con que se relacionan. See chart on page 560.

vision	visión
achromatic	acromática
binocular	binocular
blurred	nublada
central	central
chromatic	cromática
distance	a distancia
double // diplopia	doble // diplopia
in tunnel	en túnel
monocular	monocular
night	nocturna
photopic	fotopsia
stocopic	estocópica

visit *n.* visita; *v.* visitar, ir de visita.

visiting hours *n.* horas de visita.

visual *a.* visual, rel. a la visión; ___ **acuity** / acuidad ___; ___ **field** / campo ___ .

visualization, imagery *n.* visualización, proceso de crear imágenes como ayuda al tratamiento de curación.

visualize *v.* visualizar. 1. crear una imagen visual de algo; 2. hacer visible, tal como copiar la imagen de un órgano en una radiografía.

vital *a.* vital, rel. a la vida o esencial en el mantenimiento de la misma; ___ **capacity** / capacidad ___; ___ **signs** / signos ___ -es; ___ **statistics** / estadistica demográfica.

vitality *n.* vitalidad. 1. cualidad de vivir; 2. vigor mental o físico.

vitalize *v.* vitalizar, dar vida; reanimar.

vitamin *n.* vitamina, uno de los compuestos orgánicos que se encuentran en pequeñas cantidades en los alimentos y que son esenciales en el desarrollo y funcionamiento del organismo.

vitaminic *a.* vitamínico-a, rel. a las vitaminas.

vitiate *v.* viciar; infectar.

vitiligo *n.* vitiligo, trastorno epidérmico benigno que se manifiesta con manchas blancas en partes expuestas del cuerpo.

vitrectomy *n.* vitrectomía, extirpación de todo o parte del humor vítreo del ojo. Se recomienda a veces en casos avanzados de retinopatía proliferativa diabética.

vitreous *n.* fluído semejante a gelatina que llena el interior del ojo; vítreo-a, vidrioso-a, casi transparente, hialino; ___ **chamber** / cámara ___; ___ **body** / cuerpo ___; ___ **humor** / humor ___ .

vivifying *a.* vivificador, vivificante.

vivisection *n.* vivisección, corte o sección realizada en animales con fines investigativos.

vocabulary *n.* vocabulario.

vocal *a.* vocal, oral, rel. a la voz o producido por ella.

vocal cords *n., pl.* cuerdas vocales; órgano esencial de la voz; **false** ___ / ___ superiores o falsas; **true** ___ / ___ inferiores o verdaderas.

vocalization *n.* vocalización.

vocation *n.* vocación, profesión.

voice *n.* voz.

voiced *a.* dicho-a, expresado-a; producido-a por la voz.

void *a.* nulo-a, vacío-a; inválido-a, sin efecto; *v.* anular, invalidar; evacuar, eliminar.

volatile *a.* volátil, que se evapora fácilmente.

volition *n.* volición, voluntad, poder de determinación.

Volkman's contracture *n.* Volkmann, contractura de, contractura isquémica como resultado de una necrosis irreversible del tejido muscular, vista gen. en el antebrazo y la mano.

volume *n.* volumen. 1. espacio ocupado por una sustancia o un cuerpo; 2. cantidad, intensidad; **blood** ___ / ___ sanguíneo; **expiratory air reserve** ___ / ___ de reserva expiratoria o aire de reserva; **heart** ___ / ___ cardíaco; **residual** ___ / ___ residual; **stroke** ___ / ___ sistólico; **tidal** ___ / ___ de ventilación pulmonar.

volumetric *a.* volumétrico, rel. a la medida de volumen.

voluntary *a.* voluntario-a; ___ **muscle** / músculo ___ .

volunteer *a.* voluntario-a.

voluptuous *a.* voluptuoso-a, provocador-a, sensual; **-ly** *adv.* voluptuosamente.

volvulus *a.* vólvulo, obstrucción intestinal causada por torsión o anudamiento del intestino en torno al mesenterio.

vomer *n.* vómer, hueso impar que forma parte del tabique medio de las fosas nasales.

vomit *n.* vómito; *v.* vomitar.

vomiting *n.* manifestación de vómitos.

vomitive *n.* vomitivo.

Von Gierke disease *n.* Von Gierke, enfermedad de, almacenamiento anormal de glucógeno.

Von Recklinghausen's disease *n.* enfermedad de Von Recklinghausen. V. **neurofibromatosis.**

Von Willebrand's disease *n.* Von Willebrand, enfermedad de, desorden hereditario de la sangre caracterizado por episodios hemorrágicos gen. en las membranas mucosas.

voracity *n.* voracidad.

vortex *n.* (*pl.* **vortices**) vórtice, estructura de forma espiral.

voucher *n.* comprobante.

vowel *n.* vocal.

voyeur *n., Fr.* voyeur, persona que practica voyeurismo.

voyeurism *n.* voyeurismo, perversión sexual por la cual la contemplación de actos u órganos sexuales induce erotismo.

vulnerability *n.* vulnerabilidad.

vulnerable *a.* vulnerable, propenso a accidentes o enfermedades.

vulva *n. L.* vulva, conjunto de los órganos femeninos externos del aparato genital.

vulval *a.* vulvar, rel. a la vulva.

vulvectomy *n.* vulvectomía, excisión de la vulva.

vulvitis *n.* vulvitis, infl. de la vulva.

vulvovaginal *a.* vulvovaginal, rel. a la vulva y la vagina.

vulvovaginitis *n.* vulvovaginitis, infl. de la vulva y la vagina.

V

W

W *abbr.* **water** / agua; **weight** / peso.
waddle *n.* marcha tambaleante, andar anserino.
wail *v.* lamentarse; gemir.
waist *n.* cintura; talle.
waistband *n.* cinto, cinturón.
waistline *n.* cintura.
wait *v.* esperar, aguardar; **to ___ on** / servir, atender a.
waiting *n.* espera; demora; **___ room** / sala de ___ .
waive *v.* diferir, posponer.
wake *vi.* despertar; **to___up** / despertar; despertarse.
wakefulness *n.* dificultad para dormir, insomnio.
Waldenstrom's macroglobulinemia *n.* Waldenstrom, macroglobulinemia de, síndrome hemorrágico con manifestaciones de anemia y adenomegalia.
walk *n.* paseo; caminata; *v.* caminar, andar;**to ___ up and down** / caminar de un lado a otro.
walker *n.* andador, andaderas, aparato que se usa para ayudar a caminar.
walking *n.* el acto de caminar; **___pneumonia** / neumonía errante.
wall *n.* pared; tabique; **___ tooth** / diente molar.
walled-off *a.* encapsulado-a.
walleye *n.* 1. estrabismo divergente, exotropía; 2. leucoma corneal.
wander *v.* vagar; [*to lose one's way*] desviarse, perderse, extraviarse.
wandering *a.* errante, errático-a; desviado-a; **___ cell** / célula; **___ goiter** / bocio móvil; **___ pain** / dolor ___; **___ tooth** / diente desviado.
want *n.* necesidad, falta, carencia; *v.* querer, desear; necesitar; carecer de.
war *n.* guerra.
ward *n.* sala de hospital; **isolation___** / sala de aislamiento; **___ diet** / dieta hospitalaria; **___ of the state** / bajo custodia, bajo tutela del estado.
warm *a.* caluroso-a; caliente; [*lukewarm*] tibio-a; [*character*] afectuoso-a, expresivo-a; *v.* **to be ___** / tener calor, [*not very hot but feverish*] tener destemplanza; [*weather*] hacer calor; **to ___ to** / simpatizar con; **to ___ up** / calentar; **-ly** *adv.* afectuosamente, con entusiasmo.

warm-up *n.* [*physical fitness*] calentamiento.
warn *v.* prevenir, advertir, avisar.
warning *n.* advertencia; aviso; [*hard lesson*] escarmiento; **___ signal** / advertencia; señal premonitoria; **___ symptoms** / síntomas premonitorios.
warp *n.* torcedura; torcimiento; *v.* torcer; retorcer; perder la forma.
warranty *n.* garantía.
wart *n.* verruga. V. **verruca**.
warty *a.* verrugoso-a, rel. a verrugas.
was *pret.* of **to be**.
wash *n.* lavado, baño, lavadura; **mouth- ___** / enjuague; *v.* lavar; **to ___ away** / quitar con una lavadura; [*oneself*] lavarse.
washbasin *n.* lavamanos, palangana, vasija.
washcloth *n.* toallita de manos; paño de lavarse.
washed-out *a.* descolorido-a, desteñido-a.
washstand *n.* lavabo, lavamanos.
wasp *n.* avispa; **___ sting** / picadura de ___ .
Wasserman test *n.* prueba de Wasserman, análisis serológico de la sífilis.
waste *n.* desperdicio, residuo, gasto inútil; merma, pérdida; **___ of time** / pérdida de tiempo; *v.* desperdiciar, desgastar, malgastar; **to ___ away** / demacrarse, consumirse.
wastebasket *n.* cesto de basura.
wasted *a.* desgastado-a, malgastado-a; [*person*] demacrado-a; consumido-a.
wasting *n.* agotamiento, consunción, pérdida de funciones vitales.
watch *n.* reloj de pulsera o bolsillo; vigilia; *v.* cuidar, observar, esperar; tener cuidado; **to ___ one's step** / cuidarse, tener cuidado; **___out!** / ¡Cuidado!
water *n.* agua, líquidos del cuerpo; infusión;**___ bag** / bolsa de ___; **___ bed** / cama de, colchón de ___; **___ blister** / ampolla acuosa; **___ -cooled** / enfriado-a por ___; **___ faucet** / grifo, pila, llave; **___ intake** / ingestión o toma de ___; **___ level** / nivel del ___; **___ pill** / diurético; **___ pollution** / contaminación del ___; **___ purification** / purificación del ___; **___ -tight** / hermético, impermeable; **___ -soluble** / soluble en ___, que se disuelve en ___; **___ supply** / abastecimiento de ___; *v.* **to be in deep ___** / tener dificultades; **to give ___** / dar ___; **to wash with ___** / lavar con ___ [*plants*]; **to ___** / regar; humedecer; mojar.
watered *a.* aguado-a; diluido-a.
water-electrolyte balance *n.* equilibrio hidroelectrolítico.

water-electrolyte imbalance *n.* desequilibrio hidroelectrolítico

water-hammer pulse *n.* pulso en martillo de agua.

Waterhouse-Friderichsen syndrome *n.* Waterhouse-Friderichsen, síndrome de, hemorragia aguda en las glándulas suprarrenales con hemorragia en la piel asociada a un repentino choque bacteriogénico agudo.

water intoxication *n.* intoxicación acuosa, retención excesiva de agua.

watery *a.* acuoso-a, aguado-a, húmedo-a; ___ **eyes** / ojos llorosos.

wave *n.* onda, ondulación; ademán de la mano. 1. movimiento o vibración ondulante que tiene una dirección fija y prosigue en una curva de ondulación; 2. representación gráfica de una actividad tal como la obtenida en un encefalograma; **brain** ___ **-s** / ___ **-s** cerebrales; **electromagnetic** ___ **-s** / ___ **-s** electromagnéticas; **excitation** ___ / ___ de excitación; **high-frequency** ___ / ___ de alta frecuencia; **short** ___ / ___ corta; **ultrasonic** ___ **-s** / ___ **-s** ultrasónicas; ___ **length** / longitud de ___; *v.* hacer señales o ademanes con la mano.

waved *a.* ondulado-a, ondeado-a.

wavy *a.* ondulado-a.

wax *n.* cera. 1. cera producida por abejas; 2. secreción cerosa; **ear** ___ / ___ del oído; 3. cerumen, sustancia de origen animal, vegetal o mineral que se emplea en preparaciones de pomadas y ceratos; **depilatory** ___ / ___ depilatoria.

waxing *n.* el acto de encerar, aplicar o frotar cera a la piel.

waxy *a.* ceroso-a, céreo-a; [*applied wax*] encerado-a.

way *n.* vía, camino; pasaje; **by the** ___ / a propósito; **in no** ___ / de ningún modo; **out of the** ___ / fuera de curso, desviado-a; lejano-a; **that** ___ / por allí; **the other** ___ **around** / por el contrario; ___ **of life** / manera de vivir; costumbres; ___ **out** / salida; *v.* **to make** ___ **for** / abrir paso.

weak *a.* débil, flojo-a, endeble, enclenque; poco fuerte.

weaken *v.* debilitar; desfallecer; debilitarse; deteriorarse.

weakness *n.* debilidad, debilitamiento, flojera, flaqueza.

wealth *n.* riqueza, abundancia.

wealthy *a.* rico-a, acaudalado-a, adinerado-a.

wean *n.* destetar, quitar el pecho de la madre.

weaning *n.* destete.

weanling *n.* el, la recién destetado-a, desmamado-a.

wear *n.* uso, gasto, deterioro, deteriorización; *vr.* usar, llevar puesto; desgastar; **to** ___ **out** / gastar; gastarse; desgastarse.

wearing *n.* desgaste; pérdida; decaimiento.

weary *a.* cansado-a, fatigado-a.

weather *n.* [*climate*] tiempo; ___ **forecasting** / pronóstico del ___ .

web *n.* red, membrana; **pulmonary arterial** ___ / ___ -es de membranas arteriopulmonares.

webbed *n.* unido-a por una telilla o membrana.

wedge *n.* cuña.

Wegener's granulomatosis *n.* Wegener, granulomatosis de, enfermedad caracterizada por la formación de granulomas en las arterias que afecta las fosas nasales, los pulmones y los riñones.

weight *n.* peso; **birth** ___ / ___ al nacer; ___ **gain** / aumento de ___; ___ **loss** / pérdida de ___ .

welcome *n.* bienvenida; *a.* bienvenido-a; agradable; deseado-a; *v.* dar la bienvenida, recibir con agrado; **You are** ___ / De nada; para servirle; no hay de que; **a** ___ **surprise** / una sorpresa agradable.

welfare *n.* bien, bienestar; salud; asistencia; ___ **benefits** / beneficios de asistencia social; ___ **work** / trabajo de asistencia social; ___ **worker** / trabajador-a social;

well *a.* bueno-a; en buena salud; **well-being** / bienestar; *adv.* bien, favorablemente, felizmente; **all is** ___ / todo va bien.

welt *n.* verdugón, roncha.

Western Blot, immunoblot *n.* Western Blot, "inmunoblot", prueba subsecuente para confirmar la infección por el virus VIH, en pacientes con evidencia de exposición, indicada por un ensayo enzimático inmuno-sorbente (ELISA).

West Nile Virus *n.* Virus del Nilo Occidental, enfermedad causada por la picadura de un mosquito infectado por un pájaro. Es una epidemia que se manifiesta durante el verano gen. en América del Norte. Síntomas severos incluyen fiebre alta, dolor de cabeza, cuello rígido, desorientación, temblores, convulsiones, alguna pérdida de la visión, entumecimiento y parálisis; un 20% de las personas infectadas sufren síntomas benignos.

wet *a.* mojado-a, humedecido-a; *v.* mojar, humedecer.

wet dream *n.* emisión seminal nocturna.
Wharton's duct *n.* conducto de Wharton, conducto excretorio de la glándula submaxilar.
wheal *n.* roncha.
wheat *n.* trigo; ___ **germ** / germen de ___ .
wheel *n.* rueda; *v.* hacer rodar.
wheelchair *n.* silla de ruedas.
wheezing *n.* respiración sibilante.
when *pron.* cuándo; **Since** ___? / ¿Desde ___?; *conj.* cuando; si.
whenever *adv.* cuando quiera; siempre que; ___ **is needed** / siempre que se necesite; ___ **you wish** / siempre que lo desee.
while *adv.* mientras, un rato, algún tiempo; **for a** ___ / temporalmente; **not for a** ___ / por ahora no.
whimper *n.* quejido, lloriqueo; *v.* sollozar, lloriquear.
whine *n.* quejido, gemido, lamento; *v.* gemir, quejarse, lamentarse.
whiplash injury *n.* lesión de latigazo.
Whipple's disease *n.* enfermedad de Whipple, trastorno causado por la acumulación de depósitos lípidos en los tejidos linfáticos e intestinales.
whirlpool bath *n.* baño de remolino.
whisper *n.* susurro, cuchicheo; *v.* susurrar, cuchichear.
whistle *n.* silbido; *v.* silbar.
white *n.* color blanco; ___ **of the egg** / clara de huevo; *a.* blanco-a; ___ **corpuscle** / leucocito, glóbulo ___ .
white-head *n.* comedón cerrado.
whitish *a.* blanquecino-a; blancuzco-a.
white matter *n.* sustancia blanca, tejido nervioso formado en su mayor parte por fibras mielínicas y que constituye el elemento conductor del cerebro y de la médula espinal.
whiteness *n.* blancura.
whole *n.* total, conjunto; **as a** ___ / en conjunto; *a.* todo-a; **the** ___ **day** / todo el día.
wholesome *a.* sano-a, saludable.
whoop *n.* estridor, sonido que caracteriza la respiración después de un ataque de tos ferina.
whooping cough *n.* tos ferina. V. **pertussis**.
whorl *n.* espiral. 1. disposición de fibras en forma esférica, esp. las fibras cardíacas; 2. tipo de huella digital.
wide *a.* ancho-a; **three feet** ___ / tres pies de ancho; amplio-a; extenso-a; ___ **open** / muy abierto; **-ly** *adv.* ampliamente, extensamente.
widen *v.* ensanchar, extender.
widespread *a.* extendido-a; muy difundido-a; general.

widow *n.* viuda.
widower *n.* viudo.
width *n.* anchura, ancho.
wife *n.* esposa.
wig *n.* peluca.
will *n.* voluntad, determinación, deseo; testamento; *v.* querer, ordenar, mandar.
Wilms' tumor *n.* tumor de Wilms, neoplasma del riñón que se desarrolla rápidamente y usu. se ve en la infancia.
Wilson's disease *n.* enfermedad de Wilson, enfermedad hereditaria que se manifiesta con serios trastornos hepáticos y cerebrales.
win *vi.* ganar, vencer.
wind *n.* viento, aire; flato, ventosidad.
windburn *n.* quemadura por el viento.
window *n.* ventana.
windpipe *n.* tráquea; *pop.* gaznate.
wine *n.* vino.
wing *n.* ala.
wink *n.* pestañeo; *v.* pestañear.
winter *n.* invierno.
wire *n.* alambre.
wisdom teeth *n.* cordales, muelas del juicio.
wise *n.* cuerdo, prudente.
with *conj.* con.
withdraw *vi.* retirar, suprimir, descontinuar; privar de; **to** ___ **a product from the market** / descontinuar o suprimir un producto.
withdrawal *n.* supresión, retracción; introversión; privación.
withdrawal syndrome *n.* síndrome de privación de una droga adictiva como resultado de la supresión de la misma.
withdrawal treatment *n.* tratamiento de desintoxicación.
within *prep.* dentro de, en el interior de; a distancia de; al alcance de; cerca de; ___ **an hour** / ___ una hora.
without *prep.* sin, falto de, fuera de; *adv.* fuera, afuera.
withstand *vi.* resistir, soportar, sufrir.
woman *n.* (*pl.* **women**) mujer.
womb *n.* matriz, útero. V. **uterus**.
wonder *n.* maravilla, prodigio, admiración; admirarse, asombrarse.
wonderful *a.* maravilloso-a, asombroso-a, estupendo-a, excelente.
wood *n.* madera.
wool sorter's disease *n.* enfermedad de los cargadores de lana. anthrax.
word *n.* vocablo, palabra, término.
work *n.* trabajo, empleo, ocupación; *v.* trabajar.

workshop *n.* laboratorio o taller de trabajo.

workup *n.* 1. preparación del paciente para la aplicación de un tratamiento; 2. obtención de los datos pertinentes a un caso.

worm *n.* lombriz, gusano.

wormlike *a.* vermicular, vermiforme.

worsen *v.* agravarse.

wound *n.* herida, lesión; **contused** ___ / ___ contusa, lesión subcutánea; **gunshot** ___ / ___ de bala; **penetrating** ___ / ___ penetrante; **puncture** ___ / ___ de punción, con un instrumento afilado; ___ **debridement** / desbridamiento de ___ .

wrinkle *n.* arruga; *v.* arrugarse.

wrinkled *a.* arrugado-a.

wrist *n.* carpo, muñeca. **carpus;** ___ **drop** / muñeca caída.

write *vi.* escribir.

writing *n.* escritura, acto de escribir.

wrong *n.* error, falsedad; *a.* erróneo-a; incorrecto-a; ___ **treatment** / el tratamiento equivocado___; **the** ___ **side** / el lado afectado, el lado incorrecto; *v.* **to be** ___ / no tener razón; estar equivocado-a; **to go** ___ / [*to fail to understand*] interpretar mal; equivocarse; **-ly** *adv.* mal; incorrectamente, equivocadamente.

w

X

X *abbr.* **xanthine** / xantina;

xanthelasma *n.* xantelasma, manchas o placas amarillentas que aparecen gen. alrededor de los párpados.

xanthic *a.* amarillento-a, rel. a la xantina.

xanthine *n.* xantina, grupo de substancias tales como la cafeína estimulantes del sistema nervioso central y del corazón.

xanthochromia *n.* xantocromía, color amarillento visto en placas de la piel o en el líquido cefalorraquídeo.

xanthochromic *a.* xantocrómico-a, de apariencia amarillenta o relacionado-a con la xantocromía.

xanthoderma *n.* xantoderma, color amarillento de la piel.

xanthoma *n.* xantoma, formación tumoral de placas o nódulos en la piel; **diabetic** ___ / ___ diabético; **disseminated** ___ / ___ diseminado; **eruptive** ___ / ___ eruptivo; **planar** ___ / ___ plano; ___ **tendinosum** / ___ tendinoso; ___ **tuberosum** / ___ tuberoso.

xanthomatosis *n.* xantomatosis, presencia de múltiples xantomas en la piel.

xanthosis *n.* xantosis, descoloración amarillenta de la piel debida a ingestión excesiva de alimentos tales como la zanahoria y la calabaza.

x chromosome *n.* cromosoma x, cromosoma sexual diferencial que determina las características del sexo femenino.

xenograft *n.* xenoinjerto; ___ **rejection** / rechazo de ___ .

xenon *n.* xenón, elemento gaseoso, radioisótopo que se encuentra en pequeñas cantidades en el aire atmosférico.

xenon-133 *n.* xenón 133, radioisótopo de xenón usado en la fotoescanción del pulmón.

xenophobia *n.* xenofobia, temor excesivo o aversión a algo o a alguien extraño o extranjero.

xenotransplant *n.* xenotransplante, proceso de transplantar un órgano o parte de una especie a otra.

xeroderma *n.* xeroderma, piel excesivamente seca.

xerography *n.* xerografía. V. **xeroradiography.**

xeromammography *n.* xeromamografía, xerorradiografía de la mama.

xerophthalmia *n.* xeroftalmia, sequedad excesiva de la conjuntiva causada por deficiencia de vitamina A.

xeroradiography *n.* xerorradiografía, registro de imágenes electrostáticas por medio de un proceso en seco usando placas cubiertas con un elemento metálico tal como el selenio.

xerosis *n.* xerosis, sequedad anormal presente en la piel, ojos y membranas mucosas.

xerostomia *n.* xerostomía, excesiva sequedad en la boca debida a una deficiencia de secreción salival.

xiphoid *a.* xifoide, en forma de espada, similar al apéndice xifoide o ensiforme.

xiphoid process *n.* apéndice xifoide, formación cartilaginosa que se une al cuerpo del esternón.

X-linked *a.* rel. a caracteres genéticos que se relacionan con el cromosoma x.

x-rays *n.* rayos-x (equis), radiografía. 1. ondas electromagnéticas de alta energía de radiación que se usan para penetrar tejidos y órganos del cuerpo y registrar densidades en una placa o pantalla; 2. placa fotográfica o fluorescente que obtiene la imagen de estructuras internas del organismo.

y

Y *abbr.* **y/o** year-old / de un año de edad.

yaw *n.* lesión primaria de la frambesia.

yawn *n.* bostezo; *v.* bostezar.

yaws *n., pl.* frambesia.

Y chromosome *n.* cromosoma Y, cromosoma sexual diferencial que determina las características sexuales del sexo masculino.

year *n.* año; **at the beginning of the** ___ / a principios de ___ ; **at the end of the** ___ / al final del ___ ; **every** ___ / todos los ___ -s; **last** ___ / el ___ pasado; **New Year** / Año Nuevo; **once a** ___ / una vez al ___ ; **-ly** *adv.* anualmente.

years of potential life lost *n.* años perdidos de vida potencial. Medida potencial del impacto en un individuo de enfermedades y fuerzas letales sociales. Se establece teniendo en cuenta los años que la persona pudo haber vivido si una muerte prematura debido a heridas mortales, cáncer, enfermedades del corazón, etc. no hubiera ocurrido.

yeast *n.* levadura, hongo diminuto capaz de provocar fermentación que se usa en la nutrición como fuente de vitaminas y proteínas.

yell *n.* grito, alarido; *v.* gritar.

yellow *n.* color amarillo; *a.* amarillo-a.

yellow atrophy of the liver *n.* atrofia amarilla del hígado.

yellow bile *n.* bilis amarilla, uno de los cuatro humores del cuerpo según la antiguedad, que produce irritabilidad.

yellow body *n.* cuerpo amarillo. V. **corpus luteum**.

yellow fever *n.* fiebre amarilla, enfermedad endémica de regiones tropicales debida a un virus que es transmitido por la picadura del mosquito hembra *Aedes Aegypti* y que se manifiesta con fiebre, ictericia y albuminuria.

yellow fibers *n.* fibras amarillas. *Syn.* **elastic fibers.**

yellow hepatization *n.* hepatización de etapa final, en la cual las exudaciones se han convertido virulentas.

yellow jack *n. pop.* fiebre amarilla.

yellow spot *n.* mácula lútea.

yellowish *a.* amarillento-a.

yersinia *n.* yersinia. gene del tipo de especie *Yersinia pestis,* bacteria parasítica en humanos, que no forma esporas y contiene bastoncillos de células ovoides, gramma negativas.

yesterday *adv.* ayer.

yet *conj.* todavía; no obstante, sin embargo.

yield *n.* rendimiento; producción; *v.* producir, rendir.

Y ligament *n.* ligamento iliofemoral.

yoga *n.* yoga, sistema de creencias y práctica de meditación y autodominio a través del cual se trata de alcanzar un estado de unión entre el yo y el universo.

yogurt *n.* yogur, leche fermentada por la acción del *Lactobacillus bulgaricus* a la que se le atribuyen valores nutritivos y terapéuticos.

yolk *n.* 1. yema del huevo; 2. conjunto de sustancias que nutren al embrión.

young *a.* joven; juvenil.

young at heart *n.* de corazón joven (aunque la edad cronológica no lo muestre).

youngish *a.* de aspecto joven.

youngster *n.* jovencito-a, muchacho-a.

youth *n.* juventud, mocedad.

youthful *a.* juvenil, joven; **to look** ___ / parecer joven.

Z

Z *abbr.* **z zero** / cero; **zone** / zona.

zero population growth *n.* crecimiento cero de población, condición demográfica que existe en un período de tiempo determinado en el cual la población permanece estable, sin aumentar ni disminuir.

zinc *n.* zinc, elemento metálico cristalino de propiedad astringente.

zinc ointment *n.* pomada de zinc.

Zollinger-Ellison syndrome *n.* síndrome de Zollinger-Ellison, condición manifestada por hipersecreción gástrica, hiperacidez y ulceración péptica del estómago e intestino delgado.

zona *n.* zona. 1. área o capa específica; 2. herpes zóster.

zone *n.* zona, estructura anatómica en forma de banda; **comfort** ___ / ___ de bienestar; **equivalence** ___ / ___ de equivalencia; **gliding** ___ / ___ de deslizamiento; **respiratory** ___ / ___ respiratoria; **transition** ___ / ___ de transición; ___ **radiata** / ___ radiada.

zoogenous *a.* zoógeno-a, que se adquiere o deriva de animales.

zoograft *n.* zooinjerto, injerto que proviene de tejido animal.

zoophobia *n.* zoofobia, ansiedad y miedo irracional hacia los animales.

zootoxin *n.* zootoxina, sustancia venenosa que procede de un animal como el veneno de la serpiente.

zoster *n.* zóster. V. **herpes zoster, shingles**.

zoster ophthalmicus *n.* zóster oftálmico, infección herpética del ojo, que afecta esp. el nervio óptico.

zygoma *n.* cigoma, zigoma, prominencia ósea que forma un arco en la unión del hueso malar y el temporal.

zygomatic *a.* cigomático-a, rel. al cigoto; ___ **arch** / arco ___; ___ **bone** / hueso ___; ___ **egg** / óvulo ___ .

zygote *n.* cigoto, óvulo fertilizado, célula fecundada por la unión de dos gametos.

Appendix A
•Communicating with Patients
•Medications
•Emergencies and Trauma

Apéndice A
•Communicación con los pacientes
•Medicamentos
•Emergencias y trauma

Guide to Questions and Answers in English and Spanish

The following Appendices from A-E (pp. 569–769) contain questions and answers, charts, illustrations, and vital medical material to help the health care providers and staff at health institutions to establish a better communication with their Hispanic patients. By including medical information with added lay vocabulary spoken daily in a clinical facility the health provider can obtain the necessary information to engage in basic dialogues with their patients.

Following these questionnaires as a guide, you may take them as a model to write your own. Take the following steps to make a successful interview or dialogue. Keep in mind that the interviewer should identify the patient by his or her name, personalizing the interview and creating a friendly rapport.

1. Making a statement that requires a Yes/No answer. This type of question/answer, limits the respondent to answer in a negative or positive, e.g.,
   Do you have Medicare? ____Yes ____No

2. Some questions can be expanded requiring more information from the interviewer.
   Do you have children? ____Yes ____No and then, if the answer is Yes, continue to question x number:
   How many? I have __children

3. If a limited answer from the patient is needed, provide a format with multiple answers, and ask the respondent to select the answer from multiple answers, a response that is the most convenient and accurate. Choosing common useful choices:
   Instruction: Select the word(s) that describes how you feel now.
   I feel
   __completely well
   __better
   __so-so
   __ill
   __worse

Guía de preguntas y repuestas en inglés y español, guía de cuestionarios

Los siguientes apéndices de A-E (pp. 597–796) contienen cuestionarios, cuadros, ilustraciones y material médico vital para ayudar a los proveedores de atención médica y su personal en las instituciones de salud a establecer una mejor comunicación con los pacientes hispano-hablantes. Al incluir información médica así como vocabulario que se usa a diario en las facilidades médicas, el proveedor de atención médica puede obtener la referencia necesaria para entablar diálogos básicos con sus pacientes.

Tomando estos cuestionarios como guía, usted puede valerse de ellos para crear su propio modelo. Tome los siguientes pasos para poder llevar a cabo un diálogo o una entrevista con éxito.

El / la entrevistador-a debe identificar al / a la paciente por su nombre propio, personalizando la entrevista y así creando una relación amistosa.

1. Haciendo la pregunta en forma tal que ésta requiera solamente una respuesta de **Sí/No**. Este tipo de pregunta /respuesta limita a la persona a responder en forma positiva o negativa. Por ejemplo:
   ¿Tiene usted Medicare?__Sí __No

2. Algunas preguntas se pueden expandir para obtener mayor información del entrevistado:
   ¿Tiene usted hijos? __Sí __ No y si la respuesta es **Sí,** esto puede llevar a una nueva pregunta / respuesta:
   ¿Cuántos? Tengo___hijos.

3. Si se requiere una respuesta limitada del paciente, o se le quiere facilitar una respuesta, provea un formato con selecciones múltiples, y pídale al/a e trev stado-a que seleccione la repuesta más apropriad .
   Instrucción:
   Seleccione las palabras que mejor describan como usted se siente ahora. Me siento
   __completamente bien
   __mejor
   __regular, más o menos
   __mal
   __peor

4. Other questionnaires require answers that will give the interviewer information with needed facts about the patient. Ask a question and then, a follow-up question:
a) Factual information about the patient, social and economic status, medical insurance, etc. What do you do?
__I am a teacher
__I am a carpenter
__I work in an office
__I am a mechanic
__Other
b) Providing information such as symptoms and details that would describe the patient's condition
__Did you get hurt at work?
__Do you have pain?
__Where is the pain?
__On the right side?
__On the left side?
__Does it hurt you more now?

This type of dialogue will provide the interviewer with the information he/she needs, and will give the patient the opportunity to express the reason of his visit in an easy and simple manner.

4. Otras preguntas requieren respuestas que pueden proveer al investigador datos que necesita saber sobre el /la paciente. Haga una pregunta seguida de otra pertinente a:
a) información factual del paciente, estado social y económico, seguro médico, etc. e.g.
¿Cuál es su trabajo?
__ Soy maestro-a
__ Soy carpintero
__ Trabajo en una oficina
__ Soy mecánico-a
__ Otro
b) provea síntomas u otros detalles que puedan ayudar a describir la condición del paciente.
__ ¿Se lastimó usted en el trabajo?
__ ¿Tiene dolor?
__ ¿Dónde es el dolor
__ ¿En el lado derecho?
__ ¿En el lado izquierdo?
__ ¿Le duele más ahora?

Este tipo de diálogo le proveerá al entrevistador la información que necesita y al entrevistado le facilitará comunicar la razón de su visita de una manera simple y sin gran esfuerzo.

Interrogative Words

Palabras Interrogativas

ENGLISH	SPANISH
whom?	¿a quién, a quiénes?
which?	¿cuál, cuáles?
when?	¿cuándo?
how many? how much?	¿cuánto?, ¿cuántos?, ¿cuántas?
where from?	¿de dónde?
whose?	¿de quién, de quiénes?
where?	¿dónde?
why?	¿por qué?
what?	¿qué?
when?	¿cuándo?
where?	¿dónde?
where to?	¿adónde?
where from?	¿de dónde?

who?	¿quién?, ¿quiénes?
whom?	¿a quién?, ¿a quiénes?
which?	¿cuál?, ¿cuáles?
whose?	¿de quién?, ¿de quiénes?
why?	¿por qué?

QUESTIONING THE PATIENT / PREGUNTAS AL PACIENTE

Personal Data   ## Datos personales

ENGLISH	*SPANISH*
The questions are followed by one or more possible answers, other than __**Yes**__**No** and the patient is to choose the one more appropriate or the corresponding one to him or her.	Las siguientes preguntas están se uidas de dos o más posibles respuestas fuera de __**Sí**__**No** y el/la paciente debe escoger la más apropiada o la que mejor le corresponda a él/ella.

Personal Data	**Datos personales**
Name_____	nombre_____
Age____	edad____
Address_____	dirección_____
Family Member_____	familiares_____

1. Are you the patient?	1. ¿Es usted el/la paciente?
2. Who is the patient? __I am. __She is. __My mother is the patient.	2. ¿Quién es el/la paciente? __Soy yo. __Es ella. __Mi madre es la paciente.
3. What is your name? __My name is __John, __Linda.	3. ¿Cómo se llama usted? Me llamo __Juan, __Linda.
4. How old are you? __I am __twenty, __thirty, __seventy-five years old.	4. ¿Cuántos años tiene? Tengo __veinte, __treinta, __setenta y cinco años.
5. How old is the patient? He/she is __forty, __fifty, __seventy-five years of age.	5. ¿Cuántos años tiene el/la paciente? Él/Ella tiene __cuarenta, __cincuenta, __setenta y cinco años.
6. What is your telephone number? It is 323-4197 (three, two, three, four, one, nine, seven).	6. ¿Cuál es su teléfono? 323-4197 (tres, dos, tres, cuatro, uno, nueve, siete)
7. What is your address? My address is 43 N. (forty-three North) Elm.	7. ¿Cuál es su dirección? Mi dirección es 43 N. (cuarenta y tres Norte) de Elm.
8. Is this your permanent address?	8. ¿Es ésta su dirección permanente?
9. What is your present address? It is 789 S. (seven, eight, nine, South) Paseo del Monte.	9. ¿Cuál es su dirección actual? Es 789 S. (siete, ocho, nueve, Sur) Paseo del Monte.
10. How long have you lived at the present address? __three months __one year __five years	10. ¿Qué tiempo hace que vive en su dirección actual? __tres meses __un año __cinco años
11. Are your parents living? __My mother is living. __My father is deceased.	11. Sus padres viven? __Mi madre vive. __Mi padre murió.
12. What is your father's name? Peter Smith.	12. ¿Cómo se llama su padre? __Pedro Smith.

Personal Data

Datos personales

ENGLISH

SPANISH

13. What is your mother's name? __Her name is Rose. __My mother's name is Rose.	13. ¿Cómo se llama su madre? __Su nombre es Rosa. __Mi madre se llama Rosa.
14. Are you __ single? __ married? __ divorced? __ separated? __ living with partner? __ a widow? __ a widower?	14. ¿Es usted __ soltero-a? __ casado-a? __ divorciado-a? __ está separado-a? __ convive con alguien? __ viudo-a?
15. What is your spouse's name? __His name is Henry Pritchard. __Her name is Sylvia Pritchard.	15. ¿Cómo se llama su esposo-a? __Su nombre es Enrique Pastor. __Ella se llama Silvia Pastor.
16. Do you have children? How many? I have __one child, __three children.	16. ¿Tiene hijos? ¿Cuántos? Tengo __un hijo, __tres hijas.
17. Do they live with you?	17. ¿Viven con usted?
18. Do you live alone?	18. ¿Vive solo-a?
19. Can you give us the name, address, and telephone of a person that can be notified in case of an emergency.	19. ¿Nos puede dar el nombre, dirección y teléfono de alguien a quien podamos notificar en caso de emergencia?

Financial Facts

Finanzas y pagos

- ▶ medical insurance
- ▶ occupation
- ▶ paying the bill

- ▶ seguro médico
- ▶ ocupación
- ▶ pago de la cuenta

ENGLISH

SPANISH

1. What is your occupation? __teacher __mechanic __dentist __painter __doctor	1. ¿Cuál es su trabajo o profesión? __maestro-a __mecánico __dentista __pintor __doctor
2. Where do you work? __at home __in a garage __in a warehouse __in an office	2. ¿Dónde trabaja? __en mi casa __en un garaje __en un almacén __en una oficina
3. What is the name and address of your employer? __His name is Mark Smith and his address is 3967 E. (three, nine, six, seven East) Swan.	3. ¿Cuál es el nombre y dirección de la persona para quien trabaja? __Es el señor Marcos Smith y su dirección es 3967 E. (tres, nueve, seis, siete Este) de Swan.
4. What is your Social Security number? __It is 415-493-8765 (four, one, five, four, nine, three, eight, seven, six, five).	4. ¿Cuál es el número de su Seguro Social? __Es el 415-493-8765 (cuatro, uno, cinco, cuatro, nueve, tres, ocho, siete, seis, cinco).
5. Do you receive any workman's compensation?	5. ¿Recibe usted alguna compensación laboral?
6. Are you self-supporting?	6. ¿Se mantiene usted con sus propios recursos?
7. Do you have medical insurance?	7. ¿Tiene usted seguro médico?
8. Do you have Medicare?	8. ¿Tiene usted Medicare?
9. Do you have supplementary insurance?	9. ¿Tiene usted seguro suplementario?
10. May I have your insurance cards in order to copy them? __I don't have them with me.	10. ¿Me permite sus tarjetas de seguro médico para copiarlas? __No las tengo conmigo.
11. How would you like to pay your bill? __by cash __by check __with a credit card	11. ¿Cómo quiere pagar su cuenta? __en efectivo __con cheque __con tarjeta de crédito
12. Will you pay for this bill in a lump sum or would you like to make other arrangements? __I would like to pay the full amount. __I need to make other arrangements.	12. ¿Va usted a pagar esta cuenta en su totalidad o quisiera hacer otros arreglos? __La voy a pagar en su totalidad. __Tengo que hacer otros arreglos.

AT THE DOCTOR'S OFFICE / EN EL CONSULTORIO MÉDICO

ENGLISH	SPANISH
1. Please indicate if you have seen the doctor before.	1. Por favor indique si ha visto al doctor anteriormente.
2. Please fill out this form.	2. Por favor, llene esta planilla.
3. Please sit down, and we will call you shortly.	3. Siéntese, por favor, y le llamaremos dentro de un ratico.
4. Follow me, please.	4. Sígame, por favor.
5. Please get on the scale.	5. Por favor, súbase a la báscula.
6. Now I am going to take your blood pressure.	6. Ahora le voy a tomar la presión arterial.
7. Please undress and put on this gown.	7. Por favor, desvístase y póngase esta bata.
8. Would you like to use the bathroom?	8. ¿Quisiera usar el servicio?
9. The doctor will be here shortly.	9. El doctor vendrá dentro de poco.
10. Breathe __ normally __ deeply __hold your breath	10. Respire __ normalmente __ profundamente __ aguante la respiración
11. Cough lightly.	11. Tosa ligeramente.
12. Does it hurt here when I touch you?	12. ¿Le duele aquí cuando le toco?
13. Show me where it hurts.	13. Indíqueme donde le duele.
14. You may get dressed now.	14. Ya se puede vestir.
15. The doctor would like to see you in __ a week __ a month __ 6 months __ a year	15. El doctor le quiere ver dentro de: __ una semana __ un mes __ 6 meses __ un año
16. You can make an appointment now.	16. Puede hacer una cita ahora.
17. You may take care of your bill now.	17. Puede saldar su cuenta ahora.

Indications and Recommendations

Indicaciones y recomendaciones

ENGLISH

SPANISH

1. I will prescribe some medication that should:
   __ alleviate the discomfort
   __ relieve the pain
   __ help us determine the problem

1. Le voy a recetar una medicina que le va a:
   __ aliviar el malestar
   __ mejorar el dolor
   __ ayudar a determinar cual es el problema

2. Take the medicine
   __ twice a day
   __ three times a day
   __ four times a day
   __ before meals
   __ after meals
   __ first thing in the morning
   __ before going to bed
   __ with some solid food
   __ with milk or juice

2. Tome la medicina
   __ dos veces al día
   __ tres veces al día
   __ cuatro veces al día
   __ antes de las comidas
   __ después de las comidas
   __ al levantarse
   __ al acostarse
   __ con algo de comer
   __ con leche o jugo

3. Always shake the bottle well.

3. Siempre agite bien la botella.

4. Apply to the area
   __ an ice pack
   __ a heating pad

4. Póngase en la parte afectada
   __ una bolsa de hielo
   __ una almohadilla eléctrica

5. Take a warm Sitz bath
   __ once a day
   __ twice a day
   __ three times a day

5. Dése un baño de asiento caliente
   __ una vez al día
   __ dos veces al día
   __ tres veces al día

6. When you lie down, raise the feet above the level of the heart.

6. Cuando se acueste, levante los pies por encima del nivel del corazón.

7. You should
   __ lose weight
   __ exercise more
   __ stop smoking
   __ avoid salt in your diet
   __ eat a more balanced diet
   __ eat more vegetables
   __ eat more fruit and fiber

7. Usted debe
   __ bajar de peso
   __ hacer más ejercicio
   __ dejar de fumar
   __ no comer comidas con sal
   __ hacer una dieta más balanceada
   __ comer más vegetales
   __ comer más fruta y fibra

8. We still don't know what is causing your illness.

8. No hemos podido determinar todavía la causa de su enfermedad.

9. It is necessary that you have
   __ a blood test
   __ some laboratory tests
   __ a urinalysis
   __ a mammogram
   __ a sonogram
   __ an x-ray
   __ a scan
   __ therapy

9. Es necesario que se haga
   __ un análisis de sangre
   __ unas pruebas de laboratorio
   __ un análisis de orina
   __ un mamograma
   __ un sonograma
   __ una radiografía
   __ un escán
   __ terapia

10. We will make the necessary arrangements with
  __ the laboratory
  __ the hospital
  __ the therapist
	10. Nosotros haremos los arreglos necesarios con
	  __ el laboratorio
	  __ el hospital
	  __ el (la) terapista

11. Take the written orders with you.	11. Lleve las órdenes médicas consigo.
12. It is advisable to put you in the hospital for further tests.	12. Es conveniente hospitalizarlo-a para hacerle pruebas adicionales.
13. You will need an operation.	13. Usted va a necesitar una operación.

14. The operation is
  __ not serious
  __ somewhat serious
	14. La operación
	  __ no es seria
	  __ es de cierta gravedad

15. Take your hospitalization and insurance papers with you.	15. Lleve consigo al hospital las órdenes del médico y la póliza de seguro.
16. We still do not have the results of the tests.	16. Todavía no tenemos el resultado de las pruebas.
17. Are you taking any medication?	17. ¿Está tomando alguna medicina?
18. Are you taking any sedatives?	18. ¿Está tomando algún calmante?

19. Do you have nausea?
  __once in a while
	19. ¿Tiene náuseas?
	  __de vez en cuando

20. Have you fainted at any time?
  __never
	20. ¿Se ha desmayado alguna vez?
	  __nunca

21. Have you felt dizzy or fainted after eating or exercising?	21. ¿Se ha desmayado o mareado después de comer o de hacer ejercicio?

22. Do you suffer from headaches?
  __sometimes
	22. ¿Padece de dolores de cabeza?
	  __algunas veces

23. Have you ever suffered from convulsions or seizures?	23. ¿Ha sufrido alguna vez de convulsiones o ataques repentinos?

CHIEF COMPLAINT / QUEJA PRINCIPAL

▶ PRESENT ILLNESS
▶ DATE AND TIME OF ONSET OF ILLNESS
▶ CHARACTERISTICS OF ILLNESS
▶ FREQUENCY OF ILLNESS

▶ ENFERMEDAD ACTUAL
▶ COMIENZO DE LA ENFERMEDAD
▶ CARACTERÍSTICAS DE LA ENFERMEDAD
▶ FRECUENCIA DE LA ENFERMEDAD

ENGLISH	*SPANISH*
1. What brings you here? __my yearly check-up __I have not been feeling well __I have a constant headache __This is a follow-up appointment	1. ¿Cuál es la causa de su visita? __mi chequeo anual __No me he estado sintiendo bien. __Tengo un dolor de cabeza constante. __Esta es una visita de seguimiento
2. How do you feel right now? __not well __fair __not too good __well	2. ¿Cómo se siente en este momento? __no me siento bien __regular, __más o menos __no muy bien __bien
3. When did this problem begin? __It began about a month ago __It has been going on for quite a while __I can't remember	3. ¿Cuando le comenzó este problema? __Empezó hace como un mes. __Empezó hace bastante tiempo __No recuerdo
4. Have you lost any weight recently? __some	4. ¿Ha bajado de peso recientemente? __algo
5. Is this problem preventing you from working? __sometimes __once in a while	5. ¿Este trastorno (problema o condición) le impide trabajar? __algunas veces __de vez en cuando
6. Is this problem affecting your regular activities? __up to a point	6. ¿Este problema afecta sus actividades diarias? __hasta cierto punto
7. Are you able to do housework? __only light chores	7. ¿Puede hacer los quehaceres de la casa? __solamente los más simples
8. Have you had this problem (symptom or discomfort) before?	8. ¿Ha tenido este malestar, (síntoma, trastorno) antes?
9. Did it start suddenly or gradually? __suddenly, __gradually	9. ¿Le empezó de pronto o gradualmente? __de pronto, __gradualmente
10. Do you have this problem constantly? __when I get up in the morning __after meals	10. ¿Tiene este trastorno continuamente? __cuando me levanto por las mañanas __después de las comidas
11. Every day? __almost every day __not every day, but very frequently	11. ¿Todos los días? __casi todos los días __no todos los días, pero muy frecuentemente

ENGLISH	SPANISH
12. How many times a day? __once a day __a few times a day __two, three, four times a day __when I get up __in the afternoons __after I walk more than 1/2 hour	12. ¿Cuántas veces al día? __una vez al día __varias veces al día __dos, tres, cuatro veces al día __cuando me levanto __por las tardes __después que camino por más de 1/2 hora__
13. When do you feel worse? __in the evenings	13. ¿Cuándo se siente peor? __ por la noche
14. Does it make you feel __weak __tired __exhausted?	14. ¿Le hace sentirse __débil __cansado-a __exhausto-a?
15. Do you have a fever?	15. ¿Tiene fiebre?
16. Are you in pain now? __Not at this time __I am in a lot of pain	16. ¿Tiene dolor ahora? __no en este momento __Tengo mucho dolor.
17. Have you seen a doctor since you became ill?	17. ¿Ha visto a algún doctor desde que se enfermó?
18. Is your family aware of this problem?	18. ¿Está su familia al tanto de su problema?
19. Are you taking medication now? __only pain killers	19. ¿Está tomando alguna medicina ahora? __solamente pastillas para el dolor
20. Have you taken or done anything that seems to help you? __I have taken some aspirin __I do some stretching excercises	20. ¿Ha hecho o tomado algo que le mejore? __he tomado aspirina __hago algunos ejercicios de estiramiento
21. Have you ever been hospitalized on account of this problem?	21. ¿Ha tenido que ingresar alguna vez en el hospital debido a este problema?

MEDICAL HISTORY / HISTORIA CLÍNICA

General Questions	Preguntas Generales
ENGLISH	*SPANISH*
1. Have you gained weight recently? __a little bit, some	1. ¿Ha aumentado de peso últimamente? __un poco
2. Have you lost weight recently?	2. ¿Ha bajado de peso recientemente?
3. Do you have any pain?	3. ¿Tiene dolor?
4. Where does it hurt? __here __in the neck __in the chest	4. ¿Dónde le duele? __aquí __en el cuello __en el pecho
5. Is the pain __ sharp __ severe __ mild __ dull?	5. ¿Es el dolor __ agudo __ fuerte __ leve __ sordo?
6. Do you tire easily? __sometimes	6. ¿Se cansa fácilmente? __algunas veces
7. Do you feel dizzy?	7. ¿Se siente mareado-a?
8. Do you generally sleep well? __pretty well	8. ¿Duerme bien generalmente? __bastante bien
9. How many hours do you sleep? __I sleep about three, five, seven hours	9. ¿Cuántas horas duerme durante la noche? __Duermo como tres, cinco, siete horas
10. Do you sleep during the day? __once in a while	10. ¿Duerme durante el día? __a veces
11. Do you take any pills to help you to sleep?	11. ¿Toma alguna pastilla para dormir?
12. How long have you had this pain? __for about two months __for about a week __since my last period	12. ¿Cuánto tiempo hace que tiene el dolor? __hace como dos meses __hace como una semana __desde mi último periodo

Family History; Past Medical History

Historia familiar; historia clínica previa

> **Note:** Questions from the section **Personal Data** at the beginning of this section can be included in this interview as well as for more complete data. / Las preguntas de la sección **Datos personales** que se encuentran al principio de este cuestionario se pueden usar en esta entrevista también para obtener una información más completa.

ENGLISH	SPANISH
1. Do you have any children?	1. ¿Tiene hijos?
2. How old were you when you had your first child? __I was twenty-one, __thirty-three, __forty years old.	2. ¿Cuántos años tenía cuando nació su primer/a hijo/a? Yo tenía __veintiún, __treinta y tres, __cuarenta años.
3. Do your children live with you?	3. ¿Viven sus hijos con usted?
4. Are your parents living?	4. ¿Viven sus padres?
5. Are they in good health? __fair	5. ¿Tienen buena salud? __regular
6. Is your father living? [if the answer is Yes]	6. ¿Vive su padre? [Si la respuesta es sí]
7. What is his health like? __good__ __not too good __fair [If the answer is No]	7. ¿Cómo está de salud? __bien __no muy bien __regular [Si la respuesta es no]
8. What did he die from? __from a heart attack __from a stroke __from surgery complications __from natural causes	8. ¿De qué murió? __de un ataque cardíaco __de una embolia cerebral __de complicaciones de cirugía __de muerte natural
9. How old was he when he died? __He was __sixty-two, __seventy, __eighty-two years old.	9. ¿Qué edad tenía cuando murió? __Tenía __sesenta y dos, __setenta, __ochenta y dos años.
10. Is your mother living?	10. ¿Vive su madre?
11. What is her health like? __fair __bad	11. ¿Cómo está de salud? __regular, más o menos __mal
12. What did she die of? __from breast cancer __from ovarian cancer	12. ¿De qué murió ella? __de cáncer de la mama (cáncer del seno) __de cancer ovárico

Family History; Past Medical History

Historia familiar; historia clínica previa

> **Note:** Questions from the section **Personal Data** at the beginning of this section can be included in this interview as well as for more complete data. / Las preguntas de la sección **Datos personales** que se encuentran al principio de este cuestionario se pueden usar en esta entrevista también para obtener una información más completa.

ENGLISH	SPANISH
13. Did any of your parents, grandparents, or close relatives die of or have had any of the following diseases? __ cancer __ blood disease __ diabetes __ epilepsy __ glaucoma __ heart disease __ high blood pressure __ mental retardation __ insanity __ tuberculosis	13. ¿Murió o padeció alguno de sus padres, abuelos o familiares inmediatos de una de estas enfermedades? __ cáncer __ enfermedad de la sangre __ diabetes __ epilepsia __ glaucoma __ enfermedad del corazón __ la presión alta __ retraso mental __ demencia, locura __ tuberculosis
14. Have you ever been hospitalized?	14. ¿Ha estado hospitalizado-a alguna vez?
15. What for? __for surgery __to deliver a baby __for acute respiratory problems	15. ¿Debido a qué? __para operarme __por estar de parto __por un problema respiratorio agudo
16. For how long? __a week __fourteen days __a month	16. ¿Por cuánto tiempo? __una semana __catorce días __un mes
17. How many times? __one, __two, __three times	17. ¿Cuántas veces? __una, __dos, __tres veces

Family History; Past Medical History

Historia familiar; historia clínica previa

Note: Questions from the section **Personal Data** at the beginning of this section can be included in this interview as well as for more complete data. / Las preguntas de la sección **Datos personales** que se encuentran al principio de este cuestionario se pueden usar en esta entrevista también para obtener una información más completa.

ENGLISH	SPANISH

18. Have you ever had any of the following illnesses?
  __ amebic dysentery
  __ allergies
  __ anemia
  __ appendicitis
  __ arthritis
  __ asthma
  __ cancer
  __ chicken pox
  __ chorea
  __ chronic laryngitis
  __ chronic tonsilitis
  __ cirrhosis
  __ conjunctivitis
  __ cystitis
  __ diabetes
  __ diphteria
  __ ear infections
  __ emphysema
  __ epilepsy
  __ gallbladder attack
  __ gallstones
  __ goiter
  __ gonorrhea
  __ hay fever
  __ heart disease
  __ hepatitis
  __ high blood pressure
  __ jaundice
  __ measles; German measles
  __ mononucleosis
  __ mumps
  __ scarlet fever
  __ syphilis
  __ tuberculosis
  __ typhoid fever

18. ¿Ha tenido alguna de las enfermedades siguientes?
  __ disenteria amebiana
  __ alergias
  __ anemia
  __ apendicitis
  __ artritis
  __ asma
  __ cáncer
  __ varicela
  __ corea
  __ laringitis crónica
  __ amigadalitis crónica
  __ cirrosis
  __ conjuntivitis
  __ cistitis
  __ diabetes
  __ difteria
  __ infecciones de los oídos
  __ enfisema
  __ epilepsia
  __ ataque vesicular
  __ cálculos en la vejiga
  __ bocio
  __ gonorrea
  __ fiebre del heno
  __ enfermedad del corazón
  __ hepatitis
  __ presión arterial alta
  __ ictericia
  __ sarampión, sarampión alemán, rubéola
  __ mononucleosis
  __ paperas
  __ fiebre escarlatina
  __ sífilis
  __ tuberculosis
  __ fiebre tifoidea

Family History; Past Medical History

Hístoria familiar; hístoria clínica previa

Note: Questions from the section **Personal Data** at the beginning of this section can be included in this interview as well as for more complete data. / Las preguntas de la sección **Datos personales** que se encuentran al principio de este cuestionario se pueden usar en esta entrevista también para obtener una información más completa.

ENGLISH	SPANISH
19. Have you or any of your immediate relatives been addicted to __alcohol __tobaco __drugs?	19. ¿Usted o algún familiar cercano ha sido adicto a __alcohol __tabaco __drogas?
20. Has anyone in your family died of a heart attack?	20. ¿Algún familiar cercano ha muerto de un ataque al corazón?
21. Is there any sickness that seems to be repeated in your family? __cardiac disease __diabetes	21. ¿Hay alguna enfermedad que se repite en su familia? __enfermedad del corazón __diabetes
22. Have any of your siblings died?	22. ¿Ha muerto alguno de sus hermanos-as?
23. How old was he/she? He/she was __twenty-three, __thirty-five, __forty years old.	23. ¿Qué edad tenía? Él/ella tenía __veintitrés, __treinta y cinco, __cuarenta años.
24. Where have you lived most of your life? __here in the United States __abroad __in my native country	24. ¿Dónde ha vivido la mayor parte de su vida? __aquí en los Estados Unidos __fuera del país __en mi país natal

REVIEW OF SYSTEMS/ REPARO POR APARATOS

Eyes, Ears, Nose, and Throat

Ojos, oídos, nariz y garganta

ENGLISH	SPANISH
1. Have you noticed any bleeding from your gums or mouth?	1. ¿Ha notado si las encías o la boca le sangran?
2. Does your tongue feel sore? Is any part of your mouth sore?	2. ¿Siente la lengua adolorida? ¿Le duele otra área de la boca?
3. Do you have swelling or lumps in the mouth?	3. ¿Tiene alguna hinchazón o bola en la boca?
4. Do you have difficulty swallowing?	4. ¿Tiene dificultad al tragar?
5. Do you suffer from sore throats? how frequently? __about once a month __several times a year	5. ¿Padece de dolor de garganta? ¿con qué frecuencia? __como una vez al mes __varias veces al año
6. Do you have any dripping or drainage in the back of the throat?	6. ¿Tiene alguna supuración o flema en la parte posterior de la garganta?
7. Are you often hoarse?	7. ¿Tiene ronquera frecuentemente?
8. Have you noticed any swelling in your neck?	8. ¿Ha notado alguna hinchazón en el cuello?
9. Have you ever had nosebleeds?	9. ¿Ha tenido sangramiento por la nariz?
10. Do you have any difficulty hearing?	10. ¿Tiene alguna dificultad para oír?
11. Do you have ringing in your ears? __ right ear __ left ear __ both	11. ¿Tiene zumbido o tintineo en los oídos? __ en el derecho __ en el izquierdo __ en ambos
12. Have you noticed any secretion from your ears?	12. ¿Ha notado alguna secreción por los oídos?
13. Do you have earaches?	13. ¿Padece de dolor de oído?
14. Have you noticed any change in your vision?	14. ¿Ha notado algún cambio en la vista?
15. Do you wear glasses or contact lenses? __ for close-up __ for distance __ for reading __ all the time	15. ¿Usa espejuelos o lentes de contacto? __ para ver de cerca __ para distancia __ para leer __ siempre
16. Have you noticed any redness or swelling in your eyes?	16. ¿Se ha notado los ojos enrojecidos o hinchados?
17. Do you have double vision?	17. ¿Tiene visión doble?
18. Do you see spots or flashes of light?	18. ¿Ve alguna vez manchas o luces?
19. Have you had pain in your eyes?	19. ¿Ha tenido dolor en los ojos?
20. Do you have any discharge from your eyes?	20. ¿Le supuran los ojos?

Eyes, Ears, Nose, and Throat

Ojos, oídos, nariz y garganta

ENGLISH	SPANISH
21. Have your eyes ever been affected by any sickness or accident?	21. ¿Ha sido su vista afectada por alguna enfermedad o accidente?
22. Do you have blurred vision?	22. ¿Se le nubla la vista?
23. Do you have a burning feeling in your eyes?	23. ¿Le arden los ojos?
24. Do you have to strain your eyes to see better?	24. ¿Tiene que forzar la vista para ver mejor?
25. When was your last vision test? __it has been a year __two years ago __since I was a child	25. ¿Cuándo fue la última vez que se hizo un examen de la vista? __hace un año __dos años atrás __desde niño

Cardiopulmonary System | Sistema cardiopulmonar

ENGLISH	SPANISH
1. Have you ever had an electrocardiogram?	1. ¿Se le ha hecho alguna vez un electrocardiograma?
2. Have you ever noticed rapid heartbeats?	2. ¿Ha notado alguna vez si tiene palpitaciones?
3. Have you ever had chest pain?	3. ¿Ha tenido alguna vez dolor en el pecho?
4. How long did it last? __a couple of hours __all day yesterday __almost a week	4. ¿Cuánto tiempo le duró? __un par de horas __todo el día de ayer __casi una semana
5. In what part of the chest? __the upper chest __the lower chest	5. ¿En qué parte del pecho? __en la parte superior del pecho __en la parte inferior del pecho
6. Does it radiate to any part of your body? __ arm __ shoulder __ neck __ back	6. ¿Se le corre a alguna parte del cuerpo? __ al brazo __ al hombro __ al cuello __ a la espalda
7. Do you cough? __ a little __ a lot __ a dry cough	7. ¿Tiene tos? __ poca tos __ mucha tos __ una tos seca
8. Does your chest hurt when you cough?	8. ¿Le duele el pecho cuando tose?
9. Do you have any swelling in your legs or ankles?	9. ¿Se le hinchan las piernas o los tobillos?
10. Do you have high blood pressure?	10. ¿Tiene la presión alta?
11. Do you bleed easily?	11. ¿Tiene tendencia a sangrar?
12. Do you smoke? For how long have you smoked? __for five years __for one year __for a long time	12. ¿Fuma? ¿Cuánto tiempo hace que fuma? __durante cinco años __un año __hace mucho tiempo
13. How many cigarettes per day? __five, __ten, __a pack a day	13. ¿Cuántos cigarros al día? __cinco, __diez, __un paquete al día
14. Have you tried to stop?	14. ¿Ha tratado de dejar de fumar?
15. Have you ever had lung disease?	15. ¿Ha tenido alguna enfermedad de los pulmones?
16. Have you ever had any heart trouble?	16. ¿Ha tenido algún problema del corazón?
17. Do you have frequent colds?	17. ¿Tiene catarros frecuentes?
18. Do you cough up any phlegm?	18. ¿Tose con flema?

Cardiopulmonary System

Sistema cardiopulmonar

ENGLISH	SPANISH
19. What does it look like? __viscous __bloody __watery	19. ¿Cómo es la flema? __viscosa __sangrienta __líquida
20. What color is it? __ clear __ white __ yellow __ green __ dark __ brown	20. ¿De qué color es la flema? __ clara __ blanca __ amarilla __ verde __ oscura __ marrón o chocolate
21. Have you ever coughed up blood?	21. ¿Alguna vez ha tenido sangre al toser?
22. Have you had any trouble breathing?	22. ¿Ha tenido dificultad para respirar?
23. Are you short of breath __ at night __ after meals __ when you exercise __ when you walk __ even resting?	23. ¿Le falta la respiración __ por la noche __ después de comer __ al hacer ejercicio __ cuando camina __ aún si descansa?
24. Have you noticed any particular sound in your breathing?	24. ¿Ha notado algún sonido diferente al respirar?
25. Is there any position that makes your breathing __ easier __ worse?	25. ¿Hay alguna posición que le haga respirar __ mejor __ peor?

Gastrointestinal System

Aparato o sistema digestivo

ENGLISH	SPANISH
1. Is there any food that disagrees with you? __fried foods __acid fruits __dairy foods	1. ¿Le cae mal algún alimento? __comidas fritas __frutas ácidas __comidas lácteas
2. Do you have heartburn?	2. ¿Tiene ardor en el estómago?
3. Do you suffer from stomachaches? __ before eating __ while eating __ after eating	3. ¿Padece de dolores de estómago? __ antes de comer __ mientras come __ después de comer
4. Do you suffer from indigestion?	4. ¿Padece de indigestión?
5. Do you drink or eat between meals?	5. ¿Come o toma líquidos entre las comidas?
6. Do you drink coffee? How many cups a day? __one, __two, __three or __four cups	6. ¿Toma café? ¿Cuántas tazas al día? __una, __dos, __tres o __cuatro tazas
7. Do you eat fried or fatty foods?	7. ¿Come comidas fritas o grasosas?
8. Do you burp a lot?	8. ¿Eructa mucho?
9. How much milk do you drink? What kind? __ 2% __ skim __ whole milk	9. ¿Cuánta leche toma? ¿De qué clase? __ desnatada __ natural __ completa
10. At what time do you eat breakfast?	10. ¿A qué hora se desayuna?
11. At what time do you eat your last meal of the day?	11. ¿A qué hora hace su última comida del día?
12. Do you try to eat a balanced meal every day?	12. ¿Trata de comer una comida balanceada todos los días?
13. What kind of food do you generally eat more? __ meats __ vegetables __ bread and cereals __ fruits	13. ¿Qué clase de alimentos generalmente come más? __ carnes __ vegetales __ panes y cereales __ frutas
14. Do you eat a good breakfast every day?	14. ¿Toma un buen desayuno todos los días?
15. Are you constipated?	15. ¿Padece de estreñimiento?
16. Do you have a bowel movement every day?	16. ¿Elimina (obra, está al corriente) todos los días?
17. Are your stools normal?	17. ¿Sus evacuaciones son normales?

Gastrointestinal System

Aparato o sistema digestivo

ENGLISH	SPANISH

18. What color and consistency are they?
   __normal
   __hard and dark
   __bloody
   __greasy
   __dark and viscous
	18. ¿Qué color y consistencia tienen?
	   __normal
	   __oscuras y duras
	   __con sangre
	   __grasientas
	   __oscuras y viscosas

19. Do you have diarrhea?	19. ¿Tiene diarrea?
20. Have you noticed any blood or mucous in the stools?	20. ¿Ha notado sangre o mucosidad en las heces fecales?

Musculoskeletal System

Sistema musculoesquelético

ENGLISH	SPANISH
1. Do you have pain in your joints?	1. ¿Le duelen las articulaciones?
2. Do you have pain in the neck or back?	2. ¿Tiene dolor en el cuello o la espalda?
3. Do your muscles hurt?	3. ¿Le duelen los músculos?
4. Do you feel general muscle weakness?	4. ¿Siente debilidad muscular general?
5. Have you noticed any swelling on a bone?	5. ¿Ha notado hinchazón en algún hueso?
6. Do you have pain in your bones?	6. ¿Siente dolor en los huesos?
7. Have you ever had a fracture or a sprain?	7. ¿Ha tenido alguna vez una fractura o luxación?
8. How long ago? __last year __five years ago __a long time ago	8. ¿Cuánto tiempo hace? __el año pasado __hace cinco años __hace mucho tiempo
9. What bone or part was affected? __I fractured the Achilles tendon. __I broke the femur. __I had a hip fracture.	9. ¿Qué hueso o parte le afectó? __Me fracturé el tendón de Aquiles __Me partí el fémur __Me fracturé la cadera.

Neurological System

Sistema neurológico

ENGLISH	SPANISH
1. Do you have any feeling of tingling or numbness?	1. ¿Tiene alguna sensación de hormigueo o entumecimiento?
2. Do you forget things easily?	2. ¿Olvida las cosas con facilidad?
3. Is your memory worse than before?	3. ¿Tiene la memoria peor que antes?
4. Do you have good balance?	4. ¿Tiene buen equilibrio?
5. Do you have any difficulty walking?	5. ¿Tiene alguna dificultad para caminar?
6. Do you have difficulty moving __ towards the right __ towards the left?	6. ¿Tiene dificultad en moverse __ hacia la derecha __ hacia la izquierda?
7. Have you ever lost consciousness?	7. ¿Ha perdido el conocimiento alguna vez?
8. More than once?	8. ¿Más de una vez?
9. Do you walk without difficulty?	9. ¿Camina sin dificultad?
10. Do you need any walking device to maintain your balance? __ cane __ walker	10. ¿Necesita alguna ayuda para mantener el equilibrio? __ bastón __ caminador
11. Do you feel sometimes like you are going to fall?	11. ¿Siente algunas veces como si fuera a caerse?
12. Have you had any seizures or convulsions?	12. ¿Ha tenido ataques o convulsiones de algún tipo?
13. Is your memory __ good __ bad __ not as good as it used to be?	13. ¿Es su memoria __ buena __ mala __ no tan buena como antes?
14. Can you feel this?	14. ¿Puede sentir esto?
15. Can you smell this?	15. ¿Puede oler esto?
16. Does any particular food taste different to you?	16. ¿El sabor de algún alimento en particular le parece diferente?

Skin   ## Piel

ENGLISH	SPANISH
1. Do you have any sores or blisters?	1. ¿Tiene algunas llagas o ampollas?
2. Do you have any mole that is red or itchy?	2. ¿Tiene algún lunar que se pone rojo o le pica?
3. Do you have a skin rash?	3. ¿Tiene alguna erupción?
4. Since when have you had this eruption?	4. ¿Desde cuándo ha tenido esta erupción?
5. Have you noticed any change?	5. ¿Ha notado algún cambio?
6. Have you noticed any unusual spots in your skin?	6. ¿Ha notado alguna mancha peculiar en la piel?
7. Do you use any cosmetics that cause redness or swelling to your skin?	7. ¿Usa cosméticos que le causen enrojecimiento o hinchazón en la piel?
8. Have you had any severe burns?	8. ¿Ha tenido alguna vez una quemadura grave?
9. Does anything make you itchy?	9. ¿Hay algo que le da picazón?
10. Is your skin very sensitive to the sun's rays?	10. ¿Es su piel muy sensitiva a los rayos del sol?
11. Do you use any sunblockers (creme or lotion) if you are going to be exposed to the sun?	11. ¿Usa algún bloqueador de rayos del sol (crema o loción) si va a estar expuesto-a a los rayos del sol?
12. Have you noticed any discoloration on your skin?	12. ¿Ha notado algún cambio de color en la piel?

Genitourinary System

ENGLISH

(TO FEMALE PATIENTS)

1. How old were you when you had your first period?
   I was __ten, __thirteen, __fourteen years old.

2. When was your last period?
   __one, __three weeks ago
   __two, __six months ago

3. Are your periods difficult?

4. How long does your period last?
   __three to four days
   __a week
   __eight to nine days

5. Do you ever bleed between periods?

6. Do you have any discharge from the vagina?

7. What does it look like?
   __viscous
   __yellowish
   __bloody

8. Do you have any itching or burning in the genital area?

9. Have you ever had a venereal disease?

10. Have you ever had any trouble with your breasts?
    __ secretion
    __ pain
    __ swelling
    __ a lump

11. Have you learned how to examine your breasts?

12. Do you examine your breasts regularly?

13. Do you have any discharge from your breasts?

14. Have you noticed any mass or lump in your breasts?

15. Are you pregnant?

16. Have you ever been pregnant? How many times?
    __two, __four, __seven times

Aparato genitourinario

SPANISH

(PARA LOS PACIENTES FEMENINOS)

1. ¿Qué edad tenía cuando tuvo la primera regla (periodo)?
   Yo tenía __diez, __trece, __catorce años de edad.

2. ¿Cuándo tuvo la última regla?
   hace __una, __tres semanas
   hace __dos, __seis meses

3. ¿Son sus periodos difíciles?
   (¿Es la regla dificultosa?)

4. ¿Cuántos días le dura el periodo?
   __tres o cuatro días
   __una semana
   __ocho a nueve días

5. ¿Tiene algún sangramiento entre reglas?

6. ¿Tiene algún flujo o secreción de vagina?

7. ¿Cómo es?
   __viscosa
   __amarillenta
   __con sangre

8. ¿Tiene alguna picazón o ardor en alguna parte interior?

9. ¿Ha tenido alguna enfermedad venérea?

10. ¿Ha tenido alguna vez algún trastorno en los senos?
    __ secreción
    __ dolor
    __ hinchazón
    __ una bolita, un bulto

11. ¿Ha aprendido a examinarse los senos?

12. ¿Se autoexamina los senos regularmente?

13. ¿Tiene alguna secreción de los senos?

14. ¿Ha notado algún bulto o bolita en los senos?

15. ¿Está embarazada, (en estado? encinta?)

16. ¿Ha estado embarazada alguna vez? ¿Cuántas veces?
    __dos, __cuatro, __siete veces

Genitourinary System

ENGLISH

Aparato genitourinario

ENGLISH

SPANISH

(TO FEMALE PATIENTS)

(PARA LOS PACIENTES FEMENINAS)

17. Have you ever had a miscarriage? How many times?
    __one, __two, __three times

17. ¿Ha tenido alguna vez un malparto? ¿Cuántas veces?
    __una, __dos, __tres veces

18. Have you ever had an induced abortion? How many times?
    __once
    __twice

18. ¿Ha tenido alguna vez un aborto inducido? ¿Cuántas veces?
    __una vez
    __dos veces

19. Do you have any problem during intercourse?

19. ¿Tiene algún problema o dificultad durante las relaciones sexuales?

20. Do you have any pain during intercourse?

20. ¿Tiene dolor durante las relaciones sexuales?

21. Do you use any type of birth control?

21. ¿Usa algún tipo de anticonceptivo?

22. How many live births have you had?

22. ¿Cuántos embarazos se le han logrado?

23. Did you have any stillbirths?

23. ¿Tuvo algún parto no logrado?

(TO MALE PATIENTS)

(PARA PACIENTES MASCULINOS)

1. Do you have any discharge from the penis?

1. ¿Tiene alguna secreción por el pene?

2. Do you have pain in the testicles?

2. ¿Tiene dolor en los testículos?

3. Do you have pain or swelling in the scrotum?

3. ¿Tiene dolor o hinchazón en el escroto?

4. Are you unable to have an erection?

4. ¿Se le dificulta tener una erección?

5. Do you have a satisfactory sex life?

5. ¿Está satisfecho con su vida sexual?

6. Have you had any venereal disease?

6. ¿Ha tenido alguna enfermedad venérea?

7. Have you fathered any children?

7. ¿Ha tenido hijos?

Urinary System

ENGLISH

Aparato o sistema urinario

SPANISH

1. Do you have any trouble urinating?	1. ¿Tiene dificultad cuando orina?
2. Do you have to get up to urinate during the night? How many times? __two, or __three times __many times	2. ¿Tiene que levantarse por la noche a orinar? ¿Cuántas veces? __dos o __tres veces __muchas veces
3. Do you have back or flank pain?	3. ¿Tiene algún dolor en la espalda o en el costado?
4. Do you have pain or burning when urinating?	4. ¿Tiene dolor o ardor cuando orina?
5. Is the color of the urine __ yellow __ murky __ milky __ pale __ reddish?	5. ¿Es la orina __ amarilla __ turbia __ lechosa __ sin color __ rojiza?
6. Do you have blood in the urine?	6. ¿Tiene sangre en la orina?
7. Are you unable to control your urination?	7. ¿No puede controlar la salida de orina?
8. Do you urinate too often?	8. ¿Orina con demasiada frecuencia?
9. Do you pass a little or a lot of urine regularly?	9. ¿Orina mucho o poco regularmente?
10. Do you have difficulty starting to urinate?	10. ¿Tiene dificultad para comenzar a orinar?
11. Do you have difficulty maintaining a continuous flow of urine?	11. ¿Tiene dificultad en mantener el chorro?
12. Do you have any urine leakage?	12. ¿Tiene pérdida de orina?
13. When does it usually occur? __when I change positions while I am sitting down __when I cough	13. ¿Cuándo ocurre generalmente? __cuando cambio de posición mientras estoy sentado-a __cuando toso
14. Have you ever had any kidney problem?	14. ¿Ha padecido de los riñones?
15. Have you ever passed stones?	15. ¿Ha expulsado cálculos?
16. Have you had a vasectomy?	16. ¿Se ha hecho una vasectomía?
17. Do you examine your testicles regularly ?	17. ¿Usted se examina los testículos regularmente?
18. Have you had a PSA test? When? __about six months ago __I have never had the test.	18. ¿Se ha hecho la prueba del PSA? ¿Cuándo? __hace como seis meses __nunca me he hecho la prueba.

LABOR AND DELIVERY / LABORES DEL PARTO

ENGLISH	*SPANISH*
1. When is the expected date of delivery? __the fourteenth of July __it is past, it was the day before yesterday __next week, on the eighteenth	1. ¿Cuál es la fecha supuesta del parto? __el catorce de julio __ya pasó, fue antes de ayer __la próxima semana, el dieciocho
2. Are you having pains?	2. ¿Tiene ya dolores?
3. When did they start? __an hour ago __since noon __early this morning	3. ¿Cuándo le comenzaron? __hace una hora __desde el mediodía __temprano en la mañana
4. Are your pains spaced at regular intervals?	4. ¿Ocurren los dolores a intervalos regulares?
5. How long does the pain last? __five, __ten, __fifteen minutes __half hour __about forty-five minutes	5. ¿Cuánto le dura el dolor? __cinco, __diez, __quince minutos __media hora __como cuarenta y cinco minutos
6. How much time is there between pains?	6. ¿Cuánto tiempo pasa entre cada dolor?
7. Has your water broken?	7. ¿Se le rompió la fuente (la bolsa de aguas)?
8. Push. Push more. Do not push.	8. Puje. Puje más. No puje más.
9. Do not push until we tell you.	9. No puje hasta que le digamos.
10. Breathe in and out.	10. Respire para adentro y para afuera.
11. Breathe slowly when you have the contractions.	11. Respire lentamente cuando tenga las contracciones.
12. Breathe normally.	12. Respire normalmente.
13. Breathe slowly and then rapidly.	13. Respire lenta y luego rápidamente.
14. Are you going to breastfeed your baby?	14. ¿Va a darle el pecho al nene?
15. We are going to prepare you for the delivery.	15. Vamos a prepararla para el parto.
16. I am going to do a vaginal examination to determine the progress of the labor.	16. Voy a hacerle un examen vaginal para determinar el progreso del parto.
17. I am going to have to do a cesarean section.	17. Le vamos a tener que hacer una cesárea.
18. You have a fine baby.	18. Tiene un bebé precioso. Tiene una bebita preciosa.

THE NEWBORN / EL RECIÉN NACIDO

Practical vocabulary including characteristics, health care, anomalies, and the most common congenital disorders.	**Vocabulario práctico referente a características, cuidado de la salud, anomalías, y trastornos congénitos más comunes.**
CHARACTERISTICS	CARACTERÍSTICAS
ENGLISH	*SPANISH*
full-term	nacido(-a) a término completo
premature	prematuro
body weight at birth	peso al nacer
body length	largo del cuerpo
body temperature at birth	temperatura tomada al nacer
normal breathing	respiración normal
vital signs normal	signos vitales normales
face features	rasgos faciales
breastfed	(lactante) toma el pecho de la madre
bottle-fed	toma el biberón
normal patterns of sleep	patrones normales de sueño
normal cry	llanto normal
nurses well	toma el pecho bien
crying when hungry or wet	llora cuando tiene hambre o está mojado-a
weight gain normal	aumento de peso normal
normal growth and development	crecimiento y desarrollo normales
weight loss	pérdida de peso
time sleeping	tiempo durmiendo
time awake	tiempo despierto
movements	movimientos
alertness	expresión viva
lifts his/her head	levanta la cabeza
umbilical cord drop	caída del cordón umbilical
taking vitamins with formula	toma vitaminas en la fórmula
suckling well from breast or bottle	toma bien el pecho o chupa bien el biberón

ANOMALIES	ANOMALÍAS
abdominal swelling	inflamación abdominal
blood in the stools	sangre en las deposiciones
cyanosis	cianosis
colic	cólico
constipation	estreñimiento
convulsions	convulsiones
cradle cap	costra láctea
diaper rash	eritema, erupción
diarrhea sudden and explosive	diarrea explosiva y súbita
Down syndrome	síndrome de Down
dry scales	escama seca
excessive crying	llanto excesivo
feeding problems	problemas de alimentación
inadequate gaining	aumento inadecuado de peso
increasing fussiness	mayor intranquilidad
infantile spasms	espasmos infantiles
infections	infecciones
intolerance to lactose	intolerancia a la lactosa
jaundice	ictericia
Marfan's syndrome	síndrome de Marfan
milk allergy	alergia a la leche
nasal congestion	congestión nasal
seborrheic eczema	eczema seborreico
skin irritation	irritaciones en la piel
sudden jerk	contracción brusca
vaginal bleeding	sangramiento vaginal
weight loss	pérdida de peso

The Newborn's Assessment Prenatal Assessment Including Family History.	Evaluación del recién nacido[1] evaluación incluyendo la historia médica familiar.
(See Family History pp. 583–586)	(V. historia clínica familiar, pp. 611–614)
QUESTIONS TO THE MOTHER	PREGUNTAS A LA MADRE
ENGLISH	*SPANISH*
1. Are there any health problems that the family doctor should know?	1. ¿Hay algunos problemas de salud en la familia que su doctor debe saber?
2. Did you have prenatal care?	2. ¿Tuvo usted atención médica prenatal?
3. Did you have any worries during your pregnancy about the baby's health?	3. ¿Tuvo alguna preocupación durante el embarazo sobre la salud del bebé?[2]
4. Did you have a healthy diet?	4. ¿Se alimentaba bien?
5. Did you have any sickness during the pregnancy?	5. ¿Padeció alguna enfermedad durante el embarazo?
6. Did you have any addiction?	6. ¿Tenía alguna adicción?
7. Do you smoke?	7. ¿Fuma usted?
8. Did you smoke when you were pregnant?	8. ¿Fumaba cuando estaba embarazada?
9. Do you drink?	9. ¿Toma bebidas alcohólicas?
10. Do you have an addiction to any drug, a street drug, or a legal one?	10. ¿Es usted drogadicta a alguna droga, ilegal o legal (comprada en la farmacia)?
11. When was the last time you used or took this drug?	11. ¿Cuándo fue la última vez que usó o tomó la droga?
12. Was it before you were pregnant?	12. ¿Fue antes del embarazo?
13. Did you tell the doctor about your addiction?	13. ¿Informó al médico sobre su adicción?
14. Did you have a treatment to stop your addiction?	14. ¿Siguió un tratamiento para dejar la droga?

Assessment of Feeding

Evaluación de la alimentación

ENGLISH	SPANISH
1. Is the mother nursing the baby?	1. ¿Está lactando la madre al bebé? [3]
2. Or is the baby taking a formula	2. ¿O toma la bebita una fórmula?
3. Is the mother nursing the baby too often?	3. ¿Le da la madre el pecho al bebé muy seguido?
4. Is the mother giving the bottle to the baby too often?	4. ¿Le da la madre el biberón a la bebita muy seguido?
5. Is she nursing the baby as it was indicated?	5. ¿Está ella dándole el pecho al bebé como se le indicó?
6. Does the baby have difficulty nursing?	6. Tiene dificultad la bebita para tomar el pecho?
7. How long does she/he take to breast feed?	7. ¿Cuánto tiempo pasa tomando el pecho?
8. Does he/she fall asleep and stop nursing?	8. ¿Se duerme y deja de mamar?
9. How long does the baby spend taking the bottle?	9. ¿Cuánto tiempo pasa tomando el biberón?
10. Does the baby seem to have a colic?	10. ¿Parece que tiene cólico la bebita?

Urine and Stool Patterns

Patrones de orina y defecación

ENGLISH	SPANISH
1. Is the baby constipated?	1. ¿Tiene estreñimiento el bebé?
2. Is he/she urinating normally?	2. ¿Orina normalmente?
3. Is there any bleeding present in the stools?	3. ¿Hay evidencia de sangre en el excremento?
4. What color do they have?	4. ¿Qué color tiene el excremento?
5. Does the baby have a bowel movement every time he/she nurses?	5. ¿Hace la caca[4] cada vez que toma el pecho o el biberón?

Patterns of Sleep

Patrones del sueño

ENGLISH	SPANISH
AWAKE - SLEEP	DESPIERTO-A[5] Y DORMIDO-A
1. How long is he/she awake?	1. ¿Cuánto tiempo pasa despierto?
2. How many times does he/she wake up to nurse?	2. ¿Cuántas veces se despierta a tomar el pecho?
3. How many hours does he/she sleep?	3. ¿Cuántas horas duerme?
4. Does he/she sleep longer at night or during the day?	4. ¿Duerme más por la noche o durante el día?

Recommendations / Recomendaciones

ENGLISH	SPANISH
FEEDING	**ALIMENTACIÓN**
1. Be careful in the preparation of the formula, follow the instructions carefully. Keep bottles and nipples clean and sterilized.	1. Tenga cuidado en la preparación de la fórmula siga con cuidado las instrucciones. Conserve los biberones bien lavados, y esterilizados.
2. Burp the baby after nursing.	2. Sáquele el viento, ayúdele a eructar entre las tomas del pecho o del biberón
3. Observe any changes that could indicate that the formula does not agree with the baby.	3. Observe cualquier cambio que indique que la fórmula no le hace bien.
4. Follow safety habits with bed covers, clothing, and bottle caps, so they do not cause any danger. When you put your baby to bed, position her/him on her/on his back.	4. Conserve hábitos de seguridad con las mantas, la ropita, las tapas del biberón, para que no causen ningún peligro. Acueste al bebé boca arriba.
5. Avoid overdressing the baby.	5. Evite ponerle demasiada ropa.
6. Keep the room at a moderate temperature.	6. Mantenga la habitación con una temperatura adecuada.
7. Change the baby's diapers as needed, to avoid any skin rash.	7. Cambie los pañales (culero, tapico) cuando lo necesite, para evitar cualquier erupción.
8. Check if bowel movements are normal. The first two weeks the BM is dark.	8. Observe si las defecaciones son normales. En las dos primeras semanas tienen un color oscuro.
9. Keep a regular schedule for bathing.	9. Asigne una hora especial para el baño.
10. Check the baby while he sleeps.	10. Observe al bebé mientras duerme.

First Visit To The Pediatrician / Primera consulta con el pediatra

ENGLISH	SPANISH
1. What is the baby's weight? She weighs three and a half kilos.	1. ¿Cuánto pesa el bebé? Pesa tres kilos y medio.
2. Did she gain or lose any weight? She lost six ounces, but she gained them back.	2. ¿Bajó o aumentó de peso? Bajó seis onzas pero luego las recuperó.
3. Is his/her weight normal? Yes, his weight is normal.	3. ¿Es su peso normal? Sí, su peso es normal.
4. Has he/she grown at all? No, she has the same measurement.	4. ¿Ha crecido algo? No, tiene la misma medida.
5. Is his head of a normal size? Yes, her head has a normal size and shape.	5. ¿Es la cabecita de tamaño normal? Sí, la cabecita tiene un tamaño y una forma normal.
6. How many more ounces of formula should he/she have? Now, he/she must drink three ounces.	6. ¿Cuántas onzas más de fórmula debe tomar? Ahora él /ella debe tomar tres onzas.

ENGLISH	*SPANISH*
7. When he/she should have the first immunizations? He/she must have the immunizations when he/she is two months old.	7. ¿Cuándo debe ponerse las primeras vacunas? Debe ponerse las primeras vacunas a los dos meses.

[1] The feminine form is **la recién nacida.** *pp.* of **nacer** or a.m. **nacido**; *f.* **nacida**

[2] When referring to a baby girl, say **de la bebita**.

[3] If referring to a baby girl say **lactando** (to the) **a la bebita** *f.*; (to the) **al bebé** *m.*,. appear in questions and answers to distinguish the agreement with the article in both nouns.

[4] **la caca** is a coloquial term used only referring to children's bowel movement, it can be used instead of **excremento.**

[5] The irregular *pp.* **despierto**, changes to **despierta** if qualifies the *f.* **la bebita.**

[6] Form of the reflexive verb **despertarse**, third person.

MEDICATIONS / MEDICAMENTOS

Types of Medications / Tipos de medicamentos

MEDICATION	MAIN USE	MEDICAMENTO	USO PRINCIPAL
ENGLISH		*SPANISH*	
adrenergenic	to dilate the pupil; increase heart rate; strengthen heart beat	adrenérgicos	para dilatar la pupila; dar fuerza a los latidos del corazón
aminosalicylates	to help treat inflammation	aminosalicilatos	para tratar inflamaciones
anesthetics	to reduce sensation of pain	anestésicos	para aliviar el dolor
antiarrythmics	to treat arrythmia	antiarrítmicos	para tratar la arritmia
antibiotics	to treat bacterial infections	antibióticos	para tratar infecciones bacterianas
anticholinergics	to increase heart rate	anticolinérgico	para aumentar la frecuencia cardíaca
anticoagulants	to prevent blood clotting	anticoagulantes	para prevenir la coagulación sanguínea
anticonvulsants	to prevent or treat convulsions	anticonvulsivos	para prevenir o tratar convulsiones
antidepressants	to treat depression	antidepresivos	para tratar la depresión
antidiarrheal	to treat diarrhea	antidiarreicos	para tratar la diarrea
antiemetics	to prevent nausea or vomiting	antiemético	para prevenir o tratar la náusea o vómitos
antihistaminics	to block histamine receptors	antihistamínicos	para bloquear los receptores de histamina
antihypertensives	to lower blood pressure	antihipertensivos	para bajar la presión arterial
anti-inflammatory	to reduce inflammation	antiinflamatorio	para reducir la inflamación
anti-leukotrienes	to treat allergies	anti-leucotrienes	para tratar alergias
antilipidemics	to reduce concentration of lipids in the serum	antilipidémicos	para reducir la concentración de lípidos en el suero
antioncotics	to treat tumefaction	antioncóticos	para tratar la tumefacción
antipruritics	to reduce itching symptoms	antipruríticos	para tratar síntomas de picazón
antiseptics	to inhibit infection or putrefaction	antisépticos	para impedir infección o la putrefacción
antitussive	to relieve or reduce cough	antitusivos	para aliviar o reducir la tos
barbiturics	to relieve anxiety or insomnia	barbitúricos	para reducir la ansiedad o el insomnio
bronchodilators	to expand the air passages or dilate bronchi	broncodilatador	para ampliar los conductos respiratorios o dilatar los bronquios
cathartics	to treat constipation	catárticos, purgantes	para tratar el estreñimiento

corticosteroids	to treat swelling, or glands deficiency	corticosteroides	para tratar la inchazón o la deficiencia
decongestants	to reduce congestion or swelling	descongestionantes	para reducir la congestion o la hinchazón
diuretics	to increase urine production	diuréticos	para aumentar la producción de orina
emetics	to cause vomiting	eméticos	para promover el vómito
expectorants	to promote expectoration	expectorantes	para promover la expectoración
hypnotics, soporifics	to induce sleep and treat anxiety	hipnóticos o soporíficos	para inducir el sueño y tratar la ansiedad
laxatives	to prevent or treat constipation	laxantes	para prevenir o tratar el estreñimiento
stimulants	to stimulate or produce a reaction	estimulantes	para estimular o producir una reacción
tranquilizers	to treat stress and anxiety	tranquilizantes	para traer el estrés y la ansiedad
vasodilators	to cause vasodilatación	vasodilatador	para causar la vasodilatación

A Medication may be Prescribed to:

ENGLISH

1. Prevent or diagnose a disease.

2. Relieve a physical pain or mental problem.

3. Destroy bacteria in the organism.

4. Add to the body a substance that is not produced naturally any more.

5. Create antibodies as a helper to the immune system

Se puede recetar una medicina para:

SPANISH

1. Prevenir o diagnosticar una enfermedad.

2. Aliviar un dolor físico o un problema mental.

3. Destruir bacterias en el organismo.

4. Añadir al cuerpo una sustancia que no produce ya naturalmente.

5. Como una ayuda al sistema inmunológico para crear anticuerpos.

How to Take or Administer Medicines

Administración y toma de medicinas

English	Spanish
Do you have any allergies?	¿Tiene alguna alergia?
Yes, I am allergic to penicillin and aspirin.	Sí, soy alérgico a la penicilina y la aspirina.
Any allergies to any particular food?	¿Alguna alergia a un alimento en particular?
Yes, I am allergic to shellfish.	Sí, soy alérgico a los mariscos.
Take this pill, it is an antihistaminic.	Tome esta pastilla, es un antihistamínico.
This medicine may make you sleepy.	Esta medicina le puede dar sueño.
Take this tablet, do not chew it.	Tome este comprimido, no lo mastique.

This medication will lower your blood pressure. Take it

 __ at bedtime
 __once a day
 __three times a day

Esta medicina le bajará la presión arterial. Tómela

 __ a la hora de acostarse
 __ una vez al día
 __ tres veces al día

How many times should I take the pill?

 __ every three hours
 __ with your meals
 __ before breakfast

¿Cuántas veces debo tomar la pastilla?

 __ cada tres horas
 __ con las comidas
 __ antes del desayuno

How are you feeling today?

 I am coughing very much.

¿Cómo se siente hoy?

 Estoy tosiendo mucho.

Take a spoonful of this syrup

 __ every three hours
 __ if needed to prevent coughing
 __ twice a day

Tome una cucharada de este jarabe

 __ cada tres horas
 __ si lo necesita para prevenir la tos
 __ dos veces al día

Can I take something for the pain? Take

 __ this sedative
 __ as needed for pain
 __ to alleviate the discomfort
 __ before going to bed

¿Puedo tomar algo para el dolor? Tome

 __ este sedante (calmante)
 __ cuando tenga dolor
 __ para aliviar el malestar
 __ antes de acostarse

I have a skin rash, what could I do?

 __ Do not be out when it is sunny and hot
 __ Apply this cream in the affected area
 __ Clean the affected area and apply this lotion
 __ Apply an ice pack to the affected area

Tengo una urticaria, qué puedo hacer?

 __ No salga cuando hace mucho sol y calor
 __ Aplique esta crema al área afectada
 __ Limpie el área afectada y póngase esta loción
 __ Ponga hielo empaquetado sobre el área afectada

English	Spanish
What are the results of the test?	¿Cuáles son los resultados de la prueba?
Your cholesterol is high.	Su colesterol está alto.
This tablet is a cholesterol reducer.	Este comprimido es un reductor del colesterol.
Take the capsule orally (by mouth).	Tome la pastilla oralmente.
Do not chew the pill, swallow it whole.	No mastique la pastilla, tráguela entera.

How to Take or Administer Medicines

Administración y toma de medicinas

ENGLISH	SPANISH
I feel my lungs are congested.	Siento los pulmones congestionados.
This medication is for your lung problem.	Este medicamento es para su problema pulmonar.
__ It reduces congestion	__ reduce la congestión
__ It reduces swelling and congestion	__ reduce la inflamación y la congestión
__ It dilates the lung air passages	__ dilata las vías aéreas del pulmón
What is this other prescription for?	¿Para qué es esta otra receta?
I am prescribing you a diuretic besides the blood pressure pill	Le receto un diurético además de la pastilla de la presión arterial para
__ to increase urination	__ aumentar la emisión de orina
__ take it in the morning	__ tómela por la mañana
__ take it once a day	__ tómela una vez al día
I recommend this suppository, but do not use it if you have a stomachache.	Le recomiendo este supositorio, pero no se lo ponga si tiene dolor de estómago.
Before you begin taking any medication either prescribed or over the counter, check with your doctor or pharmacist.	Antes de comenzar a tomar una medicina, por receta médica o sin ella, consulte a su médico o farmacéutio.
Before you have any dental treatment, tell your dentist that you are taking this medication.	Antes de recibir un tratamiento dental informe a su dentista que está tomando este medicamento.
Are you going to have the influenza vaccine today?	¿Se va a poner la vacuna de la influenza hoy?
This vaccine will be given by injection.	Esta vacuna se administra inyectada.
What are these drops for?	¿Para qué son estas gotas?
It is an antibiotic. You must apply one drop in each eye for three days in a row at bedtime.	Es un antibiótico. Debe ponerse una gota en cada ojo por tres días seguidos, antes de acostarse.

Warnings about Dependancy on Medications

Advertencia Sobre La Dependencia en Medicinas

ENGLISH	SPANISH
1. Is this the first time that you take this medication? Yes, it is the first time.	1. ¿Es esta la primera vez que toma esta medicina? Sí, es la primera vez.
2. You have to be careful with this medication.	2. Debe tener cuidado con esta medicina.
3. This medication is habit-forming.	3. Esta medicina es adictiva.
4. This prescription cannot be refilled without your doctor's approval.	4. Su receta no puede repetirse sin la aprobación de su médico.
5. You cannot take this medication longer than the time prescribed.	5. No puede tomar la medicina más tiempo que el indicado.
6. That is why it is important to take only the amount prescribed.	6. Por eso es importante que tome sólo la cantidad indicada.

Interactions

Interacciones

Interactions	Interacciones
ENGLISH	*SPANISH*
1. Do not drink alcohol while taking this medication.	1. No tome bebidas alcohólicas mientras esté tomando esta medicina.
2. Do not take any other medication if you are taking this pill.	2. No tome ninguna otra medicina mientras esté tomando esta pastilla.
3. This drug interferes with your blood pressure medication.	3. Esta medicina interfiere con su pastilla de la presión arterial.
4. If you are pregnant you cannot take this pill.	4. Si se encuentra embarazada no puede tomar esta pastilla.
5. If you are breast feeding do not take this medication.	5. Si está dando el pecho no puede tomar esta medicina.
6. Medication can cause to have more sensitivity to the sun.	6. Evite exponerse al sol, esta medicina puede causarle mayor sensibilidad al sol.
7. Do not take this medication if you have a fever and pain or if you vomit.	7. No puede tomar este medicamento si tiene calentura y dolor o si tiene vómitos.

Possible Reactions

Posibles reacciones

Possible Reactions	Posibles reacciones
ENGLISH	*SPANISH*
This medication may cause you to have:	**Este medicamento puede causarle:**
an allergic reaction	una reacción alérgica
cough	tos
depression	depresión
dizziness	mareo
insomnia	insomnio
lack of appetite	falta de apetito
nausea	náusea
shortness of breath	falta de respiración
weakness	debilidad

Dosage and Manipulation

Dosis y manipulación

All medications must be safely discarded when it is outdated.	Todo medicamento debe ser desechado en un lugar seguro cuando está pasado de fecha.
If you forget to take the medication do not take a double dose; wait until the next indicated time.	Si se le olvida tomar la medicina no tome una dosis doble, tome la dosis regulada en el próximo tiempo indicado.
The dosage of your medication has been regulated according to your needs; do not give your medication to another person.	La dosis de su medicina se ha graduado de acuerdo con sus necesidades; no ofrezca su medicina a otra persona.
Keep antibiotics refrigerated.	Mantenga los antibióticos refrigerados.
Make sure they are discarded safely.	Cuando los deseche hágalo con precaución.
Always shake the bottle well.	Siempre agite bien la botella.
Certain medicines should be kept at room temperature below 86 degrees F. or 30 degrees C, away from heat, moisture, and light.	Ciertas medicinas deben guardarse a una temperatura ambiental de no más de 86 grados F, o 30 grados C, lejos del calor, la humedad y la luz.

Dosage

Dosis

drops	gotas
half teaspoon	media cucharadita
one tablespoon 1 tbs	una cucharada 1 c.
one teaspoon 1 tsp	una cucharadita 1 cta
one drop	una gota
5 (five) milligrams (mg.)	5 (cinco) miligramos (mg.)
50 (fifty) milligrams (mg.)	50 (cincuenta) miligramos (mg.)
120 (one hundred and twenty) milligrams	120 (ciento veinte) miligramos
240 (two hundred and forty) milligrams	240 (doscientos cuarenta) miligramos
500 (five hundred) milligrams	500 (quinientos) miligramos
1 cubic centimeter (cm .)	1 (un) centímetro cúbico (cm^3.)
1 (one) ounce	1 (una) onza

Use of a medication

El uso de un medicamento

atomizer, spray / atomizador	Use the spray once a day. / Use el **atomizador** una vez al día.
bandage / venda	Keep the bandage clean. / Conserve la **venda** limpia.
capsule, tablet / cápsula, tableta	Chew the tablet. / Mastique la **tableta**.
cough medicine, syrup / jarabe	Shake the cough medicine before using. / Agite el **jarabe** antes de usarlo.
creme, ointment / crema, pomada	Rub in this ointment. / Póngase esta **crema (pomada)**.
drops / gotas	Apply two drops to each eye. / Ponga dos **gotas** en cada ojo.
every day / todos los días	I take the medication every day. / Me tomo la medicina **todos los días**.
glass of water / vaso de agua	I want a glass of water. / Quiero un **vaso de agua**.
habit-forming drug / droga adictiva	Be careful with habit-forming drugs. / Tenga cuidado con las **drogas adictivas**.
injection / inyección	This injection will not hurt. / Esta **inyección** no le dolerá.
intravenous injection / inyección	An intravenous injection is injected in the vein. /Una **inyección intravenosa** se inyecta en la vena.
lotion / loción	Rub the lotion in the affected area. / Frote la **loción** en el área afectada.
pill / pastilla, pildora	Put the pill under the tongue. / Ponga **la pastilla** debajo de la lengua.
powder / papelillo, polvo	Dissolve the powder. / Disuelva el **papelillo**.
water bag (cold, hot) / bolsa de agua (fría, caliente)	Apply a cold **water bag** over the leg. / Ponga **una bolsa** de agua (fría, caliente) sobre la pierna.
suppository / supositorio	Use the applicator to insert the suppository. / Use el aplicador para insertar **el supositorio**.
tonic / tónico, reconstituyente	Take a spoonful of the tonic. / Tómese una cucharada del **tónico**.
sedative / calmante	Take a **sedative** for the pain. / Tómese un **calmante** para el dolor.

Useful Verbs

Verbos útiles

to avoid mistakes	**evitar** los errores
to bring the prescription	**traer** la receta
to destroy the bacteria	**destruir** las bacterias
to discard the pills	**descartar, desechar** las pastillas
to dissolve the tablet	**disolver (ue)** la tableta
to forget, to forget the medication	**olvidar, olvidarse de la medicina**
to inject him, her	**ponerle** una inyección
to keep, put away the medication	**guardar, conservar** la medicina
to miss taking the medication	**dejar de tomar** la medicina
to relieve the pain	**aliviar, aliviarse** (oneself) el dolor
to supply the body	**abastecer** el cuerpo
to swallow the pill whole	**tragar** to swallow la pastilla entera; **trague** (command)
to take the medication (yourself)	**tomar** la medicina, **tomarse** la medicina

DRUG ABUSE / EL ABUSO DE LAS DROGAS

Prescription Drugs and Illegal Drugs "street drugs" / Drogas de prescripción y drogas ilegales "de la calle"

Drug Classification

Clasificación de las drogas

NARCOTICS

Substances derived from opium or produced artificially as analgesics. These drugs produce feelings of euphoria and relief accompanied by symptoms of drowsiness and sleepiness that provoke alterations on mood and behavior. If a narcotic is used repeatedly the user can develop a physical and psychological dependence that becomes an addiction.

OPIATES

heroin / heroína   *morphine / morfina*   *opium / opio*

Opiates: painkillers or **analgesics, antianxiety drugs**; affect the central nervous system disrupting vital functions like perception, speech, coordination and memory; its addiction could induce the addict to commit violent crimes. **Heroin** is a morphine like drug, its addiction causes withdrawal effects. In the United States the heroin is only permitted to be used legally in research. **Morphine** produces a combination of depression and excitation to the central nervous system. When it is not used in sedatives with caution, it can be addictive and become a hard drug which addiction is hard to get rid off.

BARBITURATES

Sedatives, **hypnotics**, are prescribed for insomnia, anxiety, digestive problems, taken with repetition tend to cause physical dependence, affect the respiratory system, the blood pressure, causing physical and psychological dependence, and even death when taken in an overdose.

DEPRESSANTS: DOWNERS

Alcohol, tranquilizers, barbiturates, depress the central nervous system, diminish anxiety; affect bodily function in motor and cognitive activities reducing muscular activities, coordination, and inhibition in the addicted person.

NARCÓTICOS

Sustancias analgésicas derivadas del opio o producidas artificialmente como analgésicos. Estas drogas producen una sensación de euforia y bienestar, acompañados por síntomas de somnolencia y sopor que provocan alteraciones en el estado de ánimo y la conducta. Si la dosis del narcótico se repite con frecuencia puede causar en el usuario de la droga una dependencia física y psicológica que se convierte en adicción.

OPIÁCEOS

Los opiáceos se clasifican en: **calmantes** o **analgésicos, drogas contra la ansiedad**; afectan el sistema nervioso central obstruyendo funciones vitales de la percepción, del habla, la coordinación, pueden inducir al adicto a cometer crímenes de violencia. **La heroína** es parecida a la **morfina**, su adicción provoca efectos terribles, se usa sólo legalmente en investigaciones en los Estados Unidos. **La morfina** produce una combinación de depresión y excitación en el sistema nervioso central. Si no se usa con precaución en la composición de los sedativos llega a ser una droga adictiva en los sedativos cuya adicción es muy difícil de curar.

BARBITÚRICOS

Sedativos, **hipnóticos**, son recetados para el insomnio, la ansiedad, problemas digestivos, tomados repetidas veces son adictivos afectan la respiración, la presión arterial y el sistema nervioso. Los sedativos pueden causar dependencia física y psicológica, y pueden provocar la muerte en una sobredosis.

DEPRESIVOS: SEDANTES

El alcohol, los tranquilizantes, y los **barbitúricos**, actúan como depresivos del sistema nervioso, disminuyen la ansiedad, las funciones motoras y cognitivas reduciendo la actividad muscular, la coordinación e inhibición de la persona adicta.

Drug Classification

Clasificación de las drogas

STIMULANTS:

Caffeine, **amphetamines** and **cocaine** are three stimulants that are addictive; both drugs are circulatory and respiratory stimulants and psycho-stimulant substances. **Cocaine** is a potent central nervous system stimulant, vasoconstrictor, and anesthetic. An addiction to **cocaine** can cause severe adverse physical and mental volatile effects. **Inhalants** belong to this group, inhalers are: glue, gasoline, aerosols and anesthetics that damage the exterior layer of the brain destroying nervous cells.

ESTIMULANTES

Cafeína, **anfetaminas** y **cocaína** son tres estimulantes adictivos. Las **anfetaminas** y la **cocaína** son estimulantes circulatorios, respiratorios y sustancias sicoestimulantes. La **cocaína** es un potente estimulante del sistema nervioso central, es vaso constrictor y anestésico; una adicción a la **cocaína** puede causar adversos efectos físicos y mentales. Los **inhalantes** pertenecientes a este grupo son los pegamentos, la gasolina, los rociadores y anestésicos que actúan en el cerebro destruyendo la capa exterior de las células nerviosas.

HALLUCINOGENICS

Mescaline or **peyote**, **phencyclidine** (**PCP**), the most potent of the hallucinogenic drugs, produces symptoms of an aggressive behavior with long lasting emotional problems. Lysergic acid (LSD) can produce mind alterations: colors can be heard and sounds that can be seen by the user. A high dose can cause tremors, high blood pressure, and loss of consciousness.

ALUCINÓGENOS

La mezcalina o **peyote está** entre los alucinógenos, (PCP) o **lietelmida**. El más potente de los alucinógenos produce síntomas de una conducta agresiva con problemas emocionales de larga duración. El ácido lisérgico (LSD) produce alteraciones mentales: colores pueden oírse por el adicto y los sonidos pueden verse. Altas dosis puede producir temblores, presión alta y pérdida del conocimiento.

DESIGNER DRUGS

Potentially lethal drugs, synthetically manufactured, non prescription drugs known as "street drugs", herbal ectasy: **methamphemine**, **amphemine**, **ephedrin**, **marijuana, synthetic heroin**. An overdose may cause respiratory paralysis, causing death. Other drugs such as **steroids**, **crack cocaine**, as well as **inhalants**, cause devastating psychological and physical effects, such as nausea, faintness, stroke, depression, and paranoia.

DROGAS DE DISEÑO

Drogas manufacturadas sintéticamente, potencialmente mortales, sin prescripción, conocidas por "drogas de la calle" son: éxtasis herbicida: **metanfemin**, **anfemin**, **efedrina**, **marijuana**, **heroína sintética**; una sobredosis puede causar parálisis respiratoria. Otras drogas **esteroides**, **cocaína crack**, al igual que drogas por inhalación, causan daños desvastadores, psicológicos y fisiológicos, tales como náusea, desmayos, derrame cerebral, depresión y paranoia.

Symptoms Related to Drug Abuse

Síntomas relacionados con la adicción a las drogas

anxiety	ansiedad
blisters	ampollas
blood vessel constriction	constricción de los vasos sanguíneos
chemical odor on breath	aliento con olor a sustancia química
chronic cough	tos crónica
seizures	convulsiones

Symptoms Related to Drug Abuse	Síntomas relacionados con la adicción a las drogas
damage in the brain	daño cerebral
depression	depresión
dilated pupils	pupilas dilatadas
disorientation	desorientación
elevated blood pressure	tensión alta
excitement	excitación
goose bumps	carne de gallina
heightened sexual sensations	sensaciones sexuales exaltadas
hyperactivity	hiperactividad
in the kidneys	en los riñones
in the liver	en el hígado
in the lungs	en los pulmones
in the nerves	en los nervios
increased heart rate	aumento de la frecuencia cardíaca
increased sensory perception	aumento en la percepción sensorial
increased heart beat	taquicardia
increased sweating	aumento sudorífico
liver failure	fallo hepático
rash around the mouth	erupción alrededor de la boca
rash around the nose	erupción alrededor de la nariz
reduced anxiety	ansiedad disminuída
reduced inhibición	inhibición disminuída
restlessness	inquietud
tremors	temblores

Questions and some possible answers the caller must be ready to answer if he/she calls 911 in case of an emergency.

Preguntas y algunas posibles respuestas que la persona que llama al 911 en caso de emergencia debe estar preparada para contestar.

ENGLISH	*SPANISH*
1. What is your name? My name is Andrew Smith.	1. ¿Cómo se llama usted? Me llamo Andrés Pérez.
2. Where do you live? I live at 445 (four, four, five) North Camino Mayor.	2. ¿Dónde vive? Vivo en el 445 (cuatro, cuatro, cinco) Norte de Camino Mayor.
3. Where are you calling from? __ from my home __ from Broadway and 50th street	3. ¿De dónde está haciendo la llamada? __ de mi casa __ de las calles Broadway y 50 (cincuenta)
4. Are you the person having the problem? __Yes, it is me. __ No, it is my brother. __ No, it is someone that fell down in the street.	4. ¿Es usted la persona que tiene el problema? __Sí, soy yo. __No, es mi hermano. __No, es alguién que se cayó en la calle.
5. Can you describe as best as possible what is the problem? __ I have a pain in my chest __My brother has difficulty breathing. __This man that fell on the pavement doesn't seem able to move.	5. ¿Puede usted describir lo mejor posible cuál es el problema? __Tengo dolor en el pecho. __Mi hermano tiene dificultad al respirar. __ Este señor que se cayó en el pavimento no parece poder moverse.
6. The ambulance will be there soon. Thank you.	6. La ambulancia llegará en breve. Gracias.

AMBULANCE AND EMERGENCY ROOM/ AMBULANCIA Y SALÓN DE EMERGENCIA

Questions addressed directly to the patient / Preguntas directas al paciente

ENGLISH	SPANISH
1. To what hospital do you wish to go? __ to the closest __ to St. Mary's __ I don't have a preference. __ I don't know.	1. ¿A qué hospital quiere que lo (la) llevemos? __ al más cercano __ al Santa María __ No tengo preferencia. __ No sé.
2. Do you understand what I am saying? __barely __Yes, I can understand you.	2. ¿ Entiende lo que le digo? __apenas __Sí, lo entiendo.
3. What is your name? Andrew Smith	3. ¿Cómo se llama ? Me llamo Andrés Pérez.
4. What day of the week is it? __ I don't know. __ It is Tuesday. __Today is Saturday.	4. ¿Qué día de la semana es hoy? __ No sé. __ Es martes. __ Hoy es sábado.
5. Who is your doctor? __ My doctor is Dr. Joseph Meyer. __I don't have a doctor.	5. ¿Quién es su médico? __ Mi médico es el doctor José Meyer. __ No tengo ningún médico.
6. Has someone notified your doctor? __ I think so. __ I don't know.	6. ¿Alguién le ha notificado a su médico? __ Creo que sí. __ No sé.
7. Are you in pain? __ I have some pain. __Yes, I have a lot of pain.	7. ¿Tiene dolor? __Tengo un poco de dolor. __ Sí, tengo mucho dolor.
8. Are you having any problem breathing? __ some difficulty __Yes, it is difficult to breathe.	8. Tiene alguna dificultad para respirar? __ alguna dificultad __ Sí, me resulta difícil respirar.
9. Have you fainted or lost consciousness at any time? __ No, I have not. __Yes, I have fainted.	9. ¿Se ha desmayado o ha perdido el conocimiento alguna vez? __ No, nunca. __ Sí, me he desmayado.
10. Are you taking any medication?	10. ¿Está tomando alguna medicina?
11. How many pills did you take? __two, __ four,__ six	11. ¿Cuántas pastillas tomó? __dos,__cuatro,__seis
12. Are you allergic to any medications?	12. ¿Es alérgico-a a alguna medicina?
13. When did the accident occur? __about one hour ago __yesterday __over the week-end	13. ¿Cuándo ocurrió el accidente? __ hace como una hora __ ayer __ durante el fin de semana

Questions addressed directly to the patient

Preguntas directas al paciente

ENGLISH	SPANISH
14. Where did it happen? __on this same street __at my parents' house __at the beach	14. ¿Dónde ocurrió? __ en esta misma calle __ en casa de mis padres __ en la playa
15. Have you had a tetanus shot? __I am not sure.	15. ¿Se ha inyectado contra el tétano? __ no estoy seguro-a
16. When was the last time? __about a year ago __when I was a child	16. ¿Cuándo fue la última vez? __ hace como un año __ cuando era niño-a
17. Have you been hospitalized before?	17. ¿Ha sido hospitalizado-a alguna vez?
18. When? __six months ago __last year __many years ago	18. ¿Cuándo? __ hace seis meses __ el año pasado __ hace muchos años
19. For what reason? __when I had my baby __when I had surgery __when I had a bout of vertigo	19. ¿Por qué razón? __ cuando di a luz __ cuando tuve cirugía __ cuando tuve un episodio de vértigo
20. Was it here or somewhere else? __Yes, it was here. __It was in New York, where I used to live.	20. ¿Fue aquí o en alguna otra parte? __ Sí, fue aquí. __ fue en Nueva York, donde yo vivía antes.
(to a female patient) 21. Do you know if you are pregnant? __ No, I could not be pregnant. __Yes, it is possible. __ I don't know.	*(a pacientes femeninos)* 21. ¿ Sabe usted si está embarazada? __ No, no puedo estar embarazada. __ Sí, es posible. __ No sé.

QUESTIONS RELATED TO A THIRD PARTY

PREGUNTAS REFERENTES A UNA TERCERA PERSONA

ENGLISH	*SPANISH*
Is he/she wounded?	¿Está él/ella herido-a?
Is he/she confused?	¿Está él/ella confuso-a?
Is he/she lethargic?	¿Está él/ella aletargado-a?
Is he/she coherent?	¿Está coherente?
Is he/she bleeding?	¿Está sangrando?
Does he/she have pain?	¿Tiene dolor?
Is he/she conscious or unconscious?	¿Está consciente o inconsciente?
Can he/she talk?	¿Puede hablar?
Is he/she breathing well?	¿Respira bien?
Can he/she move?	¿Puede moverse?
Is he/she agitated?	¿Muestra agitación?
Can he/she hear you?	¿Puede oirle?
Is he/she vomiting?	¿Está vomitando?
Is he/she hemorrhaging?	¿Tiene hemorragia?
Does he/she seem to be having a heart attack?	¿Parece tener un ataque al corazón?
Can he/she answer any questions?	¿Puede responder a preguntas?

HOSPITALIZATION / HOSPITALIZACIÓN

ENGLISH	SPANISH
1. Do you have the written doctor's orders with you?	1. ¿Tiene las indicaciones del doctor consigo?
2. It is necessary to complete some paper work before you are admitted.	2. Necesitamos obtener cierta información antes de ingresarlo-a.
3. Sit in this wheelchair, please.	3. Siéntese en esta silla de ruedas, por favor.
4. We are taking you to your room.	4. Lo (la) vamos a llevar a su cuarto.
5. We suggest you don't keep any valuables in your room because the hospital is not responsible for lost items.	5. Le aconsejamos que no deje objetos de valor en el cuarto ya que el hospital no se hace responsable por cualquier pérdida de objetos.
6. We need a signed consent for your surgery.	6. Necesitamos una autorización firmada para su operación.
7. Push this button for assistance.	7. Apriete este botón si necesita algo.
8. Call if you need __ to use the bedpan __ a sleeping pill __ something for the pain __ something to drink __ an extra pillow or blanket	8. Llame si necesita __ usar el bacín __ una pastilla para dormir __ algo para aliviar el dolor __ algo para tomar __ una almohada o una frazada (cobija) adicional
9. You can get out of bed.	9. Puede bajarse de la cama.
10. You must stay in bed.	10. Debe quedarse en la cama.
11. I am the nurse.	11. Soy el (la) enfermero-a.
12. I need to take your __ pulse __ temperature __ blood pressure	12. Tengo que tomarle __ el pulso __ la temperatura __ la presión arterial
13. I am going to take a sample of blood.	13. Voy a tomarle una muestra de sangre.
14. I need to give you a shot.	14. Tengo que ponerle una inyección.
15. I am going to give you an intravenous feeding.	15. Voy a ponerle un suero en la vena.
16. This will not hurt.	16. No le va a doler.
17. Someone will come to take you to __ the x-ray room __ the laboratory __ the rehabilitation room	17. Alguien va a venir a llevarlo-a __ a la sala de rayos-x __ al laboratorio __ a la sala de rehabilitación

SURGERY / CIRUGÍA

ENGLISH	SPANISH
1. I am going to prepare you for surgery	1. Voy a prepararlo-a para la operación.
2. I am going to give you an enema.	2. Voy a ponerle un lavado intestinal.
3. I am going to shave you.	3. Lo (la) voy a rasurar.
4. Your surgery is scheduled for __ later __ this afternoon __ tomorrow morning __ tomorrow afternoon	4. La cirugía va a ser __ más tarde __ esta tarde __ mañana por la mañana __ mañana por la tarde
5. The anesthetist will be here to talk to you and ask you some questions __ soon __ later __ before surgery	5. El (la) anestesista vendrá a hablar con usted y a hacerle algunas preguntas __ dentro de un ratico __ más tarde __ antes de la operación
6. We will give you a sedative before taking you to the operating room.	6. Le vamos a dar un calmante antes de llevarlo-a a la sala de operaciones.
7. Would you like us to notify your family of the time of the operation?	7. ¿Quiere que le hagamos saber a su familia a qué hora es la operación?
8. After the operation you will be taken to the recovery room.	8. Después de la operación lo (la) llevarán a la sala de recuperación.
9. When you wake up you may have __ a tube in your throat to help you breathe __ a tube in the bladder to help you urinate __ a tube in the stomach so you will not vomit	9. Al despertarse tal vez tenga __ un tubo en la garganta para ayudarlo-a a respirar __ un tubo en la vejiga para que pueda orinar __ un tubo en el estómago para que no vomite
10. An IV will be inserted before and throughout surgery until you start eating and drinking again.	10. Le van a poner un suero intravenoso antes y durante la cirugía hasta que empiece a alimentarse de nuevo.
11. Your doctor will be here __ soon __ later __ tomorrow	11. Su médico vendrá a verle __ pronto __ más tarde __ mañana
12. You will be discharged __ later __ tomorrow __ in a week	12. Le van a dar de alta __ más tarde __ mañana __ dentro de una semana
13. Call your doctor's office and make an appointment __ in a week __ in ten days	13. Llame a la consulta de su médico y pida turno para dentro de __ una semana __ diez días
14. Call us if you need help, but if it is an emergency, call 911 (nine one one).	14. Llame aquí si necesita asistencia, pero si se trata de una emergencia, llame al 911 (nueve uno uno).

ANESTHESIA / ANESTESIA

ENGLISH	**SPANISH**
1. I am the anesthetist.	1. Soy el (la) anestesista.
2. I need to ask you some questions.	2. Tengo que hacerle algunas preguntas.
3. Are you allergic to anything? To what? __to dairy products __to aerosols __I suffer from hay fever.	3. ¿Es alérgico-a a algo? ¿A qué? __a productos lácteos __a aerosoles __Yo padezco de fiebre de heno.
4. Are you allergic to any medication? Which? __to penicillin __to antibiotics in general	4. ¿Es usted alérgico-a a alguna medicina? ¿A cuál? __a la penicilina __a antibióticos en general
5. Are you taking any medication? Which? __medication for high blood pressure __an antidepressant __something for my allergy	5. ¿Está tomando alguna medicina? ¿Cuál? __medicina para la presión arterial alta __un antidepresivo __algo para mi alergia
6. How long have you been taking it? __for three months __since I had my last child __for many years	6. ¿Por cuánto tiempo la ha estado tomando? __por tres meses __desde que tuve mi último parto __durante muchos años
7. Have you been taking aspirin for any reason?	7. ¿Ha estado tomando aspirina por algún motivo?
8. Are you taking any diuretic?	8. ¿Toma algún diurético?
9. Have you had surgery before?	9. ¿Ha tenido alguna operación anteriormente?
10. What kind of an operation was it? __an appendectomy __heart surgery __a hernia operation	10. ¿Qué tipo de operación fue? __una apendectomía __cirugía del corazón __operación de una hernia
11. Do you remember what kind of anesthesia you had?	11. ¿Recuerda usted que clase de anestesia le dieron?
12. Did you have any trouble with the anesthesia?	12. ¿Tuvo alguna dificultad con la anestesia?
13. What kind of trouble? __nausea and vomiting __difficulty in walking __heart problems __lung problems	13. ¿Qué tipo de dificultad? __náusea y vómito __dificultad al caminar __problema cardíaco __problema pulmonar
14. Today we are going to give you the following anesthesia. (*V.* **anesthesia**)	14. Hoy le vamos a dar la siguiente anestesia. (*V.* **anestesia**)
15. Try to relax.	15. Trate de relajarse.

COMMANDS / ÓRDENES

Positions and Body Movements	Posiciones y movimientos del cuerpo
ENGLISH	SPANISH
1. Stand here.	1. Párese aquí.
2. Stand here and do not move.	2. Párese aquí y no se mueva.
3. Sit on the table.	3. Siéntese sobre la mesa.
4. Lie down on the table __ on your back __ face down __ on your right side __ on your left side	4. Acuéstese sobre la mesa __ boca arriba __ boca abajo __ sobre el lado derecho __ sobre el lado izquierdo
5. Put your knees against your chest and let your chin touch your chest.	5. Acerque las rodillas al pecho lo más posible y deje que la barbilla toque el pecho.
6. Put your arms around this machine.	6. Ponga los brazos alrededor de esta máquina.
7. Do not get up, remain lying down.	7. No se levante, quédese acostado-a.
8. Raise your head.	8. Levante la cabeza.
9. Raise your hands.	9. Levante las manos.
10. Raise your right hand.	10. Levante la mano derecha.
11. Raise your left hand __ higher __ lower	11. Levante la mano izquierda __ más hacia arriba __ más hacia abajo
12. Open your hand.	12. Abra la mano.
13. Close your hand.	13. Cierre la mano.
14. Extend your fingers.	14. Extienda los dedos.
15. Close your fingers one at a time.	15. Cierre uno por uno los dedos.
16. Lift your right leg.	16. Levante la pierna derecha.
17. Lift your left leg.	17. Levante la pierna izquierda.
18. Can you move the leg?	18. ¿Puede mover la pierna?
19. Bend over.	19. Dóblese.
20. Bend over backwards.	20. Dóblese hacia atrás.
21. Raise your buttocks (hips).	21. Levante las nalgas (las asentaderas, caderas).
22. Put your hands behind your head.	22. Ponga las manos detrás de la cabeza.
23. Extend your arms, and bringing them towards the front, touch the tips of your index fingers together.	23. Extienda los brazos y, trayéndolos hacia el frente, toque las puntas de los dedos índice.

Commands / Órdenes

Positions and Body Movements	Posiciones y movimientos del cuerpo
ENGLISH	*SPANISH*
24. Bend your arm.	24. Doble el brazo.
25. Extend your arm.	25. Extienda el brazo.
26. Squeeze my hand.	26. Apriéteme la mano.
27. Squeeze my hand as hard as you can.	27. Apriéteme la mano lo más fuerte que pueda.
28. Make a fist.	28. Cierre el puño.
29. Open your mouth.	29. Abra la boca.
30. Rinse your mouth.	30. Enjuáguese la boca.

TRAUMA AND EMERGENCY PROBLEMS / TRAUMA Y PROBLEMAS DE EMERGENCIA

ENGLISH		*SPANISH*	
Foreign Bodies Penetrating the Body		**Cuerpos extraños que penetran el cuerpo**	
ORGAN OR PART	CAUSE CONSEQUENCES	ÓRGANO O PARTE	CAUSA CONSECUENCIAS
abdomen	splinter	abdomen	astilla, espina
chest	abrasions	tórax	abrasiones
eye, ear,	knives	ojo, oído,	cuchillos
throat	hemorrhage	garganta	hemorragia
extremities	sharp instruments	extremidades	instrumentos afilados
skull	infections	cráneo	infecciones
	bullet		heridas de bala
	projectile wounds		laceraciones por proyectil
	scratches		rasguños

SOME COMPLICATIONS DUE TO FOREIGN BODIES		*CIERTAS COMPLICACIONES DEBIDAS A CUERPOS EXTRAÑOS*	
abdominal:	internal hemorrhage; infection	**abdominal:**	hemorragia interna; infecciones
chest:	infection complications, hemorrhage	**tórax:**	complicaciones de infecciones, hemorragia
eye:	scratches, abrasions, lacerations, infections	**ojo:**	rasguños, abrasiones, desgarros, infecciones
ear and nose:	pain and pus	**oído y nariz:**	dolor y secreción purulenta
pharynx:	occlusion of the airway	**faringe:**	oclusión del conducto respiratorio
stomach and bowel:	discomfort, pain; sharp objects when swallowed may cause vomiting, gastrointestinal hemorrhage	**estómago e intestino:**	molestia y dolor; la ingestion de objetos cortantes puede causar vómitos, hemorragia intestinal
urethral:	discharge, pain, and bleeding	**uretral:**	flujo, dolor y sangramiento
vaginal:	lacerations, infection, bleeding	**vaginal:**	laceraciones, infección, sangramiento

ENGLISH	SPANISH
PENETRATING WOUNDS	**HERIDAS PENETRANTES**
gunshot wounds, knife, dagger, blade or stab wounds, blunt instrument injury, wounds produced by animal bites: dogs, cats, rodents, wild animals, African bees, black widow spiders, snakes, scorpions, jellyfish, octopuses, sponges, etc.	heridas de bala, heridas de cuchillo o puñal, heridas de instrumento despuntado, lesiones producidas por picaduras o mordidas de animales: perros, gatos, roedores, animales salvajes, abejas africanas, serpientes, arañas negras, escorpiones, aguamala, pulpos, esponjas, etc.

Airway Foreign Bodies
Cuerpos extraños en el conducto respiratorio

VIA	SYMPTOMS	VIA	SÍNTOMAS
penetrating through puncture wounds, by swallowing	cough, chest pain, dyspnea, gasping for air, unable to speak, unable to swallow normally	penetrando a través de heridas de perforación, o al tragar.	tos, dolor en el pecho, disnea, estridor, jadeo, dificultad al hablar o al tragar

Substances Causing Toxic Effects by Inhalation, Ingestion, or by Direct Contact
Sustancias que causan efectos tóxicos por aspiración, ingestión o por contacto directo

SUBSTANCE	SUSTANCIA
alcohols (ethanol, methanol)	alcoholes (etanol, metanol)
alkalis (ammonia)	alcalíes (amoníaco)
arsenic	arsénico
boric acid	ácido bórico
carbon monoxide	monóxido de carbono
cleaners (toilet, ovens, pools)	limpiadores (de servicios, hornos, piscinas)
contaminated fish, ciguatera	pescado contaminado, ciguatera
cyanide	cianuro
herbicides	herbicidas
metals (iron, lead)	metales (hierro, plomo)
muriatic acid	ácido muriático
mushrooms	setas (hongos)
overdose of medications (salicylates, neuroleptics, antidepressants, opiates, etc.)	sobredosis de medicamentos (salicilatos, neurolépticos, tranquilizantes, opiáceos, etc.)
paint thinners, antifreeze, etc.	aguarrás, trementina, anticongelante
plants (hemlock, morning glory, daffodil, hyacinth, ivy, oleander)	plantas (cicuta, gloria de la mañana, narciso trompón, jacinto, hiedra venenosa, adelfa)
contaminated shellfish	mariscos contaminados
strong acids	ácidos fuertes

EFFECT	EFECTO
abdominal pain	dolor abdominal
airway obstruction	obstrucción del conducto respiratorio
allergies	alergias
arrhythmias	arritmias
asphyxia	asfixia
bronchospasm	broncoespasmo
burns	quemaduras
collapse	colapso

ENGLISH	SPANISH
EFFECT	*EFECTO*
coma	coma
confusion	confusión
dizziness	mareo
dehydration	deshidratación
dyspnea	disnea
edema of the pharynx and larynx	edema de la faringe y la laringe
hoarseness	ronquera
intoxication	intoxicación
muscle spasms	espasmo muscular
pulmonary edema	edema pulmonar
respiratory failure	fallo respiratorio
stridor	estridor

Intoxication—poisoning / Intoxicación—envenenamiento

alkali poisoning – ingestion of an alkali or ammoniac	**ingestión de una sustancia alcalí** – amoníaco, legía
caffeinism – excessive ingestion of products containing caffeine	**cafeinismo** – envenenamiento por ingestión excesiva de productos conteniendo cafeína
carbon monoxide – absorbing carbon monoxide causes a toxic condition that can be lethal	**monóxido de carbono** – envenenamiento por absorción e inhalación de monóxido de carbono puede ser letal
cyanide poisoning – can occur by inhaling smoke or ingesting cyanide industrial chemicals	**envenenamiento de cianuro** puede ocurrir por inhalaciones de humo o ingestión de sustancias químicas industriales
ergotism – ingesting ergot-infected grain products that cause diarrhea, vomiting and even alteration of the heart rhythm	**ergotismo** – consumiendo productos de grano infestado por ergot que pueden causar diarrea y hasta causar alteración del ritmo cardíaco
alcohol intoxication – excessive ingestion of alcohol can be habit forming and cause serious physical and psychological problems	**intoxicación alcohólica** – ingestión excesiva de alcohol puede ser adictiva y causar serios problemas físicos y psicológicos
lead poisoning – by ingestion or inhalation of paints that contain lead, or containers of water such as water pipes and water tanks	**envenenamiento por plomo** – por ingestión o absorción, causado por pinturas que contienen plomo, o por contenedores de agua tal como tuberías y tanques
mercury poisoning – poisoning by ingesting mercury could cause acute kidney damage, vomiting and diarrhea that could be lethal	**envenenamiento por mercurio** – puede causar daño severo al riñón, vómito y diarrea que pueden ser letales
nicotine poisoning – inhalation and ingestion of great amounts of nicotine	**envenenamiento por nicotina** – inhalación e ingestión de una gran cantidad de nicotina
overdose of drugs – salicylates, neuroleptics, antidepressants, and opiates prescribed or obtained illegally	**sobredosis de drogas** – salicilatos, neurolépticos, antidepresivos, opiados, prescritos u obtenidos ilegalmente
contaminated shellfish	**mariscos contaminados**

ophidism – poisoning by snakes, bees, ants, spiders, producing an injected venom	**ofidismo** – envenenamiento causado por la ponzoña de una abeja, hormiga, avispa, o araña negra o el veneno de una serpiente
strong cleaning substances – mixed with strong acids	**sustancias limpiadoras** – mezcladas con ácidos fuertes

Burns

Quemaduras

acid burns	quemaduras por ácido
fire burns	quemaduras por fuego
frostbite	quemadura de frío
radiation burns	quemaduras por radiación
sunburns	quemadura de sol

SKIN BURNS	POSSIBLE EFFECTS	QUEMADURAS DE LA PIEL	EFECTOS POSIBLES
first-degree burns (scalds)	painful erythema, scalds	quemaduras de primer grado (escaldadura)	eritema doloroso, escaldaduras
second-degree burns (damage to the lower layer of the skin; superficial or deep)	blisters, scars	quemaduras de segundo grado: (daño a la segunda capa cutánea; superficial o profundo)	ampollas
third-degree burns (go into the subcutaneous layer; destruction of epidermis and posible dermis)	hard and charred burns, inhalation of vapors, shock, possible airway obstruction	quemaduras de tercer grado (penetran la capa subcutánea; destrucción de la epidermis y posiblemente la dermis)	quemaduras duras y carbonizadas, inhalación de vapores, choque, posible obstrucción del conducto respiratorio
fourth-degree burns (involving skin, muscle and bones)	same damage as third-degree burns, involving a higher % of the body	quemaduras de cuarto grado (comprenden la piel, músculos y huesos)	el mismo daño que las quemaduras de tercer grado; pero cubriendo un por ciento mayor del cuerpo

Chest Pain

POSSIBLE CAUSES	SYMPTOMS
myocardial infarction, heart attack	chest pain in the center of the chest behind the sternum; sweating, possible nausea and vomiting
angina pectoris	chest pain with a sensation of pressure, sweaty brow, pain radiates to the left shoulder, and sometimes to the arm
pericarditis	chest pain, dull or sharp, rapid breathing, cough

Dolor en el pecho

CAUSA POSIBLE	SÍNTOMAS
infarto del miocardio, ataque al corazón	dolor en el pecho que puede correrse al cuello, al maxilar y al brazo; sudor y posibles náuseas y vómitos
angina de pecho	dolor en el pecho con sensación de presión, sudores en la frente; el dolor se irradia al hombro izquierdo y a veces al brazo
pericarditis	dolor sordo o agudo en el pecho, respiración rápida, tos

Loss of Consciousness

CAUSED BY SEIZURES

alcohol or other drug withdrawal
drug abuse
epilepsy
febrile convulsions
head trauma
metabolic problems

CAUSED BY COMA

diabetic
traumatic: head, massive hemothorax
hyperglycemic
hypoglycemic
drug overdose

Pérdida del Conocimiento

DEBIDO A CONVULSIONES

privación de alcohol o de otra droga
adicción a las drogas
epilepsia
convulsiones febriles
contusión cerebral
problemas metabólicos

DEBIDO A COMA

diabético
traumático: cerebral, hemotórax masivo
hiperglicémico
hipoglicémico
sobredosis

Eye Emergencies

SYMPTOM

abrasion, scrape
perforating injury
swelling and pain
chemical penetration
foreign body piercing
eye discharge with pus and redness
severe constant pain
sudden red or pink colored vision
sudden blindness or double vision

Other Emergencies

cardiopulmonary resuscitation
overdose
emergency delivery
vaginal bleeding
hypertension
child abuse
sexual assault
drowning
suicide

Emergencias de la vista

SÍNTOMA

abrasión o desgarramiento
herida con perforación
hinchazón y dolor
penetración de una sustancia química
penetración de cuerpo extraño
enrojecimiento y supuración del ojo con pus
dolor constante y fuerte
visión súbita de color rojo o rosada
ceguera súbita o visión doble

Otras emergencias

reanimación cardiopulmonar
sobredosis
parto de emergencia
sangramiento vaginal
hipertensión
niños maltratados
violación sexual
ahogo
suicidio

Appendix B
- Signs and Symptoms
- Medical Tests
- Surgical Procedures

Apéndice B
- Señales y síntomas
- Pruebas o estudios médicos
- Procedimentos quirúrgicos

SIGNS AND SYMPTOMS IN MOST COMMON DISORDERS AND DISEASES / SEÑALES Y SÍNTOMAS DE TRASTORNOS Y ENFERMEDADES MÁS COMUNES

ENGLISH	*SPANISH*
abscess in	**absceso**
brain	cerebral
breast	de la mama
kidney	del riñón
throat (tonsilar)	amigdalino (garganta)
abnormal color in feces, stools	**color anormal en las heces fecales o excremento**
black	ennegrecido
pale	pálido
red	rojizo
white	blanquecino
abnormal color in the urine	**cambios anormales en el color de la orina**
coffee	pardo-negrusco
pale	casi sin color
pink, reddish	rosáceo, rojo
yellow-orange	amarillo-anaranjado
abnormal fatigue	**cansancio excesivo**
abnormal odor in urine	**olor anormal en la orina**
aromatic	aromático
foul	fétido
abnormal walking	**marcha, andar anormal**
accummulation of fluids in	**acumulación de líquido en**
abdomen	el abdomen
joints	las articulaciones
tissues	los tejidos
absent periods	**falta de menstruación**
aging, premature	**envejecimiento prematuro**
anxiety	**ansiedad**
apathy	**apatía**
atrophy of muscles	**atrofia muscular**
asphyxiating episodes	**ataques de asfixia**
attention span, limited	**capacidad de atención limitada**
backache	**dolor de espalda**
low	en la parte baja
bad breath, halitosis	**mal aliento, halitosis**
baldness	**calvicie**
behavior	**conducta**
belligerent	agresiva, violenta
excited	excitada

635

ENGLISH	SPANISH
belching	eructos, eructación
black-and-blue marks	morados, moretones
blackheads	espinillas
bleeding from	sangramiento [sangrado de]
the ear	el oído
the gums	las encías
the mouth	la boca
the nose	la nariz
the vagina	la vagina
under the skin	debajo de la piel (sangrado subcutáneo)
a wound	una herida
blemishes	manchas
blindness	ceguera
blind spots	puntos ciegos
blisters	ampollas
blood clot	coágulo
blood flow	flujo de sangre
copious	abundante
scanty	escaso
blood in	presencia de sangre en
the feces	las heces fecales
the urine, spotty	la orina, con manchas
bloodshot eye	ojo inyectado
bluish skin	piel amoratada
blurring	vista nublada
body odor	olor fuerte a sudor
boil	grano, comedón
bones	huesos
calcium loss	pérdida de calcio
deformity	deformidad
fractures	fracturas
spontaneous fractures	fracturas espontáncas
bowlegs	piernas arqueadas
breathing	respiración
abnormal breathing	respiración anormal
choking sensation	sensación de ahogo
difficulty in exhaling	dificultad al exhalar
difficulty in inhaling	dificultad al aspirar
bronzed skin	piel bronceada
bruised body	contusiones en el cuerpo
bulbous red nose	nariz roja y bulbosa

ENGLISH	SPANISH
burning feeling	ardor; sensación quemante
cardiac arrest	paro cardíaco
cardiac arrythamia	arritmia cardíaca
change in bowel habits	cambio en el hábito de defecar, obrar
chapped lips	labios resecos
chills	escalofríos
severe	intensos
cleft lip	labio leporino
cleft hands	manos en garra
clenched teeth	dientes apretados
clotting of blood	coagulación de la sangre
clubbed fingers	dedos en maza
coated tongue	lengua pastosa
coldness in extremities	frialdad de manos y pies
collapse	colapso
collapsing	colapso
knee	de la rodilla
lung	del pulmón
coma	coma
common cold	catarro, resfriado
constipation	estreñimiento
extended, chronic	continuado, crónico
constriction of the penis	constricción del pene
contractions of	contracciones
a muscle	de un músculo
the uterus	del útero
convulsions	convulsiones
coordination loss	pérdida de la coordinación
corns	callos
cough	tos
dry	seca
excessive	excesiva
coughing up blood	expectoración de sangre
coughing up bloody phlegm	expectoración de flema sanguinolenta
crack in the corner of the mouth	grieta en la comisura del labio
cracked lips	labios agrietados
cramps	calambre
cross-eye	estrabismo, bizquera

ENGLISH	SPANISH
cyanosis	cianosis
cyst	quiste
dandruff	caspa
deafness	sordera

deformity of
    the bones
    the fingers
    the joints
    the muscles
	deformidad de
	    los huesos
	    los dedos
	    las articulaciones
	    los músculos

dehydration	deshidratación
delirium	delirio
depression	depresión
desintegration of nails	desintegración de las uñas
diaper rash	eritema de los pañales

diarrhea
    bloody
    constant
    explosive
    light colored
    frothy
    ten to twenty times daily
    severe
	diarrea
	    con sangre
	    constante
	    explosiva
	    de color pálido
	    espumosa
	    de diez a veinte veces al día
	    grave

difficulty in
    breathing
    defecating
    urinating
    swallowing
	dificultad al
	    respirar
	    defecar, obrar
	    orinar
	    tragar

dilated pupil	dilatación de la pupila
dimpling	formación de depresiones u hoyuelos

discharge from
    the ear
    the eye
    the nipples
    the penis
    the vagina
	supuración por
	    el oído
	    el ojo
	    los pezones
	    el pene
	    la vagina

discoloration around the eye	cambio de color de la piel alrededor del ojo
discomfort	molestia
discomfort in passing water	dificultad, molestia al orinar
distended abdomen	abdomen, vientre distendido

ENGLISH	SPANISH
distortion of (visual)	**distorsión visual de**
color	color
size	tamaño
shape	forma
dizziness	**mareo**
double vision	**visión doble**
dribbling	**goteo**
drowsiness	**amodorramiento**
dry mouth	**boca seca**
dyspepsia	**dispepsia**
earache	**dolor de oído**
echoing sounds	**repetición de sonidos**
edema	**edema**
emaciation	**emaciación, enflaquecimiento**
emotional instability	**inestabilidad emocional**
empty bladder	**vejiga vacía**
enlarged	**agrandamiento, engrosamiento**
abdomen	del abdomen
eyeball	del globo del ojo
feet	de los pies
heart	del corazón
lymph nodes	de los nódulos linfáticos
erection difficulty	**dificultad en la erección**
euphoria	**euforia**
excessive urination	**micción excesiva**
exhaustion	**agotamiento**
eyeball	**globo ocular**
rolled upward	virado hacia arriba
palsied	paralizado
protruding	protuberante
failure to gain weight	**no poder aumentar de peso**
failure to lose weight	**no poder adelgazar**
fainting	**desmayo**
false labor pains	**dolores de parto falsos**
fatigue	**cansancio excesivo**
feminization	**feminización**

ENGLISH	SPANISH
fever	**fiebre, calentura**
erratic	errática
high	alta
intermittent	intermitente
persistent	persistente
recurrent	recurrente
fissured tongue	**lengua fisurada**
fixed pupil	**pupila fija**
flabby skin	**piel flácida**
flatfoot	**pie plano**
flushing	**rubor**
foul breath	**aliento fétido**
foul taste	**sabor (muy) desagradable**
fragility of bones	**fragilidad de los huesos**
freckles	**pecas**
frigidity	**frigidez**
frostbite	**quemadura de frío, congelación**
furred tongue	**lengua saburral**
growing pains	**dolores del crecimiento**
hard nodules	**nódulos endurecidos**
in the face	en la cara
in the head	en la cabeza
hardening of the skin	**endurecimiento de la piel**
harelip	**labio leporino**
headache	**dolor de cabeza**
excrutiating and throbing	agudísimo y palpitante
pounding	demoledor
hearing loss	**pérdida de la audición**
heart attack	**ataque al corazón**
heartbeat	**latido del corazón**
extra, repeated	extra, repetido
irregular	irregular
skipped	intermitente
slow	lento
heartburn	**ardor en el estómago**
heart pain	**dolor en el corazón**
heart palpitations	**palpitaciónes cardíacas**
heavy breasts	**senos pesados**
height loss	**disminución en la estatura**

ENGLISH	SPANISH
hemorrhage after menopause	hemorragia después de la menopausia
hiccups	hipo
hissing in the ear, ringing	zumbido en los oídos
hoarseness	ronquera
hot flashes	fogaje, bochorno
incontinence of feces of urine	incontinencia de heces focales de la orina
indigestion	indigestión
inflammation	inflamación
insensibility	insensibilidad
insensitivity to heat or cold	insensibilidad térmica al frío o al calor
insomnia	insomnio
intercourse, painful	coito doloroso
irregular periods	menstruación irregular
jaundice	ictericia
lack of appetite	falta de apetito
large head limbs tongue	agrandamiento de la cabeza de las extremidades de la lengua
lesion	lesión
lethargy	letargo
limping	cojera
listlessness	falta de ánimo, apatía
locked jaw	mandíbula bloqueada
locked knee	rodilla bloqueada
loose teeth	dientes flojos

ENGLISH	SPANISH
loss of	**pérdida**
appetite	del apetito
balance	del equilibrio
bladder control	del control de la vejiga
consciousness	del conocimiento
control of muscle tonicity	del control del tono muscular
muscular coordination	de la coordinación muscular
feeling	del sentido del tacto
libido	del libido
luster in hair	del brillo del pelo
luster in nails	del brillo de las uñas
peripheral vision	de la visión periférica
smell	del olfato
voice	de la voz
low birth weight	**peso bajo al nacer**
lumps in	**bultos, masa en**
breast	el seno, la mama
joints	las articulaciones
neck	el cuello
pubic area	el pubis
magenta tongue	**lengua magenta**
malocclusion	**maloclusión**
masculinization	**masculinización**
memory loss	**pérdida de la memoria**
menstruation problems	**problemas de la menstruación**
mental ability impairment	**deterioro de la habilidad mental**
moles	**lunares**
mouth breathing	**respiración por la boca**
muscular incoordination	**falta de coordinación muscular**
nasal speech	**habla nasal**
night blindness	**ceguera nocturna**
night urination	**micción nocturna**
numbness	**entumecimiento**
obstruction	**obstrucción**
odor	**olor, aroma**
oozing	**excreción**

ENGLISH	SPANISH
pain	**dolor**
dull	sordo
fulminant	fulminante
gripping	opresivo, con sensación de agarrotamiento
lancinating	lancinante
intense	intenso, agudo
irradiating	que se irradia, que se corre
mild	leve
persistent	persistente
severe	severo
painful gums	**encías dolorosas**
painful swelling	**hinchazón dolorosa**
paleness	**palidez**
paleness around the mouth	**palidez alrededor de la boca**
pallor	**palidez**
palpitations	**palpitaciones**
palsy	**parálisis**
paralysis	**parálisis**
peeling of the skin	**peladura, descamación de la piel**
pimples	**granos, barros**
pins and needles sensation	**cosquilleo, hormigueo**
polyps	**pólipos**
postnasal drip	**goteo postnasal**
premature aging	**envejecimiento prematuro**
premature beat	**latido prematuro**
premature ejaculation	**eyaculación prematura**
premature menopause	**menopausia prematura**
premenstrual tension	**tensión premenstrual**
profuse sweating	**sudor excesivo**
prominence of blood vessels	**prominencia de vasos capilares**
prostration	**postración**
protrusion from vagina	**protrusión a través de la vagina**
puffiness	**hinchazón, intumescencia, abotagamiento**
of the face	de la cara
of the legs	de las piernas

ENGLISH	SPANISH
pulmonary	**pulmonar**
abscess	absceso
edema	edema
embolism	embolia
infarction	infarto
tuberculosis	tuberculosis
pyorrea	**piorrea**
rapid heartbeat	**latidos rápidos**
rapid loss of vision	**pérdida percipitada de la visión**
rapid loss of weight	**rápida pérdida de peso**
rapid pulse	**pulso rápido**
rash	**erupción, ronchas**
red spots (tiny)	**pequeñas manchas rojas**
red and swollen joints	**articulaciones inflamadas y enrojecidas**
relapse	**recaída**
restlessness	**intranquilidad**
retraction of the nipple	**retracción del pezón**
rigidity	**rigidez**
ringing in the ears	**zumbido en los oídos**
salivation, excessive	**salivación excesiva**
salivation and difficulty in swallowing	**salivación excesiva y dificultad al tragar**
scaled ulcer	**llaga con costra**
scanty urine	**escasez de orina**
seizures	**ataques, episodios**
semiconscious state	**estado seminconsciente**
shock	**shock, choque**
shortness of breath	**falta de respiración**
skin	**piel**
clammy	pegajosa
cold	fría
moist	húmeda
skin discoloration	**cambio de color de la piel**
ashen	cenicienta
brownish	cetrina
darkening	oscurecida
pale	pálida
pallor (face)	palidez (en la cara)
reddening	enrojecimiento
reddening (flushing)	rubor
yellow-white	blanco-amarillenta

ENGLISH	SPANISH
slow clotting blood	coagulación lenta
slow growth	crecimiento retardado
slow loss of vision	pérdida gradual de la visión
slow pulse	pulso lento
slow speech	habla despaciosa
smarting	escozor
sneezing	estornudo
snoring	ronquido

softening of
    the bones
    the nails
	reblandecimiento de
	    los huesos
	    las uñas

soft ulcerating tumor	tumor ulceroso blando
sore	llaga
sore, hard crusted	llaga de costra dura
to be sore	estar adolorido-a
sore throat	dolor de garganta
spasm	espasmo
spastic gait	marcha espástica
spasticity	espasticidad
speech difficulties	trastornos del habla
split nails	uñas partidas
sticky mucus	mucosidad pegajosa
stiffening	rigidez
stiff neck	cuello rígido

stools
    hard and dark
    clay-colored
    bulky and greasy
    black and tarry
    pencil shaped
    persistently bloody
	heces fecales
	    oscuras y duras
	    de color arcilloso
	    deposición abundante y grasienta
	    oscuras y viscosas
	    heces fecales largas y finas
	    con persistente presencia de sangre

stuttering	tartamudeo
subnormal temperature	temperatura subnormal
sudden stoppage of flow (urine)	paro súbito del chorro (orina)
swallowing difficulty	dificultad al tragar

ENGLISH	SPANISH
swelling	**hinchazón**
inside the mouth	dentro de la boca
of the ear canal	del conducto auditivo
of face; of eyes	de la cara; de los ojos
of feet	de los pies
of hands	de las manos
of the lymph nodes	de los ganglios
tachycardia	**taquicardia**
tingling	**cosquilleo**
total lack of urination	**ausencia total de orina**
tremor of	**temblor en**
the fingers	los dedos
the hands	las manos
the lips	los labios
tumor	**tumor**
twitch	**sacudida nerviosa, "tic nervioso"**
ulcer	**úlcera, llaga**
unawareness of surroundings	**no saber donde uno se encuentra**
unconsciousness	**pérdida del conocimiento**
unresponsiveness	**sin dar una respuesta sensible; sin dar de sí**
urgent urination	**micción imperiosa**
urination, decreased	**deficiencia de orina**
urination, weak stream	**chorro de orina débil**
vaginal bleeding	**sangramiento vaginal**
vaginal discharge	**flujo vaginal**
varicose veins	**venas varicosas**
vertigo	**vértigo, vahido**
vomiting	**vómitos, náuseas**
black	de color oscuro
occasional	ocasionales
bloody	sanguinolentos, con sangre
waddling gait	**marcha, andar tambaleante**
warts	**verrugas**
weak muscles	**debilidad en los músculos**
weakness	**debilidad**
weight	**peso**
loss	pérdida de
gain	aumento de
wheezing	**respiración sibilante**

ENGLISH	*SPANISH*
worms	**gusanos, lombrices, parásitos**
in instestine	en el intestino
in stool	en el excremento
wrist fracture	**fractura de la muñeca**
yawning	**bostezo**

VITAL SIGNS / SIGNOS VITALES

Temperature (T)

ENGLISH

The measurement can be:
    a) Oral. Average normal temperature is 98.6 degrees Fahrenheit, 37.0 degrees Centigrade. It is the most common form of measurement. Glass mercury thermometer.

    b) Rectal. Usually one degree higher than oral temperature. It is the least preferred by patients, and it is not to be used in patients following rectal surgery or suffering from seizure or cardiac disorders. Glass mercury thermometer.

    c) Axillary. Usually one degree lower than the oral temperature. When properly done, it is considered a very accurate measurement. Glass mercury thermometer.

    d) Tympanic or aural. Obtained through insertion of a tympanic thermometer in the ear. It is a very common and preferred method to measure the temperature, although still used mostly in hospitals.

Pulse

The pulse is evaluated by its *rate, rhythm,* and *volume.* Pulse is usually measured at *pulse points,* points where the artery can be pressed against a bone or some other firm surface, the most common one being the radial artery at the wrist. Palpation for obtaining the pulse is done by placing the index and middle finger, the middle finger and ring finger, or the three fingers over a *pulse point.*

Respiration

Measured through auscultation or by the use of a stethoscope. The two variables that are measured are *rate* and *depth.* The average rate in a normal adult is between 14 and 20 breaths per minute.

Weight

Weight is required for all patients, from the prenatal, to the elderly.

Temperatura (T)

SPANISH

Se puede medir por vía:
    a) Oral. La temperature media normal es 98.6 grados Fahrenheit, 37.0 grados Centígrados. Es la vía más usada para la medición. Termómetro de vidrio y mercurio.

    b) Rectal. Generalmente marca un grado más alto que la temperatura oral. Es el menos preferido por los pacientes, y su uso está contraindicado en casos de cirugía rectal postoperatoria, o en pacientes que sufren de trastornos convulsivos o trastornos del corazón. Termómetro de vidrio y mercurio.

    c) Axilar. Generalmente marca un grado más bajo que la temperatura oral. Cuando se administra propiamente, se considera un tipo de medición muy preciso. Termómetro de vidrio y mercurio.

    d) Del tímpano o aural. Se obtiene introduciendo un termómetro timpánico en el oído. Es uno de los métodos más usados y preferidos por los pacientes para medir la temperatura, aunque todavía se emplea mayormente en los hospitales.

Pulso

El pulso se evalúa de acuerdo con el *índice, ritmo y volumen.* El pulso se mide generalmente en *puntos de pulsación*, puntos en los cuales la arteria se puede presionar contra un hueso o alguna otra superficie firme. La arteria más común para medir el pulso es la arteria radial de la muñeca. La palpación para tomar el pulso se hace colocando el dedo índice y el medio, el dedo medio y el anular, o los tres dedos sobre el *punto de pulsación.*

Respiración

Se mide por medio de la auscultación o del uso de un estetoscopio. Las dos características que se evalúan son la *frecuencia cardíaca* y la *profundidad.* La frecuencia cardíaca en un adulto normal es de 14 a 20 respiraciones por minuto.

Peso

Se requiere registrar el peso de todos los pacientes, desde la fase prenatal hasta la edad avanzada.

Height

ENGLISH

Height can be measured using several devices and can be registered in inches, or centimeters, depending on the physician's preference.

Altura

SPANISH

La altura se puede medir por medio de varios mecanismos y se puede registrar en pulgadas o en centímetros de acuerdo con la preferencia del médico.

WARNING SIGNS OF A HEART ATTACK / SEÑALES DE ADVERTENCIA DE UN ATAQUE AL CORAZÓN

ENGLISH

Most heart attacks start slowly, with mild pain or discomfort.

The mild signs that are ignored in many cases, could be the onset of an imminent heart attack. The *American Heart Association* indicates the importance of these and other signs:

▶ **Chest discomfort.** You may feel certain discomfort in the center of the chest that could last more than a few minutes. This symptom could go away and then come back. It will change to feel like a big pressure, squeezing, with feeling of fullness or pain. Some patients describe it as "an elephant sitting on my chest."

▶ Other parts of the upper body could be affected. You may feel discomfort or pain in the stomach, in one or both arms, the back, neck, and the jaw.

▶ **Shortness of breath**. This symptom appears regularly with the chest discomfort although it may occur before the feeling of tightness in the chest.

▶ **Other Signs:** Nausea and lightheadedness could be other symptoms, accompanied by breaking out in a cold sweat.

If the above signs are present, it is necessary to call 911 immediately and request an ambulance.

SPANISH

La mayor parte de los ataques al corazón comienzan lentamente, con un dolor leve o malestar.

Las señales benignas que son ignoradas en muchos casos pueden constituir el comienzo de un inminente ataque al corazón. La Asociación Americana del Corazón nos indica la importancia de estas señales y otros síntomas:

▶ **Malestar en el pecho.** Se puede sentir cierto malestar en el centro del pecho que sólo dura unos pocos minutos. Este síntoma puede desaparecer y volver. Puede sentirse una presión irresistible que aprieta el pecho con sensación de llenura y un dolor muy fuerte. Algunos pacientes lo describen como "un elefante sentado en el pecho".

▶ Otras partes superiores del cuerpo pueden ser afectadas. Puede sentirse malestar o dolor en el estómago, en uno o ambos brazos, en la espalda, el cuello y la mandíbula.

▶ **Falta de respiración.** Este síntoma se manifiesta con regularidad al mismo tiempo que el malestar en el pecho, aunque puede ocurrir antes de sentirse la presión en el pecho.

▶ **Otras señales:** Náusea o mareo pueden manifestarse acompañados de sudores fríos.

Si las señales antes indicadas se presentan, es necesario llamar al teléfono 911 inmediatamente y pedir una ambulancia.

STROKE WARNING SIGNALS / SEÑALES DE UN DERRAME CEREBRAL

ENGLISH	SPANISH
The following stroke warning signals are indicated by the American Stroke Association:	La Sociedad Americana de Estudios sobre el Derrame Cerebral indica las siguientes señales de advertencia de una embolia o derrame cerebral:

▶ Sudden numbness or weakness in the face, arm or leg present especially on one side of the body

▶ Sudden confusion and inability to speak coherently, faulty understanding

▶ Difficulty seeing in one or both eyes

▶ Sudden trouble walking, dizziness, loss of balance or coordination

▶ Sudden severe headache with no known cause

▶ Entumecimiento o debilidad repentina en la cara, el brazo o la pierna, especialmente en un lado del cuerpo

▶ Confusión repentina, dificultad en hablar coherentemente, entorpecimiento del entendimiento

▶ Dificultad para ver con uno o ambos ojos

▶ Dificultad repentina al andar, mareo, pérdida de equilibrio o de coordinación

▶ Fuerte y repentino dolor de cabeza, sin causa conocida

A person that suffers a stroke is almost totally helpless requiring immediate professional attention. It is extremely important that THE TIME when symptoms started is recorded or remembered by the person attending the victim and he or she should communicate it to the paramedics and to the staff at the emergency room.

Una persona que sufre un derrame cerebral está totalmente desvalida y requiere atención profesional inmediata. Es extremadamente importante que la persona que asista a la víctima recuerde con seguridad LA HORA en que se presentaron los síntomas y lo comunique a los paramédicos y al personal de emergencia del hospital.

▶ The drug TPA (tissue plasminogen activator, a protein used as a thrombolitic agent), is a life saver to stroke victims, as long as it can be successfully administered within three hours of the onset of the stroke. TPA is commonly known as "clog buster."

▶ La droga conocida por TPA (activador de plasminógeno en el tejido, proteína usada como agente trombolítico) es una droga que puede salvar la vida o reducir la posibilidad de invalidez permanente en víctimas de derrame cerebral. El medicamento TPA es comúnmente llamado "estirpador de coágulo."

If you notice that these symptoms are present, either of a heart attack or stroke, do not waste time, call 911 and request an ambulance. The paramedics will start the necessary help as soon as they arrive, and will continue to do so on the way to the hospital. A patient taken to the hospital by ambulance receives faster care than if he/she is taken by a private car.

Si nota que estos síntomas están presentes, de un ataque al corazón o de un derrame cerebral, no pierda tiempo, llame al teléfono 911 y pida una ambulancia. Los paramédicos comenzarán a atender a la víctima apenas lleguen y continuarán haciéndolo mientras la trasladan al hospital. Un paciente que es transportado al hospital en ambulancia generalmente recibe una atención más rápida que si es llevado en un automóvil particular.

MEDICAL TESTS / PRUEBAS MÉDICAS

Diagnostic and Clinical Tests	Pruebas y estudios de diagnósticos

Cardiovascular Tests	Pruebas Cardiovasculares
Tests marked below may also be indicated in pulmonary studies.	Las pruebas señaladas abajo también pueden ser indicadas en estudios pulmonares.

ENGLISH		SPANISH	
Angiography (Coronary)	**Procedure**	**Angiografía (Coronaria)**	**Procedimiento**
A method to visualize the interior of an artery and blood vessels with a series of x-rays, to determine vascular disease and neoplasms, and to find the region of coronary occlusion in patients with chest pains.	Consent form is required. Complications are minimum. After catheter is in place the cardiac pressure and volume are taken; radiopaque iodinated dye injected as a contrast medium to take pictures and visualize the arteries that supply the heart muscle.	Método de visualización del interior de una arteria y vasos sanguíneos con una serie de rayos-x, para determinar enfermedades vasculares y neoplasmas y encontrar la región de oclusión coronaria en pacientes con dolores en el pecho.	Firma de consentimiento es necesaria. Complicaciones son mínimas. Después de poner el catéter en su lugar se toman las medidas cardiacas de presión y volumen; se inyecta una sustancia radioopaca yodurada para visualizar las arterias que abastecen el corazón.
Aortography	**Procedure**	**Aortografía**	**Procedimiento**
Imaging of the ascending aorta, the aortic arch with the supraaortic branches, and the descending aorta	Use of selective injection of a contrast medium and catheter to be able to trace and visualize the course of the artery.	Imágenes de la aorta ascendente, el cayado de la aorta, con las ramas supraaórticas, y la aorta descendiente	Uso de medio de contraste y catéter para poder rastrear y visualizar el trayecto de la arteria.
Cardiac Catheterization	**Procedure**	**Cateterización Cardíaca**	**Procedimiento**
Insertion of catheters that measure the pressures within the chambers of the heart, and assessment of how much blood the heart is pumping to the rest of the body; it visualizes and evaluates the function of the heart. Anesthetic is used.	Computer assisted test to register the cardiac output and other functions of the heart; insertion of catheters passing the contrast medium to the heart through a vein or artery to assess diseased valves, congenital heart disease, and do a calculation of the cardiac function.	Inserción de catéteres que miden la presión dentro de las cámaras del corazón y determinan por evaluación la cantidad de sangre que el corazón bombea al resto del cuerpo; visualizan y evalúan la cualidad del funcionamiento cardíaco. Se administra anestesia.	Prueba asistida por computadora para registrar el gasto cardíaco y otras funciones del corazón; inserción de catéter a través de una vena o arteria para evaluar válvulas afectadas, cardiopatias congénitas, y para calcular el funcionamiento cardíaco.

Cardiovascular Tests

Chest Films, X-Rays	Procedure
Series of x-rays taken for evaluation of the cardiac system.	X-rays of the thorax as a diagnostic test to indicate the heart size, and to show the degree of calcification of major vessels in adults.

Echocardiography	Procedure
Non invasive ultrasound procedure used as special detector of a beating heart; the patient can see his own heart in action.	A diagnostic test used in emergencies of patients with chest pain; detects valvular heart disease, stenosis, infarction, aneurysm, and congenital heart disease.

Enzyme Test or Biomarker's Test	Procedure
Blood test of the enzymes Troponin T and I, chemical substances released in the blood indicating by their high levels if there is damage to the heart muscle; the troponins will rise after 6 hours; the tests are done to detect myocardial ischemia and unstable angina.	Fasting or avoiding certain foods; after a heart attack a blood test of the enzymes is indicated to find out the amount of damage to the heart; the test verifies if the heart attack occurred; several blood samples are taken intravenously during the day of hospitalization.

Cardiac Exercises Test	Procedure
A method to visualize the interior of an artery and blood vessels with series of x-rays, to determine vascular disease and neoplasms, and to find the region of coronary occlusion in patients with chest pains.	Consent form is required. Complications are minimum. After catheter is in place the cardiac pressures and volumes are taken; radiopaque iodinated dye injected as a contrast medium to take pictures and visualize the arteries that supply the heart muscle.

Pruebas Cardiovasculares

Radiografías del Tórax	Procedimiento
Serie de radiografías tomadas para una evaluación del sistema cardíaco.	Radiografías del tórax, una prueba de diagnóstico que indica el tamaño del corazón y muestra el grado de calcificación en los grandes vasos.

Ecocardiografía	Procedimiento
Procedimiento de ultrasonido no invasivo que usa un detector especial del corazón latiendo; el paciente puede visualizar la acción de su propio corazón.	Prueba de diagnóstico usada en emergencias de pacientes con dolor en el pecho; detecta enfermedad de las válvulas, estenosis, infarto, aneurismo, y cardiopatías congénitas.

Pruebas de Enzima o de Biomarcadores	Procedimiento
Pruebas sanguíneas Troponina T y Troponina I, sustancias químicas o enzimas liberadas en la sangre indicadoras en niveles altos cuando existe daño al músculo cardíaco; las troponinas se elevarán después de 6 horas; las pruebas se hacen para detectar isquemia del miocardio y angina inestable.	Se indica ayuno o restricción de algunos alimentos; después de un ataque al corazón se ordena un análisis de sangre de las enzimas para evaluar el daño hecho al corazón, y verificar un ataque cardíaco; se toman varias muestras sanguíneas intravenosas sangre durante el día de la hospitalización

Pruebas Cardíacas de Esfuerzo	Procedimiento
Método de visualización del interior de una arteria y vasos sanguíneos con una serie de rayos-x, para determinar enfermedades vasculares y neoplasmas y encontrar la región de oclusión coronaria en pacientes con dolores en el pecho.	Firma de consentimiento es necesaria. Complicaciones son mínimas. Después de poner el catéter en su lugar se toman las medidas cardíacas de presión y volumen; se inyecta una sustancia radioopaca yodurada para visualizar las arterias que abastecen el corazón.

Work-ups

Estudios, radiografías y análisis

ENGLISH	SPANISH
arterial blood gases	tensión de gases en sangre arterial
biochemical profile	pruebas selectivas bioquímicas
biopsy (lung)	biopsia pulmonar
complete blood count	recuento hemático total
chest films	radiografías torácicas
electrocardiogram	electrocardiograma
erythrocyte sedimentation rate	índice de eritrosedimentación
hematocrit	hematócrito
protein electrophoresis	electroforesis proteica
serum creatinine	creatinina sérica
serum potassium	potasio sérico
urynalisis	análisis de orina

Respiratory Tests and Studies

TEST	
ENGLISH	
acid-fast stain	
bronchography	
bronchoscopy	
gammagraphy (lung)	
Gram stain	
lung scan	
needle aspiration biopsy	
respiratory function tests	
serologic studies	
serum electrolytes	
skin testing	
sputum culture	
Wright stain	

Pruebas y estudios respiratorios

PRUEBA
SPANISH
tinción fijada en ácido
broncografía
broncoscopía
gammagrafía pulmonar
tinción de Gram
escán pulmonar
biopsia de aspiración con aguja
pruebas de función respiratoria
estudios serológicos
electrólitos en suero
pruebas cutáneas
cultivo de esputo
tinción de Wright

Reflex Tests

ENGLISH

Motor neurons are the messengers of the brain and spinal cord that tell the muscles to contract or relax and stimulate the glands into action. Reflexes are predictable and involuntary responses to a specific stimulus.

1) The Knee-Jerk Reflex

In resting position, with the leg hanging over the edge of the bed, at a right angle with the thigh, strike the patellar tendon with the hammer below the kneecap; as a response the lower leg extends automatically.
If there is no knee-jerk, or if the extension is not complete, there may be a dysfunction with connections to the spinal cord.

Pruebas de reflejo

SPANISH

Las neuronas motoras son mensajeras del cerebro y de la médula espinal que transmiten a los músculos la orden de contraerse o relajarse y de estimular la acción de las glándulas. Los reflejos constituyen respuestas involuntarias predecibles a un estímulo determinado.

1) Reflejo patelar o rotuliano

En posición de descanso, con la pierna colgando sobre el borde de la cama en ángulo recto con el muslo, golpee levemente con el martillo el tendón patelar, debajo de la rodilla y por respuesta, la pierna se extiende automáticamente.
Si no ocurre el reflejo automático de la pierna es posible que exista alguna anormalidad con las conexiones a la espina dorsal.

Reflex Tests

ENGLISH

2) Babinski reflex

An infantile reflex, normal in children under 2 years old, which disappears as the nervous system develops. How is it tested? With a blunt object or a flick of the finger, strike (stimulus) the outside of the sole of the foot; a normal response is done if after striking the sole of the foot it causes (response) the big toe to flex upward and the other toes to fan out. The Babisnki reflex tests if there is impairment of the nerves of the spinocortical track.

3) Achilles reflex or ankle reflex

The calf muscles contract when the calcaneous tendon is sharply struck with a small hammer.

4) The Corneal Reflex or Lid Reflex

The corneal reflex or lid reflex is a contraction of the eyelids produced by gentle palpation of the lateral aspect of the cornea.

5) Brachioradialis Reflex

With the arm supinated to 45°, a tap near the lower end of the radius causes contraction of the brachiradialis muscle.

6) Biceps reflex

Contraction of the biceps muscle of the arm when its tendon is struck with the hammer. This reflex is normal, but when greatly increased it indicates a dysfunction similar to an increased knee jerk.

All tests marked above are done in addition to tests administered for specific problems.

Pruebas de reflejo

SPANISH

2) Reflejo de Babinski

Un reflejo infantil que es normal hasta los dos años, desaparece al desarrollarse el sistema nervioso. ¿Cómo se pone a prueba? Con un objeto romo o con el dedo se golpea la parte exterior de la planta del pie; una respuesta normal resulta si el golpe o presión en el dorso del pie (estímulo) causa una flexión inmediata hacia arriba del dedo grande y los otros dedos del pie se despliegan en abanico (respuesta). El reflejo de Babinski prueba si hay debilitamiento de los nervios del tracto corticoespinal.

3) Reflejo de Aquiles o del tobillo

Los músculos de la pierna se contraen cuando el tendón calcáneo se golpea con un pequeño martillo.

4) Reflejo de la córnea o del párpado

El reflejo de la córnea se obtiene al palpar levemente el borde del revestimiento lateral de la córnea, lo cual cierra automáticamente el párpado.

5) Reflejo braquioradial

Con el brazo en posición hacia arriba a 45°, un golpe leve en la parte inferior del radio causa una contracción del músculo braquioradial.

6) Reflejo del bíceps

Contracciones del músculo del bíceps del brazo cuando el tendón se golpea con el martillo. Este reflejo es normal, pero si es exagerado indica una disfunción similar al tirón de la rodilla.

Todas las pruebas señaladas arriba se hacen además de pruebas administradas por problemas específicos.

Other Tests for Specific Problems

Otras pruebas de problemas específicos

ENGLISH	*SPANISH*
barium x-ray examinations	radiografía con bario
bone marrow biopsy	biopsia de la médula ósea
bone scan	escán óseo
cervical smear test	prueba de unto
cholecistography	colecistografía
chromosome analysis	análisis cromosomático
coagulation time	tiempo de coagulación
colonoscopy	colonoscopía
gastroscopy	gastroscopía
hysterosalpingography	histerosalpingografía
intravenous pyelography	pielografía intravenosa
kidney imaging	imágenes renales
laparoscopy	laparoscopía
liver function tests	pruebas de función hepática
liver scan	escán hepático
mammography	mamografía
mediastinoscopy	mediastinoscopía
occult blood (fecal)	sangre oculta (fecal)
pregnancy tests	pruebas de embarazo
prostatic specific antigen	antígeno prostático específico
semen analysis	análisis del semen
thyroid function tests	pruebas de función tiroidea
ultrasound scanning	escán de ultrasonido
HIV serology	serología de VIH

X-ray and Laboratory Examination

INDICATIONS FOR LABORATORY AND X-RAY EXAMINATION

ENGLISH

1. You cannot drink or eat anything before the test.

2. You can brush your teeth, but do not drink water.

3. Before the test you should not
   __ eat
   __ drink water or any other liquid
   __ smoke
   __ chew gum
   __ take any medicine
   __ suck any pills or candy

4. You should eat at least two hours before taking a cathartic.

5. You should eat a light supper the night before the test (operation).

6. You should not eat any greasy food the day before the test.

7. You must take these tablets which are especially for this test.

8. The tablets contain a substance that we can trace during the test and that will help make a diagnosis.

9. You must follow these directions exactly as you are told.

WHEN YOU ARRIVE FOR YOUR TEST, YOU MAY BE REQUESTED:

1. __to indicate what type of test you are there for

2. __to give them the written orders of the doctor

3. __to indicate if you have had anything to eat or drink that morning

4. __to indicate if you ate or drank anything after midnight

Examen radiológico y de laboratorio

INDICACIONES PARA PRUEBAS DE LABORATORIO Y RADIOGRAFÍAS

SPANISH

1. Tiene que estar en ayunas (sin beber ni comer nada) antes de la prueba.

2. Se puede lavar los dientes, pero no tome agua.

3. Antes del examen no debe
   __ comer
   __ tomar agua ni ningún otro líquido
   __ fumar
   __ masticar chicle
   __ tomar ninguna medicina
   __ chupar ninguna pastilla o caramelo

4. Debe comer por lo menos dos horas antes de tomar un purgante.

5. Debe comer una comida ligera la noche antes de la prueba (operación).

6. No debe comer comidas grasosas el día antes del examen.

7. Debe tomarse estas pastillas que son especialmente para la prueba.

8. Las tabletas contienen una substancia que se puede rastrear durante la prueba y que ayudará a hacer el diagnóstico.

9. Debe seguir estas instrucciones al pie de la letra.

CUANDO USTED LLEGUE PARA HACERSE LA PRUEBA, LE PUEDEN PEDIR:

1. __que indique que clase de prueba (análisis) se vino a hacer

2. __que les dé la orden escrita del médico

3. __que indique si ha comido o bebido algo esa mañana

4. __que indique si ha comido o bebido algo después de la medianoche

X-ray and Laboratory Examination

Examen radiológico y de laboratorio

ENGLISH

5. __to indicate if you ever had an x-ray examination that required
   __an injection
   __swallowing any pills
   __special medication
   __catheterization
   before the x-ray was taken

6. __to tell them if you are allergic to any medication

7. __to tell them if you are presently taking any medication

8. __to let them know if you suffer from or have ever suffered from asthma

9. __to let them know if you suffer from any allergies

POSSIBLE INDICATIONS DURING THE EXAM

1. You may use this room to remove your clothes and put on the gown that is on the chair.
   Tie the gown __in the front, __in the back.

2. I have to take an x-ray.

3. Breathe deeply.

4. Breathe deeply and hold your breath.

5. You can breathe normally.

6. I have to take one more x-ray.

7. Please wait but do not put on your clothes yet to make sure I don't need to take another x-ray.

8. We are going to take a series of x-rays.

9. After the first x-rays, we will give you a liquid to drink.

10. Drink this liquid, please.

11. After the test, you can have something to eat.

12. We are going to give you a barium enema.

13. We are going to turn off the light.

14. This is not going to hurt you, but it may be unpleasant.

SPANISH

5. __que indique si le han hecho alguna vez una radiografía que haya requerido
   __una inyección
   __tomar alguna pastilla
   __un medicamento especial
   __cateterización
   antes de hacerse la placa

6. __que les deje saber si es alérgico a algún medicamento

7. __que les deje saber si está tomando actualmente algún medicamento

8. __hacerles saber si padece o ha padecido alguna vez de asma

9. __hacerles saber si padece de alguna alergia

POSSIBLES INDICACIONES DURANTE LA PRUEBA

1. Puede usar este cuarto para desvertirse y ponerse la bata que está en la silla.
   Amárrese la bata __en el frente, __por atrás.

2. Tengo que tomarle una placa.

3. Respire profundamente.

4. Respire profundamente y aguante la respiración.

5. Puede respirar normalmente.

6. Tengo que sacarle una placa más.

7. Por favor, espere un momento pero no se vista todavía para comprobar si tengo que tomar otra placa.

8. Le vamos a sacar una serie de placas.

9. Después de las primeras placas le daremos a tomar un líquido.

10. Tómese este líquido, por favor.

11. Después de la prueba puede comer algo.

12. Le vamos a poner un enema de bario.

13. Vamos a apagar la luz.

14. Esto no le va a causar dolor, pero puede causar cierta molestia.

15. This light is used to examine your intestine.

15. Esta luz es para examinarle el intestino.

16. You can use the bathroom here.

16. Puede usar el servicio (el baño) aquí.

17. I am going to inject this into your vein.

17. Voy a inyectarle esta sustancia en la vena.

18. In this test I am going to take fluid from your spine.

18. En esta prueba le voy a sacar líquido de la columna.

19. This is a cold solution.

19. Esta es una solución fría.

20. This machine is to take the mucus from your lungs.

20. Esta máquina es para extraer mucosidades de los pulmones.

21. I am going to insert this tube to
__ take out the phlegm that is bothering you
__ help you void

21. Voy a ponerle esta sonda
__ para sacarle la flema que le molesta
__ para ayudarle a orinar

22. We are going to draw some blood from
__ the vein
__ the finger
__ the ear

22. Le vamos a extraer sangre
__ de la vena
__ del dedo
__ de la oreja

23. Leave the cotton (the Band-aid) in place for a few minutes.

23. Déjese el algodón (la curita) puesto-a por unos minutos.

24. Call tomorrow to find out the results of the test.

24. Llame mañana para saber el resultado de la prueba.

25. We will call to notify you.

25. Le llamaremos para notificarle.

Diagnostic Tests and Studies

CT SCAN COMPUTERIZED TOMOGRAPHY	Definition	Contrast Medium	Patient Care	Abnormal Findings
Diagnostic test done to find the location of tumors, infections, congenital anomalies; in the CT, certain studies require x-rays in series monitoring and staging a disease in evolution.	The conventional tomography is in many tests an invasive x-ray that produces cross-sectional images for the study of blood, internal tissues, and organs.	Water-soluble iodine or another contrast medium is administered orally, by injection, or by catheters to opacify the electron x-ray beams in order to obtain a better image.	Consent is required. The patient must remain still during the test; emission of radiation. The patient must not carry in his body any metallic objects that could interfere with the mechanism and could harm him/her. Fasting may be required.	Tumor, cysts, cancer; tracking perforation, bleeding, hemorrhage, inflammatory bowel disease, urethral obstruction.

CEREBRAL ANGIOGRAPHY	Definition	Contrast Medium	Patient Care	Abnormal Findings
Visualization of the cerebral vascular system with use of subsequent x-ray films in timed sequence.	To test anormalities of the cerebral vascular system with identification of malformations.	Administration of injection of radiopaque dye into the carotid or vertebral arteries to observe the arteries and anomalies in blood vessels.	Informed consent is necessary. Anticoagulants should not be taken; NPO from 2 to 8 hours before test; risk of stroke; bed rest after test.	Aneurysm, vascular occlusion, vascular tumor, abscess or tumor, hematoma appearing like a mass; risk of allergic reaction to the contrast medium.

Pruebas de diagnóstico y estudios clínicos

CAT ESCÁN (TOMOGRAFÍA COMPUTARIZADA)	Definición	Medio de Contraste	Atención del Paciente	Hallazgos Anormales
Examen de diagnóstico para localizar tumores, infecciones, anomalías congénitas; en la prueba TAC ciertos estudios requieren radiografías en serie para monitoreo y estadificación de una enfermedad en evolución.	La tomografía convencional de rayos-x es gen. invasiva; TAC produce imágenes de corte transversal para el estudio de la sangre, de los tejidos y de los órganos internos.	Uso de yodo soluble en agua, u otro medio de contraste que se administra oralmente, en forma inyectada, o por medio de catéteres, para opacar el haz de luz radiográfico y lograr una imagen visible más perfecta.	Firma de consentimiento; el paciente debe permanecer inmóvil durante la prueba; emisión de radiación; el paciente no debe llevar objetos metálicos en su cuerpo que interfieran con el mecanismo, y puedan dañarle; ayuno puede ser requerido.	Tumor, quistes, cáncer, rastreo de perforación, sangramiento, hemorragia, enfermedad inflamatoria intestinal, obstrucción uretral.

ANGIOGRAFÍA CEREBRAL	Definición	Medio de Contraste	Atención del Paciente	Hallazgos Anormales
Visualización del sistema vascular cerebral con toma de rayos-x en una secuencia de tiempo calculado.	Prueba que detecta enfermedades del sistema vascular, neoplasmas cerebrales e identifica malformaciones.	Se administra una inyección de contraste radioopaco dentro de la arteria carótida y se toman rayos-x para observar las arterias y anormalidades en vasos sanguíneos.	Firma de consentimiento requerida; no deben tomarse anticoagulantes; ayunar de 2 a 8 horas antes de la prueba; existe riesgo de embolia.	Aneurisma, oclusión vascular, tumor vascular, absceso o tumor, hematoma aparece como un bulto o masa, riesgo de reacción alérgica al medio de contraste.

Diagnostic Tests and Studies

BRONCHOSCOPY	Definition	Contrast Medium	Patient Care	Abnormal Findings
Used to locate and remove a foreign body or to inspect where bleeding comes from, and to diagnose pulmonary diseases.	Endoscopy for direct visualization of the larynx, trachea, and bronchi for diagnostic or therapeutic purposes.	Local anesthetic is sprayed into the throat before inserting bronchoscope; no contrast medium is used.	Informed consent is required; fasting for 8 hours is necessary; cleaning teeth and rinsing mouth is advisable before the test.	Inflammation, tuberculosis, hemorrhage, cancer, abscess, infection, foreign body.

GALBLADDER CHOLESCINTIGRAPHY	Definition	Contrast Medium	Patient Care	Abnormal Findings
Evaluation of the biliary tract in a non-invasive safe way.	Evaluation to determine gallbladder-function in a numeric non-invasive manner.	Technetium-99, radionuclide dye injected; identification of the radionuclide in the biliary tree indicates the bile duct obstruction.	Preferable fasting 2 hours before test; gallbladder visualized 60 min. after injection, or as long as 4 hours later.	Obstruction of the cystic duct, acute cholecystitis, bile duct obstruction; biliar calculi.

GASTROINTESTINAL ENDOSCOPY	Definition	Contrast Medium	Patient Care	Abnormal Findings
Visualization of the tract (GI) with a flexible fiberoptic-lighted scope.	Visualization for evaluation of the esophagus, stomach, duodenum, colon, and rectum.	By using a laser beam passing through the endoscope, corrective surgery can be performed. No contrast medium is used.	Fasting since midnight; sedation is applied. For lower GI endoscopy, preparation is needed to clean the bowel a day before the test.	Tumors, benign or malignant, chronic pancreatitis, colorectal cancer, colorectal polyps, diverticulosis, duodenum cancer, peptic ulcer, and bleeding cysts.

Pruebas de diagnóstico y estudios clínicos

BRONCOSCOPÍA	Definición	Medio de Contraste	Atención del Paciente	Hallazgos Anormales
Usada para localizar y extirpar una cuerpo extraño y para inspeccionar un sangrado, y diagnosticar enfermedades pulmonares.	Endoscopía con visualiza- ción directa de la laringe, tráquea y bronquios para diagnóstico o propósito terapéutico.	Anestésico local rociado dentro de la garganta antes de insertar el broncoscopio, no se usa medio de contraste.	Firma de con- sentimiento necesaria; ayuno de 8 horas anterior a la prueba; se aconseja asepsia de la boca y dientes antes de la prueba.	Inflamación tuberculosis, hemorragia, cáncer, absceso, infección, cuerpo extraño.

COLESCINTIGRAFÍA DE ES VESÍCULA BILIAR	Definición	Medio de Contraste	Atención del Paciente	Hallazgos Anormales
Evaluación del conducto biliar, no invasivo.	Método numérico no invasivo para determinar la función de la vesícula.	Talio-tecnecio- 99 radionúclido inyectado; si el radionúclido es identificado en el árbol biliar indica obstrucción en el conducto biliar.	Preferible ayunar 2 horas antes de la prueba; la vesícula se visualiza 60 min. después de la inyección, pero también se puede visualizar al cabo de 4 horas.	Obstrucción del conducto cístico, colecistitis aguda, obstrucción del conducto biliar, cálculos biliares.

ENDOSCOPÍA GASTROINTESTINAL	Definición	Medio de Contraste	Atención del Paciente	Hallazgos Anormales
Visualización directa del tracto gastrointestinal (GI) con un mirador flexible de fibra óptica iluminado.	Visualización para evaluación del esófago, estómago duodeno, colon y el recto por medio de un endoscopio, con el que también se puede visualizar la bilis y los conductos pancreáticos.	Uso de un rayo láser que pasa a través del endoscopio para hacer cirugía correctiva; no se usa medio de contraste.	Permanecer en ayunas desde la medianoche del día anterior; se inyecta un sedativo; en endoscopías del tubo digestivo el paciente debe ingerir una preparación el día anterior para limpiar el intestino.	Tumores benignos o malignos, pancreatitis crónica, cáncer colorectal, pólipos colorectales, diverticulosis colorectal, cáncer del duodeno, úlcera péptica, sangramiento de quistes.

INTRAVENOUS PYELOGRAPHY (IVP)	Definition	Contrast Medium	Patient Care	Abnormal Findings
X-ray study to visualize the kidneys, renal pelvis, ureters, and bladder to evaluate the traumatic effect to the urinary system.	X-rays taken every 5 minutes following the course of the dye; after patient voids the empty bladder is visualized. If the renal artery is blocked, the image of the kidney cannot be taken.	Use of radiopaque dye. The dye will indicate an abnormal renal function.	Patients allergic to shellfish or iodine should be screened; laxative should be given the night before; abstinence of food may be necessary except for children.	Cysts, congenital defects, kidney tumor, trauma to the kidneys, renal or uretral calculi, hydronephrosis, bladder tumor, enlargement of the prostate.

MAMMOGRAPHY	Definition	Contrast Medium	Patient Care	Abnormal Findings
X-ray exam to diagnose breast cancer.	An x-ray examination of the breast to identify cancers and other diseases of the breast.	No contrast medium used; minimal radiation and compression of the breast.	No fasting is required; minimum exposure to radiation. The patient must delay or cancel the test if she is pregnant.	Breast cancer, benign tumor, cyst, fibrocystic changes, breast abscess, suppurative mastitis.

ULTRASOUND MAMMOGRAPHY	Definition	Contrast Medium	Patient Care	Abnormal Findings
Breast ultrasound. Non invasive exam that is generally done after a mammography to identify the nature of a malignant tumor.	Test to determine if an abnormality observed in the breast, such as a lump, is a cyst or a tumor and whether it is malignant or benign.	No contrast medium is used; a conductive gel is applied to the breast as a contact with the transducer which produces the ultrasound waves; there is no radiation emitted from this test.	One breast at a time is immersed in heated and chlorinated water; the ultrasound transducer is placed in the water; a conductive gel is applied to the breast.	Hematoma, cysts, breast cancer, fibroadenoma, fibrocystic illness.

Pruebas de diagnóstico y estudios clínicos

PIELOGRAFÍA INTRAVENOSA (PIV)	Definición	Medio de Contraste	Atención del Paciente	Hallazgos Anormales
Estudio radiográfico para visualizar los riñones, la pelvis renal, los uréteres y la vejiga y para evaluar el efecto traumático en el sistema urinario.	Rayos-x tomados cada 5 minutos siguiendo el curso del tinte; después de orinar se visualiza la vejiga vacía; si la arteria renal está bloqueada la imagen del riñón no se puede captar.	Uso de tinte radioopaco. La sustancia yodurada puede afectar si se tiene una función renal anormal.	Pacientes alérgicos a mariscos o al yodo deben ser descartados; es necesario tomar un laxante la noche anterior; pacientes adultos deben ayunar; no en el caso de un menor.	Quistes, defectos congénitos, tumor del riñón, trauma cálculos renales o ure- trales, hidro- nefrosis, tumor en la vejiga, agrandamiento de la próstata.

MAMOGRAFÍA	Definición	Medio de Contraste	Atención del Paciente	Hallazgos Anormales
Técnica radiográfica para diagnosis del cáncer de la mama.	Examen de rayos-x del seno para identificar el cáncer y otras enfermedades.	Sin uso de un medio de contraste; compresión del seno y radia- ción mínima.	No se necesita ayunar; mínima exposición de radiación; la paciente debe suprimir la prueba si está embarazada.	Cáncer de la mama,tumor benigno, quistes, cambios fibroquísticos, abscesos mamarios, mastitis supurativa.

MAMOGRAFÍA POR ULTRASONIDO	Definición	Medio de Contraste	Atención del Paciente	Hallazgos Anormales
Examen de diagnóstico no invasivo que se hace generalmente después de una mamografía para identificar la naturaleza de un tumor canceroso.	Prueba de ultrasonido para determinar si una masa observada en el seno es un quiste o un tumor y si éste es maligno o benigno.	No se usa medio de contraste; se aplica un tipo de jalea a cada seno que sirve de contacto con el transductor, el cual produce las ondas ultrasónicas; no se aplica radiación alguna en esta prueba.	Un seno a la vez se sumerge en agua templada clorinada; el transductor de ultrasonido se coloca en el agua y se aplica una jalea conductiva a cada seno.	Hematoma, quiste, cáncer de la mama, fibroadenoma, enfermedad fibrocística.

CAT Scan

ENGLISH

1. You cannot eat or drink anything 4 to 8 hours before the test.

2. Change into a hospital gown.

3. You will be secured on the table by a strap.

4. You will receive a contrast medium by mouth or by injection.

5. Sometimes you may receive the contrast medium before your test.

6. You will be moved into the scanner; it will scan your body in about 15 minutes.

7. You must remain still to prevent the images from blurring.

8. During the scan you may be asked to hold your breath for a few seconds.

9. You may hear some noises made by the x-ray machine.

10. Remain still. They may need more images to complete the exam.

11. During the test you can usually talk to the technician over an intercom if necessary.

12. If you get nervous and cannot continue the test, you can press a button and let them know and the test will stop.

Escán (exploración) de TAC

SPANISH

1. No puede comer o beber líquidos de 4 a 8 horas antes de la prueba.

2. Póngase esta bata.

3. Le ayudarán a sujetarse a la mesa con un cinturón de seguridad.

4. Le administrarán un medio de contraste oralmente o inyectado si es necesario.

5. A veces se administra el medio de contraste oralmente o inyectado antes de la prueba.

6. Pasará al interior del escáner (explorador), el cual explorará su cuerpo en unos 15 minutos.

7. No se mueva para evitar que las imágenes salgan borrosas.

8. Durante la exploración es posible que le indiquen que aguante la respiración por unos segundos.

9. Es posible que oiga los ruidos que hace la máquina de rayos-x.

10. No se mueva. Es posible que necesiten tomar más imágenes para completar el examen.

11. Durante la prueba generalmente puede hablar con el/la técnico-a por el intercomunicador.

12. Si se pone muy nervioso-a y no puede continuar el examen, puede apretar un botón y el examen se descontinúa.

MRI

ENGLISH

The MRI (Magnetic Resonance Image) test is an imaging technique used to produce clear images of the inside of the human body. This test may require signing a consent form.

INSTRUCTIONS TO THE PATIENT

1. The day of your test appointment, you will be taken to the room where you will change your clothing into a hospital gown.

2. You will be assigned a locker to keep your belongings. Make sure you leave at home or in your locker: pens, coins, credit cards, your watch or any type of jewelry or metal objects. Such objects may interfere with the magnets of the machine and create a distorted image. Furthermore, the magnets may damage these objects in a way that may cause harm.

ANY PATIENT AS DESCRIBED IN THE FOLLOWING CATEGORIES MAY NOT TAKE THE TEST:

1. An extremely obese patient, weighing as much as three hundred pounds. The space inside the cylinder-tube is limited. (A patient is tested in a cylinder which is approximately 60 cm / 24 inches in diameter.)

2. A patient who cannot remain still during the whole procedure.

3. A pregnant woman. In some extreme cases when the woman's life is at risk, and she is advised and aware of the danger to the fetus, some hospitals will allow the MRI to take place if necessary.

4. Any patient who is agitated and unstable. Patients who need life support equipment, such as a pacemaker, which stops functioning in the magnetic field.

5. A patient who cannot endure the machine thumping noise. (To avoid it, earplugs are available or the patient may listen to music.)

6. Patients who have metal fillings or implants, clips or pins, which are ferromagnetic and interfere with the magnetic field.

Exploración de IRM

SPANISH

La IRM (Imagen de Resonancia Magnética) es una prueba para reproducir visualmente imágenes de alta calidad del interior del cuerpo humano. Esta prueba puede requerir que el paciente firme un consentimiento.

INSTRUCCIONES AL PACIENTE

1. El día de la prueba le llevarán a un cuarto donde se cambiará la ropa y se pondrá una bata de hospital.

2. Le asignarán una casilla con llave para guardar sus pertenencias. Deje en su casa o en la casilla plumas, monedas, tarjetas de crédito, su reloj de pulsera, joyas u objetos metálicos que lleve consigo. Estos objetos pueden interferir con los imanes y causar una imagen distorsionada. Además el campo magnético puede dañar los objetos y causarle daño.

UN PACIENTE QUE PERTENEZCA A ALGUNA DE LAS SIGUIENTES CATEGORÍAS NO PODRÁ HACERSE LA PRUEBA:

1. Un paciente extremadamente obeso que pesa trescientas libras o más. El espacio dentro del tubo en forma de cilindro es limitado. (La prueba se hace dentro de un cilindro que tiene aproximadamente 60 cm / 24 pulgadas de diámetro).

2. Un paciente que no puede permanecer sin moverse durante todo el proceso.

3. Una mujer embarazada. En casos extremos cuando la vida de la paciente está en peligro y ella ha sido informada y tiene conocimiento del riesgo que corre el feto y lo acepta, algunos hospitales permiten que la prueba se lleve a cabo.

4. Cualquier paciente inestable que esté agitado. Todo paciente que necesita equipo de soporte vital, tal como un marcapasos, que dejare de funcionar en un campo magnético.

5. Un paciente que no puede soportar el fuerte sonido de la máquina. (Para evitar esto, el paciente puede usar tapones para los oídos o escuchar música.)

6. Pacientes que tienen empastes o implantes, ganchos o alfileres, los cuales son ferromagnéticos e interfieren con el campo magnético.

MRI

ENGLISH

7. Patients who are claustrophobic.

8. Patients allergic to iodine or any of the contrast agents that may be needed as part of the test.

Information by the MRI Professional Team

▶ The MRI personnel has your doctor's orders and will ask you some questions to determine if you can be safely imaged.

▶ The test may require a medication or contrast agent depending on the part of the body that is going to be examined.

▶ When the test begins you will be placed on a table that will slide into the tube-cylinder.

▶ Your position in the tube-cylinder will depend on the part of the body that will be imaged.

▶ If your shoulder, chest, or head is imaged, your feet will not be inside the magnet.

▶ If your feet and knees are imaged, your head will be outside the magnet.

▶ At all times you will be able to press a button located next to your hand to indicate that you want to communicate with the technician.

Exploración de IRM

SPANISH

7. Pacientes que padezcan de claustrofobia.

8. Pacientes alérgicos al yodo o a algún agente de contraste que es necesario como parte de la prueba.

Información por el Equipo Profesional de IRM

▶ El personal del equipo de IRM tiene las indicaciones de su médico y le hará algunas preguntas para determinar si usted puede hacerse la prueba de IRM.

▶ Es posible que la prueba requiera que le administren algún medicamento o agente de contraste de acuerdo con la parte del cuerpo que va a ser examinada.

▶ Cuando comience la prueba, lo colocarán en una mesa que se desliza dentro del tubo cilíndrico.

▶ Su posición en el tubo cilíndrico depende de la parte del cuerpo que necesita ser reproducida en la imagen.

▶ Si su hombro, tórax o cabeza van a ser reproducidos en imagen, sus pies no estarán dentro del imán.

▶ Si sus pies y rodillas van a ser reproducidas en la imagen, su cabeza quedará fuera del imán.

▶ En cualquier momento podrá presionar un botón colocado al lado de su mano para indicar que desea comunicarse con el técnico.

SURGICAL PROCEDURES / PROCEDIMIENTOS QUIRÚRGICOS

DEFINITION	PROCEDURE	WARNINGS	DEFINICIÓN	PROCEDIMIENTO	ADVERTENCIAS
ENGLISH			*SPANISH*		
Bone marrow transplantation: Transplant of a healthy bone marrow into a patient whose bone marrow is not functioning well, or as a transplant to correct genetic blood cell problems.	After matching the patient tissue's type with the donor's, the patient is ready to receive the donated part of bone marrow; the transplant's material needed is transfused through an IV line and it will grow to replace the depleted BM.	Immune system disorders, high risk of infection; convalescence from 4 to 6 months; it may take up to 6 months or more for the immune system to recuperate.	**Trasplante de la médula ósea:** Transplante de una médula ósea sana a un paciente de médula ósea deficiente; o un transplante para corregir problemas de origen genético en células sanguíneas.	Después de emparejar el tipo de tejido del donante con el del paciente, éste está listo para recibir la parte de la médula ósea donada; la infusión intravenosa de la médula donada reemplaza la médula ósea deficiente.	Trastornos del sistema inmune, alto riesgo de infección; convalecencia de 4 a 6 meses, puede tardar de 6 o más meses para que el sistema inmune se recupere.
Corneal Transplantation, Keratoplasty: Partial or total replacement of the sick cornea; insertion in its place of a healthy cornea of which a piece or the whole cornea will be adapted of the same size and shape as the sick cornea.	Surgery done under general or local anesthesia; a round shape button is cut of the corneal tissue of the required size, the diseased cornea is removed and the graft is precisely placed in the empty place.	Observe carefully for signs of infection, inflammation, redness in the operated eye, headache and fever; other serious complicatios such as glaucoma, cataract and retinal detachment could occur.	**Trasplante de la córnea, Keratoplastia:** Extirpación de una porción o reemplazo total de la córnea enferma; inserción en su lugar de una parte o la córnea sana completa del mismo tamaño y forma que la córnea enferma.	La cirugía se hace con anestesia local o general; se corta en forma de botón el tejido de córnea donado del tamaño del injerto y se reemplaza la córnea enferma en el lugar vacio dejado por ésta.	Observe con cuidado si hay señales de infección, inflamación, enrojecimiento en el ojo operado, dolor de cabeza, o estado febril, o complicaciones de glaucoma, catarata, y desprendimiento de retina que se presenten.

DEFINITION	PROCEDURE	WARNINGS	DEFINICIÓN	PROCEDIMIENTO	ADVERTENCIAS
Lumpectomy: Surgical removal of a cancerous lump; the procedure is normally done on women with small breast cancers, performed to treat ductal carcinoma, carcinoma in situ, stage I, II or III.	Removal of the tumor and the adjacent normal breast tissue; the axillary lymph nodes may be removed; a study of the marginal tissue revealing if all the cancer has been taken out will be done while the patient is in the operating room.	Watch for a recurrence; after removal of lymph nodes a side effect of chronic swelling, pain and redness of the arm are signs of lymphedema; report symptoms as soon as they occur.	**Tumorectomía:** Excisión de un bulto o tumor canceroso; el procedimiento se hace normalmente en mujeres con pequeños tumores, para tratar carcinoma ductal, carcinoma in situ o de etapas I, II, ó III.	Excisión del tumor y de tejido normal del seno, los ganglios linfáticos de la axila pueden ser extraídos; se estudia en seguida el tejido marginal que revela si todo el cáncer se ha sacado.	Vigile una recaída; la extracción de los ganglios linfáticos puede traer una secuela de dolor, hinchazón y enrojecimiento del brazo llamada linfedema; reporte los síntomas en seguida que ocurran.

Cataract Removal

ENGLISH

Surgery done to remove a cataract, followed by implantation of a plastic artificial lens. It is an outpatient procedure. Surgery is short unless complications occur.

1. Preparations for the surgery:

   ▶ Three days before the surgery the patient will administer in the eye to be operated two different types of eye drops as prescribed

   ▶ The patient cannot eat or drink anything after midnight the day before the surgery

   ▶ The patient should be at the clinic or the designated outpatient place two hours before the surgery

Extirpación de una catarata

SPANISH

Cirugía para extirpar una catarata seguida por el implante de un lente articicial plástico. No requiere hospitalización. Normalmente la operación es breve a menos que hayan complicaciones.

1. Preparación para la cirugía:

   ▶ Tres días antes de la operación el paciente debe administrar en el ojo que será operado, dos tipos de gotas diferentes, de acuerdo con lo indicado

   ▶ El paciente debe ayunar desde las doce de la noche del día anterior a la operación

   ▶ El paciente debe estar en la clínica o lugar indicado dos horas antes de la hora señalada para la cirugía

Cataract Removal	Extirpación de una catarata

2. The Day of the Operation

▶ The nurse takes the vital signs and prepares the patient for the surgery. She/he keeps on hand while the anesthetist administers the anesthesia.

▶ Drops are administered to dilate the pupil.

▶ The procedure begins. The surgeon makes an incision around the margin of the cornea.

▶ After the cataract lens is removed the intraocular lens is slipped in with an injector which is taken out when the plastic lens is in place.

▶ A plastic lens is implanted.

▶ Sutures are very fine and will not leave scars.

▶ The operation is completed and the patient is taken to the recovery room where he/she remains until he/she becomes fully rested and strong enough to go home.

3. Precautions

▶ Do not rub your eyes at any time

▶ To avoid infections, continue using prescribed eye drops

▶ Use a patch over the operated eye at night while sleeping

▶ Bright sunlight, strenuous exercise and swimming should be avoided for at least two to three weeks

▶ Dark glasses are recommended to avoid sunlight

4. Complications

▶ Dislocation of the lens

▶ Redness of the eye or inflammation

▶ Cloudiness of the cornea

▶ Possible development of glaucoma

▶ Possible correction of the lens

▶ Possible double vision

Call your opthalmologist immediately if any of the above complications occur.

---

2. El día de la operación

▶ La enfermera le tomará los signos vitales al paciente y lo preparará para la operación; estará con élla mientras el/ella anestesista administra la anestesia.

▶ Se administran gotas para dilatar la pupila.

▶ La operación comienza. El cirujano hace una incisión alrededor del margen de la córnea.

▶ Después que se extirpa la catarata, se coloca el lente intraocular plástico con un inyector que se saca una vez que el cristalino plástico está colocado.

▶ Se implanta un lente de cristalino artificial.

▶ Las suturas son mínimas y no dejan cicatrices.

▶ Cuando la operación termina el/la paciente es trasladado-a al cuarto de recuperación donde permanece hasta que se sienta con fuerzas para irse a su casa.

3. Precauciones

▶ No se frote los ojos en ningún momento

▶ Para evitar una infección, continúe usando las gotas indicadas

▶ Póngase un parche sobre el ojo por la noche mientras duerma

▶ Evite la luz del sol; no haga ejercicios extremos; no nade por lo menos durante dos o tres semanas

▶ Se recomienda usar gafas de lentes oscuras para evitar la luz directa del sol

4. Complicaciones

▶ Dislocación del cristalino artificial

▶ Enrojecimiento o inflamación del ojo

▶ Nubocidad de la córnea

▶ Posible desarrollo de glaucoma

▶ Posibilidad de corrección del cristalino artificial

▶ Posibilidad de visión doble

Consulte al oftalmólogo lo antes posible si ocurre alguna de las complicaciones mencionadas arriba.

Appendix C
- Diseases
- Bioterrorism
- Consent Forms
- Nutrition

Apéndice C
- Enfermedades
- Terrorismo biológico
- Formularios
- Nutrición

ALZHEIMER DISEASE / LA ENFERMEDAD DE ALZHEIMER

Different Stages of Alzheimer Disease /
Diferentes Fases de la Enfermedad de Alzheimer

Phases 1 and 2 / Primera y Segunda fase	Mild dementia that precedes senility may come to an end; forgetfulness, no significant brain change; the patient is able to perform most of his daily activities; most significant early symptom is loss of short-term memory.	Estado leve de demencia que precede a la de senilidad y que puede dejar de avanzar; falta de memoria sin producirse cambios mayores en el cerebro; continuación con las actividades diarias; el síntoma más significativo es la pérdida de la memoria inmediata.
Phase 3 / Tercera fase	Moderate dementia. Still able to perform many of the daily living activities; frustration and anger start to set in as the inability to remember names, facts, and faces becomes progressively more acute; patient is still aware of what is happening to him.	Demencia moderada. El paciente todavía puede desempeñar muchas de las actividades diarias; comienza a sentir frustración e ira al no poder recordar muchos nombres, hechos y caras; todavía está consciente de lo que le está sucediendo.
Phase 4 / Cuarta fase	Mild Alzheimer. The patient is very confused and starts to misplace things as memory is getting worse; difficulty in carrying out daily activities; although patient is aware of a problem, he does not seem to think it is of major concern.	Estado leve de Alzheimer. El paciente está muy confuso y empieza a situar cosas fuera de su lugar común; la memoria se va empeorando; tiene dificultad en llevar a cabo actividades cotidianas; reconoce que existe un problema, pero no le concierne.
Phase 5 / Quinta fase	Moderate Alzheimer. Patient needs custodial care; early dementia will cause him/her to be very disoriented; anger and frustration increase due to severe lapses of memory.	Estado moderado de Alzheimer. El paciente requiere estar bajo custodia; la incipiente demencia le desorienta grandemente; largos lapsos de la memoria aumentan la ira y la frustración.
Phase 6 / Sexta fase	Moderately severe Alzheimer's. The patient has almost a total loss of memory; unable to take care of himself in any way; increased anger, hostility;patient may become combative and develop fear of water.	Alzheimer moderadamente severa. Casi total pérdida de la memoria; el paciente no puede desempeñar las actividades diarias; incremento en la ira y hostilidad; en esta fase se vuelve combativo y muestra fobia al agua.

Techniques for reducing the effects of cognitive impairments / Técnicas empleadas para reducir los efectos de impedimentos mentales

Reality Orientation / Orientación a la realidad	Patients remain tuned in to their environment, to time and to themselves; forms of reality orientation could be marking off days in a calendar, setting a patient's watch to the correct time, or cleaning his glasses.	Los pacientes se mantienen en contacto con su medio ambiente, con el tiempo y consigo mismos; algunas formas de orientación a la realidad incluyen marcar los días en un calendario, ajustar su (el/la paciente) reloj a la hora correcta y limpiar sus lentes.
Validation therapy / Terapia de validación	The idea behind this form of therapy is to try to search for the meaning and feelings behind the confused words or behavior of the patient; this will help preserve the patient's dignity and self-esteem.	Este tipo de terapia se basa en tratar de encontrar el verdadero significado y los sentimientos detrás de las palabras confusas del paciente; esto ayudará a preservar la dignidad del paciente aumentando la confianza en sí mismo.
Reminiscing / Recordar el pasado	Reminiscing means encouraging the patient to talk about his past, specially about good times; allows the patient to enjoy those past experiences and feel good about himself/herself.	Recordar el pasado consiste en estimular al paciente a recordar el pasado, especialmente experiencias y sucesos felices; el paciente goza esas experiencias de nuevo aumentando la confianza en sí mismo.

ETIOLOGY OF COMMON DISEASES

Disease	Transmission	Incubation	Contagion Period	Symptoms
Chicken pox, Varicella	by direct contact or by respiratory droplets	7-21 days	from onset of symptoms until pocks are gone	fever, discomfort, patches of red spots that appear first in the upper part of the body and then, to a lesser degree, on the arms and legs; the vesicles fill with fluid rupture, and disappear without leaving any scars
Diphtheria	by contact with carrier or by contaminated milk	2-6 days	from onset of symptoms to 4-6 weeks thereafter	weakness, sore throat, fever, rapid pulse, grayish membrane covering the throat and tonsils
German measles, Rubella	by direct contact or by inhaling infected droplets	2-3 weeks	one week before rash appears	slight fever, swelling of the neck glands, and a rash of flat, pink spots
Measles	by direct contact or by inhaling infected droplets	7-14 days	10-14 days before symptoms appear until rash is gone	high fever, nasal congestion, conjunctivitis, dry cough, tiny red spots, first in mouth, then spreading throughout the body
Mumps, parotitis	by direct contact or by inhaling infected droplets	12-24 days	one day before symptoms appear until swelling goes down	from medium to high fever, headache, swelling of the parotid glands (below and in front of the ear), painful chewing and swallowing, sudden high fever that lasts for about three days and that may cause convulsions, rash, and swelling of the lymph glands

Roseola infantum	undetermined, believed to be caused by a virus	undetermined	undetermined	sudden, high fever that lasts for about three days and that may cause convulsions, rash, and swelling of the lymph glands
Scarlet fever, scarlatina	contact with carrier	24 hours to 3 days	from onset to one day after antibiotic treatment begins	sudden onset of fever, sore and infected throat, rash on neck and chest, strawberry tongue
Viral colds	contact with carrier or infected secretion	1-2 days after exposure	for duration	headache, nasal congestion, cough, sneezing, hoarseness, watering eyes

ETIOLOGÍA DE ENFERMEDADES COMUNES

Enfermedad	Transmisión	Incubación	Período de contagio	Síntomas
La china, varicela	por contacto directo o destilación o aspiración de microgotas infectadas	7-21 días	desde la aparición de los síntomas hasta que las pústulas desaparecen	fiebre, malestar, grupos de pápulas rojizas que surgen primero en la porción superior del cuerpo y, en menor grado, en las piernas y brazos; las pápulas se llenan de fluido, revientan y no dejan cicatriz
Difteria	por contacto directo o a través de leche contaminada	2-6 días	desde el momento en que aparecen los síntomas hasta 4-6 semanas después	debilidad, dolor de garganta, fiebre, pulso rápido, membrana grisácea que cubre la garganta y las amígdalas
Sarampión alemán, Rubéola	por contacto directo o por destilación o aspiración de microgotas infectadas	2-3 semanas	una semana antes de la erupción	fiebre ligera, infl. de las glándulas del cuello y erupción de pequeñas máculas rosáceas

Enfermedad	Transmisión	Incubación	Período de contagio	Síntomas
Sarampión	por contacto directo o por destilación o aspiración de microgotas infectadas	7-14 días	de 10-14 días antes de la aparición de los síntomas hasta que éstos desaparecen	fiebre alta, congestión nasal, conjuntivitis, tos seca, pequeñas máculas rojas que surgen en la boca y luego se difunden por todo el cuerpo
Paperas, parotiditis	por contacto directo o por destilación o aspiración de microgotas infectadas	12-24 días	un día antes de la aparición de los síntomas hasta que la hinchazón desaparece	fiebre alta, dolor de cabeza, hinchazón de las glándulas parótidas (debajo y por delante de la oreja), dolor al masticar y al tragar
Roséola infantil	indeterminada, se cree que es de origen viral	indeterminada	indeterminada	fiebre alta súbita que dura unos tres días y que puede dar lugar a convulsiones, erupción cutánea e infl. de los ganglios
Fiebre escarlata, Escarlatina	por contacto con el (la) portador-a	desde 24 horas hasta 3 días después	desde que aparecen los síntomas hasta un día después de empezar el tratamiento con antibióticos	fiebre súbita, garganta adolorida y enrojecida, erupción cutánea en el cuello y pecho, lengua aframbuesada
Catarros virales	contacto con el (la) portadora o con cualquiera secreción infectada	1-2 días después de estar expuesto	durante todo el curso del catarro	dolor de cabeza, congestión nasal, tos, estornudos frecuentes, ronquera, ojos aguados y llorosos

SEXUALLY TRANSMITTED DISEASES (STD) / ENFERMEDADES VENÉREAS

Sickness	Transmission	Enfermedad	Contagio
candidiasis *Candida albicans*, fungus, yeast infection; thick, creamy discharge	Sexual contact, use of towels or clothing belonging to an infected person, or caused by a low pH in the vagina	**candidiasis** *Cándida albicans*, infección fungosa caracterizada por flujo cremoso	Contacto sexual, ropa de toallas o ropa interior de una persona infectada, o pH bajo de la vagina
chlamydia *Chlamydia Trachomatis*, causative agents of urethritis, lymphogranuloma, prostatitis, salpingitis, newborn conjunctivitis	Sexual contact; newborns may be infected during childbirth	**clamidia** *Chlamydia Trachomatis*, agente causante de uretritis, linfogranuloma, prostatitis, salpingitis, conjuntivitis del neonato	Contacto sexual rectal, oral o vaginal, o de la madre al feto durante el parto
condyloma acuminatum Venereal warts	By sexual contact or by using towels belonging to an infected person	**condiloma acuminatum** Verrugas venéreas	Por contacto sexual o por el uso de toallas de una persona infectada
genital herpes virus type 2 causing blisters and sores on the genitals	anal, oral, vaginal sexual contact at the outbreak of the disease; touching blisters and sores; can be transmitted to the newborn at birth	**herpes de los genitales, virus de tipo 2** causante de ampollas y ulceraciones en los genitales	contacto sexual anal, oral o vaginal; de la madre a la criatura durante el parto; por contacto con ampollas y ulceraciones
gonorrhea *gonococcus Neisseria*, infection invading the genitourinary tract, pharynx, anus	anal, oral, vaginal sexual contact; from mother to child during childbirth; period of incubation from 3 to 5 days	**gonorrea** *gonococo Neisseria*, infección que invade el tracto genitourinario, la faringe y el recto	contacto sexual rectal, oral o vaginal; de la madre a la criatura durante el parto; período de incubación de 3 a 5 días
hepatitis: A-, B-, C-, and D-type viruses inflammation of the liver; other serious disorders are also present	sexual contact, transfusion of contaminated blood; contact through abrasions, tiny cuts, or wounds with the blood of an infected person; or by the mother at childbirth or through breastfeeding	**hepatitis: víruses de tipo A, B, C y D (delta)** inflamación del hígado, manifestándose en otros trastornos serios	por contacto sexual, transfusión de sangre contaminada; contacto a través de heridas o abrasiones con la sangre de una persona infectada; por la madre durante el parto o durante la lactancia
hepatitis B	usually involves oral-anal sex	**hepatitis B**	generalmente resulta de contacto sexual oral-anal
HPV virus human *papillomavirus,* considered a strong cocarcinogen; generally present with other STD diseases	venereal disease, characterized by warts, can expand by autoinoculation in the genitals and anus	**HPV virus** *papilomavirus* humano, considerado un posible cocarcinógeno; generalmente presente con otras enfermedades venéreas	enfermedad venérea, caracterizada por verrugas o condilomas en los genitales y el ano que se expanden por autoinoculación

Sickness	Transmission	Enfermedad	Contagio
pubic lice, crabs, *pthirus pubis* discomfort produced by itching	sexual contact, transmitted in bed linen, towels, toilet seats	**el piojo púbico** *pthirus pubis*, malestar por intensa picazón	contacto sexual, transmitido en toallas, y ropa de cama y asiento de retrete, (inodoro)
syphilis *Treponema pallidum*, 10 to 90 day incubation period; ulceration, warts in the genital area; invades the bloodstream to different organs	anal, oral, vaginal sexual contact, by sores through mucous membranes or abrasions or by touching a chancre; from mother to child; in pregnancy can cause stillbirth or congenital syphilis	**sífilis** *Treponema pallidum*, de 10 a 90 días de incubación; úlcera primera, verrugas en el área genital; se extiende por vía sanguínea a diferentes órganos	contacto sexual rectal, oral, vaginal, por contacto con ulceraciones a través de membranas mucosas o al tocar un chancro; durante el embarazo puede causar sífilis congénita o muerte al feto
trichomoniasis *Trichomonas vaginalis*, causes foul-smelling vaginal discharge, itching, burning	sexual activity, infected semen on washcloths, bedclothes	**tricomoniasis** *trichomonas vaginalis*, causa flujo vaginal de olor desagradable, picazón, ardor	actividad sexual, semen infeccioso en toallas o ropa de cama

Testing of HIV should be administered to patients that have genital ulcers caused by *T. palidum* or *H. ducreyi*, which are cases of genital herpes, chancroid and syphilis. When chancroid is diagnosed, testing of HIV would be a precaution, and 3 months later the patient should be retested for syphilis and HIV if the test of chancroid was negative.

STD testing is available for sexually active men and women:

▶ HIV serology
▶ syphilis serology
▶ urethral culture or urine test for chlamydia
▶ pharyngeal culture for gonorrhea and chlamydia
▶ rectal gonorrhea and chlamydia culture

HIV AND AIDS / EL VIH Y EL SIDA

Questions and Answers on HIV and AIDS

Preguntas y respuestas sobre el VIH y el SIDA

ENGLISH	SPANISH
1. What causes AIDS (*acquired immune deficiency syndrome*)? The retrovirus HIV(*human immunodeficiency* virus)[1] causes AIDS. AIDS is a late manifestation of HIV.	1. ¿Qué causa el SIDA (*síndrome de inmunodeficiencia adquirida*)? El VIH (*virus de la inmunodeficiencia humana*[2]) es el retrovirus causante del SIDA. VIH es una manifestación tardía de SIDA.
2. How does an HIV infection occur? HIV is transmitted through four body fluids: a) blood b) semen c) vaginal fluid d) breast milk	2. ¿Cómo ocurre una infección de VIH? El VIH es transmitido a través de cuatro líquidos corporales: a) sangre b) semen c) secreción vaginal d) leche materna
3. How does HIV attack the body system? The infecting virus HIV attacks the immune system that protects the body against infections. It overpowers the immune cells CD4 and reproduces itself in them, thus debilitating the immune system. This evolution opens the door to "opportunistic" infections that attack a body already low in antibodies. When the body is at its lowest level count of CD4, or T cells, it is vulnerable to AIDS.	3. ¿Cómo ataca el VIH el organismo? El virus VIH ataca el sistema inmunológico que protege el organismo contra las infecciones. Comienza a dominar las células CD4 y se reproduce en ellas; de esta manera debilita el sistema inmune. Esta evolución abre la puerta a infecciones "oportunistas" que atacan un organismo bajo en anticuerpos. Cuando el organismo presenta el nivel más bajo de células CD4, o T, es vulnerable al SIDA.

Questions and Answers on HIV and AIDS

Preguntas y respuestas sobre el VIH y el SIDA

ENGLISH	SPANISH
4. How a transmission occurs: a) HIV is transmitted by having intercourse (vaginal or anal) with an infected partner. If one of the partners is infected by HIV, the virus is transmitted to his or her partner during intercourse by introducing the infected semen or vaginal secretion through the mucous membranes or through a small cut or sore hardly visible. b) By direct blood contact such as injection with exchanged drug needles and syringes between drug addicts infected by AIDS; in direct transmission by tainted blood transfusions, or by accident if it enters the system through a percutaneous lesion when handling infected blood.[3] c) Transmission from hemophiliacs who had been treated with Factor VIII[5] (contaminated platelets) to their sexual partners without knowing that they were carriers. d) The transmission of HIV from the infected mother to the fetus (perinatal or vertical transmission)[7] during pregnancy, or during labor and birth to the newborn has approx. 20% probability of transmission if she has not received a drug treatment to reduce this probability.	4. Cómo ocurre una transmisión de VIH: a) VIH se transmite por medio del acto sexual (vaginal o anal). Si uno de los contrayentes está infectado por VIH el/ella puede transmitir al otro el semen o secreción vaginal a través de las membranas mucosas o de una pequeña cortada apenas visible. b) Por contacto sanguíneo directo tal como una inyección con agujas y jeringas intercambiadas entre drogadictos infectados por SIDA; en transfusión de sangre contaminada, o por accidente si sucediera una exposición durante el manejo de sangre infectada[4] a través de una lesión percutánea. c) Transmisión por hemofílicos que habían sido tratados con Factor VIII[6] (de plaquetas infectadas) a su pareja sexual sin saber que eran portadores de virus VIH. d) La transmisión de la madre infectada por VIH al feto (transmisión perinatal o vertical) durante el embarazo, o en las labores del parto, es aprox. de un 20% si ella no ha recibido tratamiento para evitar la probabilidad de transmisión.
5. What is done today to avoid PNT /(TMH)[8]? Clinical studies have indicated that if the delivery is done by caesarean section before labor begins, it would be possible to reduce the probability of HIV-1 infection to the newborn. This is a procedure that is done in combination with AZT[9] therapy.	5. ¿Qué se ha hecho para evitar la transmision perinatal (TMH)? Estudios clínicos verificados con este fin han indicado que si antes de comenzar la labor del parto se realiza una cesárea combinada con un tratamiento de terapia de AZT[10] que se hace durante el embarazo, la transmisión perinatal disminuye considerablemente.

Questions and Answers on HIV and AIDS

Preguntas y respuestas sobre el VIH y el SIDA

ENGLISH	SPANISH
6. What is the HIV transmission probability to an infant through the mother's milk? The infected mother's milk contains HIV-1 virus, which is a viable means of infection with approx. 12% of probability of transmission. If the mother is not following any treatment to avoid transmission during pregnancy, the risk is very high. In 1994 a clinical analysis "076" determined that women who submitted voluntarily to AZT therapy would diminish considerably the probability of HIV infection to their children.	6. ¿Cuál es la probabilidad de un neonato infectarse con VIH a través de la leche materna? La leche infectada de la madre que contiene el virus VIH, es una fuente de infección que proporciona un12% de probabilidad de transmisión. Si la madre no sigue ningún tratamiento para evitar transmisión durante el embarazo, el riesgo es muy alto. En 1994 el análisis clínico "076" determinó que las mujeres que se sometieron voluntariamente a la terapia de AZT disminuyeron considerablemente la probabilidad de infección a su hijo-a.
7. What recommendations are given to HIV infected pregnant women? ▶ To submit voluntarily to a therapy of drug inhibitor's program. ▶ To follow a therapeutic regimen of antiretroviral drugs reducers of VIH and perinatal transmission. ▶ To keep visits and therapy with their physician as regularly as recommended. ▶ To take her medication accordingly ▶ To request assistance to monitor the progress of the disease in herself and her baby. ▶ To be aware of any drug interaction effect and report it to their doctors.	7. ¿Qué recomendaciones se han dado a mujeres embarazadas infectadas por VIH? ▶ Someterse voluntariamente a una terapia de medicamentos de inhibidores de retrovirus. ▶ Seguir un régimen terapéutico de fármacos antiretrovíricos reductores de VIH y de la transmisión perinatal. ▶ Asistir regularmente a las citas con el médico y seguir con regularidad la terapia recomendada. ▶ Estar al tanto de cualquier efecto inesperado de las medicinas que tome y reportarlo al personal médico que le atiende. ▶ Pedir asistencia para poder seguir el progreso del embarazo y la evolución del virus.

[1] Also called human T-lymphotrophic virus.

[2] También llamado virus T-linfotrófico humano

[3] There is a very small percentage of health providers who have been infected by accident with HIV.

[4] Existe un porciento muy bajo de asistentes de salud que se han infectado accidentalmente por HIV.

[5] Factor VIII made by donated blood from various donors is now treated to avoid transmission.

[6] El Factor VIII hecho por sangre donada por varios donantes se trata ahora para evitar transmisión.

[7] PNT perinatal transmisión / transmisión perinatal

[8] TMH transmisión de madre a hijo / TMC transmisión of mother to child.

[9] An analog inhibitor of replication of HIV virus.

[10] Análogo inhibidor de replicación del VIH.

Questions Commonly Asked About HIV

Preguntas hechas regularmente sobre VIH

ENGLISH	SPANISH
1. Can one get the virus from food prepared by an infected person? That has not been considered to be so.	1. ¿Se puede contraer la infección a través de comida preparada por una persona infectada? No, no se cree que sea una forma de contagio.
2. Can one be infected by using the same utensils (glasses, spoons, or other objects) used by an infected person? Unless the infected person that uses the objects has left a trace of blood and the other person has an open wound in the mouth or gums, only that way, could there be a possibility of infection.	2. ¿Se puede contraer la infección a través del uso de los mismos utensilios (vasos, cucharas u otros objetos) que han sido usados por una persona infectada? Solamente ocurre si la persona infectada de SIDA dejara sangre que penetrara una herida o en la boca, o las encías de otra persona.
3. Can one be infected by the bite of a mosquito or by any other type of bite? It is not possible unless a person infected with AIDS would be the biter.	3. ¿Se puede contraer el virus a través de la picadura de un mosquito o de cualquier otro tipo de picada o mordedura? No es posible, a no ser la mordedura de una persona infectada con SIDA.
4. Is the use of condoms a safe protection? It is not totally safe.	4. ¿Es el uso de condones una protección segura? No es totalmente segura.
5. Is AIDS transmitted by kissing? The answer given is that HIV is a fragile and dangerous virus which produces AIDS; contagion may occur when the person infected and the person who is not have bleeding gums or sores in the lips or mouth. But given the cleansing properties of the saliva, there is a very small possibility for HIV infection.	5. ¿Se transmite el SIDA en un beso? La respuesta que se da es que el VIH es un virus muy frágil y peligroso que produce el SIDA; el contagio sólo ocurre cuando la persona infectada y la persona no contagiada tienen encías sangrantes o llagas en la boca, o en los labios. Aun así, debido a las propiedades naturales de limpieza de la saliva, es muy difícil que ocurra el contagio del virus VIH.
6. Is there any other type of protection? Not to be associated with persons who belong to a *"high risk"* group as described next.	6. ¿Hay algún otro tipo de protección? No asociarse a personas que pertenezcan a un grupo de *"alto riesgo"* tal como se menciona a continuación.

INCLUDED IN "*HIGH-RISK*" GROUPS ARE:	INCLUÍDOS EN GRUPOS DE "ALTO RIESGO" SON:
▶ Sexually active adults who do not not follow a safe sexual conduct.	▶ Personas sexualmente activas que no siguen una conducta sexual protegida.
▶ Drug addicts who inject drugs and exchange infected needles.	▶ Drogadictos infectados que intercambian agujas y jeringas.
▶ Hemophiliacs who receive tainted blood products from infected donors.	▶ Hemofílicos que reciben productos contaminados por donantes infectados.
▶ Infants exposed to their infected mothers during gestation, delivery and breast feeding.	▶ Niños de pecho infectados por la madre portadora del virus durante el embarazo, el parto y la lactancia.
▶ Heterosexuals who engage in sexual activity with multiple partners who might belong to any of the above groups.	▶ Heterosexuales que tienen contacto sexual con múltiples compañeros sexuales que pueden pertenecer a alguno de los grupos descritos.
▶ Adolescents who have unsafe sex with multiple partners.	▶ Adolescentes que tienen relaciones sexuales sin protección con múltiples compañeros.

Protection Against Infection

Protección contra la infección

ENGLISH	SPANISH
1. What are the safe sex rules to follow? ▶ Abstinence or to follow a safe sexual conduct. ▶ Have a single partner who does not belong to any of the described *"high risk"* groups.	1. ¿Cuál sería un comportamiento sexual sin riesgo? ▶ Abstinencia o seguir una conducta sexual no arriesgada. ▶ Elegir una pareja que no tenga una conducta sexual arriesgada.

Questions About Testing for HIV and AIDS

Preguntas sobre pruebas de VIH y SIDA

ENGLISH	*SPANISH*
1. What does a positive test result mean? It means that the patient may have AIDS.	1. ¿Qué significa un resultado positivo a la prueba? Significa que el paciente puede tener SIDA.
2. Is the test always right? No, it's not always right.	2. ¿Es siempre definitivo el resultado de la prueba? No, el resultado no es siempre definitivo.
3. Are the first results definite? No, they are not.	3. ¿Son los primeros resultados definitivos? No, no la son.
4. Will test results be confidential? Yes, they will be confidential.	4. ¿Son confidenciales los resultados de las pruebas? Sí, son confidenciales.
5. Is there a special test to confirm if a person is infected by HIV? Yes, the EIA (enzyme immunoassay) validated by the Western Blot (immunofluorescense assay), is one of the tests. Repeat testing is required in 3 to 6 months. ELISA (enzyme-linked immunosorbent assay) for HIV and antibody tests for antibodies in serum or plasma. It is not possible to affirm that ELISA detects the presence of HIV antibodies in the blood stream at an early stage. But it is 99% effective after 3 to 6 months of the virus infection when the HIV antibodies are present in the system.	5. ¿Hay alguna prueba o análisis para confirmar si una persona está infectada por el virus del VIH? Si, la prueba EIA (cimoinmunoanálisis) confirmada por el Western Blot (inmunoblot) no debe ser considerada la primera vez negativa o positiva, la repetición de la prueba debe ser efectuada de 3 a 6 meses. ELISA (análisis inmunosorbente enzimático), es una prueba o análisis que se realiza para detectar anticuerpos de VIH presentes en el suero o plasma de la sangre. No es posible afirmar que ELISA detecte la presencia de anticuerpos de VIH en la corriente sanguínea en una etapa primaria de la enfermedad. Pero es un 99% efectiva después de 3 a 6 meses de la infección del virus con la presencia de los anticuerpos de VIH en el organismo.

Questions About Testing for HIV and AIDS

6. Does a test result show immediately that the person is infected?
A person infected with HIV recently, may not show HIV antibodies in their bloodstream for months. A person that may have been exposed to the virus should do repeated tests to find the best results.

   ▶ P24 (antigen capture assay) detects the viral protein p24 in the peripheral blood of persons infected with HIV, which may be detected just 2 to 6 weeks after infection.
   ▶ Lymphocyte immunophenotyping is a type of test that determines the amount of CD4 lymphocytes responsible for immunity present in the body. These cells are attacked by the HIV virus. When the remaining amount of these cells is less than 300 cells mm.^{3}, it is an indication that there is a strong probability of having "opportunistic infections" invading the body and causing AIDS.

7. Is there a cure for HIV or AIDS patients? A definite cure for HIV or AIDS has not been found.

Treatment and Therapy of HIV

1. Is any preventive treatment for HIV available?
Constant research is being done on the treatment and evolution of the disease. The use of protease inhibitors in combination with antiretrovirus drugs, such as in AZT therapy, have been administered in the last decade and have been effective in reducing the levels of HIV in the blood. These results have improved the quality of life of AIDS's patients. Also, in some cases, the infection has been prevented when the drug treatment was administered to non infected HIV partners in the first few hours or days after the exposure to the virus.

Preguntas sobre pruebas de VIH y SIDA

6. ¿Muestran los resultados inmediatamente si la persona está infectada?
Una persona infectada con VIH recientemente es posible que no presente anticuerpos VIH en la corriente sanguínea por varios meses. Para obtener mejores resultados, una persona expuesta al virus VIH debe repetir la prueba sucesivamente.

   ▶ P24 (análisis de captura de antígeno) detecta la proteína vírica p24 en la sangre periférica de personas infectadas con VIH, la cual se puede detectar sólo de 2 a 6 semanas después de ocurrir la infección.
   ▶ La prueba de fenotipificación inmunológica de linfocitos se usa para determinar el número de linfocitos CD4 responsables por la inmunidad presente en el organismo. El VIH ataca estas células y se posesiona de ellas. Cuando el número de células CD4 que queda es menos de 300 mm.^{3}, es una indicación probable que las enfermedades oportunistas se encuentran invadiendo el organismo y causando la enfermedad del SIDA.

7. ¿Existe alguna cura para los pacientes de VIH o SIDA? Una cura definitiva no se ha encontrado.

El tratamiento y terapia de VIH

1. ¿Hay algún tratamiento preventivo contra HIV?
Se hacen constantes estudios sobre el tratamiento, la evolución y el progreso de la enfermedad. El uso de inhibidores de protease usados en combinación con otras drogas antiretrovíricas tal como en la terapia de AZT en la década pasada, han sido efectivos en reducir los niveles de VIH en la sangre. Los resultados obtenidos han mejorado la calidad de vida de los pacientes de SIDA. La infección ha llegado a prevenirse en algunos casos de personas no infectadas por HIV con tratamiento de inhibidores de protease y otras potentes drogas horas o días después de estar expuestos al virus.

Observations Related to HIV and AIDS

ENGLISH

Observaciones generales en relación con VIH y el SIDA

SPANISH

HIV *seronegative* means that the test does not show HIV antibodies in the bloodstream.

VIH *seronegativo* quiere decir que la prueba no indica la presencia de anticuerpos VIH en la corriente sanguínea.

---

1. Why should you be tested for HIV?:
   a) you think you may have had any kind of sexual contact with an infected person.
   b) you have used intravenous drugs and exchanged needles or syringes with an infected person.
   c) you had sexual contact with a person who belongs to a "*high risk*" group.
   d) you are pregnant and have doubts about whether your sexual partner belongs to a "*high risk*" group.

1. ¿Cuándo debe usted hacerse la prueba del VIH?:
   a) ha tenido cualquier tipo de contacto sexual con una persona infectada.
   b) ha usado drogas intravenosas o compartido agujas o jeringuillas con personas infectadas.
   c) ha tenido contacto sexual con una persona que pertenece a un grupo de "*alto riesgo*".
   d) está embarazada y tiene dudas si su compañero está asociado a un grupo de "*alto riesgo*".

HIV *seropositive* means that there are HIV antibodies in the bloodstream.

VIH *seropositivo* quiere decir que existen anticuerpos de VIH en la corriente sanguínea.

---

2. It is very important to follow a safe sexual conduct.

2. Es sumamente importante evitar una conducta sexual arriesgada.

---

3. You are capable of being infected by the virus even if you are exposed only once.

3. Usted puede ser infectado-a por el virus aunque haya estado expuesto-a una sola vez.

---

4. Does the health laboratory official have the obligation to report the results of the test to the health authorities?
   Yes, it has to be reported to the health authorities and also it has to be registered in the infected person's medical record. Other persons who also have had sexual contact with the infected person should be notified in order to have a serologic test and determine if there is infection.

4. ¿Tiene el profesional de salud o director del laboratorio que reportar resultados de la prueba a las autoridades de salubridad?
   Sí, se debe reportar a las autoridades los casos de VIH y de SIDA, y también debe ser registrado en el expediente médico de la persona infectada. Otras personas que tuvieron contacto sexual con la persona infectada deben ser notificadas para que se hagan una prueba serológica y puedan determinar si hay contagio.

---

serostatus unknown refers to any person that has never been tested for HIV infection.

seroestado desconocido indica el estado de una persona que nunca se ha hecho una prueba de VIH.

---

5. If the results of your tests are positive, you should be right away under the care of an immunologist or an AIDS knowledgeable health professional.

5. Si el resultado de las pruebas es positivo, usted debe estar en seguida bajo el cuidado de un inmunólogo o profesional de salud con conocimientos del tratamiento del SIDA.

Observations Related to HIV and AIDS

Observaciones generales en relación con VIH y el SIDA

ENGLISH	SPANISH
6. It would be helpful if you would join a support group.	6. Sería beneficioso que usted se asociara a un grupo de apoyo.

Note: Concerning questions 4 and 5. All AIDS clinics observe confidentiality, some observe total anonymity; the patient is observed and identified only by a code number. Results of the test are only given to the patient by his doctor.

Nota: Respecto a las preguntas 4 y 5. Todas las clínicas de SIDA observan confidencialidad, algunas observan completa anonimidad; el paciente es asistido y se identifica por un número o código. Los resultados de las pruebas son entregados solamente al paciente por su médico.

BIOTERRORISM / TERRORISMO BIOLÓGICO

|

Definition / Definición

A biological agent is genetically produced, resistant to known vaccines and drugs, highly contagious and able to harm thousands of people. Bioterrorism is the release of such potentially lethal biological agents in the air with the intent to cause mass destruction.

Un agente biológico es producido genéticamente, resistente a vacunas y drogas conocidas, sumamente contagioso y capaz de dañar a miles de personas. El terrorismo biológico es la liberación de estos agentes potencialmente letales en el aire con la intención de causar destrucción masiva.

Selected list of agents that could pose the greatest risk in the event of a terrorist attack. / Lista selecta de agentes que pueden presentar el mayor riesgo en el caso de un ataque terrorista

Anthrax (*Bacillus anthracis*)
Botulism (*Chlostridium botulinum toxin*)
Plague (*Yersinia pestis*)
Radiation Emergencies

Ricin
Smallpox
Mustard Gas (Sulfur Mustard)
VX

Antrax (*Bacillus anthracis*)
Botulismo (*Chlostridium botulinum toxina*)
Peste (*Yersinia pestis*)
Emergencias como resultado de estar expuesto a radiación

Ricina
Varicela
Gas mostaza (Mostaza sulfúrica)
VX

Characteristics of two of the most commonly known agents / Características de dos de los agentes más comúnmente conocidos

ANTHRAX / ANTRAX

Origin and where it is mostly found / *Origen y donde se encuentra más comúnmente*

Anthrax is caused by a spore-forming bacterium, *Bacillus anthracis,* that can affect both humans and animals. The bacteria is found mostly in agricultural areas of the world.

El Antrax es causado por una bacteria, *Bacillus anthracis*, que forma esporas y puede afectar a seres humanos y a animales por igual. Las bacterias se encuentran mayormente en las áreas agrícolas del mundo.

Types or forms of Anthrax / *Tipos o clases de Antrax*

The three forms of Anthrax are determined by how the bacteria enter the body.

a) skin or cutaneous, the most common naturally occurring type of infection
b) inhalational, the most deadly of the three
c) gastrointestinal

Los tres tipos de Antrax se determinan por la forma en que las bacterias penetran en el cuerpo.

a) de la piel o cutánea, tipo de infección que ocurre más comúnmente en forma natural
b) por inhalación, el más mortal de los tres
c) gastrointestinal

Symptoms of the three forms of Anthrax

a) **Cutaneous:** Usually starts after skin contact with contaminated meat, wool, hides, or leather from infected animals. The infection begins with an itchy bump that develops into a fluid-filled ulcer. A depressed, black scab develops in the middle of the ulcer. This scab will eventually fall in about two to three weeks. The lesion is usually painless, but the affected person may develop symptoms of fever, headache, and infl. of the lymph nodes around the ulcer. Incubation period ranges from 1-12 days.

b) **Inhalational:** It is the most lethal form of Anthrax; spores may be aerosolized in order to cause the disease. The first phase of the disease presents flu-like symptoms. In the more deadly second stage which may come within hours or days, the symptoms of sore throat, mild fever, and muscle aches may develop into respiratory failure, shock and a possible development of meningitis. Incubation period is not clear, but some reports indicate a range from 1-7 days, possibly ranging up to 60 days.

c) **Gastrointestinal:** It can cause two types of illnesses. The more common of the two affects the large or small intestine with manifestations of loss of appetite, nausea, vomiting, and fever. The symptoms can develop into severe and/or bloody diarrhea, abdominal pain, vomiting blood, and signs of septicemia. The less severe form is characterized by sore throat, fever, and sometimes lesions at the base of the tongue and back of the throat.

Treatment

Anthrax can be treated with antibiotics. The two most used presently are Cipro (ciprofloxacin) and the generic Doxycycline.

Testing

There is no test that can determine exposure to anthrax, but there is a blood culture test that can determine actual infection.

Síntomas de los tres tipos de Antrax

a) **Cutánea:** Gen. empieza después de haber contacto con carne, lana, o piel de animales infectados. La infección comienza desarrollando un bulto con picazón que se convierte en una úlcera llena de fluido. En el centro aparece una depresión con pústula negra que se cae a las dos o tres semanas. La lesión no suele ser dolorosa, pero la persona afectada puede tener fiebre, dolor de cabeza e hinchazón de los ganglios linfáticos alrededor de la úlcera. El período de incubación es de 1-12 días.

b) **Por inhalación:** Es la forma más letal de Antrax y las esporas se pueden aerosolizar para causar la enfermedad. La primera fase de la enfermedad presenta síntomas parecidos a la gripe. La segunda fase, mucho más mortal, puede brotar a las pocas horas o días más tarde; los síntomas como dolor de garganta, fiebre baja y dolor en los músculos pueden progresar y causar un fallo respiratorio, shock y posiblemente meningitis. El período de incubación es incierto pero algunos informes indican de 1-7 días, pudiéndose extender hasta 60 días.

c) **Gastrointestinal:** Puede causar dos tipos de enfermedad. La más común de las dos afecta el intestino delgado o grueso con síntomas de pérdida de apetito, náusea, vómito y fiebre que se pueden convertir en diarrea severa y/o sangrienta, dolor abdominal, vómitos de sangre y signos de septicemia. La forma menos severa se presenta con dolor de garganta, fiebre y a veces lesiones en la base de la lengua y la parte de atrás de la garganta.

Tratamiento

El Antrax puede ser tratado con antibióticos. Los dos más usados actualmente son Cipro (ciprofloxacina) y el producto genérico Doxiciclina.

Pruebas

Aunque no existe una prueba definitiva que determine si se ha estado expuesto o no al Antrax, hay una prueba sanguínea que puede determinar la infección.

ENGLISH	SPANISH

Vaccine

The anthrax vaccine is given to military personnel and workers who by the nature of their work may be exposed to the anthrax bacterium. For example, such would be the case of veterinarians handling potential infected animals, or persons who handle animal products that may come from areas where the disease is more common. The vaccine is scarce and it is not available to the public at large. New vaccines are currently being developed that will hopefully be abundant and easier to administer.

Frequently asked questions about Anthrax

Is Anthrax contagious?
No, Anthrax is not contagious; the illness cannot be transmitted from person to person.

Can the presence of anthrax spores be detected by their appearance, odor or taste?
No. The spores are too small to be seen by the naked eye and have no odor, but can be mixed with powder to transport them.

How can we know when a cold or flu is not Anthrax?
Gen. Anthrax is distinguished from the flu or cold because these diseases present additional symptoms.

SMALLPOX

Origin and where it is mostly found

Smallpox is an infectious disease caused by the variola virus. Unlike Anthrax and other possible bioterrorist agents, smallpox does not occur naturally in soil or animals. After a world wide campaign launched by the World Health Organization (WHO) in 1967, the disease was totally eradicated. Today, the only known stores of smallpox are two approved research labs, the CDC in Atlanta and the Institute of Virus Preparations in Moscow. Nevertheless, in the war against bioterrorism, there is an increased concern that the variola virus may be used as a bioterrorist agent.

Vacuna

Una vacuna contra el Antrax se le suministra actualmente a personal militar, y a trabajadores cuyo tipo de trabajo los puede exponer a la bacteria del Antrax. Por ejemplo, ese sería el caso de veterinarios que pueden estar en contacto con animales potencialmente infectados o personas que manipulan productos animales que provienen de áreas donde la enfermedad es más común. El número de vacunas es limitado, y no está al alcance del público en general. Se están desarrollando actualmente nuevas vacunas que se espera sean suficientes y más fáciles de administrar.

Preguntas más frecuentes sobre el Antrax

¿Es contagioso el Antrax?
No, el Antrax no es contagioso; la enfermedad no se transmite de una persona a otra.

¿Se puede detectar la presencia de Antrax por apariencia, olor o sabor?
No. Las esporas son demasiado pequeñas para verse a simple vista y son inodoras, pero pueden mezclarse con polvo para ser transportadas.

¿Cómo podemos saber cuando un catarro o influenza no es Antrax?
Gen. el Antrax se distingue de un catarro o influenza porque éstos presentan síntomas adicionales.

VIRUELA

Origen y dónde se encuentra más comúnmente

La viruela es una enfermedad infecciosa causada por el virus variola. A diferencia del Antrax y otros posibles agentes del terrorismo biológico, la viruela no se encuentra en forma natural en la tierra o en animales. Después de una campaña mundial iniciada por la Organización Mundial de Salud (OMS) en 1967, la viruela ha sido totalmente erradicada. Hoy en día, los únicos dos lugares donde hay almacenamiento del virus es en dos laboratorios aprobados, el CCE en Atlanta y el Instituto de Preparaciones de Virus en Moscú. Sin embargo, en la lucha contra el terrorismo biológico hay de nuevo la preocupación de que el virus variola sea empleado como agente terrorista biológico.

ENGLISH	SPANISH
Types or forms of Smallpox	*Tipos o clases de viruela*

a) variola major, the more lethal of the two	a) variola mayor, la más letal de las dos
b) variola minor, much less severe	b) variola menor, mucho menos severa
c) some unusual forms of the disease such as hemorrhagic and malignant smallpox	c) algunas formas poco usuales de la enfermedad, e.g. la viruela hemorrágica y la viruela maligna

Symptoms and characteristics of variola major	*Síntomas y características de la variola mayor*
Exposure to the virus is followed by an incubation period during which the affected person shows no symptoms and may feel fine; incubation period about 12 to 14 days, can also be between 7 and 17 days. The first symptoms include fever, malaise, head and body aches, and sometimes vomiting. The fever is usually high and within 2 to 4 days there may be a total physical collapse. The pox (rash) appears about 2 to 3 days after the incubation period in the form of very small pink spots in the mouth and the throat; at this time the person becomes most contagious. Rash spreads to the face and extremities, and occurs on the palms of the hands and the soles of the feet (one of the characteristics that differentiates the smallpox from the chicken pox). Rash develops into painful vesicles that eventually fill with pus; a scab forms and when it falls leaves some characteristic scarring. Usually the rash spreads to all parts of the body within 24 hours and once the rash appears, the fever usually drops and the person may start to feel better.	La exposición al virus es seguida de un período de incubación durante el cual la persona afectada no presenta síntomas y puede sentirse bien; el período de incubación dura de 12 a 14 días, pero también puede extenderse de 7 a 17 días. Los primeros síntomas son fiebre, dolor de cabeza y en el cuerpo, malestar general y a veces vómito; la fiebre es gen. alta y entre los 2 y 3 primeros días puede ocurrir un colapso físico total. La erupción aparece como dos o tres días después del período de incubación en forma de pequeñas manchitas rosadas en la boca y el cuello; este es el momento más contagioso de la enfermedad. La erupción se extiende a la cara y las extremidades y ocurre en las palmas de las manos y las suelas de los pies (una de las características que distingue la viruela de la varicela). La erupción se convierte en pústulas dolorosas que se llenan de pus y forman postillas que cuando finalmente se caen dejan marcas características de la enfermedad. Gen. el sarpullido se extiende a todas las partes del cuerpo en 24 horas y una vez que aparece, la fiebre usualmente baja y la persona empieza a sentirse major.

Contagion	*Contagio*
Smallpox is acquired primarily through aerosols or respiratory droplets from an infected person, and only persons that come very close to the infected person are in danger of contracting the disease. It can also be spread through direct contact with infected bodily fluids, and in some extreme cases clothing or bedding can also spread contagion. The infected carrier remains contagious until all the vesicles have scabbed and these have fallen.	La viruela se contrae mayormente por aspiración de microgotas o partículas respiratorias aéreas de la persona infectada, y solamente individuos que se encuentran muy cerca de la persona infectada están en peligro de contraer la enfemedad. También se puede contraer por contacto directo con fluidos corporales infectados, y en algunos casos extremos, la ropa personal y ropa de cama de la persona infectada también pueden resultar elementos de contagio. El contagio continúa hasta que todas las pústulas forman postillas y éstas se caen.

Testing	*Pruebas*
Samples of fluid from skin lesions can be tested for the virus, but these tests have to be done in very specialized laboratories with adequate protection and procedures.	Actualmente, se pueden hacer pruebas de muestras del fluido de las lesiones de la piel, pero sólo se pueden llevar a cabo en laboratorios muy especializados con un alto grado de seguridad y procedimientos.

ENGLISH	SPANISH

Vaccine and Treatment

Vacuna y Tratamiento

There is a vaccine against smallpox, the vaccinia vaccine, which can protect from the disease if given between one and four days after exposure. Even if the person has already fallen ill, prompt vaccination may greatly ameliorate the effects of the sickness. A quick diagnosis and prompt vaccination is of essence.

Existe una vacuna contra la viruela, que contiene el virus vaccinia, que puede proteger contra la enfermedad si se aplica entre uno a cuatro días después de la exposición al virus. Incluso si la persona ya está enferma, la aplicación rápida de la vacuna puede mejorar bastante los efectos de la enfermedad. Un diagnóstico rápido y una pronta vacunación son esenciales.

Frequently asked questions about bioterrorism

Preguntas más frecuentes sobre terrorismo biológico

Is it helpful to have a family plan and supply kit?

¿Sirve de ayuda tener un plan familiar de emergencia y tener suministros a mano?

Yes, because terrorist attacks will likely occur covertly, without previous notice and it can prove to be helpful to make provisions such as:

Sí, porque un ataque terrorista probablemente ocurrirá en secreto, sin aviso previo y puede resultar provechoso hacer planes en cuanto a :

Who would be included in the plan, only the family in the house, other family members, neighbors, etc. and what to do with the pets?

¿Quiénes estarían incluídos en el plan, la familia que habita la casa nada más, otros miembros de la familia, vecinos. etc. y cómo se dispondría de los animals?

Where would it be? The home will probably be the cornerstone of any family emergency plan, but if it's not a possibility, alternate locations should be considered?

¿Dónde llevarlo a cabo? La casa propia sería probablemente el centro de cualquier plan de emergencia, pero si la casa no fuese una posibilidad, se deben considerar otras alternativas.

Responsibility. It is important to assign the person who will be responsible for carrying out the plan.

Responsabilidad. Es importante asignar la persona que va a poner el plan en efecto.

Children. Plans should be discussed with children, age permitting, and they should be encouraged and reassured to follow the instructions of their teachers if the attack should occur during school hours.

Niños. Los niños deber ser alertados de todos los planes si la edad lo permite y se les debe asegurar y alentar a que sigan las instrucciones de sus maestros si el ataque ocurre durante las horas de clase.

Does sealing windows with duct tape and sheeting help?

¿Puede servir de ayuda sellar las ventanas con cinta adhesiva y cubiertas plásticas?

No. Even if the attack could be anticipated, the tape and the sheeting would only slow the air from outside, but would not stop it altogether.

No, aunque se pudiese anticipar el ataque, la cinta adhesiva y la cubierta plástica solamente demorarían la entrada del aire, pero no la detendrían por completo.

Should we keep masks (disposable or otherwise) as part of a plan of readiness?

¿Sería conveniente tener a mano máscaras (ya sean desechables o de otro tipo) como parte de un plan de preparación?

A mask is helpful only if it is worn at the exact moment of a terrorist attack, and this is likely to occur without notice. Nevertheless, in some cases, like in the case of an explosion, a simple mask may be helpful, in which case it is possible to improvise some barrier between the air and the mouth and the nose. A heavy-weave cotton material can help filter fine debris and toxic gases, as well as a simple cloth facemask.

Una máscara ayudaría solamente si se usa en el momento mismo del ataque, y lo más probable es que éste ocurra sin aviso previo. No obstante, hay situaciones, como en el caso de una explosión, cuando una máscara ayudaría, en cuyo caso siempre se puede improvisar alguna barrera entre el aire y la boca y la nariz. Un tejido grueso de algodón puede ayudar a filtrar las pequeñas partículas de detrito, así como una simple careta de tela.

Should we keep a supply of antibiotics in case there should be a terrorist attack?

No. Although many antibiotics are available, no single antibiotic is effective against every disease. Also, antibiotics are not effective against viruses; they have expiration dates and should be taken only by medical advice as some of them have serious side effects.

What is the best way to protect our families and our community from a terrorist attack?

At the present time much of the help following a terrorist attack would come from the government, health care institutions, and public health departments. Local health departments are responsible for protecting their communities against terrorist attacks, and should be able to assist a community with all bioterrorist-related concerns. Individuals and families can also address the federal government through their congressional respresentatives as to what assistance is being given to local authorities to better deal with threats of bioterrorism.

¿Se deben tener antibióticos a mano en caso de un ataque terrorista?

No. A pesar de que existen muchos antibióticos no hay ningún antibiótico que sea efectivo contra todas las enfermedades. Además, no son efectivos contra gérmenes de virus; tienen fecha de caducidad y solamente deben tomarse por indicación médica, ya que algunos tienen efectos secundarios serios.

¿Cuál es la mejor manera de proteger a nuestras familias y a la comunidad de un ataque terrorista?

Por el momento mucha de la ayuda que sigue a un ataque terrorista debe provenir del gobierno, instituciones y departamentos de salud pública. En última instancia, las instituciones locales son las que tienen la responsabilidad de proteger a la comunidad contra ataques terroristas, y deben poder ayudar a la comunidad en todo lo que concierne al terrorismo biológico. Individuos y familias también pueden dirigirse al gobierno federal a través de sus representantes en el Congreso para informarse en cuanto a que tipo de ayuda el gobierno le está dando a las autoridades locales para mejor combatir las amenazas del terrorismo biológico.

BIOTERRORISM INFECTION CONTROL PRECAUTIONS / PRECAUCIONES CONTRA INFECCIÓN POR TERRORISMO BIOLÓGICO

STANDARD PRECAUTIONS	PRECAUCIONES BÁSICAS
Wash hands before and after patient contact.	Lávese las manos antes y después de tener contacto con el paciente.
Wear gloves when touching blood, body fluids, secretions, excretions, and contaminated items.	Use guantes cuando se esté en contacto con sangre, líquidos corporales, secreciones o excreciones y objetos contaminados.
Wear protective gown, mask, and eye protection during procedures likely to generate splashes or sprays of blood, body fluids, secretions, and excretions.	Use batas protectoras, máscara y protección sobre los ojos durante procedimientos donde pueda haber salpicaduras o rociadas de sangre, líquidos corporales, secreciones y excreciones.
Handle used patient-care equipment and linen in a manner that prevents the transfer of microorganisms to other people or equipment.	Maneje cualquier equipo o ropa de cama que se haya usado en el paciente de manera tal que prevenga la transferencia de microorganismos a otras personas o equipo.
Use care when handling sharps and place disposable sharps in a sharp's container.	Tenga cuidado en el manejo de objetos agudos y disponga de ellos en un recipiente designado para eso.
Use a mouthpiece or other ventilation device when giving mouth-to-mouth resuscitation, when practical.	Use un tapabocas u otro dispositivo ventilado cuando esté dando resuscitación de boca a boca, si resulta práctico.
Standard precautions are required for the care of ALL patients.	Las precauciones básicas se deben implementar con TODOS los pacientes.

CONTACT PRECAUTIONS	PRECAUCIONES CON EL CONTACTO
Use all standard precautions plus:	**Emplée todas las precauciones básicas y además:**
Place patient in a private room or cohort them with someone with the same infection, if possible.	Ponga al paciente en un cuarto privado o de compañero con alguien que sufre de la misma enfermedad, si es possible.
Wear gloves and protective gowns when entering the room, and change gloves and/or gown after contact with infectious material.	Use guantes y bata protectora cuando entre al cuarto, y cámbiese de guantes y/o bata después de contacto con material infectado.
Limit the movement or transport of patient from the room.	Limite el movimiento o transporte del paciente fuera del cuarto.
Ensure that the patient care items, bedside equipment, and frequently touched surfaces receive daily cleaning.	Asegúrese de que todos los objetos que se emplean en la asistencia al paciente, efectos de cama, y superficies que se tocan a menudo, se limpien todos los días.
Non critical patient-care equipment (e.g., stethoscope) should be limited to a single patient or cohort of patients with same pathogen. If not feasible, adequate disinfection of equipment between patients is necessary.	El material médico (ej., estetoscopio) se debe limitar a un solo paciente o a compañeros de cuarto que sufren del mismo patógeno. Si eso no es posible, los instrumentos médicos se deben desinfectar a-decuadamente cada vez que se utilicen en un paciente.

Taken from the Arizona Department of Health Services. Tomado del Departamento de Servicios de Salud del estado de Arizona.

Where to obtain information:	Dónde se puede obtener información:
Center for Disease Control and Prevention (CDC) www.bt.cdc.gov/	Centro para el Control y Prevención de Enfermedades (CCE) www.bt.cdc.gov/
American Medical Association (AMA) www.ama-assn.org	Asociación Médica Americana (AMA) www.ama-assn.org
American Red Cross www.redcross.org (can give information on specific actions to take during each threat level)	La Cruz Roja www.redcross.org (puede dar información sobre medidas a tomar en cada situación específica)
Department of Homeland Security www.ready.gov (has a full list of items, foods, water, and medical supplies that should be kept on hand for the worst-case scenario)	Departamento de Seguridad Nacional www.ready.gov (tiene una lista completa de artículos, alimentos, agua y suministros médicos que se deben tener a mano cuando se contempla la peor situación posible)

HIPAA (HEALTH INSURANCE PORTABILITY AND ACCOUNTABILITY ACT) / HIPAA

This legislation is concerned with many areas of health care, including research.	**Esta legislación atañe áreas de la salud incluyendo proyectos de investigación.**
The most important principles of this legislation concerning the process of informed consent on the part of the investigators and the participants are the following:	Los puntos principales de esta legislación concerniente al proceso de consentimiento informado por parte de los investigadores y participantes son los siguientes:
1. Protection of human subjects.	1. Protección de sujetos humanos.
2. Voluntary consent of the human subject to participate in a research project.	2. Consentimiento voluntario del participante en un proyecto de investigación.
3. Right to refusal without any repercussions to the medical care of the participant.	3. Derecho de rechazo sin repercusiones al cuidado médico del participante.
4. Right to withdraw from the research project at any time.	4. Derecho del participante a dejar de ser parte del proyecto en cualquier momento.
5. Identification of the person authorized to do the research.	5. Identificación de la persona autorizada para realizar el proyecto.
6. Confidentiality as to the participant's identity and health information.	6. Confidencialidad en cuanto a la identidad del participante y de su historial médico.
7. Authorization by signature of validity of participation.	7. Autorización firmada de validez de participación.
8. Participant's acknowledgment of having received information as to the nature, risks, and benefits involved in the project.	8. Conocimiento por parte del participante de haber recibido información en cuanto a la naturaleza, riesgos, y beneficios del proyecto.

CONSENT AND AUTHORIZATION FORMS / FORMULARIOS DE CONSENTIMIENTO Y AUTORIZACIÓN
Research Project with Human Subjects Participants

SUBJECT AUTHORIZATION

Before giving my consent to participate in this project by signing this form, the methods, inconveniences, risks, and benefits have been explained to me. I have received a satisfactory answer to all my questions, and I have been informed that I may continue to ask questions related to the project whenever I consider it necessary.

If in the course of this project there is any reason that may cause me to withdraw, I am free to do so without causing bad feelings. My participation in the project may be ended by the sponsor or by the investigator for reasons that they will explain to me. I will be given, as it becomes available, any new information developed during the course of this study that may affect my willingness to continue as a participant.

Federal regulations require information and a written informed consent prior to participation in this research study so I can know the nature, risks, and benefits of my participation and can decide to participate or not in a free and informed manner.

It is my understanding that this consent form will be filed in an area designated by

_____

(ORGANIZATION AUTHORIZING THE PROJECT)

with access only to the principal investigator: _____,

or an authorized representative of

_____.

I do not give up any of my legal rights by signing this form.
I will receive a copy to keep of this consent form signed by me.

_____   _____
Subject's Signature   Date

_____   _____
Legal Guardian Signature   Date

INVESTIGATOR'S AFFIDAVIT

I have carefully explained to the subject the nature of the above project. I hereby testify that to the best of my knowledge the person who is signing this consent form understands clearly the nature, demands, benefits, and risks involved in his/her participation and his/her signature is legally valid. A medical problem or language or educational barrier has not precluded this understanding.

_____   _____
Investigator's Signature   Date

700

Proyecto de investigación con sujetos humanos

AUTORIZACIÓN DEL PARTICIPANTE

Antes de dar mi firma de consentimiento, me han explicado los métodos, inconvenientes, riesgos y beneficios tratados en este proyecto. Me han contestado las preguntas que tenía satisfactoriamente. Me han informado que puedo hacer preguntas relacionadas con el proyecto en cualquier momento, y estoy en libertad de dejar de participar en el proyecto cuando lo decida sin causar ningún mal entendido. Mi participación en este proyecto puede ser terminada por la persona investigadora o por el patrocinador por razones que se me explicarán. Me comunicarán cualquier nueva información que se desarrolle durante el curso de este estudio que pueda afectar mi deseo de continuar como participante en este proyecto.

De acuerdo con requisitos federales se requiere dar información y un consentimiento previo por escrito antes de participar en este estudio de investigación de manera que se sepa la naturaleza, riesgos y beneficios de mi participación y que yo pueda decidir si deseo participar o no voluntariamente.

ENTIENDO QUE ESTE CONSENTIMIENTO SERÁ ARCHIVADO EN UN LOCAL

designado por _____ con acceso restringido

al investigador principal_____,

o a una persona autorizada de_____.

NO RENUNCIO A NINGUNO DE MIS DERECHOS CIVILES AL DAR MI FIRMA EN ESTE DOCUMENTO

Recibiré una copia firmada de este consentimiento.

_____   _____
Firma del participante   Fecha

_____   _____
Firma del tutor o guardián   Fecha

AFFIDÁVIT DEL INVESTIGADOR:

He explicado claramente al participante la naturaleza de este proyecto. Atestiguo al presente que según mi entender la persona que firma este consentimiento comprende con claridad la naturaleza, demandas, beneficios y riesgos comprendidos en su participación, y que su firma es legalmente válida. Ningún problema médico, barrera educacional o lingüística ha impedido este consentimiento.

_____   _____
Firma del investigador   Fecha

Request by Physician for Retrovirus (HIV) Testing

Patient: _____ **is not able** or is incompetent to provide informed consent for a test or anlysis of retrovirus (HIV) which is necessary for an appropriate diagnosis, treatment, or care. Any other authorized persons to give consent for this patient are not available. There is a reasonable suspicion that this patient has an HIV infection, therefore, it is my medical judgement that the above mentioned test is necessary to obtain an appropriate diagnosis, care, or treatment, of this patient to improve his/her quality of life.

_____   _____
Physician's Signature   Date

M D Code: _____

Petición facultativa para realizar una prueba de retrovirus VIH

Paciente: _____ por no estar capacitado, o estar impedido de proporcionar un consentimiento informado para hacerse una prueba o análisis de Retrovirus (VIH), lo cual es necesario para obtener una diagnosis acertada, tratamiento o atención de su caso. Otras personas autorizadas para dar el consentimiento no se encuentran disponibles. Existe una sospecha razonable que el paciente mencionado sufre de una infección de VIH. Por lo tanto, es mi criterio médico que el análisis antes mencionado es necesario para obtener una diagnosis apropiada, para atenderle y tratarle, y mejorar la calidad de su vida.

_____   _____
Firma del facultativo   Fecha

Código Médico o Licencia: _____

Patient's Request To Be Tested For Retrovirus (HIV)

I request that _____ hospital and its physicians test my blood for antibodies to HIV. I understand that HIV is the virus that causes AIDS. I also understand that this test will determine whether the blood contains antibodies to the virus. I am told that antibodies generally appear 1-6 months after infection has occurred. I understand that I will be informed of the results whether they are negative or positive and that test results will be placed in my medical record. I agree that if a confirmed positive result is found, it will be reported to the Health Authorities of the State of _____.

_____
Patient's signature

_____
Date

_____
Witness

_____
Date

Petición del paciente para la prueba de retrovirus (VIH)

Solicito que el hospital _____ y sus médicos me hagan la prueba de sangre de anticuerpos para el VIH. Me han informado que VIH es el virus que causa el SIDA. Entiendo que la prueba determina si la sangre contiene anticuerpos contra el virus VIH. Los anticuerpos aparecen generalmente de 1-6 meses después que la infección ocurre. Entiendo que seré informado-a del resultado ya sea negativo o positivo, y que este resultado será registrado en mi expediente médico. Entiendo también y confirmo que si el resultado es positivo, éste será reportado a las autoridades de Salud del Estado de _____.

_____
Firma del participante

_____
Fecha

_____
Firma del testigo

_____
Fecha

Parent's Consent to the Participation of a Minor

Before giving my consent for my child to participate in this project by signing this form, the methods, inconveniences, risks, and benefits have been explained to me, and my questions have been answered satisfactorily. I may ask questions at any time in the course of the project, and my child is free to withdraw at any time without causing bad feelings. My child's participation in this project may be ended by the investigator or by the sponsor for reasons which would be explained to me.

New information developed during the course of this study which may affect my willingness to have my child continue as a participant in this research project will be given to me as it becomes available.

Federal regulations require a written informed consent prior to participation in this research study so I can know the nature and risks of my participation and can decide to participate or not in a free and informed manner.

I understand that this consent form will be filed in an area designated by _____with access restricted to the principal investigator_____or an authorized representative of the _____ department.

I do not waive any of my legal rights by signing this form.

A copy of this signed consent form will be given to me.

_____   _____
Parent or Legal Guardian   Date

_____   _____
Witness   Date

INVESTIGATOR'S AFFIDAVIT:

I have carefully explained to the subject the nature of the above project. I hereby testify that to the best of my knowledge the person who is signing this consent form fully understands the nature, demands, benefits and risks involved in his/her participation and his/her signature is legally valid. A medical problem or language or educational barrier has not precluded this understanding.

_____   _____
Investigator's Signature   Date

Consentimiento del progenitor a la participación de un menor de edad

Antes de dar mi firma para el consentimiento de participación de mi hijo-a en este proyecto, personas autorizadas me han explicado los métodos, inconvenientes, riesgos y beneficios que se refieren a este proyecto. Me han contestado las preguntas que tenía y me han informado que puedo hacer todas las preguntas necesarias respecto al proyecto cuando lo desee.

Mi hijo-a está en libertad de dejar de participar en el proyecto si así fuera su deseo sin causar ningún mal entendido. La participación de mi hijo-a puede ser terminada por la persona investigadora o por el patrocinador por razones que se me explicarán.

Es posible que durante el curso del estudio reciba nueva información cuando esté disponible que afecte mi deseo o el de mi hijo-a de continuar como participante en este proyecto. En ese caso, si decido que mi hijo-a deje de participar, se me ha afirmado que él/ella no dejará de recibir el cuidado médico ofrecido.

De acuerdo con requisitos federales se requiere un consentimiento previo por escrito antes de participar en este estudio de investigación de manera que yo sepa la naturaleza, riesgos y beneficios y mi hijo-a pueda decidir si desea participar o no voluntariamente.

Entiendo que este consentimiento será archivado en un local designado por_____con acceso restringido al investigador principal_____, o a una persona autorizada de_____.

No renuncio a ninguno de mis derechos civiles al dar mi firma en este documento. Recibiré una copia de este consentimiento que he firmado.

TESTIMONIO DEL INVESTIGADOR:

He explicado claramente al participante la naturaleza del proyecto. Atestiguo al presente que según mi entender, la persona que firma este consentimiento comprende con claridad la naturaleza, demandas, beneficios y riesgos comprendidos en su participación y que su firma es legalmente válida. Ningún problema médico, o barrera educacional o lingüística ha impedido este conocimiento.

_____   _____
Firma del investigator   Fecha

_____   _____
Firma del testigo   Fecha

705

Authorization for Surgical Procedures

In signing this consent form I authorize the following surgical procedure: _____

Acting surgeon and assistants_____

I consent to the use of anesthetics, blood transfusions (if necessary), and the procedures that are normal to the operation that Dr._____ will perform.

I also consent to any additional procedures that my surgeon and his/her assistants may deem necessary during the course of the surgery because of unforeseen circumstances.

I also consent to the technical use of instruments and cameras that would be needed, if necessary, to study different parts and organs of my body for medical, scientific, or educational purposes, provided that my identity is not revealed.

I also consent to the attendance of other professional observers in the operating room.

I give my permission to the hospital authorities for the examination and disposal of any tissue or part of my body that may have to be removed during this operation, if that should be necessary.

By signing this form, I acknowledge that the advantages, benefits, and risks of this operation have been explained to me and that I understand the reason for this treatment, and give my authorization and consent to have the operation performed.

I have also been informed that there can be no guarantee or assurance as to the results of this operation.

_____   _____
Patient's name: Date

_____
Patient or guardian's signature

_____
Witness signature

Autorización para procedimientos quirúrgicos

Al dar mi firma a este consentimiento autorizo al procedimiento quirúrgico siguiente:

Cirujanos y asistentes_____
Consiento el uso de anestésicos, transfusiones de sangre (si son necesarias) y los procedimientos que son normales a la operación que el Dr._____ llevará a cabo.

También consiento a cualquier procedimiento adicional que mi cirujano y sus asistentes consideren necesario durante el curso de la operación debido a circunstancias imprevistas.
También consiento al uso técnico de instrumentos y cámaras que se necesiten, para el estudio de distintas pa y órganos del cuerpo con fines médicos, científicos o educacionales, con la condición de que mi identidad no se revele.

También consiento en que otros observadores profesionales estén presentes en la sala de operaciones.

Doy mi permiso a las autoridades hospitalarias para examinar o disponer de cualquier tejido y parte del cuerpo que tengan que ser extraídos durante la operación.

Al dar mi firma a este documento, reconozco que las ventajas, los riesgos y los beneficios de esta operación han sido explicados, entiendo la decisión tomada para este tratamiento, y doy mi autorización y consentimiento para que la operación se lleve a cabo.

También se me ha informado y reconozco que no existe garantía ni certeza en el resultado de la operación.

_____   _____
Firma del / de la paciente   Fecha

_____
Firma del guardián

_____
Firma del /de la testigo

Informed Consent for Surgery Procedure
Surgeon Statement of Informed Consent

The patient has been informed by me of possible risks and complications, as well as benefits and alternate treatments. I have also answered any questions the patient may have had. The patient/guardian has agreed to the procedure in question.

If blood transfusion is a possibility, I have answered the patient's questions and informed his/her guardian of possible risks associated with blood transfusions. I have discussed the risks and benefits as well as the advantages and disadvantages for autologous blood donation and directed or undirected donation of blood by volunteers.

The patient has been allowed adequate time before surgery to make necessary arrangements for donation of blood. Exceptions to this would be a) if the patient waives his/her right; b) if there are medical contraindications; c) if a life-threatening emergency should occur.

I have verbally discussed and verified with the patient/guardian the correct site where surgery will take place.

_____   _____
Surgeon performing procedure   Date

If anesthesia is required, the following should be completed:

Informed Consent for Anesthesia

I have discussed the risks, benefits, and complications of anesthesia with the patient, as well as some of the rare complications that may occur. I have answered all the questions asked by patient/guardian and he/she agrees to the use of anesthesia.

I have verbally verified with the patient/guardian the correct site of surgery.

_____   _____
Anesthesiologist   Date

Consentimiento para un procedimiento quirúrgico
Informe de Consentimiento del Cirujano

El paciente ha sido informado por mí de los posibles riesgos y complicaciones, así como de los beneficios y tratamientos alternativos.

También he contestado a todas las preguntas del paciente y éste está de acuerdo con el procedimiento.

Si se anticipa la posibilidad de una transfusión de sangre, he contestado a todas las preguntas del paciente/guardián y he informado de los posibles riesgos asociados a la transfusión. También le he explicado los riesgos y beneficios así como las ventajas y desventajas de donación de sangre autóloga y de donación directa o indirecta de sangre de voluntarios.

Se le ha otorgado al paciente el tiempo adecuado antes de la cirugía para hacer los arreglos necesarios para la donación de sangre. La excepción a esto sería a) si el paciente renuncia a este derecho; b) si hay contraindicaciones médicas; c) si surge una situación de emergencia que ponga en riesgo la vida del paciente. He discutido y verificado con el paciente/guardián el sitio donde se llevará a cabo la cirugía.

_____   _____

Ferma del cirujano que lleva a cabo la operación   Fecha

Si se require anestesia para la operacíon:

Consentimiento para recibir anestesia

He explicado los riesgos, beneficios y complicaciones de la anestesia con el paciente, así como algunas complicaciones poco usuales que pueden ocurrir.

He contestado a todas las preguntas del paciente/guardián y él/ella está de acuerdo con el uso de la anestesia.

He establecido verbalmente con el paciente/guardián el lugar donde se va a llevar a cabo la cirugía.

_____   _____

Firma del Anestesista   Fecha

THE RIGHTS OF THE PATIENT

The rights of the patient, and the rights of the health providers are instituted by the Federal Government in all health centers providing health care.

The Bill of Rights of the patient, of hospitals, and health care centers, informs that the patients have the following rights:[19]

1. **Quality of care.** To receive respectful and careful care.
2. **Knowledge about his/ her own case.** To be able to request information about the patient's own diagnosis, treatment and prognosis, at anytime during his/her illness.
3. **Identity of attending personnel.** To be informed about the identity of doctors, nurses, technicians or any health care providers in attendance of his/her case.
4. **Treatment Cost**. To know the immediate and long term cost of the treatment as far as it is possibly to be known, and to have a plan to pay for them.
5. **Information and decisions about the treatment**. To make decisions about the treatment received or that is to be given. To be informed of the risks and benefits of any medication or treatment that is to be received.
6. **Refusal of treatment.** To refuse to be treated and be advised of any other treatment or care available to him/her by the health institution or health care provider. To be advised by the health care institution of any limitations to this effect.
7. **The Living Will.** To have on file on his/her record, a Living Will written and legalized concerning specific directions of treatment, in case the patient is incapacitated to do it. To this effect, the patient has the right to designate a surrogate person that would follow the patient's decision. The health institution must instruct the patient about the availability of such a document.
8. **To have privacy**. Any consultations, examinations, case considerations done by physicians and other health care providers have to comply with the patient's privacy. The record of each patient has to be kept with complete confidentiality. Reporting of any facts from the patient's record can only be done if permitted by law.
9. **Revision of records.** The patient has the right to review his or her own medical records and be assisted by health care personnel if necessary, to fully understand the treatments and state of his or her health care. Limitations to his/her review of the records are only those required by law.
10. **Confidentiality.** The right to expect that the health care institution in charge of his/her records will preserve their confidentiality and will release them only to other interested parties that are legally authorized to review the information .
11. **The right to transfer.** The patient has the right to continue to receive treatment, and to be transferred to another institution, if permitted by such institution, if the institution where he or she is treated is not able to continue the necessary care and has advised him or her to receive a treatment that the other institution can provide.
12. **The right to decline or consent.** The patient should have complete information about the risks, inconveniences and benefits of proposed research studies or in human experimentation that require patient participation and may affect his or her treatment. The patient can exercise the right to consent or decline participation in such projects without affecting in any way the medical treatment or medical care that is received.

---

[19]This incomplete summary of the Bill of Rights of the Patient contains the most repeated rights of the patient. Este extracto de la Declaración de Derechos del Paciente contiene los derechos más repetidos del paciente.

LOS DERECHOS DEL PACIENTE

Los derechos del / de la paciente y los derechos del personal de salud que le asisten, son derechos instituidos por ley por el Gobierno Federal en todos los centros de salud.

La Ley de Derechos del paciente, hospitales y centros de salud informa que los pacientes tienen los siguientes derechos:

1. **Calidad de atención.** Recibir cuidado médico con consideración y respeto.
2. **Conocimiento sobre su caso.** Pedir información en todo momento sobre el diagnóstico, tratamiento y prognosis de la enfermedad que sufre.
3. **Identidad del personal a cargo del caso.** Ser informado sobre la identidad de médicos, enfermeras, técnicos o personal médico a cargo de su caso.
4. **Costo del tratamiento.** Conocer el costo inmediato y a largo plazo del tratamiento, de lo que es posible saber, y tener un plan para su pago.
5. **Información y decisiones sobre el tratamiento.** Hacer decisiones sobre el tratamiento recibido, o sobre el que se le dará. Ser informado de los riesgos y beneficios de cualquier medicamento o tratamiento a que se le someta.
6. **Rehusar tratamiento.** Negarse a recibir tratamiento médico, y ser informado de otro tratamiento o servicio médico ofrecido por la institución médica o el profesional de salud que le atiende. La institución de salud debe advertirle sobre cualquier otra limitación al respecto.
7. **Testamento en Vida.** Tener archivado con su expediente un Testamento en Vida legalizado, con órdenes específicas del tratamiento que desea recibir en caso de que se encuentre incapacitado para comunicar sus deseos. Si fuera así, el / la paciente tiene derecho a autorizar a una segunda persona que haga cumplir su decisión. La institución de salud debe informarle al/a la paciente sobre la disponibilidad de este documento.
8. **El derecho de privacidad.** Las consultas, exámenes y deliberaciones médicas del caso hechas por médicos y cualquier otro personal de salud se deben tratar teniendo en cuenta la privacidad del/de la paciente. El expediente médico de cada paciente debe guardarse con completa confidencialidad. Sólo podrá darse información registrada en el expediente del / de la paciente si es permitido legalmente.
9. **Revisión del expediente.** El paciente tiene el derecho de revisar su expediente y ser asistido por un miembro del personal de salud si fuera necesario, para entender su tratamiento y conocer el estado de su salud. Las limitaciones a su revisión del expediente son solamente las establecidas por la ley.
10. **Confidencialidad.** El derecho de confiar en que la institución de salud a cargo de su expediente guardará la confidencialidad del mismo y sólo será abierto a las personas que estén autorizadas para revisar la información.
11. **Derecho a ser transferido.** El paciente tiene derecho a continuar su tratamiento y ser transferido a otra institución, si dicha institución así lo permite, siempre que el centro de salud donde se encuentra ingresado no pueda continuar asistiéndole y le recomiende un tratamiento que la institución que le recibirá puede proporcionarle.
12. **El derecho de rehusar o dar consentimiento.** El paciente debe tener completa información sobre los riesgos, inconveniencias y beneficios de los estudios de investigación o de experimentación humana que requieran su participación y que puedan afectar su tratamiento. Por lo que, si invitado a participar, el paciente puede aceptar o rehusar participación, sin que afecte en ninguna manera su tratamiento o atención médica.

LIVING WILL

A Living Will is a written directive issued by a person regarding the treatment he or she wishes to receive in the event of mortal illness, and is unable to communicate his or her desire to the attending health care providers.

In this document the patient designates a surrogate person or guardian to make decisions in his/her regard. It is the duty of the health care institution or provider to carry out the wishes of the patient who has filed and made a Living Will, following legal advice.

The Living Will is effective only when the person is unable to communicate his or her own health care decisions in the event of death.

1. The wish and desire not to have his/her life artificially prolonged just to receive comfort care.
2. The patient has the doctors decide if his/her condition is incurable, terminal, or in a vegetative state, and to provide only the necessary care to keep comfortable.
3. The patient refuses cardiopulmonary resuscitation, electric shock, drugs, artificial breathing or food and fluids artificially administered, and to avoid to be taken to a hospital.
4. In case of a pregnant woman, the patient requests to be provided with life-sustaining treatment if the embryo/fetus is viable to the point of live birth.
5. The patient requires all the medical care necessary until the doctors determine that his/her condition is terminal, with a persistant vegetative state.
6. The patient simply states to want all medical treatment necessary to be kept alive as long as possible.

TESTAMENTO EN VIDA

Un Testamento en Vida es un documento de autorización por escrito del tratamiento que una persona desea recibir en caso de sufrir una enfermedad terminal o condición mortal, y se encuentre impedida de poder comunicar sus últimos deseos a los facultativos que le asisten. El paciente en este documento designa a un familiar o guardián aquien autoriza para tomar las decisiónes necesarias en su lugar. La institución de salud tiene el deber de llevar a cabo la voluntad expresada por el/la paciente en el Testamento en Vida registrado legalmente en su expediente.

El Testamento en Vida es efectivo únicamente si la persona se encuentra incapacitada para comunicar las decisiones a seguir si se encuentra en peligro de muerte.

1. Expresa la voluntad de no prolongar su vida artificialmente y de sólo recibir un cuidado adecuado que provea alivio.
2. Es la voluntad del/de la paciente que los médicos decidan si su estado es terminal o vegetativo, y que sólo le proporcionen un cuidado paliativo para evitar sufrimiento.
3. Rehusa recibir resucitación cardiopulmonar, choque eléctrico, drogas o respiración artificial, y que eviten su traslado a un hospital.
4. En el caso de estar embarazada, su voluntad es de recibir tratamiento si el embrio/feto es capaz de sobrevivir hasta el momento de su nacimiento.
5. Requiere todo el cuidado médico necesario hasta que los médicos determinen que su condición es terminal y su estado es vegetativo persistente.
6. El/la paciente declara su voluntad de recibir todo el tratamiento médico necesario para prolongar su vida lo más posible.

LIVING WILL STATEMENT

CHOICE DETERMINED BY THE PATIENT: _____, on her/his own behalf, without assistance by anyone, relative, friend, or any health care professional connected with this case.

1. ___ If I have a terminal condition I do not wish that my life be artificially prolonged. I desire only comfort care.

2. ___ If my doctors decide that I am in irreversible or permanent coma, a terminal condition, or an unchangeable vegetative state, I wish to have only the medical treatment necessary to provide care that would keep me comfortable. I do not want the following:

   a) Cardiopulmonary resuscitation, use of drugs, electric shock and artificial breathing or any means to prolong my life.

   b) Artificially administered food and fluids.

   c) To be taken to a hospital if at all avoidable.

3. ___ In the event that I am pregnant, I do not want life-sustaining treatment withheld or withdrawn if it is at all possible that the embryo / fetus can develop to the point of live birth.

4. ___ Until my doctors conclude after carefully studying my case that it is terminal, or I am in a persistent vegetative state, I desire to have the use of all medical care necessary to treat my condition.

5. ___ I want all the medical treatment necessary to keep me alive as long as possible.

Signature of patient: _____

_____   _____   _____
Location City   State   Date

_____   _____
Name and Signature of Witness   Date

DECLARACIÓN VOLUNTARIA DE TESTAMENTO EN VIDA

ELECCIÓN DETERMINADA DE TRATAMIENTO:_____, por propia voluntad y sin interferencia de familiares, amigos o personal de salud relacionado con este caso, elijo lo siguiente:

1. ___ Si me encontrara en una condición terminal no deseo que mi vida se prolongue artificialmente. Sólo deseo que se me dé la atención necesaria que me provea alivio.

2. ___Si los médicos que me atienden deciden que me encuentro en un estado de coma permanente, en una condición terminal o irreversible, o en un estado vegetativo, sólo deseo la atención médica necesaria para mantenerme confortable. No deseo lo siguiente:

   a) Resucitación cardiopulmonar, choque eléctrico, respiración artificial, uso de medicamentos o cualquier otra forma para prolongar mi vida artificialmente.

   b) Alimentación artificial en forma sólida o líquida.

   c) Ser trasladado a un hospital si se puede evitar.

3. ___ que dejen de darme el tratamiento necesario para sostener mi vida en caso de estar embarazada, si hay posibilidades de que el embrio/feto se desarrolle hasta que pueda ser viable. Pero sí deseo:

4. ___ que si los médicos que me atienden después de haber estudiado mi caso deciden que mi estado es terminal, irreversible o incurable, o que me encuentro en un estado vegetativo, me dén toda la atención médica necesaria para tratar mi condición.

5. ___tener todo el tratamiento médico necesario que prolongue mi vida lo más posible.

_____
Firma del/de la paciente

_____   _____   _____
Localidad Ciudad   Provincia o   Estado

_____   _____
Nombre y firma de testigo   Fecha

MUSCLES AND ACTIONS / MÚSCULOS Y ACCIONES

Muscle	Action	Músculo	Acción
occipitofrontal	draws scalp backward and forward; raises the eyebrows	occipitofrontal	mueve el cuero cabelludo hacia atrás y hacia adelante; levanta las cejas
buccinator	compresses the cheek and retracts the angle of the mouth	buccinador	comprime el cachete y retracta el ángulo de la boca
sternocleidomastoid	flexes the vertebral column and rotates the head to the opposite side of the muscle that is being contracted	esternocleidomastoideo	flexiona la columna vertebral y rota la cabeza hacia el lado opuesto del músculo que se contrae
trapezius	draws back the head of the humerus; rotates the scapula	trapecio	mueve la cabeza del húmero hacia atrás; rota la escápula
deltoid	abducts, flexes, and extends the arm	deltoides	abduce, flexiona y extiende el brazo
biceps (of arm)	flexes the articulation of the elbow and turns the forearm	bíceps (braquial)	flexiona la articulación del codo y gira el antebrazo
triceps (of arm)	extends the forearm and the arm	tríceps (braquial)	extiende el antebrazo y el brazo
latissimus dorsi	adducts, extends, and rotates the arm	dorsal ancho	aduce, extiende y rota el brazo
pectoral, greater	adducts, flexes, and rotates the arm medially	pectoral mayor	aduce, flexiona y rota el brazo hacia adentro
pectoral, smaller	draws shoulder forward and downward, raises the ribs, and acts as an inhaling muscle	pectoral menor	baja y lleva el hombro hacia adelante, eleva las costillas y actúa como músculo inspirador
psoas, greater	flexes, adducts, and rotates the thigh	psoas mayor	flexiona, aduce y rota el muslo
psoas, smaller	assists the greater psoas	psoas menor	asiste al psoas mayor
oblique of abdomen, external	lowers the ribs, flexes the thorax, and presses the abdominal viscera	oblicuo del abdomen, externo	baja las costillas, flexiona el tórax y comprime las vísceras abdominales
gluteus maximus	extends and rotates the thigh	glúteo mayor	extiende y rota el muslo
gluteus medius	abducts and rotates the thigh	glúteo mediano	abduce y rota el muslo
gluteus minimum	abducts and extends the thigh	glúteo menor	abduce y extiende el muslo

715

Muscle	Action	Músculo	Acción
quadriceps	extends the leg and flexes the muscle over the pelvis	cuadríceps	extiende la pierna y flexiona el muslo sobre la pelvis
soleus	extends and rotates the foot	sóleo	extiende y rota el pie
abductor pollicis brevis	abducts the thumb	abductor corto del pulgar	abduce el pulgar
abductor pollicis longus	abducts and flexes the thumb	abductor largo del pulgar	abduce y flexiona el pulgar
anconeus	extends the forearm stabilizing the elbow joint	ancóneo	extiende el antebrazo estabilizando la articulación del codo
sacrococcygeus, anterior and posterior	protrudes the coccyx forwards and backwards	sacrococcígeo, anterior y posterior	empuja el cóccix hacia adelante y hacia atrás
diaphragm	breathing and expulsive acts	diafragma	respiración y actos expulsivos
obliquus internus and externus abdominis	flex and rotate the vertebral column ; compress the abdominal viscera	oblicuo interno y externo del abdomen	flexionan y rotan la columna vertebral; comprimen las vísceras abdominales
gastrocnemius	flexes ankle when knee is extended; raises heel when walking; flexes leg at knee joint	gastrocnemio	flexiona el tobillo cuando se extiende la rodilla; levanta el talón al caminar y flexiona la pierna en la articulación de la rodilla
sternocleidomastoideus	flexes the trunk and the head	esternocleidomastoideo	flexiona la columna vertebral y la cabeza
quadriceps femoris	extends the leg over the thigh	cuadríceps crural	extiende la pierna sobre el muslo
tensor *fascia latae*	flexes and abducts the thigh; helps to keep knee extended	tensor de la *fascia lata*	flexiona y abduce el muslo; ayuda a mantener la rodilla extendida
sartorius	flexes the thigh and the knee	sartorio	flexiona el muslo y la rodilla
pyramidalis	tenses abdominal wall	piramidal del abdomen	tensa la pared abdominal

PHYSICAL FITNESS / ACONDICIONAMIENTO FÍSICO

Vocabulary	Vocabulario
aerobic	aeróbico-a
cardiovascular	cardiovascular
cool down	enfriarse, enfriamiento
endurance	resistencia
equipment	equipo
exercise	ejercicio
flexibility	flexibilidad
muscle tone	tono muscular
strengthening	fortalecer, fortalecimiento
strength training	programa de fortalecimiento
stretching out	estirarse, estiramiento
treadmill	rueda de andar
warm up	calentarse, calentamiento
weights	pesas
workout	programa de ejercicio

General Observations and Recommendations	Observaciones y Recomendaciones Generales
Exercise helps in many ways.	El ejercicio es beneficioso de muchas maneras.
It keeps the lungs and heart healthy.	Mantiene los pulmones y el corazón saludables.
It helps the blood flow in the body.	Ayuda la circulación de la sangre.
It improves muscle tone.	Aumenta la tonicidad muscular.
It alleviates arthritic pain.	Alivia el dolor artrítico.
It strengthens bones and stimulates the production of hormones.	Fortalece los huesos y estimula la producción de hormonas.
It helps to keep weight down.	Ayuda a mantener un buen peso.
It makes one feel good.	Le hace sentirse bien.
Do exercises that you like.	Haga ejercicios que le gusten.
Exercise a few times a week.	Haga los ejercicios varias veces a la semana.
Talk to your doctor about a good exercise program for you.	Consulte con su médico sobre un programa de ejercicios que sea beneficioso para Ud.

Warming up and Cooling Down Exercises

Ejercicios de calentamiento y de enfriamiento

rotating the neck	girando el cuello
raising the shoulders	alzando los hombros
making a fist	cerrando el puño
stretching the calves and arms	estirando las pantorrillas y los brazos
rotating the ankles	girando los tobillos
breathing deeply	respirando profundamente

Common Exercises and Sports

Ejercicios y deportes comunes

neck stretches	estiramiento del cuello
arm stretches	estiramiento de los brazos
arm circles	rotación de los brazos
rise on your toes	pararse de puntillas
waist bends	doblamiento de la cintura
weight lifting	levantamiento de pesas
bicycling	ciclismo
jogging	correr rítmicamente
swimming	natación
walking	caminar o andar
brisk walking	caminata rápida

Taking Care of Your Back

El cuidado de la espalda

Maintain a good posture.	Mantenga una postura correcta.
When lifting, allow the legs to do the work.	Cuando levante algún peso, deje que las piernas hagan el esfuerzo.
Bend your knees, not your back.	Doble las rodillas, no la espalda.
Don't stand or sit in the same position for long periods of time.	No mantenga la misma posición, sentado-a o parado-a, por largo tiempo.
Sleep on your side with legs pulled in towards the chest.	Duerma sobre el costado con las piernas dobladas hacia el pecho.
Watch your weight.	Mantenga un buen peso.
Talk to your doctor about a good exercise program for you.	Consulte a su médico sobre un programa de ejercicios que sea adecuado para usted.

Calories Burned per hour / Calorías que se queman por hora

Exercise	Ejercicio	Burnt Calories per Hour / Calorías que se queman por hora
aerobics	aeróbica, aerobic	360-480
bicycling	ciclismo	410
jogging	correr	650-700
swimming	nadar	275-500
walking	caminar	300-440
weight lifting	levantar peso	480

NUTRITION / NUTRICIÓN

USDA PYRAMID WITH FOOD GROUPS AND PROPORTIONS / USDA PIRÁMIDE DE GRUPOS ALIMENTICIOS Y RACIONES DIARIAS[1]

Food Guide Pyramid
A Guide to Daily Food Choices

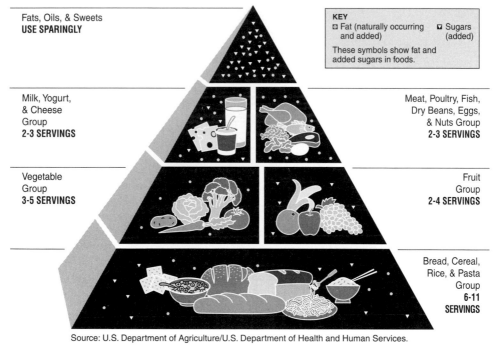

Fats, Oils, & Sweets
USE SPARINGLY

KEY
▫ Fat (naturally occurring   ▪ Sugars
  and added)   (added)
These symbols show fat and
added sugars in foods.

Milk, Yogurt,
& Cheese
Group
2-3 SERVINGS

Meat, Poultry, Fish,
Dry Beans, Eggs,
& Nuts Group
2-3 SERVINGS

Vegetable
Group
3-5 SERVINGS

Fruit
Group
2-4 SERVINGS

Bread, Cereal,
Rice, & Pasta
Group
**6-11
SERVINGS**

Source: U.S. Department of Agriculture/U.S. Department of Health and Human Services.

Note: Many of the serving sizes given above are smaller than those on the Nutrition Facts Label.
For example, 1 serving of cooked cereal, rice, or pasta is 1 cup for the label but only ½ cup for the Pyramid.

[1]The pyramid created by the U.S. Department of Agriculture (USDA) has served as a model for a good healthy diet. It is divided
  into six groups, each of which indicates the recommended portions of that food to be eaten daily.

La Guía Pirámide de Alimentos
Una Guía Para la Selección Diaria de Alimentos

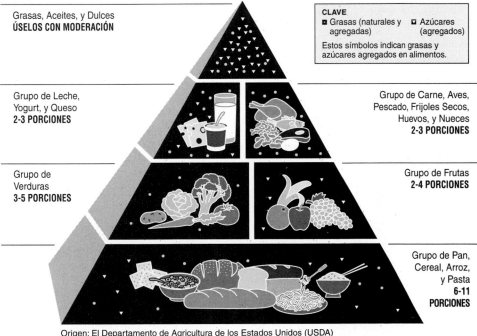

Grasas, Aceites, y Dulces
ÚSELOS CON MODERACIÓN

CLAVE
◪ Grasas (naturales y   ◪ Azúcares
   agregadas)   (agregados)

Estos símbolos indican grasas y
azúcares agregados en alimentos.

Grupo de Leche,
Yogurt, y Queso
2-3 PORCIONES

Grupo de Carne, Aves,
Pescado, Frijoles Secos,
Huevos, y Nueces
2-3 PORCIONES

Grupo de
Verduras
3-5 PORCIONES

Grupo de Frutas
2-4 PORCIONES

Grupo de Pan,
Cereal, Arroz,
y Pasta
**6-11
PORCIONES**

Origen: El Departamento de Agricultura de los Estados Unidos (USDA)
y el Departamento de Salud y Servicios Humanos (DHHS), agosto de 1992

[1]La Pirámide creada por el Departamento de Agricultura de los Estados Unidos (USDA) ha servido de modelo para seguir una dieta buena y saludable. Se divide en seis grupos, cada uno de los cuales indica las porciones diarias que se deben comer de dicho alimento.

GROUPS	GRUPOS	SERVINGS PER DAY / RACIONES POR DÍA
1. fats, oils, sweets	grasas, aceites, dulces	Use sparingly / uso moderado
2. milk, yogurt, and cheese	leche, yogurt y queso	2 – 3
3. meat, poultry, fish, dry beans, eggs, and nuts	carne, aves, pescado, frijoles secos, y nueces	2 – 3
4. vegetables	vegetales	3 – 5
5. fruits	frutas	2 – 3
6. breads, cereal, rice, pasta	pan, arroz, cereal, pasta	6 – 11

FOOD DISTRIBUTION / DISTRIBUCIÓN DE ALIMENTOS

1. **Fats, Oils, and Sweets** Grasas, Aceites, y Dulces	use sparingly uso moderado	restriction in the consumed amount restricción en la cantidad consumida
2. **Milk, Yogurt, and Cheese** Leche, Yogurt y Queso	1 cup of milk or yogurt 1 ½ oz. of natural cheese 2 oz. of processed cheese	1 taza de leche o yogurt 1 ½ oz. de queso natural 2 oz. de queso procesado
3. **Meat, Poultry, Fish, Dry Beans, Eggs, and Nuts** Carne, aves, pescado, frijoles secos, huevos, y cacahuate (maní)	2 or 3 oz. cooked lean meat, poultry, or fish 1 oz. meat = 1 egg or ½ cup of dry beans or 2 Tsp. of peanut butter, or 1/3 cup nuts = 1 oz. of meat	2 o 3 oz. de carne desgrasada, aves o pescado cocinados, 1 huevo = 1 oz. de carne ó ½ taza de frijoles secos ó 3 cucharadas de mantequilla de cacahuate, ó 1/3 taza de nueces
4. **Vegetables** Vegetales	1 cup raw leafy vegetables or a cup of chopped cooked vegetables or chopped raw vegetables	una taza de vegetales de hoja ó una taza de vegetales de hortaliza crudos o cocinados
5. **Fruit** Fruta	1 medium apple, banana, orange or, ½ cup of chopped, cooked or canned fruit	¾ taza de zumo o jugo de fruta, media manzana, ½ taza de fruta, picada, cocinada, o de lata
6. **Bread, Cereal, Rice, and Pasta** Pan, cereal, arroz, y pasta	1 slice of bread ½ cup of cooked cereal, rice, or pasta 1 cup of ready to eat cereal	1 rebanada de pan ½ taza de cereal, arroz, o pasta preparados 1 taza de cereal

VITAMINS AND MINERALS–SOURCES / VITAMINAS Y MINERALES–FUENTES

Vitamin A: fish, liver, egg yolk, butter, yellow fruits

Vitamina A: pescado, hígado, yema de huevo, mantequilla, frutas amarillas

Vitamin D: fish liver oils, liver, egg yolk, butter

Vitamina D: aceite de hígado de pescado, yema de huevo, mantequilla

Vitamin E: vegetable oil, wheat germ, leafy vegetables, margarine, egg yolk, legumes

Vitamina E: aceite vegetal, hojas de vegetales, margarina, yema de huevo, legumbres

Vitamin K, K_1, K_2: pork, liver, vegetable oils

Vitamina K, K_1, K_2: cerdo, hígado, aceites vegetales

Vitamin B_6 group: spinach, organ meats, fish, legumes, whole-grain cereals, sweet potatoes, avocado

Grupo de B_6: espinaca, carne de órganos, pescado, cereales de grano, legumbres, boniato, aguacate

Vitamin B_{12}: liver, meats, egg yolk, milk and dairy products

Vitamina B_{12}: hígado, carnes, yema de huevo, leche y derivados

Vitamin C (ascorbic acid): citric fruits, tomatoes, green peppers, cabbage

Vitamina C (ácido ascórbico): frutas cítricas, tomate, ají verde, repollo

Fatty Acids: vegetable oils (sunflower, corn, canola), margarine

Acidos grasos: aceites vegetales (de maíz, girasol, canola), margarina

Folic Acid: fresh green vegetables, fruits, gizzards, kidneys, liver

Ácido Fólico: vegetales frescos, frutas, molleja de ave, hígado, riñones

Biotin: legumes, liver, nuts, cauliflower, egg yolk

Biotina: legumbres, hígado, nueces, repollo, yema de huevo

Niacin (niacinamide, nicotinic acid): dried yeast, liver, meat, fish, legumes, whole grain cereal

Niacina (niacinamida, ácido nicotínico): levadura en polvo, hígado, legumbres, cereales de grano

Thiamine (vitamin B_1): potatoes, legumes, pork, liver, enriched cereals

Tiamina (vitamina B_1): papas, legumbres, cerdo, hígado, cereales enriquecidos

Riboflavin (Vitamin B_2): milk, cheese, liver, eggs, enriched cereals

Riboflavina (vitamina B_2): leche, quesos, huevos, cereales enriquecidos

Potassium: bananas, apricots, peaches, prunes, raisins, milk

Potasio: plátanos, albaricoque, durazno (melocotón), ciruelas pasas, pasas, leche

Calcium: milk, milk products, meat, fish, eggs, beans, fruits, vegetables

Calcio: leche y sus derivados, carnes, pescado, huevos, frijoles, vegetales, frutas

Copper: liver, shellfish, whole grains, nuts, poultry

Cobre: mariscos, hígado, granos enteros, carne de ave

Magnesium: dark green vegetables, dairy products, nuts, meat, whole grain cereals

Magnesio: vegetales de color verde oscuro, productos lácteos, nueces, carne, cereales de granos enteros

Phosphorus: dairy products, meat, fish, poultry, legumes, grains, nuts

Fósforo: productos lácteos, carne, pescado, carne de ave, legumbres, granos enteros, nueces

Iron: Meats, spinach, radishes

Hierro: Carnes, espinaca, rábanos

Sodium: Beef, pork, cheese, olives, sauerkraut

Sodio: carne de res, cerdo, queso, aceitunas, col agria

Zinc: dairy products, liver, wheat bran, shellfish

Zinc: productos lácteos, salvado, mariscos

WHY VITAMINS ARE ESSENTIAL?	¿POR QUÉ SON ESENCIALES LAS VITAMINAS?
Vitamin A: helps to have good vision, healthy hair, skin and nails; fights infection	**Vitamina A:** ayuda a tener buena visión, pelo, piel y uñas saludables; combate infecciones
Vitamin D: calcium absorbent, helps to maintain healthy bones and teeth	**Vitamina D:** absorbente del calcio, ayuda a mantener los huesos y dientes.
Vitamin E: important in the formation of red blood cells, building tissues, and muscle development	**Vitamina E:** importante en la formación de glóbulos rojos y en el desarrollo de los tejidos y en el desarrollo muscular
Vitamin K, K_1, K_2: intervene in the formation of prothrombin and other coagulation factors	**Vitamina K, K_1, K_2:** intervienen en la formación de protrombina y otros factores de coagulación
Vitamin B_6 group: of great importance in the metabolism and absorption of proteins	**Grupo de B_6:** de gran importancia en el metabolismo y en la absorción de las proteínas
Vitamin B_{12}: effective in pernicious anemia, aids in formation of genetic materials (DNA and RNA)	**Vitamina B_{12}:** efectiva en la anemia perniciosa, ayuda a la formación de materiales genéticos (DNA y RNA)
Vitamin C (ascorbic acid): aids in the formation of collagen, helps prevent infection and bleeding of the gums	**Vitamina C (ácido ascórbico):** ayuda a la formación de colágeno, ayuda a prevenir infecciones y sangramiento de las encías
Fatty Acid: precursors of prostaglandins, builders of many lipids	**Ácidos Grasos:** precursores de prostaglandinces, constructores de varios lípidos
Folic Acid: maturation of RBCs, helpful to prevent anemia, intervenes in the formation of genetic material	**Ácido Fólico:** maturación de RBCs, ayuda a prevenir la anemia, necesario en la formación de elementos genéticos
Biotin: aids in body growth, amino acid and fatty acid metabolism	**Biotina:** ayuda al crecimiento, metabolismo de ácidos aminos y ácidos grasos
Niacin (niacinamide, nicotinic acid): helps in carbohydrates metabolism	**Niacina (niacinamida, ácido nicotínico):** ayuda en el metabolismo de carbohidratos
Thiamine (vitamin B_1): aids in peripheral and central nerve cell functions, and in metabolizing carbohydrates into energy	**Tiamina (vitamina B_1):** esencial en la funciones de las células nerviosas y periféricas, y en el metabolismo de carbohidratos
Riboflavin (Vitamin B_2): aids to metabolize carbohydrates, proteins and fats	**Riboflavina (vitamina B_2):** ayuda a metabolizar carbohidratos, proteínas y grasas
Potassium: necessary to keep acid-base balance, muscle activity, water retention	**Potasio:** necesario al balance ácido-básico, a la actividad muscular, en la retención de agua
Calcium: blood coagulation, bone and teeth formation, transmission of nerve impulses	**Calcio:** coagulación de la sangre, formación de dientes y huesos, transmisión de impulsos nerviosos
Copper: necessary in the synthesis of hemoglobin, component of digestive enzymes	**Cobre:** necesario en la síntesis de hemoglobina, componente de enzimas digestivas
Magnesium: aids to synthesize protein, formation of bones and teeth	**Magnesio:** ayuda en la síntesis de las proteínas, formación de huesos y dientes
Phosphorus: aids metabolize calcium, protein and glucose, formation of bones and teeth	**Fósforo:** ayuda a metabolizar el calcio, las proteínas y la glucosa; esencial en la formación de huesos y dientes
Sodium: acid-base balance, blood pH, muscle activity	**Sodio:** balance ácido básico, actividad muscular, pH sanguíneo
Iron: Needed to maintain the correct level of hemoglobin in the blood	**Hierro:** Necesario para mantener el nivel correcto de hemoglobina en la sangre
Zinc: It aids metabolism of proteins	**Zinc:** ayuda en el metabolismo de las proteínas

WATER VALUES

► Contains important minerals

► Acts as a regulator of body temperature

► Plays an important roll in digestion

► It is a major component of plasma

► It is a provider of nutrients to the cells

► Works as a helper to empty body waste

It comprises about two thirds of the human body

VALORES DEL AGUA

► Contiene minerales importantes

► Actúa como reguladora de la temperatura corporal

► Desempeña un papel importante en la digestión

► Es un componente principal del plasma

► Provee de nutrientes a las células

► Trabaja como ayudante en vaciar el gasto corporal

Comprende cerca de las dos terceras partes del cuerpo humano

Methods of Food Preparation / Métodos de preparación

baked	asado, horneado
boiled	hervido
broiled	asado a la parrilla
canned	enlatado, en conserva
cooked; well done	cocinado; bien cocinado
cut	cortado, tajado
defrosted	descongelado
drained	secado; colado
enriched	enriquecido; aumentado con
fried	frito
grilled	a la brasa
homogenized	homogeneizada
pasteurized	pasteurizada
peeled	pelado; (*naranja*) mondada
pickle	en encurtido, escabeche
raw	crudo; sin cocinar; (*fruta*) verde
salted	salado
scraped	raspado
skimmed	descremada
sliced	en rebanadas, en tajadas
steamed	cocinado al vapor
stewed	guisado, estofado
sweeten	endulzado, azucarado
unpeeled	sin pelar
unsalted	sin sal
unsweetened	sin azúcar
well done	bien hecho, bien cocinado

FOOD ADDITIVES	ADITIVOS A LOS ALIMENTOS	FOOD PROCESSING	PROCESAMIENTO DE ALIMENTOS
allergens	alérgenos	baking	asado, horneo
chemicals	sustancias químicas	blanching	blanqueado
color	color	canning	enlatado
contaminants from natural sources	contaminantes de fuentes naturales	dehydration	dehidratación
minerals	minerales	freezing	congelación
natural toxins	toxinas naturales	homogenization	homogeneización
nutrients	sustancias nutritivas	pasteurization	pasteurización
preservatives	preservativos	refining	refinando
toxicants	tóxicos producidos en la elaboración		

NUTRITION VOCABULARY

FOODS FRUITS, VEGETABLES, MEATS, BREADS, AND BEVERAGE		ALIMENTOS FRUTAS, VEGETALES, CARNES, PANES Y BEBIDAS	
FRUITS		**FRUTAS**	
Fruits are rich in potassium, carbohydrates, fiber, and vitamins A and C.		Las frutas son ricas en potasio, carbohidratos, fibra y vitaminas A y C.	
VEGETABLES	**VEGETALES**	**FRUITS**	**FRUTAS**
asparagus	espárrago	avocado	aguacate
basil	mejorana	apple	manzana
bean	frijol; S.A. habichuela	apricot	albaricoque
beets	remolacha, betabel	banana	plátano
brussel sprouts	colecita de Bruselas	blueberry	mora azul
broccoli	brocol	blackberry	zarzamora
cabbage	repollo	cantaloupe	cantalúp /melón
capers	alcaparras	coconut	coco
carrot	zanahoria	cranberry	arándano
cauliflower	coliflor	cherry	cereza
celery	apio	date	dátil
coriander	cilantro	fig	higo
cumin	comino	grape	uva
corn	maíz, elote	guava	guayaba
cucumber	pepino	grapefruit	toronja
eggplant	berenjena	lemon	limón

FOODS		ALIMENTOS	
FRUITS, VEGETABLES, MEATS, BREADS, AND BEVERAGE		*FRUTAS, VEGETALES, CARNES, PANES, Y BEBIDAS*	
VEGETABLES	**VEGETALES**	**FRUITS**	**FRUTAS**
endive	escarola, endivia	mango	mango
fennel	hinojo	melon	(verde) sandía
garlic	ajo	nectarine	nectarina
ginger	gengibre	orange	naranja
green bean	habichuela	papaya	papaya
kale	col rizada	peach	melocotón, durazno
leek	puerro	pear	pera
lentil	lenteja	pineapple	piña
lettuce	lechuga	plum	ciruela
mushrooms	hongos, champiñones	prune	ciruela pasa
olives	aceitunas	raisins	pasas
onions	cebollas	raspberry	frambuesa
parsley	perejil	strawberry	fresa
peas	guisantes, arvejas	tangerine	mandarina
potato	papas, patatas	watermelon	melón de agua
rice	arroz		
rosemary	romero		
spinach	espinaca		
squash	calabaza		
sweet potato	camote, boniato		
tomato	tomate		
yam	batata, boniato		
watercress	berro		

BEEF	RES	SHELLFISH	MARISCOS, FRUTAS DE MAR
chicken, hen	pollo, gallina	clams	almejas, mejillones
lamb	carnero	crab	cangrejo
pork	cerdo, puerco	lobster	langosta
fish	pescado	oysters	ostras
turkey	pavo	shrimp	camarón
duck	pato	scallops	venera
goat	cabra	squid	calamar

BREADS – CEREALS	PANES – CEREALES	MILK PRODUCTS	PRODUCTOS LÁCTEOS
barley	cebada	butter	mantequilla
buttermilk bread	pan de suero	cheese	queso
egg bread	pan de huevo	condensed milk	leche condensada
cookies	galleticas	cottage cheese	requesón
cheese bread	pan de queso	cream	crema
oat bran	salvado de avena	evaporated milk	leche evaporada
rolls	panecitos	goat cheese	queso de cabra
sweet rolls	panecitos dulces	goat milk	leche de cabra
corn bread	pan de maíz	ice cream	helado
potato bread	pan de papas	lactaid	leche sin lactosa
crackers	galletas	margarine	margarina
French bread	pan francés	skim milk	leche desnatada
tortillas	tortillas	yogurt	yogur
white bread	pan blanco		
whole-grain bread	pan de grano entero		
whole-wheat toast	pan de trigo, pan negro		

BEVERAGES	BEBIDAS	BEVERAGES	BEBIDAS
beer	cerveza	water (mineral)	agua mineral
bouillon	caldo	water (spring)	agua de manantial
broth	caldo	wine	vino
carbonated drinks	sodas	white wine	vino blanco
chocolate	chocolate	red wine	vino tinto
coffee	café	juice	jugo, zumo
consomme	consomé	apple juice	zumo de manzana
fruit juices	jugos de fruta	prune juice	jugo de ciruelas
gelatin	gelatina		
ice	hielo		
lemonade	limonada		
milk	leche		
condensed milk	leche condensada		
evaporated milk	leche evaporada		
skim milk	leche descremada		
sherbet	sherbet		
tea; herbal tea	té negro; té de hierbas, infusión		
thirst-quencher beverages	bebidas que matan la sed		

THERAPEUTIC DIETS	DIETAS TERAPÉUTICAS	FOOD QUALITIES	CUALIDADES DE LOS ALIMENTOS
balanced	balanceada	acid	ácido
bland	blanda	bitter	amargo
carbohydrate-free	libre de carbohidratos	bloody	algo crudo, con sangre
cholesterol free	libre de colesterol	cold	frío
dried	limitada en líquido	dry	seco, escurrido
diabetic	diabética	enough	suficiente
fat free	libre de grasa	healthy	saludable
gluten-free	libre de gluten	spoiled	dañado, contaminado
high-calorie	rica en calorías	fresh	fresco
high-fiber	alta en fibra	frozen	congelado
high-potency	con vitaminas	ground	molido
liquid	líquida	highly priced	muy caro
low calorie	baja en calorías	light	ligero
low carbohydrate	baja en carbohidratos	nutritious	nutritivo
low salt	baja en sal	liquified	licuado
mashed	en puré	kneeded	amasado
macrobiotic	macrobiótica	mashed	en puré; machacado
sodium-restricted	limitada en sodio (sal)		
soft	semisólida		
weight reduction	de reducción de peso		
with proteins	con proteínas		

Note: Adjectives ending in -o form the feminine by dropping the -o and adding -a.

FAT	
fatty acids	ácidos lípidos
unsaturated fats	grasas no saturadas
saturated fats	grasas saturadas

Calculation of the % of Fat in Foods	**Cálculo del % de Grasa en los Alimentos**
fat grams $\times$ 9 (calories) = #	gramos de grasa $\times$ 9 (calorías) = #
# divided by 235 calories = % of fat	# dividido por 235 calorías = % de grasa

Negative Factors

▶ Saturated fats increase the danger of building up cholesterol in the artery walls

▶ Fat production of calories is more than double of that of protein or carbohydrates. If the production of calories is not consumed (i.e. exercise), body fat will be increased.

Factores Negativos

▶ Las grasas saturadas aumentan el peligro de almacenar colesterol en las paredes de las arterias.

▶ La producción de calorías de las grasas es más del doble que la producida por las proteínas o los carbohidratos. Si la producción de calorías no se consume (p.ej. ejercicios, trabajo activo) la grasa en el cuerpo aumenta.

Appendix D
•Medical Phrases
•Idiomatic Expressions
•Verb Tables

Apéndice D
•Frases médicas
•Expresiones idiomáticas
•Tablas de verbos

IDIOMATIC EXPRESSIONS AND USEFUL PHRASES / EXPRESIONES IDIOMÁTICAS Y FRASES ÚTILES

ENGLISH	*SPANISH*
a close relative	un pariente cercano
a long time	mucho tiempo
a long time ago	hace mucho tiempo
above all	sobre todo
according to	de acuerdo con
after meals	después de las comidas
again	otra vez
all at once	de una vez
all over the body	por todo el cuerpo
anyone else	alguien más
anything else	algo más
as a matter of fact	en realidad, de hecho
as early as possible	lo más temprano posible
as much as	tanto como
as often as necessary	tan a menudo como sea necesario
as soon as possible	tan pronto como sea posible
as well as	lo mejor posible, tan bien como
at any rate	en cualquier caso
at bedtime	a la hora de acostarse
at first sight	a primera vista
at least	por lo menos
at the earliest	lo más temprano
at the latest	a más tardar
at the same time	a la vez
at night	de noche, por la noche
at once	en seguida, ahora mismo
birth certificate	partida o certificado de nacimiento
can I have?	¿puedo tener?
can you show me?	¿me puede enseñar, mostrar?
classified information	información confidencial o secreta
come back in a week	regrese en una semana
complete this questionnaire	responda a este cuestionario

ENGLISH	SPANISH
cost effectiveness	rentabilidad
day off	día libre
deep freezing	ultracongelación
do you know where you are?	¿sabe dónde está?
don't be afraid	no tenga miedo
don't hurry	no se apure
don't worry	no se preocupe
each day	cada día
each time	cada vez
ease one's mind	tranquilizarse
every day	todos los días, cada día
every other day	un día sí y un día no, un día de por medio
every two hours	cada dos horas
everything is going fine	todo va bien
far away	lejos, distante
far cry	gran diferencia
fill out this form	llene esta planilla
from bad to worse	de mal en peor
from now on	de aquí en adelante
full name	nombre y apellido
get off from work	ausentarse del trabajo
get out	váyase
get up, please	levántese, por favor
getting old	envejeciendo
go on	siga
hardly ever	casi nunca
hourly	a cada hora
how often?	¿cuán a menudo?
how old are you?	¿cuántos años tiene?
I am sorry	lo siento
I like it	me gusta
in a short time	en breve
in effect	en efecto, en realidad
in order to, in order that	para que

Idiomatic Expressions and Useful Phrases / Expresiones idiomáticas y frases útiles

ENGLISH	SPANISH
instead of	en vez de
it can't be helped	no tiene remedio
it is convenient	es conveniente
it is difficult for him/her	le resulta difícil, le cuesta trabajo
it is important	es importante
it is necessary	es necesario
it is difficult for him, her	le cuesta trabajo
it is possible	es posible
jet-lag	desajuste de horario
just now	ahora mismo, en este momento
later on	más tarde, después
last night	anoche
may I come in?	¿puedo entrar?
may I see you?	¿puedo verlo-a?
my name is	me llamo
never mind	no importa
next of kin	parientes cercanos
not as much as before	no tanto como antes
of course	por supuesto, claro, desde luego
on account of	debido a, a causa de
on and off	a intervalos; a veces sí, a veces no
on edge	irritable, impaciente, nervioso-a
on foot	a pie
on the contrary	al contrario
on the other hand	por otro lado
on time	a tiempo
once	una vez
once in a while	de vez en cuando
one must	uno debe, se debe
otherwise	de lo contrario
participant assent form	forma de asentimiento del (de la) participante
perhaps	quizás, tal vez
presence of mind	presencia de ánimo
right away	en seguida

ENGLISH	SPANISH
sanitary facilities	instalaciones sanitarias
shake the bottle	agíte la botella
so far	hasta ahora, hasta aquí
sometimes	a veces
stand up, please	párese, por favor
the other one	el otro, la otra
the whole day	todo el día
there is, there are	hay
things are not going well	las cosas no van bien
to agree	estar de acuerdo
to ask a question	hacer una pregunta
to be against	oponerse
to be aware of	darse cuenta de, estar al tanto, tener conocimiento de
to be calm	calmarse
to be careful	tener cuidado
to be cold	tener frío
to be hot, warm	tener calor
to be hungry, thirsty, sleepy	tener hambre, sed, sueño
to be in a jam	estar en un aprieto
to be in good hands	estar en buenas manos
to be in the habit of	tener la costumbre de
to be on the go	estar activo-a
to be out of breath	faltar el aliento
to be patient	tener paciencia
to be ready	estar listo
to be relieved	aliviarse, sentirse mejor
to be right	tener razón
to be unaware of	no tener conocimiento de
to be (20, 30, 40) years old	tener (20, 30, 40) años de edad
to bear in mind	tener en cuenta
to break the news	dar la noticia
to breast-feed	dar el pecho, dar de mamar
to carry out	llevar a cabo
to conduct an interview	hacer una entrevista

ENGLISH	SPANISH
to do one's best	hacer lo mejor posible
to feel like	tener ganas de
to feel sorry for	compadecerse de
to gargle	hacer gárgaras
to give birth	dar a luz
to go away	irse
to harm	hacer daño
to hold one's breath	aguantar la respiración
to hurry	darse prisa
to kick the habit	*(drugs)* dejar la adicción, curarse
to kill time	pasar el tiempo
to make a fist	cerrar el puño
to move about, around	caminar, andar, dar una vuelta (caminando)
to move away	irse, trasladarse, mudarse
to pay attention	prestar atención
to put in	poner dentro de, meter en
to put off	aplazar, posponer
to put on	*(clothes)* vestirse
to put out	*(light or fire)* apagar
to save time	ahorrar tiempo
to shake hands	dar la mano
to the best of my knowledge	a mi entender
to this effect	en ese sentido
too much	demasiado
turn over	voltéese, dé la vuelta
(two, three, four) times (a day, week, month)	(dos, tres, cuatro) veces (al día, a la semana, al mes)
(two, three) out of (twenty, a hundred)	(dos, tres) de cada (veinte, cien)
unless	a menos que
you need to	necesita, tiene que
what is happening?	¿qué sucede? ¿qué pasa?
what is the matter?	¿qué pasa, qué ocurre?
what is your name?	¿cómo se llama?
what time is it?	¿qué hora es?
whatever is necessary	lo que sea necesario

ENGLISH	SPANISH
where am I?	¿dónde estoy?
with the naked eye	a simple vista
within reach	al alcance
who is next?	¿quién es el (la) próximo-a?
youthful appearance	apariencia juvenil

MEDICAL PHRASES / FRASES MÉDICAS

access to medical records	acceso al expediente médico
acquired immunity	inmunidad adquirida
admission and discharge date	fecha de ingreso y fecha de alta del hospital
admitting diagnosis	diagnóstico de ingreso
age of consent	mayor de edad
alcohol-related brain damage	incapacidad cerebral por consumo de alcohol, incapacidad cerebral debida a alcoholismo
ambulatory care	cuidado ambulatorio
amniotic fluid embolism	embolia amniótica
aqueous shunting device	mecanismo acuoso de desviación
attending physician	médico de cabecera
average duration of hospitalization	promedio de estancia en el hospital, tiempo promedio de hospitalización
bladder examination, cytoscopy	citoscopía
blind study	estudio con anonimato
blood-air barrier	barrera alveocapilar
blood bank	banco de sangre
blood clot	coágulo de sangre
blood count	hemograma
blood culture	hemocultivo
blood donor	donante de sangre
blood transfusion	transfusión de sangre
calcium channel blocker	antagonista del calcio
cardiac depressants	agentes antiarrítmicos
care unit	unidad de cuidado
case-control study	estudio de casos y testigos
casualty	víctima de un accidente
chemotherapeutic agents	antineoplásticos

ENGLISH	SPANISH
chronic illness	enfermedad crónica
collapse of the lung	atelectasia pulmonar
congestive heart failure	colapso o fallo cardíaco
control group	grupo de referencia
cough drops	pastillas para la tos
current medications	medicamentos actuales
custodial parent	progenitor o guardián de los hijos
day on leave	día de salida con permiso de ausencia
day of admission	día de ingreso
decreased sperm count	descuento en el esperma
deteriorating eyesight	visión en proceso de deteriorización
diet-related disease	enfermedad relacionada con la dieta
differential blood count	fórmula leucocítica
dimmed vision	visión disminuida
discharge abstract or summary	informe de alta
discharge date	fecha de alta hospitalaria
discharge form	planilla de alta hospitalaria
discharged and sent to another hospital	dado de alta y transferido a otro hospial
discharged and sent home	dado de alta y enviado a su casa
disease-free area	zona indemne
distended bladder	distensión vesical
doctor on call	médico de guardia
dosage interval	intervalo de administración de la dosis
elderly	de edad avanzada
electroshock therapy	terapia electroconvulsiva
electrolyte balance	equilibrio hidroelectrolítico
electrosurgical knife	bisturí eléctrico
emergency center ward	centro de emergencia
entrapment neuropathy	neuropatía compresiva
entry wound	orificio de entrada de un proyectil
epileptic seizure	ataque epiléptico
essential hypertension	hipertensión (arterial) idiopática
estrogen replacement therapy	terapia de reemplazo de estrógeno

ENGLISH	SPANISH
evaluation of a disorder	evaluación de un trastorno
expected date of delivery	fecha prevista del parto
exudating wounds	heridas con supuraciones
feeding tube	tubo de alimentación
fetal movement (quickening)	movimiento fetal (animación)
fever blisters	herpes labial
film-coated tablet	comprimido recubierto
fluid balance chart	hoja de balance hídrico
fluid depletion	deshidratación
follow-up appointment	turno de seguimiento
food additives	aditivos alimenticios
fresh fracture	fractura reciente
full blood count	hemograma completo
gastrointestinal bleeding	hemorragia digestiva
gastrointestinal disorders	trastornos digestivos
general condition	estado general
generic name	nombre genérico
genital area	zona inguinal
gestational psychosis	psicosis gravídica
gonadotropin	gonadoliberina
gonadotropin	gonadotropina
gray or grey matter	sustancia gris
gross exam	examen macroscópico
gross findings	resultados del examen macroscópico
gross pathology	anatomía patológica macroscópica
guarded condition	estado de gravedad
health certificate	certificado de salud
health care	atención a la salud
health food	comida saludable
health services	servicios de salud
health services for the aged	cuidado de la salud de los ancianos
heart rate	frecuencia cardíaca
heavy smoker	fumador empedernido
high calorie diet	dieta hipercalórica

ENGLISH	SPANISH
high resolution imaging	imagen de alta resolución
high risk	alto riesgo
home health	cuidado de la salud en el hogar
homologous insemination	inseminación artificial, con semen del marido
host cells	células anfitrionas
immune response	respuesta o reacción inmune
impaired lung function	función pulmonar disminuida
impaired short memory	memoria inmediata impedida
impaired thought processes	proceso cognitivo dañado
impaired vision	vista defectuosa
in urgent need of treatment	urgente necesidad de recibir tratamiento
inapparent infection	infección asintomática
independent group	grupo independiente
industrial disease	enfermedad profesional laboral
infirmities of old age	achaques de la vejez, achaques de la edad
influenza-like syndrome	síndrome seudogripal
initial bleeding	hematuria inicial
inpatient accommodations	facilidades del paciente hospitalizado
inpatient discharge	alta del paciente hospitalizado
intestinal malabsorption	hipoabsorción intestinal
intracranial pressure monitoring	monitoreo de presión intracraneal
invasive devices	dispositivos invasores
isolation ward	sala de aislamiento
joint motion	movilidad articular
joint pain	dolor en las coyunturas
kidney stone	cálculo renal
killed vaccine	vacuna inactivada
killer cell	linfocito citolítico
labyrinthine concussion	conmoción laberíntica
laboratory findings	datos analíticos del laboratorio
language skills	habilidad lingüística
left-sided chest pain	dolor precordial
legal rights	derechos legales
length of stay in hospital	tiempo de hospitalización

ENGLISH	SPANISH
life expentancy	esperanza de vida; expictativa de vida
light wound	herida leve
living related donor transplantation	trasplante de un órgano de un pariente vivo
logic ability	capacidad para aplicar la lógica
long term care facility	institución de atención médica a largo plazo
low blood pressure	hipotensión arterial
low-grade lymphoma	linfoma de escasa malignidad
low-grade tumor	tumor bien diferenciado
lymphatic spread	diseminación por vía linfática
mass hysteria	histeria colectiva
memory assessment	evaluación de la memoria
mental disorders	trastornos psíquicos
mental impediment	impedimento mental
metabolic defect or error	trastorno o alteración metabólica
metabolic disturbances	trastornos metabólicos
minor illness	enfermedad leve benigna
missed abortion	aborto retenido, retención fetal
mottled skin	piel veteada
narrowing of joint space	pinzamiento del espacio articular
negative feedback	retroinhibición
noninvasive diagnostic tool	instrumento diagnóstico no-invasivo
normal disease progression	evolución natural o espontánea de una enfermedad
normal skin markings	pliegues naturales de la piel
nurse in charge	enfermero-a jefe, jefe de sala
onset of labor	comienzo del parto
operating surgeon	cirujano a cargo de la operación
osteoporosis of disuse	osteoporosis por inactividad
outpatient	paciente externo
outpatient clinic	clínica para pacientes externos
over the counter medication	medicamento de venta sin receta
overt hyperglycemia	hiperglucemia franca
oxygen tent	cámara de oxígeno
packed cells	concentrado de eritrocitos
participant assent form	forma de asentimiento del participante

ENGLISH	SPANISH
patient in need of urgent treatment	paciente con necesidad de atención urgente
patient's care	cuidado del/de la paciente[20]
patient's discharge	alta del/de la paciente
patient's record	expediente del/de la paciente
patient's rights	derechos del/de la paciente
pericardial effusion	derrame pericardíaco
physical assessment	evaluación física
physical changes	cambios físicos
plain film	radiografía simple
positive feedback	retroactivación
primary adhesion	cicatrización por primera intención
primary diagnosis	diagnosis principal
primary lesion	lesión elemental
prolapsed disc	hernia de disco, hernia discal
protein requirements	necesidades proteínicas
public health	salud pública
public health facilities	instituciones de salud pública
recovery room	sala de recuperación
referred to another provider	referido a otro proveedor
rehabilitation center	centro de rehabilitación
right to receive treatment	derecho a recibir tratamiento
root curettage	raspado radicular
rough murmur	soplo rudo áspero
sexual arousal	excitación sexual
shallow breath	respiración poco profunda
short of breath	falto de aire
short term memory impairment	memoria inmediata impedida
shoulder or thoracic girdle	cintura escapular
signs and symptoms	signos y síntomas
silent bleeding	hemorragia oculta
single all-purpose vaccine	vacuna única polivalente
sore throat	dolor de garganta
speech defect	defecto en el habla
spinal cord transection	transección medular completa

ENGLISH	SPANISH
stellate ganglion	ganglio estrellado
state of mind	estado de ánimo
stuffy nose	nariz tupida
support group	grupo de apoyo
surgical procedure	procedimiento quirúrgico
target group	grupo elegido como objetivo
telephone follow-up	seguimiento por teléfono
temperature range	variación de la temperatura
test run	serie analítica
testamentary capacity	capacidad testamentaria
therapeutic services	servicios terapéuticos
tightness of the chest	opresión en el pecho
to discharge	dar de alta
to leave against medical advice	salir sin consentimiento médico
to lose consciousness	perder el conocimiento
to pass a stone	eliminar un cálculo a través de la orina
to pass out	desmayarse, desvanecerse
to refuse treatment	rehusar tratamiento
to remain in bed	guardar cama, permanecer en cama
to worsen	agravarse, empeorar
traffic accident	accidente de tráfico
treatment and monitoring of wound	tratamiento y monitoreo de la herida
triggering point	punto de desencadenamiento
under age	menor de edad
undescended testicle	testículo no descendido
upper gastrointestinal bleeding	hemorragia digestiva alta
unpredictable behaviour	conducta incierta
unsatisfactory treatment	tratamiento sin resultado positivo
urgent care	tratamiento urgente
uterine curettage	raspado del útero, raspado de la matriz
vaginal examination	tacto vaginal
verbal simple ability	capacidad verbal limitada
visiting hours	horas de visita
vital signs	signos vitales

ENGLISH	SPANISH
voluntary admission	ingreso voluntario
water pollution	contaminación del agua
water bag	bolsa de agua
water bed	cama de colchón de agua
water soluble	soluble en agua
white matter	sustancia blanca
withdrawal symptoms	síntomas de abstinencia
X-ray film	radiografía o película radiográfica,

[20]The preposition **de** and the masculine definite article **el** contract when the preposition **de** precedes a masculine singular noun; this contraction does not occur when **de** precedes the feminine article.

PHRASES RELATED TO HEALTH INSURANCE POLICY CLAIMS / FRASES RELATIVAS A RECLAMOS DE PÓLIZAS DE SEGURO DE SALUD

ENGLISH	*SPANISH*
accumulation period	días deducibles de beneficio
allocated benefits	beneficios alocados
benefits coordination	coordinación de beneficios
cancellation of insurance	cancelación de la póliza
claim	reclamación de beneficios
copayment of not covered expenses	pago por la porción de servicios no cubiertos
deductible amount	cantidad deducible
disability insurance	seguro por incapacidad
exclusion of coverage	exclusión de cobertura
explanation of benefits	explicación de beneficios
grace period	tiempo de gracia
hospital insurance	póliza de hospitalización
indemnity policy	póliza de indemnización
insurance effective date	fecha de comienzo de la póliza
lapsed policy	póliza vencida
personal injury	delito de lesiones
policy limit	límite de la póliza
potential benefits	beneficios potenciales
premium	prima de la póliza
to pay by medical insurance	pago por seguro médico
work related accident	accidente de trabajo

REGULAR VERBS / VERBOS REGULARES

Simple Tenses

INFINITIVE	TOMAR	COMER	ADMITIR
	to take, to drink	to eat	to admit
-NDO FORM (GERUND)	tomando	comiendo	admitiendo
-DO FORM (PP.)	tomado	comido	admitido
INDICATIVE *PRESENT*	tomo	como	admito
	tomas	comes	admites
	toma	come	admite
	tomamos	comemos	admitimos
	tomáis	coméis	admitís
	toman	comen	admiten
PRETERIT	tomé	comí	admití
	tomaste	comiste	admitiste
	tomó	comió	admitió
	tomamos	comimos	admitimos
	tomasteis	comisteis	admitisteis
	tomaron	comieron	admitieron
IMPERFECT	tomaba	comía	admitía
	tomabas	comías	admitías
	tomaba	comía	admitía
	tomábamos	comíamos	admitíamos
	tomabais	comíais	admitíais
	tomaban	comían	admitían
FUTURE	tomaré	comeré	admitiré
	tomarás	comerás	admitirás
	tomará	comerá	admitirá
	tomaremos	comeremos	admitiremos
	tomaréis	comeréis	admitiréis
	tomarán	comerán	admitirán

CONDICIONAL	tomaría	comería	admitiría
	tomarías	comerías	admitirías
	tomaría	comería	admitiría
	tomaríamos	comeríamos	admitiríamos
	tomaríais	comeríais	admitiríais
	tomarían	comerían	admitirían

SUBJUNCTIVE PRESENT	tome	coma	admita
	tomes	comas	admitas
	tome	coma	admita
	tomemos	comamos	admitamos
	toméis	comáis	admitáis
	tomen	coman	admitan
IMPERFECT (-RA)	tomara	comiera	admitiera
	tomaras	comieras	admitieras
	tomara	comiera	admitiera
	tomáramos	comiéramos	admitiéramos
	tomarais	comierais	admitierais
	tomaran	comieran	admitieran
IMPERFECT (-SE)	tomase	comiese	admitiese
	tomases	comieses	admitieses
	tomase	comiese	admitiese
	tomásemos	comiésemos	admitiésemos
	tomaseis	comieseis	admitieseis
	tomasen	comiesen	admitiesen

Root-Vowel Changing Verbs

INFINITIVE	APRETAR	MOSTRAR	ENTENDER
	to squeeze	to show	to understand
-NDO FORM (GERUND)	apretando	mostrando	entendiendo
-DO FORM (PP.)	apretado	mostrado	entendido

Regular Verbs / Verbos regulares

INDICATIVE PRESENT			
	aprieto	muestro	entiendo
	aprietas	muestras	entiendes
	aprieta	muestra	entiende
	apretamos	mostramos	entendemos
	apretáis	mostráis	entendéis
	aprietan	muestran	entienden
SUBJUNCTIVE PRESENT			
	apriete	muestre	entienda
	aprietes	muestres	entiendas
	apriete	muestre	entienda
	apretemos	mostremos	entendamos
	apretéis	mostréis	entendáis
	aprieten	muestren	entiendan

Note: Use **apretar** as a model to conjugate: **cerrar** / to close: **comenzar** / to begin; **despertar** / to wake up; **empezar** / to begin; **pensar** / to think; **sentar** / to settle, to fit; **sentarse** / to sit down.
Other verbs like **mostrar** are: **acordar** / to agree; **acordarse** / to remember; **acostarse** / to lie down; **apostar** / to bet; **encontrar** / to find; **encontrarse** / to run across, to meet; **probar** / to test; to taste; **recordar** / to remember; **rogar** / to beg; **volar** / to fly.
Other verbs like **entender** are: **atender** / to attend; **defender** / to defend; **encender** / to light, to set fire to; **perder** / to lose.

IRREGULAR VERBS / VERBOS IRREGULARES

INFINITIVE	VOLVER	SENTIR	DORMIR	REPETIR
	to return	to feel	to sleep	to repeat
-NDO FORM (GERUND)	volviendo	sintiendo	durmiendo	repitiendo
-DO FORM (PP.)	vuelto	sentido	dormido	repetido
INDICATIVE PRESENT	vuelvo	siento	duermo	repito
	vuelves	sientes	duermes	repites
	vuelve	siente	duerme	repite
	volvemos	sentimos	dormimos	repetimos
	volvéis	sentís	dormís	repetís
	vuelven	sienten	duermen	repiten
SUBJUNCTIVE PRESENT	vuelva	sienta	duerma	repita
	vuelvas	sientas	duermas	repitas
	vuelva	sienta	duerma	repita
	volvamos	sintamos	durmamos	repitamos
	volváis	sintáis	durmáis	repitáis
	vuelvan	sientan	duerman	repitan

Note: Other verbs that follow the same changes: **mover** / to move; **disolver** / to dissolve; **doler** / to hurt; **moler** / to grind; **morder** / to bite; **promover** / to promote; and other verbs formed by adding a prefix to **volver. Volver** and its derivatives have an irregular past participle as does **disolver (disuelto).**

Verbs conjugated like **sentir: advertir** / to advise, to take notice; **consentir** / to consent; **convertir** / to convert; **digerir** / to digest; **divertirse** / to have a good time; **herir** / to wound, hurt, stab; **hervir** / to boil; **mentir** / to lie; **preferir** / to prefer; **referir** / to refer. Like **dormir** are: **dormirse** / to fall asleep, and **morir** / to die.

Use **repetir** as a model verb for: **competir** / to compete; **concebir** / to conceive; **derretir** / to melt; **conseguir** / to obtain; **medir** / to measure; **pedir** / to ask, to request; **reir** / to laugh.

The following verbs and their compound forms have irregularities that do not allow their inclusion in any of the previous classifications. For the twenty irregular verbs listed here only the tenses with irregular forms are given. Apply the rules for regular verbs to tenses not given here. Only the singular forms are given when the ordinary rules of those tenses are followed in their formation. The auxiliary verb **haber** belongs to this group.

Irregular Verb Conjugations / Conjugación de los verbos irregulares

INFINITIVE: ANDAR / TO WALK

PRESENT PARTICIPLE: andando

PAST PARTICIPLE: andado

INDICATIVE		SUBJUNCTIVE
PRESENT	PRETERIT	IMPERFECT
ando	anduve	anduviera
andas	anduviste	anduvieras
anda	anduvo	anduviera
andamos	anduvimos	anduviéramos
andáis	anduvisteis	anduvierais
andan	anduvieron	anduvieran

INFINITIVE: CAER / TO FALL

PRESENT PARTICIPLE: cayendo

PAST PARTICIPLE: caído

INDICATIVE		SUBJUNCTIVE
PRESENT	PRETERIT	IMPERFECT
caigo	cayó	cayera
cayeron		cayeras
		cayera
		cayéramos
		cayerais
		cayeran

INFINITIVE: DAR / TO GIVE

PRESENT PARTICIPLE: dando

PAST PARTICIPLE: dado

INDICATIVE		SUBJUNCTIVE	
PRESENT	PRETERIT	PRESENT	IMPERFECT
doy	di	dé	diera
das	diste	des	dieras
da	dió	dé	diera
damos	dimos	demos	diéramos
dais	disteis	deis	dierais
dan	dieron	den	dieran

INFINITIVE: DECIR / TO TELL

PRESENT PARTICIPLE: diciendo

PAST PARTICIPLE: dicho

	INDICATIVE		SUBJUNCTIVE		CONDITIONAL
PRESENT	PRETERIT	FUTURE	PRESENT	IMPERFECT	
digo	dije	diré	diga	dijera	diría
dices	dijiste	dirás	digas	dijeras	dirías
dice	dijo	dirá	diga	dijera	diría
decimos	dijimos	diremos	digamos	dijéramos	diríamos
decís	dijisteis	diréis	digáis	dijerais	diríais
dicen	dijeron	dirán	digan	dijeran	dirían

INFINITIVE: ESTAR / TO BE

PRESENT PARTICIPLE: estando

PAST PARTICIPLE: estado

	INDICATIVE	SUBJUNCTIVE	
PRESENT	PRETERIT	PRESENT	IMPERFECT
estoy	estuve	esté	estuviera
estás	estuviste	estés	estuvieras
está	estuvo	esté	estuviera

INFINITIVE: HACER / TO DO, MAKE

PRESENT PARTICIPLE: haciendo

PAST PARTICIPLE: hecho

	INDICATIVE		SUBJUNCTIVE		CONDITIONAL
PRESENT	PRETERIT	FUTURE	PRESENT	IMPERFECT	
hago	hice	haré	haga	hiciera	haría
	hiciste	harás	hagas	hicieras	harías
	hizo	hará	haga	hiciera	haría

INFINITIVE: IR / TO GO

PRESENT PARTICIPLE: yendo

PAST PARTICIPLE: ido

	INDICATIVE		SUBJUNCTIVE	
PRESENT	PRETERIT	IMPERFECT	PRESENT	IMPERFECT
voy	fui	iba	vaya	fuera
vas	fuiste	ibas	vayas	fueras
va	fue	iba	vaya	fuera
vamos	fuimos	ibamos	vayamos	fuéramos

vais	fuisteis	ibais	vayáis	fuerais
van	fueron	iban	vayan	fueran

INFINITIVE: OIR / TO HEAR

PRESENT PARTICIPLE: oyendo

PAST PARTICIPLE: oído

INDICATIVE		SUBJUNCTIVE	
PRESENT	PRETERIT	PRESENT	IMPERFECT
oigo	oí	oiga	oyera
oyes	oíste	oigas	oyeras
oye	oyó	oiga	oyera
oímos	oímos		
oís	oísteis		
oyen	oyeron		

INFINITIVE: PODER / TO BE ABLE

PRESENT PARTICIPLE: pudiendo

PAST PARTICIPLE: podido

INDICATIVE			SUBJUNCTIVE		CONDITIONAL
PRESENT	PRETERIT	FUTURE	PRESENT	IMPERFECT	
puedo	pude	podré	pueda	pudiera	podría
puedes	pudiste	podrás	puedas	pudieras	podrías
puede	pudo	podrá	pueda	pudiera	podría
podemos	pudimos	podremos	podamos	pudiéramos	podríamos
podéis	pudisteis	podréis	podáis	pudierais	podríais
pueden	pudieron	podrán	puedan	pudieran	podrían

INFINITIVE: PONER / TO PUT

PRESENT PARTICIPLE: poniendo

PAST PARTICIPLE: puesto

INDICATIVE			SUBJUNCTIVE		CONDITIONAL
PRESENT	PRETERIT	FUTURE	PRESENT	IMPERFECT	
pongo	puse	pondré	ponga	pusiera	pondría
pones	pusiste	pondrás	pongas	pusieras	pondrías
pone	puso	pondrá	ponga	pusiera	pondría
	pusimos		pongamos		
	pusisteis		pongáis		
	pusieron		pongan		

INFINITIVE: QUERER / TO WANT

PRESENT PARTICIPLE: queriendo

PAST PARTICIPLE: querido

	INDICATIVE		SUBJUNCTIVE		CONDITIONAL
PRESENT	PRETERIT	FUTURE	PRESENT	IMPERFECT	
quiero	quise	querré	quiera	quisiera	querría
quieres	quisiste	querrás	quieras	quisieras	querrías
quiere	quiso	querrá	quiera	quisiera	querría
queremos	quisimos	querremos	queramos	quisiéramos	querríamos
queréis	quisisteis	querréis	querráis	quisierais	querríais
quieren	quisieron	querrán	quieran	quisieran	querrían

INFINITIVE: SABER / TO KNOW

PRESENT PARTICIPLE: sabiendo

PAST PARTICIPLE: sabido

	INDICATIVE		SUBJUNCTIVE		CONDITIONAL
PRESENT	PRETERIT	FUTURE	PRESENT	IMPERFECT	
sé	supe	sabré	sepa	supiera	sabría
sabes	supiste	sabrás	sepas	supieras	sabrías
sabe	supo	sabrá	sepa	supiera	sabría

INFINITIVE: SALIR / TO LEAVE

PRESENT PARTICIPLE: saliendo

PAST PARTICIPLE: salido

	INDICATIVE		SUBJUNCTIVE		CONDITIONAL
PRESENT	PRETERIT	FUTURE	PRESENT	IMPERFECT	
salgo		saldré	salga		saldría
		saldrás	salgas		saldrías
		saldrá	salga		saldría

INFINITIVE: SER / TO BE

PRESENT PARTICIPLE: siendo

PAST PARTICIPLE: sido

	INDICATIVE		SUBJUNCTIVE	
PRESENT	PRETERIT	FUTURE	PRESENT	IMPERFECT
soy	fui	era	sea	fuera
eres	fuiste	eras	seas	fueras
es	fue	era	sea	fuera
somos	fuimos	éramos	seamos	fuéramos

sois	fuisteis	erais	seáis	fuerais
son	fueron	eran	sean	fueran

INFINITIVE: TENER / TO HAVE

PRESENT PARTICIPLE: teniendo

PAST PARTICIPLE: tenido

INDICATIVE			SUBJUNCTIVE		CONDITIONAL
PRESENT	PRETERIT	FUTURE	PRESENT	IMPERFECT	
tengo	tuve	tendré	tenga	tuviera	tendría
tienes	tuviste	tendrás	tengas	tuvieras	tendrías
tiene	tuvo	tendrá	tenga	tuviera	tendría
tenemos	tuvimos	tendremos	tengamos	tuviéramos	tendríamos
tenéis	tuvisteis	tendréis	tengáis	tuvierais	tendríais
tienen	tuvieron	tendrán	tengan	tuvieran	tendrían

INFINITIVE: VENIR / TO COME

PRESENT PARTICIPLE: viniendo

PAST PARTICIPLE: venido

INDICATIVE			SUBJUNCTIVE		CONDITIONAL
PRESENT	PRETERIT	FUTURE	PRESENT	IMPERFECT	
vengo	vine	vendré	venga	viniera	vendría
vienes	viniste	vendrás	vengas	vinieras	vendrías
viene	vino	vendrá	venga	viniera	vendría
venimos	vinimos	vendremos	vengamos	viniéramos	vendríamos
venéis	vinisteis	vendréis	vengáis	vinierais	vendríais

Appendix E
•Weights and Measures
•Numbers
•Time

Apéndice E
•Pesos y Medidas
•Números
•Tiempo

WEIGHTS AND MEASURES / PESOS Y MEDIDAS

All equivalents are approximate. / Todas las equivalencias son aproximadas.

Liquid Measure doses	Líquidos: Capacidad dosis (sistema métrico)
1 quart / cuarto = 0.946 liter / litro	1000 cc.[a]
1 pint / pinta = 0.0473 liter / litro	500 cc.
8 fluid ounces / onzas	240 cc.
3.5 fluid ounces / onzas	100 cc.
1 fluid ounce / onza	30 cc.
4 fluid drams / dracmas	4 cc.
15 minims, drops / gotas	1 cc.
1 minim, drop / gota	0.06 cc.
1 teaspoonful / cucharadita de café	4 cc.
1 teaspoonful / cucharadita de postre	8 cc.
1 tablespoonful / cucharada sopera	15 cc.
1 teacupful / media taza	120 cc.
1 cup / taza	240 cc.
½ grain / grano	30 mg.

a.cc. **abbr**. cubic centimeters / centímetros cúbicos

Solids	Sólidos
1 pound / libra	373.24 grams / gramos
1 ounce / onza	30 grams / gramos
4 drams / dracmas	15 grams / gramos
1 dram / dracma	4 grams / gramos
60 grains / granos = 1 dram / dracma	4 grams / gramos
30 grains / granos = 0.5 dram / dracma	2 grams / gramos
15 grains / granos	1 gram / gramo
10 grains / granos	0.6 grams / gramos
1 grain / grano	60 milligrams / miligramos
¾ grain / grano	50 mg.[a] ½ grain / grano
¼ grain / grano	15 mg.
1/10 grain / grano	6 mg.

[a]mg. **abbr**. milligrams / miligramos

Other Liquid Measures

Otras medidas líquidas

1 barrel / barril	119.07 liters / litros
1 gallon / galón = 8 pints / pintas (*Ingl.*) 3.785 L[a]	4 quarts / cuartos 3.785 L
1 liter / litro	2.113 pints / pintas
1 quart / cuarto	0.946 L
1 pint / pinta	0.473 L

a.L *abbr*. liter / litro.

Avoirdupois Weights

Peso avoirdupois (comercio)

1 ton / tonelada	1016 kilograms / kilos
1 hundredweight = 112 pounds / libras	50.80 kilograms / kilos
2.20 pounds / libras	1 kilogram / kilo
1 pound / libra = 16 ounces / onzas	0.453 kilograms / kilo
1 ounce / onza	28.34 grams / gramos

Length

Longitud

1 mile / milla	1.60 kilometers / kilómetros
1 yard / yarda = 3 feet / pies	0.914 meters / metros
1 foot / pie = 12 inches / pulgadas	0.304 meter / metro
1 inch / pulgada	25.4 millimeters / milímetros
0.04 inch / pulgada	1 millimeter / milímetro
0.39 inch / pulgada	1 centimer / centímetro
39.37 inches / pulgadas	1 meter / metro

CARDINAL NUMERALS / NÚMEROS CARDINALES

Cardinal Numerals	Números cardinales
0 cero / zero	30 treinta / thirty
1 uno (un, una) / one	40 cuarenta / forty
2 dos / two	50 cincuenta / fifty
3 tres / three	60 sesenta / sixty
4 cuatro / four	70 setenta / seventy
5 cinco / five	80 ochenta / eighty
6 seis / six	90 noventa / ninety
7 siete / seven	100 ciento, cien / one hundred
8 ocho / eight	101 ciento uno / one hundred and one
9 nueve / nine	110 ciento diez / one hundred and ten
10 diez / ten	200 doscientos / two hundred
11 once / eleven	300 trescientos / three hundred
12 doce / twelve	400 cuatrocientos / four hundred
13 trece / thirteen	500 quinientos / five hundred
14 catorce / fourteen	600 seiscientos / six hundred
15 quince / fifteen	700 setecientos / seven hundred
16 diez y seis, dieciséis / sixteen	800 ochocientos / eight hundred
17 diez y siete, diecisiete / seventeen	900 novecientos / nine hundred
18 diez y ocho, dieciocho / eighteen	1,000 mil / one thousand
19 diez y nueve, diecinueve / nineteen	1,010 mil diez / one thousand and ten
20 veinte / twenty	1,500 mil quinientos / one thousand five hundred
21 veinte y uno, veintiuno / twenty-one	2,000 dos mil / two thousand
	1,000,000 un millón / one million

Note: **Uno** and **ciento** and its multiples are the only cardinal numbers that change form. **Uno** drops the -o when it precedes a masculine singular noun: one liter of water / **un litro de agua**; but it does not drop the -o in: one out of ten / **uno de cada diez**.

Ciento changes to **cien** before nouns and before **mil** and **millón**: one hundred cases / **cien casos**; one hundred thousand cases / **cien mil casos**.

ORDINAL NUMERALS / NÚMEROS ORDINALES

Multiples of **ciento** agree in gender and number with the nouns they modify: two hundred cases / **doscientos casos**; two hundred pills / **doscientas píldoras.**

The Ordinals First to Tenth

ENGLISH	MASCULINE	FEMININE
first	$1^{\underline{o}}$ primero	primera
second	$2^{\underline{o}}$ segundo	segunda
third	$3^{\underline{o}}$ tercero	tercera
fourth	$4^{\underline{o}}$ cuarto	cuarta
fifth	$5^{\underline{o}}$ quinto	quinta
sixth	$6^{\underline{o}}$ sexto	sexta
seventh	$7^{\underline{o}}$ séptimo	séptima
eighth	$8^{\underline{o}}$ octavo	octava
ninth	$9^{\underline{o}}$ noveno	novena
tenth	$10^{\underline{o}}$ décimo	décima

Primero and **tercero** drop the -o before masculine singular nouns.

the first year / **el primer año**
the third day / **el tercer día**

Note: If a cardinal number and a numeral are used to qualify the same noun, the cardinal always precedes the ordinal.

the first three patients / **los tres primeros pacientes**
Take the first two pills now. / **Tome las dos primeras pastillas ahora.**

In reference to dates, the ordinal **primero** is used for the first day of the month; the cardinal is used for the other dates.

FRACTIONS / FRACCIONES

½	a, one half / medio, la mitad
1/3	a, one third / un tercio, una tercera parte
¼	a, one fourth / un cuarto, una cuarta parte
1/5	a, one fifth / un quinto, una quinta parte
1/6	a, one sixth / un sexto, una sexta parte
1/8	a, one eighth / un octavo, una octava parte
1/10	a, one tenth / un décimo, una décima parte
3/5	three fifths / tres quintos
5/8	five eighths / cinco octavos
7/10	seven tenths / siete décimos
0.1	a, one tenth / un décimo
0.01	a, one hundredth / un centésimo
0.001	a, one thousandth / un milésimo

TEMPERATURE / TEMPERATURA

Fahrenheit (°F)	Centígrado (°C)
32°F freezing point (sea level)	0°C punto de congelación (nivel del mar)
212°F boiling point	100°C punto de ebullición
Normal Body Temperature	Temperatura normal del cuerpo
Children: 99°F	Niños: 37.2°C
Adults: 98.6°F	Adultos: 37.0°C

Conversion to °C		Conversión a °F	
subtract 32	−32	multiplique por 9	× 9
multiply by 5	× 5	divida entre 5	÷ 5
divide by 9	÷ 9	añada 32	+32

TIME / EL TIEMPO

Days of the Week — Días de la semana

Days of the Week	Días de la semana
Monday	lunes
Tuesday	martes
Wednesday	miércoles
Thursday	jueves
Friday	viernes
Saturday	sábado
Sunday	domingo

You must return on Monday. / **Debe volver el lunes.**
On Thursdays the office is closed. / **Los jueves la consulta está cerrada.**
The test will be next Friday. / **La prueba será el próximo viernes.**

Note: Days of the week and months of the year are not capitalized in Spanish. / **En inglés los días de la semana y los meses del año se escriben con mayúscula.**

Seasons and Months of the Year / Estaciones y meses del año

SPRING	PRIMAVERA
March	marzo
April	abril
May	mayo

Your operation will be in May. / Su operación será en mayo.

SUMMER	VERANO
June	junio
July	julio
August	agosto

It is very hot in the summer. / Hace mucho calor en el verano.

AUTUMN	OTOÑO
September	septiembre
October	octubre
November	noviembre

Make your next appointment for May. / Haga la próxima cita para mayo.
April is a bad month for allergies. / Abril es un mes malo para las alergias.
I saw the patient last September. / Vi al paciente el pasado mes de septiembre.

WINTER	INVIERNO
December	diciembre
January	enero
February	febrero

Do you have many colds in the winter? / ¿Tiene muchos resfriados en el invierno?

Time of Day — La hora

What time is it?	¿Qué hora es?
At what time?	¿A qué hora?
It is ...	Es la ... (Son las...)
At	a la, a las
in the morning	por la mañana
in the afternoon	por la tarde
in the evening (at night)	por la noche

Es la una	**A la una** tomo la medicina. / I take the medication **at one.**
Son las dos	**A las dos** llegaré al hospital. / I will arrive at the hospital **at two.**
Son las dos y media	**A las dos y media** tengo una consulta. / I have an appointment **at two-thirty.**
Son las cuatro	**A las cuatro** voy a la farmacia. / I am going to the pharmacy **at four.**
Son las once	**A las once** hablé con la enfermera. / I spoke to the nurse **at eleven.**
Son las doce	**Al mediodía** como el almuerzo. / I eat lunch **at noon.**

Expressions of time / Expresiones de tiempo

GENERAL TERMS	TÉRMINOS GENERALES	GENERAL TERMS	TÉRMINOS GENERALES
night	noche	daily	diario, diariamente
midnight	medianoche	2 weeks	dos semanas, quince días
mid-morning	media mañana	annual	anual
evening	tardecita	bimester	bimestre
sunset	atardecer	century	siglo
morning	mañana	date	fecha
day	día	decade	década
sunrise, dawn	amanecer, la aurora	monthly	mensual, mensualmente
afternoon	tarde	trimester	trimestre
night	noche	twice a day	dos veces al día
noon	mediodía	weekly	semanal, semanalmente

Phrases / Frases

after lunch	después del almuerzo	at bedtime	al acostarse
at dinner time	a la hora de la cena	before breakfast	antes de desayunar
during meals	durante las comidas	one week from today	en una semana, en siete días

Timing Tests and Medications / Tiempo marcado en pruebas y medicinas

liquid intake 24 hours	toma líquida de 24 horas
first morning specimen	espécimen de primera hora en la mañana
timed specimen	espécimen de tiempo marcado
fasting blood test	prueba sanguínea en ayunas
one teaspoon every three hours	una cucharadita cada tres horas
one pill a day	una pastilla al día

Stages of Life / Etapas de la vida

AGES	EDADES
pre-born, fetus	prenacido(a), feto
newborn	neonato, recién nacido(a)
parvulum	párvulo(a)
toddler	el pequeño, la pequeña
child, childhood	niño(a), la niñez
puberty, adolescence	la pubertad, la adolescencia
adult	adulto(a), mayor de edad
young man, young woman, youth	el joven, la joven, la juventud
maturity, middle age	la madurez, la mediana edad
old man, old woman; old age	el anciano, el señor mayor, la anciana, la señora mayor; la vejez
date of birth	fecha de nacimiento
date of death	fecha de fallecimiento

Contents: Color Anatomy Images
Contenido: Imágenes de Anatomía en color

Anterior region of the neck
Región anterior del cuello o la nuca

Sternocleidomastoid region
Región esternocleidomastoidea

Lateral region of the neck
Región lateral del cuello o la nuca

Deltoid region
Región deltoidea

Clavipectoral triangle
Triángulo clavículo-pectoral

Presternal region
Región preesternal

Pectoral region
Región pectoral

Mammary region
Región mamaria

Axillary region
Región axilar

Anterior region of arm
Región anterior del brazo

Inframammary region
Región inframamaria

Anterior region of elbow,
cubital fossa
Región anterior del codo,
fosa cubital

Epigastric region
Región epigástrica

Hypochondriac region
Región hipocondríaca

Posterior region of forearm
Región posterior del antebrazo

Umbilical region
Región umbilical

Anterior region of forearm
Región anterior del antebrazo

Lateral abdominal region
Región lateroabdominal

Inguinal region
Región inguinal

Dorsum of hand
Dorso de la mano

Pubic (hypogastric) region
Región púbica (hipogástrica)

Femoral triangle
Triángulo femoral

Urogenital region
Región urogenital

Anterior region of thigh
Región anterior del muslo

Anterior region of knee
Región anterior de la rótula (rodilla)

Posterior region of leg
Región posterior de la pierna

Anterior region of leg
Región anterior de la pierna

Dorsum of foot
Dorso del pie

A2

Regions of the Human Body–Posterior View
Regiones del cuerpo humano–Vista posterior

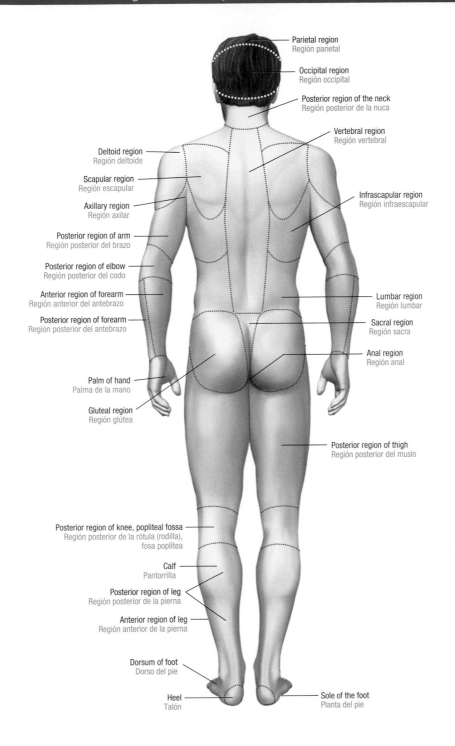

Parietal region
Región parietal

Occipital region
Región occipital

Posterior region of the neck
Región posterior de la nuca

Vertebral region
Región vertebral

Deltoid region
Región deltoide

Scapular region
Región escapular

Axillary region
Región axilar

Infrascapular region
Región infraescapular

Posterior region of arm
Región posterior del brazo

Posterior region of elbow
Región posterior del codo

Anterior region of forearm
Región anterior del antebrazo

Lumbar region
Región lumbar

Posterior region of forearm
Región posterior del antebrazo

Sacral region
Región sacra

Anal region
Región anal

Palm of hand
Palma de la mano

Gluteal region
Región glútea

Posterior region of thigh
Región posterior del muslo

Posterior region of knee, popliteal fossa
Región posterior de la rótula (rodilla),
fosa poplítea

Calf
Pantorrilla

Posterior region of leg
Región posterior de la pierna

Anterior region of leg
Región anterior de la pierna

Dorsum of foot
Dorso del pie

Heel
Talón

Sole of the foot
Planta del pie

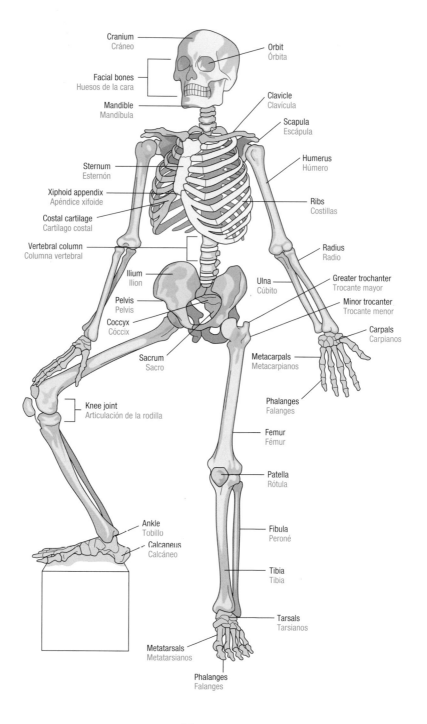

Cranium
Cráneo

Orbit
Órbita

Facial bones
Huesos de la cara

Mandible
Mandíbula

Clavicle
Clavícula

Scapula
Escápula

Sternum
Esternón

Humerus
Húmero

Xiphoid appendix
Apéndice xifoide

Costal cartilage
Cartílago costal

Ribs
Costillas

Vertebral column
Columna vertebral

Radius
Radio

Ilium
Ilion

Greater trochanter
Trocante mayor

Ulna
Cúbito

Minor trocanter
Trocante menor

Pelvis
Pelvis

Coccyx
Cóccix

Carpals
Carpianos

Metacarpals
Metacarpianos

Sacrum
Sacro

Phalanges
Falanges

Knee joint
Articulación de la rodilla

Femur
Fémur

Patella
Rótula

Ankle
Tobillo

Calcaneus
Calcáneo

Fibula
Peroné

Tibia
Tibia

Tarsals
Tarsianos

Metatarsals
Metatarsianos

Phalanges
Falanges

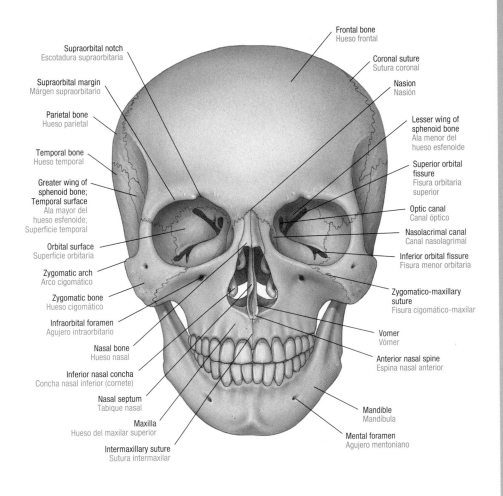

Supraorbital notch
Escotadura supraorbitaria

Supraorbital margin
Márgen supraorbitario

Parietal bone
Hueso parietal

Temporal bone
Hueso temporal

Greater wing of
sphenoid bone;
Temporal surface
Ala mayor del
hueso esfenoide;
Superficie temporal

Orbital surface
Superficie orbitaria

Zygomatic arch
Arco cigomático

Zygomatic bone
Hueso cigomático

Infraorbital foramen
Agujero intraorbitario

Nasal bone
Hueso nasal

Inferior nasal concha
Concha nasal inferior (cornete)

Nasal septum
Tabique nasal

Maxilla
Hueso del maxilar superior

Intermaxillary suture
Sutura intermaxilar

Frontal bone
Hueso frontal

Coronal suture
Sutura coronal

Nasion
Nasión

Lesser wing of
sphenoid bone
Ala menor del
hueso esfenoide

Superior orbital
fissure
Fisura orbitaria
superior

Optic canal
Canal óptico

Nasolacrimal canal
Canal nasolagrimal

Inferior orbital fissure
Fisura menor orbitaria

Zygomatico-maxillary
suture
Fisura cigomático-maxilar

Vomer
Vómer

Anterior nasal spine
Espina nasal anterior

Mandible
Mandíbula

Mental foramen
Agujero mentoniano

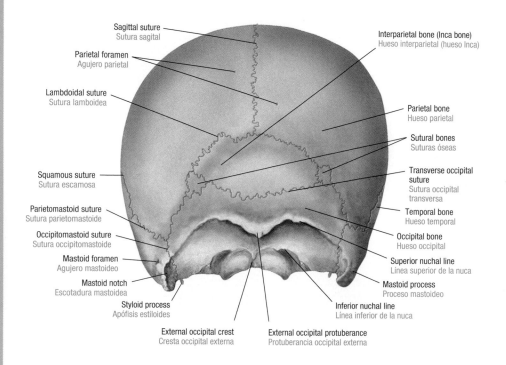

Sagittal suture
Sutura sagital

Parietal foramen
Agujero parietal

Lambdoidal suture
Sutura lamboidea

Squamous suture
Sutura escamosa

Parietomastoid suture
Sutura parietomastoide

Occipitomastoid suture
Sutura occipitomastoide

Mastoid foramen
Agujero mastoideo

Mastoid notch
Escotadura mastoidea

Styloid process
Apófisis estiloides

External occipital crest
Cresta occipital externa

External occipital protuberance
Protuberancia occipital externa

Interparietal bone (Inca bone)
Hueso interparietal (hueso Inca)

Parietal bone
Hueso parietal

Sutural bones
Suturas óseas

Transverse occipital suture
Sutura occipital transversa

Temporal bone
Hueso temporal

Occipital bone
Hueso occipital

Superior nuchal line
Línea superior de la nuca

Mastoid process
Proceso mastoideo

Inferior nuchal line
Línea inferior de la nuca

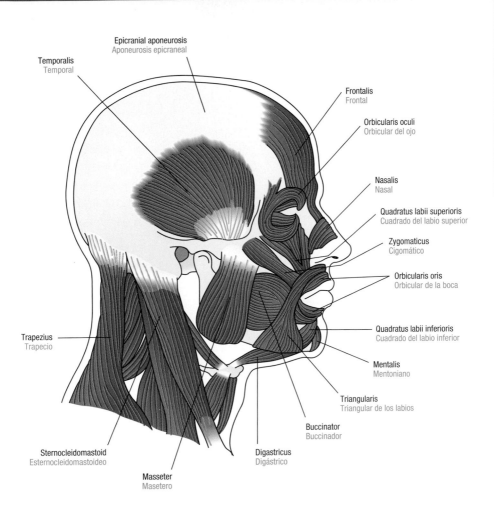

Epicranial aponeurosis
Aponeurosis epicraneal

Temporalis
Temporal

Frontalis
Frontal

Orbicularis oculi
Orbicular del ojo

Nasalis
Nasal

Quadratus labii superioris
Cuadrado del labio superior

Zygomaticus
Cigomático

Orbicularis oris
Orbicular de la boca

Quadratus labii inferioris
Cuadrado del labio inferior

Trapezius
Trapecio

Mentalis
Mentoniano

Triangularis
Triangular de los labios

Buccinator
Buccinador

Sternocleidomastoid
Esternocleidomastoideo

Digastricus
Digástrico

Masseter
Masetero

A7

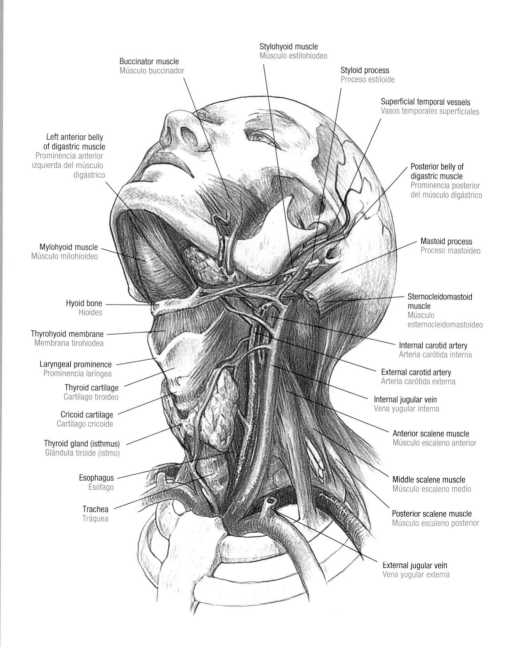

Stylohyoid muscle
Músculo estilohiodeo

Buccinator muscle
Músculo buccinador

Styloid process
Proceso estiloide

Superficial temporal vessels
Vasos temporales superficiales

Left anterior belly
of digastric muscle
Prominencia anterior
izquierda del músculo
digástrico

Posterior belly of
digastric muscle
Prominencia posterior
del músculo digástrico

Mylohyoid muscle
Músculo milohioideo

Mastoid process
Proceso mastoideo

Hyoid bone
Hioides

Sternocleidomastoid
muscle
Músculo
esternocleidomastoideo

Thyrohyoid membrane
Membrana tirohiodea

Internal carotid artery
Arteria carótida interna

Laryngeal prominence
Prominencia laríngea

External carotid artery
Arteria carótida externa

Thyroid cartilage
Cartílago tiroideo

Internal jugular vein
Vena yugular interna

Cricoid cartilage
Cartílago cricoide

Anterior scalene muscle
Músculo escaleno anterior

Thyroid gland (isthmus)
Glándula tiroide (istmo)

Esophagus
Esófago

Middle scalene muscle
Músculo escaleno medio

Trachea
Tráquea

Posterior scalene muscle
Músculo escaleno posterior

External jugular vein
Vena yugular externa

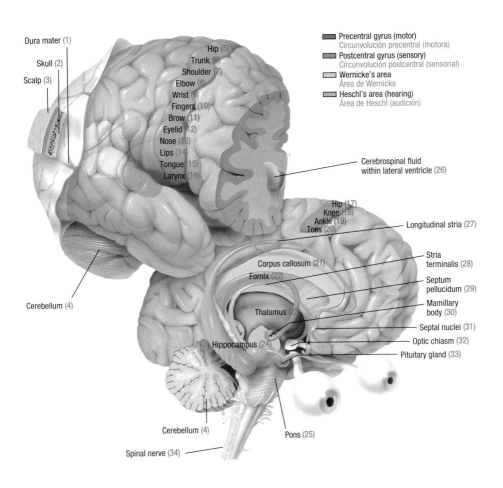

Dura mater (1)

Skull (2)

Scalp (3)

Hip (5)
Trunk (6)
Shoulder (7)
Elbow (8)
Wrist (9)
Fingers (10)
Brow (11)
Eyelid (12)
Nose (13)
Lips (14)
Tongue (15)
Larynx (16)

Precentral gyrus (motor)
Circunvolución precentral (motora)
Postcentral gyrus (sensory)
Circunvolución postcentral (sensorial)
Wernicke's area
Área de Wernicke
Heschl's area (hearing)
Área de Heschl (audición)

Cerebrospinal fluid
within lateral ventricle (26)

Hip (17)
Knee (18)
Ankle (19)
Toes (20)

Longitudinal stria (27)

Stria terminalis (28)

Corpus callosum (21)
Fornix (22)

Septum pellucidum (29)

Mamillary body (30)

Thalamus (23)

Septal nuclei (31)

Hippocampus (24)

Optic chiasm (32)

Pituitary gland (33)

Cerebellum (4)

Cerebellum (4)

Pons (25)

Spinal nerve (34)

Key/Translations Llave/Traducciones

(1) Dura mater	(11) Ceño	(21) Cuerpo calloso	(29) Tabique pelúcido
(2) Cráneo	(12) Párpado	(22) Fórnix	(30) Cuerpo mamilar
(3) Cuero cabelludo	(13) Nariz	(23) Tálamo	(31) Núcleo septal
(4) Cerebelo	(14) Labios	(24) Hipocampo	(32) Quiasma óptico
(5) Cadera	(15) Lengua	(25) Pons	(33) Glándula pituitaria
(6) Tronco	(16) Laringe	(26) Fluido cerebroespinal	(34) Nervio espinal
(7) Hombro	(17) Cadera	dentro del ventrículo	
(8) Codo	(18) Rodilla	lateral	
(9) Muñeca	(19) Tobillo	(27) Estría longitudinal	
(10) Dedos de la mano	(20) Dedos de los pies	(28) Estría terminal	

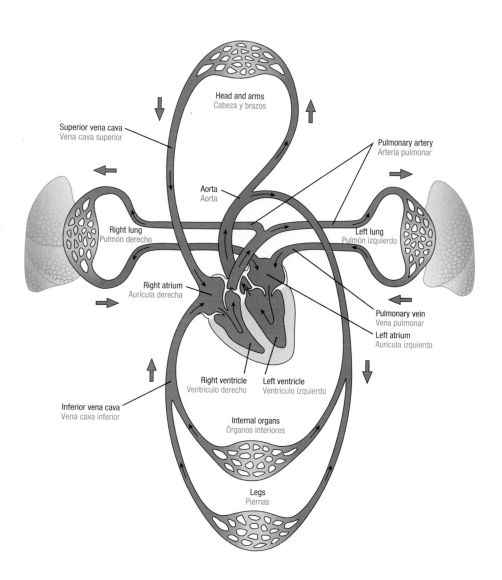

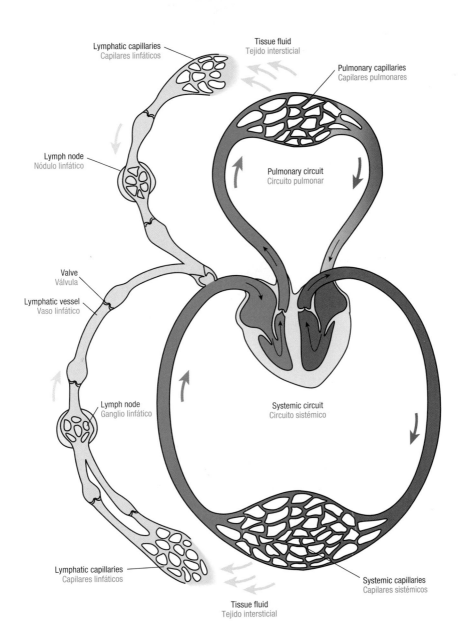

Lymphatic capillaries
Capilares linfáticos

Tissue fluid
Tejido intersticial

Pulmonary capillaries
Capilares pulmonares

Lymph node
Nódulo linfático

Pulmonary circuit
Circuito pulmonar

Valve
Válvula

Lymphatic vessel
Vaso linfático

Lymph node
Ganglio linfático

Systemic circuit
Circuito sistémico

Lymphatic capillaries
Capilares linfáticos

Systemic capillaries
Capilares sistémicos

Tissue fluid
Tejido intersticial

In relation to the cardiovascular system
En relación al sistema cardiovascular

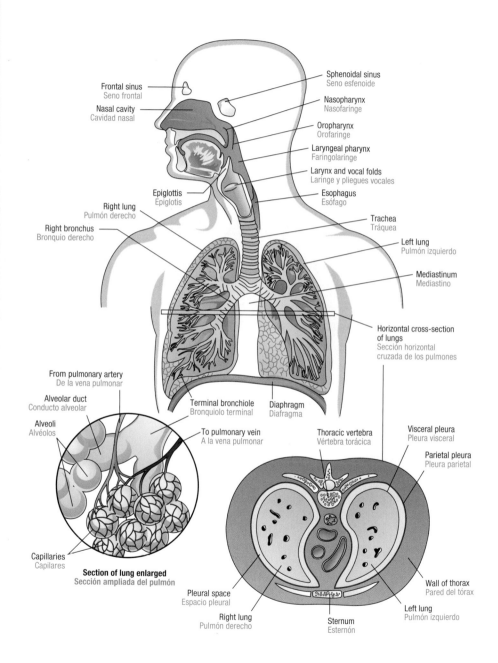

Frontal sinus
Seno frontal

Nasal cavity
Cavidad nasal

Sphenoidal sinus
Seno esfenoide

Nasopharynx
Nasofaringe

Oropharynx
Orofaringe

Laryngeal pharynx
Faringolaringe

Larynx and vocal folds
Laringe y pliegues vocales

Epiglottis
Epiglotis

Esophagus
Esófago

Right lung
Pulmón derecho

Right bronchus
Bronquio derecho

Trachea
Tráquea

Left lung
Pulmón izquierdo

Mediastinum
Mediastino

Horizontal cross-section of lungs
Sección horizontal cruzada de los pulmones

From pulmonary artery
De la vena pulmonar

Alveolar duct
Conducto alveolar

Alveoli
Alvéolos

Terminal bronchiole
Bronquiolo terminal

Diaphragm
Diafragma

To pulmonary vein
A la vena pulmonar

Thoracic vertebra
Vértebra torácica

Visceral pleura
Pleura visceral

Parietal pleura
Pleura parietal

Capillaries
Capilares

**Section of lung enlarged
Sección ampliada del pulmón**

Pleural space
Espacio pleural

Right lung
Pulmón derecho

Sternum
Esternón

Left lung
Pulmón izquierdo

Wall of thorax
Pared del tórax